Handbook of
Mouse Auditory Research

From Behavior
to Molecular Biology

James F. Willott, Ph.D.
University of South Florida
Tampa, Florida
and
The Jackson Laboratory
Bar Harbor, Maine

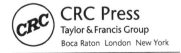
CRC Press
Taylor & Francis Group
Boca Raton London New York

CRC Press is an imprint of the
Taylor & Francis Group, an **informa** business

CRC Press
Taylor & Francis Group
6000 Broken Sound Parkway NW, Suite 300
Boca Raton, FL 33487-2742

First issued in paperback 2019

© 2001 by Taylor & Francis Group, LLC
CRC Press is an imprint of Taylor & Francis Group, an Informa business

No claim to original U.S. Government works

ISBN-13: 978-0-8493-2328-7 (hbk)
ISBN-13: 978-0-367-39732-6 (pbk)
Library of Congress Card Number 00-068879

Library of Congress Cataloging-in-Publication Data

Handbook of mouse auditory research : from behavior to molecular biology / edited by James F. Willcott.
      p.   cm.
   Includes bibliographical references.
   ISBN 0-8493-2328-2 (alk. paper)
   1. Hearing--Research--Metholdogy--Handbooks, manuals, etc. 2. Mice as laboratory animals. I. Willott, James F.

QP461 .H26 2001
573.8′91935—dc21
                                                                          00-068879

Visit the Taylor & Francis Web site at
http://www.taylorandfrancis.com

and the CRC Press Web site at
http://www.crcpress.com

Dedication

This book is dedicated to the students and colleagues who worked in my laboratory over the past 24 years.

Preface

It has been almost two decades since I edited *The Auditory Psychobiology of the Mouse* (Charles Thomas, Springfield, Illinois, 1983). That book covered the field of mouse auditory research quite adequately with only a third as many chapters as this one. Things have changed dramatically during the last two decades, and truly exciting developments have emerged in areas of molecular biology, genetics, and mouse models of human hearing disorders. Many of the topics and techniques reviewed here were not even a gleam in the eye of the authors writing in the early 1980s. But make no mistake; familiar areas of research such as auditory behavior and psychophysics, development, physiology, and anatomy have not been standing still, and equally exciting, cutting edge work is being done in these areas as well. There is a growing interest in mouse auditory phenotypes for their own sake, as well as to inform the molecular and genetic research. Fortuitously, the various disciplines fuel activity in one another. Behavioral and psychophysical research identifies the mouse models that are worthy of study at more molecular levels, whereas molecular biology helps to explain the properties of interesting auditory phenotypes. This mutual, integrative aspect of mouse auditory research is evident throughout the chapters of this book.

This book brings together as much information about these areas as is physically possible within the covers of a reasonably sized volume. The authors have done a marvelous job of presenting general background along with the current mouse research to present the state of the art of many diverse disciplines. There are always omissions in a handbook, and for those I am sorry. Every topic cannot be covered, but not many have been excluded here.

The list of contributors is close to my dream team: a mix of seasoned leaders in the field who have been well known for decades, as well as a number of rising young stars. Some of the authors were also involved with *The Auditory Psychobiology of the Mouse*, including John Nyby, Jim Saunders, and David Ryugo. Despite my begging, two other original contributors, Karen Steel and Guenter Ehret, were unable to write chapters this time because of other commitments. Their fine work on mice has continued over the last two decades and is well represented in various chapters.

It is hoped that the reader will come away from this handbook with an appreciation for the value and power of mouse auditory research, while being brought up to date on many topics for which mice are important subjects. We have tried to provide a mixture of reviews of the literature, current research (much of it not previously published), along with insights into the various methodologies being used. Several "focus" chapters deal with specific topics as well.

MICE AS RESEARCH ANIMALS

Of course, the use of mice in research has a long history. As reviewed recently by Pennisi (2000), it essentially began in 1664, when Robert Hooke made the first known scientific observations on mice. In 1909 Clarence Little (who would later found The Jackson Laboratory in 1929) began to develop the first inbred strain, DBA (dilute, brown, non-agouti), followed by BALB/c (Bagg albino) from 1913 to 1916, and the C57BL strain (BL = black) in 1921. Interestingly, all three of these now widely used strains possess a gene that results in progressive hearing loss, making them valuable animal models, as evidenced throughout this book. Whereas the availability of these inbred strains as models was fortunate, it has become possible to intentionally generate a variety of new models with the development of techniques to produce transgenic mice in the 1980s and knockout mice in 1987. Indeed, progress in genetic engineering of mice continues to accelerate in the 21st century, with the development of techniques that were unheard of only a few years ago.

As Davisson (1999) notes, mice have several unique advantages as animal models. First, they possess the best characterized genome of any experimental vertebrate, soon to be fully sequenced. As of 1999 about 4000 human gene homologies had already been identified and hundreds of targeted mutations had been made. Second, the variety and power of genetic techniques are unrivaled among vertebrates. Recombinant and congenic strains of various types have been produced; genes can be transferred from one genetic background to another to identify modifying genes; it is relatively easy to find polymorphic markers and phenotypic variability; sophisticated computer analysis programs are available; and others. Third, mice are practical; they are cost-efficient, easy to handle (excepting a few strains that are well known to exasperated researchers), and they reproduce rapidly. Added to this is the substantial support for mouse research provided by the NIH and other funding agencies.

The backbone of mouse research is the use of inbred strains. Many inbred strains of mice have interesting and useful auditory phenotypes themselves, but they also serve as hosts for myriad mutations and genetically engineered traits that are invaluable for auditory research. The occurrence of spontaneous mutations, and nowadays, induced-mutagenesis, provide congenic mutations that can be studied within the homogeneous inbred background. Pure-inbred strains of mice can be studied and reproducibly compared for virtually any characteristics of development, anatomy, physiology, or behavior.

Given any documented differences among the inbred strains, those strains can be crossed to produce F1 hybrids which are also genetically homogenous; that is, genetically identical except for the sex differences. All truly F1 hybrids will be either homozygous (AA or bb) or heterozygous (Cc, Dd), according to the parental inbreds. In fact, the F1 hybrids often exhibit "hybrid vigor," or advantage(s) over their respective inbred parents.

As Dr. Larry Erway (one of our contributors) notes, the greatest advantage of inbred and F1 hybrid strains of mice is that the F1 hybrids can be backcrossed to either of the parental strains for detection of: (1) equal segregation of alleles, (2) independent assortment among loci, and (3) linkage-recombination between genes. In the current age of genetic mapping, this includes some ten thousand microsatellite DNA markers closely linked among the genetic loci. Given any F1 hybrids, they can be backcrossed to either of the parent inbreds, thus the possibility of detecting equal segregation or recombination among linked genes. By crossing F1 males and females derived from the same inbred stains, the F2 progeny also provide the advantages of comparing the expression of all three genotypes (AA, Aa, aa). Potentially such comparisons can be extended to the interaction of two loci, including all nine genetic combinations: e.g., AA;BB;cc, Aa;bb;cc, and aa;Bb;cc.

As many as 25 million mice may be raised worldwide in the year 2000, accounting for more than 90% of mammals used in research (Malakooff, 2000). Whereas this is twice as many mice as were used a decade ago, the rate of use is expected to continue growing by 10 to 20% annually. Only a relatively small portion of these animals are used as subjects in research on the auditory system. However, our share of the pie is becoming larger all the time. Auditory research on mice will only continue to grow and, in all likelihood, the best is yet to come.

James F. Willott

Contributors

Stuart Apfel
Kennedy Center
Albert Einstein College of Medicine
Bronx, New York

James F. Battey, Jr.
NIDCD
NIH
Bethesda, Maryland

James Bell
Departments of Psychiatry and Pharmacology
SUNY at Stony Brook
Stony Brook, New York

Lynne M. Bianchi
Neuroscience Program
Oberlin College
Oberlin, Ohio

Nenad Bogdanovic
Karolinska Institute
Stockholm, Sweden

Barbara A. Bohne
Washington University School of Medicine
Department of Otolaryngology
Head and Neck Surgery
St. Louis, Missouri

Robert Burkard
Center for Hearing and Deafness
SUNY at Buffalo
Buffalo, New York

Barbara Canlon
Department of Physiology II
Karolinska Institute
Stockhom, Sweden

Stephanie Carlson
Department of Psychology
Bethel College
Mishawaka, Indiana

Donald M. Caspary
Department of Pharmacology
Southern Illinois University School of
  Medicine
Springfield, Illinois

E. Bryan Crenshaw III
Department of Neuroscience
University of Pennsylvania
Philadelphia, Pennsylvania

Mark A. Crumling
Department of Otorhinolaryngology HNS
University of Pennsylvania School of Medicine
Philadelphia, Pennsylvania

Thomas M. Daly
Department of Pathology
Washington University School of Medicine
St. Louis, Missouri

Rickie R. Davis
Hearing Loss Prevention Section, Engineering
  and Physical Hazards Branch
Division of Applied Research and Technology
National Institute for Occupational Safety and
  Health
Cincinnati, Ohio

Dalian Ding
Center for Hearing and Deafness
SUNY at Buffalo
Buffalo, New York

Blanca Durand
Center for Hearing and Deafness
SUNY at Buffalo
Buffalo, New York

Lawrence C. Erway
Department of Biological Science
University of Cincinnati
Cincinnati, Ohio

William Falls
Department of Psychology
The University of Vermont
Burlington, Vermont

Michael J. Ferragamo
Department of Biology
Gustavus Adolphus College
Saint Peter, Minnesota

Robert D. Frisina
Otolaryngology Division
University of Rochester Medical Center
Rochester, New York

Gary W. Harding
Washington University School of Medicine
Department of Otolaryngology — Head and
  Neck Surgery
St. Louis, Missouri

Henry E. Heffner
Department of Psychology
University of Toledo
Toledo, Ohio

Rickye S. Heffner
Department of Psychology
University of Toledo
Toledo, Ohio

Robert Hitzemann
Department of Behavioral Neuroscience
Oregon Health Sciences University
Portland, Oregon

Esma Idrizbegovic
Department of Audiology
Huddinge University Hospital
Huddinge, Sweden

James R. Ison
Department of Brain and Cognitive Sciences
University of Rochester
Rochester, New York

Jennifer Jeskey
Department of Psychology
Northern Illinois University
DeKalb, Illinois

Kenneth R. Johnson
The Jackson Laboratory
Bar Harbor, Maine

Matthew Kelley
Unit on Developmental Neuroscience
National Institute on Deafness and Other
  Communication Disorders
National Institutes of Health
Rockville, Maryland

Duck O. Kim
Department of Neuroscience
University of Connecticut Health Center
Farmington, Connecticut

Gimseong Koay
Department of Psychology
University of Toledo
Toledo, Ohio

Verity A. Letts
The Jackson Laboratory
Bar Harbor, Maine

Charles J. Limb
Center for Hearing Sciences
Johns Hopkins University School of Medicine
Baltimore, Maryland

James McCaughran, Jr.
Department of Psychiatry
SUNY at Stony Brook
Stony Brook, New York

Sandra L. McFadden
Center for Hearing and Deafness
SUNY at Buffalo
Buffalo, New York

JoAnn McGee
Developmental Auditory Physiology Laboratory
Boys Town National Research Hospital
Omaha, Nebraska

D. Kent Morest
Department of Neuroscience
Center for Neurological Sciences
University of Connecticut Health Center
Farmington, Connecticut

Lina M. Mullen
Department of Surgery
University of California San Diego
La Jolla, California

Alfred L. Nuttall
Oregon Hearing Research Center
Department of Otolaryngology
Head and Neck Surgery
Oregon Health Sciences University
Portland, Oregon

John G. Nyby
Department of Biological Sciences
Lehigh University
Bethlehem, Pennsylvania

Donata Oertel
Department of Physiology
University of Wisconsin — Madison Medical
  School,
Madison, Wisconsin

Kevin K. Ohlemiller
Research Department
Central Institute for the Deaf
St. Louis Missouri

William E. O'Neill
Department of Neurobiology and Anatomy
University of Rochester Medical Center
Rochester, New York

Henry C. Ou
Department of Otolaryngology
University of Washington
Seattle, Washington

Kourosh Parham
Division of Otolaryngology
Department of Surgery
University of Connecticut Health Center
Farmington, Connecticut

De-Ann M. Pillers
Department of Pediatrics
Oregon Health Sciences University
Portland, Oregon

Paul Pistell
Department of Psychology
The University of Vermont
Burlington, Vermont

Erik Rasmussen
Department of Psychiatry
SUNY at Stony Brook
Stony Brook, New York

Allen F. Ryan
Division of Otolaryngology
University of California San Diego
LaJolla, California

David K. Ryugo
Center for Hearing Sciences
Johns Hopkins University School of Medicine
Baltimore, Maryland

Richard J. Salvi
Center for Hearing and Deafness
SUNY at Buffalo
Buffalo, New York

Mark S. Sands
Departments of Internal Medicine and Genetics
Washington University School of Medicine
St. Louis Missouri

James C. Saunders
Department of Otorhinolaryngology HNS
University of Pennsylvania School of Medicine
Philadelphia, Pennsylvania

Carrie Secor
Center for Hearing and Deafness
SUNY at Buffalo
Buffalo, New York

Hanna M. Sobkowicz
Department of Neurology
University of Wisconsin School of Medicine
Madison, Wisconsin

Hinrich Staecker
University of Maryland School of Medicine
Division of Otolaryngology
Head and Neck Surgery
Baltimore, Maryland

Xiao-Ming Sun
Department of Speech Pathology and Audiology
University of South Alabama
Mobile, Alabama

Victoria Sundin
Department of Psychology
Northern Illinois University
DeKalb, Illinois

Joseph Trettel
Department of Neuroscience
Center for Neurological Sciences
University of Connecticut Health Center
Farmington, Connecticut

Dennis R. Trune
Oregon Hearing Research Center
Department of Otolaryngology
Head and Neck Surgery
Oregon Health Sciences University
Portland, Oregon

Thomas R. Van De Water
Kennedy Center
Albert Einstein College of Medicine
Bronx, New York

Carole A. Vogler
Department of Pathology
St. Louis University School of Medicine
St. Louis, Missouri

Edward Walsh
Developmental Auditory Physiology Lab
Boys Town National Research Hospital
Omaha, Nebraska

Joseph P. Walton
Otolaryngology Division
University of Rochester Medical Center
Rochester, New York

James F. Willott
Department of Psychology
University of South Florida
Tampa, Florida
and The Jackson Laboratory
Bar Harbor, Maine

Qing Yin Zheng
The Jackson Laboratory
Bar Harbor, Maine

Contents

SECTION I

AUDIOLOGY, AUDITORY BEHAVIOR, AND PSYCHOPHYSICS...................................1

Chapter 1

Auditory Communication among Adults...3
John G. Nyby

Chapter 2

Behavioral Assessment of Hearing in Mice...19
Henry E. Heffner and Rickye S. Heffner

Chapter 3

Focus: Sound-Localization Acuity Changes with Age in C57BL/6J Mice....................................31
Rickye S. Heffner, Gimseong Koay, and Henry E. Heffner

Chapter 4

Noninvasive Assessment of Auditory Function in Mice: Auditory Brainstem Response and
Distortion Product Otoacoustic Emissions..37
Kourosh Parham, Xiao-Ming Sun, and Duck O. Kim

Chapter 5

The Acoustic Startle Response: Reflex Elicitation and Reflex Modification by Preliminary
Stimuli...59
James R. Ison

Chapter 6

Modulation of the Acoustic Startle Response by Background Sound in C57BL/6J Mice............83
Stephanie Carlson and James F. Willott

Chapter 7

Focus: Learning and the Auditory System — Fear-Potentiated Startle Studies 91
William A. Falls and Paul J. Pistell

SECTION II

PERIPHERAL AUDITORY SYSTEM **97**

Chapter 8

The Outer and Middle Ear..99
James C. Saunders and Mark A. Crumling

Chapter 9

The Development of the GABAergic Innervation in the Organ of Corti of the Mouse..............117
Hanna M. Sobkowicz

Chapter 10

Development and Neuronal Innervation of the Organ of Corti.......................137
Matthew W. Kelley and Lynne M. Bianchi

Chapter 11

The Role of Neurotrophic Factors in the Development and Maintenance of Innervation
in the Mouse Inner Ear...157
Hinrich Staecker, Stuart Apfel, and Thomas R. Van De Water

Chapter 12

Preparation and Evaluation of the Mouse Temporal Bone.........................171
Barbara A. Bohne, Gary W. Harding, and Henry C. Ou

Chapter 13

Cochlear Hair Cell Densities and Inner-Ear Staining Techniques................189
Dalian Ding, Sandra L. McFadden, and Richard J. Salvi

Chapter 14

Effects of Exposure to an Augmented Acoustic Environment on the Mouse Auditory System.....205
James F. Willott, Victoria Sundin, and Jennifer Jeskey

Chapter 15

Cochlear Blood Flow..215
Alfred L. Nuttall

Chapter 16

Development of the Endbulbs of Held..225
Charles J. Limb and David K. Ryugo

SECTION III
THE CENTRAL AUDITORY SYSTEM 237

Chapter 17

Focus: Diversity of the Mouse Central Auditory System..........................239
James F. Willott

Chapter 18

Neuroanatomy of the Central Auditory System.....................................243
Robert D. Frisina and Joseph P. Walton

Chapter 19

Cytoarchitectonic Atlas of the Cochlear Nucleus of the Mouse 279
Joseph Trettel and D. Kent Morest

Chapter 20

Functional Circuitry of the Cochlear Nucleus: *In Vitro* Studies in Slices................297
Michael J. Ferragamo and Donata Oertel

Chapter 21

Focus: GABA and Glycine Neurotransmission in Mouse Auditory Brainstem Structures 317
Donald M. Caspary

Chapter 22

Calcium Binding Proteins in the Central Auditory System: Modulation by Noise Exposure
and Aging 321
Esma Idrizbegovic, Nenad Bogdanovic, and Barbara Canlon

Chapter 23

Auditory Neurons in the Reticular Formation of C57BL/6J Mice...331
Stephanie Carlson

Chapter 24

Aging of the Mouse Central Auditory System..339
Robert D. Frisina and Joseph P. Walton

Chapter 25

Focus: Elicitation and Inhibition of the Startle Reflex by Acoustic Transients: Studies of
Age-Related Changes in Temporal Processing 381
James R. Ison, Joseph P. Walton, Robert D. Frisina, and William E. O'Neill

SECTION IV

GENETICS AND THE MOUSE AUDITORY SYSTEM **389**

Chapter 26

Human Hereditary Hearing Impairment: Research Progress Fueled by the Human Genome
Project and Mouse Models 391
James F. Battey, Jr.

Chapter 27

Genetic Analyses of Non-Transgenic Mouse Mutations Affecting Ear Morphology or
Function..401
Kenneth R. Johnson, Qing Yin Zheng, and Verity A. Letts

Chapter 28

Inbred Strains of Mice for Genetics of Hearing in Mammals: Searching for Genes for
Hearing Loss 429
L.C. Erway, Q.Y. Zheng, and K.R. Johnson

Chapter 29

Mapping the Genes for the Acoustic Startle Response (ASR) and Prepulse Inhibition of
the ASR in the BXD Recombinant Inbred Series: Effect of High-Frequency Hearing
Loss and Cochlear Pathology 441
Robert Hitzemann, James Bell, Erik Rasmussen, and James McCaughran, Jr.

Chapter 30

Transgenic Mice: Genome Manipulation and Induced Mutations 457
Lina M. Mullen and Allen F. Ryan

SECTION V
MURINE MODELS OF DISEASES OR CONDITIONS AFFECTING THE
AUDITORY SYSTEM...475

Chapter 31
Noise-Induced Hearing Loss 477
Rickie R. Davis

Chapter 32
The Role of Superoxide Dismutase in Age-Related and Noise-Induced Hearing Loss:
Clues from SOD1 Knockout Mice 489
Sandra L. McFadden, Dalian Ding, Kevin Ohlemiller, and Richard J. Salvi

Chapter 33
Mouse Models for Immunologic Diseases of the Auditory System............................505
Dennis R. Trune

Chapter 34
Focus: Muscular Dystrophy Mouse Models and Hearing Deficits...............................533
De-Ann M. Pillers and Dennis R. Trune

Chapter 35
Hypothyroidism in the TSHR Mutant Mouse...537
Edward J. Walsh and JoAnn McGee

Chapter 36
Mouse Models for Usher and Alport Syndromes 557
JoAnn McGee and Edward J. Walsh

Chapter 37
Preventing Sensory Loss in a Mouse Model of Lysosomal Storage Disease 581
Kevin K. Ohlemiller, Carole A. Vogler, Thomas M. Daly, and Mark S. Sands

Chapter 38
Auditory Brainstem Responses in CBA Mice and in Mice with Deletion of the RAB3A
Gene 603
Robert Burkard, Blanca Durand, Carrie Secor, and Sandra L. McFadden

Chapter 39
Focus: Mutations of the *Brn4/Pou3f4* Locus 617
E. Bryan Crenshaw, III

References 621

Index 717

Section I

Audiology, Auditory Behavior, and Psychophysics

This section presents what is currently known about mouse auditory behaviors and abilities, and how to measure these in the laboratory. This is the best way to begin a book on the mouse auditory system, because one needs to know what mice hear and how they use auditory information, before one can address biological mechanisms and processes. In addition to reviewing past and current literature, methodological issues are discussed when appropriate.

Chapter 1 (Nyby) makes it clear that (unlike some other laboratory species) mice are highly vocal animals, for which auditory communication is of great importance; mice make great use of their auditory system for social and other purposes. The various ways researchers can assess hearing behaviorally in mice are reviewed by Drs. Heffner in Chapter 2, with a focus on auditory localization as well (Chapter 3, Heffner, Koay, and Heffner).

The method of choice for measuring hearing thresholds is the auditory brainstem response (ABR), while otoacoustic emissions are finding increasing use for evaluation of the mouse cochlea. The literature and methodology are the topic of Chapter 4 (Parham, Sun, and Kim).

With the growing interest in evaluation of mouse auditory phenotypes in mutagensis and other programs of research, the acoustic startle response and its modification by preceding sounds (prepulse inhibition) are showing up in most phenotype screening protocols. One suspects that many researchers who use these methods do not have a thorough appreciation of the rich history of research on these topics or the complexity of these "simple" behaviors. Such deficiencies should be remedied by Chapter 5, written by James Ison, one of the pioneers in the field. Chapter 6 (Carlson and Willott) provides additional information on variables that influence the startle response in mice. Chapter 7 (Falls and Pistell) takes a different turn, focusing on the relationship between the auditory system and fear conditioning.

1 Auditory Communication among Adults

John G. Nyby

INTRODUCTION

Any comprehensive understanding of mouse hearing should be informed by an understanding of the sounds that the mouse auditory system has evolved to detect. All sensory systems, including the auditory system, have evolved because they allow an organism to process sensory inputs important for survival and reproduction. In the case of the mouse, the sounds that mice produce as part of their social behavior have likely contributed to the evolution of the mouse auditory system. This conclusion would seem warranted by auditory sensitivity in normal-hearing house mice roughly corresponding to frequencies at which mice emit audible and ultrasonic sounds. This chapter examines the auditory communication of adult mice.

While mice can certainly vocalize at frequencies audible to the human ear, a great deal of mouse vocalizing occurs at ultrasonic frequencies. This chapter examines both the ultrasonic and audible signals produced by mice, the factors that regulate and modulate their production, and what is known of their role in mouse communication. Because much of the seminal research describing infant rodent vocalizations was performed some time ago and has been ably reviewed by others (rodents in general [Brown, 1976; Noirot, 1972; Okon, 1972; Sales and Pye, 1974] and mice in particular [Haack, Markl, and Ehret, 1983]), the present review concentrates on communication in adult mice.

MECHANISM OF RODENT VOCALIZING

A great deal of evidence (reviewed by Nyby and Whitney, 1978) supports the hypothesis that both audible and ultrasonic vocalizations in rodents are produced in the larynx by air passing over the vocal cords. While audible vocalizations are produced by vibrating vocal cords (Roberts, 1975), ultrasonic vocalizations are produced when the vocal cords are constricted so tightly that they can no longer vibrate. In so doing, the vocal cords are thought to provide the plates and aperture of a whistle mechanism. In fact, all of the sonographic features of rodent ultrasounds can be duplicated by passing air through a bird whistle at physiological pressures (Roberts, 1975). A laryngeal mechanism for both audible and ultrasonic vocalizations would also account for the occasional instantaneous transitions from audible to ultrasonic calls and vice versa seen in rodents (Roberts, 1972).

As expected, mouse ultrasonic vocalizations are severely disrupted by transecting the nerves that control the laryngeal musculature. One group of investigators (Nunez, Pomerantz, Bean, and Youngstrom, 1985) found that the best strategy for devocalizing mice was to transect unilaterally the inferior laryngeal nerve. However, such males remained devocalized for less than a week. Thus, a relatively short window of opportunity exists for using such devocalized mice experimentally. On the other hand, bilaterally cutting the inferior laryngeal nerve was usually fatal because of breathing difficulties, while bilateral superior laryngeal nerve cuts had only minor effects in reducing ultrasounds.

0-8493-2328-2/01/$0.00+$.50
© 2001 by CRC Press LLC

ULTRASONIC VOCALIZATIONS

Adult mice, like virtually all myomorph rodents, emit ultrasonic vocalizations during adult social interactions. Among rodents in general, such vocalizations are emitted mainly in reproductive or agonistic situations. Anderson (1954), the discoverer of rodent ultrasounds, speculated that such vocalizations also might be used for echolocation although little evidence has since been found to support this hypothesis.

For earlier reviews of adult rodent ultrasonic vocalizations, see Sales and Pye (1974), Brown (1976), and Nyby and Whitney (1978). The reader is also directed to earlier reviews of mouse ultrasonic communication (Whitney and Nyby, 1983) and of the stimuli that elicit mouse ultrasonic vocalizations (Whitney and Nyby, 1979).

MALE ULTRASONIC VOCALIZATIONS

Much research has focused on the ultrasonic vocalizations emitted by male mice in response to females. While females have the capability to vocalize ultrasonically (Sales, 1972b), and under certain circumstances vocalize quite a lot (Maggio and Whitney, 1985), they rarely vocalize in male/female pairs. Thus, males are responsible for most of the vocalizations when a male and female are placed together. This conclusion has been supported by anesthetizing (Whitney, Coble, Stockton, and Tilson, 1973) or by devocalizing (Nunez et al., 1985; Warburton, Sales, and Milligan, 1989; White, Prasad, Barfield, and Nyby, 1998) one member of a male/female pair. If the male was either anesthetized or devocalized prior to pairing, few or no ultrasounds were detected. However, if the female was devocalized or anesthetized prior to pairing, the resulting high level of ultrasound was similar to that in unmanipulated male/female pairs.

In contrast to the results of Whitney et al. (1973), Warburton et al. (1989) reported that males emitted few vocalizations to anesthetized females. The likely explanation for this difference is that the act of anesthetizing a mouse can induce variable degrees of stress. In Warburton's experiments, the stress may have been sufficient to cause the release of an alarm pheromone (Abel, 1991; 1992; 1994)) that stimulated male responses incompatible with ultrasonic vocalizations. Consistent with the findings of both groups, this author has observed considerable variability in the effectiveness of anesthetized females to elicit vocalizations from one experiment to the next (unpublished observations).

Mice are different from rats (White and Barfield, 1987) and hamsters (Floody and Pfaff, 1977b), where both the male and the female vocalize during reproductive behavior. Mice are also unusual among rodents in that they do not normally emit ultrasounds during agonistic situations (Sales, 1972b). In mice, the only social context that involves male ultrasonic vocalizations is reproduction. Sales (1972a) detected ultrasounds on occasion in male/male pairs but only when one male was investigating or mounting the other. Thus, such ultrasounds would appear misguided and usually disappear at the first sign of intermale agonistic behavior (Whitney and Nyby, 1983).

Sonagraphic Analysis of Male Mouse Ultrasounds

Adult mice emit ultrasonic vocalizations as short pulses, with each exhalation typically containing one pulse. Each individual pulse is typically from 50 to 300 ms in duration, with approximately 200 ms between pulses. A train of ultrasonic pulses may contain from 3 to 80 such pulses in quick succession, with the total train of pulses lasting from about 0.5 s up to about 30 s in duration. These trains of pulses are most frequent just after a male and female are placed together (Sales, 1972b). Although substantial individual variability exists, up to 450 of these pulses have been detected in the 3-min period immediately after pairing (Nyby and Whitney, 1978). Male mice clearly expend more effort emitting ultrasonic vocalizations during reproductive behavior than do male rats (Sales, 1972b) or hamsters (Floody and Pfaff, 1977a).

While audible mouse squeals typically have a major frequency plus harmonically related minor frequencies (as would be expected from vibrating vocal cords), ultrasonic vocalizations are quite often pure tones with no harmonics. Most of these ultrasonic calls can be detected from adults with an ultrasonic receiver tuned to 70 kHz (with a bandwidth of ±10 kHz). Hence, these calls are sometimes referred to as 70-kHz calls. However, sonagraphic analysis reveals frequency modulation with frequency drifts, rapid frequency changes, and instantaneous frequency steps up to 60 kHz (Sales, 1972b). Sales' sonograms also provide evidence for some ultrasounds at frequencies that do not include 70 kHz.

A more recent study (White et al., 1998) systematically followed sonagrams of ultrasonic vocalizations across a mating bout. This work confirmed Sales' observations of the relationship between 70-kHz vocalizations and male-typical courtship and sexual behavior. However, once the male began mounting the female, a second ultrasonic vocalization of about 40-kHz call was interspersed among the 70-kHz calls. Both types of vocalizations declined across intromissions. The 40-kHz calls were louder, more variable in length, and less variable in frequency.

The suggestion was made that perhaps the 40-kHz and 70-kHz calls are serving different functions (White et al., 1998). Because the 70-kHz calls occurred at their highest rates during investigatory behavior and early in the mating sequence, these calls may be involved in communicating information during courtship and the early stages of copulation. On the other hand, the 40-kHz calls occurred mainly during mounting and were suggested to play a role during copulation only.

Ethographic Analysis of Male Mouse Ultrasounds

One way of obtaining a first approximation of the functional significance of male vocalizations has been to observe exactly what the male is doing when his ultrasonic vocalizations are detected. Sales (1972b) found that in male/female pairs of C3H, T.O. Swiss, and E.N. mice, ultrasounds correlated better with the behaviors of the male than with those of the female. The ultrasounds were most common immediately after the male and female were placed together when the male was engaging in olfactory investigation of the female. However, the ultrasounds continued, although at a lower level, after investigatory behavior had ceased and sexual behavior had begun. Once mounting began, the ultrasounds occurred mainly during the mounting attempts. Relatively few ultrasounds were detected between mounts when the male and female were separated and not interacting. Sales also reported that for some male/female pairs, the ultrasounds correlated with the pelvic thrusts of the male during mounts both with and without intromissions. The ultrasounds declined across intromissions, and in males that ejaculated, no ultrasounds were detected during and immediately after ejaculation.

In general, the ultrasounds of male mice correlated well with other male behaviors indicative of sexual arousal. These observations led Sales to conclude that ultrasounds themselves can serve as a good index of male sexual arousal. On the other hand, audible squeals, when they occurred, correlated best with the nonreceptive behaviors of the female, suggesting that audible sounds were most often female-produced.

Ejaculation by male mice is usually followed by a postejaculatory refractory period of about 15 to 30 min in duration (Mosig and Dewsbury, 1976; Nyby, 1983; but see also McGill, 1962). At the end of this refractory period, many males reinitiate another mating sequence leading to a second ejaculation, which then generally leads to sexual exhaustion (Mosig and Dewsbury, 1976). In rodents, such a postejaculatory refractory period is further subdivided into an absolute refractory period when the male is physiologically incapable of mating and a relative refractory period when mating is physiologically possible but normally does not occur (Barfield and Geyer, 1972).

Nyby (1983) quantified levels of 70-kHz ultrasonic vocalizations through the first ejaculation, the postejaculatory refractory period, and into a second mating bout. The cessation of vocalizations at the time of ejaculation continued for about the first 75% of the refractory period. The vocalizations began again and continued for about the last 25% of the refractory period, generally coincident with male investigation of the female. Once the refractory period ended and the male resumed mounting, the patterning of male mouse vocalizations was similar to that preceding ejaculation with an even stronger temporal relationship to mounting. The period of ultrasonic silence following ejaculation was hypothesized to demarcate the absolute refractory period, while the resumption of ultrasounds during the latter portion of the refractory period was hypothesized to index that the male had entered the relative refractory period. The period of ultrasonic silence during the postejaculatory refractory period appears analogous to the emission of 22-kHz postejaculatory ultrasounds by male rats which similarly demarcate the absolute refractory period in that species (Barfield and Geyer, 1975).

In summary, male mice emit substantial amounts of 70-kHz ultrasound immediately preceding and during the time that they are engaging in either olfactory investigation or mounting of the female. On the other hand, males typically emit fewer ultrasounds when disengaged from the female between investigatory or sexual encounters and emit no ultrasounds at all for much of the postejaculatory refractory period. These findings support the hypothesis that male ultrasounds index immediate sexual motivation on the part of the male.

Genetic Basis for Motivation to Vocalize

Early work (described in Nyby and Whitney (1978)) examined a number of inbred, hybrid, and outbred strains of mice for their latency to emit 70-kHz vocalizations in response to a female. Although strain differences were evident, males of all strains emitted at least some ultrasound, indicating that such vocalizing is likely a general phenomenon among male mice. Males from a "low-vocalizing" strain (A/J) in which less than 10% of the males vocalized during a 3-min test were later found to reliably emit ultrasound when tested over a longer time period (Nyby, 1983). The low levels of ultrasound originally attributed to this strain simply reflected that this strain was slower to begin vocalizing. Thus, conclusions about vocalization levels obtained from short time-sampling periods can sometimes be misleading, as has also been pointed out by others (Warburton, Stoughton, Demaine, Sales, and Milligan, 1988).

The latency of male mice to vocalize to a female does exhibit the genetic property of heterosis. That is, hybrid mice are generally quicker to begin vocalizing than males of their progenitor inbred strains. Such a relationship is indicative of directional dominance. In addition, in an unpublished doctoral dissertation, Coble (1972) found that the realized heritability for latency to vocalize from one generation of bi-directional selection in a genetically heterogeneous population was not significantly different from zero. Directional dominance and a low heritability represent the genetic architecture of a trait that has undergone strong directional selection and is closely related to reproductive fitness (Falconer, 1960). Thus, genetic work is certainly consistent with male vocalizations subserving some important biological function.

Androgenic Regulation of Male Mouse Ultrasounds

Androgenic hormones are generally hypothesized to influence behavior by acting upon the brain in two fashions. Androgens can exert organizational effects early in development during sensitive periods where they permanently and irreversibly masculinize target tissues (particularly the brain). On the other hand, androgens can also exert activational effects, mainly in adulthood, that produce reversible effects. While this dichotomy is not absolute (Arnold and Breedlove, 1985), it has nonetheless proven a useful heuristic for guiding a great deal of research examining hormone effects upon the brain and behavior (Breedlove, 1992). While considerable evidence supports the idea that testosterone exerts activational effects upon the production of male vocalizations, the evidence that testosterone organizes the neural substrate underlying this behavior is not very compelling.

Activational Effects

Several early observations indirectly suggested that male vocalizations might be activated by male-typical sex hormones. For example, infant mice emit ultrasonic distress calls that stimulate retrieval and reduce maternal aggression (Noirot, 1972). By 14 to 16 days of age, these ultrasounds cease. However, ultrasounds, similar in frequency to the infant ultrasounds, reappear in C57BL/6J x BALB/cJ male mice sometime after 35 days of age, at roughly the time of puberty (Whitney et al., 1973). In a more systematic study (Warburton et al., 1989), the time of reappearance of vocalizations in male T.O. Swiss mice was between 30 and 40 days of age, the approximate age of puberty. The exact age at which the ultrasounds reappeared depended on the amount of previous experience that young males had with females. Despite this variation, the reappearance of vocalizations in young males clearly correlated with the endogenous increase in androgenic hormones at puberty.

Another observation suggesting hormonal control of male vocalizations was that dominant DBA/2J males were quicker to begin emitting ultrasound and emitted more ultrasound in response to females than did subordinates (Nyby, Dizinno, and Whitney, 1976). Because dominant male mice generally have higher reproductive fitness than subordinates (Horn, 1974), this finding again raised the possibility that ultrasounds might be regulated by androgenic hormones.

Dizinno and Whitney (1977) provided the first direct evidence that androgens regulate male ultrasounds. In that work, castrated hybrid males (C57BL/6J x DBA/2J) emitted substantially fewer ultrasounds to females than gonadally intact males. However, ultrasounds were restored in castrates by treatments with testosterone propionate. The positive role of testosterone in activating male ultrasounds has since been confirmed in DBA/2J (Nunez, Nyby, and Whitney, 1978), Swiss-Webster (Nunez and Tan, 1984), and Tucks Swiss T.O. (Warburton et al., 1989) strains and thus appears as a general phenomenon among mice.

A widely used approach to determine the receptor system by which testosterone (T) regulates male-typical behaviors involves assessing the behavior-restorative properties of estradiol (E2) and dihydrotestosterone (DHT), the major CNS metabolites of T (Larsson, 1979; Luttge, 1979). Estrogen receptors are assumed to mediate the effectiveness of E2 while DHT (a nonaromatizable androgen) is thought to be specific for androgen receptor activation.

Initial work with DBA/2J mice (Nunez et al., 1978) was consistent with testosterone activating male-typical reproductive behavior following aromatization to estradiol and then binding to estrogen receptors in the brain. In contrast, subsequent work with Swiss-Webster mice (Nunez and Tan, 1984) and with C57BL/6J x AKR/J mice (Bean, Nyby, Kerchner, and Dahinden, 1986b) demonstrated that both E2 and DHT were effective in restoring ultrasonic vocalizations in males of these strains. This work suggests that mice possess redundant neural receptor mechanisms for androgenic responsiveness, both of which are present in some genetic strains but not in others. Work on copulatory behavior in mice and rats similarly finds that all strains uniformly show estrogenic responsiveness but show much more variation in their degree of androgenic responsiveness (Nyby and Simon, 1987).

A later study (Nyby and Simon, 1987) demonstrated that ultrasounds could be restored in castrated DBA/2J males (the DHT insensitive strain) with high (900 µg) but not lower doses (600 µg and 300 µg) of methyltrienolone (R1881). R1881 is an artificial nonaromatizable androgen thought to be even more specific for androgen receptors than DHT (Doering and Leyra, 1984). However, in contrast to expectations, the 900-µg dosage that restored behavior also showed significant binding with estrogen receptors in the brain (Nyby and Simon, 1987). This finding raised the possibility that the restorative effects of R1881 in this study, and perhaps DHT in the previous studies (Bean, Nunez, and Wysocki, 1986a; Nunez and Tan, 1984) were mediated by these androgens binding estrogen receptors. Because estrogens restored ultrasounds in all studies at much lower dosages than androgens, the estrogen receptor system is clearly important in regulating sex hormone activation of ultrasonic vocalizations. Establishing unequivocally that the androgen receptor system can also mediate responsiveness clearly requires further work.

Female mice also respond to androgen treatment with increased levels of ultrasonic vocalizations (Nyby, Dizinno, and Whitney, 1977a). In fact, ovariectomized DBA/2J females were quite similar to castrated males of this genotype in their responsiveness to testosterone. In contrast, C57BL/6J x AKR/J females did not respond quite as quickly to repeated testosterone injections as castrated males of their own strain. However, with extended treatment over several weeks, their amount of ultrasound eventually became indistinguishable from that of males. Such androgenic treatments also increased the females' incidence of male-typical mounting of other females in both strains (Nyby et al., 1977a). Thus, females appear to possess the same potential as males for showing male-typical courtship and mounting behavior and will quite reliably express this potential following extended androgenic stimulation.

Organizational Effects

One approach to demonstrate organizational effects is simply to administer male hormones to females in adulthood. If parts of the female brain have been organized differently from those of males, then females should respond differently to androgens. As noted above (Nyby et al., 1977a), females were either similar to or slightly slower in responding to androgenic treatment. Whether the delayed female response reflects an organizational difference or whether females were simply more refractory because of lower initial androgen levels is not clear. However, if a sex difference in hormone responsiveness exists, it is not profound.

Another strategy to demonstrate organizational effects examines whether phenotypic differences between animals of the same sex can be accounted for by their intrauterine position. Specifically, individuals developing *in utero* between two males (2M mice) are exposed to more androgen early in development than individuals developing between two females (0M mice) (Clemens, Gladue, and Coniglio, 1978; vom Saal, 1981). As a result, 2M female mice should be more masculinized in adulthood than 0M females for traits organized by the early effects of androgens. Consistent with this hypothesis, adult 2M female mice were more aggressive (Gandelman, Vom Saal, and Reinisch, 1977; Kinsley, Miele, Konen, Ghiraldi, and Svare, 1986; Quadagno et al., 1987; Rines and vom Saal, 1984) and more likely to engage in male-typical copulatory behavior (Quadagno et al., 1987; Rines and vom Saal, 1984) than 0M females.

However, Jubilan and Nyby (1992) found intrauterine position to have little influence on the ultrasonic vocalizations of either adult females or adult males to either a female mouse or her urine. Thus, this approach also did not support an early organizational influence of androgens upon ultrasonic vocalizations. In conclusion, females have much the same potential to vocalize as males, and the sex difference in adulthood is likely due to a sex difference in androgen titers.

Neural Regulation of Male Mouse Ultrasounds

Because 70-kHz ultrasounds appear to be a male-typical courtship behavior, research examining their neural regulation has focused on areas of the brain known to be important in male reproductive behavior. One such area is the medial preoptic area (MPOA). Bilateral lesions of the MPOA cause severe impairment or abolishment of male-typical copulatory behavior in other mammals (Hart and Leedy, 1985). Bean, Nunez, and Conner (1981) demonstrated that mouse copulatory behavior was similarly impaired by MPOA lesions but that ultrasonic vocalizations, either to adult females or to female bedding, were relatively unaffected. These results suggested that while male copulatory behavior is regulated by the MPOA, ultrasonic vocalizations are regulated by other parts of the brain.

In contrast, other studies have consistently implicated the MPOA as the important site at which androgens activate male vocalizations (Matochik, Sipos, Nyby, and Barfield, 1994; Nyby, Matochik, and Barfield, 1992; Sipos and Nyby, 1996; 1998). In these studies, cannula implants of either testosterone or testosterone propionate into the MPOA were highly effective in restoring ultrasonic vocalizations in castrated male C57BL/6J x AKR mice. However, implants into the anterior hypothalamus (Nyby et al., 1992), ventromedial hypothalamus (Nyby et al., 1992), septum (Nyby, 1992; Matochik, 1994), medial amygdala (Matochik et al., 1994; Nyby et al., 1992), and ventral tegmental area (Sipos and Nyby, 1996) were without effect.

Perhaps the reason that MPOA lesions did not eliminate ultrasounds (Bean et al., 1981) was that not enough of the MPOA was lesioned. While plausible, this hypothesis may be difficult to test because large bilateral lesions of the MPOA are often lethal. Nonetheless, androgenic implant work clearly implicates the MPOA as an important site for the neural regulation of male ultrasonic vocalizations.

It seems likely that other areas of the brain also participate in the regulation of male mouse ultrasonic vocalizations. Newman (1999) hypothesized that all social behaviors (including sexual, aggressive, and parental behaviors) may be regulated by a common neural network (the medial extended amygdala) that includes the corticomedial amygdala, lateral septum, ventromedial hypothalamus, midbrain central gray and tegmentum, anterior hypothalamus, as well as the medial preoptic area. While testosterone implants demonstrated the involvement of the medial preoptic area, other strategies will be necessary to examine the importance of these other areas, since most of them are androgenically unresponsive for the activation of ultrasounds (Matochik et al., 1994; Nyby et al., 1992; Sipos and Nyby, 1996; 1998). In addition, the parts of the nervous system that control motor output to the larynx should also be involved.

At the same time, estradiol implants restored ultrasounds in the MPOA, ventromedial hypothalamus, anterior hypothalamus, and lateral septum (Nyby et al., 1992). These results could reflect the greater activity of this treatment, more diffusion of hormone from the implant site, or that the distribution of estrogen-responsive neurons was not identical to that of androgen-responsive neurons. Further research is necessary to choose among these alternatives.

Pheromonal Elicitation of Male Mouse Ultrasounds

Not only are female mice good stimuli for eliciting ultrasonic vocalizations from males, the odors of females are also quite effective. Early work showed, for example, that the soiled cage shavings of females were good stimuli (Whitney, Alpern, Dizinno, and Horowitz, 1974). Subsequent work revealed that female urine (Nyby, Wysocki, Whitney, and Dizinno, 1977b), female saliva (Byatt and Nyby, 1986), and female vaginal fluids (Nyby et al., 1977b) were also effective. Whether these different body fluids all contain the same ultrasound-eliciting chemosignal or whether they contain different female chemosignals, all of which elicit ultrasounds, has not been determined.

However, most of the research on the chemosensory elicitation of male ultrasounds has focused on female urine. One reason was to keep the work as comparable as possible to a much larger body of research examining pheromonal communication in mice. For example, in addition to eliciting ultrasonic vocalizations, female urine causes a reflexive release of luteinizing hormone in male mice (Maruniak and Bronson, 1976), promotes male copulatory behavior (Dixon and Mackintosh, 1971), and reduces intermale aggression (Mugford and Nowell, 1971). In recent unpublished work, we (Sipos, Nyby, Snyder, and Kerchner, 1999) present evidence that all of these different effects of female urine upon males, including ultrasound elicitation, may be mediated by the same urinary chemosignals. In addition, work in my laboratory provided evidence that two different urinary chemosignals of female mice elicit ultrasounds from male mice. In what follows, some of our earlier work on pheromonal elicitation of ultrasounds is reinterpreted in light of these newer findings.

Freshly voided urine of female mice contains a potent ultrasound-eliciting chemosignal that in most ways fits the most rigorous definitions of a pheromone (Beauchamp, Doty, Moulton, and Mugford, 1976). This pheromone is salient even to sexually naïve adult males (Sipos, Kerchner, and Nyby, 1992), remains a potent stimulus for eliciting vocalizations with repeated testing (Sipos et al., 1992), and can even serve as an unconditioned stimulus for causing neutral stimuli to acquire ultrasound-eliciting properties (Sipos et al., 1992). At the same time, this chemosignal is ephemeral; its activity is normally destroyed by oxidation within 15 to 18 h after voiding (Sipos, Nyby, and Serran, 1993). This chemosignal is not present in urine collected overnight (12 h) in a metabolic cage, indicating that this method of urine collection likely hastens the oxidation that destroys the pheromone.

Because urine aged well beyond 24 h (up to 30 days) also elicits ultrasounds under certain circumstances (Nyby and Zakeski, 1980), a second ultrasound-eliciting chemosignal must exist as well. However, aged urine elicits ultrasounds only under limited circumstances. First, males do not vocalize to aged urine unless they are sexually experienced (Dizinno, Whitney, and Nyby, 1978; Sipos et al., 1992). Although such males initially vocalize at high levels to aged urine, their vocalizations rapidly habituate following three to four exposures (Dizinno et al., 1978; Sipos et al., 1992). Furthermore, repeatedly pairing a neutral stimulus with aged urine does not result in vocalizations to the neutral stimulus (Sipos et al., 1992).

Although the chemosignal in aged urine elicits ultrasounds in certain circumstances, its properties do not fit the original narrow definition of a pheromone (Beauchamp et al., 1976). However, some workers subscribe to a broader definition to include chemosignals where the roles of learning and contextual cues are important in establishing the signal value of the chemosignal (reviewed by Albone, 1984). As such, we (Sipos et al., 1992) have referred to these two chemosignals as the "ephemeral pheromone" and the "stable pheromone," respectively. We believe that both chemosignals are probably present in freshly voided urine and that, when a male encounters such urine, their association permits aged urine to acquire the property to elicit male vocalizations. Moreover, the relative concentrations of these two chemosignals in a female scent mark may also provide important information about how recently a female has been in the area. However, attempts to chemically characterize these chemosignals have not been successful, and it is not known whether these chemosignals are single molecules or chemical mixtures. We have hypothesized, however, that oxidation may turn the ephemeral pheromone into the stable pheromone.

Other work has demonstrated that males can learn to vocalize not only to the stable pheromone in aged female urine, but also to other odors that normally do not elicit ultrasounds. For example, by pairing the following with repeated exposures to a female, males acquired the capacity to vocalize to some degree to: urine from female rats (Kerchner, Vatza, and Nyby, 1986), urine from hypophysectomized females (Maggio, Maggio, and Whitney, 1983), perfume (Nyby, Whitney, Schmitz, and Dizinno, 1978), foenugreek (Kerchner et al., 1986), clean cotton swabs (Sipos, Wysocki, Nyby, Wysocki, and Nemura, 1995), and plastic bags (Nyby, Wysocki, Whitney, Dizinno, and Schneider, 1979). In fact, some males will vocalize to the entry of a human experimenter into the colony room if the male has been paired repeatedly with females by an experimenter (unpublished). Almost any stimulus that allows a male to anticipate an encounter with a female would appear to acquire the property of eliciting ultrasounds. However, some constraints must exist on the cues that can elicit ultrasounds because attempts to train males to vocalize to the urine of other males were not successful (unpublished).

How male mice learn to vocalize to stimuli that normally do not elicit vocalizations has been the subject of some research. Although previous work suggested that encountering a novel odor during a socio/sexual encounter with a female provided the best learning, others (Marr and Gardner, 1965; Müller-Schwarze and Müller-Schwarze, 1971) have hypothesized that the salience of sex odors is acquired as a result of neonatal imprinting on the mother. Using a perfume that normally does not elicit vocalizations, we systematically explored whether male experience with such perfume during infancy (associated with the dam) or during adulthood (associated with a female during sexual encounters) was most important in causing the perfume to acquire ultrasound-eliciting properties (Nyby et al., 1978). Very briefly, adult experience with an odorized female was far more important than infant experience with an odorized dam. However, some synergy appeared to exist between the two experiences, suggesting that imprinting might enhance the learning of novel signals in adulthood. At the same time, males that had seen only perfumed females at these two developmental periods nonetheless exhibited high levels of ultrasonic responsiveness to normal female urine (Nyby et al., 1978). Thus, responsiveness to perfume, when it occurred, was superimposed upon, and did not replace, normal ultrasonic responsiveness to female urine.

Whether male vocalizations to the ephemeral chemosignal in freshly voided urine are "learned" as a result of neonatal imprinting or are simply an innate response is not known.

Sensory Detection of Ultrasound-Eliciting Pheromones

Potential nasal chemosensory systems for mediating responsiveness to ultrasound-eliciting chemosignals include the main olfactory system, the accessory olfactory or vomeronasal system (Jacobson's organ), the terminal nerve system, and the trigeminal nerve system (Wysocki, 1979; Wysocki and Lepri, 1991). In addition, some investigators classify the septal organ system as an additional chemosensory system separate from the main olfactory system. However, work on ultrasound elicitation in mice has centered on the relative contributions of the main olfactory system and the vomeronasal system.

Early work (Bean, 1982; Wysocki, Nyby, Whitney, Beauchamp, and Katz, 1982), which involved deafferenting all of the nasal chemosensory systems of male mice by olfactory bulbectomy, greatly reduced ultrasonic vocalizations to female mice. However, vocalizations to the female herself were not totally eliminated in all bulbectomized males, particularly if the male was sexually experienced prior to olfactory bulbectomy (Wysocki et al., 1982). This finding was consistent with sexually inexperienced males relying more on chemosensory input for vocalization elicitation, while experienced males were better able to use non-chemosensory cues in making this determination. On the other hand, vocalizations of sexually experienced male mice to the soiled cage shavings of females (perceived mainly by chemosensory input) were eliminated by bulbectomy (Wysocki et al., 1982). Thus, olfactory bulbectomy did not eliminate the motivation to vocalize, but rather eliminated the detection of pheromonal cues that normally elicit vocalizations.

Earlier work (Wysocki et al., 1982) indicated that sexually inexperienced males required a functioning vomeronasal organ to learn to vocalize to the stable chemosignal in aged urine. However, sexually experienced males vocalized to the stable chemosignal after vomeronasalectomy. Thus, the ability of a male to recognize the stable chemosignal based upon non-vomeronasal chemoreception required previous experience with such cues in the presence of a functioning vomeronasal organ (Wysocki et al., 1982). Again, the deficits in vocalizing following vomeronasal removal were sensory rather than motivational deficits.

Another line of research (Sipos et al., 1995) examined the relative roles of the main and accessory olfactory systems in vocalizing to the potent but ephemeral pheromone in recently voided urine. In one experiment, selectively deafferenting the accessory system (by surgically removing the vomeronasal organ) or selectively deafferenting the main olfactory system (by intranasal irrigation with $ZnSO_4$) each had only minor effects in reducing ultrasounds to freshly collected urine. However, if both chemosensory systems were simultaneously deafferented, ultrasounds to fresh urine were eliminated. Thus, for this pheromone, both chemosensory systems were approximately equally important and appeared redundant for pheromone detection. For a chemosignal carrying biologically important information, it is not surprising that redundant sensory systems exist for its detection.

Function of Male Mouse Ultrasounds

Most hypotheses on the function of male mouse ultrasounds have focused on the 70-kHz calls. Sales [nee Sewell (Sewell, 1967; 1968)] first suggested that male vocalizations serve to signal females that the male is sexually and not aggressively motivated. Sales further suggested that ultrasounds also serve both to reduce female aggression and to promote female sexual motivation. Whitney (1973) developed this hypothesis further by suggesting that ultrasounds may, in fact, be a ritualized courtship display in which the male is mimicking ultrasounds emitted by infant mice of both sexes. Because infant ultrasounds are attractive to the dam and reduce rough parental handling, adult male vocalizations may similarly attract adult females and reduce their aggression. Such ritualized use of infantile behaviors in adult male courtship occurs in a variety of birds and mammals (Eibl-Eibesfeldt, 1970).

The hypothesis that male ultrasounds serve to reduce female aggression becomes more plausible in light of the fact that most mouse matings in nature occur during the female's postpartum estrus (Whitney et al., 1973). At this time, the female is very protective of her pups and very aggressive toward strange males. Perhaps male ultrasounds are particularly important in reducing female aggression at this time.

Various indirect lines of evidence are certainly consistent with a courtship/reproductive function for 70-kHz ultrasounds. As described earlier, ultrasound production is hormonally and neurologically regulated very similar to other components of male-typical reproductive behavior. This phenotype also exhibits the genetic architecture (directional dominance and low heritability) of a trait closely related to reproductive fitness. At the same time, some strains of laboratory mice are deaf in adulthood and yet clearly mate without obvious difficulty. While ultrasonic vocalizations likely promote reproductive behavior, such vocalizations are clearly not essential. The effects of ultrasounds may be subtle. For example, in hamsters, male ultrasonic vocalizations promote female receptivity through the prolongation of lordosis (Floody and Pfaff, 1977c); and in rats, male ultrasounds increase the female proceptive behaviors of darting and hopping (Thomas, Howard, and Barfield, 1982).

However, attempts to experimentally demonstrate functional significance for male mouse ultrasounds have been mixed. One approach (Pomerantz, Nunez, and Bean, 1983) gave females access to tethered males in adjoining compartments that were either vocalizing or not and observing which male they preferred. The rate of vocalizing was manipulated by either devocalizing only one of the males or by devocalizing both males and using an ultrasound generator to associate artificial vocalizations with only one of the males. While neither natural nor artificial ultrasounds caused more entries into a compartment, once the female entered a compartment containing ultrasounds, she stayed in that compartment longer. Thus, one possible function of 70-kHz ultrasounds may be to keep the female in close proximity.

Although performed in the context of mother/infant communication, it is also quite interesting that female mice are more attracted to infant ultrasounds if they can hear them with their right ear than their left ear (Ehret, 1987). Such a finding suggests that the decoding of ultrasonic vocalizations is a left-hemisphere phenomenon, providing certain parallels to human speech. If female processing of male-produced ultrasounds is similarly lateralized, indirect evidence would certainly be provided for functional significance.

If male vocalizations serve a courtship function, one might predict that devocalized males would be less successful in initiating reproductive behavior. However, attempts to demonstrate such a relationship were not successful (Nunez et al., 1985). Devocalized males readily mated and did not show an impairment in their latency to begin mounting. Thus, while male ultrasounds may play a role in mating, they clearly are not required for successful mating.

Recognizing that mating with an ovariectomized female in hormone-induced receptivity may not entirely reflect mating situations in nature, Bean et al. (1986a) looked at the ability of male vocalizations to reduce aggression in lactating females (when estrus occurs most often in natural situations). In contrast to expectations, the lactating females attacked vocalizing males even more quickly than devocalized males. At the same time, these lactating females were likely not experiencing postpartum estrus, which may have been necessary to show an effect of male ultrasounds in reducing female aggression.

An alternative hypothesis for why it has been difficult to experimentally demonstrate functionality for male ultrasounds is that perhaps ultrasonic vocalizations have no communicatory significance. Such an explanation was postulated for Mongolian gerbils by Thiessen and colleagues (Thiessen and Kittrell, 1979; Thiessen, Kittrell, and Graham, 1980), who were unable to find any evidence that ultrasonic vocalizations serve as a form of communication in this species. These workers further observed that about 90% of gerbil ultrasonic vocalizations occur during hopping movements when the forepaws hit the ground. Other situations that involved ultrasounds included turning, stretching, compression of the upper body, and hind-foot thumping. What all of these behaviors had in common was the physical compression of the thorax and lungs, which forced air out of the lungs, through the larynx, and out the nose. Thiessen suggested that the ultrasonic vocalizations produced by gerbils are simply an incidental by-product of bodily movements and have no communicatory significance.

Blumberg (1992) critically evaluated this hypothesis for rodents in general and concluded that house mice, rats, woodrats, hamsters, and gerbils are indeed often engaging in behaviors that promote thoracic compression while emitting ultrasounds. In mice, the correlation between ultrasound production and pelvic thrusting during mounting was seen as particularly consistent with this idea.

However, Blumberg (1992) also makes additional important points in favor of ultrasonic vocalizations possessing communicatory significance. For example, even if an ultrasound is produced as an incidental by-product of thoracic compression, it could still acquire communicatory significance during evolution if it reliably predicts a particular behavioral or physiological state. As already noted, male mouse ultrasounds clearly correlate with male sexual arousal and thus could clearly communicate the male's motivational state to other nearby mice. Blumberg (1992) also points out that not all rodent ultrasounds can be related to biomechanical strain alone. For example, training rats to hop (and thereby compress their thorax) did not cause them to emit ultrasonic vocalizations (Blumberg, 1992).

With regard to mice, I have observed high levels of 70-kHz ultrasounds when a male is stationary and have even noted repeated vocalizations from males hanging by their front paws from the top of a mouse cage. While thoracic compression may accompany and perhaps even aid in the emission of some mouse ultrasonic vocalizations, thoracic compression is not essential. Whether the 40-kHz calls of male mice better fit the thoracic compression hypothesis is not clear. More work on the 40-kHz call is clearly necessary.

Two additional caveats are necessary for investigators interested in experimentally examining the functional effects of male mouse ultrasounds on female behavior. The first is that while male ultrasounds may play a communicatory role in wild mice, such a role may have been altered in domesticated mice by years of selective breeding. Clearly, domesticated mice have been bred, either on purpose or inadvertently, to readily engage in reproductive behavior. As a result, perhaps female reproductive behavior in domesticated mice does not require the same degree of ultrasonic facilitation as it does for wild mice (possibly accounting for the difficulty that experimenters have had in demonstrating function). The second caveat is that many domesticated mouse strains (particularly inbred strains) have high-frequency hearing loss during development and in some cases become deaf in adulthood (Nyby and Whitney, 1978) (see Chapters 5, 6, 13, 24, 28). For either of these reasons, studying the functional aspects of male mouse vocalizations in domesticated mice can present problems of interpretation. On the other hand, studying the function of ultrasonic vocalizations using wild mice, which in many ways would be more desirable, has its own attendant difficulties.

ULTRASONIC VOCALIZATIONS BY FEMALE MICE

Although most of the work on adult mouse ultrasonic vocalizations has concentrated on male-produced vocalizations, normal females clearly have the capability to vocalize. For example, Sales in an early paper (Sales, 1972b) reported two cases in which 70-kHz ultrasounds were detected from female/female pairs. Maggio and Whitney (1985) subsequently confirmed that the best stimulus for eliciting ultrasounds from female mice was indeed another female.

Similar to findings from males, females vocalized not only to awake females but also to anesthetized females (Maggio and Whitney, 1985). Anesthetized males, however, were not good stimuli for ultrasound elicitation. Such findings might suggest that the females were vocalizing to odor cues from other females. However, attempts to verify the importance of odors were not successful: very few females vocalized either to female-soiled cage shavings or to female urine

(Maggio and Whitney, 1985). Moreover, giving the females increased experience with females (which promotes male vocalizations to female odors) was without effect in promoting female vocalizations to female odors (Maggio and Whitney, 1985). Maggio and Whitney (1985) also found that a brief exposure to a male inhibited vocalizing to other females for at least 48 hours.

Genetics of Female Vocalizing

Two strain surveys indicated that while females of all inbred and hybrid strains emitted ultrasonic vocalizations, strain differences clearly existed (Maggio and Whitney, 1985). In fact, the propensity of females of a given genotype to vocalize and their levels of vocalizations were similar to that of males of the same genotype. Moreover, female vocalizing exhibited the genetic property of heterosis, with hybrids generally vocalizing more than their inbred progenitors.

Function of Female Ultrasounds

Maggio and Whitney (1985) saw little evidence that females were also engaging in male-typical behaviors while vocalizing to other females, suggesting that these vocalizations were not simply an inappropriate male-typical behavior. As a result, these authors hypothesized that female vocalizations may contribute to the establishment of social dominance hierarchies among females within demes (i.e., breeding groups).

However, a result that complicates this interpretation was that brief exposure to an anesthetized male greatly inhibited female vocalizations to other females for at least several days (Maggio and Whitney, 1985). The social structure of mice usually involves females living in a deme that includes one or more males (Bronson, 1979). Thus, if the presence of a male inhibits female vocalizing, females would be unlikely to vocalize under naturalistic conditions. This finding raises the possibility that female vocalizations are just a laboratory artifact that arises when females are kept isolated from males. Clearly, more work is necessary on vocalizations by females to determine whether these vocalizations are functionally important or simply an epiphenonmenon.

Alternatively, perhaps female ultrasonic vocalizations are an adaptive facultative response to isolation from males. If the males in a deme leave or die, it may be necessary for a female to assume some role normally performed by males. In the absence of a male, perhaps one of the females in the deme (perhaps the most dominant female) would take over this function. This line of reasoning is highly speculative and further research certainly is necessary to test this and other hypotheses about female vocalizations.

AUDIBLE SOUNDS OF ADULT MICE

Audible mouse sounds during social behavior have not received nearly the attention of ultrasonic vocalizations. However, audible sounds are common and often index a distinct emotional state in the vocalizer. As such, they clearly convey information that could potentially be useful to another mouse. Two audible sounds that could have communicatory significance during social behavior include squealing (also referred to as squeaking) and tail rattling (also called tail lashing).

SQUEALING

Both adult male and female mice squeal during normal social/sexual and agonistic encounters. For example, males often squeal during intermale aggression, while females are likely to squeal during reproductive behavior in response to the sexual advances of a male. However, in response to human handling, male and female mice squeal with about equal probability (Whitney, 1969). Thus, it seems likely that this vocalization is indexing the same emotional state in both sexes. Mice of both sexes also squeal in response to a predatory attack (Blanchard et al., 1998).

Sonagrams of Mouse Squealing

Houseknect (1968) examined the fundamental frequencies and durations of squeals produced by adult house mice during aggressive interactions (both intraspecific and interspecific) and when being held by the tail. During aggressive interactions, the subordinate mouse always appeared to be the vocalizer. Squeals were much more common in male/male interactions than in female/female interactions. However, the sonagrams of mouse squealing were similar regardless of sex and context, with a fundamental frequency of about 4 kHz, a secondary frequency of about 8 kHz, and a duration of about 125 ms.

Female Squealing

In male/female pairs, squealing is observed most often when a sexually motivated male is interacting with a nonreceptive female. I have observed that nonreceptive females often squeal not only to the mounting attempts of a male, but also, in some cases, to mere tactile contact by the male. Thus, the squeals index not only painful interactions, but also the anticipation of such interactions.

Whether female squealing has any impact on the male's sexual behavior has not been rigorously tested. I have observed that males often reduce their sexual advances to nonreceptive squealing females. Whether the reduction in male sexual behavior is caused by the squealing itself or by other aspects of the female's nonreceptivity (not presenting the genital region to male and pushing the male away) is not clear.

Note in this regard that female mice are more difficult to bring into reliable behavioral estrus through exogenous hormone treatment than female rats or hamsters. Thus, to ensure the availability of sufficient receptive females in an experiment, it is often desirable to screen females for receptivity with stud males prior to their use. In this context, repeated squealing by a female in response to the male's advances is a clear indication of nonreceptivity. In fact, McGill (1962) has used amount of squealing as a major component in defining a five-point scale of female sexual receptivity.

Male Squealing

In male/male encounters, squeals are often emitted by the subordinate member of the pair when attacked by the dominant member and are usually associated with defensive, escape, or submissive behaviors of the subordinate (Scott, 1966; Scott and Fredericson, 1951). Squealing is occasionally seen in a subordinate simply in response to being sniffed or approached by a dominant (Clark and Schein, 1966; Scott, 1966). Thus, males squeal not only during painful interactions but also in anticipation of such interactions. Whether the squeals reduce aggression is not clear. Many dominant males are relentless in their aggression toward a subordinate and do not appear affected by the subordinate's squeals. However, the types of experimental studies that would be necessary to definitively test this hypothesis have not been performed.

Squealing has been used to index the occurrence of agonistic behavior among male mice (Morgret, 1973; Morgret and Dengerink, 1972). Using an electronic monitoring device, Morgret and Dengerink (1972) found that the number of squeals during an encounter between two males correlated with time fighting ($r = 0.76$), and number of attacks ($r = 0.72$). Moreover, the conditional probability of a squeal occurring during a fight was $p = 0.83$, while during periods of no fighting the conditional probability of a squeal was $p = 0.03$. The authors concluded that although squealing directly measures one mouse's painful stimulation during an agonistic encounter, it indirectly provides a good measure of the occurrence of aggression. Another group of investigators (Brain, Benton, Cole, and Prowse, 1980) built a similar device to monitor mouse squealing over extended periods of time and presented evidence of similar impressive relationships between the amount of squealing and various indices of aggression.

By monitoring squealing as an index of fighting, some variables that influence fighting in mice have been examined. Male mice showed an increase in fighting around the time of puberty and more fighting occurred at night than during the day (Morgret, 1973). Morgret also found evidence of fighting between female mice although the incidence was much lower than for males. The rate of aggression between male mice (as indexed by squealing) was also reduced by alcohol administration (Bertilson, Mead, Morgret, and Dengerink, 1977).

Genetics of Squealing

As noted earlier, male and female mice are equally likely to squeal when picked up by the tail by a human experimenter. Whitney (Whitney, 1969; 1970; 1973; Whitney and Nyby, 1983) provided evidence for a single gene accounting for much of the strain variation observed. Picking up a domesticated mouse by the tail is a relatively mild stressor and, accordingly, less than 5% of mice from most strains squeal under this circumstance. However, in mice of one strain (IsBi), approximately 50% of males and females squealed when picked up by the tail. Whitney examined this phenotypic difference using a variety of different genetic approaches and concluded that a single dominant gene with 50% penetrance best accounted for high levels of squealing. While work by St. John (1978) was consistent with much of Whitney's interpretation, an unexpected age effect suggested that the genetics might be somewhat more complicated than originally hypothesized. Nonetheless, squealing by domesticated mice may be a naturally occurring model system for examining the effects of single genes upon behavior.

Squealing as an Index of Nociception

Because squealing usually occurs in response to painful stimulation, pharmacologists have used this behavior to screen analgesic drugs (Winter, 1965). The general paradigm involves testing whether various drugs can affect the latency to begin squealing as increasing shock levels are delivered through a metal grid floor. This "grid-shock analgesia test" has been validated as a reliable test for antinociception and agrees well with drug data obtained by other methods (Swedberg, 1994). Moreover, by using freely moving animals, this test has the advantage of eliminating the confounding effects of restraint-induced analgesia present in several other analgesic testing methods.

Function of Squealing

Although squealing is usually caused by either a painful experience or the anticipation of such an experience, only anecdotal evidence bears on whether such squeals affect the behavior of other animals. As mentioned, squeals may serve to inhibit agonistic and sexual advances. Note in this regard that the squeals are very disorienting to a novice human experimenter trying to inject a mouse with a drug or anesthetic. Perhaps the squeals function to temporarily disorient the listener, thus allowing the squeaking mouse to escape. If true, the response to squealing would likely depend on past experience with squealing mice. Again, the types of experimental studies required to test whether other animals are behaviorally affected by squeals have not been done.

Tail Rattling

Another mouse sound with potential communicatory significance is tail rattling (also called tail lashing). In this situation, the mouse rapidly lashes its tail back and forth. As the tail rubs the substrate, a distinctive sound is produced that can easily be heard by a human observer and presumably by other mice as well. While this sound has audible components, ultrasonic components, detectable by an ultrasonic receiver, exist as well (unpublished observations). However, to my knowledge, no one has ever produced a sonagram of tail rattling.

Situations where Tail Rattling is Observed

Tail rattling is seen most often during agonistic behavior, although conflicting observations exist about whether a dominant or subordinate male is most likely to perform the behavior. Clark and Schein (1966) observed tail rattling more often in dominant mice just after dominance had been established. Tail rattling was typically seen by the dominant just before attacking a subordinate. However, tail rattling was also observed in both males prior to the establishment of dominance, by a mouse approaching another mouse, by a mouse after grooming another, and occasionally by a subordinate animal when being attacked or chased. Beilharz and Beilharz (1975) similarly observed tail rattling most often after initial aggressive interactions. However, according to these investigators, the male performing the tail rattling was usually tending toward submission. Once the mouse had clearly become submissive, tail rattling was usually replaced by squealing in intermale encounters. Whether tail rattling normally occurs most often in dominant or subordinate males may simply reflect that mice of different strains possess different thresholds for the activation of this behavior.

Beilharz and Beilharz (1975) also observed tail rattling more often in domesticated mice than in wild mice. Wild mice were more likely to flee agonistic situations before either tail rattling or squealing could occur. Tail rattling can also be elicited by electric shock (St. John, 1973).

Genetics of Tail Rattling

St. John (1973) examined a number of inbred strains as well as some of their hybrid crosses for amount of tail rattling in response to shock. Clear strain differences were apparent and, in general, hybrid strains were more likely to tail rattle than their progenitor inbred strains. Such heterosis is indicative of directional dominance and is reflective of a trait that has been directionally selected by natural selection. Thus, genetic evidence favors the hypothesis that tail rattling serves some adaptive function.

Function of Tail Rattling

R.Z. Brown (1953) interpreted tail rattling as a manifestation of extreme excitement in mice. Scott and Fredericson (1951) interpreted tail rattling as a threat produced in agonistic situations in which the mouse is considering attacking an opponent. In a later paper, Scott (1966) analogized tail rattling in mice to growling in dogs. Clark and Schein (1966) similarly believe it to be a threat behavior, particularly when the mouse is undecided about whether to attack or retreat. However, no strong evidence exists that other mice respond to tail rattling as a threat. While tail rattling may be an attempt to threaten other mice, experimental research to test this hypothesis is necessary to reach definitive conclusions.

CONCLUDING REMARKS

Much research has examined the mechanisms by which mice produce sounds, the physical characteristics of the sounds, the eliciting stimuli and contexts in which the sounds are produced, and in the case of ultrasounds, the physiology and neuroscience related to their production. While much remains to be learned in these different domains, one area of inquiry that has been much less successful than others is in experimentally establishing the functional significance of mouse sounds. While many in this field feel confident that mouse sounds play an important role in mouse social communication, work on the functional significance of mouse sounds will ultimately be necessary to validate much of the other work that has been performed. Such functional work, while fraught with difficulties, should be a high priority for future research in this field.

However, independent of their communicatory significance, mouse ultrasounds have been validated as an excellent index of male sexual motivation with a number of advantages over using copulatory behavior. In addition to the greater speed and ease of obtaining data, it is also possible to observe this behavior without the confounding presence of a sexual partner. Thus, this behavior may provide a purer measure of sexual motivation than copulatory behavior itself. In addition, it is a naturally occurring behavior that is part of the normal species repertoire that provides certain advantages over operant measures of sexual motivation.

ACKNOWLEDGMENTS

The author thanks Murray Itzkowitz and Peter James for reading and commenting on an earlier version of this manuscript.

2 Behavioral Assessment of Hearing in Mice

Henry E. Heffner and Rickye S. Heffner

INTRODUCTION

The domestic house mouse (*Mus musculus*) has become an important animal model for the study of genetic hearing loss. Not only are there strains with naturally occurring hearing impairments, but genetically engineered mice can be used to identify the specific genes involved in hearing disorders. To fully understand the effects of genetic mutations on hearing, however, it is necessary to determine with some precision the hearing abilities of these mice. This includes not only absolute thresholds, but other aspects of hearing such as frequency and intensity discrimination, the effect of masking, and sound localization acuity.

There are two general approaches to assessing hearing in mice: electrophysiological and behavioral. A popular way of assessing hearing in mice is to use an electrophysiological measure; specifically, the auditory brainstem response or ABR (e.g., Q.Y. Zheng et al., 1999b). The popularity of this technique stems from the fact that it is relatively easy to learn and can provide rapid results, with measurements usually taking no more than an hour or so. However, the ABR is actually a measure of neural synchrony — not auditory sensitivity — and at best can only be used to infer absolute sensitivity (Hood, 1998). In addition, it cannot provide information regarding an animal's ability to discriminate sounds. In the clinic, the ABR is useful in diagnosing auditory disorders, but has not supplanted behavioral tests of hearing. Indeed, it is known on occasion to significantly overestimate and underestimate the effect of auditory malfunctions on sensory thresholds (Hood et al., 1994; Starr et al., 1996). Thus, although the ABR is a useful tool in assessing hearing disorders, it is necessary to employ behavioral procedures to obtain valid measures of auditory function. The ABR method is discussed in detail in Chapter 4.

The behavioral procedures available for assessing hearing in animals can be divided into two types: those that train an animal to respond to sound using conditioning procedures, and those that make use of unconditioned or reflexive responses to sound. Conditioning procedures have been considered to be more sensitive than reflexive measures, because the animals are carefully trained to be reliable observers. Moreover, these procedures are easily adapted to testing the ability of animals to discriminate between, as well as to detect sounds. However, conditioning procedures can be difficult to use, and an animal may require lengthy training before it is ready for testing. This has led to the development of procedures involving unconditioned reflexes that are simpler to administer and involve no training of the animal. Although most tests that make use of unconditioned reflexes are limited to determining an animal's ability to hear loud sounds, one procedure, prepulse inhibition, is able to determine both an animal's ability to hear low-level sounds and to discriminate between sounds (see Chapter 5 for a detailed discussion).

The essential feature of any auditory test is that the animal makes a clearly defined response when one stimulus is presented and a different response when either no stimulus or a different stimulus is presented. Although it is possible to determine an animal's response through direct observation, it is preferable to use an automated recording system to rule out the possibility of observer bias. The animal should respond reliably to obviously suprathreshold stimuli, and decreasing the stimulus level or the difference between the stimuli must eventually result in chance performance, indicating that the animal is not using some extraneous cue to perform the task. In addition, it is commonly observed in conditioning procedures that the thresholds of naïve animals improve as the animals become experienced observers, suggesting that it may be necessary for animals to learn to listen for sounds near threshold (Stebbins, 1970). Finally, the ideal test is one that is easy to use, works with all individuals, and provides reliable and valid results in a short period of time.

The acoustic environment is also important. Test procedures should be capable of fixing an animal's head within the sound field so that the sound reaching the ears can be precisely specified. Reflections from the walls of a cage should be avoided by constructing the test cage of sound-transparent material (e.g., wire mesh) and any necessary response or reward mechanisms kept small and out of the path of the sound. For example, a water reward can be delivered through a thin vertical water spout that comes up through the cage floor and is thus well below the level of the animal's ears (Heffner and Heffner, 1995). Sounds to be detected or discriminated should be carefully checked for distortion as well as for onset and offset artifacts that may occur when sounds are turned on and off abruptly.

There are a number of behavioral procedures available for assessing animal hearing (cf., Klump et al., 1995), and it is the purpose of this chapter to describe and evaluate those that have been, or could be, used with mice. It is not our intention to provide a manual on how to conduct these tests, but to describe them in sufficient detail that one might choose between them. Anyone interested in using a particular procedure should contact investigators who use them because no written description can cover all details, and procedures are constantly being updated and refined.

PROCEDURES USING CONDITIONED RESPONSES

It is not uncommon to divide conditioning procedures into (1) those using operant (or instrumental) conditioning, in which an animal emits a response to obtain a reward or avoid a punisher, and (2) those using classical conditioning, in which a stimulus elicits a response. However, whether or not a particular procedure is true classical conditioning is a technical issue that does not affect its use in sensory testing, and the main issue in this chapter is the ease of use and validity of the results.

All conditioning procedures involve either a reward, a punisher, or both. Rewards used for mice have included sweetened water and milk (Birch et al., 1968; Sidman et al., 1966). However, water by itself works well and can be reliably delivered with a commercial syringe pump or water dipper (e.g., Markl and Ehret, 1973; Chapter 3). Electric shock is commonly used in both avoidance and classical conditioning with the levels kept relatively low, because high levels can interfere with performance by causing the animals to develop a fear of the test apparatus (Heffner and Heffner, 1995).

CONDITIONED SUPPRESSION/AVOIDANCE

In devising a psychophysical procedure for use with animals, it is helpful to choose a task that utilizes an animal's natural responses, thus making the task easier to learn. One response common to all mammals is to suppress ongoing behavior (i.e., freeze) upon detection of a stimulus that might signal danger. The suppression of behavior as a procedure for testing hearing was originally developed for mice and has since been adapted for auditory testing in other animals (Heffner and Heffner, 1998; Ray, 1970; Sidman et al., 1966). The current procedure consists of allowing an animal to make steady contact with a water spout to obtain water, and then training it to momentarily break contact whenever it hears a sound that signals impending shock. Because this procedure involves avoidable shock, we have previously referred to it as "conditioned avoidance" to distinguish it from earlier conditioned suppression procedures that used unavoidable shock (cf., Heffner and Heffner, 1995; Sidman et al., 1966). However, because the suppression of ongoing activity is the key feature, we refer to it here as "conditioned suppression/avoidance."

To determine absolute thresholds, a thirsty mouse is placed in a test cage where it drinks from a water spout that delivers water as long as the animal is in contact with the spout. Next, a tone is presented for 2 s, after which a mild electric shock is delivered through the water spout. The animal quickly learns to associate the tone with the shock and breaks contact with the spout whenever it detects the tone in order to avoid the shock. The use of avoidable, as opposed to unavoidable shock, significantly increases the number of trials that can be given.

Test sessions are divided into 2-s trials with 1.5-s intertrial intervals. Tone or "warning" trials are presented on a random schedule with approximately 22% of the trials containing a tone. The response of an animal is scored as a "hit" if the animal breaks contact during the last 150 ms of a trial that contains a tone. Breaking contact during a trial that does not contain a tone (a "safe" trial) is scored as a "false alarm" (FA). The hit rate is then corrected for the false alarm rate; one common correction is: Corrected Hit Rate = Hit rate – (Hit rate × FA rate). Another is: Corrected hit rate = Hit rate – FA rate. The intensity of the tone is lowered until the animal's performance falls to statistical chance (i.e., the hit and false alarm rates are not significantly different), and threshold is defined as the intensity yielding a corrected hit rate of 0.50. Sessions last approximately 20 min, during which 25 to 30 warning trials can be given.

There are four features of the conditioned suppression/avoidance procedure that give it an advantage over other conditioning procedures. First, the animal's head is held in a fixed position by requiring it to make contact with the water spout. This not only allows the sound pressure level at the animal's ears to be specified with precision (e.g., ±1 dB), but is essential for sound localization tests in which the azimuth of a sound source relative to an animal's head must be specified. Second, the procedure incorporates a "ready" or "observing" response in that trials are not presented unless the animal is in contact with the spout during the preceding intertrial interval. This requirement avoids presenting trials when an animal is grooming or otherwise not attending to the task. Third, the false alarm rate is easily controlled by changing the shock level and/or the reward rate. Thus, a high false alarm rate can be quickly lowered by reducing the level of the shock and/or changing the water flow rate. Finally, the procedure is easily adapted for testing any auditory discrimination, such as frequency discrimination, intensity discrimination, or sound localization acuity, and can even be used to assess an animal's ability to categorize sounds (e.g., Heffner and Heffner, 1986; Chapter 3). Tests of auditory discrimination are conducted by presenting one stimulus during safe trials (e.g., a sound from the right) and a different stimulus during warning trials (e.g., a sound from the left).

In summary, conditioned suppression/avoidance is a simple procedure for an animal to learn and has been used to test hearing in more species than any other method, including wild house mice (Heffner and Heffner, 1998; Heffner and Masterton, 1980). Given a water spout of appropriate size and height for mice and a reliable syringe pump to deliver the 0.5 to 2 ml of water that a domestic mouse will drink in one session, it takes 5 to 10 sessions for a naive mouse to become accustomed to the test cage and learn to reliably respond to suprathreshold stimuli. The time required for testing depends on the number of data points to be collected and thresholds may be most efficiently obtained by using a tracking procedure (Ray, 1970; Sidman et al., 1966).

Go/No-go

The standard procedure for assessing hearing in humans is to ask subjects to raise a hand when they hear a tone. The equivalent approach in animals is a go/no-go procedure that requires an animal to wait patiently until a stimulus is presented and then respond within a fixed amount of time.

The first go/no-go procedure to obtain a complete audiogram for mice employed a test cage that was divided in half by a barrier (Birch et al., 1968). The animals were required to wait underneath a loudspeaker on one side of the barrier (a "listening" compartment) and to cross over to the other side and press a lever within 10 s of tone onset to receive a sweetened water reward. Trials were presented at random intervals and the intensity of the tone was reduced to obtain a threshold. Requiring the animals to wait under the loudspeaker positioned them in the sound field, although the intensity of the sound at the animal's ears varied depending on where the mouse stood and whether or not its ears were directed up at the loudspeaker. The false alarm rate was monitored, and thresholds were retested if the rate was too high. The animals learned to respond reliably to a suprathreshold tone in an average of 20 sessions consisting of 10 to 20 trials per session.

Although a complete audiogram was successfully obtained using this procedure, there was considerable variability in the animals' thresholds. One factor contributing to this was the variation in the intensity of the sound reaching an animal, which depended both on where the animal was standing and whether its head was oriented toward or away from the loudspeaker. Another factor was the lack of an effective observing or ready response, and an animal would often fail to respond to a tone if it was grooming or otherwise engaged, although it was in the listening compartment.

A simpler version of the go/no-go procedure, one that dispenses with the listening compartment, has been used successfully to assess the ability of mice to perform a number of auditory discriminations (Ehret, 1975a; Markl and Ehret, 1973). In this procedure, a mouse is placed in a small test cage with a water spout and loudspeaker located in one corner. Variation in the sound pressure level is minimized by confining the animal to a small area, in this case a 10×10-cm platform, and presenting tones when the animal is facing the loudspeaker. Tones are presented at random intervals, and the animal is required to maintain contact with the spout for 3 s while a tone is on in order to obtain a water reward. Because the animals reportedly do not lick the water spout for more than 2 s in the absence of a tone, false positives are not a problem. Sessions last approximately 10 min, during which 20 tone presentations are made.

This procedure has been used to assess absolute thresholds, frequency and intensity difference limens, temporal integration, and masking (Ehret, 1983). Because it is not necessary to train the animal to enter a listening compartment, initial conditioning is accomplished in 8 days. However, the procedure works best with tame mice; that is, animals that have been handled so they are not overly shy or nervous. As a result, not all animals can be successfully trained with this procedure, especially when the task involves discriminating between two different sounds rather than simply detecting a sound (Ehret, 1975b; 1976b).

Because an animal's head is not fixed, this procedure cannot be used for sound-localization testing. However, this could be corrected by adding a second water spout to serve as an observing response. For example, an animal could be trained to place its mouth on one water spout while waiting for a tone and to contact a second water spout located directly below it when a tone is presented (a similar procedure has been used with other species; e.g., Heffner and Heffner, 1983). This modification would both fix an animal's head within the sound field and allow for the automated presentation of trials and the recording of responses. In addition, the inclusion of an observing response might increase the success rate, although the amount of time needed to train an animal would increase.

Recently, a modification of the procedure used by Birch and colleagues has appeared that contains several new features (Prosen et al., 2000). Photocells are used to determine the location of an animal, and trials start automatically once it has entered the listening side of the test cage. Instead of requiring the animal to press a lever when it hears a tone, a response is counted as soon the animal crosses over to the side of the cage containing the water reward. Errors — both false alarms and failure to respond to a tone (misses) — are punished by a time-out, which requires the animal to wait an additional 5 s before testing resumes. Finally, the detection rate is corrected for false alarms. Unfortunately, these modifications do not seem to have solved the problems of the earlier version, as the animal's head is still not fixed within the sound field and the procedure results in false alarm rates of 20% and higher, well above the rate generally considered acceptable (Stebbins, 1970). Moreover, this version involves a complicated training procedure that requires a month or more before an animal is ready to test, making it the slowest procedure of all.

CONDITIONED EYEBLINK

Auditory thresholds have been obtained in mice by conditioning them to close their eyes when a sound signaling impending shock is presented (Ehret, 1976a). It is important to note, however, that this is not the standard eyeblink reflex used by others as the aversive stimulus is delivered to an animal's feet, not to one of its eyes (cf, Martin et al., 1980). Thus, the response of closing the eyes is most likely part of a larger pattern of behavior in which the animal reacts to the anticipated shock.

For testing, the animal is placed in a small cage with a floor constructed of metal bars. Tones are presented at random intervals for a duration of 1 s and are followed immediately by a brief electric shock delivered through the cage floor. Sessions last about 10 min, during which 20 trials are given. The interval between trials varies from 3 to 60 s, depending on the behavior of the animal, because good responses can only be obtained when the animal is not moving. This procedure is a simple method for assessing hearing, and those mice that are able to learn it respond reliably after eight training sessions.

The eyeblink procedure can give good results, and audiograms generated by it are virtually identical to those obtained using the go/no-go procedure (Markl and Ehret, 1973). In addition, it has the advantage that it is not necessary to deprive an animal of food or water. However, it requires the animal to sit motionless during testing, and only about 50% of mice can be trained to respond reliably (e.g., Ehret, 1976a). Moreover, the response is determined subjectively by the experimenter and does not lend itself to automation, opening the possibility of observer bias. Finally, the procedure has not been used to test auditory discriminations, most likely because discrimination tests tend to have high false positive rates and this procedure has no means to control them.

AVOIDANCE CONDITIONING

Two procedures have made use of avoidance conditioning to obtain auditory thresholds in mice. The first procedure used a shuttle box, also known as a double grill box, to obtain absolute thresholds (Schleidt and Kickert-Magg, 1979). This procedure consists of placing an animal in a test cage consisting of two compartments (the shuttle box). The animal is then required to cross from one compartment to the other whenever it hears a tone in order to avoid an electric shock applied to the bars of the cage floor. This task is basically a go/no-go procedure in which the animal makes a response to avoid shock, as opposed to obtaining a positive reward as in the go/no-go procedures described above.

The second procedure trained mice to jump onto a platform to avoid electric shock in response to a change in the frequency of a tone (Kulig and Willott, 1984). The animals were placed in a box with a grid floor and trained to jump onto a small platform whenever an ongoing train of tone pips of the same frequency was replaced by a train of tone pips that alternated in frequency. The animals were given 5 s to respond to the change in frequency, after which electric shock was delivered through the grid floor. Jumping onto the platform when the tone pips were all the same frequency (false alarms) was punished by allowing the platform to collapse.

Although the shock avoidance procedure has an advantage in that it is not necessary to deprive an animal of food or water, it does not appear to work well with mice. The animals tested in the shuttle box required 3 months of training, and the investigators were only able to train 6 out of the 15 animals. Furthermore, an animal's head is not fixed in the sound field and the animal can continuously cross back and forth between the two compartments to avoid the shock, thus rendering it untestable. Similar problems were encountered in the test in which the animals jumped onto a platform to avoid shock. Although only 1 of the 12 animals failed to reach criterion, the false positive rates were high (usually exceeding 20%) and performances even at large frequencies differences tended to be poor. As better procedures are now available for testing mice, there is no longer any reason to consider using shock avoidance.

Approach the Source of a Sound

An attempt was made to assess the ability of mice to localize sound by training them to approach the source of a sound (Ehret and Dreyer, 1984). In this procedure, the mice were placed in a circular test cage and trained to initiate trials by contacting a water spout located in the center of the cage, which turned on a sound from one of three loudspeakers placed at the edge of the test cage 120° apart. The animals were then required to approach the active loudspeaker and contact the water spout located in front of it. However, the animals never performed the task well and failed to respond if the sound was turned off before they reached the water spout. Even if the sound was left on until they completed their response, they often did not directly approach the loudspeaker.

It is not clear why this procedure did not work well with mice, as it has been used successfully to assess sound localization in other species, including rats and gerbils (e.g., Heffner and Heffner, 1988b; Masterton et al., 1975). As used by others, the procedure ensures that an animal's head is precisely oriented with respect to the loudspeakers by requiring the animal to stand on a platform to reach the center spout. A contact switch then detects when the animal is in the proper position and turns on the sound (Thompson et al., 1974). One possible explanation for the inability of mice to do well in this task is that small prey animals may have a general reluctance to approach the source of a sound, especially if they have to cross a large open area. If so, then mice might perform better in a smaller test cage than the 1.55 m-diameter cage used by Ehret and Dreyer (1984).

It should be noted that sound localization ability can also be assessed using the conditioned suppression/avoidance procedure in which an animal ceases to drink when a sound comes from one direction, but not from another (Chapter 3). Indeed, the two procedures (approaching the source of a sound and suppressing to a change in the location of a sound source) have been shown in other mammals to give similar results (Heffner and Heffner, 1988a; 1992b). However, the suppression technique, which allows an animal to respond immediately, may be a more accurate measure of sensory ability because an animal that is required to approach the source of a sound may become distracted before it can complete its response.

Galvanic Skin Response (GSR) Audiometry

The galvanic skin response (GSR) is a measure of skin conductance and is a popular measure of autonomic arousal (e.g., Woodworth and Schlosberg, 1965). It occurs as an *un*conditioned response to a sudden loud sound that habituates with repeated presentation. However, a GSR can be obtained to low-intensity sounds by pairing the sounds with electric shock. In this way, the GSR has been used to obtain absolute thresholds in mice (Berlin, 1963).

For testing, a mouse is sedated to reduce extraneous movements and to allow it to be restrained. Shock electrodes are attached to the animal's front paws and recording electrodes to its hind paws. For conditioning, 1-s tones are presented at random intervals accompanied by an electric shock that is turned on 0.5 s after tone onset. Because the GSR occurs 0.5 to 3.5 s after tone onset, a GSR response to the tone itself can only be observed for tone presentations not followed by shock. Therefore, tones are followed by shock 40% of the time to maintain conditioning, with the tone-only trials analyzed to determine if a response occurred. Control trials are used in which no tone or shock is presented so as to obtain a measure of the animal's false alarm rate. The tones are attenuated to obtain the lowest intensity that yields a detectable response.

An audiogram for mice, derived by taking the lowest 10% of the thresholds obtained from a group of 50 mice, showed reasonable sensitivity at low and middle frequencies, although they appeared to be less sensitive to high frequencies than indicated by another audiogram that used the same strain of mice (CBA/J). This difference raises the possibility that GSR conditioning may not give accurate results at high frequencies (cf., Berlin, 1963; Birch et al., 1968). In addition, the animals showed extreme variation, differing by as much as 80 dB at some frequencies. Moreover, the animals failed to condition to a tone approximately 25% of the time and pregnant and estrous females proved too variable to be used. Thus, as noted by the investigator, although GSR conditioning may be of interest in its own right, it does not appear to be a good method for assessing auditory sensitivity in individual animals (Berlin, 1963).

SUMMARY OF PROCEDURES USING CONDITIONED RESPONSES

Of the six behavioral conditioning procedures reviewed here, the conditioned suppression/avoidance procedure appears to be the most effective for the following reasons: it has the shortest training time; it allows the most trials to be given; it holds the animal's head fixed in the sound field, thus permitting accurate specification of the auditory stimulus reaching the animal; and it works with animals considered difficult to test. Although go/no-go and eyeblink procedures can also give good results, these two procedures do not fix an animal's head within the sound field and will not work with all animals, especially those that are overly active.

UNCONDITIONED RESPONSE PROCEDURES

The simplest methods for assessing hearing in mammals take advantage of an animal's unconditioned responses to sudden loud sounds. As a result, it is possible to show that an animal can detect a sound without having to engage in lengthy training. In most cases, such tests are limited in that animals show an unconditioned response only to sounds that are very loud, the response habituates, and the procedures cannot be used to measure an animal's ability to discriminate between sounds. However, there is one unconditioned procedure that may have overcome these limitations — prepulse inhibition — which takes advantage of the fact that the acoustic startle reflex to a loud sound can be modified by preceding it with another sound.

ACOUSTIC STARTLE REFLEX

Mice, like other mammals, show an unconditioned motor reaction to sudden loud sounds, a response referred to as the acoustic startle reflex (e.g., Hoffman and Ison, 1980). The sound used to produce the startle reflex must be loud (e.g., 100 dB re 20 µPa) and have a near instantaneous onset time because sounds with onset times much greater than 10 ms may not elicit a startle. In addition, the startle reflex is best elicited when the animal is sitting quietly, because a moving animal may not show a startle response (see Chapter 5 for a detailed review).

The reflex is measured by placing an animal in a cage and presenting a startle sound at random intervals when the animal is not moving (e.g., Parham and Willott, 1988). The response of the animal to the startle sound is detected with an accelerometer attached to the test cage. A variety of startle sounds have been used, including noise (e.g., 10 to 25 ms noise burst, 100 to 115 dB, 1 to 5 ms rise/fall time) and tones (e.g., 4 to 24 kHz tone burst, 70 to 110 dB, 10 ms duration, 1 ms rise/fall time). Although habituation of the startle reflex does occur, it is generally possible to obtain a large number of trials (e.g., 60) within a single session.

Because the startle reflex occurs only to relatively loud sounds, it cannot be used to determine absolute sensitivity. However, it can provide information that may be used to supplement threshold measurements (e.g., Parham and Willott, 1988). For example, a normal startle to loud sounds in an animal with a hearing loss might indicate the occurrence of recruitment, a phenomenon in which absolute thresholds are elevated, but the apparent loudness of sounds at suprathreshold levels is unchanged (e.g., Moore, 1997). Thus, the acoustic startle reflex can provide additional information about an animal's hearing ability.

PREPULSE INHIBITION

Although the acoustic startle reflex itself can only determine an animal's ability to respond to loud sounds, the latency or amplitude of the response can be modified by a less intense sound that precedes the startle sound, but which does not itself cause a startle (e.g., Hoffman and Ison, 1980). Thus, the ability of an animal to detect a particular sound can be investigated by determining if presenting that sound before the startle sound modifies the resulting reflex, a procedure referred to as reflex modification or prepulse inhibition (see Chapter 5 for a detailed review).

As in the startle reflex test described above, a mouse is placed in a cage that has an accelerometer attached to it to detect the animal's movements (e.g., Ison et al., 1998; Willott and Turner, 1999). A startle sound, such as a 25-ms noise burst at 115 dB with a near-instantaneous rise/fall time, is presented at random intervals when the animal is sitting quietly. The startle stimulus is preceded on most trials (e.g., 75%) by a prepulse stimulus, such as a 40-ms tone, with the startle stimulus presented alone on the remaining trials for comparison. A typical interval between the two stimuli is 100 ms, although the optimal interval must be determined empirically. The effect of the prepulse stimulus is expressed as a percent reduction of the unmodified startle response. Test sessions may last 1 h, during which about 50 to 100 trials are presented.

Prepulse inhibition can be used to measure both absolute thresholds and the ability to discriminate between different sounds. Absolute thresholds are determined by reducing the intensity of the prepulse stimulus until it no longer has an effect on the startle reflex. The ability to discriminate between stimuli is determined using a change in an ongoing sound as the prepulse stimulus. For example, the ability to discriminate continuous noise from noise containing a gap is determined by presenting ongoing noise interrupted by a gap that occurs just before the presentation of the startle stimulus, that is, the gap serves as the prepulse stimulus. This procedure has produced reasonable gap detection thresholds in mice (Ison et al., 1998), and there appears to be no reason that it cannot be used for other auditory discriminations. That is, frequency- and intensity-difference thresholds, as well as sound-localization thresholds, could be determined by using a prepulse stimulus that consists of a change in the frequency, intensity, or location of an ongoing sound.

Although prepulse inhibition appears to be ideal for sensory testing, the question arises as to whether it is as sensitive as conditioned response procedures. First, experience with conditioning procedures suggests that animals must learn to listen before they becomes reliable observers; that is, initial thresholds are generally higher than those obtained in later sessions (e.g., Stebbins, 1970). Because prepulse inhibition does not involve any training for vigilance, it might not reflect an animal's best sensitivity. Second, the current method for fixing an animal's head in the sound field involves tranquilizing the animal and holding its head in place with a wooden Q-tip glued to the skin of its head (e.g., Ison and Agrawal, 1998), raising the question of whether sedation would affect thresholds.

At present, there is reason to believe that prepulse inhibition can yield sensitive thresholds. Specifically, a reflex modification study using rats obtained thresholds as low as those found using conditioned response procedures, at least for the frequencies in the midrange of the audiogram (Fechter et al., 1988a). However, the issue of validity is best settled by comparing thresholds obtained using this procedure to those obtained for the same animals in the same acoustic environment using a conditioned response procedure. Moreover, the entire audiogram should be determined to ensure that the procedure is equally sensitive at all frequencies because at least one procedure — the conditioned GSR — appears to underestimate high-frequency hearing (see above).

In summary, prepulse inhibition appears to be a simple and rapid method for assessing hearing. Because it uses a natural reflex, an animal requires no training and usable results can be obtained in the first session. However, it should be noted that tests are sometimes carried out with 2 to 4 days between sessions to avoid habituation, with the result that some tests require as much as 2 months to conduct (e.g., Ison and Agrawal, 1998). Moreover, the optimal parameters may vary with the particular task, making it necessary to conduct pilot studies before detailed testing can begin. For example, it is helpful to know the optimal startle stimulus and interval between the prepulse and startle stimuli that yield the best results, as well as the maximum number of trials that can be given without causing excessive habituation.

Pinna Movements

Because mammals with mobile ears will move their pinnae when presented with an unexpected sound, one of the first tests of animal hearing was to look for pinna movements in response to sound. One type of pinna movement is the Preyer reflex, which is a movement of the pinna in response to loud sounds (Ehret, 1983; Francis, 1979). This response is considered to be a startle reflex because it occurs only in response to loud sounds, and thresholds obtained with it are about 60 to 90 dB above those obtained with conditioning procedures (e.g., Hack, 1968; Markl and Ehret, 1973).

Another type of response is the pinna movements that occur in reaction to sounds as low as 25 dB (re 20 μPa), much lower than the sounds that elicit a Preyer reflex (Ehret, 1976a; 1983). In this case, the animal appears to be making use of the directional filtering properties of its pinnae to search its auditory environment. Although the response rapidly habituates, it can be reinstated by briefly handling the animals, which probably has the effect of sensitizing them (Ehret, 1976a).

Although both of these responses are of interest in their own right, the Preyer reflex occurs only in response to very loud sound, and it is unknown whether pinna movements to less intense sounds are a measure of absolute threshold. In other words, the absence of a response does not indicate that the animal cannot hear the sound, only that it is not responding to it. The best demonstration of the usefulness of pinna movements elicited by less intense sounds has been in studies of the development of hearing in young mice (Ehret, 1976a; 1977). However, it may now be possible to study hearing, even in young mice, using other techniques such as the acoustic startle reflex modification procedure and even, perhaps, the conditioned suppression/avoidance procedure.

Freezing Response

An animal that is moving about may stop or freeze when it hears an unexpected sound. This reaction has been used to demonstrate hearing in mice under 12 days of age, at which time the pinna detaches from the scalp and pinna movements can be observed (Ehret, 1976a; 1977). As with the pinna movements discussed above, the freezing response is probably not a measure of absolute sensitivity, although it can provide useful information in the absence of other measures. More sensitive procedures, such as the acoustic startle reflex modification procedure or conditioned suppression/avoidance procedure, should be tried first before using this procedure.

Galvanic Skin Response (GSR)

As previously noted, galvanic skin response (GSR) occurs as an unconditioned response to loud sounds. The unconditioned GSR has been used to study the relative response of mice to tones from 2 to 40 kHz delivered at a constant sound pressure level of 100 dB (Berlin et al., 1968). As in the conditioned GSR procedure, the mouse is sedated to reduce extraneous movements and GSR recording electrodes attached to its hind feet. The magnitude of the GSR appears to parallel its audiogram, suggesting that the unconditioned GSR might provide an equal loudness contour. However, given the uncertainty as to whether the GSR is an accurate indicator of high-frequency hearing (see above), other estimates of loudness (e.g., the acoustic startle reflex) might provide more accurate results.

Summary of Unconditioned Response Procedures

Of the five unconditioned procedures reviewed here, prepulse inhibition appears to hold the most potential for auditory testing. Not only is this procedure capable of demonstrating an animal's ability to detect sounds of low intensity, but it can also be used to determine the ability to discriminate between sounds. All that is required is to verify that the thresholds obtained with this procedure are as sensitive as those obtained with procedures using conditioned responses. In addition, the acoustic startle reflex itself is a useful indicator of an animal's responsiveness to loud sounds and is therefore an important adjunct to tests of absolute threshold. Both prepulse inhibition and the acoustic startle reflex have been the subject of numerous studies, with the result that much is known about them (see Chapter 5). Moreover, the acoustic startle response is measured objectively, whereas most other unconditioned procedures rely on the subjective report of the experimenter. Therefore, these two procedures are to be preferred when assessing hearing with unconditioned procedures.

CONCLUSION

Because mice play a key role in the study of the genetics of hearing, it is important to develop procedures that can quickly and accurately measure their hearing. Not only should a procedure be capable of assessing absolute sensitivity, but it also should be able to determine an animal's ability to discriminate between sounds.

Of the procedures reviewed here, two hold the most promise for testing mice. The first, conditioned suppression/avoidance, is a relatively simple procedure because the animals need only stop drinking when they hear a sound that signals impending shock. As a result, it is possible to train animals in a minimum amount of time. In addition, requiring an animal to drink from a water spout fixes its head within a sound field, which allows for precise measurement of the sound reaching the animal and makes it possible to test sound localization. Indeed, this is one of the few procedures that can be used to test any auditory discrimination.

However, the current conditioned suppression/avoidance procedure can be improved by increasing the speed with which thresholds are assessed. For example, current practice for assessing absolute thresholds is to present tones of a particular intensity in blocks of five or more trials, calculate the animal's performance, and then change to a new intensity. Because mice require little water and thus work for only 15 to 20 min, only one threshold can be obtained per daily session using this procedure. However, the speed with which thresholds are determined could be increased using an automated tracking procedure in which the intensity of the tone is changed from trial to trial, as originally recommended by Sidman and co-workers (1966), instead of collecting information in blocks of trials. Other changes that might also increase the speed of testing would be to optimize the test apparatus by determining the size and shape of the water spout and water reward rate that work best for mice.

The other behavioral procedure that holds great promise is prepulse inhibition. Because this procedure makes use of an unconditioned reflex, it is potentially the fastest of all procedures for assessing hearing in mice because the animals need not be trained. However, it remains to be determined whether absolute thresholds obtained with this procedure are as sensitive as those obtained with conditioned response procedures. In addition, it is important to find a good way to keep an animal's head fixed within the sound field because there is the possibility that the current technique, which involves sedation, might affect thresholds. Should prepulse inhibition prove to provide valid thresholds, it could easily supplant conditioned response procedures for assessing hearing in mice and other animals. Despite the fact that it may be necessary to space test sessions several days apart to reduce habituation, prepulse inhibition is simpler to use and would be able to test more animals in the same amount of time than any of the conditioned response procedures, including conditioned suppression/avoidance.

SUMMARY

Six conditioned and five unconditioned response procedures for assessing hearing in mice are reviewed. The six conditioned response procedures include conditioned suppression/avoidance, go/no-go, eyeblink conditioning, avoidance conditioning, approaching the source of a sound, and

GSR conditioning. Of these, the conditioned suppression/avoidance procedure is the most effective because it has the shortest training time, allows the most trials to be given, holds the animal's head fixed in the sound field, and is successful with animals considered difficult to test. The five unconditioned procedures are the acoustic startle reflex, prepulse inhibition, pinna movements, freezing response, and GSR. Of these, the prepulse inhibition procedure holds the most promise for auditory testing; unlike other unconditioned response procedures, it is it capable of demonstrating an animal's ability to detect low-intensity sounds as well as discriminate between sounds.

ACKNOWLEDGMENTS

We thank G. Koay and I. Harrington for their comments on an earlier draft of this chapter. Many of the ideas expressed here were developed in work supported by NIH grants NS 30539, DC 02960, and DC 03258.

3 Focus: Sound-Localization Acuity Changes with Age in C57BL/6J Mice

Rickye S. Heffner, Gimseong Koay, and Henry E. Heffner

INTRODUCTION

C57BL/6J mice show a progressive high-frequency hearing loss beginning about 2 to 3 months of age (Chapters 13, 24, 28; Mikaelian, 1979). Because mammalian high-frequency hearing (i.e., above the 10-kHz limit of other vertebrates) evolved under strong selective pressure for sound localization, such a hearing loss should affect not only the ability of mice to detect sound, but also to localize it (R. Heffner and Heffner, 1992a; H. Heffner and Heffner, 1998). Specifically, high frequencies are necessary for two of the three basic locus cues: the binaural intensity difference of a sound at the two ears and the monaural pinna cues that arise from the directionality of the pinnae (the third cue being the binaural time difference, primarily a low-frequency cue). The two high-frequency cues require sounds that are effectively shadowed by the head and/or pinnae because low frequencies bend around small obstacles with little attenuation. Just how high an animal must hear to be able to use these cues depends on the size of its head and pinnae — the smaller the animal, the higher it must hear, which is why mice can hear above 80 kHz (H. Heffner and Masterton, 1980; Markl and Ehret, 1973). Thus, the loss of high-frequency hearing should have a detrimental effect on the ability of mice to localize sound, especially because they may not be able to compensate by relying on binaural time cues because the maximum interaural delay their small heads generate is so small (about 60 μs).

We performed a study to observe the effect of age-related, high-frequency hearing loss in C57BL/6J mice by determining their sound-localization acuity at two different ages. An additional goal was to assess the ability of mice to localize brief sounds because previous research had only been able to demonstrate an ability to home in on sounds that were continuously repeated (Ehret and Dryer, 1984). Sound-localization thresholds and the ability to localize filtered noise bursts were determined for three C57BL/6J mice using an avoidance procedure involving suppression of drinking (for details, see H. Heffner and Heffner, 1995). The animals were then retested later, at which time their absolute thresholds for 16- and 32-kHz tones were also determined. The animals had free access to food in their home cages and received water during daily test sessions.

The mice were tested in a small, sound-transparent, wire mesh cage ($15 \times 8 \times 10$ cm) mounted on a camera tripod in the center of a carpeted, double-walled acoustic chamber, the walls and ceiling of which were lined with eggcrate foam to reduce sound reflections. The animals were trained to make steady contact with a water spout that came up through the floor of the cage in order to receive a slow but steady trickle of water dispensed via a syringe pump located outside the chamber. Drinking from the spout served to fix the animal's head in the center of a perimeter bar (1-m radius) on which loudspeakers were mounted. A typical test session lasted approximately 20 min, during which a mouse consumed 0.5 to 1.5 mL of water.

The mice were trained to drink in the presence of a 100-ms noise burst emitted from a loudspeaker to their right, but to break contact with the water spout whenever a sound was emitted

0-8493-2328-2/01/$0.00+$.50
© 2001 by CRC Press LLC

from a loudspeaker to their left in order to avoid a mild electric shock delivered through the spout. A 100-ms noise burst was presented once every 2.3 s from the left or right side on a quasi-random schedule in which about 22% of signals were from the left. An animal's response on each trial was determined by recording whether it was in contact with the spout during the last 200 ms of a trial (which was 1.8 s in duration). Breaking contact following a sound from the left was recorded as a hit, whereas breaking contact following a sound from the right was recorded as a false alarm.

Performance was quantified by determining hit and false alarm rates for a particular stimulus or angle in blocks of trials (typically 6 left and 25 right sounds). A performance measure was determined by correcting the hit rate according to the following formula: Performance = Hit rate − (Hit rate × False alarm rate). Threshold, defined as the angle at which performance equaled 0.50, was determined by progressively reducing the separation between the loudspeakers until performance fell to chance (i.e., the hit and false alarm rates did not differ significantly).

Sound-localization thresholds were determined using a 100-ms broadband noise burst containing measurable frequencies from 3 to 80 kHz (6 to 48 kHz ± 3dB), covering most of the hearing range of the domestic mouse (which, for sounds of 60 dB sound pressure level (SPL) ranges from 900 Hz to 79 kHz; Markl and Ehret, 1973). The intensity of the noise was varied randomly from 63 to 70 dB SPL to prevent the animals from using possible intensity differences between the loudspeakers as a cue.

A second test investigated the importance of high frequencies for localization by determining average performance for localizing low-pass filtered noise (48 dB/octave) at a fixed angle of 60° (±30° left and right of midline). The five low-pass filter settings used (and the signal intensities re 20 µPa) were: 80 kHz (70 dB), 60 kHz (70 dB), 40 kHz (69 dB), 20 kHz (71.5 dB), and 10 kHz (67 dB). The filtered noise was presented with a 50-ms rise/fall time to avoid generating high-frequency onset and offset artifacts. (For the sound production and measurement equipment, see R. Heffner, Heffner, and Koay, 1995). Blocks of six left trials (and the associated right trials) were given at four different filter settings each day until 36 left trials had been given for each noise band. Finally, absolute thresholds for 16- and 32-kHz pure tones were determined at the end of testing to verify that the animals had a high-frequency hearing loss. In this case, the animals were trained to break contact with the spout whenever they heard a tone presented from a loudspeaker located in front of the cage (3 pulses, 400 ms on, 100 ms off, 10 ms rise/decay). The intensity of the tone was reduced in 5-dB increments until performance fell to chance and threshold was defined as the level at which performance equalled 0.50.

LOCALIZATION ACUITY

The mice had little difficulty learning to localize single, brief noise bursts. Initial training and detailed testing for localizing the 100-ms broadband noise required 21 and 25 sessions, respectively. During final threshold determination at 2.4 to 2.5 months of age, all three mice were performing well at angles of 90° or larger, and their mean threshold was 33° (Figure 3.1). Retraining and testing after more than a 3-month break required only 14 sessions, as the mice were now experienced with the test. Each animal's threshold, determined between 6.9 and 7.1 months of age, had increased on average by 13° to a new average of 46° (Figure 3.1). The increased thresholds cannot be attributed to an inability to hear the noise burst, nor to any deterioration in motivation, intellect, or general localization ability because performance at large angles remained normal.

LOCALIZATION OF LOW-PASS NOISE

Determination of the ability of the mice to localize low-pass noise bursts (60° separation) required six to eight sessions. Initial performance was determined at 2.5 to 2.7 months of age, and retesting took place at 7.2 to 7.4 months (Figure 3.2). Performance declined progressively as the high frequencies were removed, demonstrating the importance of high frequencies for azimuthal localization in mice. Animals A and B fell to chance when the filter was set at 20 kHz low-pass, and

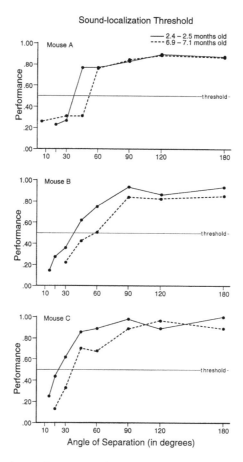

FIGURE 3.1   Sound-localization performances of the three mice at 2.4 to 2.5 months of age (solid lines) and 6.9 to 7.1 months (dashed lines). Thresholds increased with age from 37° to 51° for mouse A, 38° to 59° for mouse B, and 23.5° to 37° for mouse C.

all three mice were unable to localize above chance when the filter was set at 10 kHz low-pass although the noise burst was clearly audible. The animals showed a mild performance decrement as they aged, even when the signal contained high frequencies, presumably because a high-frequency hearing loss prevented the mice from making full use of them.

PURE-TONE THRESHOLDS

Detection thresholds at 16 and 32 kHz were completed when the mice were 7.7 months of age. Compared with NMRI mice (Markl and Ehret, 1973), the C57BL/6J mice showed hearing losses at 16 kHz of 16 to 54 dB and at 32 kHz of 52 to 59 dB (Table 3.1). Thus, these animals had an obvious hearing loss by 7.7 months of age.

DISCUSSION

TEST PROCEDURE

The use of an avoidance procedure in which an animal ceases responding when it detects a sound is a natural response that all three of the mice easily learned. Moreover, the animals could easily shift from one task (discriminating locus) to another (detecting tones) with little difficulty. Indeed,

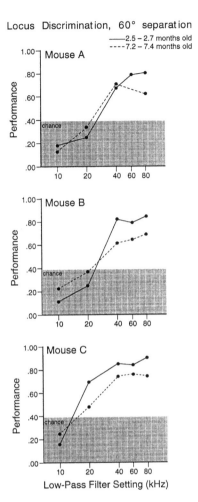

Locus Discrimination, 60° separation

—— 2.5 – 2.7 months old
---- 7.2 – 7.4 months old

Low-Pass Filter Setting (kHz)

FIGURE 3.2   Sound localization performances of the three mice at 2.5 to 2.7 months of age (solid lines), and 7.2 to 7.4 months (dashed lines) with 100-ms low-pass filtered noise bursts presented 30° to the left or right of midline.

TABLE 3.1
Detection Thresholds (dB SPL) at 16 and 32 kHz for Three C57BL/6J Mice at the End of Sound Localization Testing (7.7 months old)

	Frequency	
Strain	**16 kHz**	**32 kHz**
NMRI (average)[a]	4 dB	22 dB
C57BL/6J (7.7 mo)		
Mouse A	20 dB	74 dB
Mouse B	41 dB	80 dB
Mouse C	58 dB	81 dB

[a] *Source:* From Markl and Ehret, 1973. With permission.

this procedure has proven successful in assessing hearing in a wide variety of animals (e.g., H. Heffner and Heffner, 1995; 1998), and it probably accounts for the success in demonstrating that mice can localize brief sounds when previous studies have failed (Ehret and Dryer, 1984). Moreover, the combination of this task with the response of eating or drinking from a spout, which fixes an animal's head in the sound field, makes it ideal for auditory testing.

SOUND LOCALIZATION CHANGES ACCOMPANYING AGING

From 2.7 to 7.4 months of age, the average localization thresholds of the mice increased from 33° to 46°. Because this strain of mice is known to show a progressive high-frequency hearing loss beginning at 2 to 3 months of age, and because the mice tested here demonstrated a large high-frequency hearing loss at 7.7 months, it is probable that the increased locus thresholds were due to their hearing loss. That the mice did not suffer from any general deterioration in localization ability is suggested by the observation that their localization performance at large angles was essentially normal (Figure 3.1).

The loss of high frequencies does not affect left-right sound localization acuity in all species. For example, humans with high-frequency sensorineural hearing loss retain good left-right acuity, presumably because binaural time differences, which use low frequencies, are sufficient to maintain good localization (Colburn, Zurek, and Durlach, 1987; Noble, Byrne, and Lepage, 1994). Similarly, the left-right localization acuity of chinchillas is not degraded by filtering out high frequencies, as it is in mice. However, it should be noted that both humans and chinchillas require high frequencies to discriminate the elevation of sound and to prevent front-back reversals (Belendiuk and Butler, 1975; R. Heffner et al., 1994; 1995). The fact that mice require high frequencies for left-right localization, however, suggests that they may not use the binaural time-difference cue for locus. This would not be unique because at least one other small mammal, the big brown bat, appears to have relinquished the use of the binaural time cue, relying solely on interaural intensity differences and monaural pinna cues for passive localization (Koay et al., 1997).

COMPARISON OF MICE TO OTHER MAMMALS

The 33° mean threshold for these mice at 2.5 to 2.7 months of age is larger than that of most mammals, but comparable to that of gerbils, kangaroo rats, horses, and cattle (H. Heffner and Heffner, 1998). Although some investigators have suggested that there may be small high-frequency losses in C57BL/6J mice at 2 months of age (Li and Borg, 1991), it is likely that the explanation for the comparatively poor locus acuity in these mice lies in the relationship between hearing and vision — the primary function of sound localization is to direct the eyes to the source of a sound for visual examination (R. Heffner and Heffner, 1992c; Koay et al., 1998). Just how accurately the ears must direct the eyes depends on the width of an animal's field of best vision. Specifically, animals with narrow fields of best vision (e.g., humans and elephants) require better locus acuity than animals with broad fields of best vision (e.g., kangaroo rats and cattle). Because the density of the ganglion cells in the mouse retina indicates that it has a relatively broad field of best vision of 114° (based on retinal ganglion-cell density gradients, R. Heffner, unpublished), its comparatively poor localization acuity is not unexpected.

ACKNOWLEDGMENTS

This research was supported by NIH Grant R01 DC 02960. We thank J. Willott for suggesting this experiment and for providing the mice. In addition, we thank Terry Donnel for help in testing the animals.

4 Noninvasive Assessment of Auditory Function in Mice: Auditory Brainstem Response and Distortion Product Otoacoustic Emissions

Kourosh Parham, Xiao-Ming Sun, and Duck O. Kim

INTRODUCTION

In the 1960s and early 1970s, mouse auditory function was physiologically characterized by "near-field" responses that were invasive. For example, exposure of the round window through the bulla, and the auditory nerve or inferior colliculus through the cranium were required to record summating and compound action potentials (SP and CAP, respectively) (e.g., Alford and Ruben, 1963; Mikaelian and Ruben, 1964; Willott and Henry, 1974). The development of hearing and usually hearing loss are progressive processes, and because no two ears are alike, longitudinal study of auditory function in the same ear is often preferred. With advances in computer averaging of signals and introduction of "far-field" recording techniques (Jewett, 1970), it became possible to nontraumatically monitor auditory function in mice (e.g., Henry and Haythorn, 1978; Henry and Lepkowski, 1978; Henry, 1979a). This development allowed examination of the same mouse over several testing sessions separated by days to months. Furthermore, the new techniques were less taxing on the animal subjects and less demanding in terms of experimental preparation and time.

This chapter offers an overview of two noninvasive tools used to assess auditory function. The chapter begins by reviewing the auditory brainstem response (ABR), which has become the tool of choice for many investigations of the mouse auditory system, and then examines a relatively newer tool that allows a more focused assessment of cochlear outer hair cells (OHCs) using distortion product otoacoustic emission (DPOAE) (Kemp, 1979; Kim, 1980) and its application to investigations of the mouse auditory function. To the extent possible, various properties of ABR and DPOAE are illustrated using examples from studies of the mouse. Emphasis is placed on how studies of ABR and DPOAE in mouse have advanced our understanding of the auditory system. In addition to reviewing previously published data, this chapter also presents new data (not previously published).

AUDITORY BRAINSTEM RESPONSE

BACKGROUND

ABR has numerous applications both in the clinical and research settings. These include estimation of auditory threshold, auditory screening, and lesion localization (Weber, 1994). ABR is a type of auditory evoked potential (AEP). Excellent reviews of ABR and AEP are available elsewhere (e.g.,

Ferraro and Durrant, 1994; Musiek et al., 1994). Briefly, the AEP represents electrical potentials recorded at various levels of the auditory system in response to auditory stimulation.

There are a number of AEP classification schemes. For example, AEPs can be classified according to electrode placement (i.e., near- vs. far-field), latency (i.e., short, middle, or long), or anatomic origin (e.g., cochlear, brainstem, or cortical). Short, middle, and long latency responses are recorded about <10, 10 to 50, and >50 ms, respectively. The latency of an AEP is reflective of the level of the auditory system contributing to the bulk of electrical activity for a given response. For example, short latency responses include electrocochleogram (ECochG) and ABR, whereas long latency responses are cortically generated.

NEURAL SUBSTRATE OF ABR

Anatomically, the term ABR implies a brainstem origin for the recorded electrical activity. However, the ABR includes a significant peripheral contribution, the early components. A peripheral evoked potential, the ECochG, consists of several components, including SP (originating from cochlear hair cells) and CAP (originating from the auditory nerve). These peripheral evoked potentials are believed to contribute to the first wave of the ABR (see below).

A number of experimental studies using murine (Henry, 1979b) and non-murine (e.g., Buchwald and Huang, 1975; Achor and Starr, 1980; Gardi and Bledsoe, 1981; Pratt et al., 1991; Zaroor and Starr, 1991a; b) species have attempted to elucidate the central generators of the ABR using lesions of various structures in the auditory pathway. Henry (1979b), using a combination of ABR latency comparisons with near-field evoked potentials and lesion techniques, concluded that the first peak (P1) had a cochlear origin, and the next four peaks (P2 to P5) corresponded to cochlear nucleus, contralateral superior olivary complex, lateral lemniscus, and contralateral lateral inferior colliculus, respectively. A thorough investigation in the cat using kainic acid lesions, which spared fibers of passage, conducted by Melcher et al. (1996a; b) indicated that cells in the cochlea, cochlear nucleus, and ipsilateral and contralateral superior olivary complex are the main generators of the ABR. Using a mathematical model relating the ABR to underlying cellular activity, Melcher and Kiang (1996) suggested that P1 was generated by the spiral ganglion cells, P2 by globular bushy cells of posterior anteroventral cochlear nucleus (AVCN), P3 by spherical bushy cells of the anterior AVCN and cells of the contralateral medial nucleus of the trapezoid body, P4 by the principal cells of the ipsilateral and contraleral medial superior olivary nuclei, and P5 by cells in the nuclei of the lateral lemniscus and/or inferior colliculus. Based on their results, Melcher and Kiang (1996) concluded that the ABR primarily reflects cellular activity in two parallel pathways originating in AVCN, one with globular cells (high-frequency pathway) and the other with spherical cells (low-frequency pathway). They further speculated that in the mouse, a species with "high-frequency hearing," the ABR features are generated by the high-frequency globular pathway. This would be consistent with the substantially diminished size of the medial superior olivary nuclei in the mouse (Willard and Ryugo, 1983).

ABR RECORDING SYSTEM

Recording ABRs in the mouse is simple and requires minimal instrumentation. AEPs, in general, are dependent on computer-based summating and signal averaging to extract evoked activity by fixed and synchronous stimuli from background spontaneous electrical activity (i.e., electroenceph-alogram — EEG). Stainless-steel needle electrodes placed on the vertex, together with a ground electrode on the body of an anesthetized mouse, are sufficient at the animal end of the instrumentation. The recorded signals are bandpass filtered (300 to 3000 Hz) and amplified with a differential amplifier. Multiple repetitions of the stimuli are required to yield an averaged waveform. ABRs can be recorded in response to broadband stimuli, such as clicks or tone bursts. ABR waveforms recorded in response to clicks are shown in Figure 4.1. One limitation of the broadband stimuli is

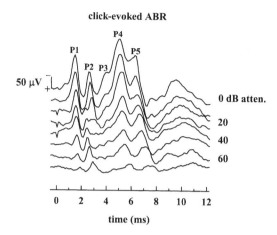

FIGURE 4.1 Click-evoked ABR waveforms recorded in a young C57BL/6J mouse as a function of click level. The five major peaks (P1 to P5) of the averaged waveform are identified. (Previously unpublished data.)

that they provide little frequency-specific information. Filtered noise pips in mouse (e.g., Hunter and Willott, 1987) have improved on this limitation, but these stimuli still lack sufficient resolution. Tone bursts, on the other hand, have the advantage of providing frequency-specific information, but usually require much longer recording times. Data acquisition is shortened by presentation of stimuli at faster rates, although rates above 10/s result in adaptation evident as increased response latencies and decreased response amplitudes (e.g., Burkard et al., 1990a). Mitchell et al. (1999) have developed a method for rapid acquisition in the mouse by using a 56-tone-burst stimulus train (seven stimulus frequencies, multiple levels in 5 to 10 dB steps). The stimuli are presented at a rate of 1.57/s using frequencies in a descending order and with separation of 0.5 to 1 octave to minimize stimulus overlap on the basilar membrane and hence adaptation.

ABR Measures

A number of measures have been utilized in mouse studies. These include threshold, waveform morphology (i.e., presence or absence of a peak), peak amplitude, and latency, such as absolute latencies of peaks and the interpeak latencies (e.g., P1 and P3). Examples of studies utilizing above ABR measures in mice are cited below.

ABR and Middle Ear Function

Reliable, accurate ABR requires healthy middle ear function. We have found a 40-dB elevation in ABR thresholds to clicks in CBA/J mice with otitis media (OM). McGinn et al. (1992) have reported a high incidence (reaching 90%) of OM in CBA/J mice over 400 days of age. We compared ABR thresholds of 10 normal and 20 OM ears in CBA/J mice to click stimuli (unpublished data). Mean threshold for the normal ears was 32 vs. 71.5 dB SPL in OM ears.

Mitchell et al. (1997) noted that C3H/HeJ mice have a genetic defect that prevents them from mounting the appropriate immune response to bacterial lipopolysaccharide and therefore are susceptible to opportunistic bacterial infections. They found that 33% of C3H/HeJ mice had middle ear disease and increased ABR thresholds to tone bursts by 15 to 40 dB, lowered peak amplitudes, and increased latencies compared to the normal C3H mouse.

ABR and Phenotyping Auditory Function

A popular application of the ABR in investigating the mouse auditory system has been phenotyping auditory function in mouse strains and mutants. The best-known example is characterization of

tone-evoked ABR

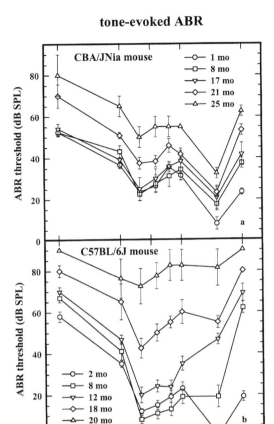

FIGURE 4.2   Age-related pattern of change in mean ABR thresholds of CBA/JNia (panel a) and C57BL/6J (panel b) mice as a function of pure tone burst frequency. Error bars represent standard error of the means (SEMs). (CBA data from Figure 1, Parham et al., 1999, and C57 data are from Figure 1, Parham, 1997.)

age-related hearing loss (AHL) of mouse models of presbycusis by recording ABR thresholds of the CBA mouse (Henry and Lepkowski, 1978; Hunter and Willott, 1987; Wenngren and Anniko, 1988; Sjostrom and Anniko, 1990; Li and Borg, 1991; Shone et al., 1991a; Parham et al., 1999;), an animal model of late onset presbycusis, and the C57BL/6J mouse (C57; Henry and Lepkowski, 1978; Hunter and Willott, 1987; Li and Borg, 1991; Shone et al., 1991a; Parham, 1997; Ichimiya et al., 2000), an animal model of early onset presbycusis. Figure 4.2 shows the pattern of age-related ABR threshold elevation in several age groups of the CBA and C57 mice documenting the progressive nature of hearing loss in these two strains. Table 4.1 provides a partial listing of mice that have been investigated using the ABR, but due to space limitations are not discussed in the remainder of this chapter (see also Chapters 28 and 38).

INFLUENCE OF EXTRINSIC FACTORS ON ABR

Auditory function is vulnerable to numerous environmental variables, and the ABR has been used to assess the impact of a wide range of such variables on the auditory system of the mouse. For example, Johnson (1993) demonstrated that toluene accelerated AHL in the C57 mouse using the ABR. Katbamna et al. (1993) examined the effect of hyperthermia on ABR in mouse. They found that hyperthermia shortened latencies of all ABR waves and altered amplitudes of P1 and P2.

TABLE 4.1
Partial Listing of Mouse Strains/Mutants Whose Auditory Functions
Have Been Assessed by ABR

Study (-ies)	Strain
Henry (1982a)	AU/SsJ
	A/J
	AKR/J
	C57BR/cdJ
	LP/J
	SJL/J
Horner et al. (1985)	*Deafness* (*dn/dn*)
Huang et al. (1995)	
Henry and Buzzone (1986)	RB/1bg, RB/3bg, and their F1 hybrid
Kitamura et al. (1991)	C3H/He spontaneous mutations
Shone et al. (1991b)	CD/1
Henry et al. (1992)	F1 hybrid of AU/SsJ × CBA/CaJ
Sjostrom and Anniko (1990; 1992a; 1992b)	*Jerker*
Saitoh et al. (1994; 1995)	SAMP1 and SAMR1
Shvarev (1994)	BALB/c
Willott et al. (1998)	
Mathews et al. (1995)	mdx and myodystrophy (myd)
Raynor and Mulroy (1997)	(mouse models of dystrophin disorders)
Trune et al. (1996)	C3H/HeJ
	C3H/HeSnJ
Hultcrantz and Spangberg (1997)	DBA/2 spontaneous mutation
Parham et al. (2000)	*Purkinje cell degeneration* (*pcd/pcd*)

Note: Studies not cited in text.

Katbamna et al. (1993) promoted the ABR monitoring as a premonitory signal of permanent damage secondary to hyperthermia. Hultcrantz (1995) examined the impact of prenatal irradiation on mouse ABRs and concluded that prenatal irradiation does not appear to cause mutations leading to impaired hearing in second-generation mice.

ABR AND NOISE-INDUCED HEARING LOSS (NIHL)

ABR has also been utilized to document NIHL in mice and its interaction with aging. Shone et al. (1991a), Li and colleagues (Li, 1992a; Li and Borg, 1993; Li et al., 1993), and Miller et al. (1998) evaluated ABR threshold shifts in C57 and CBA/Ca mice of various ages exposed to loud broadband noise. They found that the auditory system of the aging C57 mice remains highly susceptible to acoustic trauma. The findings regarding the aging CBA mice varied and ranged from resistance (Li and colleagues) to increasing susceptibility (Miller et al., 1998) to acoustic trauma. Based on these results, it has been concluded that the interaction of noise trauma and aging effects depends on the susceptibility of the individual to acoustic trauma (see Chapters 28 and 31).

Henry (1992) examined ABR thresholds for NIHL in CBA/CaJ and AUS/sJ inbred mice and their F1 hybrid offspring. He found the F1 line had an intermediate degree of loss compared to its parental strains. Ohlemiller et al. (1999b) demonstrated a permanent ABR threshold shift in C57 mice exposed to 1-h intense broadband noise. This threshold shift was associated with elevated cochlear reactive oxygen species (ROS; i.e., hydroxyl radicals) and ROS-mediated injury, thus shedding light on the peripheral mechanisms mediating NIHL.

ABR and Amelioration of Hearing Loss

Slowing down or minimizing hearing loss is a long-term objective of hearing research. A number of efforts toward that goal have utilized ABR recordings in mice. For example, Fowler et al. (1995) found that ABRs of CBA/Ca mice exposed to training exposures of moderate intensity noise did not protect ABRs from temporary and permanent threshold shifts after exposure to the same, but more intense noise. Studies of the effects of an augmented acoustic environment on hearing loss have also used ABRs (see Chapter 14).

The role of drugs in preserving auditory function in the face of insults has also been investigated. For example, methylprednisolone appears to be protective of NIHL in mice (Henry, 1992); however, naloxone (Henry, 1992) and nimodipine (Ison et al., 1997a) do not appear to affect the amount of mouse ABR threshold elevations following noise exposure.

ABR, Genetics, and Molecular Biology of Hearing

In unraveling the genetics of hearing, ABR has been the tool of choice in assessing auditory function in gene manipulation, and these are discussed in detail in Section IV of this book. Several studies are considered below, with the latter studies having influence of thyroid function on auditory system as the unifying theme. For a listing of other studies, the reader is referred to Table 4.2.

Zhou et al. used the ABR (1995a) and electrically evoked ABR (EABR) (1995b) to evaluate *Trembler J* (*Tr^J*) and P_0-*DT-A* mice, which have a deficit of their peripheral myelin. In *Tr^J* mice, the defect is due to a mutated PMP-22 gene. In P_0-*DT-A* mice, the defect is produced by a transgene using the rat P_0 promotor to direct the expression of gene encoding for the bacterial diphtherial toxin A chain (DT-A). ABR measurements exhibited differences in threshold, latency, and slope of the ABR growth function between myelin-deficient mice and their littermate controls. Figure 4.3 shows that the averaged ABR latencies for P1 to P3 of the myelin-deficient were longer than their littermate controls. There was no significant difference in P1 to P3 interpeak latency, consistent with the peripheral location of the lesions.

EABRs were recorded with a vertex electrode, but were evoked by passing rectangular electrical pulses through a bipolar stimulating electrode inserted through a small hole in the apex of the cochlea (Zhou et al., 1995b). The EABRs showed prolonged latency, decreased amplitude, and elevated threshold of P1 evoked by short-duration stimuli (20 ms/phase). A two-pulse stimulation paradigm was used to evaluate refractory properties. Myelin-deficient mice exhibited slower recovery from the refractory state than controls. Long-duration stimuli (4 ms/phase) were used to assess integration properties. Myelin-deficient mice demonstrated prolonged P1 latency and more gradual latency changes with current level, implying impaired integration.

Fujiyoshi et al. (1994) demonstrated the restoration of ABR by gene transfer in shiverer mice. Shiverer mice are homozygous for an autosomal recessive mutation (deletion) in the gene for myelin basic protein (MBP), a major protein component of the myelin sheath in the CNS. MBP-transgenic mice were produced by microinjection of an MBP cosmid clone into the pronucleus of fertilized eggs from shiverer mice. This resulted in recovery of MBP levels in the transgenics up to 25% of that of normal mice. A greater number of axons in the transgenic mice were myelinated than in the shiverer mice, but the myelin sheath was not as thick as in normal controls. Every interpeak latency of the ABR was prolonged in the shiverer mice and improved in the transgenic mice.

Congenital thyroid disorders are often associated with profound deafness, indicating a requirement for thyroid hormone and its receptors in the development of hearing (see Chapter 35). The congenital hypothyroid (*hyt/hyt*) mouse has a homozygous recessive mutation of a single locus on chromosome 12 (an amino acid substitution in a transmembrane domain of the thyrotropin receptor) that results in significant endocrine hypofunction and retarded growth. O'Malley et al. (1995) assessed hearing thresholds by ABR testing and noted a 40 to 45 dB elevation in the *hyt/hyt* mouse compared to littermate heterozygote (*hyt/+*) animals and normal progenitor controls BALB/cByJ

TABLE 4.2
Partial Listing of Studies Examining Auditory Function in Transgenic/Mutant Mice

Study (-ies)	Transgenic/Mutant Mouse	ABR Finding(s)
Rauch and Neuman (1991); Rauch (1992)	mos proto-oncogene linked to retroviral a transcriptional control sequence	No detectable ABR waveform
Motohashi et al. (1994)	Melanin-deficient (c2J/c2J)	Normal
	Microphtalmic (mibw/mibw) (dysgenesis of melanocytes)	Severe hearing loss
Reimer et al. (1996)	Pax5-deficient (underdeveloped midbrain)	Delayed development of auditory sensitivity and response latency, but normal ABRs
Muller et al. (1997)	Mpv17-negative (inner ear degeneration/nephrotic syndrome) Human Mpv17 insertion	Severe hearing loss Normal ABR audiograms
Nishi et al. (1997)	Knock-out mice lacking nociceptin receptor (a member of the opioid receptor group, subfamily of the G-protein-coupled receptor superfamily)	Normal click-evoked ABR thresholds, but higher thresholds 60–90 min after intense 1-kHz tone exposure
Pieke-Dahl et al. (1997)	rd3 (recessive gene causing retinal degenration in RBF/DnJ mouse) homozygotes (model for Usher syndrome type IIa)	High-frequency threshold elevation
Kozel et al. (1998)	Plasma membrane Ca^{2+}-ATPase isoform 2 (expressed on deficient OHCs and ganglion cells)	Homozygotes deaf heterozygotes hearing impaired
Munemoto et al. (1998)	N-methyl-D-aspartate receptor (excitatory amino acid transmitter) epsilon 1 or 4 subunit defect	Elevated thresholds in epsilon 4 mutants; normal in epsilon 1
D'Hooge et al. (1999)	Arylsulfatase A-deficient (model for metachromatic leukodystrophy)	Absent ABRs
Keithley et al. (1999)	Brn-3.1 (a hair cell transcription factor) gene deletion	Homozygotes deaf heterozygotes with threshold elevations
McFadden et al. (1999b)	Cu/Zn superoxide dismutase knock-out (free-radical scavenger)	Threshold elevations
Ohlemiller et al. (1999a)	Cu/Zn superoxide dismutase knock-out	Increased threshold elevations after noise exposure
Airaksinen et al. (2000)	Calbindin-D28 k (cytosolic Ca-binding protein) null mutant	Similar to controls even after noise-induced trauma
Zhang et al. (2000)	Multidrug-resistant 1a knock out (mdr1a(–/–))	Impaired after p-glycoprotein transported drug administration (e.g., doxorubicin)

Note: Studies not cited in text.

(+/+). The elevation of ABR thresholds was correlated with consistent morphologic abnormalities of the stereocilia on both inner and outer hair cell systems.

Two thyroid hormone (T3) receptor genes, Tr alpha1 and Tr beta, are differentially expressed, although in overlapping patterns, during development. Forrest et al. (1996) demonstrated that Tr beta-deficient (Thrb–/–) mice exhibit greatly diminished ABR waveforms, suggesting that the primary defect resides in the cochlea. Tr alpha1-deficient (Tr alpha1–/–) mice display a normal ABR (Forrest et al., 1996; Rusch et al., 1998). The abnormal ABRs of Thrb–/– mice are associated with the retarded expression of a fast-activating potassium conductance, $I_{K,f}$, on inner hair cells (IHCs) (Rusch et al., 1998). At the onset of hearing, IHCs in wild-type mice express the $I_{K,f}$ that transforms the immature IHC from a regenerative, spiking pacemaker to a high-frequency signal transmitter.

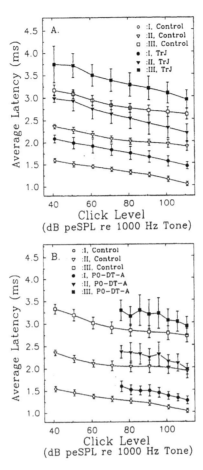

FIGURE 4.3 Averaged ABR latencies in myelin-deficient mice, *Trembler* (*Tr^J*) (panel a) and *P_0*-DT-A (panel b), compared to littermate controls. Averaged latencies are shown as a function of level for the first three peaks of click-evoked ABR (I = P1, II = P2, III = P3). ABR latencies decreased with level for all mice, but myelin-deficient mice consistently had longer latencies than control mice. Vertical bars represent standard deviations. (From Zhou, R., Abbas, P.J., and Assouline, P.G., 1995, *Hear. Res.*, 88, 98-106. With permission.)

These results suggested that the physiological differentiation of IHCs depends on a Tr beta-mediated pathway.

ABR and Forward Masking

The ABR can be used in various stimulus paradigms to explore auditory function. For example, Walton et al. (1995) and Duan and Canlon (1996) examined ABRs in forward masking paradigms. Walton et al. (1995) examined the effect of sensorineural hearing loss (SNHL) on short-term adaptation in hearing-impaired C57 mice. They used 12-kHz probe and masker tones and varied the masker-probe tone intervals (ΔT) between 0 and 100 ms. The probe tone was 20 dB above ABR threshold and the masker level was adjusted until the P5 amplitude was reduced by 50% (masked threshold). Time constants were computed from an exponential fit to the recovery functions (plots of the masked threshold vs. ΔT). They found that hearing-impaired mice had a significant increase in time constants. This suggested impairment of recovery from short-term adaptation in ears with SNHL.

Duan and Canlon (1996) measured ABR thresholds of the Bronx waltzer mouse, a mutant possessing an IHC defect, and normal CBA/CBA mice in a forward masking paradigm. They used a probe tone at 10 dB above ABR threshold and a masker tone of the same frequency, whose level was adjusted until the amplitudes of ABR peaks were reduced to a threshold criterion, thus determining the threshold of the masker. The ΔT was varied between 0 and 12 ms. Duan and Canlon (1996) found that the slope of the forward masking curve was significantly reduced compared to the control group, particularly at ΔT between 0 and 4 ms. Based on these results, Duan and Canlon (1996) suggested that the slope of the forward masking curve could be used for the detection of IHC damage.

SUMMARY

Since the introduction of signal averaging techniques, the ABR has emerged as the most commonly used tool in assessment of auditory function in mice. The noninvasive character and the simplicity of ABR recording have elevated ABRs to the tool of choice in the investigation of the mouse auditory system. Its effectiveness has been demonstrated by numerous studies aimed at character-izing various mouse strains and mutants and evaluating hearing loss due to various intrinsic (e.g., genes, autoimmune processes, and aging) and extrinsic (e.g., NIHL and ototoxicity) processes.

DISTORTION PRODUCT OTOACOUSTIC EMISSION

BACKGROUND

In the healthy ear, the OHCs are believed to act as biomechanical gain control effectors (Kim, 1984). The electromotile properties of the OHCs (e.g., Brownell, 1983; Brownell et al., 1985) appear to give rise to the active, nonlinear properties of the healthy cochlea, evident in its sharp mechanical tuning and sensitivity (Sellick et al., 1982). The unique properties of the OHCs are also thought to be associated with otoacoustic emissions (OAEs). OAEs are low-intensity sounds emanating from the cochlea which are propagated in reverse through the ossicular chain and the tympanum (Kemp, 1978). The association of OAEs with OHC function is supported by animal experiments demonstrating that electrical stimulation of the crossed-olivocochlear bundle (efferent fibers originating in the brainstem and innervating mostly the OHCs) altered OAE properties (e.g., Mountain, 1980; Siegel and Kim, 1982). Also, excessive noise exposure (e.g., Kim et al., 1980; Siegel et al., 1982; Zurek et al., 1982; Schmiedt, 1986; Lonsury-Martin et al., 1987) and ototoxic drugs (e.g., Anderson and Kemp, 1979; Anderson, 1980; Kemp and Brown, 1984; A.M. Brown et al., 1989) which damaged OHCs abolished or reduced OAE levels.

Another line of supporting evidence for the association of OAEs and OHCs emerged from studies conducted in mutant mice. Horner et al. (1985) and Schrott et al. (1991) provided the earliest reports of OAEs in normal CBA and mutant (*deafness, viable dominant spotting, quivering, Wv/Wv,* and *Bronx waltzer*) mice. Their key finding was that in *Bronx waltzer* mice (mutants that have a full complement of OHCs but up to 80% of IHCs are missing), $2f_1 - f_2$ DPOAE (see below) was clearly recordable with a 10 to 20 dB lower magnitude as compared to normal CBA control mice. The homozygous *Wv/Wv* mutant mice, on the other hand, have selective OHC loss as a constant defect and an essentially normal IHC population. The $2f_1 - f_2$ DPOAE could not be detected in *Wv/Wv* mice. Based on these results, it was concluded that the OHCs are critically involved in the production of DPOAEs.

DPOAE RECORDING SYSTEM

Traditionally, evoked OAEs have been subdivided according to the stimulus used to elicit them: stimulus frequency (i.e., pure tone), transient (e.g., click), or distortion products (e.g., two tones). Although transient evoked OAEs are recordable in mice (Khvoles et al., 1999), DPOAEs have the advantage of higher testable frequencies than click-evoked OAEs. DPOAE stimuli are generated via two separate D/A channels of a digital signal processor and delivered to the ear canal via two speakers, presenting two stimulus frequencies (e.g., the primaries, f_1 and f_2, where $f_2 > f_1$). This approach avoids artifactual, nonphysiological intermodulation distortions. A microphone, placed in the ear canal, is used to record the DPOAEs. The microphone and speakers are coupled together, and the tip of the coupler is fitted within the opening of the ear canal to form a closed acoustic system. The output of the microphone is averaged in the time domain over the duration of the stimulus and its fast Fourier transform yields an amplitude and phase spectrum.

Most studies of mouse DPOAEs have utilized the same instrumentation as that used in human studies. Thus, the ability to measure DPOAEs was limited to primary frequencies below 20 kHz (e.g., Huang et al., 1996; Parham, 1997; Le Calvez et al., 1998a; b; Parham et al., 1999). Using the Greenwood function (Greenwood, 1990) and assuming the mouse cochlea is 7 mm long (Ehret, 1983) and has an upper frequency limit of 120 kHz (Ehret, 1975a), the reported DPOAE measures excluded a basal region of about 2.5 mm. Recently, Jimenez et al. (1999) extended the testable primary frequency range up to about 50 kHz. This extended the distance along the cochlear partition examined by DPOAEs, excluding only about 1.1 mm in the base.

An important assumption in recording OAEs is that middle ear function is intact. OAEs depend on both anterograde (i.e., stimuli) and retrograde (e.g., DPOAEs) transmission of energy. Therefore, any disruption of middle ear function can alter OAEs and confound the results.

DPOAE Measures

DPOAEs are related to the primaries above and below the primary frequencies by $nf_2 - (n - 1)f_1$ and $nf_1 - (n - 1)f_2$, respectively. The magnitude and number of DPOAE components change, depending on the stimulus parameters (Figures 4.4a and b; also see below). The largest DPOAE is usually the $2f_1 - f_2$ component. The $2f_1 - f_2$ DPOAE level increases with stimulus level (Figure 4.4c), but may show a nonmonotonic growth, including a notch (Figure 4.4d). When DPOAE level vs. primary level (the input-output function) has a notch, the region of level notch is characteristically associated with a rapid DPOAE phase change of about π radians (e.g., Whitehead et al., 1992b; Fahey and Allen, 1997) (Figure 4.4d). DPOAE detection threshold, conventionally defined as the lowest primary level that produces an emission level exceeding the noise floor by a criterion amount (e.g., 3 dB), can be measured from an input-output (I/O) function (Figure 4.4c).

Applications of some of the above measures are demonstrated in Figure 4.5 to characterize DPOAEs in the DBA/2J mouse (unpublished data, previously reported in abstract form by Parham et al., 1997). The audiogenic-seizure-susceptible DBA/2J mouse, shortly after the onset of hearing, exhibits progressive elevation of auditory thresholds that becomes severe by 3 to 4 months of age (Ralls, 1967; Willott et al., 1984; Erway et al., 1993; Willott et al., 1995). This early-onset hearing loss is due in part to the *Ahl* gene (see Chapter 28). DPOAE I/O functions, obtained from DBA mice between 17 and 73 days of age, are shown in Figures 4.5a and b. With increasing age, I/O functions shifted initially to the left and then to the right. The amount of change in DPOAE detection threshold and DPOAE level, relative to those of the 17-day-old mice, are shown in Figures 4.5c and d, respectively. DPOAE detection threshold decreased with age across all frequencies tested, but began to increase after 24 days of age, first at higher frequencies, then progressing toward lower frequencies with postnatal age (Figure 4.5c). DPOAE level also increased across all frequencies, but by 31 days of age, while DPOAE level continued to increase for low frequencies ($f_2 < 12$ kHz), it started to decline for higher frequencies ($f_2 > 12$ kHz) (Figure 4.5d). These results suggest that the progressive hearing loss observed in the DBA strain is associated with a disruption of the development of OHC function.

DPOAE Sources

It was concluded from experimental and theoretical studies that the DPOAE is generated in the primary frequency region of the cochlea where both the f_1 and f_2 components are large (e.g., Kim et al., 1980; Siegel et al., 1982). One characteristic of the DPOAE is that its level often shows

Distortion Product Otoacoustic Emissions

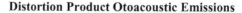

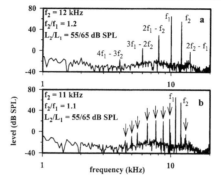

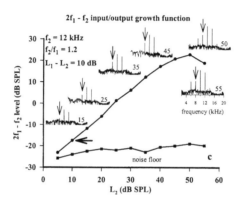

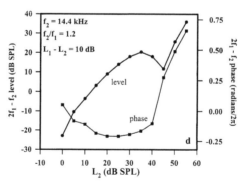

FIGURE 4.4 Spectra of microphone output from the ear of a young C57 mouse (panels a and b). The number and level of distortion product otoacoustic emissions (DPOAEs) change as the two primary frequencies are brought closer together. The input/output (I/O) growth function of $2f_1 - f_2$ DPOAE recorded from another C57 ear (panel c). The spectra of microphone output are shown for some levels (L_2 in dB SPL is noted in the right lower corner of each spectrum) with the position of the $2f_1 - f_2$ DPOAE marked by a vertical arrow. DPOAE detection threshold is identified with a horizontal arrow. $2f_1 - f_2$ DPOAE level and phase as a function of primary level recorded from the ear of a young C57 mouse (panel d). Non-monotonicity in the growth of the DPOAE level as a function of L_2 was associated with a rapid change in DPOAE phase. Primary stimulus parameters are shown in each panel.

closely spaced peaks and troughs (called the "lobing phenomenon" or "fine structure") when measured with a sweep of primary frequencies in one of several ways, such as a sweep of f_1 with fixed f_2, or a sweep of f_2/f_1 with fixed $2f_1 - f_2$ (e.g., Kim, 1980; He and Schmiedt, 1993). The interpretation that the phenomenon arises from an interaction of two sources of DPOAE, one at

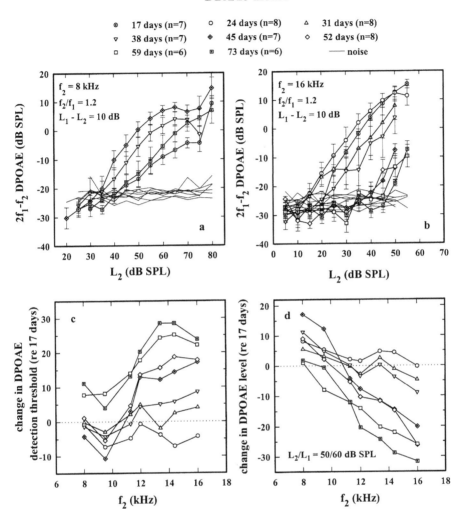

FIGURE 4.5   The $2f_1 - f_2$ DPOAE of the DBA/2J mouse with early-onset progressive sensorineural hearing loss. Mean DPOAE I/O functions (n = 10 ears) for two primary frequencies separated by an octave (panels a and b) and change in DPOAE detection threshold (panel c) and level (panel d) relative to those of a 17-day-old DBA mouse. (Previously unpublished data, reported in abstract form by Parham et al., 1997.)

the primary frequency place and the other at the distortion frequency place, was originally suggested by Kim (1980). Kemp and Brown (1983) and Brown and Kemp (1984) made the same suggestion from reasoning that a distortion signal, which is mechanically propagated from the primary frequency place to the distortion-frequency place, may give rise to stimulus frequency emission from the latter place. Many subsequent studies support the concept and provide further information about interaction of the two sources (e.g., Kummer et al., 1995; Heitmann et al., 1998; Talmadge et al., 1998; Shera and Guinan, 1999; Stover et al., 1996; Knight and Kemp, 2000; Moulin, 2000). Shera and Guinan (1999) characterized how the properties of the DPOAE contributions from the primary place (nonlinear distortion emission) and those from the distortion place (reflection emission) are different. Thus, the latter DPOAE contribution is expected to be similar to other reflection-type emissions (i.e., stimulus frequency and click-evoked emissions). Kemp and colleagues (e.g., Knight and Kemp, 2000) refer to the distortion and reflection emissions as "wave-fixed" and "place-fixed"

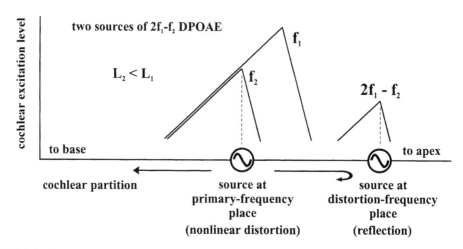

FIGURE 4.6 Schematic illustration of spatial patterns of cochlear excitation level for the two primary frequencies, f_2 and f_1, and $2f_1 - f_2$ distortion product. Two sources of $2f_1 - f_2$ DPOAE are also shown, one at the primary frequency place (the f_2 place in this case) and the other at the distortion frequency place. The stimulus level of the f_2 tone (L_2) is lower than that of the f_1 tone (L_1). (Previously unpublished.)

emissions, respectively. The relative contribution of the two DPOAE sources vary, depending on stimulus condition (Shera and Guinan, 1999; Knight and Kemp, 2000).

Figure 4.6 schematically describes cochlear excitation patterns corresponding to two primary frequencies and $2f_1 - f_2$ DPOAE, and the locations of two sources of DPOAE discussed above. It illustrates an example where the level of the f_2 tone (L_2) is lower than that of the f_1 tone (L_1), such that the cochlear excitation levels for the two primary frequency components overlap each other in a region basal to the f_2 place. For the purpose of assessing the functional status of various regions of the cochlea, a plot of DPOAE level (or DPOAE threshold) is often used with an abscissa of some measure of f_1 and f_2; $[f_1 \times f_2]^{0.5}$ (e.g., Lonsbury-Martin et al., 1990; Jimenez et al., 1999), or f_2 (e.g., Kimberley et al., 1994; Parham, 1997), where the two measures imply that the center of DPOAE generation region is located between the two primary frequencies or the f_2 place, respectively.

Which of the above two measures of primary frequencies is more appropriate? The difference would be negligible for f_2/f_1 near unity. For a large f_2/f_1, however, the difference would be more noticeable. If the apical slope of the cochlear excitation pattern is steeper than twice the basal slope, as depicted in Figure 4.6, one theoretically predicts that the center of the DPOAE generation region is close to the f_2 place for cochlear nonlinearity, where the locally generated amplitude of $2f_1 - f_2$ component is proportional to the product of the square of the f_1 component amplitude and the f_2 component amplitude. A number of papers in the literature express the view that the center of the DPOAE generation region is expected to be at the f_2 place (e.g., Allen and Fahey, 1993; Kummer et al., 1998). Regardless of which primary frequency abscissa is used, given a likelihood that DPOAEs arise from two separate sources, caution should be taken to note that a change in DPOAE may arise from impairment in either the primary frequency place or the distortion frequency place (L.J. Stover et al., 1999). Suppressing the contribution from the distortion frequency place source by the addition of a third primary tone with frequency near the distortion product (Heitmann et al., 1998) may yield DPOAE results that are better correlated with the status of the primary frequency place.

DPOAE I/O FUNCTION AND HEARING LOSS

DPOAE I/O functions of mice are altered with elevation of thresholds. Parham (1997) reported the following trends observed in aging C57 mice. When hearing loss was mild (<20 to 30 dB), I/O functions were compressed, and nonlinearities in the form of "notches" were attenuated or abolished. When hearing loss was moderate (30 to 40 dB), I/O functions were sharply altered, exhibiting broad plateaus in response to a moderate range of primary levels and steep slopes at higher primary levels. When hearing loss was severe (>40 dB), I/O functions were essentially flat at or near noise-floor level, then grew steeply at high primary levels. Similar trends, albeit without consistent findings of steeper I/O slopes with hearing loss, have been observed in other mouse studies (see Figures 4.5a and b; Sun, 1998; Jimenez et al., 1999; D. Li et al., 1999; Parham et al., 1999). Behavior of the DPOAE in I/O functions is believed to be influenced by multiple sources; for example, two sources located at different places along the cochlear partition, sometimes giving rise to phase cancellations apparent in the form of notches (e.g., Kim, 1980; Zwicker, 1986; A.M. Brown, 1987). Absence of notches and steeper slope of I/O functions with hearing loss is interpreted as an alteration of interaction between various sources, including an interaction between a low-level source and a high-level source (Norton and Rubel, 1990; Whitehead et al., 1992a; b; Mills and Rubel, 1994). The rapid growth of DPOAE I/O functions has been attributed to an unmasked high-level source of DPOAEs, under conditions where the more vulnerable low-level source has been disrupted (e.g., Lonsbury-Martin et al., 1987; Mills et al., 1993). Any relationship between the low- and high-level DPOAE sources and the primary frequency place source and distortion frequency place source of DPOAEs remains to be determined.

DPOAE DIFFERENCES BETWEEN HUMANS AND ANIMALS

Features of the mouse $2f_1 - f_2$ DPOAE are comparable to those described for other laboratory mammals in the literature with respect to fine structure, I/O functions, and DPOAE behavior as a function of f_2/f_1 and $L_1 - L_2$ (see Parham, 1997). There are differences between the behaviors of DPOAEs in mice and humans (e.g., Parham, 1997) analogous to those noted between other animals and humans (e.g., A.M. Brown, 1987; Lonsbury-Martin et al., 1997). These include animals exhibiting higher DPOAE level, less pronounced DPOAE fine structure, and less pronounced spontaneous and reflection-type OAEs (i.e., transient-evoked and stimulus frequency OAEs) than humans. One possible approach to explain these differences between humans and animals is to postulate the following hypotheses: (1) the reflection-type emission source (including the distortion place source under two-tone stimulation) is more prominent in humans than in animals; and (2) the reflection source at the distortion frequency place makes a negative contribution to DPOAE level in the ear canal under most conditions. Independent of what mechanisms may underlie the above differences, caution is needed when one applies OAE results from non-primate animals to humans (Lonsbury-Martin et al., 1997).

OPTIMAL DPOAE STIMULUS PARAMETERS

In manipulating $2f_1 - f_2$ DPOAE measures, four independent parameters of the primary stimuli can be varied: f_1, f_2, L_1, and L_2. Examples of combined parameters are stimulus frequency ratio (f_2/f_1) and level difference ($L_1 - L_2$). Varying the primary parameters has substantial effects on the level of the DPOAE recorded from normal ears. The complex mechanisms that underlie the dependence of DPOAE level on primary stimulus parameters have been extensively investigated (e.g., Kim, 1980; Gaskill and Brown, 1990; Whitehead et al., 1992a; Mills et al., 1993; He and Schmiedt, 1993; Talmadge et al., 1998; Shera and Guinan, 1999; Knight and Kemp, 2000) but have yet to be fully elucidated.

Under conditions of experimentally induced acute cochlear insults, certain combinations of stimulus frequency ratio and level difference were observed to detect changes in DPOAE level more sensitively. For example, in gerbils exposed to furosemide, stimuli with $f_2/f_1 = 1.28$, $L_2 = 50$ dB SPL re 20 µPa, and $L_1 - L_2 = 5$ dB were observed to produce a decrease of DPOAE level most consistently as an effect of the ototoxic drug (Mills and Rubel, 1994). In a study of humans exposed to acoustic overstimulation, where f_2/f_1 was 1.22 and L_1 55 or 60 dB SPL, stimuli with $L_2 = 30$ dB SPL and $L_1 - L_2 = 25$ dB produced DPOAE that was more sensitive to the exposure than stimuli with $L_1 - L_2 = 0$ dB (Sutton et al., 1994). In noise-exposed rabbits and hearing-impaired humans, where f_2/f_1 was near 1.2, and L_1 ranged from 35 to 75 dB SPL, increasing $L_1 - L_2$ from 0 up to 20 dB increased the amount of DPOAE level reduction below those of pre-exposure or normal ears (Whitehead et al., 1995). In another study of humans with SNHL, where f_2/f_1 was about 1.2 and $L_1 = 65$ dB SPL, stimuli with $L_2 = 50$ dB SPL and $L_1 - L_2 = 15$ dB had better test performance (that is, higher sensitivity and specificity) and larger area under the receiver operating characteristic curve, as well as better correlation with audiometric pure-tone thresholds, than stimuli with $L_1 - L_2 = 0$ dB (Sun et al., 1996).

In the mouse, a few investigations have examined the effects of varying selected stimulus parameters on DPOAE level in normal and impaired ears (Parham, 1997; Huang et al., 1998; Le Calvez et al., 1998b). In a recent study, we have investigated the dependence of DPOAE level of young and aged mice on stimulus parameters in greater detail. While measuring DPOAE level, we explored systematically a wide range of three-dimensional stimulus-parameter space as follows: f_2/f_1 from 1.05 to 1.40 in steps of 0.05, and L_1 and L_2, each from 0 to 75 dB SPL in steps of 5 dB with f_2 fixed at certain frequencies (e.g., 11.3 kHz). We conducted the study in four age groups of CBA/J mice (2, 17, 22, and 26 months) and in three age groups of C57 mice (2, 10, and 12 months) (unpublished data, previously reported in abstract form by Sun et al., 1997; 1998; and in a Ph.D. thesis by Sun, 1998).

Figure 4.7a shows iso-DPOAE-level contours in an L_2/L_1 plane for 2-month-old CBA mice, where a peak of DPOAE level is seen at $L_2/L_1 = 45/65$ dB SPL. Relative to the condition with $L_2/L_1 = 40/40$ dB SPL, increasing L_1 from 40 to 65 dB SPL significantly enhanced DPOAE level, but decreasing L_2 from 40 to 10 dB SPL did not substantially reduce DPOAE level. Figure 4.7b shows a contour plot of DPOAE level for 22-month-old CBA mice analogous to Figure 4.7a. Compared with Figure 4.7a, the iso-response contours of Figure 4.7b were shifted upward and to the right, indicating a decrease of DPOAE level with age. Figure 4.7c shows the difference in DPOAE level between 22- and 2-month-old mice.

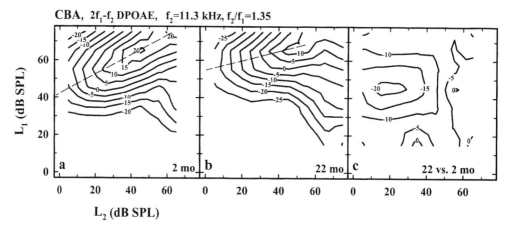

FIGURE 4.7   Mean iso-DPOAE-level contour plots as a function of primary stimulus levels (L_1 and L_2) for 2- (panel a, n = 11 ears) and 22-month-old (panel b, n = 10 ears) CBA/JNia mice. The difference between DPOAE levels of the two age groups is shown in panel c. The number associated with each contour represents DPOAE level in dB SPL for panels a and b, or the difference between DPOAE levels of the two age groups for panel c. (Previously unpublished data, reported in abstract form by Sun et al., 1998, and in a Ph.D. thesis by Sun, 1998.)

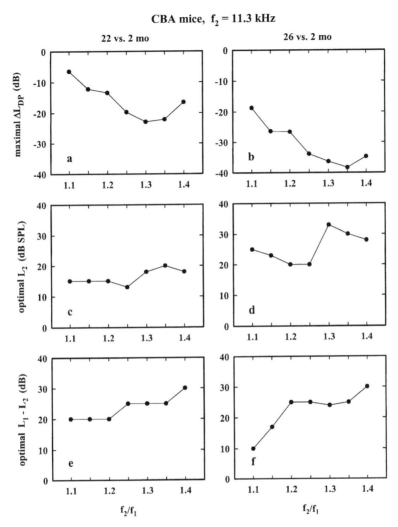

FIGURE 4.8 Maximal change in $2f_1 - f_2$ DPOAE level (max. ΔL_{DP}) relative to young mice (panels a and b), optimal L_2 (panels c and d), and optimal $L_1 - L_2$ (panels e and f) as a function of f_2/f_1 for 22- (left column) and 26-month-old (right column) CBA/JNia mice. Data are derived from plots similar to and including Figure 4.7c. (Previously unpublished data, reported in abstract form by Sun et al., 1998, and in a Ph.D. thesis by Sun, 1998.)

A well-circumscribed area in the L_2/L_1 plane, centered at 20/45 dB SPL, is identified in Figure 4.7c as the condition that produced the deepest trough of DPOAE level change (about –20 dB). This interesting new finding was not fully anticipated because the pattern of contours in Figure 4.7c is not easily predictable if one only examines the two sets of contour patterns of the normal and impaired ears described in Figures 4.7a and b, respectively. It is important to note that the location of L_2/L_1 that produced the maximal reduction in DPOAE level in impaired ears as compared with normal ears (20/45 dB SPL) was quite different from that which produced the maximal DPOAE level in normal ears (45/65 dB SPL).

Figure 4.8 summarizes results for optimal stimulus parameters for 22- and 26-month-old CBA mice. In Figures 4.8a and b, each ordinate value represents the maximal change of DPOAE level observed at a particular f_2/f_1 by varying both L_2 and L_1 in an L_2/L_1 plane as illustrated in Figure 4.7.

The largest change in DPOAE level occurred at $f_2/f_1 = 1.3$ or 1.35 (Figures 4.8a and b). Optimal L_2 was 18 or 30 dB SPL for $f_2/f_1 = 1.3$–1.35 (Figures 4.8c and d). Optimal $L_1 - L_2$ increased with increasing f_2/f_1, having a value of 25 dB for $f_2/f_1 = 1.3$–1.35 (Figures 4.8e and f). Results from C57 mice were consistent with those from CBA mice, and are not described here.

In impaired ears such as those of old subjects, optimal stimulus parameters for assessing cochlear impairment are those yielding: (1) the largest reduction in DPOAE level in impaired ears as compared with normal ears, and (2) DPOAE level reduction that is correlated with the degree of impairment of a cochlear place specifically associated with the f_2 primary frequency. Based on the results of Figures 4.7 and 4.8, and other related results, we conclude that the stimulus parameters that are optimally sensitive to cochlear impairment in CBA mice are as follows: $f_2/f_1 = 1.35$, $L_2 = 20$ to 30 dB SPL, and $L_1 - L_2 = 25$ dB.

DPOAE LEVEL VS. f_2/f_1

DPOAE level as a function of f_1 swept over a constant f_2 has been investigated in C57BL/6J (Parham, 1997; Sun, 1998); CBA (Le Calvez et al., 1998b; Sun, 1998); CD1 (Le Calvez et al., 1998b); and heterozygous deafness (+/dn) (Huang et al., 1998) mice. In normal mouse ears, as in non-murine species, the DPOAE level displays bandpass behavior. In general, the f_2/f_1 corresponding to the maximum DPOAE level is near 1.2 when $L_1 - L_2$ is 0 to 10 dB, but is >1.25 when $L_1 - L_2 > 10$ dB.

In the presence of hearing loss, the results are less consistent. In CD1 mice, with $L_1 = L_2$, the f_2/f_1 corresponding to the maximum DPOAE level shifted toward higher ratios as hearing thresholds increased. In contrast, in the C57 mouse, $L_1 - L_2 = 10$ dB, the f_2/f_1 corresponding to the maximum DPOAE level showed little change, despite elevation of hearing thresholds. In C57 and CBA mice, with $L_1 - L_2 = 20$ dB, the f_2/f_1 corresponding to the maximum DPOAE level shifted toward lower ratios with elevation of hearing thresholds.

Some investigators interpreted the bandpass characteristic as an indication of a "second filter" within cochlear micromechanics (e.g., Fahey and Allen, 1986; A.M. Brown and Gaskill, 1990; Le Calvez et al., 1998b), possibly related to the coupling of OHCs to the tectorial membrane (Allen and Fahey, 1993; A.M. Brown et al., 1992). The reason for divergence of results with respect to the f_2/f_1 corresponding to the maximum DPOAE level with elevation of hearing thresholds is unclear. A key difference, in addition to mouse strains, appears to be different $L_1 - L_2$ values used. It is important to note that from a theoretical point of view, a bandpass behavior of DPOAE level as a function of f_2/f_1 does not necessarily require a second filter. For example, a modeling study of DPOAE was able to replicate the bandpass characteristic by utilizing a single filter (Matthews and Molnar, 1986).

DPOAE GROUP DELAY

The phase gradient of $2f_1 - f_2$ DPOAE, when f_2 is kept constant and f_1 is swept over a narrow interval around its mean values, has been used to estimate group delay of DPOAE. The group delay, $\tau = \Delta\phi/2\pi\Delta f$ (ϕ = DPOAE phase; f = DPOAE frequency), is related to DPOAE onset latency — the sum of anterograde propagation of stimuli into the cochlea, nonlinear interaction processes between their traveling waves involving the local active filtering processes that are responsible for cochlear amplification and retrograde transmission of sound energy at $2f_1 - f_2$ from inside the cochlea. DPOAE group delays have been derived for CBA/J and CD1 mice (Le Calvez et al., 1998b). In normal CBA/J mice, the mean group delay is 0.73 ms. In CD1 mice, group delays shorten from 0.73 to 0.66 ms with ABR threshold elevations of 10 to 35 dB. Larger threshold increases led to significant shortening of group delays such that it could not be distinguished from instrumental distortion and transducer delays. Shortening of the group delay has been attributed to decreased local active filtering properties in a pathological cochlea.

DPOAE as a Tool in Auditory Phenotyping

The DPOAE has been promoted as a tool for phenotyping investigations. The *deafness* mouse, a recessive mutant of the curly-tail (ct) stock, are deaf from birth. The *dn* locus maps to mouse chromosome 19, and the heterozygous mice (+/*dn*) have been proposed as an animal model for studying auditory function of carriers of a gene for recessive, non-syndromic hearing impairment (Keats et al., 1995). Huang et al. (1995) used DPOAEs to identify sound-responsive or deaf mice carrying the *dn* gene as accurately as the click-evoked ABR. They found that DPOAE amplitude function was in good agreement with the ABR threshold for stimulus frequencies between 1 and 16 kHz. Huang et al. (1996) extended this work using DPOAE for auditory phenotyping of five strains: CBA/J, MOLF/Rk, ct (homozygous normal mice of the curly-tail stock), and F1: CBA/J × *dn/dn* and MOLF/Rk × *dn/dn*. They found that DPOAE of CBA and ct were similar, but different from MOLF/Rk, with the latter having lower DPOAE levels. The F1 hybrids had significantly higher DPOAE levels than their hearing parent strains, MOLF/Rk and CBA/J.

DPOAE and Aging

The DPOAE has been used to characterize age-related changes in mouse models of presbycusis (Parham, 1997; Jimenez et al., 1999; Parham et al., 1999). Inbred strains examined include C57BL/6J (Parham, 1997; Jimenez et al., 1999); CBA substrains (CBA/J, Parham et al., 1999; CBA/CaJ, Jimenez et al., 1999); BALB/cByJ; and WB/ReJ mice (Jimenez et al., 1999). DPOAEs have proven useful in assessing the effects of age on the cochlea, as the OHCs appear to be either primary and/or secondary (e.g., through disruption of stria vascularis function) targets of aging. The DPOAE levels of mouse models of presbycusis developed a pattern of age-related increase in DPOAE detection thresholds (Figure 4.9) and decrease in DPOAE levels from high to low frequencies (Figure 4.10).

Morphological Correlates of DPOAE Changes

Correlations between hair cell histology and DPOAE changes have been investigated in an animal model of progressive hearing loss, the CD1 mouse (Le Calvez et al., 1998a). Although DPOAE level changes were consistent with ABR threshold changes, mean DPOAE levels of CD1 mice were significantly lower than those of control (CBA) mice in frequency regions where ABR thresholds were normal. Interestingly, changes in DPOAEs were present before surface preparations of the organ of Corti using phalloidin staining (for filamentous actin) showed detectable changes in light microscopy. A subsequent histological examination by scanning electron microscopy showed that these CD1 DPOAE changes may be associated with disarray in OHC stereocilia, whereas absence of DPOAEs tended to be associated with missing OHCs (Le Calvez et al., 1998b).

In hypothyroid (*hyt/hyt*) mice, which have congenital SNHL (see above), DPOAE detection thresholds were increased and DPOAE levels decreased. This was consistent with click-evoked ABR threshold changes (Li et al., 1999). These changes were associated with the uniform lack of mature-appearing stereocilia on examination with scanning electron microscopy and the presence of a contiguous membrane covering the apex of the ciliary bundles (Li et al., 1999).

Efferent-Mediated Adaptation of DPOAE

The phenomenon of efferent-mediated adaptation of $2f_1 - f_2$ DPOAE has been investigated in two strains of mice (CBA and C57) of various ages using stimuli presented monaurally or binaurally (Sun and Kim, 1999). Medial olivocochlear neurons in the brainstem make descending projections onto OHCs of the cochlea, providing negative feedback (suppression of cochlear responses). Liberman et al. (1996) introduced a method of assessing the ipsilateral effect of this system on DPOAEs in cats, demonstrating adaptation of the DPOAE level over a few seconds. Sun and Kim

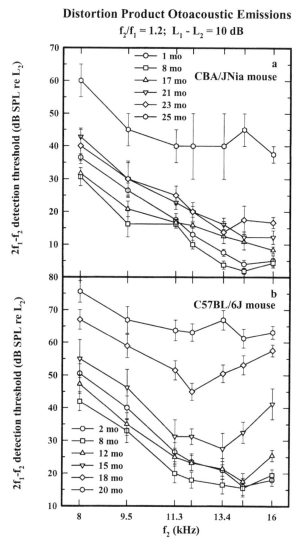

FIGURE 4.9 Age-related pattern of change in mean $2f_1 - f_2$ DPOAE detection thresholds of CBA/JNia (panel a) and C57BL/6J (panel b) mice as a function of f_2. Error bars represent SEMs. (CBA data from Figure 4, Parham et al., 1999, and C57 data are from Figure 9, Parham, 1997.)

(1999) demonstrated the existence of the DPOAE adaptation phenomenon in mice comparable to that previously reported in cats (Figure 4.11a). Furthermore, they reported that by changing primary levels relative to one another DPOAE level behavior changed from a decreasing to an increasing pattern with time (Figure 4.11b). Sun and Kim (1999) fitted their data with one- or two-exponential functions. With one-exponential fit, the average adaptation magnitude was 0.5 to 1.6 dB, and time constant of 0.5 to 2.3 s in 2-month-old mice. With two-exponential fit, the shorter time constant was 0.3 to 1.7 s. The adaptation magnitude and time constant were similar between the monaural and binaural stimulations. Sun and Kim reported that there was a statistically significant decrease of adaptation magnitude in older CBA mice (22 months) with AHL when compared with young adult mice. Because older CBA mice demonstrate ABR threshold elevations, Sun and Kim attributed their finding of reduced DPOAE adaptation in the aged mice to reduced sensation level, alteration of the olivocochlear system, and/or cochlear distortion-generation process.

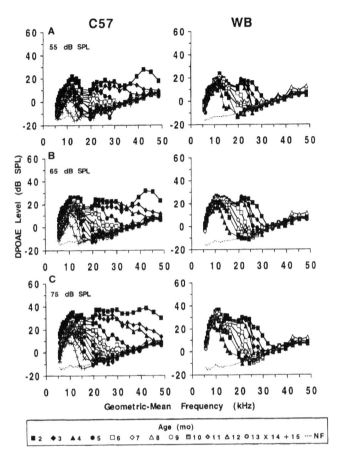

FIGURE 4.10   Age-related pattern of change in the mean $2f_1 - f_2$ DPOAE level of C57BL/6J (left column) and WB/ReJ (right column) mice. Results are shown for equilevel primaries at 55 (top row), 65 (middle row), and 75 (bottom row) dB SPL. Decreased DPOAE levels in response to high-frequency primaries (>30 kHz) in the young C57 and WB mice is consistent with the early onset of progressive hearing loss. (From Jimenez, A.M., Stagner, B.B., Martin, G.K., and Lonsbury-Martin, B.L., 1999, *Hear. Res.,* 138, 91-105. With permission.)

The effects of the olivocochlear system may be mediated by α-9 nACh receptors (Vetter et al., 1999). OHCs express α-9 nACh receptors and are contacted by descending, predominantly cholinergic, efferent fibers from CNS. Knock-out mice carrying a null mutation for the nACh α-9 gene fail to show suppression of DPOAEs during efferent activation (Vetter et al., 1999).

COMPARISON OF DPOAE MEASURES TO ABR THRESHOLD

DPOAE detection threshold or level as a function of primary frequency shows trends consistent with ABR measures when the DPOAE measures are referred to f_2 (Parham, 1997; Le Calvez et al., 1998a; Parham et al., 1999). The strength of the correlation between DPOAE measures (i.e., level or threshold) and ABR thresholds vary, depending on the mouse strain investigated. In CD1 mice, a non-inbred strain showing early-onset hearing loss (Shone et al., 1991b), DPOAE levels (obtained with $L_1 = L_2$ at 60 or 70 dB SPL) showed modest correlations with ABR thresholds obtained in the same ears, accounting for <40% of the variance (Le Calvez et al., 1998a). Increasing $L_1 - L_2$ seemed to minimally change the DPOAE levels in CD1 mice. In C57BL/6J mice, the mean increase in ABR threshold at an old age (18 months) was comparable to the change in mean DPOAE detection threshold and level ($L_2 = 40$ dB SPL, $L_1 - L_2 = 10$ dB) (Parham, 1997). In the CBA/J mice, mean ABR threshold elevations of the 25-month-old mice were more consistent with mean

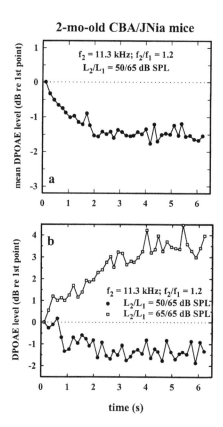

FIGURE 4.11 Adaptation of $2f_1 - f_2$ DPOAE. Time course of mean DPOAE level relative to the first point as a function of time following the onset of monaurally presented primary tones in the ears of 2-month-old CBA/JNia mice (panel a). Mean DPOAE level decreased in response to monaural stimulation. The DPOAE levels in an individual CBA ear in response to a binaural stimulation at two primary level conditions (panel b). The direction of adaptation of DPOAE level after primary tone onset was dependent on primary level difference. (From Figures 1B and 6, Sun and Kim, 1999.)

DPOAE detection threshold elevations than mean DPOAE level reduction, regardless of primary level ($L_2 = 10$ to 40 dB SPL, $L_1 - L_2 = 10$ dB) (Parham et al., 1999).

A difference between DPOAE measures and ABR thresholds is not surprising, because DPOAEs primarily reflect OHC function, whereas ABRs represent the combined function of the peripheral and central auditory elements, including the OHCs. However, given that the two measures provide consistent trends, and the difference between the various DPOAE measures is one of quantity, seeking other explanations is warranted. Among possibilities to consider are the choice of DPOAE stimulus parameters, DPOAE measure chosen, and differences in the mouse strain (i.e., inbred or non-inbred). The relationship between ABR and DPOAEs is an area that needs further investigation.

SUMMARY

DPOAE serves as a noninvasive tool to assess cochlear function, specifically that of the vulnerable OHCs. Function of OHCs appears to be disrupted by a numerous intrinsic (e.g., aging and genetics) and extrinsic (e.g., noise exposure and ototoxic drugs) processes. Although studies of mouse DPOAEs are still in an early phase, the DPOAE literature and our understanding of its underlying mechanisms are rapidly expanding. Given the diversity of mouse strains and mutants, as well as the availability of genetic manipulation techniques, DPOAE studies in the mouse have the potential to significantly advance our understanding of auditory function.

CONCLUSION

Since its introduction as a tool for noninvasive assessment of hearing, ABR has become the tool of choice in evaluating the mouse auditory function. It has been effectively used to characterize the auditory system of numerous mouse strains and mutants. Furthermore, it has helped advance our understanding of how various processes, such as aging, noise-induced hearing loss, autoimmune diseases, and gene manipulation, can alter auditory function. It is also becoming clear that, while many of the above processes have central effects, most have their primary effects in the periphery, exhibiting direct damage to OHCs or indirect disruption of OHC function by disruption of the stria vascularis. Therefore, although the ABR has been used as the main method of assessing auditory function in these mouse models, DPOAEs, by assessing OHC function, can provide more direct means of assessing peripheral functional changes. Recent investigations of peripheral function that have used both ABRs and DPOAEs in mouse models have significantly advanced our understanding of the impact of the underlying processes on the auditory system. The combined use of ABR and DPOAE is an effective strategy for further noninvasive investigation of mouse auditory function.

ACKNOWLEDGMENT

The preparation of this chapter was supported in part by NIDCD, NIH grant DC 00360 to D.O.K.

5 The Acoustic Startle Response: Reflex Elicitation and Reflex Modification by Preliminary Stimuli

James R. Ison

INTRODUCTION

The study of the behavioral effects of apparently irrelevant sensory and motoric events on reflex expression in the alert and behaving animal began toward the end of the nineteenth century, when it was becoming understood that reflex activities are not driven by stimuli acting through fixed and isolated sensory-neural pathways, but are very sensitive to subtle events of psychological significance and, thus, by complex neural activities in the brain. These early experiments on reflex modification (described in Ison and Hoffman, 1983) studied the basic phenomena of reflex modification and also its application, and demonstrated the strength and ubiquity of prestimulus effects in species as disparate as frogs (Yerkes, 1905) and humans (Lombard, 1887; Bowditch and Warren, 1890). These workers showed that both facilitation of reflex expression and its inhibition can be produced by near-threshold stimuli and by the initiation of voluntary movements, the outcome depending on small differences in the timing between their onset and subsequent reflex elicitation. Some variables that affect the strength of these reflex phenomena are important in other research domains, notably sensation and perception (L.H. Cohen et al., 1933), emotion (J.S. Brown et al., 1951), and aspects of psychopathology in humans (Braff et al., 1978). The comparability of reflex findings in rats and humans has supported the development of animal models in these areas that prove useful in understanding both normal function and disease, and this has extended the scope and the importance of research on reflex behavior. Recent advances in molecular biology have made inbred, transgenic, and knock-out mice the most powerful animal models for analyzing the functional effects of gene expression. The purpose of this chapter is to review the research on reflex elicitation and modification in mice, in order to extend these models for the more fruitful neurobehavioral analysis of genetic manipulation.

Much of the recent development in this field began with the large and systematic body of empirical work in rats and in humans published over the years by Howard Hoffman and his colleagues and students, beginning with their rediscovery of prepulse inhibition and prepulse facilitation in the acoustic startle reflex of the rat (Hoffman and Fleshler, 1963). These researchers provided an extensive series of integrated parametric experiments on the various phenomena of reflex inhibition and reflex facilitation in rats, pigeons, frogs, and humans. Among them, for example, Cohen et al. (1983) demonstrated the inhibitory effects of knowledge of stimulus presentation on the startle reflex in humans; DelPezzo and Hoffman (1980) described the increased inhibitory effect of prestimuli to which humans attend; Hoffman and Searle (1965) analyzed the time course of prepulse inhibition of acoustic startle in the rat; Leitner et al. (1981) discovered a role for the reticular formation in prepulse inhibition; Marsh et al. (1973) showed the effects of binaural interactions on reflex inhibition in humans; and Stitt et al. (1976) described startle inhibition of a light-induced reflex in pigeons by noise prepulses. Other work included the application of reflex augmentation in newborn children to the study of audition and sensorimotor control in the neonatal clinic (e.g., Anday et al., 1991).

Hoffman studied reflex elicitation and reflex modification variously in human subjects, rats, pigeons, and frogs, but never in mice. Given that the basic principles of reflex modification have been demonstrated in these several and diverse species, it seems very likely that research on the mouse should now yield a similar set of findings. But rather than assume their similarity, it may be instructive to catalogue different reflex phenomena in mice in order to describe their normative reflex behavior and its similarities and differences with other species, as well as begin to compare that behavior across inbred strains. This investigation of the conditions important for reflex elicitation and modification in mice should help us to better use these animal models, and in addition, further study of the basic phenomena in these mice may help solve the intrinsic problem of how neural processes of excitation and inhibition are organized in sensorimotor control.

THE STARTLE REFLEX

The study of reflex modification depends first on the reliable presence of a behavioral response, which can then be modified. Thus, it is not surprising that a program of research intended to study reflex modification should begin with an investigation of the important conditions for reflex elicitation. One of the first projects in Hoffman's laboratory was taken on by Morton Fleshler (1965) in a doctoral dissertation intended to determine "the adequate acoustic stimulus for [the] startle reaction in the rat." In a series of three experiments, Fleshler determined the threshold of the response with variation in the age of the rat (40, 130, and 270 days); in the rise time of his startle tones (2.5, 10, 25, and 50 ms); in their spectral frequency (720, 6380, and 13250 Hz); and in their duration (6, 12, 24, and 48 ms). His overall empirical findings were that threshold sensitivity first slightly increased, then more substantially declined with age; that reflex expression was high and about equal at rise times of 2.5 and 10 ms, and then low and about equal at rise times of 25 and 50 ms; that reflex sensitivity increased markedly with the frequency increase from 720 to 6380 Hz, and then modestly with the further increase to 13250 Hz; and that response thresholds did not vary with duration. Overall, the lowest threshold recorded for the rat was about 95 dB SPL, obtained with a 13,250-Hz stimulus presented at a rise time of 2.5 ms.

There is no single study that examines all of these variables in mice, but several experiments jointly suggest the importance of the same variables. In the first experiment concerned with the parametric control of startle thresholds in the mouse, Shnerson and Willott (1980) studied startle responding in three age groups of preweanling inbred C57BL/6J mice, 12 to 13 days old, 13 to 14 days, and 15 to 17 days, for a total of 150 trials in which the startle tones varied in their spectral frequency (5, 7, 10, 15, and 20 kHz) and their level (80, 90, and 100 dB SPL). Startle incidence increased with age and with stimulus level, and non-monotonically with stimulus frequency, being more likely for mid-frequencies. It is interesting that the threshold for startle defined as 50% incidence was less than 80 dB for the mid-frequency stimuli. This is much less than the 95 dB reported by Fleshler, but his transducer may have filtered out slow reactions that would count as startle responses in the mouse study (see below). One very informative subtlety in the developmental data presented by Shnerson and Willott was that the age-related increase in response incidence was seen at its earliest at low frequencies and lagged behind for 15-kHz and especially 20-kHz stimuli. This reveals the presence of a maturational delay in sensitivity for the higher compared to the lower frequencies, which, as the authors note, had been previously seen in other sorts of experiments by Hack (1968) and by Ehret (1976a). That age-related differences in a "startle response audiogram" confirmed these earlier observations is testimony to the ease with which objective differences in startle reflex elicitation can be used to assess certain aspects of sensory function in mice.

The C57BL/6J mouse is a frequent participant in auditory research because it has a slowly developing, progressive age-related hearing loss that appears in the animal around 2 months of age and then continues for perhaps another 12 months or so. The initial work demonstrating this sensory loss in behavioral experiments and then beginning to trace out its electrophysiological and anatomical correlates was reported by Mikaelian (1979). In interesting contrast to the C57BL/6J, the DBA/2J mouse shows a remarkably rapid degeneration in the ear that becomes evident as early as 2 to 3 weeks of age. To contrast changes in sensorimotor function in C57BL/6J and DBA/2J mice, Willott, Kulig, and Satterfield (1984) provided a near-replication of the experiment of Shnerson and Willott (1980) but tested the mice at the slightly older ages of 22 and 29 days (which is an important window on the auditory system of the DBA/2J but not the C57BL/6J mouse). Response amplitude rather than incidence was the dependent measure in this study. Both strains showed the expected increasing response amplitude with an increase in stimulus level over a range of 80 to 100 dB and, in the young mice, peak responding occurred at 12 kHz. The response then fell off from 12 kHz to 8 kHz and 4 kHz on one side, and 16 kHz and 24 kHz on the other. An interesting and not unexpected age by strain interaction resulted as response amplitudes tended to increase with age in C57BL/6J mice but showed a pronounced decrease in DBA/2J mice, consistent with their more rapid peripheral degeneration.

A later study reported by Parham and Willott (1988) focused on the development of the less rapid age-related degeneration in the C57BL/6J mouse. They contrasted the effect of age on startle response amplitudes in the C57BL/6J with those of the CBA/J mouse, which maintains normal hearing until well into its second year of life. To demonstrate hearing loss in the C57BL/6J mouse, they extended the age range beyond those used earlier and compared groups tested at 1, 6, and 10 months with CBA/J mice tested at 1, 12, and 24 months. Again, the response in the young mice was most sensitive to the mid-frequency of 12 kHz, with thresholds as low as 70 to 75 dB SPL. These response thresholds increased with age in both mouse strains, thus echoing the age-related loss of reflex sensitivity found in the rat by Fleshler; but, as expected, the decline in startle expression was most pronounced for the high-frequency stimuli in the C57BL/6J strain. These findings are exactly those anticipated on the basis of their deteriorating sensory thresholds at 6 months and especially at 10 months of age. However, more recent data (Ison et al., 2000; and below) reveal that under some conditions sensory loss can yield a transient increase in acoustic reflex sensitivity in the middle-aged C57BL/6J mouse. This finding, combined with data from other research paradigms, provides an interesting description of a shifting balance of excitatory and inhibitory processes that may accompany the withdrawal of afferent sensory input from central auditory structures.

Even in the Parham and Willott experiment, as the authors note, while the progressive change in the response to high-frequency stimulation in C57BL/6J mice is entirely compatible with their hearing loss, it is curious that there were similar if milder changes for low-frequency stimuli as well as high frequencies in the middle-aged mice, low frequencies where the ABR shows no threshold change. There are perhaps two quite different reasons for this broad behavioral effect of an apparent narrow-band hearing loss, which are not mutually exclusive. One is based on the fact that that a startle tone presented at the high intensities and brief rise times characteristic of startle experiments produces a transient click at tone onset. The low spectral frequencies present within the main body of the startle tone are thus surrounded by the broad-band frequencies of the click at tone onset, and these surrounding features could contribute to startle expression even if they do not provide much of the energy in the long-duration stimulus. Any high-frequency transients occurring at onset would be less audible for mice with a high-frequency hearing loss, and thus reflex expression could be reduced in these mice even for startle stimuli with mostly a low-frequency content. While this is a plausible and testable hypothesis, an alternative is much more interesting. It may be that central changes in suprathreshold levels of excitation and inhibition develop in the hearing impaired mouse in partial compensation for peripheral sensory loss, and thus the startle response may be revealing a central effect of peripheral hearing loss that is not apparent at the

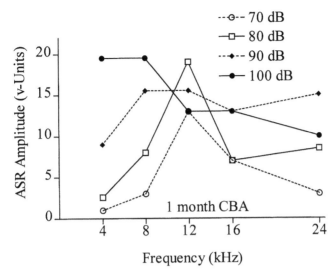

FIGURE 5.1   Mean amplitudes of the acoustic startle reflex in a group of young CBA mice as a function of the spectral frequency of tone pips and their level. (Adapted from K. Parham and J. F. Willott, 1988, *Behav. Neurosci.*, 102, 881-886. With permission.) Copyright 1988 by the American Psychological Association.

sensory threshold. This hypothesis is consistent with the observed changes in the low-frequency receptive fields in many central auditory structures following peripheral loss, beginning with Willott et al. (1982), and is interesting in its showing again that changes in reflex elicitation can generate interesting hypotheses for subsequent research.

Fleshler had concluded that the differences obtained in startle thresholds across frequency are most easily accounted for by the "sensitivity of the ear" rather than by "some special startle stimulus-sensing mechanism which has a unique sensitivity function." The data obtained by Willott and colleagues reveal a similar process working in the mouse, or at least working to affect startle expression in the young mouse with normal hearing. Their data in fact do raise questions about the extent to which sensory thresholds as defined by the ABR audiogram are predictive of startle thresholds in hearing-impaired mice, and there will be further examples of separation of sensory thresholds and suprathreshold behavioral measures in middle-aged C57BL/6J mice provided in a later discussion. However, there are some other indications in the data provided by Parham and Willott that reflex expression for stimuli at levels over the threshold for reflex elicitation may follow quite a different path from those seen in sensory thresholds even in young mice with normal hearing, and these effects are quite important in understanding the ways in which the nervous system deals with high levels of sensory input. The basic observation is that in some conditions, startle in the mouse first increases with an increase in stimulus level above its threshold, but a further increase results in a terminal loss of response strength. This effect is seen in Figure 5.1. These authors did not take any special notice of this aspect of their data, perhaps because non-monotonic rate-level functions are common in their studies of neural activity in the central auditory system; but, in contrast, they are at least unusual and, prior to this report, perhaps even unknown in the startle literature.

For example, the rat's startle reaction has been shown to be monotonically related to startle level up to 140 dB (Hoffman and Searle, 1968; and see below); but for Parham and Willott, the youngest group of CBA/J mice responded most vigorously for an 80-dB stimulus at their optimal frequency of 12 kHz, but then in an abrupt reversal the response dropped at 90 dB and again at 100 dB. Their data for the youngest C57BL/6J mice was not quite as unusual as this, but were strange enough — when presented at the best frequency of 12 kHz, startle-tone pips ranging in level from 70 dB to 100 dB were all equally effective in eliciting the response. Most certainly, this effect would never be seen in either rats or in human subjects. In fact, in these mouse studies, the prototypical monotonic increasing functions were evident only in two conditions: in the responses of older mice overall and in those of younger mice specifically for low-frequency tone pips away from the most sensitive hearing region.

It might be that not too much should be made of an isolated finding in one experiment, but to the reader conditioned to expect a monotonic increasing function between stimulus level and response amplitude, this observation was very surprising. For this reason, we ran a small experiment on this behavioral "rate/level" function to see for ourselves what might happen in a direct comparison of rats vs. mice. A total of just 9 animals were run, 5 naïve Long Evans hooded rats (3 months old), and 4 naïve C57BL/6J mice (10 weeks old), all female. The apparatus and the procedures were the same for the two species, save that the test cage for the mouse was much smaller than that of the rat, and weighed about 100 compared to about 600 g. The eliciting stimuli were different from those of Parham and Willott, but stimuli with which we were more familiar, namely, white noise bursts, 25-ms duration with 5-ms rise and decay times. They were presented at seven levels (76, 85, 94, 103, 112, 121, and 130 dB SPL), randomized in order within each of 11 blocks of trials that included a no-stimulus trial. The details of the standard procedures used are given, for example, in Ison et al. (1998a). The experiment was run under computer control, with trials scheduled every 20 s on average. The test cage is in a sound-attenuating room, and is placed on a flexible shelf over an accelerometer that records the force of a flinch response to the sound burst. The response is integrated for 100 ms after stimulus onset, and the means of the integrated responses calculated for each subject for each condition.

The results of this experiment are shown for each of the nine subjects in Figure 5.2, with the individual means for the rats above, the mice below. The two groups were similar in showing some slight increase in activity to 76- and 85-dB noise bursts, but then a sharp increase in responding at 94 dB (except for one mouse that had a shallow response function). Examining the tracings of the small responses obtained at 76 and 85 dB revealed that their fundamental frequency was lower than that provided by the larger responses to higher levels of stimulation. A careful reading of the description of the response sensor built by Hoffman and Fleshler (1965, especially p. 308) suggests that it would be insensitive to slow-wave input from non-impulsive responses to low-level stimuli. This may provide an explanation of the threshold differences described above in rats and mice, because consistent with this interpretation, it is observed that both species respond with small responses at 76 dB, about the level reported for mice, and with large responses at 94 dB, about the level reported by Fleshler in rats.

The similarity of the response amplitudes within the group of rats is striking, especially in contrast to the much greater variation between the four mice, which may be an indication that their age-related hearing loss had already had some effect. These mice were older than those in the earlier reports, and we have found that the age of onset of hearing loss can be quite variable even in this inbred strain. It is also interesting that two of the mice were jumping as vigorously as the rats for the lower stimulus levels, and it should be noted that the gain on the recording amplifier was the same for mice and rats. The rats outweighed the mice by about 10 to 1, and thus must have exerted a substantially greater force on the accelerometer. However, both the mouse and the mouse cage weigh much less than the rat and the rat cage, and therefore the point is really that the startle reflexes in the small mouse and the large rat are about equally able to quickly dislodge the animal from its normal posture, and thus provide our measuring instrument with about the same impulsive accelerative response. All of these effects are of some interest, but in context, the most important observation in this experiment is that while the rats showed a steady increase in response amplitude over this range of stimulus levels (with but two small reversals across all of them combined), for every mouse the reflex amplitudes first increased with the initial increase in stimulus level and then exhibited a terminal decline. This non-monotone effect of startle stimulus level on reflex expression is one consistent difference between the startle reactions of mouse and rat, and the terminal flattening or reversal of the reflex in mice appears again in this report.

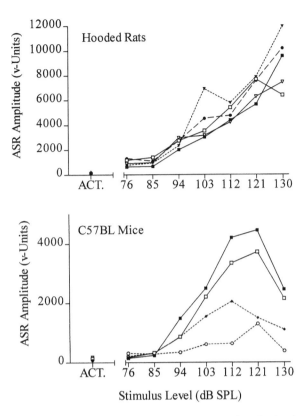

FIGURE 5.2   A comparison of startle amplitudes in rats (n = 5; above) and mice (n = 4; below) elicited by noise bursts of different levels (76 to 130 dB SPL).

The rise time of the eliciting stimulus appears to be a variable that is likely to be important for startle elicitation in the mouse, especially given that the "suddenness" of the stimulus is traditionally thought of as being with "unexpectedness" one of its two defining attributes (Landis and Hunt, 1939). Fleshler reported for the rat that while the threshold expression of the startle reaction was related to the rise time of the eliciting 4350-Hz tone burst, the actual function was essentially two-valued, with the thresholds for the two lower values of 2.5 and 10 ms being about indistinguishable, and much different from the two higher values of 25 and 50 ms. Fleshler concluded that the critical variable was not rise time as such; instead, "the stimulus must reach some critical intensity within the first 12 or so ms, but the manner in which it achieves this criterion probably has no substantial effect" (1965, p. 204). No similar parametric experiment has been published for mice, although Willott et al. (1979) showed in a single comparison that having a brief rise time is important for startle in the young C57BL/6J mouse. They reported that if an 80-dB, 10-kHz tone had a 5-ms rise time, then the mice responded over 90% of the trials and the responses had an overall mean of about 16 mV; but if the rise time was 20 ms, then the mice responded 52% of the time with a mean response of 2 mV. To determine whether a more detailed rise time function for the mouse would show further similarities with the rat data of Fleshler, we ran an experiment with 8-week-old male CBA/CaJ mice (n = 8), using 110-dB SPL noise bursts as the eliciting stimuli and jointly varying their (linear) rise and decay times (RDT) and total stimulus duration (SD) so as to roughly match the energy in each of six types of noise burst: 0 ms RDT and 30 ms SD; 2 ms RDT and 32 ms SD; 5 ms RDT and 35 ms SD; 10 ms RDT and 40 ms SD; 20 ms RDT and 50 ms SD; and 30 ms RDT and 60 ms SD. A total of 60 trials was given in 10 blocks. The data are presented in Figure 5.3, the group means (of individual medians) in the top graph and each trial in each condition for one mouse in the lower graph. The ASR data agree largely with Fleshler in

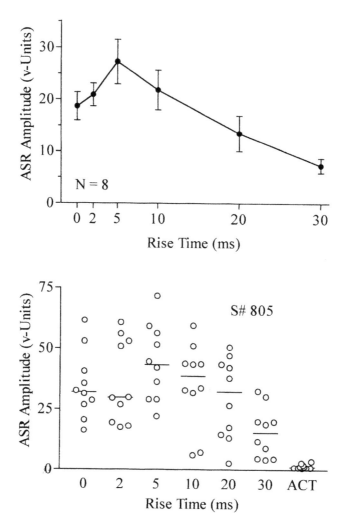

FIGURE 5.3   Group mean startle response amplitudes (±SEM) in mice to 110 dB SPL noise stimuli varying in rise time (above), and the amplitudes of all trials in each rise time condition for one mouse, showing the condition means.

finding major differences between short rise times vs. long rise times, but there is an important difference in detail arising probably because of procedural differences, namely that Fleshler used tonal stimuli that "click" at short rise times, while our noise bursts provide a click-like stimulus at all rise times. Our data show that there is a peak ASR within the short rise times that occur at 5 ms, $t = 3.75$, $df = 7$, $p < 0.01$, rather than a flat function from 0 to 10 ms. Thus, ASR amplitude in mice seems determined largely by the intensity reached within about 10 ms of onset, but there is an advantage to small, compared to 0 ms, rise times.

Fleshler concluded that the rat ASR was unaffected by stimulus duration, but his minimal duration was 6 ms. A larger study by Marsh et al. (1973) found ASR integration for brief durations. There is one experiment that studied this variable in mice (Hogan and Ison, 2000). In one of several conditions run in this experiment, young normal-hearing F1 hybrid mice (male, 6 weeks of age, n = 8) from a CBA X C57BL mating, received 144 noise bursts, presented for durations of 1, 2, 4, 8, or 16 ms, and levels of 105, 115, and 125 dB. Each stimulus condition was given in random order within blocks of trials that included a "no-stimulus" activity condition. The mouse data from Hogan and Ison is presented in the lower graph of Figure 5.4, and for comparison the rat data from

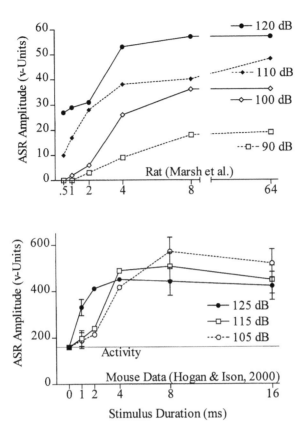

FIGURE 5.4   Mean startle responses in the rat to stimuli varying in level (90 to 120 dB SPL) and duration (0.5 to 64 ms), above; and in mice (±SEM), with levels of 105 to 125 dB SPL, and durations of 1 to 16 ms. (Adapted from R. Marsh, H.S. Hoffman, and C.L. Stitt, 1973, *J. Comp. Physiol. Psych.*, 82, 507-511; and from Hogan and Ison, 2000. With permission.)

Marsh et al. are presented at the top. The two sets of data agree in showing a rapid increase in amplitude with an increase in stimulus duration up to about 4 ms at all stimulus levels. In addition, for the lowest stimulus level of 105 dB in our data, and for the two lower levels of 90 and 100 dB in the data of Marsh et al., there is a further increase in response amplitude with an increase in duration to 8 ms. Regardless of stimulus level, there was no further increase beyond about 8 ms in either the mouse or rat data. In most respects, the findings for the mouse are very similar to those obtained in the rat, despite notable differences in the experimental procedures, such as, for example, our use of a noise stimulus in contrast to the tone burst in Marsh et al. The one difference is again an observation of a reversal in the effect of stimulus level on response output in the mouse. In contrast, the rat provides the very simple and readily explicable monotone relationship between startle reflex amplitude and stimulus level at all durations. This function is entirely consistent with the notion that the excitatory drive for the startle reflex is directly related to the greater amount of excitatory neural activity engendered by more intense acoustic stimuli. In this simple view of stimulus-driven neural activity in the reflex pathway, the behavior of the young mouse is an almost completely anomalous finding — although as mentioned previously, it is not an uncommon attribute of input/output functions in the central auditory system. It is interesting that a significant positive relationship between startle amplitude and stimulus level can be seen in the young mouse with good hearing, but one that is entirely confined to the very brief stimulus durations of 1 and 2 ms. At a 4-ms duration, stimulus level had no effect (as it had no effect in the young C57BL/6J mice in the experiment of Parham and Willott, described above). At the longer durations of 8 and 16 ms, the functions reversed so that the more intense the stimulus, the lower the response amplitude (just as it reversed at the best-frequency of young CBA/J mice in Parham and Willott).

Overall, the data on temporal integration of the startle reflex in the mouse suggest a complex dynamic balancing of positive and negative interactive effects of stimulus levels and durations, which occur over such a small period of time that they are likely to be intrinsic components of the startle mechanism itself. Thus far, this type of response/level reversal has appeared in three experiments, counting Parham and Willott, our pilot experiment, and Hogan and Ison. While the formation of a testable hypothesis to explain this effect remains elusive, it does invite speculation that perhaps in the mouse, but not so apparent in the rat or human, the massive acoustic input of a startle-eliciting stimulus engages both immediate excitation and then a briefly delayed inhibition that limits reflex expression.

In most respects, startle elicitation in the mouse is similar to that seen in the rat and the human in its substantial dependence on the intrinsic characteristics of the eliciting stimulus. But the nicety of these functional relationships is always conditioned on our aggregating groups of trials within similar conditions, a necessary stratagem that was immediately apparent to Lombard when he began his research in 1887. In fact, the expression of startle reflex behavior in both rats and mice, as well as humans and frogs, is affected by other less evident variables. As much as we all may have tried to present clean and well-controlled stimuli in a constant environment, response amplitudes always vary from one moment to the next, and the range of variation can be considerable. There is no doubt that some of this variation is produced by differences in what the animal happens to be doing at the time of the stimulus, just as the knee-jerk is affected by the Jendrassik maneuver in the early work of Lombard and Bowditch and Warren. A similar mixed excitatory/inhibitory effect of extraneous movement has been reported for the various components of the cutaneous eyeblink EMG in humans (Sanes, 1984), where there is also a pronounced mixed effect of voluntary stimulus presentation that is very precisely timed (Ison et al., 1990). Consistent with these findings, the startle reflex in the rat is substantially depressed if the rat is active at about the time of stimulus (Wecker and Ison, 1986a), and it is also reasonable to think that these movements would facilitate the startle reflex if they could be sufficiently well-synchronized with the response (Ison and Krauter, 1975). Thus, it may be suggested that one appropriate way to reduce trial-to-trial variability in the response would be to closely observe the subject and refrain from presenting stimuli while the animal is moving or fidgeting in the test cage. This was common practice in the days before computer control; but to prevent any chance of experimenter bias, it is a procedure that at best requires the continuous attention of two experimenters, one to set up the stimulus condition unbeknown to the other, who was then responsible for delivering the trial. Currently, we usually leave control over the procedure to the completely unbiased computer, but it probably leaves us more vulnerable to unwanted levels of variability. Variability might be reduced if the computer detected the presence of extraneous movement and delayed stimulus presentation until the baseline returned to normal, but we have not yet put this hypothesis to the test.

REFLEX MODIFICATION

The attempt to understand and control the sources of trial-to-trial variability leads us to the study of reflex modification, in the search for extrinsic stimulus conditions and internal state-like conditions that can alter the function of the reflex pathways, without themselves being part of the intrinsic reflex arc. The first contemporary study of startle modification by preliminary stimuli was that of Hoffman and Fleshler (1963). Figure 5.5 is adapted from their data showing the amplitude of the startle reaction to the first 60 presentations of a brief but very loud click, given in blocks of 10 trials (10 s inter-trial interval), each block in either ambient background noise (an average of 58 dB SPL, but of unknown spectral content); a steady wide-band noise (85 dB SPL); or in pulsed wide-band noise, cycled every 0.5 s. In ambient noise, the response was moderately large overall but variable from trial to trial; it was completely eliminated on almost all trials in the pulsed noise condition,

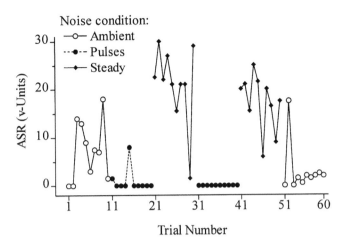

FIGURE 5.5 Startle response amplitudes for 60 trials for one rat in different blocked background noise conditions. (Adapted from H.S. Hoffman and M. Fleshler, 1963, *Science*, 141, 928-930. With permission.)

but was substantially exaggerated in the steady background noise condition. There are some incidental findings that are also interesting, one being the robust appearance of habituation but only in the aggregate; note that the first two trials for this rat had zero amplitude. Another was a brief description of an experiment done with a steady vs. pulsating light that had no effect on startle, but this conclusion was later overturned by further developments.

The next series of experiments from Hoffman's laboratory provided ever more careful control over the specification of the important stimulus conditions for these facilitatory and inhibitory effects. Most notably, they included a rediscovery of the critical importance of the temporal relationships between the stimuli to the strength of inhibition (Hoffman and Searle, 1965). Much of the early development of this work and its theoretical significance was reviewed by Hoffman and Ison (1980), but here our specific concern is how these phenomena of reflex modification might appear in the behavior of the mouse. As can be clearly seen in Figure 5.5, the presence of a steady background noise has a very powerful facilitative effect on the behavior of the rat: does this variable affect startle in the mouse? The effect in the rat came to be seen as being more complicated than Figure 5.5 reveals. Later parametric variation in background level showed that facilitation increases up to some optimal level of wide-band noise and then is reduced in strength (Ison and Hammond, 1971). Further, the optimal noise level depends in part on the relative spectral compositions of the noise and the eliciting stimuli (Gerrard and Ison, 1990), and noise with a low-frequency composition tends to facilitate startle, but with a relatively high-frequency composition tends to suppress the response. Davis (1974) also demonstrated that the optimal level of background noise varied with the intensity of the eliciting stimulus and, further, on the degree to which the response has been habituated to that stimulus. These complicated positive and negative effects of noise interacting with past experience were shown in rats, and now the available evidence, although not as rich in parametric detail, indicates that they are also found in startle reactions in mice.

In one experiment, we examined startle in a group of seven young CBA/CaJ mice (10 weeks old, all male) with the reflex elicited by wide-band noise bursts, 25 ms in duration (including 5 ms RDT) presented at levels of 94, 103, 112, 121, 130, and 139 dB SPL. These were presented in a quiet background or in a 70-dB wide-band noise (which had a broad peak at 8 kHz to 16 kHz and varied by ±6 dB over a range of 2 to 100 kHz). Trials were given in 11 blocks, which included each condition presented in random order. Figure 5.6 gives the means across all conditions; and in accord with the findings of Davis, it is clear that the effect of the noise depended on the intensity of the startle stimulus: the noise partially suppressed the response elicited by the weaker stimuli of 94 and 103 dB, had no effect at 112 dB, but enhanced the reflex elicited by stimuli of 121, 130,

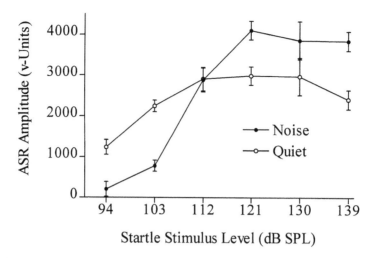

FIGURE 5.6   Startle response means (±SEM) for a group of mice to noise bursts ranging in level from 94 to 139 dB, in quiet or in the presence of a 70-dB noise.

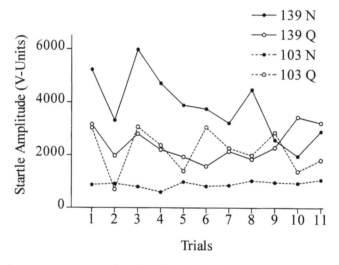

FIGURE 5.7   Startle response means on the 11 trials of a day for a group of mice to noise bursts of 103 and 139 dB, in quiet and in the presence of a 70-dB noise.

and 139 dB. An additional confirmation of the similarity between mouse and rat is given in the changing effects of the noise across the test session. Figure 5.7 gives the group means across each trial block, comparing quiet vs. the noise conditions for just the 103-dB and 139-dB stimuli. As in Figure 5.8, the 103-dB stimulus was more effective when it was presented in quiet, and this was a stable effect across the experiment. In contrast, the facilitative effect of noise for the response elicited by the 139-dB stimulus was most evident at the beginning, and was completely lost in the three final blocks when habituation was most advanced. One simple interpretation of these data is that it is noise facilitation of responses that habituates, not the responses themselves; however, the hypothesis favored by Davis on the basis of his data is that habituated reflexes are less susceptible to noise potentiation.

Another point of similarity between startle in the mouse and the rat is presented in the research of Carlson and Willott, in their examination of the effects of jointly varying the spectral composition of the background and the startle stimulus in the C57BL/6J mouse at different ages (Carlson and

Willott, Chapter 6 in this volume). Their findings are consistent with those obtained by Gerrard and Ison (1990) in the rat, showing that responses are augmented when the background is lower in frequency than the startle stimulus and suppressed in the reverse condition, with both effects exaggerated with an increase in the background stimulus. Clearly, background noise can have two effects on the acoustic startle reaction in both rat and mouse, providing in both species a positive exaggeration of the response and its opposite, a negative effect in which it appears to function as a masking stimulus. The data are also convincing in showing that facilitation is most apparent (a) in the naïve animal, (b) when the animal is presented with relatively intense eliciting stimuli in which high frequencies dominate, and (c) when the animal is in a background in which low frequencies dominate. However, Carlson and Willott caution that neither the positive arousal-like effect of noise nor its masking-like effect are well understood. They do conclude that the effects of background noise on startle are rich in their theoretical implications, and they also described their practical implications that should influence our choice of experimental procedures. They suggest that its experimental analysis may yield ideas about how the auditory system assembles a shifting balance of excitatory and inhibitory mechanisms to deal with different sources of moderate to high levels of both chronic and acoustic input. It may be that our understanding of this complexity will benefit from finding a different balance of excitation and inhibition in different strains of inbred mice and different types of mutant knock-out mice.

The other effect reported by Hoffman and Fleshler (1963) and captured in Figure 5.5 was that a pulsing noise inhibited the startle reflex, and (they mentioned in passing) a flashing light did not have any such effect. Do these observations also hold for the mouse? The first experiment described here shows that contrary to their finding in the rat, in mice the acoustic startle reflex is inhibited by a flash of light. The reasons for reporting this experiment here may appear somewhat obscure, given that the text is "mouse auditory research" and that Hoffman and Fleshler reported a negative finding in the rat for light flash inhibition. However, later research showed that rat startle is inhibited by both sound pulses and light flashes (Buckland et al., 1969; Ison and Hammond, 1971; Schwartz et al., 1976), but that flashes have a shorter temporal window in which they are effective. The idea is that the light flashes used by Hoffman and Fleshler were ineffective because they were not synchronized with the startle, and thus did not fall within the necessary time period. Additionally, the question of whether mice show visual inhibition of an auditory reflex is a question about plasticity of auditory function as well as a question about vision. This question would become especially vexing, for example, if light flashes did not affect the startle reflex in mice known to possess adequate visual abilities.

In this experiment, we examined the effects of brief light flashes on the startle reflex in young C57BL/6J mice (7 female, 5 male, 10 weeks old). A 20-ms flash of light (6 ft-c) at various lead times, 10 to 220 ms, before a 115-dB wide-band noise eliciting stimulus, the usual 25-ms long noise burst including 5-ms rise and decay times. The data from this experiment are presented in Figure 5.8. Clearly, the startle reaction in these mice was inhibited by the light flash. At the lead time of 40 ms, all 12 mice showed inhibition, at least in the sense of all having a response value relative to the baseline control of less than 1.0. At 40 ms, the range of relative scores was from 48 to 97% (i.e., a range of relative inhibition scores of 52 to 3%). It is probably important that the optimal lead time for inhibition was at 40 ms in only four of these mice, the others showing their maximal scores at 50 ms (n = 3), 70 ms (n = 2), and 110 ms (n = 3). The peak of inhibition in young rats is less variable, and in rats major shifts in the function toward longer lead times are associated with retinal degeneration (Wecker and Ison, 1986b; Ison et al., 1992; and see below). It will be interesting to follow these mice as they grow older, to find out if as a group they will exhibit the pattern of delayed inhibition across lead times and then the final loss of inhibition that is characteristic of age-related retinal dysfunction in the rat.

Given this reliable inhibitory effect of pulses of light on startle reflexes in the mouse, it would be very surprising if pulses of noise did not have the same effect. In this experiment, we examined the temporal development in inhibition over various lead times, from 5 to 640 ms. Standard wide-band

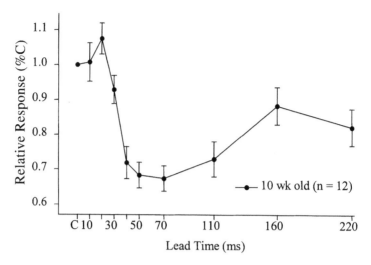

FIGURE 5.8 Mean relative response means (±SEM) for a group of mice when the startle stimulus was preceded by light flash, at intervals of 10 to 220 ms.

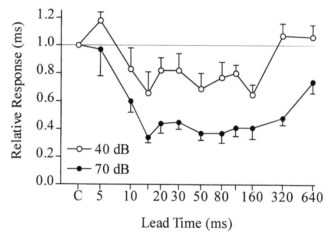

FIGURE 5.9 Mean relative response means (±SEM) for a group of mice when the startle stimulus was preceded by a noise burst of 40 dB or 70 dB, at intervals of 5 to 640 ms.

noise pulses were given at levels of 40 and 70 dB (on separate days), at 11 different lead times prior to the presentation of a 25-ms noise pulse at 115 dB. A total of 143 trials were given on each of two test days, 11 blocks of 13 trials each. Each block included one trial for each lead time plus two startle-alone control trials. The subjects were five female CBA/CaJ mice, about 2 months of age. The resulting data are presented in Figure 5.9, the amplitude measures again being converted to relative values. The data are similar to that obtained in similar conditions for the rat reported by Hoffman et al. (1980), except that inhibition developed more rapidly in the mouse. Three major effects are apparent. First, the peak strength of inhibition was greater for the more intense prepulse. Second, inhibition developed rapidly in both stimulus conditions, reaching its peak value within 15 ms. Third, inhibition persisted at that plateau for about 150 ms for the weaker stimulus and much longer for the more intense stimulus.

A more subtle effect is the slight increase in the response when the 40-dB stimulus was presented at a 5-ms lead time, which was close to significance even in this small group of subjects ($t = 2.67$, $p = 0.056$). Recent experiments have shown that early facilitation is a common finding in rats,

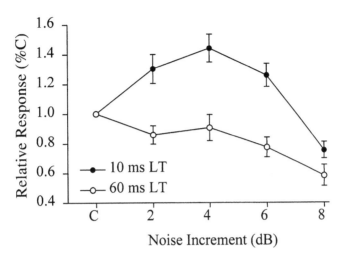

FIGURE 5.10 Mean relative response amplitudes (±SEM) for a group of mice when the startle stimuli were preceded by noise increments of 2, 4, 6, and 8 dB, at 10 ms prior to the startle stimulus, or 60 ms.

obtained usually under stimulus conditions that yield small or delayed inhibitory effects. The most powerful excitatory effects of a prepulse are seen in rats when the preliminary stimuli are small increments in a constant background noise (Ison et al., 1997). For the rat, noise increments of 3 to 6 dB facilitate startle with increasing strength as lead time increases up to about 20 to 30 ms. They may double the size of the response at the peak of effectiveness, but brief increments beyond about 10 dB tend to inhibit rather than facilitate reflex expression at this lead time. These experiments in the rat reveal that the acoustic startle reflex is governed by a dynamic balancing of excitation and inhibition in which the kinetics of excitation and inhibition are determined in large part by the intensity of the prestimulus.

We were interested in how these complex intensity- and time-dependent functions might appear in the startle reaction of the mouse under similar stimulus conditions. In the next experiment, the subjects were 10 CBA/CaJ mice, 5 to 8 months of age, 3 male, 7 female. They were run in a 58-dB background noise with 20-ms long 115-dB wide-band startle stimuli, and 0-ms rise times. Increments in the background of 2, 4, 6, and 8 dB (0-ms rise time) were presented with lead times of 10 or 60 ms, using a 10-ms duration for 10-dB lead times, and 20 ms for 60-ms lead times. The data (Figure 5.10) were very similar to those of the rat, with the exception that inhibition seems stronger in the mouse and appears earlier, although the differences are small enough that a firm conclusion should await a direct comparison of the two species. The most obvious effect is that at the 10-ms lead time, increments of 2, 4, and 6 dB were facilitatory (all $p < 0.01$), while at this same interval, the 8-dB increment was inhibitory (also $p < 0.01$). At the 60-ms lead time, the 6-dB and 8-dB incremental pulses were inhibitory ($p < 0.01$), and the 2-dB increment provided a near-miss for significant inhibition ($p = 0.051$), while the 4-ms increment did not yield significance ($p = 0.3$). The differences in the inhibitory effects of these three increments at the 60-ms interval were not significant in the analysis of variance, although the analysis of all four intensities at this lead time provided both a significant effect for intensity and a linear trend for this effect. Similarly ANOVA of the effects at 10 ms did not find overall significant differences between 2, 4, and 6 dB, although there was a significant quadratic trend.

These complicated biphasic temporal patterns raise interesting theoretical questions, but present practical problems of interpretation for those who may wish to use very simple tests for rapid screening purposes. It seems that the processes that are variously responsible for facilitation and inhibition must have different time constants, but also that they overlap in time. It is their resolution that determines the vigor in the response at any particular lead time. At any one time, our only measure of activity in the (minimally two) neural mechanisms that control reflex strength must necessarily reflect their combined action, but we cannot determine *a priori* how their separate activities vary with time, nor can we work out how they are separately affected by variables such as stimulus level. We had hoped to do a pharmacological dissection using GABA agonists to block excitation and thus isolate the effects of inhibition; but unlike background noise or fear potentiation of startle (Kellogg et al., 1991; Davis, 1979), diazepam does not affect noise increment facilitation (Ison et al., 1997b). Thus, when we find that a 6-dB stimulus facilitates startle at 10 ms but inhibits at 60 ms, we cannot tell if this results because the additional 50 ms has allowed more inhibition to accumulate, or allowed facilitation to dissipate.

There are serious implications for the practical use of reflex modification in these findings. When we use reflex inhibition as objective evidence that a prestimulus has been detected or as an index of stimulus salience (e.g., Young and Fechter, 1983), we are assuming that the stimulus is entirely inhibitory in its effect. But if stimuli simultaneously engage multiple neural mechanisms that follow independent time courses, and if one mechanism augments while another depresses reflex expression, there will be lead times at which both are active. To some extent, their joint effort will result in mutual cancellation. When there is a significant effect, whether it be facilitation or inhibition, we are assured that the stimulus was presented above the threshold: the problem is that the absence of an effect does not mean the stimulus was below threshold, because we cannot distinguish between this circumstance and that of mutual cancellation, unless our experimental designs are very clever.

An interesting example of this phenomenon and the interpretive problems to which it may lead is seen in studies of reflex inhibition by tone pips in the C57BL/6J mouse, in comparing young mice against older mice with high-frequency hearing loss. It is now well-known that receptive fields in the older mouse are reorganized following the loss of afferent input from high-frequency regions of the cochlea. The central targets of the missing hair cells are not thereafter "quiet," but instead shift in their best-frequency to become very sensitive to low-frequency input (e.g., Willott, 1984; 1986; Willott et al., 1991; 1993). Given that older mice have a larger number of low-frequency neurons, what are they able to do with low-frequency input that is beyond the ability of the young? Willott et al. (1994) used a prepulse inhibition procedure in their approach to this question, with a very positive outcome. (It is worth noting that this interesting question is also being asked of humans with high-frequency hearing loss, with mixed success: compare, for example, McDermott et al., 1998, and Buss et al., 1998.) The startle stimulus was a noise pip at 100 dB SPL, the prestimuli tones pips, variously 50 to 80 dB in level, at frequencies of 4, 8, 12, 16, and 24 kHz. The interval between S1 and S2 was a constant 100 ms. The data showed first that the inhibitory effect of high-frequency tone pips was very much reduced in 12-month-old C57BL/6J mice, and slightly reduced in 5-month-old mice, as might be expected; but in great contrast, the inhibitory effect of low-frequency tone pips was greatest in the 12-month-old mice and next in the 5-month-olds. And moreover, for the mid-frequencies, the 5-month-old mice showed the most inhibition. Similar effects were found in DBA/2J mice as well, but at an earlier age, as is consistent with their relatively rapid peripheral degeneration.

The data demonstrate a strikingly simple (but deceptive!) correspondence between the behavioral salience of low-frequency tonal input and the relative numbers of neurons in the auditory system that come to be activated by such stimuli following central reorganization. One implication of this result is that if the mechanisms of neural plasticity are similar in mice and humans, then a human listener with high-frequency hearing loss may be able to compensate by making more effective use of low-frequency input. However, the next paper published in this series showed that this behavioral effect of high-frequency loss is more complicated than a simple enhancement of reflex inhibition would suggest. In Willott et al. (1994), the experiment varied prepulse frequency and level, but maintained the lead time of the prepulse at 100 ms. Willott and Carlson (1995) used the same general procedures as Willott et al. (1994a), including their varying prepulse frequency (again 4 to 24 kHz), but now they fixed the level of the prepulse at 70 dB SPL while varying their

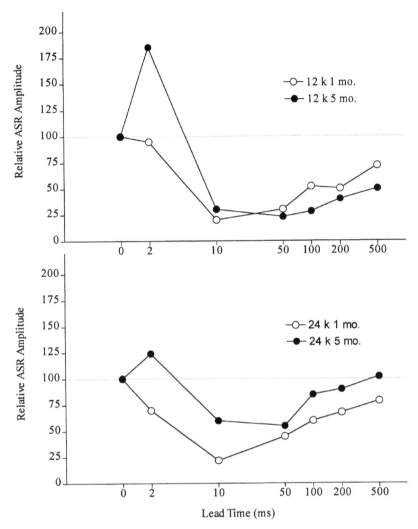

FIGURE 5.11 Mean relative startle amplitudes in two groups of C57BL mice, 1 month and 5 months old, when the 100-dB noise pulse startle stimuli were preceded at lead times of 2 to 500 ms, by 70-dB tone pips of either 12 kHz (above) or 24 kHz (below). Adapted from J.F. Willott and S. Carlson, 1995, *Behav. Neurosci.,* 109, 396-403. With permission.

lead time from 2 to 500 ms. The critical findings in this second report are represented in Figure 5.11. The data at the bottom is for the 24-kHz prepulse, revealing the reduction in peak inhibition and the retarded latency of the peak, as well, perhaps, as the suggestion of reflex augmentation at the 2-ms lead time. This is as if the stimulus had been presented to a younger mouse at a lower intensity; in this respect, peripheral damage seems reasonably described as a loss in gain at the auditory periphery. The data at the top are for the 12-kHz prepulse and agree with those previously obtained by Willott et al. (1994b) in showing that at the 100-ms lead time and beyond, the older mouse shows more inhibition that the younger mouse. But what is to be made of the differences obtained at the brief lead times of 2 ms and, to a lesser extent, at 10 ms? One thought is that this effect is simply another demonstration that the low-frequency stimulus is more effective in the older mouse, not only more effective as an inhibitor as shown here at lead times of 50 ms and beyond and also in Willott et al. (1994b), but now at very brief intervals also more effective in augmenting the startle

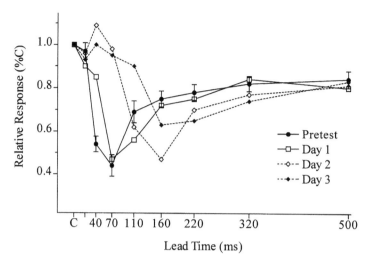

FIGURE 5.12 Mean relative startle amplitudes in groups of albino rats to a 120-dB tone startle stimulus preceded by a light flash at lead times of from 20 to 500 ms, in a pretest (mean ±95% confidence intervals), and groups exposed to light for 1, 2, or 3 days.

reflex. The paradox, however, is that while for inhibition the "more effective prestimulus" is the more intense prestimulus, for augmentation the "more effective prestimulus" is the less intense.

For this phenomenon of reflex modification, the data reveal that augmentation is strongest with small increments in a background noise (Ison et al., 1997, and above in Figure 5.10), perhaps because in this condition, delaying inhibition onset unmasks facilitation. Are there data that might support this hypothesis that sensory loss yields a delay in the development of inhibition? There are, in the changes in prepulse inhibition observed in the rat during the early stages of retinal blinding produced by light exposure. In one of our research projects, we collected baseline data on a total of 155 Fischer 344 rats at 5 to 6 weeks of age, measuring the inhibitory effects of a light flash on the acoustic startle reflex. The general procedures were exactly those we used in the experiment reported above for mice, that led to the data presented in Figure 5.8. Some of these rats (n = 18) were then exposed to fluorescent light for 1 month at 24 h/day. This procedure produces complete retinal degeneration in the rat, and, by the end of the month, results in a complete loss of light-produced reflex inhibition (accounts of this experiment are presented in del Cerro et al., 1991). We tested subgroups of these rats after 24 h of exposure (n = 5), 48 h (n = 6), and 72 h (n = 7), with the results shown in Figure 5.12, showing the data for relative responses at each lead time in the entire group of 155 rats for the pretest, and then the three subgroups with their different levels of exposure. The normal function has a sharp drop in the relative response at 40 ms, which deepens to 70 ms, and then begins a more or less exponential return toward the baseline control level. In contrast, the exposed groups show a progressive loss in inhibition, not first in the strength of its peak effect, but rather in the loss of inhibition for the brief lead times, and thus a progressive slowing of the time at which peak inhibition appeared: from peaks of 40 and 70 ms in normal rats, to 70 ms and 110 ms after 24-h exposure, 160 ms after 48 h exposure, and 160 ms and 220 ms after 72 h exposure. These changes in the kinetics of light inhibition in the rat with a degenerating retina capture the central outcome seen in Figure 5.10 for the middle-aged C57BL/6J mouse with a degenerating basilar membrane (i.e., a severe slowing of inhibition without change in peak level). This effect in the light-blinded rat cannot be simulated by manipulating the stimulus conditions, as diminished prepulse duration or power shifts both the time and the strength of peak, while light adaptation maintains the time of the peak, but reduces its strength and its persistence (Ison et al., 1992).

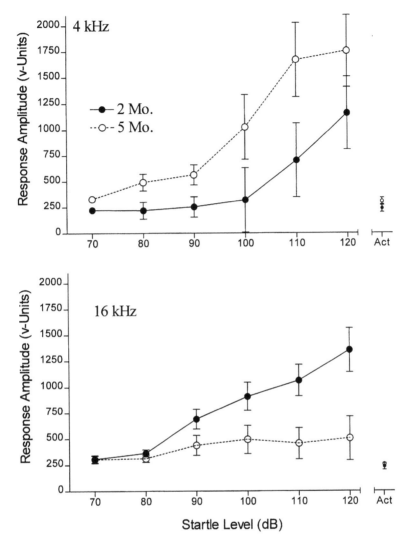

FIGURE 5.13 Mean startle amplitudes (±SEM) in two groups of C57BL/6J mice, 2 and 5 months of age, for tonal startle stimuli ranging in level from 70 to 120 dB, at 4 kHz (above) and 16 kHz (below).

Could this slowing in the kinetics of inhibition by itself be responsible for the effect of cochlear degeneration in the C57BL/6J mouse seen in Figure 5.11? This is possible; but we suspect that reflex augmentation may be a direct additional effect of the developing hearing loss, rather than a secondary effect of the change in the kinetics of inhibition. In our work on this phenomenon in the mouse (e.g., Ison et al., 2000), we have replicated the basic details of the phenomenon as reported by Willott and colleagues, but with some small but interesting differences resulting perhaps because the hearing loss in our mice appears to be more pronounced at any given age. In particular, one difference is that for our older mice, the periods of reflex facilitation for 4 and 8 kHz may last for 40 to 50 ms, rather than under 10 ms; and a second difference is that our older mice show sensitized startle responses to low-frequency tone bursts. This latter effect is evidenced in Figure 5.13. The data were collected in two groups of 12 C57BL/6J mice run at 2 or 5 months of age. The startle stimuli were 15-ms tone pips with 5-ms rise and decay times, given at levels of 70 to 120 dB and at tonal frequencies of 4 and 16 kHz. There were 11 blocks of 7 trials each

(6 levels plus a "no-stimulus" activity control) given at each frequency on different test days. For the 16-kHz stimuli in the lower graph, the data are conventional, showing that the older mice with high-frequency hearing loss jumped less. For the 4-kHz stimuli, however, the data are remarkable, as the older mice jumped more vigorously at all intensities of stimulation, except that at the highest level of 120 dB the younger mice were finally catching up. It is interesting but perhaps not surprising that for the young mice, the correlation between peak startle at 16 kHz and the ABR threshold at 16 kHz was r = –0.58; as might be expected, the young mice with the most sensitive hearing at 16 kHz responded more vigorously to the startle stimulus at 16 kHz. It is more interesting and more surprising for our conventional views of the effects of hearing loss, that for older mice the correlation between peak startle at 4 kHz and the ABR threshold at 16 kHz was r = +0.73; that is, old mice with the least sensitive hearing at 16 kHz startled more vigorously to the 4-kHz startle stimulus. The data are persuasive in showing that peripheral sensitivity changes for seeing and hearing profoundly influence both the strength and timing of central excitatory and inhibitory mechanisms.

A steady accumulation of recent electrophysiological data show that sensory loss changes receptive fields at all levels of the auditory system, as well as effecting both decrements and increments in central inhibition and excitation. This is variously seen in increased spontaneous neural noise and a combination of depressed early components and enhanced later components of auditory evoked potentials. This topic is too rich in scope to discuss here, but Willott and Carlson (1995) provide an extended discussion of research that relates it to the present context of reflex elicitation and modification. They also provide useful speculation on the potential connection between these observations and the more typical complaints of the hearing-impaired listener, which are, of course, not that their startle behavior is dysfunctional, but rather that they have problems understanding those elements of speech that depend on the precise timing among phonemes, especially in noisy and reverberant environments.

This emphasis on timing — so important in speech and also so important in understanding reflex elicitation and modification — provides the transition to the last topic of this chapter, the effects of brief gaps in noise on acoustic startle in the mouse. Temporal processing is critically important for hearing speech because of the intrinsic time-dependent nature of the speech signal, in which the fine structure of the speech envelope on a scale of some few milliseconds determines whether one phoneme or another was intended (Kewley-Port, 1983). Temporal processing is also critical for responding to startle stimuli; a drop in the envelope of a background noise lasting for these same few milliseconds can have an enormous influence on reflex expression. These powerful effects can be demonstrated (1) when a quiet period of a particular duration is inserted into the background noise and presented at various lead times, its inhibitory effect varying with lead time; or (2) if the noise is turned off prior to the startle stimulus, and its inhibitory effect varies with the length of the quiet period; or (3) if gaps of different durations are presented at a fixed interval prior to the startle and inhibition varies with gap duration. All of these effects of a gap are inhibitory, and our extensive work using decrements in noise as the preliminary stimulus we have never found them to produce reflex facilitation. In this respect, noise decrements are very different from noise increments in their effect on the startle reflex.

In the first experiment, which illustrates the temporal development of inhibition for a fixed gap as a function of lead time, a gap of 10 ms in a 80-dB background noise was presented at one of 10 intervals before a 115-dB startle stimulus: 10, 15, 20, 30, 40, 60, 100, 150, 180, and 300 ms, measured from the onset of the gap to the onset of the startle stimuli. The gaps had 0-ms rise and decay times, as did the noise startle stimuli. The subjects were 18 CBA/CaJ mice, both male and female, about 10 weeks of age. They received three test days. The data are presented in Figure 5.14, with absolute values for the mean responses at the top and relative responses below. The absolute response values are provided in part to show that young CBA/CaJ mice jump much more vigorously than C57BL/6J mice, and in part to show that the effects of habituation across days are minimal. However, these data, and also the relative data in the lower graph, show that the temporal function

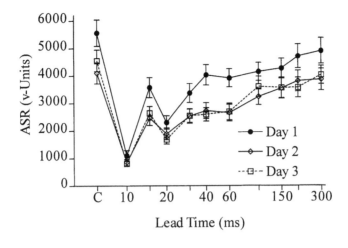

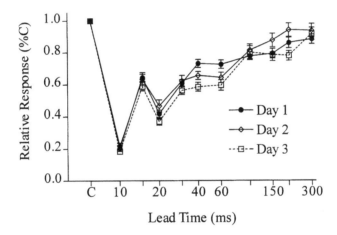

FIGURE 5.14 Mean startle amplitudes (±SEM) in a group of mice when the startle stimulus was preceded by a 10-ms gap in a 70-dB background noise at intervals of 10 to 300 ms (above), and relative response means (±SEM) (below).

for gaps is remarkable in being biphasic in the CBA/CaJ mouse (and in the rat: for example, Ison et al., 1991; Ison and Bowen, 2000). An immediate decrement is apparent when noise offset has a 10-ms lead time. The response then partly recovers at a lead time of 15 ms, but a second inhibitory trough emerges at 20 ms, and this is followed by a more gradual recovery that may last several hundred milliseconds. It can also be seen that inhibition at the later lead times is improved with training, which does not affect early inhibition; this too is evident in the rat (Ison and Bowen, 2000). In other work in rats, it was found that late inhibition is eliminated by functional decortication (Ison et al., 1991) and reduced by the systemic administration of scopolamine, a muscarinic receptor blocker (Ison and Bowen, 2000), with neither intervention affecting early inhibition. We have thought that response recovery at 15 ms reveals the transition time between the end of a first inhibitory phase and the onset of the second phase at 20 ms from more rostral mechanisms. Now we lean toward the hypothesis that the momentary increase in the response at 15 ms is a facilitatory effect produced by noise onset at the end of the gap riding on inhibition from the prior noise offset at the beginning of the gap, and that early and late inhibition partially overlap in time.

The next experimental paradigm uses noise decrements of 10, 20, 30, and 40 dB from 70 dB to inhibit the startle reflex, with their lead time equal to the duration of the gap, at 1, 2, 4, 6, 8, 10, and 15 ms. The subjects were six C57BL/6J mice, 6 weeks old, and testing continued over

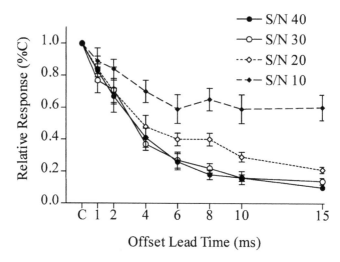

FIGURE 5.15 Mean relative startle amplitudes (±SEM) in a group of mice when the startle stimulus was preceded by decrements in a 70-dB background noise, the decrements of 10 to 40 dB, and the lead times of 1 to 15 ms.

4 days with intervening rest days. Figure 5.15 shows the relative response values for each condition. As might be expected, inhibition increased with gap depth up to an asymptote at 30 dB attenuation, and also increased with lead time with an asymptote reached at approximately 8 to 15 ms, depending on gap depth. The most remarkable aspect of the data is that noise decrements presented just 1 ms before startle onset significantly inhibit the response. With large samples (Ison et al., 1998a), 1-ms inhibition is reliable at a 10-dB S/N ratio; startle in the mouse is very sensitive to small perturbations in the background, even when they are extremely brief.

The application of reflex procedures to the study of sensory processing in some measure assumes that they provide an objective measure of "sensation" in the awake and behaving animal. These measures are expected to yield values of, for example, absolute thresholds that agree with those provided by conventional behavioral and psychophysical tests. This is a reasonable assumption, given data that, in humans, threshold measures provided by reflex inhibition agree with those of psychophysics (e.g., Reiter and Ison, 1977; Ison and Pinckney, 1982; Ison et al., 1986), as do the data collected in animals (Young and Fechter, 1983; Wagner et al., 2000). The point of this discussion is that it is unlikely that the 1-ms gaps between noise offset and startle onset are perceptible to the mouse, despite the evidence that it significantly affects startle. The gaps are brief, but moreover they are followed by an intense noise that must provide enormous backward masking. The assertion that they are not perceived would be very difficult to test in mice, but we could test it in human listeners who in other paradigms have about the same gap thresholds as mice. Three young adults were asked to discriminate the same 115-dB noise burst in a background noise from a noise burst that was preceded by noise offset, and we varied the duration between noise offset and startle onset. The detection threshold was 20 ms, not 1 ms. But how does noise offset inhibit startle if it is not perceived? We suspect that the effective mechanism is not one of the neural loops described by Koch and Schnitzler (1997) as being responsible for reflex modification, although their analysis is persuasive for prepulses with moderate and long lead times. Rather, we prefer the hypothesis that noise offset at short lead times has a direct and immediate effect on the efficiency of sensory neurons in the startle pathways. The contrary hypothesis, that it results from a complex mechanism that needs to detect noise offset and then exert inhibitory control over the startle pathways, composed of large fast-acting neurons with few synapses to slow down their activity, just seems impossible, given the brevity of the effective lead times.

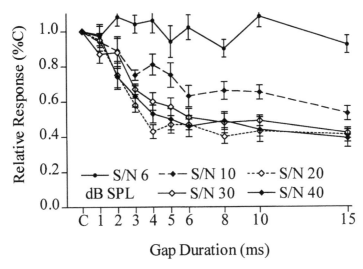

Gap Duration (ms)

FIGURE 5.16   Mean relative startle amplitudes (±SEM) in a group of mice when the startle stimulus was preceded by gaps in a 70-dB background noise, the gaps having durations of 1 to 15 ms, and ending 60 ms before the startle stimulus, and the gaps being decrements in the gap of 6 to 40 dB.

The last procedure showing the effects of gaps in noise on startle inhibition is that of presenting a gap at some moderate interval prior to the startle, in this case 60 ms from gap offset to startle onset. The subjects were 12 CBA/CaJ mice, 7 weeks old, and of mixed sex. The tests for gap detection were all given in a background of 70 dB, and the gaps were decrements in noise (6, 10, 20, 30, and 40 dB) of various durations (1, 2, 3, 4, 5, 6, 8, 10, and 15 ms). The experiment was run over 5 test days with different depths in the gap on each day, these separated by a rest day. The relative response data are presented in Figure 5.16. The inhibitory effects of the gaps are similar to those of noise offset, except that 1-ms gaps had no effect, and the functions for S/N values of 20 to 40 dB were equal in rate of growth and in asymptotic levels of inhibition. The 10-dB decrement provided less inhibition than the three larger S/N values, and there was no sign of inhibition with the 6-dB decrement. A similar study of the detection of partially filled gaps was reported by Forrest and Green (1987) in human listeners. They found that the duration threshold for partially filled gaps was minimally affected by the depth of the gap until it was less than about 4 to 5 dB. After this, gap thresholds increased rapidly from about 2 to 3 ms to about 30 s. Figure 5.17 is a scatterplot of gap thresholds of our mice, defining the behavioral threshold as the duration at which inhibition was at least 50% of its maximum. Mean gap thresholds were about equal for 20, 30, and 40 dB decrements, then increased at 10 dB, and were beyond 15 ms at 6 dB.

The power of "reflex modification audiometry" in the animal laboratory is seen in the similarity of these results and those of Forrest and Green. Thresholds in mice defined by prepulse inhibition approximate those measured in humans with the most skillful use of psychophysical techniques; and although there are quantitative differences in the relationship between gap thresholds and gap depth, both show that thresholds are minimally affected by filling the gap until the S/N ratio reaches about 5 dB for humans, and about 10 dB in mice. Psychophysical measures typically focus on the threshold, while reflex modification more naturally examines prepulse inhibition over a range of near-threshold and supra-threshold values. A single measure of threshold can be derived from these behavioral data, but this is not necessarily their primary virtue, as the differences in inhibition for stimuli above the absolute threshold provide useful information about their relative salience. For the present data, it is useful to know that both gap thresholds and asymptotic levels of inhibition are the same for gap decrements of 20 dB and beyond, as this provides further evidence of their perceptual equivalence (as do reaction times for stimulus detection in humans; Virag et al., 2000).

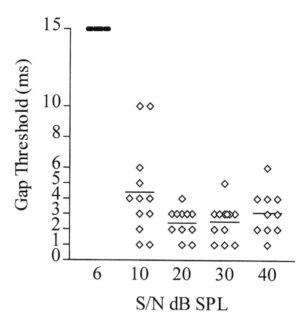

FIGURE 5.17   Gap thresholds (gaps that provide 50% of maximum inhibition) in each mouse for the gaps having different decrements, 6 to 40 dB.

CONCLUSION

We have seen that the experimental analysis of reflex elicitation and reflex modification readily yields observations comparable in their simplicity and their reproducibility to the isolated systems studied in neurophysiology. Yet in their appearance in the alert and behaving animal, they are sensitive to subtle environmental events and to the complex neural activities and their mental correlates occasioned by these events. These procedures have been applied to a range of scientific problems of great theoretical and practical importance. They have provided a unique experimental approach to the description and understanding of basic sensory and perceptual phenomena in laboratory animals, to the investigation of attention and emotionality, and to behavioral and neural plasticity. In addition, the deficit of prepulse inhibition in schizophrenia (Braff et al., 1978) has encouraged the development of an animal model of "sensory-gating deficits" based on changes in prepulse inhibition. This has extended research on startle reflex modification to animal rearing experiments and to studies of anatomical and neurochemical changes in the brain and pharmaco-logical interventions that characterize human psychosis and its treatment (e.g., Swerdlow et al., 1999).

Raymond Dodge (1931) wrote that the study of the varieties of inhibition in "normal human life …should serve as the connecting link between the nerve muscle preparation and the more elaborate processes with which the psychologist is chiefly concerned." Contemporary work has underscored the value of this linkage, going beyond the nerve muscle preparation of the physiology of that time to contemporary pharmacology and neurochemistry and neurophysiology, and now, in a new chapter, in its connection to molecular biology (Geyer, 1999). A major scientific challenge laid down by the molecular biologist is for neurobiology to uncover the functional significance of different forms of genetic expression in the brain, a new path of research that will enormously illuminate the molecular structure of the brain and its development, with great significance for all forms of normal brain function and brain function in disease and in psychopathology. The tools for this research are best provided in the mouse, in inbred strains, and in transgenic and knock-out mice, for which much genomic evidence is now available and much more soon to follow. The final consequence of brain activity is behavior and "the more elaborate processes with which the psychologist is chiefly concerned" (Dodge, 1931). The basic research described here in the mouse shows the power of the reflex elicitation and reflex modification procedures in uncovering stable behavioral phenomena with rich theoretical implications, procedures that are readily applied to the analysis of important aspects of normal perceptual, emotional, and cognitive activities in humans and in laboratory animals, to the study of aging in the auditory system, and to psychopathology. It can be expected that the continued development of these mouse models and their application will provide major contributions to our description and understanding of these complex neurobehavioral activities, of their physiological bases, and of their foundations in molecular biology.

ACKNOWLEDGMENTS

This chapter is dedicated to Howard Hoffman, on the occasion of his 75th birthday. Its preparation was aided by the U.S. Public Health Service Research Grant AG09524 and Center Support Grant EY01319. Correspondence regarding this work should be addressed to James R. Ison, Department of Brain and Cognitive Sciences, University of Rochester, Rochester, New York 14627. Electronic mail may be sent to *Ison@bcs.rochester.edu.*

6 Modulation of the Acoustic Startle Response by Background Sound in C57BL/6J Mice

Stephanie Carlson and James F. Willott

INTRODUCTION

It has been known for some time that the amplitude of the acoustic startle response can be modulated by the presence of ongoing background noise (Davis, 1974; Hoffman and Fleshler, 1963; Hoffman and Ison, 1980; Hoffman and Wible, 1969; Ison and Hammond, 1971; Ison, McAdam, and Hammond, 1973; Ison and Russo, 1990; Ison and Silverstein, 1978). This chapter contains the results of experiments that evaluated the effects of ongoing background noise and tones on the acoustic startle response in C57BL/6J (C57) mice. Additional discussion can be found in Chapter 5.

Understanding the effects of background noise on the startle response has both practical and theoretical value. On the practical level, it is important to avoid unintentional modulation of behavior by ventilation fans or noise maskers. On a theoretical level, an understanding of how and why startle behavior is modulated by backgrounds may reveal much about arousal, plasticity of auditory behavior, and the suppression or inhibition of behavior.

The processes by which startle amplitude is modulated by background sounds are apparently complex. Studies on rats have demonstrated both augmentation and reduction of startle amplitude in response to background sound. For example, when the intensity of a background noise is varied, a non-monotonic function is often in evidence (Davis, 1974; Ison, McAdam, and Hammond, 1973; Ison and Russo, 1990; Ison and Silverstein, 1978). Startle amplitudes become larger as the background intensity is increased from low to moderate levels (e.g., 50 to 60 dB SPL), but more intense background noise levels (e.g., 80 to 90 dB SPL) result in smaller startle amplitudes. These studies have suggested that the ascending limb of this function may be due to behavioral arousal elicited by the noise background, whereas the descending limb is thought to involve either auditory masking of the startle signal or some suppression mechanism that acts on the neural circuits influencing the startle reflex.

Further complicating the issue, effects of the frequency of both the background and startle stimuli are not independent. Facilitation of the startle response occurs with some frequency combinations, and inhibition of the startle response occurs with others. A study by Gerrard and Ison (1990) showed that high-frequency filtered noise backgrounds tended to reduce startle responses evoked by low- or high-frequency startle stimuli, especially when intense backgrounds were employed. Low-frequency backgrounds only reduced startles evoked by low-frequency startle stimuli. When high-frequency startle stimuli were used with low-frequency backgrounds, startle amplitudes became larger, especially when high-intensity backgrounds were used.

Given the importance of background frequency and intensity, both parameters were varied in the present series of experiments to determine their effects in C57 mice. We also investigated another issue stemming from the frequency and intensity effects — how well the animal's auditory system responds to sounds of different frequencies. For example, might high and low frequencies (of startle stimuli and/or backgrounds) have different effects because they are processed more or less effectively by the animal's auditory system? The use of C57 mice allowed this issue to be investigated in a unique manner. Young adult C57 mice (1- or 2-month-olds) have good high-frequency hearing, as do other strains of mice. By age 5 to 6 months, however, C57 mice exhibit substantial loss of high-frequency (>16 kHz) sensitivity (Henry and Chole, 1980; Mikaelian, 1979; Willott, 1986). This occurs because C57 mice possess the gene *Ahl* (*A*ge related *h*earing *l*oss), which results in damage to the basal, high-frequency region of the cochlea (Erway, Willott, Archer, and Harrison, 1993a; Johnson, Erway, Cook, Willott, and Zheng, 1997).

GENERAL METHODS

Vivarium conditions, startle-testing apparatus, and procedures have been described in detail previously (Parham and Willott, 1988; Willott, Carlson, and Chen, 1994). A mouse was placed inside a glass cylinder (the startle chamber) located in a sound-attenuated enclosure. Startle stimuli were delivered from a Radio Shack Supertweeter, mounted atop the cylinder. Movements of a mouse against the chamber floor produced voltages that were recorded on a digital storage oscilloscope as a function of time after onset of the startle stimulus. Background tones and broadband noise (BBN) were delivered via a 3-cm Sony Walkman speaker mounted on the Radio Shack Supertweeter.

The startle stimuli were 100 dB SPL (re: 20 µPa) tone pips (4 or 12 kHz) or BBN bursts (10-ms duration, 1-ms rise/fall time). Continuous backgrounds were 60, 70, or 80 dB SPL tones (4 or 12 kHz) or BBN. The BBN spectrum is shown in Figure 6.1. In quiet, the ambient sound level in the startle chamber (measured using an external filter and 6.36 mm Brüel and Kjaer condenser microphone) was 43 dB SPL for the frequencies mice hear reasonably well — 1 kHz high-pass. At all octaves within the hearing range of mice, the SPL was less than 40 dB.

A mouse was placed in the startle chamber, and testing began after initial exploratory behavior had diminished. Startle stimuli were presented when the animal was not moving or grooming itself. For each testing session, 15 startle stimuli were delivered in quiet, and 30 startle stimuli were delivered following 10 s of exposure to each background (one background frequency per day, three intensities). Presentations with and without the background were randomly intermixed through a session. Testing sessions took place at mid-day.

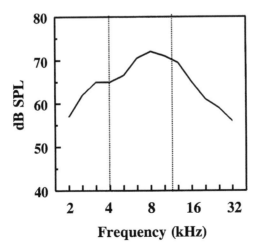

FIGURE 6.1   Frequency spectrum of the BBN as SPL per third-octave band (the abscissa indicates the upper border of each third-octave). Dotted vertical lines indicate 4 and 12 kHz, used in various experiments.

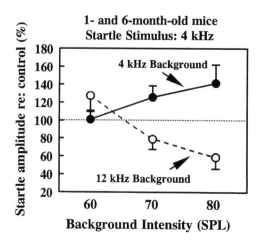

FIGURE 6.2   Relative amplitude of the acoustic startle response in the presence of 4-kHz and 12-kHz backgrounds. Startle stimulus = 4-kHz tone. Error bars = standard error of the mean.

Startle amplitude with the background on was expressed as a percentage of startle amplitude evoked in quiet. Startle amplitudes greater than 100% indicate the augmentation of acoustic startle by a background noise. Startle amplitudes less than 100% indicate suppression of the response.

EFFECTS OF BACKGROUND SOUND ON STARTLE

4-kHz STARTLE STIMULUS: TONE BACKGROUNDS

When a 12-kHz background was used with 4-kHz startle stimuli (Figure 6.2), startle amplitudes became smaller as the background intensity increased (age effects NS; data from both age groups combined). When a 4-kHz background was used (filled circles), the function was *opposite* to that seen using 12-kHz background: more intense 4-kHz backgrounds tended to increase startle amplitudes.

12-kHz STARTLE STIMULUS: TONE BACKGROUNDS

As seen in Figure 6.3, with a 12-kHz startle stimulus, 12-kHz backgrounds of higher intensities resulted in decreased startle amplitudes (open circles). In contrast, when the background was an 80-dB 4-kHz tone (filled circles), startles tended to become larger in both age groups. The results suggest that a lower frequency background tone (4 kHz) tended to facilitate the startle response, whereas a higher frequency background (12 kHz) tended to reduce startle amplitude. Also, when the startle stimulus was a 4-kHz tone, the age group difference was not significant; but when the startle stimulus was a 12-kHz tone, the background effects were more pronounced in the 6-month-old mice. In this regard, baseline startle amplitudes to 12-kHz tones were smaller in the older mice, whereas amplitudes to 4-kHz tone startle stimuli did not differ significantly.

BBN STARTLE STIMULI: TONE BACKGROUNDS

Backgrounds were tones of 4 and 12 kHz (Figure 6.4), but with a 100 dB SPL BBN startle stimulus. Results are collapsed across the two age groups (age effects NS). Both 4- and 12-kHz background frequencies produced decreases in startle amplitude (all were lower than 100%). The pattern of startle augmentation (greater than 100%) provided by 4-kHz background tones in Figure 6.3 (with tone startle stimuli) was not observed when BBN startle stimuli were employed. Consistent with Experiment 1, however, 12-kHz background tones were more effective than 4-kHz tones in decreasing startle amplitude.

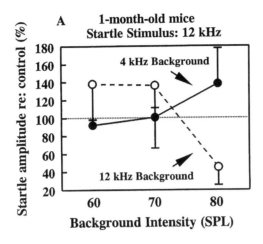

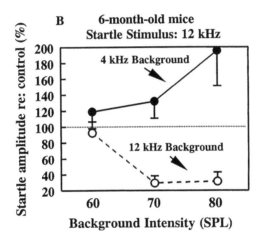

FIGURE 6.3 Relative amplitude of the acoustic startle response in the presence of 4- and 12-kHz backgrounds in 1-month-olds (A) and 6-month-olds (B). Startle stimulus = 12-kHz tone. Error bars = standard error of the mean.

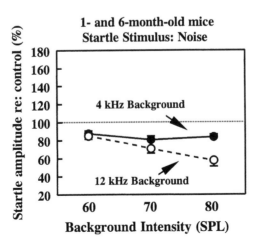

FIGURE 6.4 Relative amplitude of the acoustic startle response in the presence of 4- and 12-kHz backgrounds. Startle stimulus = BBN. Error bars = standard error of the mean.

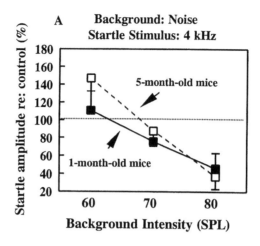

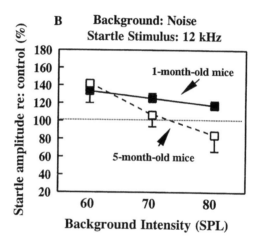

FIGURE 6.5 Relative amplitude of the acoustic startle response in the presence of a BBN background. Startle stimulus = 4-kHz tone (A) and 12-kHz tone (B). Error bars = standard error of the mean.

TONE STARTLE STIMULI: BBN BACKGROUNDS

BBN (60, 70, 80 dB SPL) was the background, and startle stimuli were 4- and 12-kHz tones of 100 dB SPL. When an 80-dB BBN background was used with a 4-kHz startle stimulus (Figure 6.5A), suppression of startle occurred for both age groups. When a 12-kHz startle stimulus was used with the BBN background (Figure 6.5B), however, inhibition was not evident, even at a level of 80 dB SPL. In 1-month-old mice, mean startle amplitudes were above 100%, regardless of the intensity of the background noise. The 5-month-old mice exhibited the typical downward-sloping pattern as background intensity increased. Thus, an age effect was present (albeit weak).

Taken together with the results in Figure 6.2, it appears that 12-kHz background tones tend to suppress the startle response whether the startle stimulus is a 4-kHz tone, a 12-kHz tone, or a BBN. On the other hand, the ability of a 4-kHz background tone to facilitate startle was not evident when the startle stimulus was a BBN. One interpretation of these findings suggests that the *relative* distribution of spectral energy between background and startle stimulus is an important factor. High frequencies in the background (relative to frequencies in the startle stimulus) tend to suppress startle, whereas low frequencies in the background tend to facilitate startle. The BBN startle stimulus has substantial spectral energy at frequencies below 4 kHz (Figure 6.1), so the 4-kHz background

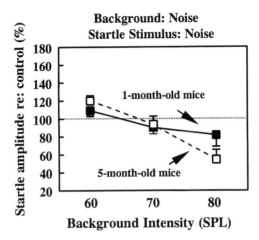

FIGURE 6.6 Relative amplitude of the acoustic startle response in the presence of a BBN background. Startle stimulus = BBN noise. Error bars = standard error of the mean.

tone is, relatively speaking, a fairly high frequency, thereby producing a degree of suppression, opposing facilitation.

As was the case for the data in Figure 6.2, when an age effect was observed with 12-kHz startle stimuli, the baseline amplitudes of startles evoked by BBN in the older mice were much less than half those observed in the young mice. Thus, the findings are consistent with the notion that "weaker" startle responses are more readily modulated by background sound.

BBN STARTLE STIMULI: BBN BACKGROUNDS

As seen in Figure 6.6, BBN background enhanced startle amplitudes slightly and a BBN background of 80 dB reduced startle amplitudes. The effect is more pronounced in 5-month-olds as indicated by the steeper slope of the intensity function and a significant Age x Background intensity interaction. The results suggest that the background intensity *per se* is a significant variable in modulation of the startle when both background and startle are a BBN.

DISCUSSION

Taken together, the results of the present series of experiments indicate that background frequency and intensity, properties of the startle stimulus, and changes in the auditory system associated with high-frequency hearing loss interact to some extent. It seems safe to conclude that the only sure way to determine the effects of background sound on startle is to measure them empirically.

One practical message of the present study has been made before (e.g., Ison and Russo, 1990): the antecedent "baseline" startle behavior may be affected substantially as a function of the acoustic background. The findings suggest that an animal placed in an experimental situation containing predominantly low frequencies (e.g., a ventilation fan) might be in a behavioral state (e.g., arousal?) that would be quite different from an animal placed in a high-frequency acoustic background or a quiet environment. Experiments using the startle response as a dependent variable obviously would be affected, but it is reasonable to expect that many behaviors (e.g., activity, habituation, conditioning) would be modulated by the background as well. The present findings, along with those reviewed above, indicate that it would behoove an experimenter to evaluate startle and other behaviors in quiet as well as in the presence of background noises which are part of the experimental setup.

The second practical implication of this study is that startle responses of all animals are not affected in the same way by background sounds. Thus, C57 mice with and without high-frequency hearing loss were affected differently, at least when the startle response had become diminished in the older mice. This is certainly an issue when using mice, because three of the most widely used inbred strains — C57BL/6J, BALB/cJ, and DBA/2J — exhibit progressive high-frequency hearing loss that begins during young adulthood (Henry, 1983; Willott, 1981; Willott, Turner, Carlson, Ding, Bross, and Falls, 1998). Other strains commonly used in genetic research also exhibit high-frequency hearing loss, including the BXD recombinant strains (Willott and Erway, 1998) and several sub-lines of the 129 strain (Zheng, Johnson, and Erway, 1999). However, strain differences are not limited to mice, and startle responses of different varieties of rats can also differ greatly (Glowa and Hansen, 1994). With respect to auditory behavior, it cannot be assumed that "a mouse is a mouse" or "a rat is a rat."

Whereas the interaction among background frequency, background intensity, and startle stimuli is complicated, several conclusions can be made from the present and earlier findings:

1. If the frequency spectrum of the background is high relative to that of the startle stimulus, suppression of startle amplitude is likely to result.
2. If the frequency spectrum of the background is low relative to that of the startle stimulus, facilitation of startle amplitude will result.
3. Both effects are augmented by increased background intensities.
4. The aforementioned observations are clear when tones are used as both background and startle stimuli.

When BBN is used as background and/or startle stimulus, however, the effects are more complicated. This presumably has something to do with the broader frequency spectrum of noise and consequent partial overlap of background and startle stimulus spectra. For example, spectral components of a BBN background may have "competing" facilitatory (low-frequency) and suppressive (high-frequency) effects. Indeed, low-intensity BBN backgrounds have a tendency to facilitate startle, whereas increasing the intensity of a BBN background causes a reduction in startle amplitudes. Despite this schizoid aspect of BBN modulation, however, the effects of the relative frequency spectra of background and startle stimuli still hold. As seen in Figure 6.5, a BBN background produces strong suppression of startles elicited by a relatively low (4 kHz) startle stimulus compared to that obtained with a relatively high (12 kHz) startle stimulus.

The mechanisms by which startle is facilitated by low-frequency backgrounds and suppressed by high-frequency backgrounds remain unknown. Facilitation of startle may represent an arousal effect (Ison and Hammond, 1971; Ison and Russo, 1990). Whether such an effect is related to fear or other emotional processes is unclear. Kellogg, Sullivan, Bitran, and Ison (1991) found that the anxiolytic compound diazepam attenuated facilitation of the startle by a background noise. However, Ison, Taylor, Bowen, and Schwarzkopf (1997b) reported that the startle-enhancing effects of a noise beginning shortly before the startle stimulus was not affected by diazepam; and when Schanbacher, Koch, Pilz, and Schnitzler (1996) destroyed the amygdala (known to interfere with fear), startle facilitation by a background noise was not altered. In any event, for the hypothesis to hold up, it must be assumed that low frequencies are arousing and/or anxiogenic, whereas high frequencies are not, or that the facilitating effect of high frequencies is counteracted by a more potent suppressive mechanism. A simple relationship between background frequency and arousal/fear is not supported by the present data because 4 kHz produced larger startles with tone stimuli (Figure 6.2), but not with BBN stimuli (Figure 6.4). Recall that Gerrard and Ison (1990) similarly observed that modulation of startle by a low-frequency background depended on the startle stimulus.

A mechanism proffered to explain suppression of startle is masking of the startle stimulus by the background (M. Davis, 1974; Hoffman and Searle, 1965; Ison and Hammond, 1971). The masking hypothesis would seem to have difficulty accounting for some of the present findings. Consider Figure 6.4a, for example. It seems unlikely that a 70- or 80-dB 12-kHz background tone would be able to mask a 100-dB SPL BBN startle stimulus. Moreover, a 4-kHz background would be expected to be a more effective masker of a 4-kHz startle, yet *facilitation* occurred under this condition. A modified version of the masking hypothesis has been proposed by Gerrard and Ison (1990). They suggested that it is high-frequency cochlear distortions associated with the abrupt, intense startle stimulus that are masked. If this aspect of the intense sound were masked, it would be less effective as a startle stimulus. The high-frequency components would be more effectively masked by a high-frequency background, accounting for the reduction of startle amplitude. Whereas this hypothesis can account for the results in Figures 6.2 and 6.3, it is more difficult to apply it to the results in Figure 6.5. Background BBN did not effectively suppress startles evoked by a 12-kHz stimulus (Figure 6.5, lower panel), but did suppress startles evoked by 4 kHz (Figure 6.5, upper panel). The 12-kHz startle stimulus had a good deal of high frequencies (e.g., for our 100-dB SPL stimulus: 97 dB in the 12- to 24-kHz octave), yet these were apparently not masked very well. In comparison, the SPL above 12 kHz for our 4-kHz startle stimulus was only about 70 dB — not enough high-frequency spectral content to contribute significantly to startle.

An alternative approach to the arousal and masking hypotheses is to consider the auditory properties of neural circuits that modulate the startle response (e.g., Ison and Russo, 1990). The key output neurons for the startle response circuit are large cells located in the caudal pontine reticular nucleus (PnC); their axons descend into the spinal cord, activating motor neurons that trigger the startle (see Carlson and Willott, 1998, for a recent review). The PnC neurons are presumed to receive excitatory synaptic input via the lower auditory brainstem, and it is through this basic circuit that the startle is triggered by sound (Davis, Gendelman, Tischler, and Gendelman, 1982; Lingenhöl and Friauf, 1994). Modulation of the startle is also likely to involve synaptic inputs to the PnC neurons. When PPI occurs, the PnC neurons are inhibited by the descending circuits, interfering with the excitatory input associated with the startle stimulus (Carlson and Willott, 1996; Koch and Friauf, 1995; Kodsi and Swerdlow, 1995). In the fear-potentiated startle paradigm (Chapter 7), the PnC neurons receive input from a circuit that includes the IC and amygdala (Davis, Campeau, Kim, and Falls, 1995), and this facilitates the excitatory input of the startle circuit. In other words, the size of the startle response is a function of the interaction between excitatory synapses of the startle circuit that drive the response and excitatory and inhibitory inputs from descending modulating circuits.

ACKNOWLEDGMENTS

This research was supported by NIH grant R37 AG-007554. We are grateful to Dr. William Falls for helpful comments on the manuscript.

7 Focus: Learning and the Auditory System — Fear-Potentiated Startle Studies

William A. Falls and Paul J. Pistell

INTRODUCTION

Learning is often defined as a relatively permanent change in behavior that is the result of some experience. For example, a field mouse may only pause when it hears the rustling of an approaching cat. However, if the mouse survives the attack, it is likely that on hearing the rustling a second time, it will engage in species-specific behaviors such as fleeing for the safety of its nest. Learning in the wild can occur in any number of circumstances and may affect foraging, maternal behavior, reproduction, and social behavior. In each of these, learning has obvious functional value. To scientists, the fact that mice learn in a variety of circumstances provides the opportunity to examine the behavioral, neurobiological, and genetic correlates of various types of learning.

With the recent advances in mouse genetics, there has been a renewed interest in learning in mice. Learning paradigms previously only used in rats are now being adapted to mice (cf, Crawley, 2000). Consequently, the database on learning in mice is growing rapidly. Sounds are routinely used in many of these learning paradigms. However, despite all this, relatively few studies have considered the relationship between the mouse auditory system and learning. It is reasonable to expect that the characteristics of the mouse auditory system would impact learning about sounds in some way, and that any differences in the auditory systems between strains would contribute to differences in learning about sounds across these strains. The goal of this chapter is to briefly review data that examine Pavlovian conditioned fear in inbred strains of mice. These data suggest that attributes of the mouse auditory system can have an impact on fear conditioning, and that fear conditioning may provide an unexplored opportunity to investigate characteristics of the mouse auditory system.

PAVLOVIAN CONDITIONED FEAR PROCEDURES

Pavlovian conditioned fear procedures are routinely used to examine the behavioral and neurobiological basis of learning in rodents. In a typical Pavlovian conditioned fear procedure, a neutral conditioned stimulus (CS), such as a tone or experimental context, is paired with an aversive unconditioned stimulus (US), such as foot shock. As a result of just a few of these pairings, the CS comes to elicit a constellation of behavioral responses that are indicative of fear. These include freezing, potentiation of the acoustic startle response (fear-potentiated startle), hypoalgesia, bradycardia, and increased blood pressure. This type of learning is rapidly acquired, maintained over the life of the organism, and easily and objectively quantified.

Pavlovian conditioned fear is measured in our laboratory using the fear-potentiated startle procedure (Davis and Astrachan, 1978). In the fear-potentiated startle procedure, the acoustic startle reflex is elicited in the presence and absence of a CS that was previously paired with shock.

0-8493-2328-2/01/$0.00+$.50
© 2001 by CRC Press LLC

Conditioned fear is operationally defined as elevated startle amplitude in the presence vs. the absence of the CS. The fear-potentiated startle procedure has been used successfully to investigate the behavioral (Davis, Falls, Campeau, and Kim, 1993) and neurobiological basis of conditioned fear (Davis, 1992).

Prior to our work, fear-potentiated startle had not been examined in mice. However, studies had shown robust conditioned fear in mice as measured by freezing (e.g., Paylor, Tracy, Wehner, and Rudy, 1994). In rats, freezing and fear-potentiated startle are positively correlated (Leaton and Borscz, 1985), suggesting that it might be possible to measure fear-potentiated startle in mice as well.

EVALUATING FEAR-POTENTIATED STARTLE IN MICE

Our laboratory has begun a series of experiments designed to evaluate fear-potentiated startle in mice. In rats, fear-potentiated startle can be measured to both auditory and visual CSs (Campeau and Davis, 1992; Falls and Davis, 1994). Thus, in an initial experiment, separate groups of 1-month-old C57BL/6 mice were given training in which either a tone (12 kHz, 70dB) or a light CS was paired with foot shock (Heldt, Sundin, Willott, and Falls, 2000). Fear-potentiated startle was assessed prior to training and after 20, 40, and 60 CS + shock training trials. Separate groups were given explicitly unpaired CS and shock training to assess the nonassociative effects of the CS and shock presentations. With this method, we could not only determine if fear-potentiated startle could be measured in C57BL/6 mice, but we could also determine the number of training trials required to produce fear-potentiated startle. The results of this experiment are shown in Figure 7.1. For both the tone and the light CSs, paired, but not unpaired, CS + shock training produced robust fear-potentiated startle. However, fear-potentiated startle to the tone was evident after 20 training trials, whereas fear-potentiated startle to the light was evident only after 60 training trials. This later result was unexpected. In rats, fear-potentiated startle to auditory and visual CSs is comparable (Falls and Davis, 1994) and is typically asymptotic within 20 training trials (Kim and Davis, 1993). In the present experiment, fear-potentiated startle to the light, as measured both by an increase in potentiated startle over pre-training levels and by an increase over levels measured in an unpaired control, was not evident until after the 60 light + shock trials. Fear-potentiated startle to the tone was evident much earlier in training. Indeed, in a separate experiment, robust fear-potentiated startle was obtained in as few as 5 tone + shock training trials (Figure 7.2). Because all other variables were held constant in these experiments, it must be concluded that differences in the CSs had an impact on fear-potentiated startle. Confirming the observation that visual CSs produce poor fear-potentiated startle, McCaughran, Bell, and Hitzemann (2000) have recently shown that C57BL/6 mice show no fear-potentiated startle following 40 light + shock training trials. However, unlike our study, McCaughran et al. discontinued training at 40 training trials and did not evaluate fear-potentiated startle following training with an auditory CS.

It is well known that CS salience is positively correlated with rate of learning as well as its asymptotic level (Kamin, 1965). A CS that is of low salience will produce little or no learning, whereas a CS of high salience will produce more rapid and robust conditioning. A tone frequency above or below the hearing range of a particular mouse should not serve as an effective CS. Similarly, one might expect that the most sensitive frequencies in the mouse auditory system (perhaps those with the lowest threshold) might serve as the most effective CSs. In fact, the studies we have conducted thus far have used middle-frequency (12-kHz) tones because these frequencies are well represented in the mouse auditory system. It also reasonable to assume that alterations in the mouse auditory system brought on by injury, mutagenesis, or aging would produce changes in stimulus salience (either a loss or gain of function) that would consequently affect learning. In rats, damage to the inferior colliculus or medial geniculate nucleus results in a loss of fear-potentiated startle to auditory but not visual CSs (Campeau and Davis, 1995; Heldt and Falls, 1998), indicating the importance of these structures for processing the auditory CS (LeDoux, Iwata, Pearl, and Reis,

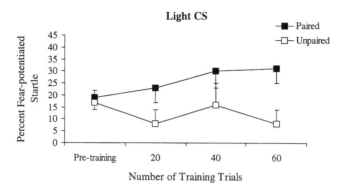

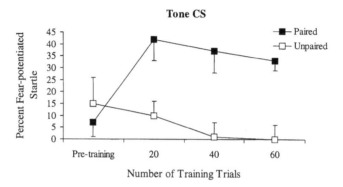

FIGURE 7.1   Fear-potentiated startle to visual and auditory conditioned stimuli in C57 mice. Mice were given training in which a 30-s light or tone (12 kHz, 70 dB) was paired with a 0.5-s, 0.6-mA foot shock. Mice were tested for fear-potentiated startle before (0) and after 20, 40, and 60 training trials. Mice in the unpaired groups were given the same number of training trials except that the conditioned stimulus and shock were explicitly unpaired. Conditioned fear is acquired to both the light and the tone. However, conditioned fear to the tone is acquired in fewer training trials.

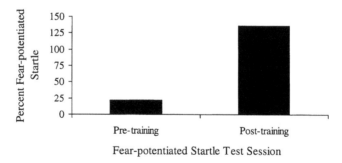

FIGURE 7.2   Fear-potentiated startle to an auditory conditioned stimulus following five tone + shock training trials. C57BL/6 mice were given five tone + shock training trials, consisting of a 30-s, 12-kHz, 70-dB tone and a 0.5-s, 0.6-mA foot shock. Twenty-four hours later, they were tested for fear-potentiated startle. Conditioned fear to the tone is acquired in as few as five training trials.

1986; LeDoux, Sakaguchi, Iwata, and Reis, 1985; LeDoux, Sakaguchi, and Reis, 1983). C57BL/6 mice possess a gene that results in high-frequency hearing loss (Erway, Willott, Archer, and Harrison, 1993a) between 1 and 6 months of age that is accompanied by enhanced neural responses to middle-frequency tones (i.e., 12 to 16 kHz) (Willott, 1984; and Chapter 24). The enhanced neural

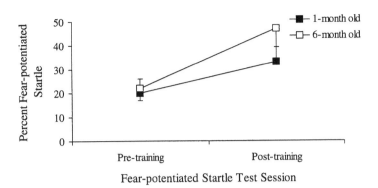

FIGURE 7.3   Fear-potentiated startle to a visual conditioned stimulus in 1-month-old and 6-month-old C57BL/6 mice. Mice were given 60 tone + shock training trials, consisting of a 30-s, light and a 0.5-s, 0.6-mA foot shock. Twenty-four hours later, they were tested for fear-potentiated startle. Six-month-old and 1-month-old mice show similar amounts of fear-potentiated startle.

responses are associated with increased behavioral salience of these tones as measured by prepulse inhibition of acoustic startle (Carlson and Willott, 1996; Willott, Carlson, and Chen, 1994b; and Chapters 5 and 14). When 1-month-old and 6-month-old C57BL/6 mice were compared on fear-potentiated startle following training to a 12-kHz tone, the 6-month-old C57BL/6 mice showed *more robust* fear-potentiated startle (Willott, Carlson, Falls, Turner, and Webster, 1996). This result is not likely due to age-related differences in learning because 6-month-old and 1-month-old C57BL/6 mice showed comparable fear-potentiated startle to visual CS (Figure 7.3; Heldt et al., 2000). These results once again indicate the importance of auditory structures in processing the CS and suggest that gain of function in the auditory system may result in a gain of function in learning.

Strain-related differences in the auditory system may also have an impact on learning. We compared fear-potentiated startle in 1-month-old C57BL/6 and DBA/2 mice following training with a 12-kHz, 70-dB tone (Falls, Carlson, Turner, and Willott, 1997). Like C57BL/6 mice, DBA/2 mice undergo high-frequency hearing loss that is accompanied by enhanced neural responses to middle-frequency tones (Willott, Kulig, and Satterfield, 1984). However, the hearing loss in DBA/2 mice occurs much earlier and is significant at 1 month of age. Following 20 tone + shock training trials, DBA/2 mice showed much greater fear-potentiated startle to the tone than the like-aged C57BL/6 mice (Figure 7.4). These strains are known to differ on a number of neurobiological variables in

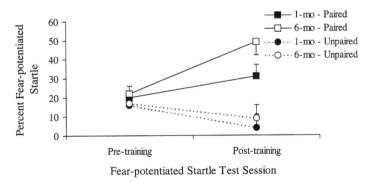

FIGURE 7.4   Fear-potentiated startle to an auditory conditioned stimulus in C57BL/6 and DBA/2 mice. Mice of both strains were given 20 tone + shock training trials consisting of a 30-s, 12-kHz, 70-dB tone and a 0.5-s, 0.6-mA foot shock. Twenty-four hours later, they were tested for fear-potentiated startle. DBA/2 mice show greater fear-potentiated startle than C57BL/6 mice.

addition to hearing loss, and have been shown to differ in other learning tasks (McCaughran et al., 2000; Paylor, Baskall, and Wehner, 1993; Paylor, Baskall-Balindi, Yuva, and Wehner, 1996; Paylor et al., 1994). Although we do not know whether greater fear-potentiated startle in DBA/2 mice can be directly attributed to a gain of function in the auditory system, these data are consistent with data indicating increased behavioral salience of middle-frequency tones in DBA/2 mice (Willott et al., 1994b).

CONCLUSION

Learning about stimuli inevitably requires the ability to process the CS. Individual or strain differences in the ability to process these stimuli will affect learning. Thus, scientists interested in studying learning should consider stimulus salience and, when auditory stimuli are to be used, the characteristics of the auditory system of the mouse under investigation. Likewise, scientists interested in studying the auditory system should consider investigating learning because it will lead to new insights into the functional significance of the auditory system.

ACKNOWLEDGMENTS

The fear-potentiated startle data shown here were collected in collaboration with James Willott in the Department of Psychology, Northern Illinois University, DeKalb.

Section II

Peripheral Auditory System

This section covers the route linking the acoustic environment to the brain — the peripheral auditory system. We begin, in Chapter 8, with a detailed description of the outer ear and middle ear (Saunders and Crumling) and end, in Chapter 16, at the interface between peripheral and central portions of the auditory system, the terminals of auditory nerve fibers (Limb and Ryugo). Much of this section focuses on development, maintenance, and degeneration of the cochlea — very important topics of research, for which mouse models are well-suited. One of the ways mouse tissue can be used to advantage in studies of development is in tissue culture, as is quite evident from the elegant work of Dr. Hanna Sobkowicz and colleagues (Chapter 9). The varied, state-of-the-art approaches to developmental auditory research are reviewed by Kelley and Bianchi (Chapter 10), while Chapter 11 (Staecker, Apfel, and Van De Water) addresses the exciting area of neurotrophins.

Research on the cochlea always has, and always must, rest on a sound foundation of histological and histopathological techniques. Chapter 12 (Bohne, Harding, and Ou) and Chapter 13 (Ding, McFadden, and Salvi) describe the modern methodological approaches, as well as exciting empirical findings derived from these methods. The material presented in these chapters makes it quite clear that a wealth of sophisticated information is being obtained from histological preparations of the cochleae of mouse models.

Progressive sensorineural cochlear degeneration is exhibited by a number of mouse strains and mutants, and having such models is one of the strengths of mouse auditory research. Thus, mice can provide an avenue to conduct research on possible ways to ameliorate such conditions. Chapter 14 (Willott, Sundin, and Jeskey) updates research showing that exposure to an augmented acoustic environment (AAE) provides one way of altering the course of progressive hearing loss.

The small size of mice imposes one of the most vexing limitations of mice as subjects for *in vivo* techniques used to study the cochlea. Measuring cochlear blood flow is an example. There are ways to measure blood flow in the mouse cochlea, however, and this challenging methodology is reviewed in Chapter 15 (Nuttall).

8 The Outer and Middle Ear

James C. Saunders and Mark A. Crumling

INTRODUCTION

The outer and middle ear of all vertebrates serve as a "sensory accessory structure" designed to focus and funnel vibratory energy from the external environment to the fluid-filled chambers of the inner ear. In the process, the efficiency of sound energy transfer from air (in the case of terrestrial animals) to the inner ear is improved. This improvement occurs through interactions between the sound field and the head, body, pinna, and ear canal (external meatus) of the outer ear, and the conducting aparatus of the middle ear (McDonogh, 1986; Chen et al., 1995).

The outer ear varies remarkably across vertebrate species. The lower vertebrates have no pinna and a small ear canal, which in some reptiles and amphibians places the tympanic membrane at the surface of the head (Saunders et al., 2000). The mammalian pinna exhibits great diversity across species, but in all cases serves as a sound-collecting device with directional selectivity (Geisler, 1998). In some species, the pinna is very mobile (e.g., bats and cats) and can actually be used to scan the acoustic field without the need for gross movements of the head.

Organization of the middle-ear system is no less diverse, extending from the single-bone ossicle found in amphibians, reptiles, and birds (Saunders et al., 2000), to the three-bone ossicular system of mammals. A three-bone conductive system is, indeed, one of the defining characteristics of the mammalian class (see Gates et al., 1974; Fleischer, 1978; Chen et al., 1995). Even in mammals, however, there are interesting specializations with two broad categories identified. These categories are the so-called "microtype" and "freely mobile" ossicular systems (Fleischer, 1978). The former is found throughout the Order Rodentia, while the latter is characteristic of other mammalian orders.

This chapter assembles information on the structure and function of the outer and middle ear of the mouse. The presentation is largely descriptive because there are ample presentations elsewhere dealing with the analytic aspects of middle-ear function (Møller, 1974; Relkin, 1988; Rosowski, 1994; 1996). Throughout this chapter, we operate under the assumption that the outer and middle ears of all mouse strains are similar. We proceed by describing the structure and function of the outer and middle ears and follow this by a consideration of the developing and aging mouse middle-ear system.

THE OUTER EAR

ANATOMY

The mouse pinna, as far as we can tell, has no obvious morphological differences across laboratory mouse strains. It is rigid in structure, mobile to a relatively small extent, and well-lateralized on the skull (Chen et al., 1995). The inner surface of the concha is fairly smooth, lacking the complex surface folds seen in other mammals. The tragus in mouse is a small protrusion in the pinna situated adjacent of the entrance to the external auditory meatus (ear canal). The pinna also exhibits a well-defined reflex twitch (the Preyer reflex) to stimulus onset, and this has been used to screen for hearing (e.g., see Phippard et al., 1999).

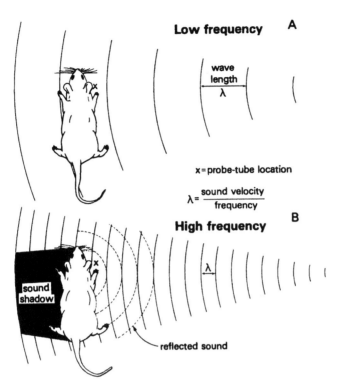

FIGURE 8.1   The interaction is seen between the mouse body and incident sound from a source at 90° for low (A) and high (B) frequencies. The head shadow produced by high frequencies is illustrated in B. (From Willott, J.F. (Ed.), 1983, *Auditory Psychobiology of the Mouse*, 131–168, Charles C. Thomas Publishers. With permission.)

The width of the skull and separation of the tympanic membranes (TM) are among the smallest in mammals, superceded only by some of the smallest bat species. The C57BL/6J mouse pup at birth has a skull width averaging only 8.6 mm. These small dimensions impose an interesting constraint on the processing of localization cues in this species. An inter-tympanic distance this small means that the interaural time difference, when a sound source is positioned at 90° (0° is directly in front of the head) is at most 25 μsec, given that sound propagation in air is approximately 344 m/s.

Similarly, sound diffraction or reflection off the head, essential for creating intensity difference cues at the two ears, is complicated in the mouse because the head is not extended from the body. The head, neck, and body represent a single obstacle to the sound wavefront. Consequently, the frequencies at which a "head shadow" develops are difficult to specify. However, given an approximate head length of 21.8 mm, the frequency with a wavelength equivalent to that size would be 15.7 kHz. The larger size of the overall body means that lower frequencies will also produce reflectance. Thus, the sound shadowing effect may extend to frequencies as low as 4.0 kHz.

Figures 8.1A and B illustrate the effect of sounds impinging upon the mouse body at low and high frequencies. If the wavelength is large relative to the head and body, (i.e., below 2 kHz), then the sound will diffract about these objects. Consequently, the SPL at the ipsilateral and contralateral meatal openings are the same. As frequency increases, the wavelength shortens (B) and sound begins to reflect off the incident surface. The interaction between incident and reflected sound can produce nodes and anti-nodes of pressure on the ipsilateral side of the head. Above 7 kHz, there is a net increase in pressure that varies with frequency, but averages about 5.5 dB (Saunders and Garfinkle, 1983). Figure 8.2A shows the consequences of sound acting on the mouse body at the contralateral ear. The SPL at the opening of the ipsi- and contralateral ear were compared for sound

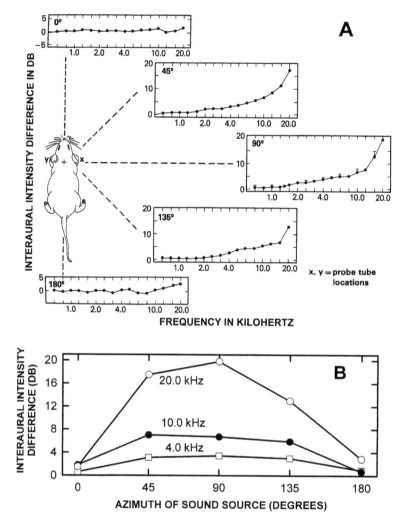

FIGURE 8.2 (A) The interaural intensity difference for sound sources at five different locations on the horizontal azimuth. (B) The intensity difference at three selected frequencies. Higher frequencies with sound sources at right angles to the body axis (90°) produce the largest interaural intensity differences. (From Willott, J.F. (Ed.), 1983, *Auditory Psychobiology of the Mouse,* 131–168, Charles C. Thomas Publishers. With permission.)

sources placed at 0°, 45°, 90°, 135°, and 180° in the right auditory field. As can be seen, SPL at the two ears is approximately the same when the sound sources are located at 0° and 180°. Similarly, for low-frequency sounds at 90°, the SPL at both ears is approximately the same. With rising frequency, the interaural intensity difference increases with a 20-kHz sound at 90° exhibiting an intensity difference as large as 19 dB. Figure 8.2B summarizes the frequency and location relationship, showing small interaural differences at 90° and 4 kHz that increase dramatically into the higher frequencies (Saunders and Garfinkle, 1983).

The ear canal length in a sample of adult C57BL/6J mice was 6.25 mm, and this was similar to that measured in several adult CBA mice (Saunders and Garfinkle, 1983). The concha exhibits the shape of an exponential horn, from its most lateral extent at the opening of the pinna, toward the tympanic membrane (TM). The shape of the adult ear canal in front of the TM is approximately oval, being 3.3 mm long and 2.0 mm wide. The canal is not straight, but exhibits a slight rostral curve. It is possible to observe the anterior portion of the TM by looking down the canal from the pinna. An otoscope with a 1.5-mm speculum can be "shimmied" into the canal so that most of the

TABLE 8.1
Dimensions of the External and Middle Ear

Measure	Sample Size	Average (mm)	S.D.[a] (±mm)
Inter-tympanic distance	4	8.6	1.0
Tip of snout to back of head	5	21.8	0.72
Ear canal length; tragus of TM[b]	10	6.25[c]	0.88
TM area			
Pars tympani	5	2.75[d]	0.08
Pars flaccida	4	1.23	0.06
Stapes footplate area	4	0.093[e]	0.01
Lever arm of the malleus	5	0.85	0.04
Lever arm of the incus	5	0.45	0.04

Note: All data obtained on C57BL/6J mice 100 days or older.

[a] S.D. refers to the standard deviation.
[b] The resonant frequency based on the ¼ wavelength hypothesis is 14.0 kHz.
[c] Ehret (unpublished) found lengths of 0.36 to 0.42 cm measured from the entrance of the ear canal to the middle of the tympanic membrane (NMRI mice).
[d] Ehret (unpublished) found the area of the entire tympanic membrane to be 3.73 mm^2 (NMRI mice).
[e] Ehret (unpublished) found a mean area of 0.136 mm^2 in NMRI mice.

Modified from Saunders and Garfinkle, 1983.

TM surface can be observed. The canal consists of a soft-tissue (cartilaginous) portion laterally, and a rigid walled (bony) portion medially. The TM sits in a bony cup, the so-called "terminal zone" (DiMaio and Tonndorf, 1978), which may serve to protect the TM. Table 8.1 shows the dimensions of various outer-ear morphological parameters in adult C57BL/6J mice.

FUNCTION

Like all mammals, the epithelium of the external meatus secretes cerumen, or "ear wax." The exact role of this material is not clear, but may serve to capture debris in the canal. Ear wax is a mixture of dead epidermal cells and secretions from sebaceous and ceruminous glands lining the canal wall. Hairs in the canal wall appear to prevent foreign objects from entering the canal, but may also retard cerumen removal from the canal. Even so, the epithelial tissue layer appears to migrate out of the meatus, and this may act as a "conveyor belt," transporting cerumen out of the canal and maintaining its patency (Johnson and Hawke, 1988; Michaels and Soucek, 1991; Kakoi and Anniko, 1996). We have not observed mice with ear canals impacted with cerumen. The absence of blocked ear canals may mean that mice do not secrete a great deal of cerumen or that they have an efficient transport system.

The external meatus has unique acoustic properties. The diameter of the ear canal, its length, and the compliance of the canal walls constitute factors that determine canal acoustics and contribute to the phenomenon of resonance in the canal. The resonance of the canal serves as a passive amplifier, increasing the SPL measured at the TM over that measured at the opening of the meatus. The resonant frequency and gain in SPL at the TM are determined by the factors noted above. As a general rule-of-thumb, the longer the canal, the lower the resonant frequency and the more compliant the canal walls, the lower the gain at resonance (a softer wall absorbs sound energy).

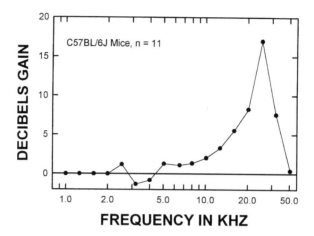

FIGURE 8.3   The gain of sound pressure at the tympanic membrane over that measured at the opening of the external meatus is depicted. The resonant peak occurs at 25 kHz. (From Willott, J.F. (Ed.), 1983, *Auditory Psychobiology of the Mouse*, 131–168, Charles C. Thomas Publishers. With permission.)

The gain of the external meatus is shown for C57BL/6J mice in Figure 8.3 (Saunders and Garfinkle, 1983). These data were obtained in cadaver preparations by placing a probe microphone at the opening to the canal and another immediately in front of the tympanic membrane. The difference between the SPLs detected at the two microphones (meatus microphone response minus the TM microphone response), across frequency, describes how sound is transferred through the ear canal to the surface of the TM. A resonant peak of 17 dB occurs at approximately 25 kHz. The ear canal from tragus to TM is 6.25 mm in this strain (Table 8.1), and the quarter wavelength equation (used with closed-end pipes) would theoretically predict a resonance at 14 kHz. The exponential horn-like curvature of the concha as it blends into the ear canal makes it difficult to specify exactly the beginning of the canal and hence its length. The meatus may be functionally shorter than our anatomical estimate. If this were the case, the predicted and measured resonance would be nearly identical.

THE MIDDLE EAR

ANATOMY

Most rodent species exhibit middle-ear structures with microtype organization (Fleischer, 1978). This design is one of two radically different lines of middle-ear evolution adapted from the ancestral form (Greybeal et al., 1989; Rosowski and Greybeal, 1991; Rosowski, 1992). The other, called the "freely mobile" type, is distinguished by the fact that the ossicles are completely suspended by ligaments in the middle-ear cavity (Fleischer, 1978). The human conductive apparatus (e.g., the TM, ossciles, suspensory ligaments, and middle-ear muscles) is an example of the freely mobile type. Key features of the microtype design are the *orbicular apophysis* and the *gonial* (Cockerell et al., 1914). The orbicular apophysis is an approximate spheroid bony mass found at the head of the malleus. This structure serves to shift the center of mass of the malleus-incus complex to a more lateral location on the malleus. The gonial is a bony fusion between the transverse process of the malleus and the tympanic ring. By firmly attaching the malleus to the bony structure of the skull, the stiffness of the ossicular system is significantly increased which, in turn, improves the high-frequency response of the middle ear (Fleisher, 1978).

The conductive apparatus is located in a bony cavity, the bulla. The bulla is an extension of the temporal bone and forms a shell around the conductive apparatus. A circular opening on the lateral wall forms the tympanic ring and supports the tympanic membrane. The organization of the mouse conductive apparatus appears in the three panels of Figure 8.4. Figure 8.4A presents a

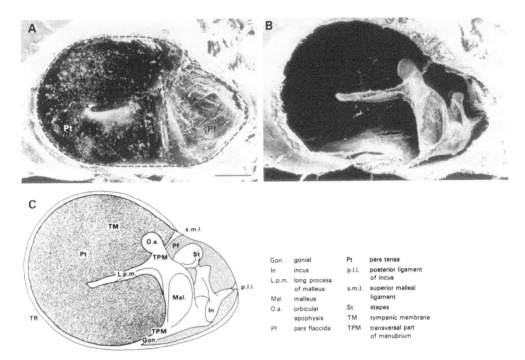

FIGURE 8.4   The tympanic membrane (A), middle ear ossicles (B) and a line drawing of the ossicular system (C) in the C57BL/6J mouse, as seen from the ear canal. (Modified from Saunders, J.C. and Garfinkle, T., 1983, Peripheral Physiology II. In J.F. Willott (Ed.), *Auditory Psychobiology of the Mouse,* 131–168, Charles C. Thomas Publishers.)

scanning electron micrograph (SEM) of the outer surface of the tympanic membrane (TM). The total surface area of the 45-day-old C57BL/6J mouse is 2.67 mm^2 (Huangfu and Saunders, 1983). The TM can be divided into two sections, and the larger of the two on the left is called the *pars tensa*. This region of the TM gains its name because of an inward pull exerted on the malleus by the tensor tympani muscle. When viewed from the side, pars tensa has a concave shape, and appears to be somewhat stretched and under tension. Yet, if the tensor tympani is cut, the TM does not suddenly spring to a flat shape. Rather, it becomes flaccid, but retains its cone-like shape. Pars tensa articulates with the long process of the malleus along its entire length (seen running down the center of pars tensa). The long process of the malleus is also known as the manubrium, and the end-point or the tip is referred to as the umbo. This tip is the deepest point on the concave surface of the TM. The organization of pars tensa has been described in detail (Lim, 1968a; 1970) and consists of three layers. The outer or epidermal layer is continuous with the epidermis of the external meatus. The inner layer is continuous with the respiratory epithelium lining the inner surfaces of the middle-ear cavity. The respiratory epithelium consists of ciliated cells, secretory cells, and supporting cells. The secretory cells produce mucus that forms the mucoid layer sitting on top of the epithelium. The ciliated cells transport this mucus down the eustachian tube, where it is eventually deposited in the nasopharynx (Bernstein, 1988). The middle layer of the TM, the *lamina propria*, contains a rich vascular supply of microcapillaries, free nerve endings associated with the trigeminal pain system, and collagen fibers arrayed in a circular or radial pattern (Shimada and Lim, 1971). Each of these parts of lamina propria are well-segmented within the middle layer.

The second portion of the TM is called the *pars flaccida*. It is continuous with the pars tensa but about half as large (1.26 mm^2 in 45-day old C57BL/6J; Huangfu and Saunders, 1983). The vertical dashed line in Figure 8.4A indicates the division between pars tensa and pars flaccida (to the right). Pars flaccida has a common structural organization across mammals and has been

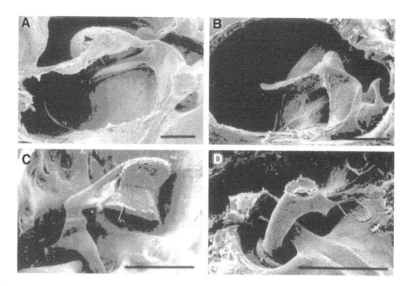

FIGURE 8.5 The four panels present various views of the ossicles in the C57 middle ear. (A) The malleus is viewed from the medial side, and the muscle mass of the tensor tympani muscle can be seen with its tendon attached to the malleus. (B) The ossicles are viewed from lateral side. (C) The spatial joint between the incus and stapes is seen, as is the surface of the incus joint with the malleus. (D) The crura of the stapes with the stapedial artery coursing through is visualized. The tendon of the stapedius muscle lies just below the head of the stapes and projects to the right. (Modified from Willott, J.F. (Ed.), 1983, *Auditory Psychobiology of the Mouse,* 131–168, Charles C. Thomas Publishers.).

described in detail elsewhere (Lim, 1968b). It is readily recognized by its limp and tension-free appearance. The epithelial and respiratory layers are the same as described above. The middle layer, however, is largely devoid of collagen but rich in elastin. Evidence in the rat suggests that pars flaccida may act to release sudden pressure changes in the middle-ear cavity by bulging out or retracting inward (Stenfors et al., 1979). This would serve to prevent damage to the ossicular chain. It has also been suggested that the size of pars flaccida varies inversely with middle-ear cavity volume (Vrettakos et al., 1988).

Figure 8.4B illustrates the underlying appearance of the ossicles after the TM is removed. The ossicles are further identified in the line drawing of Figure 8.4C. The orbicular apophysis and the bony fusion between the malleus and the tympanic ring at the gonial characterize the malleus. The ossicular bones are supported at three points: the gonial and two ligaments, the posterior ligament of the incus, and the superior malleal ligament. The joint between the malleus and incus is firmly bonded, and is fused by a cartilaginous synchondrosis that allows the two ossicles to move as a single unit. The joint between the incus and stapes is a true diarthrosis and connects the bones at approximately right angles to each other. Applying steady but gently increasing force against the joint can disarticulate these bones.

Figure 8.5 shows a series of SEM micrographs of the ossicular bones (Huangfu and Saunders, 1983; Saunders and Garfinkle, 1983). Figure 8.5A presents the malleus as seen from the medial wall of the middle-ear cavity. The large mass attached to the underside of the transverse process of the malleus (TPM), adjacent to the apophysis, is the body of the tensor tympani muscle. The medial lateral wall of the temporal bone normally encapsulates this muscle. Figure 8.5B shows the ossicles viewed from a different angle, while Figure 8.5C shows the surface of the incus where it would normally articulate with the malleus. To the left in this panel can be seen the incudo-stapedial junction. Figure 8.5D illustrates the stapes and the stapedial artery coursing between the crura of the stapes. *In vivo,* this vessel is not in contact with the stapes. The tendon of the stapedial muscle is seen articulating with the crura just below the head of the stapes on the right-hand side.

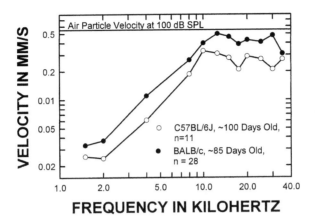

FIGURE 8.6   Tympanic membrane velocity functions for a constant input of 100 dB SPL for a group of C57BL/6J and BALB/c mice (data from Saunders and Summers, 1982; Doan et al., 1996).

FUNCTION

The transfer function of the middle ear at the tympanic membrane has been measured in C57BL/6J and BALB/c mice using capacitive probe and laser interferometry technologies. These procedures are detailed elsewhere (Saunders et al., 1993; 2000). A transfer function is measured by applying a constant stimulus to the input of a system while the magnitude and phase at the output of the system are measured. This is accomplished across a range of frequencies, and the output signal reflects the contributions of all the system elements lying between the input and output. In practice, a constant SPL across frequency, at the surface of the TM, provides a constant-velocity stimulus. If the velocity response of the system is measured, then the requirements for obtaining a transfer function are met. The open circles in Figure 8.6 show the TM velocity response averaged for 11 C57BL/6J mice as measured by a capacitive probe (Saunders and Summers, 1982; Saunders and Garfinkle, 1983). Plotted with these data are the TM velocity transfer functions obtained from 28 BALB/c mice using laser interferometry (Doan et al., 1994; 1996). Both sets of data were obtained from the tip of the manubrium. The data show that velocity of the tympanic membrane increases from about 0.022 to 0.36 mm/s between 2.0 and 12 kHz, a rate of about 8.2 dB/octave, and then declines slightly into the high frequencies. Using laser interferometry, we have seen the middle-ear response of BALB/c decline precipitously between 35 and 45 kHz (Doan et al., 1994; 1996). The velocity functions in Figure 8.6 are interpreted to indicate that the low-frequency response is dominated by the stiffness of the middle-ear system. This stiffness is most likely related to the relative incompressibility of air in the small bulla cavity of the mouse. The peak of the function around 10 to 14 kHz represents the resonant frequency of the middle ear, while the shallow decline in the high frequencies is caused by the mass of the system. The sudden decline in the BALB/c response above 40 kHz indicates the point where the conductive apparatus begins to fail. Threshold sensitivity above 40 kHz also deteriorates and becomes erratic (Ou et al., 2000).

The difference in sensitivity between the two strains could be the result of the measurement technique. The sensing head of the capacitive probe integrates mechanical activity on the TM surface over an area about 25 times larger than that detected by the focused interferometer beam (Doan et al., 1994). Moreover, the calibration methods are very different with both techniques (Doan et al., 1994). While the curves differ by approximately 6 to 8 dB across frequency, the overall shape of the TM transfer function is, nevertheless, quite similar in both strains.

Figure 8.7 illustrates the relationship between TM displacement and stimulus intensity for three different frequencies in C57BL/6J mice (Saunders and Summers, 1982). The linearity of the tympanic membrane response for stimulus levels as high as 125 and 130 dB SPL is the most

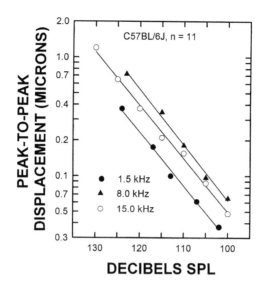

FIGURE 8.7 The displacement of the TM is plotted against stimulus SPL at three frequencies in C57BL/6J mice. The response at lower sound levels would continue to exhibit linear behavior. (Data from Saunders and Summers, 1982.)

important observation from this figure. This is a characteristic of vertebrate middle-ear systems and supports the notion that distortion in the auditory periphery is not a product of the middle ear (Relkin, 1988).

Fleischer (1978) developed an enlarged mechanical model of the microtype middle ear. From the movements of the model, it was hypothesized that the ossicles exhibit two axes of rotation, with one occurring at low frequencies and the other at high frequencies. The first axes extends through the center of the gonial, the malleo-incudo joint, the body of the incus, and the center of the posterior ligament of the incus (line AB in Figure 8.8). A second axis of rotation, perpendicular to the first, extends through the orbicular apophysis and along the transverse process of the malleus (TPM) (line CD in Figure 8.8). It is possible to test the idea of a low- and high-frequency axis of rotation. This is accomplished by measuring the tympanic membrane velocity response at the tip of the

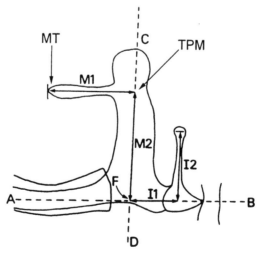

FIGURE 8.8 The lever arms (M1/I1; M2/I2) and axis of rotation (AB and CD) for the microtype middle ear are identified. (Modified from Saunders and Summers, 1982.)

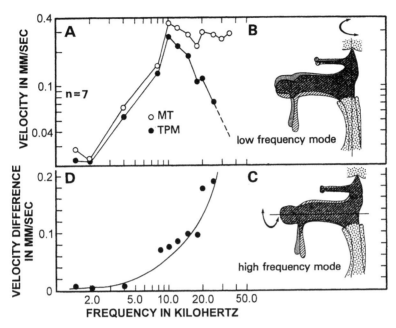

FIGURE 8.9   The transfer functions recorded from the tip of the manubrium (MT) and the transverse process of the malleus (TPM) appear in A. Panel D shows the velocity difference between MT and TPM, while panels B and C show the axis of rotation. (From Saunders and Summers, 1982. With permission.)

manubrium (MT in Figure 8.8) and at the transverse process of the malleus (TPM in Figure 8.8). If the axis of rotation is about AB at all frequencies, then the transfer function at positions MT and TPM will be the same. If the axis of rotation shifts from axis AB to CD with increasing frequency, then the transfer function (in high frequencies) should show a significant change when measured at position TPM compared to that observed at location MT. The measured velocity would be minimal at position TPM if rotation occurred about line CD. This is, indeed, what happens (Figure 8.9). As can be seen in Figure 8.9A, above 10 kHz, the response of the TPM deteriorates sharply into the high frequencies. At ~20 kHz, the response is 14 dB below that seen at MT at 20 kHz. The difference between the two curves (in mm/s) is plotted in Figure 8.9D, and increases steeply above 10 kHz (Saunders and Summers, 1982).

The data in Figure 8.6 illustrate the middle-ear response measured at the TM, but what is more important to know is the input to the cochlea. This could be accomplished by describing the transfer function at the stapes footplate. Unfortunately, it is difficult to gain access to the head of the stapes or its footplate without modifying the integrity of the middle-ear system. The lever ratio for the presumed two axes of movement in the ossicles was calculated to be approximately 1.9 (Table 8.1). If the joints between the ossicles are, indeed, fused to one another, and if the ossicles are rigid enough to resist bending, then there will be little difference in the shape of the transfer function between the TM and the stapes. However, the stapes velocity will be reduced by the lever advantage of the ossicular system. Consequently, if the transfer function at the TM is divided by the lever ratio, a very close approximation of the stapes response can be estimated (Saunders and Johnstone, 1972; Saunders et al., 1993; Saunders et al., 2000). This relationship can be tested directly. A comparison between the TPM and the tip of the long arm of the incus was made, and the results appear in Figure 8.10. The tip of the incus was exposed by removing the pars flaccida of the tympanic membrane. The transfer function at the incus is thought to reflect the response of the stapes footplate. The long arm of the incus appears to follow the TPM response, but at a reduced amplitude. The velocity of the TPM was 2.09 times greater than that of the incus when averaged

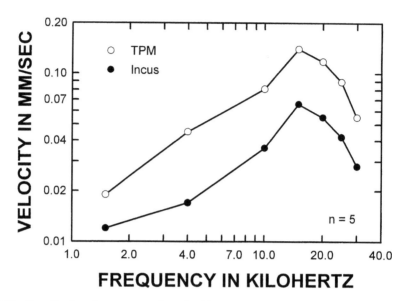

FIGURE 8.10   Transfer functions measured at the TPM and tip of the incus long arm. (Modified from Saunders and Summers, 1982.)

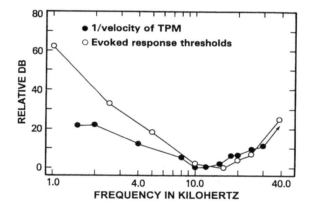

FIGURE 8.11   A comparison of the shape of the evoked response threshold curve and the inverse of the velocity transfer function is made for C57BL/6J mice. (Modified from Willott, J.F. (Ed.), *Auditory Psychobiology of the Mouse,* 131–168, 1983.)

across frequencies. This was remarkably close to the lever ratio (1.9:1) predicted from the anatomical arrangement of the middle ear in Table 8.1.

The shape of the evoked response audiogram is plotted against the inverse velocity function of the TM normalized to a common frequency (Figure 8.11). Such a relationship is justified because of the linearity of the middle-ear response (Figure 8.7). The linearity indicates that the shape of the transfer function, obtained at 100 dB SPL, can be extrapolated to that at threshold SPL levels. The two functions were normalized at 12.0 kHz, and the relative change in dB was plotted against the reference for both (Saunders and Summers, 1982).

Figure 8.11 shows that the shape of the threshold curve, measured in this case from cochlear nucleus evoked activity (Saunders et al., 1980), and the inverse velocity curve are nearly the same for frequencies between 8 and 30 kHz. Below 8 kHz, the threshold curve shows a faster decline in sensitivity than the TM velocity response. It has been suggested that the fluid pressure developed by low-frequency movements of the stapes is less effective in stimulating the cochlear partition because it is shunted through the helicotrema at the cochlear apex (Dallos, 1973). The consequence of this is that low-frequency thresholds are less sensitive than that predicted from the middle-ear velocity response. Theoretical corrections to the middle-ear response, after compensating for the shunting effect at the cochlea apex, would increase the low-frequency slope of the velocity function by about 6 dB/octave and more closely align the middle-ear response with the threshold estimate (Dallos, 1973; Saunders and Summer, 1982). The relationship between audiograms and the middle-ear transfer functions is important, and has been demonstrated in chicks, lizards, rats, guinea pigs, gerbils, and hamsters (Khanna and Sherrick, 1981; Khanna and Tonndorf, 1977; Relkin and Saunders, 1980; Saunders et al., 1993; 2000). This relationship tells us that the shape of the middle-ear transfer function determines the shape of the hearing curve, independent of any transduction processes occurring within the cochlea.

MIDDLE-EAR DEVELOPMENT

The developmental anatomy of the mouse middle ear has been examined in some detail, and targeted mutagenesis is beginning to identify the genes important to craniofacial development (Huangfu and Saunders, 1983; Saunders and Garfinkle, 1983; Saunders et al., 1983; Park et al., 1992; Saunders et al., 1993; Doan et al., 1994; Mallo and Gridley, 1996). Recent pharmacological manipulations of the developing middle ear have mapped out the morphological induction process of the outer and middle ear structures. The *Hoxa-2* and *goossecoid* genes may play a role in tympanic ring, external meatus, and malleus formation (Mallo and Gridley, 1996; Mallo, 1997; Zhu et al., 1997).

The functional development of the conductive apparatus in a variety of laboratory animal species has been investigated. The motivation behind this effort is to understand more fully the contribution of the middle-ear system to hearing maturation (Saunders et al., 1993). The onset and development of hearing relates importantly to the ontogeny of hair-cell transduction and the maturation of the auditory central nervous system. Nevertheless, the importance of the middle ear in this process cannot be discounted. The processing of signals in the peripheral ear consists largely of serial events. Sound must be conducted through the middle ear, activate the cochlear partition, stimulate hair cells, and activate the auditory nerve — in that order. The middle ear, as the "front end" of this system, may set limits on the rate of auditory development arising at more central levels. For example, regardless of how mature the hair cell and its synapse are, they would be functionally silent if the middle ear were too immature to conduct vibrational energy into the cochlea. Comparisons of the rate of middle-ear maturation with development of more centrally measured indices of auditory sensitivity test whether or not these processes proceed together.

Table 8.2 displays developmental changes in many middle-ear components. Figure 8.12A shows the changes in pars tensa and pars flaccida with increasing age in C57BL/6J mice. The TM undergoes a 292% change in total surface area reaching an adult-like size between 15 and 20 days of age (Huangfu and Saunders, 1983). The changes in the lever arm of the malleus and incus (for axis CD in Figure 8.8) are plotted as a function of age in Figure 8.12B. These lever arms reach a mature size around 10 days of age. The lever ratio appears in Figure 8.12C and shows relatively little change with age. It would appear that the lever arms are growing at about the same rate during the first 45 days of life. Finally, bulla cavity expansion is plotted in Figure 8.12D and reaches an adult-like volume by 20 days of age. Table 8.2 summarizes the time during development at which these different aspects of the middle-ear system reach 90% of their adult level (Huangfu and Saunders, 1983).

Figure 8.13 indicates the development of the TM transfer function in the BALB/c mouse from day 10 to day 45 (Saunders et al., 1993; Doan et al., 1994). The function shows an increase in the velocity of the TM response across frequency that becomes asymptotic by about days 17–18. The slope of the low-frequency portion of the curve increases with age, while the declining slope on the high-frequency side remains rather constant during development. With increasing age, the transfer function appears to have a wider bandwidth, and by 45 days of age, the velocity response

---

TABLE 8.2
Summary of Developmental Time
to Achieve 90% of Adult Value

Structure	Age (days)
Oval window area	6
Lever arm length	11.5
Area ratio	17.5
Pars tensa area	18.5
Bulla volume	19
Pars tensa concavity	10[a]
Fluid-free bulla	10[a]
Ossification of bulla	15[a]
Electrophysiological responses	
Cochlear nucleus-evoked responses	19.5[b]
Whole nerve AP (N_1)	17.5[c]

[a] Qualitative estimate.
[b] Measured for cochlear nucleus response at 20 kHz (Saunders et al., 1980).
[c] Measured for N_1 response from round window (Shnerson and Pujol, 1982).

Modified from Huangfu and Saunders, 1982.

---

is relatively constant between 10 and 25 kHz at around 0.17 mm/s. At younger ages, the response appears to peak around 20 kHz. There are slight improvements in the transfer function at 85 days of age (Doan et al., 1996). Figure 8.14 relates the developmental improvement in umbo velocity, at 16 and 20 kHz (Saunders and Summers, 1982; Doan et al., 1994), to the development of evoked response threshold sensitivity at the same frequencies (Saunders et al., 1993). Plotting velocity and threshold data as a percent change relative to the largest response normalizes the two sets of data. It is apparent that the developmental improvements in evoked response thresholds and umbo velocity are following the same time course. These results indicate that the rate of middle-ear development is controlling the rate of evoked activity threshold development. Because there is no lag between these two measures, it further indicates that the rate of functional maturation in the cochlea probably is earlier than the middle ear (Saunders et al., 1993).

THE AGING MOUSE MIDDLE EAR

Figure 8.15 illustrates histologic segments of the BALB/c mouse tympanic membrane. These segments were all harvested from the same location in front of the tip of the manubrium. The segments on the left come from different TMs in 85-day-old mice, while the samples on the right were harvested from mice about 2 years old. The magnification of the video micrographs in both sets was the same. It is apparent that the samples to the left exhibit much thicker tympanic membranes. The sections were stained with the Masson trichrome mixture (hematoxylin, Biebrich scarlet, and aniline blue), which reveals collagen fibers in a distinct sky-blue coloration (Chin et al., 1997). The most startling observation between these two age groups is the reduction in collagen fiber content in the older specimens. This is seen as a thinning of the TM in the older group. In this particular group of old animals, external signs of aging were obvious. Almost all the hair was lost, and the skin had a wrinkled appearance indicative of collagen breakdown. It would appear that this epidermal loss of collagen with aging extended to the middle layer of the TM.

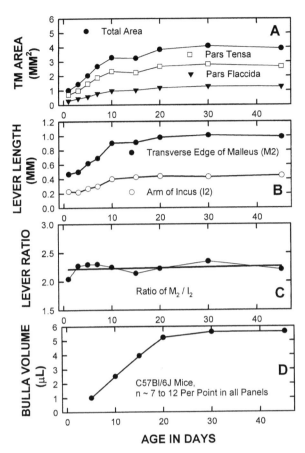

FIGURE 8.12 The development of C57 TM area (A), lever arm lengths (B), the lever ratio (C), and bulla volume (D). (Data from Huangfu and Saunders, 1983.)

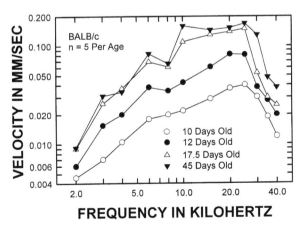

FIGURE 8.13 The development of BALB/C TM transfer functions between days 10 and 45. (Data from Saunders et al., 1993; Doan et al., 1994.)

What might be the functional consequences of this collagen loss in the TM? On visual examination, the TM presents a less tense appearance. The tip of the umbo was still under tension from the downward pull of the tensor tympani, but the TM appeared more compliant. Figure 8.16A

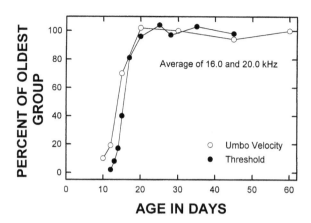

FIGURE 8.14 The development of umbo velocity as compared with the development of evoked response thresholds in BALB/C mice. The data are averaged for 16 and 20 kHz over a number of subjects. (Modified from Saunders et al., 1993).

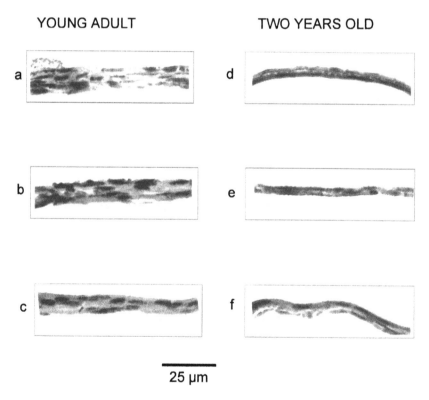

FIGURE 8.15 Tympanic membrane thickness in young adult (85 days old) and 2-year-old mice. The reduction results from a loss of collagen in the TM of older animals.

compares the average velocity transfer functions for groups of young and old BALB/c mice (Doan et al., 1996). The examples of TM thickness (Figure 8.15) were obtained from these animals. The lower panel (Figure 8.16B) shows the difference between the two groups plotted as dB change relative to the older animals. A negative value indicates that the younger animals had the larger response. The hashed areas show those frequencies where the differences were statistically reliable.

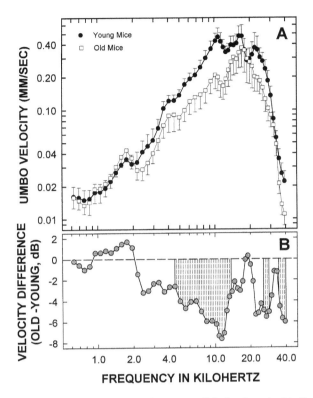

FIGURE 8.16 Umbo velocity transfer functions in young (85 days) and old (2 years) mice (A). The difference between the curves is plotted in B and the hashed areas indicate statistical significance ($p < 0.05$). (From Doan et al., 1996. With permission.)

The difference reached 7.5 dB at 12.5 kHz. With the exception of frequencies around 18 to 20 kHz, there is a consistent loss in sound transmission through the middle-ear system of the older mice. This age-related loss in sound conduction raises the interesting question of how the middle ear contributes to the age-related loss in mammalian hearing (presbycusis). Presbycusis has long been associated almost exclusively with sensorineural hearing loss arising from the progressive destruction of hair cells and auditory nerve fibers. The data in Figure 8.16 suggest that there is an unappreciated middle-ear component to the process of presbycusis. This possibility needs further investigation to see if the same results are observed in other mouse strains or other laboratory animal species.

CONCLUSIONS

This chapter has summarized a considerable amount of information about the mouse outer-ear and middle-ear systems. For a few mouse strains, the anatomy of these regions is well-understood. The generality of these observations across strains, however, has yet to be established.

The function of the mouse microtype middle ear is well-understood. The dual axis of rotation may be a unique property of this conductive system, but it appears that only one axis of rotation (CD in Figure 8.8), the one followed by the stapes, is functionally important for the conduction of sound to the cochlea. The role of the middle-ear muscles and the acoustic reflex needs to be further explored in the mouse, but if it is similar to other species, it serves to control low-frequency input to the cochlea. However, the low frequencies exhibit sufficiently poor sensitivity in this species that it is not clear what the role of the muscles might be. Perhaps in the mouse, attenuation of acoustic input to the cochlea by middle-ear muscle activation extends into frequencies above 2 kHz.

Injury to the conductive apparatus of the mouse middle ear has not received much attention, perhaps because of the difficulty in inducing specific damage or pathology to this region. In one study, the effects of TM perforations were examined. Large perforations of the TM yielded a 24 to 37 dB threshold shift (measured by evoked response activity) at frequencies below 10 kHz. Above 10 kHz, the thresholds were normal. Within 7 days, the lesion had completely healed, and the thresholds had returned to near normal levels (Rubenstein and Saunders, 1983).

The use of genetic manipulations to alter the conductive system represents a new and fruitful line of research for middle-ear studies. As noted above, it has recently been applied to identify genes controlling the normal development of the outer and middle ear. Indeed, genetic anomalies of the middle ear have until recently not been recognized (Kuratani et al., 1999). One recent observation, however, is that defects in the *Brn4/Pou34f* gene causes malformation of the stapes footplate (Phippard et al., 1999). Other genetic ossicular malformations have also been identified (Louryan et al., 1992). Given the use of the mouse as the preferred mammalian species for genetic manipulations, studies of the mouse outer and middle ear, coupled with molecular biological techniques, offer an enormous potential for the elucidation of general mechanisms at play in these peripheral ear systems across species.

ACKNOWLEDGMENTS

The authors appreciate the assistance of Amy Lieberman, Rachel Kurian, and Adam Furman. This research was supported at various times over the last three decades by The Deafness Research Foundation, The Pennsylvania Lions Hearing Research Foundation, and the NIDCD.

9 The Development of the GABAergic Innervation in the Organ of Corti of the Mouse

Hanna M. Sobkowicz

INTRODUCTION

In the adult nervous system, gamma-aminobutyric acid (GABA) is an inhibitory transmitter that regulates neuronal excitability (Barker and Nicoll, 1972; Roberts, 1986). However, in the developing nervous system, GABA is the first neurotransmitter to be expressed, and its initial role is excitatory. The release of GABA causes an elevation of ionic calcium at the synaptic site (Yuste and Katz, 1991), which is essential to the differentiation and stabilization of synapses at the time that excitatory glutamatergic connections are still immature (Hosokawa et al., 1994; for review, see Cherubini et al., 1991). GABA also plays a role as a neurotrophic factor (Spoerri, 1987; for review, see Lauder, 1993) in supporting neuronal proliferation, growth, and migration (Antonopoulos et al., 1997; Behar et al., 1998). The early developmental expression of GABA or its synthesizing enzyme, glutamic acid decarboxylase (GAD), is transitory and usually fades before the differentiation of the mature pattern of GABAergic neurons (W.-J. Gao et al., 1999; also, for review, see Sandell, 1998).

In the developing organ of Corti, the transitory expression of GAD or GABA takes place in the afferent and in the efferent innervation. In the afferent system, the GAD-65 isozyme-positive immunocytochemistry occurs early postnatally and then fades away (Nitecka et al., 1995). In the efferent system, the superfluous collaterals from the main GABAergic fibers invade the field of the incipient innervation and then dissipate. Both events recede at the accomplishment of synaptogenesis (Whitlon and Sobkowicz, 1989).

This chapter presents a series of studies performed on developing and adult ICR mice (Harlan Sprague Dawley). The light microscopical studies include mice up to 3 months old; the electron microscopical observations were followed up to 18 postnatal days (PN). Some data were obtained from organotypic cultures excised from the newborn mouse cochlea. We described the procedures for the preparation and maintenance of cultures of the newborn mouse organ of Corti, together with the corresponding segment of spiral ganglion in Sobkowicz et al. (1975; 1993). Methods for light and electron microscopy immunostaining as well as for conventional electron microscopy are described in detail in Sobkowicz et al. (1998). Cochlear mounts were stained with antibodies against GABA and its synthesizing isozyme, GAD-65. The 1440 anti serum to GAD-65 (Oertel et al., 1981) was kindly provided by Dr. Kopin, NIH.

THE DEVELOPMENTAL EXPRESSION OF GAD IN THE AFFERENT INNERVATION IN THE ORGAN OF CORTI

In vitro

Expression of GAD in the afferent innervation was initially discovered in cultures (Figures 9.1 and 9.2; see also Nitecka et al., 1995), where the organ of Corti is innervated exclusively by the afferent neurons of the spiral ganglion. A 3-day-old culture explanted from a newborn mouse showed positive staining with anti-GAD serum. GAD immunoreactivity in cultures was expressed by the neuronal soma, the peripheral fibers and their synaptic endings with the inner and outer hair cells, as well as by the growth cones of free-growing radial fibers that lost their synaptic targets. This immunoreactivity gradually faded away and was gone by 20 days *in vitro*.

IN SITU

In the intact animal, GAD immunoreactivity in the afferent innervation is expressed already in the newborn and lasts for about 6 to 8 postnatal days. It is useful to remember that, in the mouse, the litters may differ in gestation time by 24 to 48 hours; also, the "newborn" pups are received from the nursery within 24 hours after birth; furthermore, there are up to 2 days difference in innervation between the basal, mid, and apical turns. In the newborn, the peripheral fibers of spiral ganglion neurons, their growth cones, and synaptic endings, are already GAD-positive. In contrast to the *in vitro* patterns, however, the spiral ganglion neurons remain GAD-negative, and the stain is restricted to the radial and spiral fibers, usually to their distal parts and synaptic endings (Figures 9.3 to 9.5). The pattern of GAD immunoreactivity is most advanced in the middle, somewhat less in the basal turn, and the least in the apex. While the stain intensifies in the apex, it fades in the base. As the apical hair cells are the last to receive synaptic endings, they best show the sequence of the fleeting GAD expression. The inner hair cells receive their very first endings on the peripheral side (facing the stria vascularis; Figure 9.4), the next on their modiolar side and, finally, the immunoreactivity conforms to the "Y" shapes of their neurofibrillar cups (Figure 9.5). On the outer hair cells, the first endings form little round caps, also on the strial side, which later, together with the end-collaterals, appose the cells as half-moon formations (Figure 9.3). The immunoreactivity in the outer hair cell region proceeds from the first to the third row. The expression of GAD immunoreactivity already begins to weaken 48 hours postnatally, but in some neuronal endings, notably in the apical outer hair cell region, the stain may persist up to 6 to 8 days.

THE TRANSITORY PLEXUS OF GABAERGIC EFFERENT INNERVATION IN THE ORGAN OF CORTI

In the developing animal (but not in the cultured organ), GABA-positive fibers give rise to two transitory plexuses: a rich convoluted tangle running between and among the radial bundles, and a sparse network, continuous with the inner spiral bundle. The first plexus forms around 2 PN; it derives from the collaterals of GABAergic fibers destined to the inner hair cells and spreads throughout the area of growing radial bundles. Fibers that grow close to the plane of the basilar membrane beneath the hair cell region may reach as far as the outer spiral sulcus (Figures 1, 2, and 25 in Whitlon and Sobkowicz, 1989; see also Merchán-Pérez et al., 1993, rat). The second plexus is continuous with GABAergic fibers of the inner spiral bundle; it begins to grow around 6 PN, and it is confined to the upper plane of the spiral sulcus (Figure 26 in Whitlon and Sobkowicz, 1989). Both plexuses dissipate at the end of the second week.

We believe that these plexuses present true transitory formations that dissipate with the completion of growth and synaptogenesis of the GABAergic innervation. In view of the scarcity of GABA-positive innervation in the organ, it seems possible that the first GABA-positive fibers sprouting spirally along the cochlea may facilitate pathfinding for the remaining fibers (Lauder et al., 1986).

Transitory developmental expression of the GAD-65 isozyme and/or GABA has been observed in the avian retina (Hokoc et al., 1990), in cranial nerves including the cochlear ganglion neurons (von Bartheld and Rubel, 1989), and in the mammalian spinal cord (Ma et al., 1992a; b; Behar et al., 1993). It is believed that the developmental forms of GAD, even if associated with GABA synthesis, have a trophic or metabolic role (Behar et al., 1993) and may even trigger the differentiation of GABAergic receptors in the future recipient cells of the GABAergic fibers (Mandler et al., 1990).

In addition to our observations on the organ of Corti, transitory GABA expression in the mammalian auditory system was observed in the cortex of the ferret up to 20 PN (W.-J. Gao et al., 1999). Despite difficulties with the morphological identification of some of the differentiating GABAergic neurons, transitory GABA expression was unequivocally observed in the pyramidal nonGABAergic neurons up to 7 PN. Thus, both in the peripheral auditory organ as well as in the auditory cortical circuits, transitory expression of GABA correlates with the period of synaptogenesis.

DEVELOPMENT OF THE MATURE PATTERN OF GABAERGIC INNERVATION IN THE ORGAN OF CORTI

Differentiation of the mature GABAergic innervation of the olivocochlear pathway begins about 4 PN. Thus, in some preparations, both systems (afferent and efferent) may be stained simultaneously (Figure 9.6). Fortuitously, their distinctive morphology facilitates the differential identification. The "Y" formations of afferent endings on the inner hair cells are in sharp contrast to the dotted rings formed by the olivocochlear terminals (compare Figures 9.5 and 9.6). The supranuclear caps, dots, or half-moon endings of the afferent spiral fibers on the outer hair cells are very different from the round grape-like formations of olivocochlear endings (compare Figures 9.3 and 9.7). The configurations of the afferent and efferent fibers, especially those innervating the outer hair cell region, also differ. The afferent tunnel fibers show a stepwise basal shift as they pass between the inner and outer pillars and outer spiral bundles, whereas the efferent tunnel fibers [both acetylcholinesterase (AChE)- and GABA-positive] are straight vertical. The growing afferent spiral fibers are wavy and may travel through all three rows of outer hair cells (Figure 9.6 arrows), whereas the efferent spiral fibers (present only during early development) are straight and confined to their own row of outer hair cells (Figure 9.6 asterisks).

The olivocochlear fibers of the efferent system enter the cochlea around birth via two pathways: through the intraganglionic bundle and along the descending central processes of the spiral ganglion neurons. The fibers supply innervation to the inner and outer hair cells and to some of the spiral ganglion neurons (Whitlon and Sobkowicz, 1989); exceptionally, some neurons themselves express GABA immunoreactivity (see also in guinea pig: Tachibana and Kuriyama, 1974; Ylikoski et al., 1989). The early fibers from the intraganglionic bundle either enter radial bundles growing toward inner hair cells or run toward the spiral ganglion; some fibers bifurcate and give collaterals to both. The fibers destined to inner hair cells reach the inner spiral bundle in the basal turn by 2 PN. Their short varicose collaterals wrap around the lower poles of inner hair cells and begin to form a delicate plexus around them. By the end of the first week, the GABAergic fibers run through the entire length of the cochlea; they become a very prominent part of the inner spiral bundle, obscuring the fine details of synaptic connectivity in the region. The patterns of synaptic connectivity can be best demonstrated using antibody against GAD (Figure 9.7), which favors the nerve endings (Nitecka and Sobkowicz, 1996). The first efferent endings on inner hair cells may be observed by 4 PN, encircling the synaptic poles; and by 8 PN, the GAD-positive innervation encompasses each inner hair cell (Figure 9.6). It differentiates further during the second week; and by 12 PN, the GABAergic innervation of the inner hair cells is comparable to that of the mature cochlea (Figures 9.7 to 9.9).

The distinctive morphological components of the GABAergic innervation from the inner spiral plexus evolve as follows. First are the rings formed by axosomatic terminals that surround and cradle each inner hair cell; second are the lateral collaterals that pass between inner hair cells in the plane closest to the basilar membrane; and, finally, the fine straight inner pillar bundle forms along the modiolar side of the inner pillars, collects some of the tunnel fibers to outer hair cells, but also appears to send recurrent collaterals to the inner hair cells (for details, see Figures 4, 5, 8, and 9 in Nitecka and Sobkowicz, 1996).

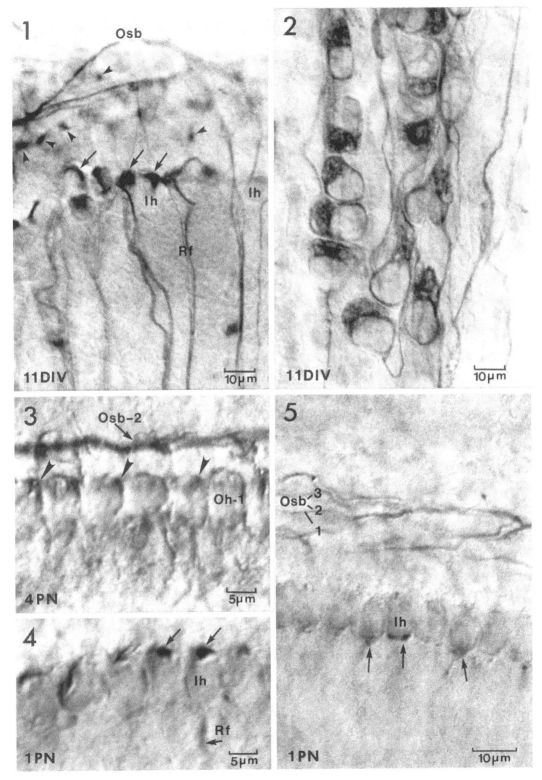

FIGURE 9.1 GAD expression in the afferent fibers and endings to inner hair cells (arrows) and outer hair cells (arrowheads). Ih, inner hair cell; Osb, outer spiral bundle; Rf, radial fiber. Culture, 11 DIV, mid turn.

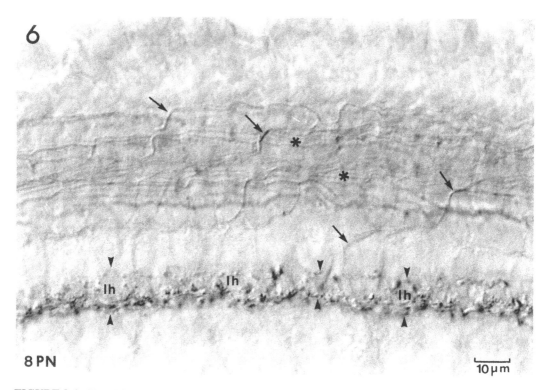

FIGURE 9.6   Transition from the developmental to the mature expression of GAD. The inner hair cells (Ih) show the mature pattern of dotted rings of GABAergic terminals (arrowheads). In the outer hair cell region, the basalward step-wise shift identifies the afferent outer spiral fibers (arrows), while spiral bundles of fine straight fibers (asterisks) denote the ingrowing efferents. The presence of efferent spiral fibers in the outer hair cell innervation is transitory as well. In the mature cochlea, the innervation in the region is exclusively radial. Compare with Figures 9.7, 9.10, and 9.11. 8 PN, apex.

The entire GABAergic innervation of inner hair cells is restricted to about 5 μm of depth and continues along the entire length of the cochlear spire. The GABA-positive innervation to outer hair cells extends throughout the mid and apical turns only (Whitlon and Sobkowicz, 1989), but GAD-positive nerve endings on outer hair cells are seen along the entire spire (Nitecka and Sobkowicz, 1996; see also in the rat Dannhof et al., 1991).

The GABAergic innervation to outer hair cells is the last to differentiate in the cochlea (see also Merchán-Pérez et al., 1990b, rat). The early tunnel fibers grow into the outer hair cell region by the end of the first week; they reach and innervate outer hair cells during the following week. The young fibers tend to ramify and send overlapping end-collaterals to segments encompassing about 6 to 8 outer hair cells in width in all three rows (Figures 9.10A and B). This is in sharp contrast to the adult pattern, in which individual fibers tend to innervate single vertical columns of outer hair cells, forming a strikingly restrictive pattern of connectivity (Figure 9.11).

FIGURE 9.2 (see page 120)   GAD-positive spiral ganglion neurons. Culture, 11 DIV, mid turn.

FIGURE 9.3   "Half-moon" endings (arrowheads) on outer hair cells (Oh). Osb, outer spiral bundle; 4 PN, apex.

FIGURE 9.4   Initial expression of GAD in inner hair cell (Ih) endings (arrows) at the outer poles on the strial side. Rf, radial fibers. 1 PN, apex.

FIGURE 9.5   Late stage of GAD expression in the endings is restricted to the neurofibrillar cups (arrows) of the inner hair cells (Ih). Osb, outer spiral bundle. 1 PN, mid turn.

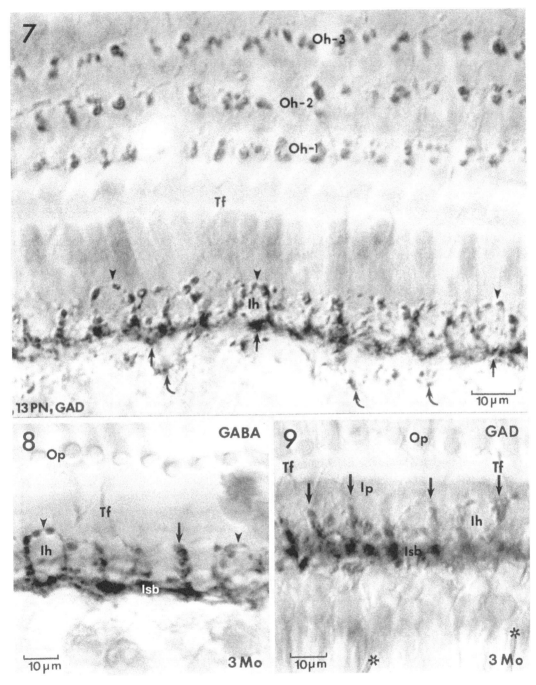

FIGURE 9.7 The mature pattern of GAD-positive innervation. The inner hair cells (Ih) are underlined by fibers and endings that directly appose the receptor poles (arrows). End-collaterals beaded with endings form a full circle around each receptor pole (arrowheads). Many collaterals also extend downward from the plexus to end within the unstained part of the inner spiral bundle (curved arrows) or as far as the oncoming radial afferents. One to three positive endings adorn each outer hair cell (Oh). Tf, tunnel fiber. 13 PN, mid. (From Nitecka and Sobkowicz, 1996, Figure 3. With permission.)

As mentioned above, some of the fibers arriving via both the intraganglionic bundle and the central bundles terminate on selective spiral ganglion neurons (Whitlon and Sobkowicz, 1989). Their end-collaterals form rings of fine endings around neuronal somas (Figure 9.12A) in a pattern corresponding to the "axonal perisomatic arrays," defined by Mugnaini and Oertel (1985) as a special class of GABAergic boutons that surround the neurons and their initial axonal segments in many cell groups in the central nervous system, that is, the ventral cochlear nucleus of the gerbil and guinea pig (Wenthold et al., 1986). The other type of GABAergic terminals on some spiral ganglion neurons are brushy endings (Figure 9.12B). These resemble the chalices of the ascending fibers of the cochlear nerve on brush cells in the central cochlear nucleus (see Figures 3.5 and 3.6 in Lorente de Nó, 1981), especially in their developmental forms (see Figure 334 in Volume I of Cajal, 1909). It is tempting to suggest that the brushy endings may derive from GABAergic cochlear neurons within the spiral ganglion.

The presence of GABAergic terminals on spiral ganglion neurons finds confirmation in ultra-structural studies of the spiral ganglion. Anniko and collaborators, in freeze fracture studies (1987; 1990), describe synaptic membrane specializations on type II spiral ganglion neurons in the mouse, some of which resemble the imprints of efferent terminals in the organ of Corti. Kimura and co-workers (1987), via transmission electron microscopy, identified diversified synaptic contacts on type II spiral ganglion neurons in the macaque monkey, some of which were evidently of efferent origin. The most common type were synaptic terminals of about 2 µm in diameter filled with small synaptic vesicles, and which resemble the GABAergic endings in the organ of Corti (Sobkowicz et al., 1998). The GABAergic nature of the efferent terminals in the spiral ganglion in our material has not been confirmed ultrastructurally. The scarcity of neurons displaying such immunocytochemical endings would suggest that they are type II.

The distinctive pattern of GABAergic innervation within the inner hair cell region is not recognized as a separate morphological entity. However, clusters or rings of GAD-positive endings around inner hair cells are shown by Fex and Altschuler (1984, Figure 7A) and by Vetter et al. (1991, Figure 8a) in the rat cochlea, stained with the same 1440 antibody (Oertel et al., 1981) as in our work, and by Engström and collaborators (1966, Figure 53) using Maillet stain in the guinea pig. Terminal fiber loops around inner hair cells formed by some lateral olivocochlear fibers were also observed by Wilson et al. (1991) after labeling with leucoagglutinin and by Warr (1992) and Warr and Beck (1995) using biotinylated dextran amine. According to Warr et al. (1997), the fiber arborizations around and below inner hair cells are formed by the intrinsic neurons of the lateral olivary complex, regardless of their neurochemical character (see also Figures 14 [CGRP], and 15 and 16 [GAP-43] in Nitecka and Sobkowicz, 1996).

To understand the development of cochlear innervation, it would be particularly important to discern the possible relationship between the AChE-/ChAT- and the GABA-/GAD-positive components in the efferent pathways. The available evidence suggests that each pathway develops

---

FIGURE 9.8 (see page 122) GABA-positive nerve endings abutting the receptor poles of inner hair cells (Ih). The focus is on the ring formations encircling each inner hair cell (arrowheads). Arrow points to a lateral collateral. Isb, inner spiral bundle; Op, outer pillar cells; Tf, tunnel fibers. 3 months, apex. (From Sobkowicz et al., 1998, Figure 1A With permission.)

FIGURE 9.9 Lateral collaterals. The focus is closer to the basilar membrane; in view are myelinated radial fibers (asterisks) within the spiral lamina. The GAD-positive fibers and endings appear as regularly spaced columns across the inner hair cell (Ih) region (arrows), stopping at the level of the inner pillars (Ip). Compare with Figure 9.25. Isb, inner spiral bundle; Op, outer pillars; Tf, tunnel fibers. 3 months, apex. (From Sobkowicz et al., 1998, Figure 1B. With permission.)

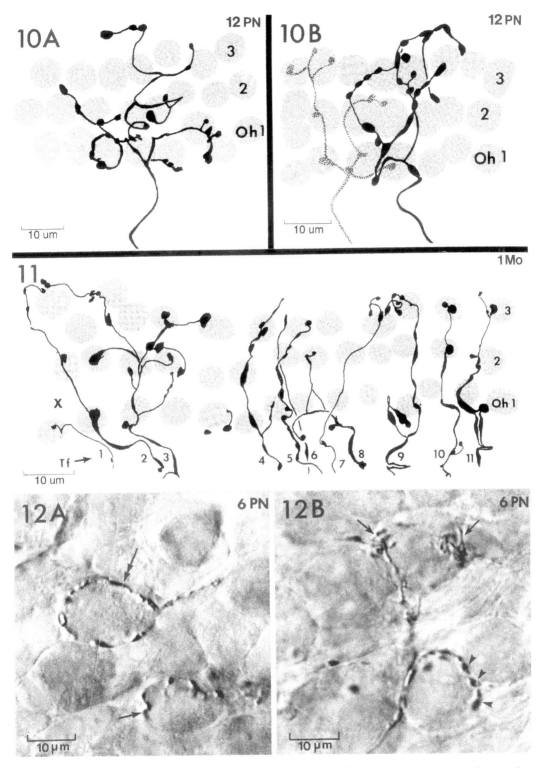

FIGURE 9.10   Arborization of two tunnel fibers in the outer hair cell region in a young mouse, drawn using a Zeiss drawing apparatus. Here, the fibers distribute endings to 4 to 6 cell wide segments of outer hair cells (Oh); adjacent fields of arborizing fibers may overlap. 12 PN, apex. (From Whitlon and Sobkowicz, 1989, Figures 6 and 8. With permission.)

independently (Sobkowicz and Emmerling, 1989; Whitlon and Sobkowicz, 1989). The GABA-positive innervation to inner hair cells arrives during the first 4 days, but the formation of the AChE-positive component of the inner spiral bundle may still be incomplete by the sixth day. The AChE-positive fibers invade the outer hair cell region by the third day and complete the innervation by 12 PN, but the GABA-positive innervation differentiates mainly during the second week. Morphologically, the AChE-positive innervation predominates in the outer hair cell region, whereas its component in the inner spiral bundle and plexus is relatively modest. Conversely, GAD- or GABA-positive innervation predominates in the inner spiral bundle, but is discrete in the outer hair cell region. Furthermore, in contrast to the stronger distribution of AChE-positive innervation to outer hair cells in the basal part of the cochlea, GABA-positive fibers are confined to the mid and apical turns. Thus, the AChE and GABA innervations appear to be separate fiber systems.

The morphological complexity of the efferent component of the inner spiral bundle is matched by its chemical composition (for a review, see Eybalin, 1993). Among neuroactive substances identified within the overall system are ChAT and AChE, GABA and GAD, dopamine, opiate peptides (enkephalins and dynorphins), CGRP, Substance P (Ulfendahl et al., 1993), NSE (Whitlon and Sobkowicz, 1989), and GAP-43 (Sobkowicz, 1992). Cholinergic and GABAergic fibers are distributed within the inner spiral bundle about evenly (Eybalin and Pujol, 1987). Not all immunoreactive systems are chemically distinctive, however. CGRP is supposed to co-localize solely with ChAT-positive fibers (Vetter et al., 1991), but some of the CGRP-positive fibers also contain enkephalins (Tohyama et al., 1990). Fibers containing opiate peptides predominate in the inner spiral bundle (Eybalin et al., 1985), but ultrastructural studies indicate that some fibers are devoid of enkephalins (Altschuler et al., 1984). The GABAergic innervation, so far, appears to be exclusive, but the abundance of fibers expressing opiate peptides in the inner spiral bundle and the tendency of these neuromodulators to link with or be co-expressed in GABAergic CNS neurons (for review, see Angulo and McEwen, 1994) may suggest some additional, not yet detected, complexity within the system.

Our investigations indicate that GABAergic terminals abutting the receptor poles of inner hair cells associate with a variety of GAD-negative nerve endings. In fortuitous stainings, CGRP-positive endings mirror the GAD-positive terminal ring configurations (see Figure 14 in Nitecka and Sobkowicz, 1996), providing indirect evidence for the participation of the cholinergic system in inner hair cell innervation.

Additionally, all morphological components of the GABAergic innervation (terminal rings around inner hair cells, lateral collaterals, long spiral fibers beneath inner hair cells and inner pillar bundle) express GAP-43 (Emmerling and Sobkowicz, 1990b; see Figures 15 and 16 in Nitecka and Sobkowicz, 1996). The GAP-43 protein is inherent in growing and regenerating neurons (Jacobson et al., 1986), but in the adult nervous system, it is expressed mainly in the limbic and integrating areas of the forebrain (for review, see Skene, 1989). The persistence of GAP-43 expression in the adult cochlea indicates the intensity of the synaptic activity and the plasticity within the immediate innervation of the primary auditory receptors — the inner hair cells — which we will presently illustrate ultrastructurally.

FIGURE 9.11 (see page 124)   Distribution of GAD-positive tunnel fibers in the adult animal, drawn using a Zeiss drawing apparatus. The innervation fields tend to narrow, often to a single vertical column of outer hair cells (Oh). The arborization within a wider segment is displayed by fiber 3. Tf, tunnel fiber. 1 month, apex. (From Whitlon and Sobkowicz, 1989, Figure 10. With permission.)

FIGURE 9.12   GABA-positive fibers and their endings in the spiral ganglion. (A) Ring-like formation of GABAergic boutons around the soma of a spiral ganglion neuron (double arrow) and a partial pericellular basket formation on the neuron below (single arrow). (B) Two brushy endings (arrows) on the upper spiral ganglion neuron and a half-ring perisomatic array of GABAergic terminals (arrowheads) on the lower neuron. 6 PN, base. (From Whitlon and Sobkowicz, 1989, Figures 21A and B. With permission.)

ULTRASTRUCTURAL DIFFERENTIATION OF THE GABAERGIC INNERVATION OF INNER HAIR CELLS

Synaptic axosomatic GABA-positive terminals appose inner hair cells around 9 PN (Figure 9.13). The GABAergic endings are morphologically distinctive: they average 1.2 µm in diameter and are uniformly packed with synaptic vesicles that group more tightly at the presynaptic densities. If there were a singular characteristic defining a GABAergic ending in the cochlea, it would be the packing density of the synaptic vesicles (Figures 9.14 and 9.15). Mize (1994), who studied the ultrastructural characteristics of GABAergic endings in the visual system, calls such constancy a "synaptic signature." Thus, in our ultrastructural studies, we used the immunocytochemical preparations to localize the endings and conventionally fixed sections to discern fine synaptic morphology. The GABAergic endings differ from the predominantly lucent endings containing scant scattered vesicles that concentrate at the presynaptic sites (compare endings 5 and 6 with 7 in Figure 11 in Sobkowicz and Slapnick, 1994); such endings were never seen stained for GAD.

Small synaptic boutons, tightly filled with synaptic vesicles, are characteristically distributed in small clusters between each pair of inner hair cells (Figure 9.16). We first identified such endings in cross-sections of 63 consecutive inner hair cells in a 12-PN apical turn (Sobkowicz and Slapnick, 1994). This surprising finding of an efferent synaptic fiber chain interconnecting possibly all inner hair cells (at least in the apical turn) demonstrates that the inner hair cells (as do the outer hair cells) receive double, afferent and efferent, innervation and, contrary to established belief, possess the ability to function in groups. Additionally, bilateral synaptic afferent endings connect adjoining inner hair cells.

The patterns of synaptic connectivity of the GABAergic terminals of the olivocochlear fibers involve both inner hair cells and their afferent dendrites in a very complex manner (Figure 9.17). Some of these relationships are discussed below.

AXOSOMATIC SYNAPSES OF INNER HAIR CELLS

Axosomatic synapses of the inner hair cells can be divided into the *main axosomatic synapses* formed on the body of sensory cells, and the *spinous synapses* made on the spine-like processes that inner hair cells extend to reach the vesiculated endings.

The main axosomatic synapses are formed by boutons that surround the lower receptor pole of inner hair cells (Figures 9.13 and 9.14). They form classical efferent synapses, characterized by postsynaptic cisternae on the sensory cell side. Several GAD-positive endings participate in synaptic chains, presumably derived from a common end-collateral. GAD-negative endings join the terminal synaptic rings (Figures 9.14 and 9.15). Characteristically, each GAD-positive bouton forms a single synapse, and their clusters are wrapped by the cytoplasmic processes of supporting cells (Figure 9.16).

Spinous synapses are formed between efferent terminals and specialized processes of inner hair cells. They are characterized — at least during development — by distinctive postsynaptic cisternae (Figures 9.18A and B). As the spinous processes differentiate (i.e., become thin and form a characteristic "lollipop" head), their cisternae decrease in size dramatically (Figures 9.19B and 9.20). Spinous synapses begin to form around 9 PN (Figure 9.13, ending 6) and persist to at least 18 PN, the oldest specimen studied thus far (Sobkowicz and Slapnick, unpublished). Their most prevalent location is on hair cell spines near the ribbon synapses of afferent dendrites (Figure 9.19A). The ability of inner hair cells to extend processes to reach synaptic targets at a distance facilitates alignment of more than one ending along the spines.

There is a trend to view the axosomatic synapses between efferent endings and inner hair cells as transitory contacts formed during the initial synaptogenesis and lasting until about 5 PN in the mouse (Pujol et al., 1978; 1979; Shnerson et al., 1982) and 14 PN in the cat (Ginzberg and Morest, 1983; 1984). Furthermore, only occasional direct axosomatic contacts have been reported in the adult (Hashimoto et al., 1990, guinea pig; Liberman et al., 1990, cat). However, in view of the fact that the spinous synapses of inner hair cells have been hitherto missed, it is conceivable that the discrepancy between the early postnatal synaptic connectivity and the mature pattern can be explained by a developmental translocation of synaptic connections from the somatic sites on inner hair cells to their specialized spines. Two such synaptic shifts occur during the differentiation of Purkinje cells: the first is the translocation of synaptic endings of the climbing fibers from somatic sites to dendritic spines in the monkey (Kornguth et al., 1968; Kornguth and Scott, 1972); and the second is the translocation of synaptic endings of the parallel fibers from dendritic shafts to spines in the mouse (Landis, 1987). In our experience, the frequency of somatic efferent synapses on inner hair cells indeed decreases postnatally; and around 14 PN, most are found on spinous processes.

COMPOUND SYNAPSES OF INNER HAIR CELLS

The efferent endings that connect with inner hair cells and their afferent endings form combined axosomatic and axodendritic synapses — serial, converging, and triadic — which are characteristic of the central nervous system (Figures 9.21 to 9.24; also, for review, see Sobkowicz et al., 1997).

Serial Synapses

A serial synapse is formed when three or more neuronal elements are closely aligned presynaptically; for example, an efferent ending synapsing on an inner hair cell, which in sequence synapses on an afferent ending (Figure 9.21). Serial synapses were initially described by Kidd (1961) in the inner plexiform layer of the retina. In the organ of Corti, an efferent somatic synapse in the neighborhood of a ribbon afferent synapse provides the means for presynaptic modulation of the auditory input.

Converging Synapses

Another configuration of the synaptic trio — efferent/inner hair cell/afferent — occurs when an afferent ending simultaneously receives synapses from an inner hair cell and an efferent fiber (Figure 9.23). Such synapses are formed by GABAergic terminals (Figure 9.24) and also by lucent efferent endings that, as a rule, are GAD-negative. Converging synapses in the central nervous system are implicated in the modulation of synaptic transmission. The most frequent locus for the synaptic convergence of morphologically or immunocytochemically different terminals is on dendritic spines (Beaulieu et al., 1992; Frotscher and Léránth, 1986; Jones and Powell, 1969). In the cochlea, the convergence of a hair cell presynaptic ribbon and a proenkephalin-positive efferent ending on an afferent dendrite was noted in the guinea pig (Eybalin et al., 1985, Figure 5). Converging synapses offer the means for immediate postsynaptic modulation of the afferent input to the peripheral fibers of the spiral ganglion neurons.

Triadic Synapses

A triadic (or triple) synaptic arrangement occurs when a presynaptic terminal synapses on two other neuronal elements that are also synaptically engaged. In the cochlea, triadic synapses are formed by efferent endings that synapse simultaneously with inner hair cells and their *synaptic* afferents (Figure 9.22). In older mice around 14 PN, serial sections are usually required to identify this type of synapse. They are especially difficult to distinguish when the efferent terminal synapses on an inner hair cell spine. As Figures 9.21 to 9.24 imply, the triadic synapse contains elements of both serial and converging synapses. Furthermore, all three synaptic types tend to cluster, forming synaptic aggregations (Jones, 1985, p. 174).

Triadic synapses are most characteristic of thalamic sensory nuclei. In the auditory system (medial geniculate nucleus), triadic synapses were identified by Morest (1975) and by Majorossy and Kiss (1976). The basic role of the triadic synapse is to integrate three different elements in a

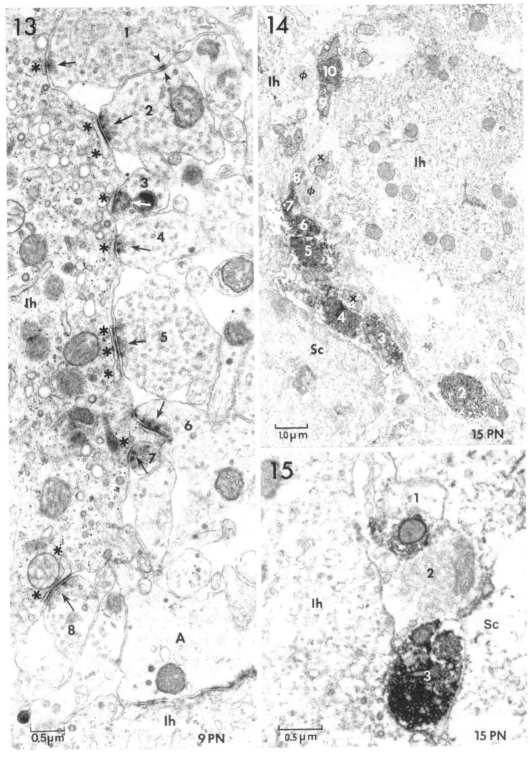

FIGURE 9.13 Eight vesiculated nerve endings (1–8) in direct axosomatic synaptic contact with an inner hair cell (Ih). Synaptic vesicles in the endings form "hot spots" along the presynaptic membrane (arrows). The postsynaptic membranes and the adjoining floor of the cisternae (asterisks) are electron-dense and straight;

semimutual relationship. The physiological role of triadic synapses depends not only on their morphological constituents, but also on their arrangements (for review, see Rapisardi and Miles, 1984). When, as in the cochlea, the GABAergic terminal is the presynaptic element, it performs an inhibitory action on two transmitting sensory elements: the inner hair cell and its afferent. Thus, the synaptic connectivity of the cochlear GABAergic terminals (or those that exhibit their morphological signature) is analogous to the integrative circuits that modulate synaptic transmission in the sensory nuclei of the central nervous system.

GABAergic INNERVATION OF TUNNEL CROSSING FIBERS TO OUTER HAIR CELLS

Olivocochlear innervation to inner and outer hair cells originates in different nuclei of the superior olivary complex. The innervation to inner hair cells originates primarily in the nuclei of the lateral superior olivary complex (LOC) of the same side, whereas the innervation to outer hair cells originates primarily in the nuclei of the contralateral medial superior olivary complex (MOC). Such a dual distribution has been confirmed in small rodents by White and Warr (1983) and by Warr et al. (1986). In the mouse, the MOC fibers originate in the ventral nucleus of the trapezoid body and provide predominantly radial innervation to the outer hair cells (Campbell and Henson, 1988; Wilson et al., 1991).

The GABAergic component of the efferent innervation, however, does not seem to conform to this scheme. Vetter et al. (1991), using the combined techniques of immunocytochemistry and HRP tracing, identified, in the rat, GAD-positive LOC neurons as possibly the unique source of the GABAergic innervation to both inner and outer hair cells. Their study confirms the initial observation of Schwarz et al. (1988), who traced retrograde transport of tritiated thymidine-labeled GABA from the perilymphatic space of the rat's inner ear to a selective subpopulation of GAD-positive neurons in the LOC. GAD-positive neurons in the LOC have also been identified in rats by Moore and Moore (1987) and in gerbils by Roberts and Ribak (1987). Thus, it is conceivable that the innervation derived from the LOC supplies innervation to both kinds of receptors, but we have no direct evidence to confirm this hypothesis. However, we found that the lateral collaterals (Figures 9.9 and 9.25) derived from the inner spiral bundle innervate afferent tunnel fibers destined to outer hair cells, and their GAD-positive endings adjoin the tunnel fibers as they cross the inner hair cell region (Figure 9.26). Most of these synaptic arrangements have associative character, incorporating into their circuitry not only several different tunnel fibers, but also the dendritic terminals of radial fibers and the inner hair cells (Figure 9.26B). Characteristically, the dense vesiculated endings synapse on afferent tunnel fibers that themselves are connected *en passant* through ribbon synapses with inner hair cells (Figure 9.27) and thus control the input from both types of receptors.

FIGURE 9.13 (continued from page 128)   the upper surfaces of the cisternae are irregular, with occasional ribosomes. Endings 1 and 2 are linked by symmetrical membrane densities of punctum adherens (arrowheads). A, afferent ending. 9 PN, mid. (From Sobkowicz et al., 1997, Figure 1. With permission.)

FIGURE 9.14   A cross-section through the infranuclear portion of an inner hair cell (Ih) receptor pole, stained for GAD. Darkly stained vesiculated nerve endings (1–10) form a semicircle. Among them are some lightly GAD-positive, nonvesiculated endings (x) and GAD-negative, vesiculated endings (Ø). Sc, supporting cell. 15 PN, apex. (From Sobkowicz et al., 1997, Figure 2. With permission.)

FIGURE 9.15   Immunocytochemical diversity of vesiculated nerve endings (1–3) within a cluster adjoining an inner hair cell (Ih). Ending 1 is a small, lightly GAD-positive, mitochondrion-containing, nonvesiculated profile. Ending 2 is vesiculated but GAD-negative, and ending 3 is vesiculated and GAD-positive. Sc, supporting cell. 15 PN, apex. (From Sobkowicz et al., 1997, Figure 3. With permission.)

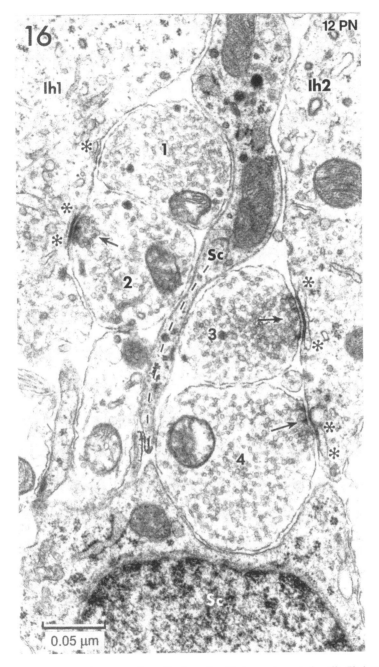

FIGURE 9.16   Four vesiculated nerve endings (1–4) wedged between inner hair cells (Ih 1 and Ih 2). Arrows point to accumulations of synaptic vesicles, and asterisks mark postsynaptic cisternae. The endings synapse in pairs with their respective hair cells. The doublets are separated by a supporting cell (Sc) process (dashed line). 12 PN, apex. (From Sobkowicz et al., 1997, Figure 4. With permission.)

The demonstration of the synaptic connectivity of the GABAergic system of the inner spiral bundle is not only a novel finding, but also contradicts the current dogma of segregation of inner and outer hair cell innervation. Spiral spans of GABAergic fibers to inner hair cells, the regular radial distribution of lateral collaterals to afferent tunnel fibers, and the integrative character of the synaptic connections bespeak this system as the major modulator of cochlear function.

17. The modes of synaptic connections between the efferent and afferent endings and the inner hair cells

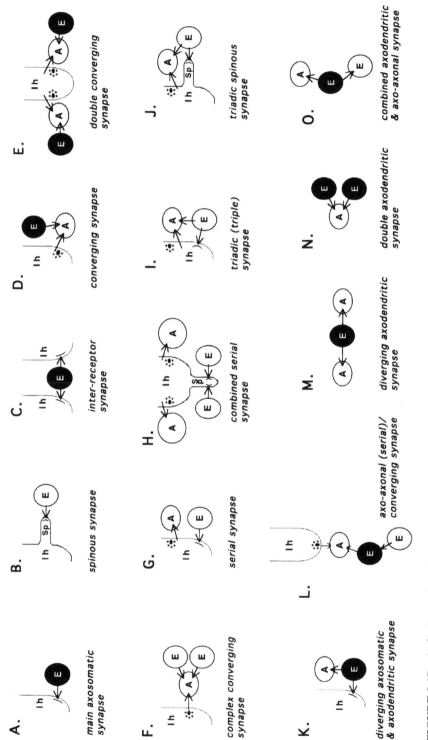

FIGURE 9.17 A–O: the modes of synaptic connections between the efferent (E) and afferent (A) endings and the inner hair cells (Ih). E in a white circle indicates an efferent seen in conventional electron microscopy; E in a black circle indicates an efferent stained for GAD. (From Sobkowicz et al., 1997, Figure 22. With permission.)

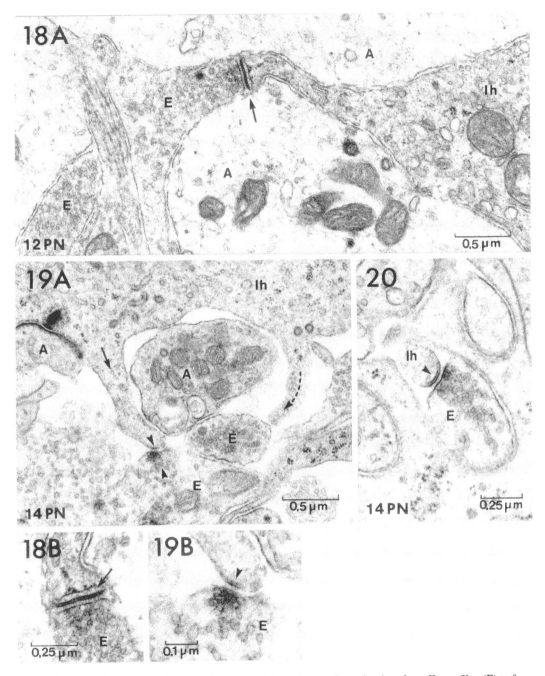

FIGURE 9.18   (A) A process of an inner hair cell (Ih) extends toward a varicosity of an efferent fiber (E) to form a spinous synapse (arrow). (B) Note a distinct postsynaptic cisterna (arrow), decorated with ribosomes, in apposition with the efferent (E). Compare with Figure 9.19B. A, afferent. 12 PN, apex.

FIGURE 9.19   (A) A specialized spinous process of an inner hair cell (Ih) synapsing with a distant efferent ending (arrow and arrowheads). Note a similar process at right (dotted arrow) reaching a different efferent ending (E). (B) High magnification of the Ih-efferent synapse in (A). Note the vestigial postsynaptic cisterna (arrowhead) of the differentiated synaptic spine in apposition with the efferent (E). Compare with Figure 9.18B. A, afferent. 14 PN, apex.

FIGURE 9.20   A cross-section through the "lollipop" head of a hair cell spine (Ih) synapsing with an efferent ending (E). Note the short synaptic apposition and the rudimentary appearance of the postsynaptic cisterna (arrowhead) as compared with the younger synapse in Figure 9.18B. 14 PN, apex.

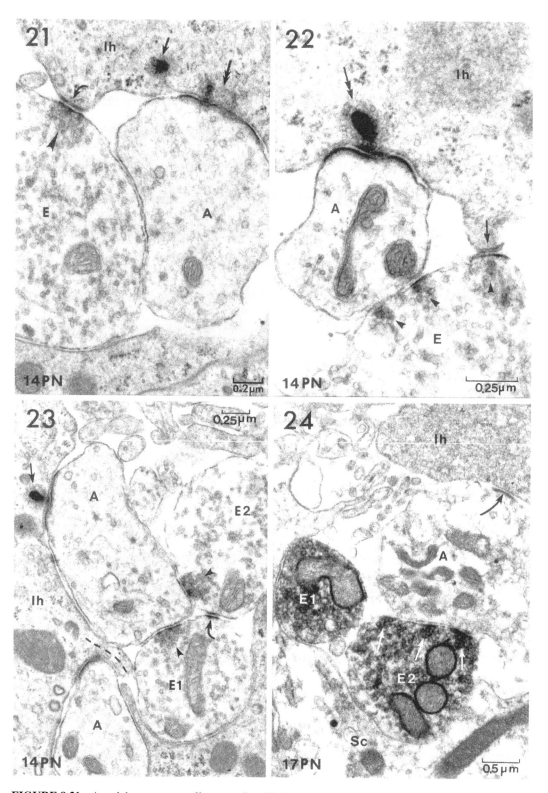

FIGURE 9.21   A serial synapse: an efferent ending (E) is presynaptic to an inner hair cell (Ih), which forms a double ribbon synapse (double arrow) with its afferent ending (A). An additional free ribbon in the vicinity is marked by a straight arrow. The efferent and afferent endings are intimately apposed; however, close serial

SUMMARY

The inner and outer hair cells both receive GABAergic innervation, and these neuronal systems are morphologically distinct. The innervation to inner hair cells is provided through the inner spiral bundle and extends along the entire cochlear spire; the spirally running fibers emit end-collaterals that distribute synaptic terminals around each inner hair cell, forming an uninterrupted chain. They also emit lateral collaterals that pass between inner hair cells and distribute endings to the afferent tunnel fibers destined to outer hair cells. The GABAergic fibers from the inner spiral bundle also provide innervation to a small population of spiral ganglion neurons. Ingrowth of the GABAergic fibers to the inner spiral bundle occurs during the first 48 hours after birth, and the innervation is complete by about 12 days.

The ingrowth of tunnel fibers to the outer hair cells occurs between 6 and 12 days. Initially, the fibers innervate segments 6 to 8 outer hair cells in width; but at maturity, they tend to restrict their innervation to single vertical columns of cells. Also early on, a transitory GAD-65 isozyme is expressed in the afferent innervation, and a transitory superfluous nerve plexiform growth sprouts from the ingrowing GABAergic fibers.

Ultrastructurally, the GABAergic terminals from the inner spiral bundle system participate in the formation of compound synapses (serial, converging, and triadic), which integrate the inner hair cells and their synaptic afferent dendrites. These synapses initially form on the somas of hair cells, but, by the second week, they appear to translocate onto specialized spinous processes. Among the GABAergic endings of the lateral collaterals, the most integrating are those that synapse on the afferent tunnel fibers that are synaptically connected with the inner hair cells.

In conclusion, the GABAergic system of the lateral olivocochlear bundle provides presynaptic control to the inner hair cells and to the afferents of both types of receptors. The integrating character of the GABAergic synaptic arrangements defines this system as the major modulator of cochlear function.

ACKNOWLEDGMENTS

The author would like to thank Susan Slapnick and Benjamin August for preparation of the illustrations and editing the manuscript. The work was supported by research grant number 5 R01 DC00517 from the National Institute on Deafness and Other Communication Disorders, National Institutes of Health.

FIGURE 9.21 (continued from page 133) sections do not reveal synaptic connections between them. The curved arrow points to the postsynaptic cisterna, and the arrowhead indicates presynaptic vesicles. 14 PN, apex. (From Sobkowicz et al., 1997, Figure 15. With permission.)

FIGURE 9.22 A triadic synapse: a presynaptic efferent ending (E) synapses on an afferent ending (A) and an inner hair cell (Ih), which in turn are both synaptically engaged through the ribbon synapse (double arrow). The presynaptic vesicles (arrowheads) collect in the same plane against the membranes of the afferent ending and of the hair cell spinous process. Arrow marks the postsynaptic cisterna. 14 PN, apex. (From Sobkowicz et al., 1997, Figure 17. With permission.)

FIGURE 9.23 Converging synapse. A hair cell ribbon (straight arrow) and two efferent axonal synapses converging on an afferent dendrite (A). Arrowheads mark presynaptic vesicles in the efferent endings (E1, E2). The curved arrow points to the punctum adherens between the efferents. Note a hair cell spine (dashed line) extending toward E1. Ih, inner hair cell. 14 PN, apex. (From Sobkowicz et al., 1997, Figure 20. With permission.)

FIGURE 9.24 Converging synapse. The inner hair cell (Ih) and GAD-positive endings E1 and E2 synapse simultaneously on an afferent ending (A). The postsynaptic density in the afferent (curved arrow) indicates the site of a nearby synaptic ribbon. Presynaptic densities with a corresponding accumulation of presynaptic vesicles (white arrows) indicate the synapse between the GAD-positive efferent (E2) and the afferent (A). Sc, supporting cell. 17 PN, mid. (From Sobkowicz et al., 1997, Figure 21. With permission.)

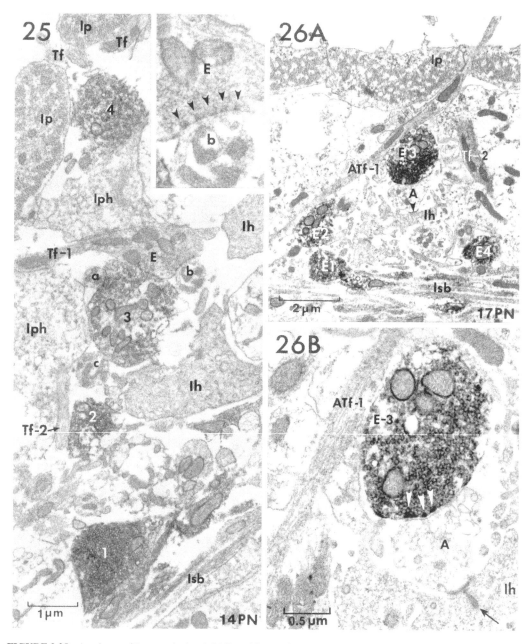

FIGURE 9.25 A column of large vesiculated GAD-positive endings (1–4) extending from the inner spiral bundle (Isb) to the inner pillars (Ip), at the point of exit of the tunnel fibers (Tf). Ending 3 is apposed to a vesiculated GAD-negative fiber (E, center). The spiral run of fiber E (Tf-1) along the inner pillar cells suggests that it is a tunnel fiber. Both efferents E and 3 are in direct contact with profiles of crosswise-cut fibers (a-c) that could be vertically running spiral afferents. Inset shows the series of presynaptic densities (arrowheads) aligned at the synaptic apposition of the efferent tunnel fiber E and the small afferent profile b. Ih, inner hair cell; Iph, inner phalangeal cell. 14 PN, mid. (From Sobkowicz et al., 1998, Figure 3. With permission.)

FIGURE 9.26 (A) In this plane of section, the tunnel fibers arrive at their exit points from the inner spiral bundle (Isb), while the inner pillar bundle is missing. The tunnel fiber at left (ATf-1) crosses the region diagonally and is apposed by two GAD-positive endings (E2 and E3). Ending 3 directly adjoins an afferent ending (A), which itself is postsynaptic to a cytoplasmic sliver of an inner hair cell (Ih); an arrowhead points to the postsynaptic mound. The synaptic details (in an adjacent section) are shown under high magnification in B. (B) The arrowheads point to the presynaptic densities of the efferent ending (E-3), and an arrow marks the presynaptic ribbon (lower right). 17 PN, apex. (From Sobkowicz et al., 1998, Figures 7A and B. With permission.)

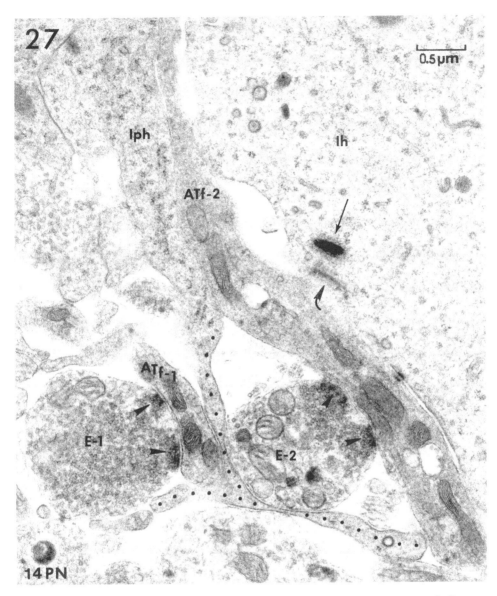

FIGURE 9.27 Two efferent endings (E1 and E2) synapsing (arrowheads) on the shafts of afferent tunnel fibers (ATf-1 and -2). The shaft of ATf-2 was followed from the inner spiral bundle to the inner pillar region. The fiber forms an *en passant* synapse with the inner hair cell (Ih); the straight arrow points to the synaptic ribbon; and the curved arrow marks the postsynaptic mound and density. The ultrastructural features of the efferent endings correspond to those of GABAergic terminals. Iph and dotted lines, inner phalangeal cell. 14 PN, mid. (From Sobkowicz et al., 1998, Figure 18. With permission.)

10 Development and Neuronal Innervation of the Organ of Corti

Matthew W. Kelley and Lynne M. Bianchi

INTRODUCTION

The mammalian organ of Corti is one of the most remarkable structures in all of the vertebrates. Our perception of the full spectrum of sounds — from simple tones through highly complex components of speech and music — is mediated through a structure that is comprised of only approximately 500,000 to 600,000 cells, of which only 3500 (the inner hair cells) are actually listening. By comparison, the mammalian retina contains six million cone photoreceptors and an additional 100 million rod photoreceptors.

As a result of selective pressures and the physical nature of sound waves, the organ of Corti has evolved into a narrow and elongated structure containing a highly ordered cellular pattern. All of the cells within the organ of Corti can be identified as one of six unique cell types (inner and outer hair cells, inner and outer pillar cells, inner phalangeal cells, or Deiters' cells). These cell types are arranged into a modular cellular unit that is repeated along the length of the organ. Organs with this degree of cellular regularity are rare in vertebrates. In fact, the structure of the organ of Corti is reminiscent of similar cellular structures from other phyla of organisms such as the compound eye of *Drosophila melanogaster*. Despite the crucial function of this organ and the remarkable nature of its structure, we still know relatively little about the cellular, genetic, and molecular factors that regulate its formation and innervation. This chapter reviews existing knowledge regarding the development of the organ of Corti and addresses some of the important issues that remain to be examined.

MORPHOLOGICAL DEVELOPMENT AND CELLULAR STRUCTURE OF THE COCHLEAR DUCT AND ORGAN OF CORTI

In the mouse, the cochlear duct can first be identified at embryonic day (E)11.5 as an outpocketing from the ventromedial region of the otocyst (Hensen, 1863; Retzius, 1884). By E12.5, the duct has extended to form a coiled tube that encompasses approximately one half a turn. As development proceeds, the duct elongates and continues to spiral such that by E17.5, the length of the duct forms a spiral of 1½ turns between its base and apex. The spiral is not flattened, but instead the apex is displaced ventrally by approximately 1.3 mm from the base (Lim and Anniko, 1985).

Differences in the epithelial composition of the dorsal and ventral walls of the developing cochlear duct are evident as early as E12.5 (Retzius, 1884; Kikuchi and Hilding, 1965a; Anniko, 1983; Lim and Anniko, 1985). The dorsal wall of the duct, which will give rise to the organ of Corti, the inner sulcus, and the spiral limbus, is comprised of a thickened epithelium that is approximately six cell layers thick (Figure 10.1). In contrast, the ventral wall that will develop as Reissner's membrane is only two to three cell layers thick. By E16, the dorsal epithelium resolves

0-8493-2328-2/01/$0.00+$.50
© 2001 by CRC Press LLC

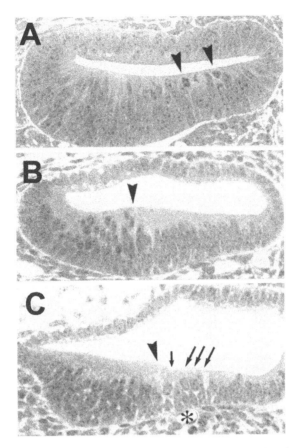

FIGURE 10.1 Development of the organ of Corti. Cross-sections from the basal turn of the cochlear duct at different developmental time points. All three micrographs have been aligned based on the position of the spiral vessel. (A) At E13, the floor of the cochlear duct is comprised of a homogeneous population of epithelial cells. Internuclear migration and proliferating cells are present throughout the epithelium. Arrowheads indicate mitotic figures. (B) By E15, the epithelium is comprised of a modiolar region in which epithelial cells continue to proliferate, and a striolar region in which most to all of the cells appear to be post-mitotic. An arrowhead indicates the border between these two regions. Based on the results of a number of morphological studies and on the position of the spiral vessel, the organ of Corti will develop from cells located in the striolar region. (C) By E17, individual cells that will develop as a single inner hair cell (arrowhead) and three outer hair cells (arrows) can be identified. The notch between the greater and lesser epithelial ridges (straight arrow) corresponds with the position of the developing pillar cells. Note the spiral vessel (asterisk) lines just beneath the pillar cells and first row of outer hair cells.

into two mounds or ridges of cells, referred to as the greater and lesser epithelial ridges (GER and LER, respectively) (Figure 10.1C). The GER comprises approximately two thirds of the dorsal wall of the duct, while the LER comprises the remaining third. Hensen (1863) originally described the GER as Kollicker's organ; however, more recently, Kollicker's organ has been used to describe the entire immature organ of Corti (Lim and Rueda, 1992). Cells within the GER will develop as the inner sulcus, spiral limbus, and probably inner hair cells, while cells within the LER will develop as outer hair cells, Deiters' cells, and the cells of the outer sulcus including Claudius, Hensen's, and Boettcher's cells. Pillar cells appear to form at the boundary between the two ridges, and it seems possible that the development of the pillar cells at this location could play a role in the development of the depression that separates the GER and LER.

The first cells to develop characteristics consistent with a specific cellular phenotype are the inner hair cells that arise in the mid-basal turn of the cochlear duct around E15 (Anniko, 1983; Lim and Anniko, 1985). These cells are characterized by nuclei that are larger than surrounding epithelial cells, a more lumenal position within the epithelium, and the apparent loss of contact with the basement membrane. As development continues, differentiation progresses in a wave that extends along both the neural (modiolar)-to-abneural (striolar) and basal-to-apical axes of the cochlea (reviewed in Rubel, 1978). However, it is important to note that differentiation is not initiated at the extreme base of the cochlea, and thus there is also a more limited gradient of differentiation that extends from the basal turn into the hook region (Bredberg, 1968).

A single row of inner hair cells and three rows of outer hair cells are present at most positions along the length of the cochlear duct, even at early developmental time points (Figure 10.1C). This observation suggests that the factors that determine the cellular pattern of the organ of Corti probably act during the initial development and specification of individual cell types. At the time that hair cells begin to differentiate, approximately three to four layers of undifferentiated cells are still present between the developing hair cells and the basement membrane (Anniko, 1983; Lim and Anniko, 1985). Some of these cells will develop as other cell types within the organ of Corti, such as Deiters' cells and pillar cells; however, some cells may also be eliminated through cell death (Kelley et al., 1995).

Initially, the cell bodies for all hair cells have a fairly cylindrical shape with a slight enlargement in the basal region of the cell as a result of the presence of a relatively larger nucleus (reviewed in Pujol et al., 1997). As development continues, inner hair cells maintain this morphology, while outer hair cells develop a much more rigorous cylindrical shape. However, the change in outer hair cell shape does not occur until the onset of hearing at approximately 14 days after birth (P14) (Pujol and Hilding, 1973). The overall size of both inner and outer hair cells continues to increase through at least P14, with the diameter of inner hair cells increasing by as much as 250% and the diameter of outer hair cells increasing by as much as 200% (Brundin et al., 1991; Pujol et al., 1992; Kaltenbach and Falzarano, 1994). In addition, there is a direct correlation between the length of outer hair cells and their position along the basal-to-apical axis of the cochlea. Hair cells located in the basal turn of the cochlea are long, while hair cells located in the apical turn are comparatively shorter. Beginning around E15, developing stereocilia can be identified on hair cells located in the mid-basal turn. The development of hair cell stereocilia has been reviewed extensively and thus will not be discussed in this chapter (see Tilney et al., 1992; Lim and Rueda, 1992; Kaltenbach et al., 1996; Hackney and Furness, 1995; Gillespie, 1996; Pujol et al., 1997).

Supporting cells become identifiable based on their position within the epithelium by E16. However, the morphological differentiation of these cells does not begin until the postnatal period (Lenoir et al., 1980; Kraus and Albach-Kraus, 1981). Beginning in the basal turn around P6, fluid spaces begin to develop between the inner and outer pillar cells, as well as between the Deiters' cells and hair cells. The opening of these fluid spaces also progresses in a basal-to-apical gradient that requires approximately 4 days to reach the apex of the cochlear duct (Sher, 1971; Kraus and Albach-Kraus, 1981).

CELLULAR PROLIFERATION AND TERMINAL MITOSIS

The dynamics of cellular proliferation and terminal mitosis within the cochlea were examined in detail in a series of studies by Ruben and colleagues in the late 1960s. Using tritiated thymidine to label mitotic cells, Ruben determined the patterns of terminal mitosis for most of the cell types within the organ of Corti, as well as for other regions within the cochlear duct (Ruben, 1967). His results demonstrated a remarkable level of coordination in the patterns of terminal mitosis for many cell types. For most of the cell types within the organ of Corti — including inner and outer hair cells, inner phalangeal cells, pillar cells, Deiters' cells, Claudius cells, and Hensen's cells — terminal mitosis occurs in a relatively small window of time that begins on E12, peaks between E13 and E14, and ends by E16. Interestingly, the majority of terminal mitoses for cells located within the inner sulcus does not occur until E16, suggesting a fundamental difference in the mechanisms that regulate the mitotic cycle of cells located in the modiolar vs. the striolar halves of the cochlear duct.

In addition to the temporal pattern of terminal mitoses, Ruben also analyzed the spatial distribution of labeled cells within the cochlea. The results indicated that terminal mitoses occur in a gradient that begins in the apical region of the cochlea and proceeds toward the base. As a result, the majority of the cells that become post-mitotic on E12 are located in the apex, while cells that become post-mitotic on E16 are located exclusively in the base. This pattern was observed for all of the cell types within the organ of Corti, including inner and outer hair cells, inner phalangeal cells, pillar cells, and Deiters' cells. Based on these results, Ruben suggested that the cells that give rise to the organ of Corti might originate in a proliferative center located near the base of the cochlea. These post-mitotic cells would then move into the cochlear duct, either through active migration or passive elongation of the duct. As a result, the first cells to become post-mitotic would be located in the apex of the cochlea, while the last cells to become post-mitotic would be located in the base. The existence of such a proliferative center, as well as its role in the development of the organ of Corti, has not been determined conclusively. However, the results of two studies have suggested that a small region (approximately 30 μm^2) of proliferative cells is located in the posteromedial wall of the otocyst in an area that corresponds with the junction between the base of the cochlea and the sacculus (Marovitz and Shugar, 1976; Khan and Marovitz, 1982). While the results of these studies are consistent with the existence of a proliferative center, they do not demonstrate that cells originating in this proliferative center give rise to the organ of Corti or that these cells ultimately become localized to apical regions of the cochlea.

The demonstration of an apical-to-basal gradient of terminal mitoses within the organ of Corti is an intriguing finding in light of the existing body of data on the relationship between terminal mitosis and differentiation. As discussed in the previous section, morphological differentiation of the organ of Corti occurs in a basal-to-apical gradient. Cellular differentiation does not begin in the base of the cochlea until approximately E15 and does not appear to begin in the apical region of the cochlea prior to E18 (Sher, 1971; Anniko, 1983; Lim and Anniko, 1985). Based on the Ruben's findings, cells located in the apical region of the cochlea become post-mitotic on E12 but do not differentiate until E18. These results suggest that these cells exist as post-mitotic progenitor cells for approximately 6 days. This is in stark contrast to most other developmental systems in which there is a close temporal correlation between terminal mitosis and the initiation of differentiation (McConnell, 1995; Stenkamp et al., 1997; Morrow et al., 1998).

The mechanisms that regulate cell cycle progression and terminal mitosis in the progenitor cells that will give rise to the organ of Corti are largely unknown. However, two recent studies have identified the cyclin-dependent kinase inhibitor (CKI) p27[kip1] as a major factor in the exit of cochlear progenitor cells from the cell cycle (Chen and Segil, 1999; Lowenheim et al., 1999). p27[kip1] and related CKIs have been implicated as negative regulators of the cyclin-dependent kinases that are required for continued progression through the G1 phase of mitosis (reviewed in Sherr and Roberts, 1995; Elledge, 1996; Harper and Elledge, 1996). Therefore, expression of CKIs such as p27[kip1] can induce an exit from the cell cycle. In the cochlear duct, expression of p27[kip1] can first be detected on E14, in the region of the duct that will develop as the organ of Corti (Chen and Segil, 1999). In contrast, p27[kip1] is not expressed in cells that will not develop as part of the organ of Corti (Chen and Segil, 1999), suggesting that different mechanisms may control progression through the cell cycle in different regions of the cochlea. Within the developing organ of Corti, p27[kip1] is initially expressed in all cells; however, p27[kip1] expression is down-regulated in those cells that will differentiate as hair cells. Interestingly, expression of p27[kip1] is maintained in all supporting cells within the organ of Corti, including Pillar, Deiters', Hensen's, and Claudius cells in both postnatal and adult animals.

To examine the possible role of p27^{kip1} in the developing cochlea, Chen and Segil (1999) and Lowenheim et al. (1999) analyzed the morphology of the organ of Corti in mice containing a targeted deletion of p27^{kip1}. Results indicated an overproduction of many cell types within the organ of Corti, including inner and outer hair cells and pillar cells. These results suggest that p27^{kip1} plays a key role in regulating the number of cells that will comprise the progenitor pool that will give rise to the organ of Corti. In addition, staining with the proliferative marker PCNA demonstrated the existence of proliferating cells within the organ of Corti as late as postnatal day 6, demonstrating that p27^{kip1} plays a key role in the regulation of terminal mitoses of cochlear progenitor cells. Despite the lack of p27^{kip1}, cells within the organ of Corti do become post-mitotic and are capable of differentiating into all of the described cell types. Therefore, while p27^{kip1} clearly plays an important role in the regulation of cell cycle progression, additional factors must also be involved.

One aspect of the role of p27^{kip1} that has not been determined is the pattern of its initial onset and whether or not this pattern correlates with the pattern of terminal mitoses. One of the most striking aspects of the pattern of terminal mitoses within the organ of Corti is the existence of a gradient that is inversely correlated with the gradient of cellular differentiation. If p27^{kip1} plays a role in the pattern of terminal mitoses, then its initial pattern of expression should be consistent with the pattern of terminal mitoses (apical-to-basal), rather than with the pattern of differentiation (basal-to-apical). Unfortunately, while the down-regulation of p27^{kip1} was shown to be correlated with the gradient of differentiation (i.e., basal-to-apical) (Chen and Segil, 1999), the gradient in the onset of p27^{kip1} has not yet been determined.

In summary, the terminal mitoses of cochlear progenitor cells occurs in a highly regulated apical-to-basal gradient. The mechanisms that mediate the formation of this gradient have not been determined However, it has been suggested that a focal source of proliferative cells located at the junction between the cochlea and sacculus may generate a pool of progenitor cells that stream away from the source as the cochlear duct extends. As a result, the oldest cells will be located at the apex of the cochlea, with relatively younger cells located at progressively more basal positions. The molecular factors that play a role in the coordinated exit of cochlear progenitor cells from the cell cycle have not been determined. However, recent evidence has demonstrated that the cell cycle inhibitor p27^{kip1} plays a key role in regulation of cellular proliferation within the cochlea.

DETERMINATION OF CELL FATE AND CELLULAR PATTERNING

One of the most striking aspects of the organ of Corti is its highly invariant cellular pattern. Along its length, the organ of Corti is comprised of a single row of inner hair cells and three rows of outer hair cells. Each inner hair cell is separated from adjacent inner hair cells by a single inner phalangeal cell, and each outer hair cell is separated from adjacent outer hair cells by single Deiters' cells. In addition, the inner and outer hair cell regions of the organ of Corti are separated by a single row of inner pillar cells and a single row of outer pillar cells. There can be some variation in the number of rows of outer hair cells in the apical region of the cochlea, with as many as five rows in some cases. In addition, inner hair cell duplications are occasionally observed. However, overall, the cellular pattern is highly invariant with a very low incidence of patterning errors (Lenoir et al., 1987; Kaltenbach and Falzarano, 1994; Zhou and Pickles, 1994).

The development of the organ of Corti probably occurs as at least three distinguishable events. Initially, a limited population of epithelial cells within the floor of the cochlear duct must become specified to develop as the organ of Corti. Because the cells within this population appear to have the ability to develop as any of the cell types found in the organ of Corti, these cells have been termed "prosensory cells" (Kelley et al., 1993; 1995). Next, individual cells within the prosensory cell population must become determined as specific cell types within the organ of Corti. Finally, these cells must be arranged into a regular geometric pattern. While it seems very likely that there may be direct relationships between the determination of individual cell types and the arrangement of those cells into a specific pattern, there is not enough information about either event to draw any strong conclusions concerning interactions.

DETERMINATION OF THE PROSENSORY CELL POPULATION

Very little is known about the cellular and/or genetic factors that determine the prosensory cell population. A number of genes that play a role in the patterning of other developing systems are expressed in the cochlea in patterns consistent with a role in the determination of this population, but experiments demonstrating that these genes are required for the formation of this population have not yet been conducted. One particularly interesting group of genes that is expressed in the cells that apparently develop as prosensory cells are members of the Notch signaling pathway. Notch is a membrane-bound receptor protein that was originally identified as a mediator of lateral inhibition between individual progenitor cells (see below, "Determination of Individual Cell Fates") (reviewed in Artavanis-Tsakonas et al., 1995; 1999). Although Notch is still believed to mediate cell-to-cell lateral inhibition, subsequent studies have suggested that it also plays a role in the formation of boundaries between cells that will develop with different fates (reviewed in Bray, 1998; Irvine, 1999). The specific mechanisms involved in the formation of this type of boundary are not completely understood; however, it has been suggested that different levels of Notch activation can be obtained between adjacent populations of cells through the co-expression of a Notch-ligand and an inhibitor of that ligand in one population of cells. The presence of a Notch-ligand will lead to activation of Notch, but only in cells that do not express the ligand-inhibitor. Because all of the cells within one population express the ligand-inhibitor, activation of Notch will only occur in cells located adjacent to that population. This type of interaction will result in the formation of a boundary between two adjacent cell populations.

The expression patterns for *Notch1* and other Notch-related genes within the cochlea suggest that this pathway may be involved in establishing the prosensory cell population. *Notch1* is expressed throughout the epithelium from the onset of otocyst formation (Lewis et al., 1998); however, beginning around E11, the Notch-ligand *Jagged1* (*Jag1*) and the ligand-inhibitor *Lunatic Fringe* (*Lfng*) are expressed within a subset of cells within the duct (Morsli et al., 1998; Morrison et al., 1999). This subset of cells is located in a region of the epithelium that appears to correlate with the cells that will develop as the organ of Corti, and examination of the expression of both *Jag1* and *Lfng* at later developmental time points indicates that expression of these genes ultimately becomes restricted to cells that will develop as supporting cells (Morsli et al., 1998; Morrison et al., 1999). These results are consistent with the hypothesis that expression of *Jag1* and *Lfng* could play a role in the formation of a boundary between prosensory and non-prosensory cells. However, this hypothesis is complicated by the observation that the pattern of *Jag1* expression changes during cochlear development (Morrison et al., 1999). In particular, between E13 and E17, the domain of *Jag1* expression appears to move from the modiolar to the striolar half of the cochlear duct (Morrison et al., 1999). Therefore, it is not clear whether the domains of *Jag1* and *Lfng* are entirely complementary throughout the development of the prosensory cell population. Finally, deletion of *Lfng* does not lead to any obvious changes in the development of the organ of Corti (Zhang et al., 2000). This result suggests that either *Lfng* is not required for the development of the organ of Corti, or that the function(s) of this gene might be replaced through compensatory expression of other fringe family members.

Another gene that is expressed in a limited population of cells within the organ of Corti and that also plays a role in cellular patterning in other systems is *Bone Morphogenetic Protein 4* (*BMP4*). *BMP4* is a member of the Transforming Growth Factor-β superfamily, which also includes *TGF-β*, *BMP2*, and the *Drosophila* protein *Dpp* (reviewed in Kawabata et al., 1998; Schmitt et al., 1999). The members of this family of genes have been shown to play a role in a number of different developmental events, including neural induction and boundary formation (reviewed in Chitnis,

1999; Podos and Ferguson, 1999). Interestingly, in the developing organ of Corti, *BMP4* is expressed in the population of cells that will develop as the outer sulcus. These cells are located adjacent to the population of cells that will develop as the organ of Corti. This pattern of expression might suggest that *BMP4* acts as an autocrine inhibitor of prosensory cell formation. Alternatively, because *BMP4* is a secreted protein, paracrine signaling by this molecule could play a role in cellular patterning within the organ of Corti. While there is no direct experimental evidence to support either of these hypotheses, it should be noted that the fates of cells that express *BMP4* are not consistent within the otocyst. *BMP4* is expressed in cells located in the anlagae for all three semicircular canal cristae, but is not expressed in the anlagea of the utricle, saccule, or cochlea (Morsli et al., 1998). In addition, *BMP4* is also expressed in all sensory anlagae in the otocyst of the chick (Oh et al., 1996). These results would suggest that expression of *BMP4* is not inhibitory for the development of hair cells and supporting cells.

In summary, one of the first steps in the formation of the organ of Corti is probably the development of a population of progenitor cells that become competent to develop as all of the cells within the sensory epithelium. While a number of genes have been shown to be expressed in patterns that are consistent with a role in the specification of this cell population, at present there is no functional evidence to indicate whether any of these candidate genes are actually required for the formation of this cell population.

DETERMINATION OF INDIVIDUAL CELL FATES

DETERMINATION OF CELLS AS HAIR CELLS

As discussed in an earlier section of this chapter, the first cells that can be identified as committed to a specific cell fate are developing inner and outer hair cells (Kikuchi and Hilding, 1965a; Sher, 1971; Rubel, 1978; Anniko, 1983; Lim and Anniko, 1985). This observation led to the suggestion that the hair cell fate might represent the preferred fate for cells within the prosensory cell population, and also to the hypothesis that subsequent cell-cell interactions might play a role in the inhibition of the hair cell fate in a subset of these cells (Lewis, 1991; Corwin et al., 1991). This hypothesis was supported by the results of laser ablation studies that demonstrated that ablation of newly developing outer hair cells leads to the development of replacement hair cells (Kelley et al., 1995). The source of these replacement hair cells are existing progenitor cells within the epithelium that would go on to develop as supporting cells in the absence of hair cell ablation. This result clearly suggests that as cells begin to develop as hair cells, these cells express inhibitory signals that prevent adjacent cells from adopting the same fate. Ablation of one of these cells leads to the loss of this signal and, as a result, to the development of replacement hair cells.

More recently, the molecular basis for both the commitment of cells as hair cells and for the subsequent inhibitory interactions that prevent adjacent progenitor cells from developing as hair cells have been examined in studies from several different laboratories. Previous work in other systems had identified a highly conserved molecular signaling loop, referred to as the neurogenic pathway, as playing a key role in regulating the number of cells within a progenitor pool that will become committed to a particular cell fate (reviewed in Kageyama and Ohtsuka, 1999). Typically, a group of progenitor cells will initially all begin to express one of the members of a family of transcription factors that positively regulate cell fate. This family is characterized by the presence of a basic helix-loop-helix (bHLH) DNA binding domain. Because most of the members of this family have been shown to play a role in the development of the nervous system, these genes are referred to as proneural genes. The expression of a proneural gene acts to initiate a determinative program that, if unaltered, will ultimately lead to the differentiation of a cell with a particular phenotype. One of the initial effects of the expression of a proneural gene is the expression of a membrane-bound ligand for the Notch receptor. Notch is a ligand-dependent, membrane-bound receptor that is expressed on many types of progenitor cells and plays a role in the inhibition of differentiation (reviewed in Artavanis-Tsakonas et al., 1999). The molecular mechanism of this inhibition is based on the induction of expression of a second class of bHLH genes that act as inhibitors of proneural genes. Because the expression of inhibitory bHLH genes is dependent on activation of Notch through cell-cell contact, this signaling pathway plays a key role in the development of alternative cellular patterns. Based on the demonstrated role of this pathway in other systems, it seemed likely that similar interactions might be involved in the development of the organ of Corti.

Two recent studies have provided strong evidence that the bHLH gene *Math1* acts as a positive regulator for the hair cell fate. First, Bermingham et al. (1999) demonstrated that *Math1* is expressed in the region of the cochlear duct that will develop as the organ of Corti, and that deletion of *Math1* leads to a complete absence of hair cells and to a disruption in the development of the organ of Corti. More recently, Zheng and Gao (2000) used electroporation to ectopically express *Math1* in cells within the developing inner sulcus of P0 mice. Results indicated that expression of *Math1* leads to the generation of hair cells in the inner sulcus region. Similarly, a preliminary report indicates that overexpression of *Math1* in cells located within the developing sensory epithelium in E13 mice leads to an increase in the density of both inner and outer hair cells (Shailam et al., 1999). These results demonstrate that *Math1* is necessary and sufficient for the development of cells as hair cells, and strongly suggest that *Math1* acts as a proneural gene, or more appropriately a prosensory gene, within the organ of Corti.

The hypothesis that the Notch-signaling pathway plays a role in the development of the alternating mosaic of hair cells and supporting cells is supported by the demonstration that *Notch1* is expressed throughout the developing cochlear duct beginning as early as E12 and continuing through at least P3 (Lewis et al., 1998; Lanford et al., 1999). In addition, beginning between E13 and E14, the Notch-ligands *Jagged2* (*Jag2*) and *Delta1* (*Dll1*) are expressed in a subset of cells within the cochlear duct. By E17, cells that express *Jag2* and *Dll1* can be identified as hair cells (Lanford et al., 1999; Morrison et al., 1999).

To determine the role of the Notch pathway during development of the organ of Corti, the effects of disruption of the pathway were determined by analysis of mice containing a targeted deletion of *Jag2* (Jiang et al., 1998). *Jag2* mutant mice were chosen because these embryos survive until the day of birth, while deletions of *Notch1* or *Dll1* lead to embryonic lethality at approximately E10 (Swiatek et al., 1994; Hrabe de Angelis et al., 1997). Results indicated that deletion of *Jag2* leads to a significant increase in the number of inner hair cells and in the total number of hair cells. The increase in the number of inner hair cells results in the formation of a nearly complete second row. These results clearly demonstrate that the Notch-signaling pathway plays an important role in the inhibition of the development of progenitor cells as hair cells and in the overall regulation of the development of the organ of Corti.

It is important to consider that although the deletion of *Jag2* leads to a significant increase in the total number of hair cells, the change in hair cell number only amounts to a 20% increase. In addition, there was no noticeable decrease in the number of supporting cells in *Jag2* mutant cochleae (Lanford et al., 1999). These results suggest several possibilities. First, it is possible that *Dll1* may be able to compensate for the loss of *Jag2*. This hypothesis is supported by a recent paper that demonstrates that deletion of *Lfng*, a gene that may inhibit the effects of some Notch-ligands (see chapter section on "Determination of Prosensory Cells"), in *Jag2* mutant mice results in a rescue of the wild-type inner hair cell phentoype (Zhang et al., 2000). As discussed in a previous section, deletion of *Lfng* alone has no apparent effect on development of the organ of Corti; however, the observed effects of deletion of *Lfng* in combination with a deletion of *Jag2* have led to the suggestion that the normal role of *Lfng* may be to suppress the activity of *Dll1*. In compound mutants, the normal inner hair cell pattern may be rescued because, in the absence of *Lfng* signaling, *Dll1* may be able to more effectively compensate for the loss of *Jag2* (Zhang et al., 2000). However, it is important to consider that a specific role for *Dll1* during the development of the organ of Corti has not been demonstrated, and because *Jag1* is also expressed in the developing cochlear duct, it is also possible that this Notch-ligand could play a role in the phenotype observed in *Jag2/Lfng* compound mutants (Zhang et al., 2000).

A second possible explanation for the limited number of additional hair cells in *Jag2* mutant cochleae would be that the number of progenitor cells that can develop as hair cells is limited. The number of progenitors with the ability to develop as hair cells is clearly greater than the number of cells that ultimately develop as hair cells, but it is not clear whether all progenitor cells have the ability to develop as hair cells. This hypothesis has not been examined extensively at this time.

In many systems, the effects of activation of the Notch pathway are mediated through the expression of members of an inhibitory class of bHLH genes that includes the *enhancer of split* genes in Drosophila and their vertebrate homologs, the *HES* genes (reviewed in Kageyama and Ohtsuka, 1999). To determine whether *HES* genes act as downstream effectors of Notch activation in the organ of Corti, the pattern of expression for *HES5* was determined (Lanford et al., 2000). Results indicated that *HES5* expression begins approximately 12 hours after expression of *Jag2*. However, *HES5* transcripts are apparently restricted to cells that will develop as supporting cells (Lanford et al., 2000). In addition, deletion of *Jag2* leads to a significant decrease in the expression of *HES5*, strongly suggesting that expression of this gene is regulated through the Notch pathway (Lanford et al., 2000).

Work in other systems has demonstrated that the main effect of expression of *HES5* is apparently the inhibition of proneural bHLH genes such as *Math1* (reviewed in Kageyama and Ohtsuka, 1999). Therefore, it seems reasonable to expect that expression of *HES5* probably leads to inhibition and down-regulation of *Math1* in the organ of Corti. While this effect has not been tested experimentally, deletion of *Jag2* does result in an increased level of *Math1* expression in a manner consistent with this hypothesis (Lanford et al., 2000).

In summary, a number of recent studies have demonstrated that the determination of cochlear progenitor cells as hair cells is apparently mediated through a signaling loop in which a population of progenitor cells initially becomes determined to develop as hair cells through expression of *Math1*. Subsequent cell-cell interactions mediated through the Notch-signaling pathway lead to the expression of *HES5* and the inhibition of *Math1* in some of those progenitors. Because *Math1* is required for the development of cells as hair cells, inhibition of *Math1* diverts these cells from the hair cell fate. While this hypothesis is consistent with existing data, there are several issues that remain to be resolved. Perhaps most intriguing is the question of how *Math1* is down-regulated in *Jag2* mutant mice. Supporting cells still develop in *Jag2* mutants, and analysis of *Math1* expression indicates that expression of this gene is down-regulated in supporting cells in these animals as well. Therefore, it seems possible that other members of the Notch-pathway could play a role in the control of *Math1* expression, or alternatively that other signaling pathways could also play a role in the regulation of hair cell vs. supporting cell fate. Finally, it is also possible that as cells begin to develop as hair cells, these cells may also produce inductive signals that recruit neighboring cells to develop as supporting cells. Once these cells begin to develop as supporting cells, expression of *Math1* could be down-regulated through mechanisms that are unrelated to the Notch-pathway.

DETERMINATION OF CELLS AS SUPPORTING CELLS

In comparison to hair cells, considerably less is known about the factors that play a role in the cellular commitment of other cell types within the organ of Corti. Progenitor cells that will develop as inner phalangeal cells and Deiters' cells can be conclusively identified by E17. However, it is not known when these cells become committed to specific fates. Results from a study in which developing inner and outer hair cells were ablated between E15 and P0 indicated that at least some of the progenitor cells located in the outer hair cell region had the potential to alter their normal phenotypic choice and to develop as replacement hair cells (Kelley et al., 1995). This result suggests that, at this time point, at least some of the cells that will develop as Deiters' cells are not committed to a specific phenotype. Similar phenotypic changes were not observed when inner hair cells were ablated even at time points as early as E16 (Kelley et al., 1995). These results led to the suggestion that cells surrounding developing inner hair cells (inner phalangeal cells and inner pillar cells) may become committed at earlier time points than Deiters' cells; however, this hypothesis has not been examined further. In fact, the results of a preliminary study in the Bronx-Waltzer mouse suggest that commitment to the pillar cell phenotype may not occur until later in development. In the Bronx-Waltzer mouse, inner hair cells start to degenerate beginning around E17 as a result of an uncharacterized mutation. However, by P0, replacement inner hair cells are observed. While the source of these replacement hair cells has not been demonstrated conclusively, the authors noted a decrease in the number of pillar cells that appeared comparable to the number of observed replacement hair cells (Bussoli et al., 1998). These results suggest that cells that will develop as pillar cells may not become committed to that fate until after E17.

An explanation for the difference in observed results between the laser ablation and Bronx-Waltzer studies is not obvious. It is possible that the mechanism of cell degeneration may play a role in the ability of neighboring cells to respond to the loss of a cell. Alternatively, while degeneration of inner hair cells may not be observed in Bronx-Waltzer mice prior to E17, it seems possible that the production of the molecular signals that mediate development of the cellular mosaic may be disrupted at earlier time points. The loss of these signals could lead to a delay in the commitment of cells that would normally develop as pillar cells.

The molecular factors that play a role in the commitment of cells as inner phalangeal cells, Deiters' cells, or pillar cells are largely unknown. However, one gene that has been implicated in the development of cells as pillar cells is *Fibroblast Growth Factor receptor 3* (*FGFr3*). In adult rats, *FGFr3* is expressed in pillar cells and Deiters' cells (Pirvola et al., 1995), and deletion of *FGFr3* results in a disruption in the development of the pillar cells (Colvin et al., 1996). However, it is not clear whether the disruption in pillar cell development is the result of a defect in cellular commitment or differentiation.

A WAVE OF CELLULAR COMMITMENT

One of the most striking aspects of the development of the organ of Corti is the observation that cellular differentiation, as determined based on morphological criteria, appears to initiate at a single position located in the mid-basal turn of the organ of Corti (Kikuchi and Hilding, 1965a; Sher, 1971; Rubel, 1978; Anniko, 1983; Lim and Anniko, 1985). From this site, differentiation proceeds in a wave that extends bi-directionally along the basal-to-apical axis. In addition, the differentiation of cells as hair cells also proceeds as a wave along the modiolar-to-striolar axis with inner hair cells differentiating prior to first row outer hair cells and first row outers differentiating prior to second row outers. Because cellular commitment and differentiation are usually tightly linked, these results suggest that specific cell types within the organ of Corti may also become committed in a wave with inner hair cells being specified first, followed by first row outer hair cells, and so forth. Although this hypothesis has not been specifically tested, several genes that apparently play a role in cellular commitment in the cochlea (see previous chapter sections) are expressed in temporo-spatial gradients that also initiate in the inner hair cell/mid-basal region and then progress along the basal-to-apical and modiolar-to-striolar axes. In particular, *Math1*, *Jag2*, and *HES5* have all been shown to be expressed in gradients that presage the gradient of differentiation (Lanford et al., 1999; 2000).

In summary, recent results have significantly increased our understanding of the genes that play a role in the determination of cells as hair cells. The bHLH gene *Math1* has been shown to be necessary and sufficient for the development of progenitor cells as hair cells, and the patterns of expression for a number of genes support the hypothesis that determination and commitment occur in a basal-to-apical gradient that presages the gradient of differentiation. A number of important questions remain to be addressed. In particular, it is not clear how progenitor cells become committed to develop as other cell types within the organ of Corti. Finally, the apparent discontinuity that exists between the patterns of terminal mitosis and cellular commitment suggests that the progenitor cells within the organ of Corti may employ unique mechanisms to maintain themselves in a post-mitotic but uncommitted state for periods of time that may be as long as 6 days.

CELLULAR DIFFERENTIATION IN THE ORGAN OF CORTI

Although cellular determination, commitment, and differentiation often occur within a narrow time span, it is important to consider that these are separable events that usually involve discreet signaling factors. With the exception of hair cells, very little is known about the factors that play a role in the commitment and determination of specific cell types within the organ of Corti. Unfortunately, although there have been extensive studies on the morphological differentiation of the organ of Corti, the amount of information regarding the molecular factors that control cellular differentiation is also somewhat limited.

Cellular determination and commitment are thought to begin in the basal turn of the cochlea around E13 (Bermingham et al., 1999; Lanford et al., 1999; 2000). Similarly, expression of early hair cell specific markers as well as morphological observations suggest that hair cell differentiation starts soon after hair cell determination, perhaps as early as E13.5 (Xiang et al., 1998). One of the first genes to be expressed in cells that will differentiate as hair cells is *Brn 3.1* (3C) (Erkman et al., 1996; Xiang et al., 1997). This gene is a member of the family of POU-domain transcription factors (reviewed in Ryan and Rosenfeld, 1997), many of which have been implicated in cellular differentiation in other systems (Veenstra et al., 1997; Latchman, 1999). *Brn 3.1* is initially expressed between E13.5 and E14 in the basal region of the cochlea and appears to extend in a characteristic basal-to-apical gradient. Deletion of *Brn 3.1* leads to the complete loss of hair cells by the early postnatal period; however, examination of the development of the cochlea during embryogenesis indicates that hair cells become committed and pass through at least the early stages of development prior to degeneration (Erkman et al., 1996; Xiang et al., 1997; 1998). In addition, some early hair cell markers such as Myosin VI and Myosin VIIa are transiently expressed in the cochleae of *Brn 3.1* mutant mice (Xiang et al., 1998). These results are consistent with the hypothesis that *Brn 3.1* is required at a specific point in the differentiation of cells as hair cells.

A second molecule that has been suggested to play a role in the differentiation of cells within the organ of Corti is GATA3. The GATA family of zinc-finger transcription factors has been shown to be required for the normal development of a number of different systems, including the hematopoietic and respiratory systems (reviewed in Warburton et al., 1998; Charron and Nemer, 1999). While a role for GATA3 in the cochlea has not been demonstrated, its pattern of expression suggests that GATA3 may act as a negative regulator of cellular differentiation (Rivolta and Holley, 1998). GATA3 is initially expressed throughout the developing sensory epithelium. However, as cells begin to differentiate as hair cells, these cells down-regulate expression of GATA3. Interestingly, GATA3 is also down-regulated in cells that will develop as supporting cells, but down-regulation in these cells is delayed in comparison to cells that will develop as hair cells. These results are consistent with the hypothesis that hair cells differentiate prior to supporting cells. The results also suggest that GATA3 might act as an inhibitor of cellular differentiation.

RETINOIC ACID AND HAIR CELL DIFFERENTIATION

The vitamin A derivative retinoic acid (RA) has been shown to play a role in a number of different developmental systems (reviewed in Morris-Kay and Ward, 1999). RA, as well as some of the enzymes required for its synthesis, have been localized to the developing organ of Corti (Kelley et al., 1993; Ylikowski et al., 1994). The cellular effects of RA are mediated through retinoic acid receptors that are members of the steroid/thyroid family of zinc-finger transcription factors (reviewed in Perlmann and Evans, 1997; Blumberg and Evans, 1998). The RA receptors are grouped into two classes (RXRs and RARs), with the formation of a functional complex requiring one RXR and one RAR. Results of *in situ* hybridization studies indicate that at least one *RAR* (*RARα*) and two *RXRs* (*RXRα* and *RXRγ*) are expressed in the developing organ of Corti (Romand et al., 1998; Raz and Kelley, 1999).

The cellular effects of RA during development of the organ of Corti have been examined in both gain- and loss-of-function experiments. Kelley et al. (1993) added exogenous RA to cochlear cultures established at specific dates between E13 and P0. Results indicated that exposure to RA leads to a significant increase in the number of cells that develop as hair cells. This effect was dependent on the dose of RA added, as well as on the timing of addition. More recently, Raz and Kelley (1999) used an RARα-specific antagonist to block the activation of RA receptors in embryonic cochlear cultures. The results were consistent with the effects of exogenous RA. Increasing concentrations of the antagonist led to increasing inhibition of hair cell formation. This effect was also dependent on the timing of addition of the antagonist, with exposure at earlier embryonic time points (E13 to E15) leading to a greater disruption of the development of the organ of Corti.

The specific effects of RA have not been completely determined. Based on the observation that addition of exogenous RA leads to an increase in both hair cells and supporting cells, Kelley et al. (1993) suggested that RA might play a role in the determination of the size of the prosensory cell population. However, Raz and Kelley (1999) demonstrated that while inhibition of RA receptor activation leads to a decrease in the number of cells that develop as hair cells, this treatment does not disrupt the expression of the early hair cell marker Myosin VI. These results suggest that RA may in fact be required for the differentiation of cells as hair cells rather than for the determination of cells as prosensory cells. The observed increase in both hair cells and supporting cells in the presence of exogenous RA might be the result of subsequent inductive interactions between hair cells and supporting cells (Raz and Kelley, 1999).

THYROID HORMONE AND COCHLEAR DEVELOPMENT

A second member of the steroid/thyroid signaling pathway that has been demonstrated to play a role in development of the organ of Corti is thyroid hormone. This topic is discussed further in Chapter 35. Classic studies by Deol (1973a; b; 1976) and Uziel et al. (1980) demonstrated significant disruptions in the formation of the organ of Corti in embryos that developed in pregnant females that were made hypothyroid through administration of the synthetic antagonist methimizole. The primary phenotypes in the cochleae of these animals were defects in the formation of the tectorial membrane, incomplete maturation of the organ of Corti, and ultimately degeneration of at least some outer hair cells. Similar results have been observed in the cochleae of *hyt* mice, which are hypothyroid as a result of a mutation in the TSH receptor (O'Malley et al., 1995). In addition, analysis of the morphology of stereociliary bundles on hair cells that are present in *hyt* mice indicates that at least some of the bundles appear deformed or absent (Li et al., 1999). These results strongly suggested that thyroid hormone plays an important role in the development of the organ of Corti. However, because hypothyroidism can have broad biological effects, it was not clear whether the effects on the development of the cochlea were direct or indirect.

More recently, the potential direct effects of thyroid hormone signaling in the ear have been examined through an analysis of the expression of thyroid hormone receptors and thyroid hormone synthetic enzymes in the cochlea. Two different thyroid receptors (*TRs*) — *TRα* and *TRβ* with two splice variants for each — have been identified (reviewed in Forrest and Vennstrom, 2000). Functional receptor complexes are comprised of a dimer pair that can be either a homodimer of TRs or a heterodimer pair of one *TR* with one *RXR* (reviewed in Perlmann and Evans, 1997; Blumberg and Evans, 1998). Results of *in situ* hybridizations for *TRα* and *TRβ* indicate that, during the late embryonic and early postnatal periods, *TRα* is expressed in all developing sensory epithelia within the ear, including the cochlea and developing ganglia (Bradley et al., 1994; Lautermann and ten Cate, 1997). Interestingly, during these same time periods, $TR\beta$ expression is restricted to the developing sensory epithelia of the cochlea (Bradley et al., 1994). In addition, a newly described deiodinase ($D2$), required for the conversion of thyroid hormone to the active T3 form, is expressed in the developing connective tissue in the cochlea in a pattern that is complementary to $TR\beta$ (Campos-Barros et al., 2000). This spatial pattern of expression suggests that local concentrations of T3 within the cochlea may be significantly increased over the concentrations in other areas of the body (Campos-Barros et al., 2000). These results clearly suggest that signaling by thyroid hormone probably plays a direct role in the development of the cochlea.

To begin to address the different potential effects of thyroid hormone during cochlear development, several labs have used molecular biological techniques to examine specific effects of thyroid signaling. Forrest et al. (1996) generated a mutant mouse with a specific deletion of the $TR\beta$ gene to examine the effects of signaling through this receptor. Results indicated that these animals develop with an approximate threshold shift of 40 dB SPL, but the overall morphology of the organ of Corti in these animals appears normal. Subsequent studies demonstrated that at least one specific defect in the $TR\beta$ mutant mice was a delay in the maturation of the $I_{K,f}$ fast-acting potassium conductance in inner hair cells (Rusch et al., 1998a; b). However, deletion of $TR\beta$ resulted in a delay of the development of this conductance, not in an absence; thus it is not clear whether the permanent threshold shift that develops in these animals is a result of this delay or of other, as yet undetermined, defects.

As discussed, although the $TR\beta$ mutant mice develop with a permanent hearing loss, the overall morphology of the cochlea in these mice appears normal (Forrest et al., 1996). In addition, mice containing a deletion of the $TR\alpha$ gene have no defects in the cochlea (Barros et al., 1998). These results contrast with the observed morphological disruptions that occur in the cochleae of hypothyroid animals (see above) and suggest that the two receptors may be able to compensate for one another (Barros et al., 1998). To begin to address this issue, Forrest and colleagues have begun to generate compound mutants that contain deletions of both TR genes, and preliminary results suggest that the morphology of the cochleae in these animals more closely resembles the morphology of the cochleae in hypothyroid mice (Rusch et al., 1998a; b). Therefore, these results are consistent with the hypothesis that thyroid hormone plays a direct role in the development of the cochlea.

While the results described above strongly suggest that signaling through thyroid hormone is required for the normal development of the cochlea, the specific effects of thyroid hormone have not been determined. However, thyroid hormone is a key regulator of the rate of cellular differentiation, and the results of several experiments suggest that this may be the main effect of thyroid hormone in the cochlea as well. As discussed with respect to hypothyroid animals, the morphology of the organ of Corti appears consistent with the hypothesis that the development of the organ of Corti has been arrested at an immature stage (Deol, 1973a; b; 1976; Uziel et al., 1980; Knipper et al., 1999). Similarly, the results of one study demonstrated that the onset of hearing is accelerated in hyperthyroid animals, suggesting that thyroid hormone may regulate the pace of cochlear development (Brunjes and Alberts, 1981). Finally, recent studies have identified at least two genes, $TrkB$ and $p75^{NGFR}$, that show a developmental delay in expression in hypothyroid animals (Knipper et al., 1999). The implications of disruptions in the expression of these genes during development will be discussed in the section on the development of cochlear innervation.

In summary, a number of genes and signaling pathways have been found to be required for the differentiation of specific cells within the organ of Corti. The roles of the POU domain gene $Brn\ 3.1$ and of the thyroid hormone signaling pathway are particularly interesting because each of these factors has been shown to play a role in congenital deafness in humans (Vahava et al., 1998). Mutations of the $Brn4/Pou3f4$ are discussed in Chapter 39. However, despite recent advances, our present understanding of the factors that interact to coordinate the differentiation of all the different cell types within the cochlea is still fairly limited (but see Chapter 35).

INNERVATION OF THE ORGAN OF CORTI

The cellular development of the organ of Corti must be intimately linked with the corresponding innervation by both afferent and efferent fibers (see also Chapter 9 for a detailed discussion). In fact, the observation that the arrival of spiral ganglion neurites coincides with morphological differentiation of cells as hair cells led to the long-held hypothesis that neurites induce hair cell differentiation. While this hypothesis has not been supported by experimental data, the precise tonotopic gradient of innervation present in the adult mammalian cochlea must be a result of complex interactions between the developing organ of Corti and entering neural fibers.

DEVELOPMENT OF THE SAG

The auditory and vestibular neurons of the eighth cranial nerve ganglia arise between E9 and E14 in the mouse (Ruben, 1967), and initially form as a single complex called the statoacoustic ganglion (SAG) or cochleovestibular ganglion (CVG). The neuroblasts form primarily along the anteroventral region of the otocyst (Li et al., 1978) where they then delaminate and migrate to form the ganglia (Hemond and Morest, 1991a; b). In contrast to the pattern of terminal mitosis described for hair cells, the spiral ganglion neurons are born in a basal-to-apical gradient within the ganglion (Ruben, 1967). The molecules that control the formation and migration of the SAG neurons are not fully understood. However, a recent report has shown that mice lacking the transcription factor *Neurogenin1* (*Ngn1*) fail to develop an SAG (Ma et al., 1998). Neurogenins appear to regulate neuroblast delamination, as well as the expression of downstream basic helix-loop-helix proteins such as *NeuroD*, *Math3*, and *NSCL1*, that are thought to ultimately regulate neuronal differentiation (Ma et al., 1998). Therefore, *Ngn1* may regulate SAG neuron migration, differentiation, or both.

FIBER EXTENSION AND GUIDANCE CUES

Soon after delamination and condensation of the SAG, individual neurons begin to extend dendritic fibers back into the developing cochlear duct. Type I spiral ganglion neurons (92 to 94% of afferent neurons) give rise to radial afferent fibers that enter the epithelium at about E16 and innervate inner hair cells near their point of innervation (reviewed by Sobkowicz, 1992). During embryonic development, fibers extend collaterals to more than one inner hair cell; but in the mature organ of Corti, these collaterals are lost and each radial nerve fiber innervates only a single inner hair cell. However, each inner hair cell may be contacted by as many as 20 afferent fibers. The afferent outer spiral fibers (6 to 8% of the afferent neurons) that innervate outer hair cells not only branch to provide collaterals to nearby inner hair cells, but also extend close to the basilar membrane, across the forming tunnel of Corti, to enter the outer hair cell region. A single such fiber can provide collateral branches to outer hair cells in the basal, middle, and apical turns of the organ of Corti (Sobkowicz, 1992). Some of these collaterals may be lost by maturity (Berglund and Ryugo, 1987); but even in the mature organ of Corti, a single outer spiral fiber can innervate five or more outer hair cells. In the adult, these outer spiral fibers can reach 200 to 470 µm in length (Bergland and Ryugo, 1987).

During their initial migration from the wall of the otic placode, the SAG neuroblasts do not appear to maintain any attachments with the differentiating sensory epithelium. Therefore, nerve fibers must extend back across the wall of the otocyst for innervation to occur (Whitehead and Morest, 1985). The otocyst itself appears to provide factors that help initiate the outgrowth of nerve fibers back across the wall of the otocyst. Tissue culture experiments demonstrated that mouse SAG fibers are able to grow into both the original otocyst as well as a second otocyst transplanted next to the SAG (Van De Water and Ruben, 1984). The otocyst also appears to be a source of survival-promoting factors. Tissue culture preparations of chick tissues show an increase in SAG survival when the otocyst and SAG are cultured intact, compared to when the SAG is cultured alone (Ard and Morest, 1985).

Subsequent *in vitro* studies demonstrated that the otocyst also releases a diffusible factor (otocyst-derived factor [ODF]) that influences the survival and outgrowth of early-stage SAG (Lefebvre et al., 1990; Bianchi and Cohan, 1991). This unidentified factor is secreted by chick, mouse, and rat otocysts during a time period that corresponds to the period of initial neurite outgrowth (E4–6 in chick; E10–12 in mouse; E11–14 in rat). In addition, ODF is not species specific, in that mouse and rat ODF can stimulate outgrowth of chick and rat SAG, and chick ODF can promote outgrowth of rat and mouse SAG (Bianchi and Cohan, 1993). Both the experiments demonstrating contacted mediated outgrowth and the studies of diffusible factors noted a limited developmental period for the outgrowth promoting effect (Van De Water and Ruben, 1984; Bianchi and Cohan, 1991).

The identity of the otocyst-derived factor (ODF) has not yet been determined. Brain-derived neurotrophic factor (BDNF) and neurotrophin-3 (NT-3), members of the neurotrophin gene family, a group of soluble factors that promote survival and outgrowth of developing neurons, have been detected in the developing inner ear at stages of initial neurite outgrowth and the time of ODF production (i.e., E11–14 mouse, rat; Pirvola et al., 1992; 1994; 1997; Ylikoski et al., 1993; Wheeler et al., 1994; Schecterson and Bothwell, 1994). In addition, mRNA for the receptors for BDNF and NT-3 (*trk B* and *trk C*, respectively) are also present in developing cochlear and vestibular ganglia at the stages of initial innervation (Pirvola et al., 1992; 1994; 1997; Ylikoski et al., 1993; Wheeler et al., 1994; Schecterson and Bothwell, 1994; Bernd et al., 1994). Therefore, BDNF and NT-3 appeared as likely candidates for ODF. However, when the biological activity of the ODF was compared to that of purified neurotrophins, the ODF was found to not contain neurotrophin-like bioactivity. None of the neurotrophins (nerve growth factor [NGF]; BDNF, NT-3; neurotrophin-4/5 [NT-4/5]) produced survival or outgrowth that was comparable to that obtained with ODF (Bianchi and Cohan, 1993). In addition, ODF did not promote outgrowth from other ganglia known to respond to one or more of the neurotrophins. Specifically, ODF failed to promote outgrowth from dorsal root, sympathetic, or trigeminal neurons at the stages that they respond to neurotrophins (Bianchi and Cohan, 1993). It is important to note that other studies have reported some outgrowth from early-stage SAG explants in response to neurotrophins (Lefebvre et al., 1990; Avila et al., 1993; Pirvola et al., 1994). However, while not directly assessed, when the outgrowth shown in these studies is compared to that seen with ODF, it appears to be less. Thus, while the addition of neurotrophins may induce some growth in some culture preparations, the existing data suggest that neurotrophins do not represent a significant component of the ODF (Bianchi and Cohan, 1993; Bianchi et al., 1998) and do not play a role in initiating SAG nerve fiber outgrowth.

The precise mechanisms that direct fiber outgrowth to the proper hair cell type and appropriate region of the organ of Corti are unknown, but it seems likely that specific guidance cues are present within the cochlea. Extracellular matrix (ECM) molecules often provide favorable substrates for neurite growth, and their location in key areas of the cochlea would presumably help to direct fiber growth to appropriate target cells. A variety of ECM and cell surface proteins have been detected in the chick and rodent inner ear and/or cochlear neurons, including fibronection, laminin, neural cell adhesion molecule (NCAM), entactin, and cytotactin/tenascin C (Richardson et al., 1987; Woolf et al., 1992; Cosgrove and Rodgers, 1997; Whitlon et al., 1999; Whitlon et al., 2000). NCAM appears to be a strong candidate for directing fiber growth in the cochlea. In mice, NCAM immunoreactivity in the cochlea is detected from E17 (the earliest stage examined) through P7 (Whitlon and Rutishauser, 1990). Immunoreactivity is noted in all of the nerve fibers surrounding the inner and outer hair cells and in the basilar membrane. Therefore, the temporospatial distribution of NCAM suggests that it may play a role in directing afferent and/or efferent fibers into the organ of Corti during the period of nerve-target recognition and early synaptogenesis (Whitlon and Rutishauser, 1990).

Tenascin C immunoreactivity is also expressed at high levels in areas of nerve fiber growth from E14 (the earliest stage examined) to P9 in the mouse (Whitlon et al., 1999). Decreased immunoreactivity was reported after the period of early synaptogenesis (after P12); however, mice lacking tenascin have auditory reflexes and cochlear anatomy appears normal. Thus, while tenascin may normally contribute to nerve fiber growth, other molecules may compensate for its absence.

In addition to ECM molecules, other cell-surface proteins are also expressed in the inner ear and may direct nerve fiber growth. Recent studies in the visual system have revealed a family of molecules that direct ingrowing retinal nerve fibers via inhibitory cues. This family, termed the Eph family (named for the first receptor from which it was cloned), consists of 14 receptor tyrosine kinases and eight ligands. The ligands in this family, termed ephrins, are all membrane anchored. One class of ligands (ephrin-A) is linked to the cell membrane by a GPI linkage. The other subclass (ephrin-B) contains transmembrane associated ligands (Gale et al., 1996). The ligands appear to function through direct cell-cell contact (S. Davis et al., 1994), and the demonstration that several Eph receptors and ephrin ligands are expressed in adjacent cells further supports a requirement for direct cell-cell contact (Gale et al., 1996). Within each subclass there is considerable binding promiscuity such that all ephrin-A ligands are able to bind to all EphA receptors, although with varying affinities. Conversely, all ephrin-B ligands can bind to all EphB receptors, again with varying affinities (Brambilla and Klein, 1995; Gale et al., 1996).

Whether Eph molecules regulate the development of tonotopic innervation to the inner ear is not yet clear. Several studies have reported Eph expression in the developing inner ear and associated cochlear and vestibular neurons (Henkemeyer et al., 1994; Ciossek et al., 1995; Ellis et al., 1995; Lee et al., 1996; Rinkwitz-Brandt et al., 1996; Pickles and van Heuman, 1997; Bianchi and Gale, 1998; Bianchi and Liu, 1999). Many Eph molecules are also located at tissue boundaries and areas separating perilymph and endolymph, suggesting they may have functions beyond nerve target interactions (Bianchi and Gale, 1998; Bianchi and Liu, 1999; Cowan et al., 2000).

At the period of initial neurite outgrowth and target innervation, several Eph receptors and ligands of both subclasses are detected in early SAG cell bodies or nerve fibers (Henkemeyer et al., 1994; Bianchi and Gale, 1998; Bianchi and Liu, 1999). Compared to the other Eph molecules studied to date, ephrin-B2 ligand appears to be the most highly expressed on SAG fibers at the period of initial target innervation (E12–14 mouse; Bianchi, 1999). The B subclass of ligands is particularly interesting because these transmembrane bound ligands contain a cytoplasmic domain that is phosphorylated on tyrosine upon binding to an EphB receptor (Holland et al., 1996; Bruckner et al., 1997). Thus, these ligands display bi-directional signaling, meaning that both the receptor and ligands are able to produce intracellular signaling events.

In the developing inner ear, EphB receptors can be used to direct ephrin-B2 expressing SAG fibers to the appropriate targets. Preliminary studies suggest that addition of EphB to eprhin-B2 expressing SAG fibers in vitro leads to a loss of neurites (Bianchi, 1999; 2000). These results suggest that EphB receptors in the cochlea may provide inhibitory cues that direct growth of SAG fibers to appropriate target cells (Bianchi and Gale, 1998; Bianchi, 1999; 2000).

One of the Eph receptors known to be highly expressed in early stages of SAG development is EphB2 (E11.5–12.5 mouse; Henkemeyer et al., 1994). However, mice lacking the kinase (signaling) portion of the EphB2 receptor show apparently normal afferent innervation to cochlear and vestibular epithelium (Cowan et al., 2000). Considering the potential for redundancy in binding of Ephs and ephrins, it is very likely that other receptors compensate for the loss of EphB2. EphB1, for example, is also expressed in the SAG at the same developmental time point (Bianchi and Gale, 1998). In contrast to afferent innervation to the inner ear, early growing vestibular efferent fibers appear to require EphB2, at least transiently. Mice engineered to lack the kinase portion of the EphB2 receptor reveal a temporary delay in the growth of efferent fibers from the brainstem to vestibular epithelium (Cowan et al., 2000). Interestingly, following a 1- to 2-day delay in growth, the efferent fibers ultimately catch up and innervate their targets.

NEUROTROPHINS AND NEURONAL SURVIVAL

Target tissues not only provide cues to promote and direct nerve fiber outgrowth, but can also provide trophic support to maintain survival of developing neurons. Nerve growth factors from the neurotrophin family have been found to be particularly important in maintaining the survival of cochlear and vestibular neurons, and this topic is discussed in some detail in Chapter 11. Both BDNF and NT-3 mRNA are detected in the otocyst and maturing cochlea and vestibular apparatus. In the cochlea, BDNF is expressed in both inner and outer hair cells and supporting cells through at least the first postnatal week (Pirvola et al., 1992; Ylikoski et al., 1993; Schecterson and Bothwell, 1994). NT-3 is initially expressed in inner and outer cochlear hair cells and supporting cells, and then becomes restricted to inner hair cells by P7–P9 (rat; Pirvola et al., 1992; Ylikoski et al., 1993). TrkB and trkC receptors, which bind BDNF and NT-3, respectively, are expressed throughout the cochlear and vestibular ganglion in an apparently overlapping fashion (Pirvola et al., 1992; Schecterson and Bothwell, 1994; Wheeler et al., 1994). The expression patterns of BDNF and NT-3 mRNA suggested that these molecules were likely to be important for regulating cochlear and vestibular neuron survival, but it was not until the production of transgenic mice lacking one or more of the neurotrophins or trk receptors that we began to understand the role of these factors in the cochlea.

Comparison of BDNF, NT-3, and compound BDNF/NT-3 knock-out mice demonstrated that by postnatal stages, mice lacking BDNF have a nearly complete loss of vestibular neurons, with only a small loss of cochlear neurons; whereas mice lacking NT-3 have a significant, although incomplete loss of cochlear neurons and only a small reduction in vestibular neurons. In addition, mice lacking both BDNF and NT-3 show a nearly complete loss of innervation to both vestibular and cochlear regions (Ernfors et al., 1995; Bianchi et al., 1996; Fritzsch et al., 1997a). Furthermore, mice lacking the receptors for these neurotrophins, trkB and trkC, respectively, also showed a reduction in cochlear and vestibular neurons (Fritzsch et al., 1995; reviewed in Fritzsch et al., 1997b). Thus, BDNF and NT-3 are critical for the survival of cochlear and vestibular neurons at some period during embryonic development. The time course for neurotrophin dependence appears to begin after E13.5. In mice lacking both trkB and trkC receptors, initial nerve fiber extension toward the inner ear is observed, but a loss of nerve fibers begins after E13.5 (Fritzsch et al., 1995). In mice lacking BDNF, the early-stage SAG shows no reduction in fiber extension; however, a progressive loss of afferent innervation to vestibular structures is detected from E13.5–E15. A decrease in vestibular ganglion volume and neuronal number is detectable by E16.5–17, and continued loss of neurons is noted through the second postnatal week (Bianchi et al., 1996). Analysis of neurotrophin protein production using bioassays and enzyme-linked immunosorbent assays further indicated that production of neurotrophins begins at mid-embryonic stages (Bianchi et al., 1998). Thus, bioasssays, transgenic mice, and protein analyses reveal that specific neurotrophins are produced by the inner ear and appear to be required for cochlear and vestibular neuron survival beginning at mid-embryogenesis.

Trophic factors may also to be required for cochlear and vestibular neuron survival at later stages of development. For example, levels of BDNF appear to increase at the time of synaptic reorganization in postnatal rats and mice (Wiechers et al., 1999); and by comparison with newborns, levels of BDNF are increased in the adult gerbil organ of Corti (Medd and Bianchi, 2000). Temporal changes in glia cell line-derived neurotrophic factor (GDNF) have also been noted. In the rat cochlea, GDNF is not detected from E16 to P5, but is first detected at P7 in both inner and outer hair cells in the basal turn of the cochlea. By P9, hair cells throughout the cochlea express GDNF. However, in the adult, only inner hair cells express mRNA for GDNF (Ylikoski et al., 1998). In vitro analysis revealed only a weak survival promoting effect of GDNF on cochlear neurons at E21, but a significant effect at P7 (Ylikoski et al., 1998). Other studies reveal that various factors can promote similar levels of cochlear neuron survival at postnatal stages. For example, survival of cochlear neurons (P5, rat) can be maintained in the presence of BDNF, NT-3, a cAMP analog, or membrane depolarization (Hegarty et al., 1997). Therefore, by postnatal stages, cochlear neuron survival may be dependent on a number of factors, provided either sequentially or in combination.

In summary, there are several soluble and membrane-associated proteins produced in the cochlea at specific stages of development that contribute to the complex, yet highly organized pattern of nerve fiber innervation. In recent years, our understanding of the cellular cues required for normal inner ear innervation has been greatly advanced, particularly through the use of *in vitro* assays and transgenic mice. As with other developing neuronal populations, innervation to the inner ear appears to rely on a variety of soluble and cell-associated cues that influence the outgrowth, guidance, and survival of SAG neurons.

SUMMARY AND FUTURE DIRECTIONS

This is an exiting time for the study of cochlear development. After years of descriptive analysis of the morphological development of the organ of Corti, we are now poised to begin to dissect the cellular and molecular interactions that dictate the formation of this exquisite structure. Based on the wealth of existing morphological data and on the general conservation of cellular signaling pathways, a working model of cochlear development has been constructed. This model suggests that progenitor cells within the cochlear duct pass through several rounds of progressive restriction that ultimately results in the partitioning of a highly regulated number of these progenitor cells into specific subsets of cellular phenotypes (Figure 10.2). At the same time, these cells produce specific signals that attract and maintain afferent and efferent projections (Figure 10.3). Finally, the cochlea and the neurons that innervate must coordinate the development of a complex tonotopic pattern.

In just the past 5 years, a number of candidate genes have been shown to be expressed in subsets of cells within the cochlea. More recently, the roles of some of these genes and gene families have been determined. In particular, examination of mice containing targeted deletions of specific genes including the neurotrophins and their receptors, *Brn 3.1*, *Math1*, *Jag2*, and *TRα* and β, have demonstrated specific roles for each of these genes.

However, a number of significant questions remain unanswered. These include: How does the cochlear duct become partitioned into prosensory and non-sensory regions? How is the coordinated exit of prosensory progenitor cells from the cell cycle controlled? What are the factors that determine progenitor cells as hair cells? As discussed, *Math1* has been shown to be necessary and sufficient for the formation of cells as hair cells, and its pattern of expression is consistent with a gene that plays a role in hair cell determination. However, it is not clear that *Math1* is the earliest determination factor for the hair cell phenotype. In addition, the factors that determine inner vs. outer hair cells are also not known. The two genes that have been shown to be required for development of hair cells, *Math1* and *Brn 3.1*, are expressed equally in both inner and outer hair cells. Therefore, it seems unlikely that these genes play a role in the determination of hair cells as either inner hair cells or outer hair cells.

Further, the number of cells that develop as hair cells is clearly regulated through cellular interactions, but it is not clear whether these interactions are solely mediated through the Notch-signaling pathway. Questions that remain to be resolved in this area include: If the Notch pathway is solely responsible, then why isn't the number of hair cells that develop in *Jag2* mutant mice even higher? If the Notch pathway is not the only factor involved in regulating the number of cells that develop as hair cells, then what other factors might be involved? Once a population of hair cells is established, how are other progenitor cells recruited to form the population of surrounding supporting cells? How are specific types of supporting cells determined?

Once cell fate is determined, how is the structural basis for frequency specificity determined? How do afferent and efferent fibers find and make synapses with frequency-matched inner and outer hair cells? Fundamental questions such as these, as well as other questions related to the overall formation of the cochlea and the maturation of the cochlea will continue to be addressed during the next several years. Our understanding of cochlear development will likely be advanced by continued identification of molecules present in the developing organ of Corti and spiral ganglion, and identification of the function of these molecules through *in vitro* and *in vivo* manipulations.

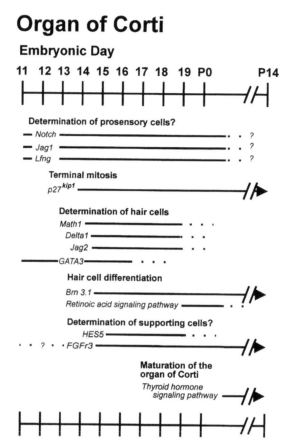

FIGURE 10.2 Timeline of gene expression in the developing organ of Corti. Important developmental events are listed based on the approximate time at which they are initiated. In addition, developmental genes that are known to be expressed or that have been shown to play a role in each event are listed below that event. Solid lines indicate known gene expression, while dotted lines indicate a gradual decrease in expression. Question marks indicate that factors that play a role in that event or the expression of a particular gene at that time point have not been determined. Functional data confirming the role of each gene have been obtained for all genes listed, except *Jag1, Dll1, Lfng, GATA3,* and *HES5.* Almost nothing is known about the determination of the prosensory cell population except that the three genes listed are expressed in prosensory cells from very early time points and ultimately become restricted to supporting cells. Similarly, with the exception of FGFr3, there is very little data regarding the factors that play a role in the determination of supporting cell fates.

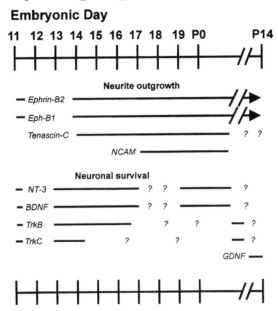

FIGURE 10.3 Timeline of expression for genes associated with neuronal pathfinding and survival. Timing of initiation of neurite outgrowth and neurotrophin-dependent survival are indicated by position of headings for each event. Solid lines indicate known expression of genes that have been implicated in either outgrowth or survivial. Question marks indicate time points where expression has not been determined. Functional data have confirmed the roles of neurotrophins and their receptors, and preliminary results indicate a functional role for ephrin-B2 as well. See text for details.

11 The Role of Neurotrophic Factors in the Development and Maintenance of Innervation in the Mouse Inner Ear

Hinrich Staecker, Stuart Apfel, and Thomas R. Van De Water

INTRODUCTION

The discovery of nerve growth factor opened a new era of understanding of neurobiology. For example, Cajal (1928) had used histologic techniques to demonstrate the capacity of a severed axon to grow back toward a target, and the discovery of trophic factors explained these observations. Nerve growth factor (NGF) has become the model for studying trophic factor function in the central and peripheral nervous system. Growth factors are now known to be involved in every step of neuronal biology, from development to maturation and phenotype determination. Many trophic factors are target derived and are responsible for maintaining healthy innervation. Loss of target and subsequent loss of growth factor production result in the degeneration of innervation through apoptosis. This effect was elegantly demonstrated in Spoendlin's studies of ototoxicity in the cat (Spoendlin, 1988).

Both the NGF family of growth factors (neurotrophins) as well as a host of other growth factors have been demonstrated to play important roles in the development and maintenance of the inner ear. The bulk of research on growth factors has been carried out in mice; however, many of the growth factors discussed in this chapter have significant homology to human growth factors, making this an important area for understanding human otologic disease. This chapter reviews the basic biology of several prominent growth factors that are active in the auditory/vestibular system and discusses their importance and potential applications in the treatment of otologic disease.

A general definition for a neurotrophic factors is a substance that will promote the survival of neurons. Included in this definition would be important metabolites such as sodium, potassium, glucose, amino acids, oxygen, etc. While these are essential for neuronal survival, they are not considered to be neurotrophic factors. Substances considered to be neurotrophic factors can do more than just promote survival. Many neurotrophic factors influence morphological differentiation (e.g., cell size and neurite elongation); others direct the physiological maturation of neurons (e.g., neurotransmitter synthesis). To clarify the definition of neurotrophic fators, we briefly review how the concept of neurotrophic factors evolved. The term "trophic" is derived from the Greek word *trophikos*, meaning nourishment; "neurotrophic" means "neuron nourishing." While studying peripheral nerve degeneration, Waller (1852) observed that nerves degenerate distal to a lesion, while new fibers originate from the "central portion," which maintained continuity with the "trophic centers" in the spinal cord. These trophic centers provided the "nourishment" necessary to maintain

0-8493-2328-2/01/$0.00+$.50

the integrity of the nerve. The distal portion of the nerve no longer in contact with the trophic center, lacked trophic support and therefore degenerated (Waller 1852; Cajal, 1928). The neurotrophic hypothesis of nerve growth began with the observation that nerve fibers from the proximal stump of a severed nerve show a preference for entering the distal stump (Forsmann, 1898). The term "tropic" is derived from the Greek word *tropikos*, meaning to turn or change direction. A "neurotropic" substance, therefore, is one that attracts a nerve, causing it to turn or change its path. Most neurotrophic substances are also neurotropics. Forsmann, experimenting with nerve regeneration, tested the hypothesis that neurotropic substances attracted the regenerating nerve fibers. He suggested that the attractive tropic substance was a lipoidal product of the degenerating myelin sheath that surrounds the nerve. Ramon y Cajal disagreed with Forsmann's suggestion. Cajal had earlier proposed a "chemotactic hypothesis" to explain a variety of phenomena that he and others in the field had observed in regenerating nerves (Cajal, 1892), preceding Forsmann's coining of the term "neurotrophic" (Forsmann, 1898). Cajal was fascinated by the observation that even nerves separated by significant distances tended to grow together toward their prospective targets (Cajal, 1928). Cajal's chemotactic hypothesis sought to explain this neural regeneration phenomenon and nerve-target interaction in developing embryos by proposing that young axons are oriented in their growth by stimuli from "attracting substances" under the form of a soluble, non-lipoidal substance, and that its elaboration is brought about by Schwann cells (Cajal, 1928). He summarized his theory in the statement that, "The neurotrophic stimulus acts as a ferment or enzyme, provoking protoplasmic assimilation...the orienting agent does not operate through attraction, as many have supposed, but by creating a favorable, eminently trophic, and stimulative of the assimilation and growth of the newly formed axons" (Cajal, 1928). In the 1930s, Hamburger (1934) excised the wing bud of a 72-hour chick embryo, and observed that both the anterior spinal cord and the spinal sensory ganglia on the operated side became severely hypoplastic. This finding suggested that neuronal survival-promoting (neurotrophic) activity was also present in the peripheral field.

THE DEVELOPMENT OF THE AUDITORY SYSTEM

To understand the mechanics of trophic factor function, it is important to first understand the sequence of auditory innervation during normal development. For simplicity, we review only the development of afferent innervation (see Chapters 9 and 10 for a detailed discussion of development). Unless specified, all research was carried out in mice. At E8 (gestation day), the otic placode, destined to become the neurosensory epithelium of both the cochlear vestibular organs, begins to invaginate to form the otic vesicle. Shortly before the completion of this step (E9), a group of cells is identifiable at the basal end of the otic flask that are destined to become the ganglion cells of both the spiral and vestibular ganglia (Ruben, 1967). These neurons can be identified by immunostaining with anti 66 kD neurofilament by E10.5. Within the next 24 hours, ingrowth into the sensory epithelium has begun. Proliferation of neurons continues to E13 (Ruben, 1967). Hair cells develop between E13 and E14, and afferent synaptogenesis occurs between E18 and 5P (postpartum day) (Sobkowitz et al., 1986). Schwann cells develop between E13 and 7P (Ruben, 1967), leading to myelination of the spiral ganglion processes between 3 and 30P (Romand and Romand, 1990). Finally, staining for various structural proteins and neurotransmitters has shown that maturation of neurons is not completed until about 60P (Sobkowitz, 1992).

THE ROLE OF CHEMOATTRACTIVE FIELDS AND FACTORS IN AUDITORY DEVELOPMENT

The mechanics of trophic fields in early embryonic sensory development were first extensively investigated by Speidel, who showed that denervated lateral line target fields attracted neurons (Speidel, 1948). By co-culturing an otocyst-statoacoustic ganglion complex with otocysts from which the ganglion had been removed, it was shown that neuronal ingrowth occurred in both otocysts (Figure 11.1). This suggested that a chemoattractant field for neurons was being produced

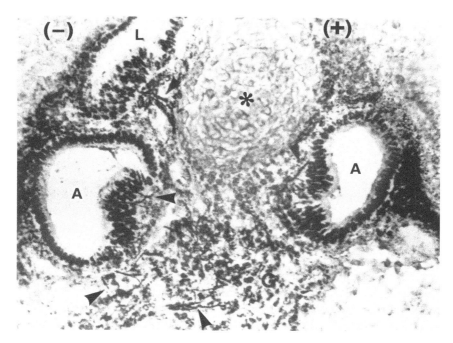

FIGURE 11.1 The trophic effect of sensory epithelium on the cohleovestibular ganglion is demonstrated in this experiment where two otocysts (A) are co-cultured with one ganglion (G). There is ingrowth of neurites into both otocysts (arrow), demonstrating that the otic epithelium produces a growth factor that acts to support and guide ingrowth of neurons.

by the developing sensory epithelium. Similar observations were made in the chick auditory system (Ard et al., 1985). In a further set of experiments, explanted ganglia were cultured alone or in the presence of peripheral (otocyst) or central (rhombencephalon) target tissues. Neuronal survival was found to depend on the presence of either central or peripheral target tissue. If both central and peripheral tissues were present, neuronal survival was even further augmented (Zhou and Van De Water, 1987). These observations led to the theory that a soluble neurotrophic factor such as NGF could be one of the factors driving auditory nerve development.

THE BIOLOGY AND FUNCTION OF NEUROTROPHINS AND OTHER NEUROTROPHIC FACTORS

NERVE GROWTH FACTOR (NGF)

Bueker (1948) investigated the nature of trophic signals released by peripheral organs. He removed embryonic chick limbs and transplanted tumor cells to act as "a uniform histogenetic tissue" substituting for the more complex developing limb. When he implanted a mouse sarcoma 180 tissue in the chick embryo at the site of the extirpated limb, he observed a marked hypertrophy of the associated sensory spinal ganglia. The sarcoma tissue was heavily innervated by ingrowing sensory fibers, but there was no ingrowth of motor nerve fibers. Bueker concluded that the sarcoma tissue possessed intrinsic physicochemical properties and mechanisms of growth that selectively caused enlargement of the spinal ganglia. The fact that spinal ganglia were enlarged, while the lateral motor column was reduced in those segments which innervated sarcoma 180, suggested that this tumor selectively favored the development of one and not the other (Bueker, 1948). Levi-Montalcini and Hamburger repeated these experiments including sarcoma 37 tissue as well (Levi-Montalcini and Hamburger, 1951). They not only confirmed the sensory ganglion hypertrophy reported by Bueker, but also observed a similar response from embryonic sympathetic ganglia. Additionally, they observed that only a select subpopulation of the sensory ganglion neurons were responding to the tumor tissue. Stanley Cohen, working with Levi-Montalcini and Hamburger succeeded in identifying the active factor as either a protein or nucleoprotein (Cohen, Levi-Montalcini, and Hamburger, 1954). Further searching among homologous tissues led them to discover potent neurotrophic activity in tissue extracts of adult male mouse salivary glands (Cohen, 1960). The active protein purified from salivary glands was given the name nerve growth factor (NGF).

OTHER NEUROTROPHINS: BRAIN-DERIVED NEUROTROPHIC FACTOR (BDNF) AND NEUROTROPHINS 3 TO 6 (NT-3, NT-4, NT-5, NT-6)

The realization that NGF does not serve as a neurotrophic factor for all neuronal populations triggered a search for additional factors. Barde, Edgar, and Thoenen (1982) discovered neurotrophic activity in glial conditioned medium that could not be inhibited by NGF antiserum. In their attempts to purify this factor, it was found to be abundant in the pig brain. The new factor was called brain derived neurotrophic factor (BDNF). It was clear from the start that BDNF was trophic for different populations of neurons than NGF. When BDNF was cloned, the structural similarity between NGF and BDNF became apparent with a greater than 50% homology in amino acid sequence (Leibrock et al., 1989). The amino acid sequence homology was most apparent in a few important regions responsible for stabilizing the three dimensional structure of these molecules. These regions contain six cysteine residues that form disulfide bonds between portions of the amino acid chain, and are essential for biological activity of these molecules.

The high degree of structural similarity between NGF and BDNF initiated a search for structurally homologous members of the same gene family, with six laboratories reporting the identification of a new member of the NGF family of neurotrophins designed as neurotrophin-3 (NT-3) (Ernfors et al., 1990; Hohn et al., 1990; Jones and Reichardt, 1990; Kaisho, Yoshuira, and Nakahama, 1990; Maisonpierre et al., 1990; Rosenthal et al., 1990). Halbook and colleagues investigated the evolutionary relationship between the three known neurotrophin molecules (i.e., NGF, BDNF, and NT-3) by constructing phylogenetic trees derived from DNA sequence analysis of the three genes (Halbook, Ibanez, and Persson, 1991). These investigators discovered another novel member of the neurotrophin family isolated from Xenopus and viper (Halbook, Ibanez, and Persson, 1991). This protein, like NGF, BDNF, and NT-3, contains the five highly conserved amino acid regions including the six cysteine residues. Following the established convention, the discoverers named it neurotrophin-4 (NT-4) (Halbook et al., 1991).

A team working at Genentech Inc. reported the discovery of yet another member of the NGF family of neurotrophins isolated from a human placental DNA library, which they designated neurotrophin-5 (NT-5). The NT-5 protein was found to have a greater homology with NT-4 from Xenopus than with the other neurotrophins (Berkemeier et al., 1991). This, together with the similarity in their biological activity, has led many investigators to conclude that NT-5 is in actuality human NT-4. Because NT-4 and NT-5 are likely to be interspecies variations of the same molecule, and have similar activities, they are commonly referred to as NT-4/5.

A new member of the NGF family called neurotrophin-6 (NT-6) has been identified in the teleost fish, Xiphophorus (Gotz et al., 1994). NT-6 is unique in that it is not naturally released into the medium; instead, this neurotrophin requires the addition of heparin. Thus far, NT-6 appears to have a profile of trophic activity similar to NGF, in that it supports both sensory and sympathetic neurons.

HIGH- AND LOW-AFFINITY RECEPTORS

A protein with a molecular weight of 75 kD (p75) was initially identified as a receptor for NGF (Johnson et al., 1986). However, this receptor bound NGF with a dissociation constant (Kd) of 10^{-9} M, which was a lower affinity than the binding affinity that appeared necessary to mediate biological activity (Kd of 10^{-11} M) (Meakin and Shooter, 1991). Other studies revealed a larger NGF receptor, about 135 to 140 kD in size, which was structurally unrelated to the 75-kD protein (Massagué et al., 1981; Meakin and Shooter, 1992). This NGF receptor had tyrosine kinase activity and was shown to bind the NGF ligand with high affinity (Meakin and Shooter, 1991).

THE TRK ONCOGENE (NGF HIGH-AFFINITY RECEPTOR)

Martin-Zanca, Barbacid, and Parada (1990) isolated an interesting oncogene from colon carcinoma cells. They named this oncogene *trk*, with the cellular homolog being the *trk* proto-oncogene. The product of the *trk* proto-oncogene was a protein receptor about 140 kD in size. At the time of its discovery, the ligand that bound the *trk* proto-oncogene receptor was unknown. A study of the pattern of expression of *trk* proto-oncogene message in mouse embryos revealed a pattern of expression in sensory neurons of neural crest origin (Martin-Zanca, Barbacid, and Parada, 1990). These were the same sensory neurons that have been shown to be responsive to NGF. Additional evidence supporting the *trk* proto-oncogene as the high-affinity receptor was provided by the observation that addition of exogenous NGF induced phosphorylation of proto-*trk* on tyrosine in PC-12 cells (Kaplan, Martin-Zanca, and Parada, 1991). The final proof was provided by demonstrating that the protein coded for by the *trk* proto-oncogene did in fact bind NGF with high affinity (Kd of 10^{-11}) (Klein et al., 1991). These results, combined with the fact that the *trk* protein product was 140 kD in size, made a compelling argument. Additional studies have demonstrated that *trk* can mediate the biological effects of NGF without the presence of the p75 low-affinity receptor (Ip et al., 1993; Nebreda et al., 1991).

OTHER NEUROTROPHIN RECEPTORS (TRKB, TRKC)

The low-affinity NGF receptor has been reported to bind BDNF with an affinity roughly equal to that of NGF (Rodriguez-Tebar, Dechant, and Barde, 1990). The high-affinity receptor, *trk*, is more discriminating and binds NGF selectively. Subsequently, it has been determined that the p75 receptor binds all members of the neurotrophin family tested to date with low affinity, but its few known activities have only been associated with NGF binding.

Klein and colleagues reported the identification of *trkB*, a second member of the tyrosine protein kinase family, which shared about 57% homology with the *trkA* gene (Klein et al., 1989a). *In situ* hybridization studies of mouse embryos revealed that *trkB* was expressed throughout the brain, spinal cord, and in some peripheral nervous system ganglia, suggesting that *trkB* may code for a cell surface receptor involved in neurogenesis. In subsequent studies, several groups reported that *trkB* bound BDNF and NT-3 with comparable high affinities (Klein et al., 1991; Soppet et al., 1991; Squinto et al., 1991). Later it was found to bind NT-4/5 as well (Klein, Lamballe, and Barbacid, 1992). All three neurotrophins can bind to *trkB*. However, NT-3 is much less efficient than NGF and BDNF in inducing biological responses through *trkB* binding (Glass et al., 1991; Squinto et al., 1991). Therefore, *trkB* probably does not serve as a receptor for NT-3. Similar findings were made with *trkA*, which also binds NT-3, but only with low biological activity. The existence of a third member of the trk family, called *trkC* was reported in 1991 (Lamballe, Klein, and Barbacid, 1991). This tyrosine kinase receptor bound NT-3 specifically, with high affinity, and mediated its biological activity efficiently, suggesting that *trkC* is the high-affinity receptor for NT-3 (Figure 11.2). Each of these tyrosine kinase receptors have multiple isoforms that are distributed throughout the CNS. *trkB* also has isoforms that lack a catalytic domain. The exact function of these proteins is unknown, but they may function to competitively bind excess growth factor.

OTHER GROWTH FACTORS WITH NEUROTROPHIC ACTIVITY

There are other growth factors that have been shown to possess neurotrophic properties. Some are localized at high concentrations in the brain or other nervous tissues, suggesting a natural role for

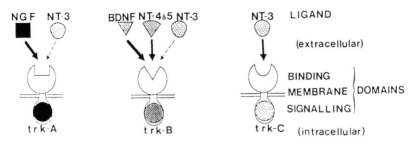

FIGURE 11.2   The neurotrophins bind to three high-affinity tyrosine kinase receptors with NGF binding *trkA*, BDNF binding *trkB*, and NT-3 binding *trkC*. There is, however, a significant overlap in binding (see text).

these factors in the nervous system. Some of these have broad systemic spectrums of action outside the nervous system, thereby rendering their administration more complicated because of the potential for excessive systemic side effects. Whether these proteins prove to be important with respect to the auditory system is unclear, but a brief mention is warranted.

Ciliary Neurotrophic Factor

Studies of ciliary ganglion-target tissues interactions revealed that the targets express a soluble protein that is trophic for the cholinergic neurons of the ciliary ganglion (Adler et al., 1979). This soluble protein was purified and represented a new neurotrophic factor from chick ocular tissues, that is, ciliary neurotrophic factor (CNTF) (Barbin, Manthorpe, and Varon, 1984). CNTF was the third neurotrophic factor to be purified, after NGF and BDNF, but was recognized as being markedly different from these neurotrophins. Additionally, CNTF was the only growth factor discovered that was trophic for parasympathetic neurons, although it had trophic activity for sensory nerves as well (Manthorpe et al., 1982).

Insulin and Its Related Peptides

Insulin is a member of a family of structurally and functionally related proteins that also includes insulin-like growth factors I and II (IGF-I and IGF-II). *In vitro* experiments have shown insulin to be capable of supporting cultured neurons in defined media without a fetal calf serum supplement (Snyder and Kim, 1980; Huck, 1983; Aizenman and de Vellis, 1988). Receptors for insulin are widely distributed in the brain (Baskin, 1987), with their highest concentration in the choroid plexus, olfactory bulb, limbic system structures, and hypothalamus. Insulin receptors in the brain are found primarily on neurons, with few receptors localized to the glia (Han, Lauder, and D'Ercole, 1987). The neurotrophic effects of insulin have been shown to directly affect the neurons without any need for mediation by glial cells (Marks, King, and Baskin, 1991). However, insulin has been demonstrated to stimulate glial cell DNA and RNA synthesis, through interactions with the IGF-I or IGF-II receptors, both of which are present on glial cells and bind insulin with biological activity (Devaskar, 1991). The insulin-like growth factors have broad somatic activities associated with the regulation of body growth during development.

Fibroblast Growth Factor

Fibroblast growth factors (FGFs) were initially isolated from crude brain homogenates that promoted mitogenic activity in cultured fibroblasts. A partial purification of what was believed to be a single FGF protein (Gospodarowicz, 1974) was later shown to be two closely related factors that could be further separated by isoelectric focusing (Lemmon et al., 1982; Thomas, Rios-Candelore, and Fitzpatrick, 1984). One FGF possessed an acidic isoelectric point, and the other FGF had a basic isoelectric point. Therefore, they were designated as acidic (aFGF) and basic (bFGF). The amino acid sequences for these two FGF proteins share about a 55% homology (Gospodarowiz et al., 1984; Esch et al., 1985; Gimenez-Gallego et al., 1986). Despite their close homology, aFGF and bFGF are the products of different genes. Both acidic and basic FGF proteins have similar systemic activities. They are both potent mitogens for cells of mesodermal and neuroectodermal derivation. The responsive cell types include fibroblasts, vascular endothelial cells, chondrocytes, osteoblasts, myoblasts, neuroblasts, and astrocytes (Gospodarowicz et al., 1987; Perraud et al., 1988). In the peripheral nervous system, bFGF enhances the survival dorsal root ganglia (Unsicker, Reichert-Preibsch, and Schmidt, 1987), parasympathetic ciliary ganglia (Dreyer et al., 1989), sympathetic neurons (Eckenstein et al., 1990), and motor neurons (Arakawa, Sendtner, and Thoenen, 1990). The ability of bFGF to promote motor neuron survival can be enhanced by CNTF (Arakawa et al., 1990). Both bFGF and aFGF are able to promote motor and sensory nerve regeneration across a nerve gap pending further evidence for their role as promoters of neural regeneration (Aebischer, Salessiotis, and Winn, 1989; Cordeiro, Seckel, and Lipton, 1989).

Glial Cell Line-Derived Neurotrophic Factor (GDNF)

GDNF is a member of the TGF β superfamily and was first identified as a trophic factor for dopaminergic neurons. The main receptor for GDNF is a glycocosylphosphatidylinositol-anchored surface receptor associated with a low-affinity transmembrane protein (ret) with tyrosine kinase activity. The distribution of ret and GFR α were studied in the rat using *in situ* hybridization. Both ret and GFR α were expressed in the inner ear (Nosrat et al., 1997). An RT PCR study of the inner ear of the rat identified mRNA for GDNF and three related growth factors that are members of the GDNF family (neuturin, artemin, and persephin) are all expressed in the adult rat cochlea and spiral ganglion (Stover et al., 2000).

THE ROLE OF NEUROTROPHINS IN AUDITORY NEURON SURVIVAL

The response of auditory neurons to NGF, as well as binding of ^{123}I-labeled NGF to the E11–14 statoaccoustic ganglion, was clearly demonstrated in cultures of E11–14 ganglia (Lefebvre et al., 1991). These observations were extended to include BDNF and NT-3, which were shown to enhanced survival and neuritogenesis of embryonic avian auditory neurons *in vitro* (Avila et al., 1993). Subsequently, the presence of BDNF and NT-3 and their tyrosine kinase receptors (*trkB* and *trkC*) were documented to be present in the developing sensory neuroepithelium of the otocyst using *in situ* hybridization (Pirvola et al., 1992; Schecterson and Bothwell, 1994).

The actions of neurotrophins were also clearly documented in the early postnatal period, during which time final development and fine-tuning of the auditory system is taking place. *In situ* hybridization studies carried out by Ylikosky et al. (1993) in the 7P rat showed that there was a high level of expression of NT-3 mRNA in the inner hair cells and a lower level of expression in the outer hair cells. BDNF expression localized to the hair cells of the early postnatal organ of Corti, but overall was expressed more strongly in the vestibular system. This study failed to detect the presence of NGF in the inner or outer hair cells. As a correlate, hybridization for neurotrophin receptors showed that both *trkB* and *trkC*, the receptors for BDNF and NT-3, localized to both postnatal spiral and vestibular ganglia (Ylikosky et al., 1993). This study failed to detect the presence of NGF or *trk* in the postnatal organ of Corti. Patterns of hybridization were found to be slightly different in the adult organ of Corti. BDNF was not found to be expressed in the adult organ of Corti, and expression of NT-3 was limited to the inner hair cells. There was also a difference in NT-3 expression levels between the base and apex of the cochlea (Ylikosky et al., 1993). Interestingly, this change in BDNF expression roughly corresponds to the timing of programmed neuronal cell death and the differentiation of a uniform neuronal population into Type I and Type II neurons.

Type I neurons comprise 90% of the neuronal cells of the spiral ganglion and innervate the inner hair cells, thus suggesting that NT-3 may exert a tropic influence on the afferent Type I neurons. A change in BDNF expression was also observed between the postnatal and adult stages. This again suggests that changes in expression of this neurotrophin may affect the process of cochlear maturation. BDNF has been shown to be a survival factor for embryonic neurons (Avila et al., 1993). Thus, a decrease in expression may once again be related to the onset of neuronal cell death.

THE EFFECTS OF NEUROTROPHINS ON THE *IN VITRO* DEVELOPMENT OF AUDITORY NEURONS

To evaluate which of the ever-expanding family of trophic factors is present in the developing ear, work in our laboratory used PCR to amplify cDNA of NGF, BDNF, and NT-3 in the E12 mouse otocyst-statoacoustic ganglion complex. Using reverse transcription of pooled mRNA extracted from 12 E mouse otocysts, we demonstrated that cDNA for NGF, BDNF, and NT-3 could be amplified with PCR. These data were confirmed by sequencing the accumulated reaction product, thus demonstrating that all three of these trophic factors are present in the otocyst during the time at which innervation is actively occurring (Sher, 1971; Galinovic-Schwartz et al., 1991). It is unclear as to why previous studies did not detect NGF. Possibly, levels of NGF mRNA are too low to be detected by *in situ* hybridization.

To more clearly identify possible functions for these trophic factors, their exact histological location was pinpointed using *in situ* reverse transcription PCR (IS-RT PCR). This technique relies on the application of the PCR reaction on a tissue section. NGF mRNA reaction product localized not only to the otic epithelium, but interestingly also to the developing otic capsule and spiral ganglion. This may suggest that NGF is not only produced by the otic epithelium and thus influences growth of neurons, but that it may also play a role in the development of the ganglion itself. Amplification of BDNF and NT-3 showed accumulation of amplification product within the otic epithelium, confirming previous *in situ* hybridization studies (Pirvola et al., 1992).

To functionally assess the role of these trophic factors, we used an organotypic organ culture system. As previously discussed, the first spiral neuronal cells are identifiable in the E10 spiral ganglion (Rugh, 1968) with mitosis continuing through E14 (Ruben, 1967). The otocyst-statoacoustic ganglion complex can be microsurgically excised from an E10 mouse embryo and cultured in defined medium, allowing observation of the developmental processes described above (Van De Water, 1986). Through the addition of trophic factors or down-regulation of their production, the development of innervation could be observed and potential roles for these growth factors determined. We chose to use antisense oligonucleotides to down-regulate neurotrophin production because they were more specific than antibodies. Specific sense and antisense oligonucleotides were synthesized against 5′ regions of NGF, BDNF, and NT-3 mRNA. Two sets of unique sense and antisense oligonucleotides were synthesized for each trophic factor to ensure specificity. Using the oligonucleotide analysis program Oligo, it was determined that there was no cross-hybridization between each of the oligos and other neurotrophins. Addition of a 5 mM concentration of NGF antisense oligonucleotide to an E10 otocyst-statoacoustic ganglion (SAG) culture resulted in an 80% down-regulation in NGF production, determined by ELISA. The effect of the other oligonucleotides on BDNF or NT-3 production could not be determined because no reliable ELISA is available (Staecker et al., 1996).

After addition of oligonucleotide, cultures were maintained for 72 hours and then fixed. The cultures were then double-labeled for laminin (present in the otocyst basement membrane) and 66-kD neurofilament, which highlighted the afferent auditory neurons of the SAG. Analysis with confocal microscopy after 3 days *in vitro* with different oligonucleotides allowed us to count the total number of neurons within a ganglion, trace and measure neuritic growth, and determine ingrowth onto the otocyst. Interestingly, inhibition of production of each of the neurotrophins resulted in a unique effect. Addition of equivalent concentrations of NGF, BDNF, or NT-3 sense oligonucleotide (5 m*M*) resulted in normal development, demonstrating that at 5 m*M*, the oligo-nucleotides have no inherent neurotoxic activity (Staecker et al., 1996).

Control cultures grown for 72 hours showed the development of a healthy SAG with a total neuron count of 15,520 ± 3760. A single dominant neuritic bundle could be traced along the path of the developing otocyst for >200 mm. On average, 7.5 neuritic bundles penetrated the basement membrane of the otocyst. Cultures treated with 5 m*M* NSF, BDNF, or NT-3 sense oligos resembled the control groups. Treatment of an E10 otocyst-SAG complex with antisense BDNF oligonucle-otide (BDNF-AS) resulted in degeneration of neurons. Average total neuron counts were 8348 ± 2218 for oligo 1. Antisense oligo 2 showed a similar average total neuron count, representing a 47% decrease in neuronal count compared to controls and sense oligo treated cultures. The neurons appeared rounded and dense, with no evidence of any neuritic outgrowth. Because some neuritic outgrowth is present at E10, decrease in BDNF production through addition of antisense oligonu-cleotide clearly resulted in neuronal degeneration, leading to the conclusion that BDNF is a survival factor in this system. The degenerative effect brought about by BDNF-AS could be reversed through the addition of exogenous recombinant BDNF protein. In these rescue cultures, the average total neuron count was 16,411 ± 3556, and a single dominant neuritic bundle that measured >200 μm could be observed growing toward the developing neurosensory epithelium of the otocyst, further suggesting that BDNF is required for survival of the SAG neurons (Staecker et al., 1996). BDNF has been demonstrated to act as a survival factor in quail dorsal root ganglia (Hofer and Barde, 1988), in the rat CNS (Knusel et al., 1992), and in motor neurons (Sendtner et al., 1992). This trophic factor has also been demonstrated to be a survival factor in trigeminal neurons (Buchman and Davies, 1993). More recently, gene knockout studies have demonstrated that postnatal rats lacking BDNF have a severe reduction of vestibular neurons and a mild reduction in auditory neurons (Ernfors et al., 1994). At the stage of development examined in this experiment, vestibular and auditory neurons have not yet separated, but it appears clear that BDNF plays an important role in early neuronal survival.

Treatment of cultures with antisense NGF oligonucleotide (NGF-AS) resulted in arrest of neuronal growth. No dominant neuritic bundle was present, and there was no penetration of neurites into the basement membrane of the otocyst. Average neuritic length measured 20 ± 5.6 mm, and average total neuronal count per ganglion was 10,105 ± 2551. Treatment with NGF-AS2 showed similar results. Overall neuronal counts were less than controls, presumably because neuronal division has not been completed at the E10 stage (Ruben, 1967). Again, the effect of NGF-AS treatment could be reversed through the addition of exogenous HrNGF. Thus, NGF probably functions to stimulate neuritogenesis (Staecker et al., 1996). This neuritogenesis effect has also been demonstrated in dissociated auditory neuron cultures, as well as in other systems (Edwards et al., 1989; Harper and Davies, 1990; Hoyle et al., 1993).

Inhibition of NT-3 through addition of antisense NT-3 oligonucleotide (NT-3 AS) showed a startlingly different result. There was no decrease in neuronal count vs. controls. However, neuritic growth within the ganglion appeared disorganized, and rather than a single large dominant neuritic bundle, the NT-3 AS treated cultures showed an average of 17 neuritic bundles penetrating the otocyst basement membrane. Application of a second unique antisense NT-3 oligonucleotide gave similar results. NT-3 must therefore play a role in organization of neuritic bundles and chemotraction of neurites. This effect could not be reversed through the addition of exogenous NT-3, indicating that NT-3 probably acts on a gradient. Recent gene knockout experiments have shown that absence of NT-3 results in a significant decrease in spiral ganglion neurons in the postnatal rat, suggesting that NT-3 may be a survival factor for auditory neurons (Farinas et al., 1994). During the early stages of development, SAG neurons may not yet be dependent on NT-3 for survival. Alternatively, the inability of neurites to reach their targets because of misdirected growth may result in degen-eration when the neuritic growth cones fail to contact their target.

These data clearly demonstrate that NGF, BDNF, and NT-3 all play important roles as neuri-togenesis, survival, and chemotactic factors during the early development of peripheral auditory innervation. However, at this early stage of development, the auditory and vestibular portions of the otocyst have not developed; thus, it is unclear whether there is any difference between auditory and vestibular neuronal response to these trophic factors.

It is apparent that the neurotrophins play an important role in the early development of the auditory system. Evidence is now available that numerous factors, both bound and soluble, cooperate in both the process of development of innervation and subsequently the maintenance of innervation. Development of the organ of Corti and its innervation, however, is far from complete after innervation of the auditory hair cells is complete. Patterns of innervation continue to change, neurons enter into a close relationship with Schwann cells, and the maturation of the organ of Corti is completed. The adult pattern of innervation is not reached until several weeks postnatal. Furthermore, as shown by several recent studies, trophic factors continue to function in adult animals as mediators of maintenance of neuronal integrity. Several groups of distinctively different trophic molecules have been identified. Among these are the neurotrophins, tissue growth factor beta (TGFβ1), basic fibroblast growth factor (bFGF) and the more recently identified CNTF. These factors act both in paracrine and autocrine mechanisms and appear to function in both normal biology and in the response to injury. Most of the data gathered to date pertain to the afferent portion of the auditory nerve and are based on *in vitro* and *in vivo* studies of rodents. The postnatal development — and even function — of efferent auditory innervation has not been completely elucidated.

During the postnatal period, several important events conclude the maturation of the cochlea. Schwann cells continue to undergo mitosis, and complete division 3 to 5 days postnatal (Ruben, 1967). Myelination of neuronal fibers occurs 4 to 5 days postnatally (Romand and Romand, 1990) and is extended to the neuronal soma at about 7 days. In the mouse, ultrastructural differentiation of spiral ganglion neurons into type I (innervating inner hair cells) and type II (innervating outer hair cells) occurs postnatally (Hafidi and Romand, 1989). Furthermore, during the postnatal period, spiral ganglion neurons undergo physiological cell death. At 5P, the rat loses 22% of spiral ganglion neurons (Rueda et al., 1987). This change corresponds to the completion of synaptogenisis. Completion and optimization of neuronal tuning is not completed until postnatal week 4, thus completing the differentiation of spiral ganglion neurons.

Observations made by Sobkowicz and colleagues in postnatal organotypic cochlear cultures (see Chapter 9) suggest that these postnatal changes are driven by the hair cells. In these cultures, the opening of the cochlear duct results in growth of the hair cells away from the ganglion. The neuronal processes subsequently elongate to maintain synaptic contact with the hair cells (Rose et al., 1977). If hair cells are destroyed by ototoxic or noise trauma, degeneration of auditory neurons results (Bichler et al., 1983), again suggesting that there is a link between the sensory cells and the spiral neurons. As discussed in previous sections of this chapter, trophic factors, both soluble and matrix bound, provide a potential mechanism for both the development and later the maintenance of spiral ganglion neurons.

In our studies, the *trkB* and *trkC* receptors could clearly be localized to the 3P spiral ganglion using immunohistochemistry, indicating that at least BDNF and NT-3 are active during the early postnatal period. The role of these trophic factors was again investigated using an organotypic culture system. At 3P, the organ of Corti along with its associated spiral ganglion can be dissected out of the otic capsule and placed into defined medium. Inner and outer hair cells survive for at least 10 days in defined medium. Neuronal survival, however, decreases after 5 to 6 days *in vitro*, despite the presence of the peripheral target cell, suggesting that central derived trophic factors are also required for neuronal survival.

Manipulation of the culture environment again allows us to examine the role of individual neurotrophins by either augmenting or decreasing their concentration *in vitro* and then observing subsequent changes in neuronal morphology. Expression of neurotrophins in culture can be specifically down-regulated through the use of antisense oligonucleotides. When antisense BDNF oligonucleotides are added to 3P organotypic organ of Corti cultures for 48 hours, neuronal degeneration ensues. This degeneration is reversible through the concomitant addition of exogenous BDNF to the cultures, showing that it is the specific withdrawal of BDNF that causes neuronal degeneration.

When 3P neuronal survival in organotypic culture is examined for a more protracted period of time, we observed that after 4 to 5 days in defined medium, a slow degeneration of neurons took place, despite the integrity of the auditory hair cells, which are presumed to produce neurotrophins, and thus support auditory neurons survival. This degeneration was not prevented by the addition of fetal calf serum 10%, NGF (5, 10, or 50 ng/ml); BDNF (5, 10, 50 ng/mL); or basic FGF (5, 10, or 50 ng/mL). Addition of NT-3 (10 ng/mL), CNTF (2.5 ng/mL), or acidic FGF (25 ng/mL) resulted in significantly increased neuronal survival. As suggested by Lefebvre et al. (1994), neurotrophins and other trophic factors may also function as central target derived trophic factors. It has been shown that cutting the afferent portion of the auditory nerve resulted in neuronal degeneration (Bichler et al., 1983). Furthermore, the emergence of NT-3 as a survival factor can be explained on the basis of maturation of the organ of Corti. As previously discussed, at 5P, expression of *trk* receptors switches from *trkB* and *trkC* to predominantly *trkC* (Ylikoski et al., 1993), indicating that NT-3 plays a much more prominent role in neuronal survival after full maturation of Corti's organ.

Application of these techniques becomes more difficult once the cochlea is mature because at this point the spiral ganglion is embedded in bone. To investigate the effect of neurotrophins on adult auditory neurons, two strategies have been used. Lefebvre initially dissociated adult auditory neurons were prepared and tested for their response to a variety of exogenously applied neurotrophins. Because no hair cells were present in these cultures, production of neurotrophins within the culture was minimal. Addition of both BDNF and NT-3 at supraphysiological levels resulted in increased neuronal survival but had little effect on neuritogenesis, whereas addition of NGF resulted only in stimulation of neuritogenesis (Lefebvre et al., 1994). Alternatively, whole spiral ganglia from which the organ of Corti had been stripped were placed *in vitro* and tested for the effect of exogenously applied neurotrophins on neuronal survival. Addition of BDNF, NT-3, and BDNF + NT-3 increased neuronal survival *in vitro*, with NT-3 demonstrating the most significant effect. These data are again consistent with the studies showing a gradual switch of neurotrophin expression in the organ of Corti from BDNF and NT-3 to NT-3 alone (Ylikoski et al., 1993). One can speculate that it is this switch in expression that brings about the final neuronal maturation of the cochlea.

KNOCKOUT STUDIES

Deletion of the gene for BDNF results in a profound decrease in vestibular ganglion neurons in newborn mice (Ernfors et al., 1994). The vestibular ganglion in the knockout mice underwent an 82% neuronal degeneration, with neurites appearing atrophic and asymmetric. The spiral ganglion did not appear to be significantly affected, thus suggesting that BDNF is the dominant trophic survival factor in the postnatal vestibular system. Currently, no data are available on the effect of this gene knockout on maturation of cochlear innervation. Deletion of NT-3 appears to have no effect on the vestibular system, but results in degeneration of the spiral ganglion. The spiral ganglion undergoes an 85% neuronal degeneration. The vestibular ganglion, on the other hand, is only mildly affected (Farinas et al., 1994). Clearly, specific neurotrophins are responsible for neuronal survival in both the vestibular and auditory systems, and it is the modulation of expression of these factors that results in maturation of the auditory and vestibular systems after birth.

Several studies have examined the effect of neurotrophin knockouts and *trk* knockouts on the auditory/vestibular system. As previously described, loss of BDNF resulted in loss of vestibular innervation, wheras knockout of NT-3 resulted in loss of cochlear innervation (Figures 11.3 and 11.4). A potential deficit in efferent innervation to the BDNF knockout mice was also noted (Ernfors et al., 1995). Analysis of corresponding *trkB* and *trkC* knockouts confirmed these findings. Deletion of *trkB* receptor resulted in initial ingrowth of neurites to the sensory epithelia during early embryogenesis. By the time auditory and vestibular hair cells had developed, degeneration of vestibular ganglion cells has taken place. Innervation to all semicircular canals is lost, and overall

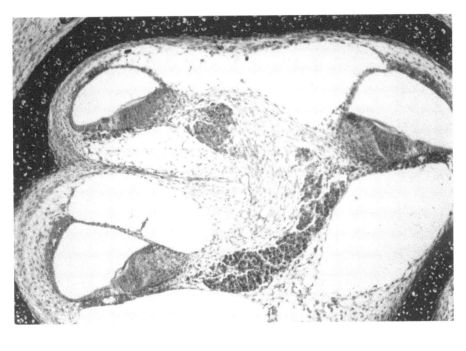

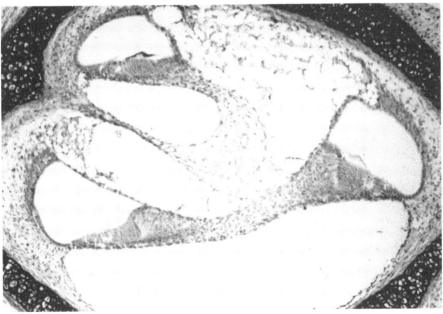

FIGURE 11.3   The importance of neurotrophins in the auditory system is demonstrated through knockout studies. Knockout of NT-3 results in loss of cochlear innervation. The wild-type is shown in (A) and the null NT-3 –/– in (B).

volume of the vestibular ganglion is reduced to 35% of control (Fritzsch et al., 1997b). In this study, *trkC* knockouts showed a reduction but not complete loss of cochlear innervation. Combination knockouts of BDNF and NT-3 or *trkB* and *trkC* led to total losses of auditory and vestibular innervation. This suggests that NT-3 is the predominant growth factor controlling survival of cochlear neurons, and BDNF is the predominant growth factor controlling survival of vestibular ganglion cells.

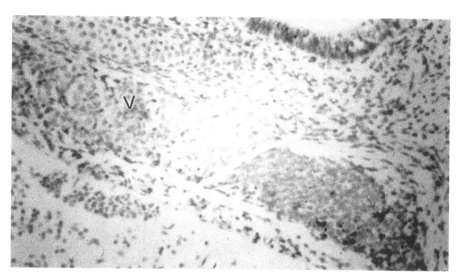

FIGURE 11.4 Loss of NT-3 production results in apoptotic cell death. Staining using the TUNEL technique shows the presence of apoptotic nuclei in the spiral ganglion (arrow) of this13.5-gd mouse cochlea. The adjacent vestibular ganglion (V) shows no signs of apoptosis.

EFFECTS OF NEUROTROPHIN WITHDRAWAL

Although placing an isolated auditory neuron *in vitro* in itself is a model of neuronal injury, very few studies specifically address the subject of injury response and neurotrophins. Recent experiments carried out in chinchillas have shown that vestibular neuronectomy results in up-regulation of the p75 low-affinity neuotrophin receptor. The high-affinity receptors for BDNF or NT-3 (*trkB* and *C*) were not affected (Fina et al., 1994). The low-affinity receptor is thought to play a role in sequestration and presentation of neurotrophins (Lee et al., 1992). This study suggests that neurotrophins may also play a role in central target derived trophic support of auditory neurons. At this time, no studies have assessed the molecular biology of neurotrophin receptor expression in response to peripheral injury.

To determine the effect of loss of peripheral target supplied growth factor on auditory neurons, Gabazideh et al. (1997) prepared a series of dissociated 3P rat auditory neuron cultures maintained in Dulbecos Modified Eagle Medium supplemented with BDNF (100 ng/mL). After 24 hours *in vitro*, BDNF was withdrawn from the cultures, and the cultures were stained with fluorescent stains that targeted reactive oxygen species (ROS) or stained for glutathione. Individual culture plates were imaged every 10 minutes for a total of 2 hours using a confocal microscope. Within 20 minutes of neurotrophin withdrawal, there was a slow increase in levels of oxygen free radicals and intracellular glutathione that was seen only in the neurtotrophin-deprived cultures. Glutathione levels than decreased and, subsequently, levels of ROS within the neurons peaked. This suggests that loss of neurotrophin support results in overwhelming oxidative stress that cellular glutathione supplies cannot keep up with (Gabaizideh et al., 1997).

The studies reviewed above have shown that the neurotrophins NGF, BDNF, and NT-3 play significant roles in the development and maintenance of auditory innervation. At the earliest stages of development, ranging from E10.5, where outgrowth of neurites is initiated from the SAG to E13, where innervation of the otocyst has occurred, BDNF appears to function as a survival factor. NT-3, on the other hand, directs neuronal growth and controls organization of neuritic fasiculization. NSF mediates initiation of neuritic outgrowth. In the postnatal period when neuronal pruning and final development of innervation is occurring, the roles of these factors change. During the early postnatal period, BDNF still appears to function as a survival factor, although it does not appear to have a strong survival effect on adult neurons in organotypic cultures. NT-3, however, plays a minimal role in the survival of early postnatal neurons but becomes a potent survival factor for adult auditory neurons. Further study of these factors and their role in the development of innervation should elucidate their function in maintenance of auditory neurons and provide vital information leading to their development as agents preventing neuronal degeneration *in vivo*.

CONCLUSIONS

The experiments reviewed above demonstrate that within the auditory and vestibular systems, the neurotrophin family of trophic factors as well as a variety of other growth factors with neurotrophic effects are intimately involved with both the development and maintenance of auditory innervation. Once the basic molecular mechanisms of the development and maintenance of auditory innervation have been defined, therapy to prevent degeneration of neurons after damage or even therapy to establish functional reinnervation will become a reality.

Over the last 50 years, significant discoveries have been made rearranging the biology of neuronal damage and recovery. Possible clinical applications for neurotrophins after injury of auditory and vestibular hair cells are numerous. Neurotrophin therapy may be useful in ameliorating overall damage to the auditory system after treatment with aminoglycosides or other ototoxic agents such as *cis*-platinum. Furthermore, neurotrophin therapy may also improve existing cochlear implant technology by improving neuronal survival or possibly even regrowth after cochlear injury. Ultimately, if mammalian cochlear hair cell regeneration becomes a reality, as has been shown in the avian system, neurotrophin treatment will be required initially to support neuronal health until a new target for innervation has been found.

12 Preparation and Evaluation of the Mouse Temporal Bone

Barbara A. Bohne, Gary W. Harding, and Henry C. Ou

INTRODUCTION

The inner ear or membranous labyrinth presents several challenges when preparing it for microscopic examination and histopathological analysis. First, it contains six separate sensory organs, one for hearing (i.e., organ of Corti [OC] in the cochlea) and five for balance and equilibrium (i.e., saccular and utricular macula, superior, lateral, and posterior crista in the vestibule). These organs are surrounded by large fluid spaces that contain either perilymph that has a high sodium concentration, or endolymph that has a high potassium concentration. The membranous labyrinth and surrounding fluid spaces are embedded in the bony labyrinth of the temporal bone. It is difficult to prepare the delicate sensory epithelia for microscopic examination without causing mechanical or dissection artifacts in the tissue. Second, within each organ, there are regional variations in the density of sensory cells, their pattern of innervation, and their responses to stimulation. Third, a number of genetic mutations that affect the auditory system also involve balance and equilibrium. Thus, to fully characterize the morphological changes in the inner ear of a new mutant mouse, cells must be analyzed at representative locations throughout all of the sensory regions.

Each sensory organ in the membranous labyrinth contains both sensory (hair) and supporting cells attached to a basal lamina that rests on subepithelial connective tissue. In the hearing portion of the ear, the subepithelial connective tissue is called the basilar membrane (BM). On the surface of each hair cell, there are a number of elongated microvilli (stereocilia) that project into an extracellular membrane (tectorial membrane for the OC; otolithic membrane for the maculae; cupula for the cristae) that covers the sensory and supporting cells. The myelinated peripheral processes of the primary cochlear neurons (spiral ganglion cells) and vestibular neurons (Scarpa's ganglion cells) approach the epithelium through the underlying connective tissue and lose their myelin sheaths before crossing the basal lamina to innervate the basolateral surfaces of the hair cells.

Because the sensory epithelia in the inner ear are difficult to access, histopathological studies generally involve preservation of the entire ear with fixative, decalcification of the bone, embedment of the specimen in a supporting medium such as paraffin, celloidin, or plastic, followed by the cutting of sections through the entire temporal bone (e.g., Schuknecht, 1993).

The intact temporal bone can also be dissected after fixation while it is immersed in liquid ("wet" dissection; e.g., Engström et al., 1966). Flat preparations of the six sensory areas are made and examined, with or without staining, by placing them in a liquid mounting medium and studying them with phase-contrast, bright-field, or fluorescence microscopy. Different levels within the epithelia can be observed using the *z*-axis of the microscope (fine-focus) to "optically section" the tissue. The flat preparations of the six sensory epithelia can also be prepared for scanning electron microscopic (SEM) study or embedded in plastic, then semi-thick or thin-sectioned for bright-field or transmission electron microscopic study (e.g., Friedmann and Ballantyne, 1984).

No single histopathological technique can be used to address all research questions, nor will it permit utilization of all the different types of examinations mentioned above. The appropriate choice of technique depends on the research question being addressed. However, it should be noted that only by preparing flat preparations can the sensory epithelium from each organ be examined in its entirety. Performing flat-preparation analyses prior to sectioning the epithelia is essential to avoid the introduction of sampling errors into the evaluation.

PREPARATION AND ANALYSIS TECHNIQUES

This chapter describes a versatile preparation technique in which the mouse temporal bone is embedded in plastic prior to dissection (Bohne and Harding, 1997). After embedding, the hearing and vestibular organs are dissected into flat preparations that are then examined at magnifications of 40 to 1250X. After the sensory epithelia have been examined in their entirety, precisely determined regions are sectioned on an ultramicrotome for examination by high-resolution light or transmission electron microscopy (TEM).

Cochleae that have been examined with the plastic-embedding technique include those from wild-type mice and several mutants (i.e., tilted [*tlt/tlt*; Ornitz et al., 1998]; viable dominant spotting [*W*^{V}/*W*^{V}; Miller, 1994]; Wheels [*whl*; Nolan et al., 1995]; fibroblast growth factor receptor 3 knockout [*fgfr3*; Colvin et al., 1996]). In this chapter, illustrative data from mouse strain 129, control and noise-exposed C57BL/CBA F1 hybrids, and tilted mice and their heterozygous (normal) litter mates are presented.

FIXATION AND ISOLATION OF THE BONY AND MEMBRANOUS LABYRINTHS

Because of the small size and fragility of mouse temporal bones, the sensory epithelia are best preserved by cardiac perfusion prior to separating the temporal bone from the skull. Vascular perfusion of a warm buffer solution (e.g., lactated Ringer's, normal saline, phosphate buffered saline) minimizes the possibility of bleeding into the middle and inner ears, which can obscure important landmarks (e.g., round window). Once the vessels are cleared of blood, the fixative is perfused through the vascular system to begin tissue preservation as soon as possible after the animal's death. Fixing the temporal bones prior to their removal from the skull toughens the soft tissue and helps to prevent mechanical damage to the sensory organs during their dissection.

Mice are anesthetized with an ip injection (0.005 mL/g body weight) of a mixture of ketamine (17.4 mg/mL) and xylazine (2.6 mg/mL). The animal has reached an appropriate depth of anesthesia when it has a negative pedal-withdrawal response. Once anesthetized, the animal is taped, ventral side up, to a solid board. Bupivacaine (0.05 mL of 0.5% solution) is injected on the right and left sides of the chest wall for local control of pain. The xiphoid process of the sternum and the rib cage are cut on both sides with a scissors and the flap reflected rostrally to expose the heart. The descending aorta is clamped with a small hemostat. The right atrium of the heart is opened with a small scissors and the left ventricle is penetrated with a 0.5 in. × 30G needle that has been covered by PE20 tubing except for 3 mm at its tip. The tubing prevents the needle from penetrating the apex of the heart during the perfusion. The needle is attached to a 12-cc syringe. Buffer is slowly infused into the vascular system until the fluid escaping from the right atrium is nearly clear (about 5 min). Another syringe-needle combination is used to infuse fixative into the vascular system for 5 to 15 min. The fixative and the duration of perfusion depend on the type of microscopic examination to be performed and the structure(s) of interest. For example, for immunohistochemical studies, either buffered 4% paraformaldehyde (PF) or PF and a low concentration of glutaraldehyde is usually best (e.g., Schulte and Steel, 1994; Pack and Slepecky, 1995). For quantitative morphological examinations, 1% buffered osmium tetroxide (OsO_4) provides excellent results (Ou et al., 2000a). The tissues for all of the illustrations in this chapter were fixed in 1% OsO_4 in Dalton's buffer containing 1.65% $CaCl_2$.

After completion of the perfusion, the animal is decapitated and the head skinned as far as the orbits, the calvarium opened along the midline, and the brain removed to reveal the temporal bones. At this point, the internal auditory meatus, seventh and eighth nerves, and superior semicircular canal are visible in the right and left temporal bones from inside the skull under 25X magnification. Suction is used to remove the paraflocculus from inside the curvature of the superior semicircular canal. Because the temporal bones of the mouse have only fibrous connections to the rest of the skull, fine-tipped forceps are used to carefully divide this fibrous tissue and separate the temporal bones from the skull.

Structures such as the ossicles (malleus, incus, stapes) in the middle-ear space (bulla) are examined under the dissection microscope after the middle and external ears are separated from the bony labyrinth along a suture line. Usually, the malleus and incus remain attached to the tympanic membrane, while the stapes stays in position in the oval window. Once opened, the middle ear is inspected for signs of pathology (e.g., fluid accumulation, thickened tympanic membrane). The ossicles are inspected for gross structural deformities. If a higher power examination of the ossicles is needed, they are decalcified for several days in 0.2 M ethylenediaminetetraacetic acid (EDTA) in 0.1 M phosphate buffer, embedded in plastic (see below) and semi-thick and thin sectioned.

A right-angle hook is used to remove the stapedial artery from the basal turn and the crura of the stapes from the oval window. Generally, the footplate of the stapes separates from the oval window when the crura are pulled away. However, if the crura break, care must be taken when removing the footplate because the saccular macula is attached to the bony labyrinth directly below the footplate. A fine-pointed steel pick (0.7-mm diameter shaft; three-sided pyramidal point) is used to make a small fenestra at the cochlear apex and in the middle of the superior semicircular canal. Using a small-tipped glass pipette (0.15 to 0.20 mm), fixative is infused into the fenestrae alternately with perfusate escaping from the oval window. After perfusing the fluid spaces of both bony labyrinths, the two inner ears from a single animal are immersed in 6 mL fixative in a scintillation vial for the appropriate length of time to ensure adequate fixation of the soft tissue (e.g., for OsO_4, 4°C for 2 h; for PF, 4°C for 4 to 16 h).

EMBEDDING AND DISSECTING THE MEMBRANOUS AND BONY LABYRINTHS

After the ears are fixed, they are washed three times (15 min each) in Hank's balanced salt solution and then placed in 70% ethanol. Each inner ear is inspected under a dissection microscope at a magnification of 40X. The facial nerve is removed from its canal with fine-tipped forceps so that the cristae of the superior and lateral semicircular canals can be visualized through the bone. Adhering muscle and soft tissue are separated from the specimen. The fine-pointed steel pick is used to create small infiltration holes in the bony labyrinth at the cochlear apex (ventral surface) and just rostral to the internal auditory meatus (dorsal surface). Extreme care is taken to avoid damaging the boundaries of the endolymphatic space. Bone chips and bubbles in the perilymphatic spaces are removed with small glass pipettes and light suction.

The inner ears are dehydrated in ethanol (80, 95, 100, and 100%; 0.5 h at each concentration) and propylene oxide (PO) (two 0.5-h changes). The specimens are embedded in plastic (Durcupan) by first infiltrating them with increasing concentrations of diluted plastic (PO:plastic ratio = 2:1, 1:1, and 1:2; 0.5 h at each dilution) and then pure plastic (four 1-h changes). All steps from dehydration through infiltration take place while the specimens are rotated at 65 rpm on a rotary shaker. Once the specimens are in pure plastic, the stopper on the vial is removed and a 100-W light is shined on the rotating vial. The heat from the light helps to volatilize any propylene oxide remaining in the tissue and keeps the plastic from becoming viscous. After infiltration, the specimens are placed in a 5-mm-thick layer of fresh plastic that is polymerized at 60°C for 48 h.

After the plastic has polymerized, each specimen is sawed out of its block and mounted in an aluminum specimen holder by a "handle" of plastic that is left below the superior canal. Under 40X magnification, the plastic outside the bony labyrinth is removed with quarter pieces of double-edged razor blades. The specimen is then thinly coated with liquid plastic to improve visibility. The fine-pointed steel pick is used to gently flake off the bony labyrinth from the membranous labyrinth and the plastic-filled perilymphatic spaces. After removal of the cochlear bone, the two perilymphatic spaces or scalae (s. vestibuli and tympani) are visible along with their communicating passage (helicotrema) at the cochlear apex. The triangular-shaped endolymphatic space (s. media) is visible between the perilymphatic spaces. The surface of the OC (reticular lamina) and BM separate s. media from s. tympani. Reissner's membrane separates s. media from s. vestibuli. The stria vascularis forms the lateral wall of s. media.

Once the scalae are visible, the cochlear duct is dissected into four half-turns. Starting at the apex, pieces of razor blade are used to make one cut through s. vestibuli and s. media, perpendicular to the OC, and another cut through s. tympani, parallel to the BM. The cuts intersect at the helicotrema (for apical half-turn) or in the modiolus (for the other half-turns) and separate that half-turn from the remainder of the specimen. With fine-tipped forceps, each half-turn is held in place in a pool of liquid plastic on the glass plate of a dissection microscope. The plastic filling s. tympani is trimmed close (~0.1 mm) and parallel to the BM. If present, bone above Reissner's membrane is carefully trimmed away. The half-turn is divided in two and the resulting quarter-turns are numbered appropriately as the apical and basal halves of that segment. In some instances, a razor blade is used to hand-cut a 50- to 100-μm-thick radial section from one edge of a quarter-turn. The trimmed quarter-turn segments from one cochlea are flat-embedded in a 2-mm-thick layer of liquid plastic with the BM side facing the bottom surface of the embedding mold (Peel-A-Way, R-40). Each thick radial section is placed in a droplet of liquid plastic on a microscopic slide, covered with a glass coverslip, and polymerized for 24 h at 60°C. When the stria vascularis needs to be examined in detail, short lengths are removed from the quarter-turns with a razor cut through s. vestibuli and media, just lateral to the OC. The strial segments are embedded flat, endolymphatic surface down, in a separate embedding mold.

The hook of the cochlear duct and the remainder of the sensory areas are separated *en bloc* from the superior canal and plastic handle. This block is placed on the glass plate of a dissection microscope in a pool of liquid plastic and firmly held with fine-tipped forceps. With bright illumination, quarter pieces of razor blade are used to divide the hook and posterior crista from the rest of the block. The individual vestibular organs are then identified and separated from one another with carefully placed razor cuts. Plastic above the epithelium of the isolated vestibular sensory organs is trimmed away, parallel to their endolymphatic surface. All vestibular organs are embedded flat, endolymphatic surface down, in another embedding mold. The plastic layers containing the dissected segments of membranous labyrinth are polymerized at 60°C for 48 h.

MICROSCOPIC ANALYSIS OF FLAT PREPARATIONS OF THE MEMBRANOUS LABYRINTH

The polymerized plastic layers containing the dissected cochlear duct and stria vascularis are examined by bright-field or phase-contrast microscopy at magnifications of 125 to 1250X. Each block is taped in a custom aluminum holder with its bottom surface facing up (BM for the OC; marginal cells for the stria vascularis). The aluminum holder permits the plastic layer to be moved precisely in the x and y dimensions. A droplet of immersion oil (R.I. = 1.515) is placed on the plastic block over each tissue segment. The oil fills up irregularities in the surface of the block that will distort the light path and make it impossible to obtain a clear view of the cells. When the tissue segments are examined with a 50 or 100X oil immersion objective lens, the lens is immersed directly in the oil droplet on the surface of the plastic block. Because the length of the mouse's outer hair cells (~10 to 20 μm) is much smaller than in other species (e.g., 25 to 45 μm for chinchillas [Smith, 1968]), they are best evaluated with a 50 or 100X objective lens; stereocilia can be seen clearly only with the 100X lens.

The lengths (in millimeters) of all dissected OC segments from a particular cochlea are measured using an imaging system interfaced to a computer. Length is measured along a curved line at the approximate junction of the heads of the inner and outer pillar cells. The millimeter length of an OC segment is converted to a percentage of the total length for that OC. To compensate for within-species variation in OC length, graphs of damage in the OC are plotted as a function of percentage distance from the cochlear (OC) apex.

The total numbers of present and missing (i.e., those replaced by phalangeal scars) inner (IHC) and outer (OHC) hair cells were counted in each OC segment from a number of C57BL/CBA F1 mice. In the OC, the density of IHCs and OHCs (number per millimeter) was determined for that strain by dividing the number present plus missing IHCs or OHCs in the segment by its length. The percentage of missing IHCs or OHCs in a segment is equal to the number of missing cells divided by the number of present plus missing IHCs or OHCs, respectively.

Except for the gross shape of the vestibular sensory organs, it is impossible to see much detail (e.g., individual hair cells) in the plastic-embedded flat preparations because of the curvature of the organs, the darkly stained nerve fibers that approach the epithelium from the underlying connective tissue and, in the case of the maculae, the thick layer of otoconia that overlies the epithelium. For this reason, the flat preparations are sawed out of their plastic layer and divided with razor blades, perpendicular to their endolymphatic surface, into several thick sections (~50 to 100 µm thick). The hand-cut razor sections are embedded, cut edge down, in 2-mm-thick layers of plastic. After polymerization, these thick sections are examined as described above for the OC and stria vascularis.

CUTTING OF SEMI-THICK AND THIN SECTIONS OF THE SENSORY ORGANS

After detailed study of the flat preparations of OC and stria vascularis, and the thick radial sections of the vestibular organs, selected areas are prepared for semi-thick or thin sectioning at a radial, horizontal, or tangential angle. In the OC, the areas chosen for sectioning correspond to regions with specific changes in auditory function (e.g., TTS; PTS), or have a specific pattern of cell loss (e.g., focal loss of IHCs) that had been identified in the flat preparations. The areas chosen for sectioning in the vestibular sensory organs are those thought to be responsible for deficits in vestibular function (e.g., maculae in tilted mice).

The tissue segments are sawed out of their plastic layer, leaving a handle to mount in a vise chuck. Using an ultramicrotome and glass knives, the tissue blocks are semi-thick sectioned at 1 to 2 µm and heat-mounted on glass slides, or thin-sectioned at 60 to 90 nm and mounted on copper grids. Semi-thick sections are stained for 30 to 45 s at 80°C (Lewis and Knight, 1977) with a 1:1 mixture of 1% methylene blue in 1% borax and 1% azure II in distilled water (Richardson et al., 1960). Thin sections are either stained with lead acetate and uranyl acetate or examined without staining.

In instances where bone closely approaches the cells of interest (e.g., hook portion of the cochlear duct), sectioning is improved if the bone is decalcified. Decalcification can be accomplished in 5 to 7 days through the plastic block by immersion in buffered 0.2 M EDTA at room temperature, changing the solution daily. After decalcification is completed, the blocks are washed in 1-h changes of phosphate buffer (×2), 50% and 70% ethanol, and then dried for 12 to 16 h at 60°C. The blocks are re-infiltrated with a 1:1 mixture of Durcupan components "A" and "B" for 1 h, followed by three 1-h changes in pure Durcupan. The decalcified blocks are embedded flat in 2-mm-thick plastic layers as described above.

EVALUATION OF PREPARATIONS

GROSS MORPHOLOGY OF THE BONY AND MEMBRANOUS LABYRINTHS

After the inner ear has been dehydrated and infiltrated with plastic, the bony labyrinth becomes nearly transparent. By studying the inner ear under a dissection microscope at 40X magnification while it is immersed in liquid plastic, its general morphology can be determined. Figure 12.1 shows the ventral surface of the right inner ear from a control mouse that had normal cochlear and

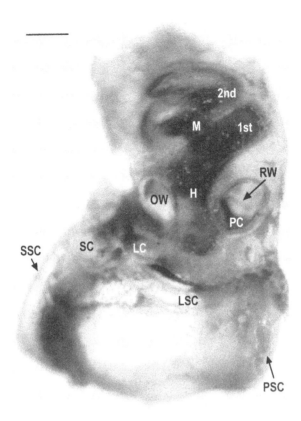

FIGURE 12.1 Ventral surface of right temporal bone from a C57BL/CBA F1 hybrid mouse that was fixed by vascular perfusion, dehydrated, and infiltrated with plastic (Durcupan). The photomicrograph was taken through liquid plastic. The cochlear duct makes approximately 2.5 turns around the modiolus (M): 2nd — second turn; 1st — first turn; H — round window hook. The oval window (OW), with its whitish margin, and the round window (RW) are clearly visible because facial nerve, stapes, and stapedial artery were removed before dehydration. The posterior crista (PC) is seen at the caudal rim of the RW. On the opposite side of the labyrinth from the PC, the cristae of the superior (SC) and lateral (LC) semicircular canals are seen close to one another. The non-sensory portion of the superior (SSC), lateral (LSC), and posterior (PSC) semicircular canals can also be seen. Bar equals 0.5 mm.

vestibular function. The bony labyrinth is light gray. The cochlear duct or s. media appears as a darkly stained structure that spirals approximately 2.5 times (i.e., 2nd = second [apical] turn; 1st = first [basal] turn; H = round window hook) around the modiolus (M) where the axons of the primary auditory neurons are located. The oval (OW) and round (RW) windows are visible near the hook of the cochlear duct. The non-sensory regions of the semicircular canals appear as rounded channels in the bone (lsc = lateral; psc = posterior; ssc = superior). The cristae of the semicircular canals (LC = lateral; PC = posterior; SC = superior) are visible as small, roundish areas that are darkly stained and into which a dark-staining band of nerve fibers project. If the specimen is rotated at different angles, the endolymphatic surface of the saccular macula can be observed through the OW on the superior wall of the vestibule. It is also possible to determine whether or not the canals are completely formed. If the specimen is rotated so that its cranial side faces the microscope lens, the internal auditory meatus, eighth nerve, common crus, endolymphatic duct and sac, and posterior crista can be inspected (view not shown). This level of analysis is performed on all specimens prior to polymerization of the plastic. At this stage, mice having morphogenetic mutations of the temporal bone such as a shortened cochlear duct or an incomplete semicircular canal can be readily identified (e.g., Nolan et al., 1995).

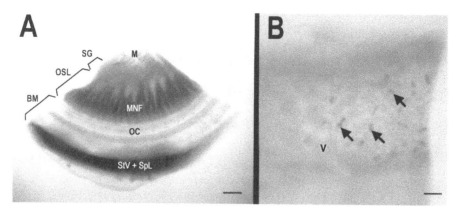

FIGURE 12.2 Bright-field images of tissue from specimen in Figure 12.1: (A) dissected segment of the cochlear duct viewed from Reissner's membrane. Cells in organ of Corti (OC) appear as gray stripes on basilar membrane (BM) near the lip of the osseous spiral lamina (OSL). Visible through the OSL are the myelinated peripheral processes (MNF) of the spiral ganglion cells (SG) or primary auditory neurons. The axons of the spiral ganglion cells are gathered in the modiolus (M) before they exit the temporal bone. The stria vascularis (StV) and spiral ligament (SpL) form the lateral wall of the cochlear duct. To the right of the segment, a portion of the stria vascularis was removed during the dissection and embedded flat (see Figure 12.2B); (B) flat preparation of stria vascularis viewed from its endolymphatic surface. Area at left is out-of-focus because of curvature of tissue. Arrows point to some melanin-containing intermediate cells. Blood vessels (V) appear light because the red blood cells were washed out of the vascular system during the fixation procedure. Bars equal 100 μm and 50 μm, respectively.

EVALUATION OF THE COCHLEA

The low-magnification appearance (10X objective lens, 2.5X eyepiece) of the cochlear duct from a control mouse is shown in Figure 12.2A. No damage is visible in the OC, nerve fibers (MNF) in the osseous spiral lamina (OSL), spiral ganglion (SG), or stria vascularis and spiral ligament (StV + SpL). The short segment of stria vascularis and spiral ligament that was removed from the cochlear duct during the initial dissection is shown in Figure 12.2B. By bright-field microscopy, a full complement of dark, melanin-filled intermediate cells is seen scattered throughout the stria vascularis. At this level of analysis, cochleae can be identified with regions of moderately or severely damaged OC, nerve-fiber and spiral-ganglion-cell degeneration, or pathology in the stria vascularis, including a paucity of melanocytes.

An overview of the different cells in the OC can be gained by examining thick radial sections of the cochlear duct such as shown in Figure 12.3. The OC, located between s. media (SM) and s. tympani (ST), is attached to the BM. The tectorial membrane (TM) extends over the surface of the OC, but is separated from the hair-cell stereocilia because of excess shrinkage during tissue processing. Visible within the OC are sensory cells (inner [IHC] and outer [1, 2, 3] hair cells with stereocilia [st]), supporting cells (inner [IP] and outer [OP] pillars, Deiters' cells [D1, D2, D3], and Hensen's cells [H]), and cross-sectioned bundles of nerve fibers (outer spiral bundles [white arrowheads]). Nerve fibers (MNF) lose their myelin sheaths before entering the OC through holes (habenulae perforata [HP]) in the spiral lamina below the IHCs. At this level of analysis, the general shape of the OC and the presence or absence of its component cells and structures can be quickly assessed.

In experimental mice, an accurate picture of the type(s) of pathological changes and their distribution within the cochlea cannot be obtained unless the entire OC from apex to base is examined at a magnification of 625 to 1250X. For example, Figure 12.4 shows photomicrographs of the OC from the second and first cochlear turns in a mouse that sustained a permanent threshold

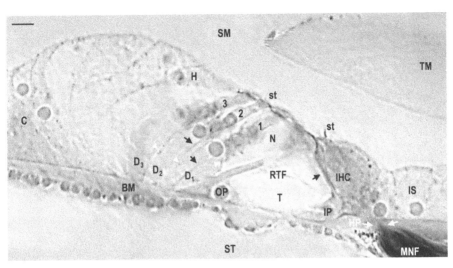

FIGURE 12.3   Thick radial section of the cochlear duct from segment #3 (~25% distance from apex) in a control mouse. The organ of Corti (OC) is attached to the s. media side (SM) of the basilar membrane (BM). The BM separates SM from s. tympani (ST). An extracellular membrane, the tectorial membrane (TM), extends over the surface of the OC. The inner (IHC) and outer (1, 2, 3) hair cells with their stereocilia (st) are found on either side of the fluid-filled tunnel space (T). Fluid-filled Nuel spaces (N) surround the bodies of the outer hair cells. Supporting cells include inner (IP) and outer (OP) pillar cells, and Deiters' cells. Each Deiters' cell body (D1, D2, D3) sends a slender process to the surface of the OC where it expands to form a phalangeal process. The pillar and Deiters' cells contain compact bundles of microtubules (black arrows) extending from the cell's base on the BM to its apex in the reticular lamina. Supporting cells that lack microtubular bundles include Hensen's cells (H). Medial and lateral to the OC, inner sulcus (IS) and Claudius' (C) cells cover the s.-media side of the BM. The peripheral processes of the spiral ganglion cells are myelinated (MNF) until they cross the BM through the habenulae perforata (HP), enter the OC, and form fiber bundles, including the radial tunnel fibers (RTF) and the three outer spiral bundles (white arrowheads). Bar equals 10 μm.

shift (PTS) for high-frequency tones following excessive noise exposure. In the second turn (A), all hair cells (IHC; OHC 1, 2, 3) and supporting cells are present. In the first turn (B), some IHCs and OHCs have degenerated as a result of the exposure. To quantify the damage, missing cells must be counted as a function of apex-to-base position in the cochlea (see below).

Knowledge of the density of IHCs and OHCs in the different cochlear turns in a given mouse strain is valuable when quantifying histopathological changes in the cochlea. To determine hair-cell density in C57BL/CBA F1 hybrid mice, the length of the OC segments in a representative sample of cochleae was measured. The total length of the second turn, first turn, and hook portion of the OC was measured in 8 control and 39 noise-exposed mice (i.e., 25 male and 22 female). The average length of each turn, along with its conversion to percentage distance from the apex, is provided in Table 12.1 (column 2). For all mice, the total length of the OC averaged 5.90 ± 0.12 mm. When OC length was determined for each sex separately, it was found to average 5.95 ± 0.11 mm for males and 5.83 ± 0.10 mm for females. An independent samples t-test indicated that this length difference is highly significant ($p < 0.0003$). A significant difference in the average OC length for human males and females was reported previously by Sato et al. (1991).

In a subset of the mice (8 control and 31 noise-exposed) used to determine OC length, the average densities for IHCs and OHCs, along with the linear regression slope and intercept, in the individual cochlear turns are presented in Table 12.1. These latter values are used to estimate the total number of hair cells that should be present in different regions of other C57BL/CBA F1 mouse cochleae. For the entire OC of these mice, the total number of IHCs and OHCs averaged 706 and 2416, respectively. These values compare favorably with those determined by Ehret (1977) for the

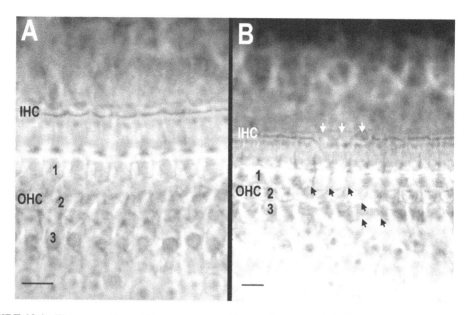

FIGURE 12.4 Flat preparations of the organ of Corti from noise-exposed C57BL/CBA F1 mouse at 1-month post-exposure. (A) At 53% distance from the cochlear apex, all inner (IHC) and outer (OHC 1, 2, 3) hair cells are intact. The stereocilia on the IHCs appear as slightly curved dark lines. (B) At 64% distance from the cochlear apex, three adjacent IHCs (white arrows) are missing. Some OHCs in all three rows (black arrows) have degenerated and have been replaced by phalangeal scars. Bars equal 5 μm and 10 μm, respectively.

TABLE 12.1
Organ-of-Corti Length and Hair-Cell Density in C57BL/CBA Mice

Turn	Turn Length (mm)		Hair–cell Density[a]	Regression		Sample
				Slope	Intercept	
Second	2.51 ± 0.13 (0–42.5%)[b]	IHC	120 ± 3	−8.875	172.069	39
		OHC[c]	418 ± 10	−40.318	656.269	39
First	1.96 ± 0.14 (42.6–75.6%)[b]	IHC	128 ± 3	−8.866	180.283	39
		OHC	425 ± 8	−9.821	483.209	39
RW hook	1.44 ± 0.18 (75.7–100%)[b]	IHC	107 ± 4	−11.094	172.229	25
		OHC	371 ± 8	−1.022	377.197	22
Ave.	5.90 ± 0.12	IHC	118 ± 2			
		OHC	405 ± 4			

Note: N = 47 for cochlear length. Data from control and noise-exposed mice were used for length and hair-cell density determinations. Counts of total hair cells could not be made in the round window (RW) hook in as many specimens as in the first and second turns because there was often moderate to severe hair-cell loss in this region.

[a] Per millimeter of organ of Corti.

[b] Percentage distance from cochlear apex.

[c] Sum of three rows of OHCs.

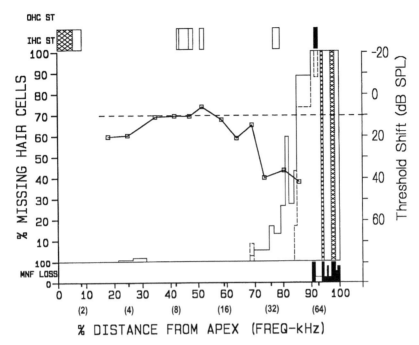

FIGURE 12.5 ABR threshold shift and cytocochleogram from C57BL/CBA F1 mouse that was exposed for 2 hours to an octave band of noise with a center frequency of 8 kHz and a sound pressure level of 100 dB. Mouse was terminated 4 weeks post-exposure. Squares connected by solid line indicate ABR threshold shift (right *y*-axis), just prior to termination. Shifts less than or equal to 10 dB (horizontal dashed line) are not considered significant. The mouse developed a 20-dB permanent threshold shift (PTS) for 3 and 4 kHz, and a 40-dB PTS for 30 to 50 kHz. The frequencies in parentheses on the *x*-axis were aligned to percentage distance from the cochlear apex using the "edges" map developed by Ou et al. (2000b). The percentages of missing hair cells (left *y*-axis, middle: IHC – dashed line; OHC – solid line), degenerated peripheral processes of the spiral ganglion cells (left *y*-axis, bottom: MNF LOSS) and location of IHC stereocilia damage (left *y*-axis, top: IHC ST) are plotted as a function of percentage distance from the cochlear apex (*x*-axis). In the apical half of the organ of Corti (OC), IHC and OHC losses are minimal but there are scattered regions where the IHC stereocilia are splayed or disarrayed (i.e., open box – slight; cross-hatched box – moderate). In the basal 20% of the OC, there is 33% IHC loss and 81% OHC loss, along with degeneration of many nerve fibers (short, black bars). At this same location, there are two small regions of total loss of the OC (tall, hatched bars).

outbred NMRI mouse with a much longer OC (6.84 mm; 765 IHCs; 2526 OHCs). By using the data in Table 12.1 and measuring OC segment length in an experimental cochlea, only missing hair cells need be counted in most regions of the OC. An estimate of the total number of hair cells in an OC segment is calculated by multiplying segment length by hair-cell density that is adjusted for total OC length. The percentage of missing hair cells is equal to the number missing divided by the calculated total times 100. These data are especially valuable when the cochlea has so much damage that phalangeal scars are not visible (e.g., when the OC has entirely degenerated). In these cases, the number of missing hair cells is determined by estimating the total, counting present cells (if any), and subtracting present from total to obtain an estimate of the number missing.

This estimation technique was used in the evaluation of the cochlea illustrated in Figure 12.5. This figure is a graphical representation (i.e., cytocochleogram) of the apex-to-base position of cochlear damage in a C57BL/CBA F1 mouse that had been exposed for 2 h to an octave band of noise with a center frequency of 8 kHz and a sound pressure level of 100 dB, and terminated 4 weeks post-exposure. The data on hair-cell loss/injury are plotted as a function of percentage distance from the cochlear apex. There is minimal hair cell loss in the apical 70% of the OC. In the basal 30%,

TABLE 12.2
Hair-Cell Losses in Control Mice (Male)

An #	Age (mo)	ABR Test	% Missing Hair Cells							
			0–50% dist[a]		50.1–100% dist		0–80% dist		80.1–100% dist	
			IHC	OHC	IHC	OHC	IHC	OHC	IHC	OHC
HO27	1.8	No	0	0	0	2.5	0	0.5	0	4.4
HO28	1.8	No	0	0.2	0	4.6	0	0.3	0	12.3
HO29	3.3	5×	0.3	0.2	0	0.2	0.2	0.2	0	0.5
HO30	3.3	No	0	0.1	0	1.1	0	0.2	0	2.2
HO42	3.3	1×	0	0.6	0	0.6	0	0.5	0	1.0
HO18	3.5	4×	0	0.6	7.7	27.4	0.5	0.8	19.9	73.4
HO43	4.0	1×	0	0.3	0	0	0	0.2	0	0
HO44	4.0	1×	0	0.3	0.3	0.4	0.2	0.3	0	0.7
Mean	3.1	—	0.0	0.3	1.0	4.6	0.1	0.4	2.5	11.8
(SD)[b]	(±0.9)	—	(±0.1)	(±0.2)	(±2.7)	(±9.3)	(±0.2)	(±0.2)	(±7.0)	(±25.2)

[a] Percentage distance from cochlear apex.
[b] Standard deviation.

there is significant loss of IHCs and OHCs, including two regions in which the OC had entirely degenerated and was replaced by squamous epithelium (tall hatched bars – middle). There is a corresponding loss of MNFs (short black bars – bottom) associated with the regions of IHC loss that equaled or exceeded 60%. This figure also shows the permanent threshold shift (PTS) for auditory brainstem response thresholds (ABR; open squares) determined 4 weeks post-exposure. Frequencies on the x-axis were assigned a percentage distance in the OC using the "edges" equation developed by Ou et al. (2000b). The mouse sustained a mild PTS at 3 to 4 kHz, and a moderate PTS at 30 to 50 kHz. The PTS at 3 to 4 kHz correlates with damage to IHC stereocilia (open and cross-hatched boxes–top), rather than a loss of hair cells. On the other hand, the PTS at 30 to 50 kHz correlates, in part, with the significant sensory-cell loss in the basal 30% of the OC.

Tables 12.2 presents summary data on hair-cell loss in eight non-noise-exposed C57BL/CBA F1 mice (male) that ranged in age from 1.8 to 4 months. The hearing (ABR thresholds) of some mice was tested prior to termination and revealed normal thresholds. The cell-loss data, obtained from the individual cytocochleograms, were averaged in the apical half (0 to 50% distance from the apex), basal half (50.1 to 100% distance from the apex), apical 80%, and basal 20% of the OC. Hair-cell loss is variable, especially in the basal 20% of the cochlea, as evidenced by the large standard deviations. This loss did not appear to be related to the mouse's age or to prior functional testing.

Figure 12.6 shows a TEM of the base of a third row OHC and Deiters' cell in OC segment #7 (~70% distance from the apex). This section was cut from a plastic-embedded flat preparation of a control mouse cochlea after its length had been measured and hair cells counted. Considerable cellular detail is visible in the hair cell (e.g., mitochondria, ribosomes), Deiters' cell (e.g., bundles of microtubules, mitochondria) and efferent nerve endings (e) (e.g., synaptic vesicles, mitochondria).

THREE-DIMENSIONAL STRUCTURE OF THE ORGAN OF CORTI

The OC is commonly diagrammed in cross-section with a single IHC and one OHC from each of the three rows lined up radially in a plane perpendicular to the BM (Slepecky, 1996). The supporting cells (pillar and Deiters' cells) are also shown as lying in this radial plane with the pillar heads in one-to-one correspondence. This is a simplified view. Examination of flat preparations of the mouse OC (e.g., Figure 12.4) shows that the third-row OHCs are directly lateral to the first-row OHCs,

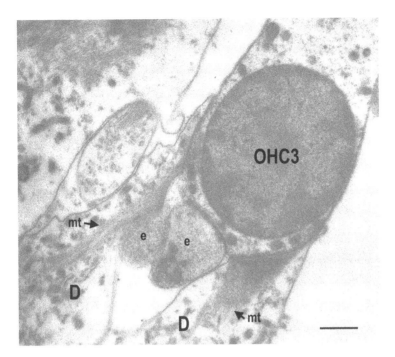

FIGURE 12.6 Transmission electron micrograph of the third outer hair cell (OHC3) in organ of Corti segment #7 (~70% distance from apex) of control mouse (strain 129). The infranuclear region of the hair cell is small and contains few mitochondria. Deiters' cell (D) forms a "V" around hair-cell base and sends processes, including microtubular bundles (mt), up to mid-nuclear region. Two efferent nerve fibers (e) are inserted into "V." Bar equals 1 μm.

while the second-row OHCs are offset by half an OHC. The head of the IP is in the same plane as its foot. Each IP headplate overlaps a portion of two adjacent OP heads. The head of the OP is basal to its foot by approximately one-half to one OHC. Each Deiters' cell base sends a slender process in an apical direction, crossing two to three OHCs, before reaching the reticular lamina and forming a phalangeal process in the reticular lamina. The organ of Corti is an engineering marvel, employing the classic triangular arrangement that provides low mass and high tensile strength.

Nerve fibers are depicted as synapsing on the hair cells directly lateral to the habenula through which they entered the OC. This depiction is true for the fibers that innervate the IHCs. Depending on the apex-to-base position in the mouse cochlea, 7 to 19 fibers take a direct radial course from habenula to nearest IHC (e.g., Ehret, 1979). On the other hand, fibers that innervate the OHCs either cross the tunnel as radial tunnel fibers (upper tunnel crossing [efferent] or basilar [afferent] fibers) and enter the outer spiral bundles between the Deiters' bases and BM. Once in the outer spiral bundles, these fibers run basally for a variable distance before synapsing on multiple OHCs. Nerve fibers to the OHCs may also enter the inner spiral bundle and run basally for a variable distance before crossing the tunnel.

The complex organization of the OC makes it impossible to obtain a semi-thick or thin radial section that contains all of its elements. To understand its three-dimensional structure, especially in malformed cochleae or those damaged by external trauma, it is important to examine the OC, both as a flat preparation and in radial sections.

EVALUATION OF THE VESTIBULAR ORGANS

At a low magnification, the general shape of the maculae can be evaluated as shown in Figure 12.7A. This mouse had normal vestibular function (i.e., normal swimming ability). The flat-preparation

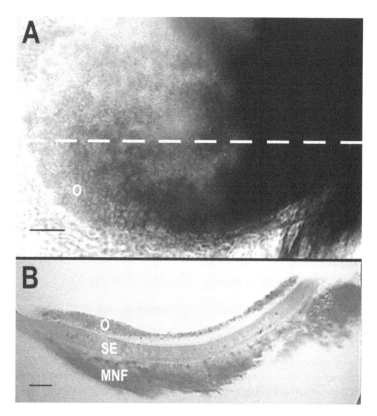

FIGURE 12.7 Utricular macula from heterozygous littermate of tilted mutant mouse. (A) Flat preparation viewed from endolymphatic surface. White dashed line indicates region from which section in (B) was taken. Individual otoconia (O) are just visible over the sensory epithelium. (B) Thick radial section view by bright-field microscopy. Otoconial layer (O) varies in thickness from periphery to center of sensory epithelium (SE). The myelinated peripheral processes (MNF) of the primary vestibular neurons are seen approaching the sensory cells in the SE. Bars equal 50 μm.

view (A), focused on the endolymphatic surface of the utricular macula, reveals a number of otoconia (O) at the periphery of the organ. The nerve fibers with their thick myelin sheaths enter the organ from the right, and then fan out beneath the epithelium. Because of the thickness of the organ and the presence of its otoconial layer, the nerve fibers are not clearly visible. The hair cells cannot be seen at all. Figure 12.7B is a thick radial section made at the position of the white dashed line in Figure 12.7A. Even at a low magnification, the otoconial layer (O), sensory epithelium (SE), and connective tissue and nerve fibers (MNF) underlying the epithelium are clearly visible. This thick section was also examined at 1250X magnification, which allowed identification of type I and type II hair cells, their stereocilia, supporting cells, and nerve chalices (data not shown).

A clearer view of the sensory epithelium of the macula and its relation to the otoconial layer can be obtained from the examination of semi-thick radial sections. Figure 12.8 illustrates stained 1-μm-thick sections of the utricular macula from a wild-type littermate with normal swimming ability (A) and a tilted mouse (B) that was unable to swim. The sensory epithelium in both mice contains type I and type II hair cells and supporting cells (SC). The sensory epithelium is separated by the basal lamina (BL) from the underlying connective tissue that contains nerve fibers (NF). The hair-cell stereocilia (st) project into the overlying gelatinous otoconial membrane (OM). The only difference in the maculae of these animals is the absence of otoconia (O) in the tilted mouse.

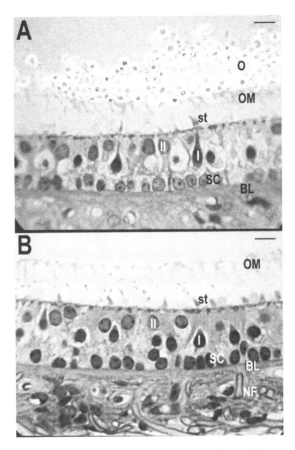

FIGURE 12.8   Stained 1-µm-thick sections of utricular macula from: (A) heterozygous littermate (see Figure 12.7); and (B) tilted (*tlt/tlt*) mouse. In both mice, sensory epithelium contains type I (I) and type II (II) hair cells with stereocilia (st) and supporting cells (SC) that rests on the basal lamina (BL). Nerve fibers (NF) lose their myelin sheaths at the BL before entering the sensory epithelium to synapse on the hair cells. A gelatinous otoconial membrane (OM) covers the sensory epithelium in both mice, but only the heterozygous littermate has otoconia (O) embedded in its otoconial membrane. Bars equal 10 µm.

Detailed examination of the cristae of the semicircular canals requires the cutting of thick, semi-thick, or thin radial sections as described for the maculae. Figure 12.9 is a low magnification photomicrograph of a thick razor section through the superior crista. The enlarged end or ampulla (A) of the semicircular canal is seen in cross-section. The sensory epithelium (SE) is divided into two parts by the septum cruciatum (SC) and is covered by the gelatinous cupula (C). The hair cells and their stereocilia can be examined at a high magnification either in the thick, semi-thick, or thin sections as shown above for the macula.

DISCUSSION AND ANALYSIS

CHOICE OF PREPARATION TECHNIQUE TO ASSESS PATHOLOGY IN INNER-EAR SENSORY EPITHELIA

The technique of decalcifying the temporal bone, embedding it in a support medium, and cutting sections parallel to the modiolus of the cochlea is useful for relating pathology in outer and middle ears and bony labyrinth to that in the membranous labyrinth (e.g., Schuknecht, 1993). However, with this technique, it is difficult to obtain an overview of gross structural anomalies of the bony

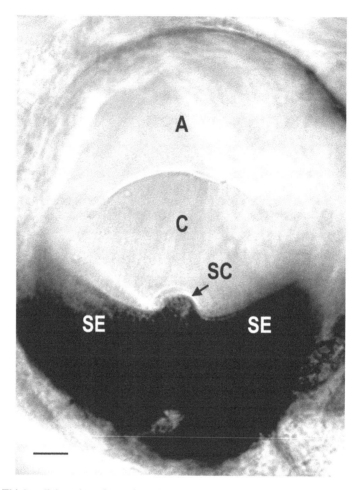

FIGURE 12.9 Thick radial section of superior crista from control mouse (strain 129). The sensory epithelium (SE) is housed in the ampullated (A) portion of semicircular canal. It is divided in two by the septum cruciatum (SC) and is entirely covered by the gelatinous cupula (C). Bar equals 50 μm.

and membranous labyrinths without performing serial reconstruction of the sections. In addition, complete quantitative data on the magnitude and location of sensory and supporting cell losses/damage cannot be obtained.

Examining the temporal bone by SEM requires that the endolymphatic space be opened and the extracellular membranes (i.e., tectorial membrane, otoconial membrane, cupula) be removed from the surface of the sensory epithelia. In well-prepared specimens, all sensory areas can be examined and quantitative data collected (e.g., Mulroy and Curley, 1982; Fredelius et al., 1987). The side- and tip-links that connect adjacent stereocilia are more easily examined by SEM (e.g., Hackney et al., 1988). However, it has been noted (e.g., Hunter-Duvar, 1978; Hackney et al., 1991) that the mechanical manipulation of the sensory epithelia that occurs during the dissection may alter certain cellular features or obscure a variable number of sensory cells. In addition, structures below the surface of the sensory epithelia (e.g., cell bodies, nerve fibers and endings) cannot be systematically examined.

If the sensory epithelia are evaluated solely by TEM, generally only a small percentage of sensory cells in a given inner ear is studied. Thus, it is not known if the examined cells contain pathological changes that are representative of those in the entire epithelia. It is known that the sensory epithelia in the inner ear are not homogeneous. There are pronounced differences in hair-cell dimensions, innervation patterns, functional properties, and response to trauma across each sensory organ (e.g., Bohne, 1976; Bohne and Carr, 1985; Ehret, 1979; Lee and Kimura, 1994; Ou et al., 2000a; Pack and Slepecky, 1995; Thalmann, 1976). For this reason, TEM findings in one region of a particular sensory organ may not be the same as those in another region.

The technique described here for plastic embedding of the temporal bone prior to its dissection protects the delicate sensory epithelia from mechanical damage during processing. Because the entire membranous labyrinth and most of the bony labyrinth are embedded in a single block, all six sensory epithelia in the inner ear can be dissected as flat preparations for examination at low and intermediate magnifications. This approach allows the sensory epithelia to be thoroughly screened in order to identify and quantify the extent of pathological changes prior to the cutting of sections for examination at higher magnifications, including by TEM.

IDENTIFICATION OF HISTOPATHOLOGICAL CHANGES IN THE TEMPORAL BONE

Many spontaneous or induced genetic mutations involving the membranous and bony labyrinths have been described for the mouse (e.g., Sidman et al., 1965; Steel, 1995). New mutations involving the mouse ear continue to be discovered or developed (e.g., Holme and Steel, 1999; and Chapters 27 and 30 in this book). A certain proportion of these mutations may involve multiple structures, including the external and middle ears, and the auditory and vestibular portions of the inner ear. Thus, it is important to perform at least a cursory examination of all relevant structures. For example, if the middle ear is grossly normal, detailed histopathological analysis can be restricted to the organ of Corti. Furthermore, if the mouse has no signs of vestibular dysfunction, the sensory epithelia from the vestibule can then serve as fixation and/or processing controls.

In some mutant mice, abnormalities may vary between an animal's two ears (e.g., Cable et al., 1992; Deol, 1964; Nolan et al., 1995). Thus, to determine the range of histopathological changes that occurs in specific mutant mice, it is necessary to examine both inner ears from a reasonable sample of animals.

It is known that sizable variations in damage may occur among individuals receiving identical exposures to ototoxic drugs or noise (e.g., Bohne and Clark, 1982; Bredberg and Hunter-Duvar, 1975; Miller et al., 1963; Santi et al., 1982). This variability was initially seen in non-inbred animals (e.g., chinchillas, guinea pigs, gerbils) and may have been due, in part, to genetic differences among the individual members of the species. We recently found that there can be sizable variation in hair-cell losses across genetically identical control (Table 12.2) and noise-exposed mice (Ou et al., 2000a) of similar ages, although other studies have reported less variability (e.g., Yoshida et al., 2000). We also found a significant difference in OC length between male and female C57BL/CBA F1 mice. Thus, some variation in noise-induced hair-cell losses could be the result of differences in susceptibility between the sexes. For this reason, studies involving noise exposure should specify the sex of the animals used, or employ equivalent numbers of males and females. The number of animals needed to obtain a representative sample of histopathological changes should be determined using an independent measure of damage (e.g., functional impairment). It should be noted, however, that the two ears of a particular animal generally have equivalent susceptibilities to external trauma (e.g., Bohne et al., 1986). Thus, the appropriate sample size should be based on number of animals, rather than number of ears.

FUNCTIONAL ASSESSMENT OF THE AUDITORY AND VESTIBULAR SYSTEMS

It is important to observe behavioral abnormalities (e.g., circling, head tilting, head tossing) and to perform some simple tests of auditory (e.g., ABRs, distortion product otoacoustic emissions; Yoshida et al., 2000; also Chapter 4 in this book) and vestibular function (e.g., swim test; Ornitz et al., 1998) prior to processing an animal's ears for histopathological analysis. For mice with genetic mutations, such data will indicate which sensory organs are likely to have pathological alterations and which organs are probably normal. This is a necessary step in identifying how the mutant gene causes disease (i.e., functional genomics [Kwitek-Black, 2000]). For aging mice or those exposed to external trauma, these data can be used to compare the susceptibility of different strains and to correlate functional losses with structural damage.

ADVANTAGES OF MICE

With respect to anatomical and histopathological studies, the mouse cochlea has thinner bone, and its organ of Corti is much shorter and contains fewer hair cells (mean 706 IHCs; 2416 OHCs) than the OCs from other rodents (e.g., chinchilla, mean 1900 IHCs; 7500 OHCs). For these reasons, dissection of the mouse cochlea and collection of quantitative data throughout its OC take much less time.

LIMITATIONS OF MICE

- Without special acoustic equipment, the highest frequency that can be tested is 32 to 50 kHz. It has been reported that the upper limit of mouse hearing is 80 to 100 kHz (Berlin, 1963; Ehret, 1974; Mikaelian et al., 1974). An anatomical-based frequency-place map of the C57BL/CBA F1 mouse OC developed by Ou et al. (2000b) assigns 32 kHz to 76% distance from the cochlear apex and 50 kHz to about 87% distance. Thus, damage in the basal 13 to 24% of the OC cannot be detected audiometrically with standard acoustic equipment. Age-related loss of hearing begins in the high frequencies for humans and mice, and is accompanied by degeneration of cochlear hair cells at the basal tip of the OC (Table 12.2; Spongr et al., 1997a). Therefore, beginning hearing loss and hair-cell degeneration cannot be detected if the highest audible frequencies are not tested.
- Unlike the chinchilla, guinea pig, and rat, it is difficult to perform survival surgery on the mouse inner ear because of its small size, the fragility of its skull and temporal bone, and the fact that the sutures between the temporal bone and the remainder of the skull are not ossified. Thus, the mouse temporal bone can easily be displaced from the skull, the middle ear disrupted, or the cochlear bone and membranous labyrinth damaged during survival surgery to insert recording electrodes, collect cochlear fluids, or inject test fluids into the perilymphatic scalae.
- The patterns of hearing loss and OC damage following excessive exposure to noise appear to be different for mice and humans. In humans and rodents, including mice, high-frequency noise produces a high-frequency hearing loss and focal losses of sensory cells at the high-frequency end of the OC (e.g., Bredberg, 1968; Bohne, 1976; Bohne and Clark, 1982; Ou et al., 2000a; Yoshida et al., 2000). Low-frequency noise initially results in OHC loss only in the low-frequency region of the human and chinchilla cochleae (e.g., Bredberg, 1968; Bohne and Clark, 1982), but no corresponding hearing loss for low-frequency pure tones. On the other hand, low-frequency noise initially damages IHC stereocilia at the apex of the mouse cochlea, while sparing OHCs and IHCs. The IHC stereocilia damage is associated with a hearing loss for low-frequency tones (Ou et al., 2000a).

ACKNOWLEDGMENTS

Funds for this work were provided by the National Organization for Hearing Research, the American Heart Association, and the Department of Otolaryngology. The authors gratefully acknowledge the excellent technical assistance provided by Ms. Rosie Saito and Mr. Thomas J. Watkins. Dr. David M. Ornitz kindly provided the tilted mice. The animal care and use protocol for functional testing of hearing and balance, anesthesia, and cardiac perfusion in mice was reviewed and approved by Washington University's Animal Studies Committee (#97329 - B.A. Bohne, P.I.).

13 Cochlear Hair Cell Densities and Inner-Ear Staining Techniques

Dalian Ding, Sandra L. McFadden, and Richard J. Salvi

INTRODUCTION

The past decade has witnessed an explosive growth in the number of new strains of mice available for scientific study, as is evident throughout this book. The introduction of new strains and phenotypes and the eventual sequencing of the mouse genome will allow auditory neuroscientists to understand how different genes influence the structure and function of the inner ear (Fritzsch et al., 1997b; Lanford et al., 1999; Lewis et al., 1998). Studies of different strains and phenotypes will undoubtedly provide important clues about the genetic factors that influence an individual's susceptibility to presbycusis, ototoxicity, and noise-induced hearing loss (Erway and Willott, 1996; McFadden et al., 1999; Richardson et al., 1997).

To appreciate the functional significance of these genetic differences and manipulations, it is important to have a basic understanding of some of the fundamental anatomical features of the mouse inner ear, such as hair cell density, cochlear length, and number of rows of inner hair cells (IHCs) and outer hair cells (OHCs). Surprisingly, a survey of the literature reveals little in the way of a systematic body of data that mouse researchers can draw upon to assess the effects of various genetic mutations. Thus, one purpose of this chapter is to provide the reader with an assessment of hair cell density, cochlear length, and hair cell loss in a number of common mouse models used in auditory research.

As the number of mice with induced mutations increases, it will become increasingly important to have reliable and efficient methods for quantifying and assessing the integrity of the sensory hair cells, nerve fibers, and spiral ganglion neurons in the mouse inner ear. In some cases, it may be sufficient to determine if the hair cell body is present or missing. In other cases, the hair cells may be present, but it may be necessary to determine if significant impairments exist in the stereocilia or if the metabolic activity of the cells is compromised. On other occasions, it may be necessary to assess the integrity of the afferent or efferent innervation of the cochlea. How can these measurements be performed accurately and efficiently when the sensory organ is extremely small and notoriously difficult to dissect because it is encased in bone? In addition to providing normative data on cochlear hair cells, this chapter describes a number of histological techniques that are particularly useful for surveying the structural integrity of the inner ear in normal and mutant mice.

NORMATIVE DATA

HAIR CELL DENSITY AND COCHLEAR LENGTH

Any quantitative assessment of the sensory hair cells in the inner ear requires an initial assessment of hair cell density along the length of the cochlea. These data are essential for evaluating sensory cell loss in damaged ears and for relating basic measures of auditory performance to the structural

TABLE 13.1
Cochlear Cell Densities in CBA/CaJ Mice

Distance	IHC	OHC1	OHC2	OHC3
0–10	131	135	131	136
11–20	125	131	130	137
21–30	125	133	133	137
31–40	125	133	132	135
41–50	131	139	140	143
51–60	134	140	139	142
61–70	127	130	131	132
71–80	118	122	122	122
81–90	111	118	118	119
91–100	106	113	112	112
Mean	123	129	129	131

Note: Density given in number of cells/mm in successive 10% segments of the cochlea beginning at the apex.

TABLE 13.2
Cochlear Cell Densities in C57BL/6J Mice

Distance	IHC	OHC1	OHC2	OHC3
0–10	115	133	134	140
11–20	114	129	129	131
21–30	120	133	134	138
31–40	122	136	136	140
41–50	120	137	137	142
51–60	135	135	139	136
61–70	123	130	131	134
71–80	117	126	125	126
81–90	109	120	119	122
91–100	104	111	110	112
Mean	116	129	129	132

Note: Density given in number of cells/mm in successive 10% segments of the cochlea beginning at the apex.

dimensions of the cochlea. Tables 13.1 to 13.4 show the density (cells/mm) of IHCs and each of the three rows of OHCs from the apex to the base of the cochlea (10% intervals) in four common inbred strains: CBA/CaJ (CBA), C57BL/6J (B6), DBA/2, and BALB/cJ. The two strains most frequently used in presbycusis research are CBA and B6 mice. CBA/CaJ and CBA/J mice show relatively little hearing loss and hair cell loss until late in their life span (Henry and Chole, 1980; Li and Borg, 1991; Spongr et al., 1997a; Willott and Mortenson, 1991). B6 mice, in contrast, develop hair cell lesions in the base of the cochlea in early adult life, which rapidly progress toward the apex of the cochlea with advancing age (Henry and Chole, 1980; Li and Borg, 1991; Mikaelian, 1979; Spongr et al., 1997a). The onset of hearing loss and hair cell loss in BALB/cJ is more rapid than in B6 mice, but less rapid than in DBA/2 mice (Willott et al., 1998).

Several differences in cell density can be seen in these four strains. First, IHC and OHC hair cell densities are more uniform along the length of the cochlea in DBA/2 and BALB/cJ mice than

TABLE 13.3
Cochlear Cell Densities in DBA/2J Mice

Distance	IHC	OHC1	OHC2	OHC3
0–10	126	126	125	125
11–20	129	140	139	140
21–30	129	145	144	145
31–40	129	145	145	145
41–50	128	144	144	144
51–60	129	145	146	145
61–70	129	144	144	144
71–80	128	146	145	146
81–90	125	144	144	144
91–100	124	144	144	144
Mean	127	142	142	142

Note: Density given in number of cells/mm in successive 10% segments of the cochlea beginning at the apex.

TABLE 13.4
Cochlear Cell Densities in BALB/cJ Mice

Distance	IHC	OHC1	OHC2	OHC3
0–10	127	136	135	134
11–20	129	141	141	141
21–30	127	143	143	143
31–40	128	147	146	147
41–50	127	144	146	144
51–60	126	146	146	146
61–70	126	144	144	144
71–80	124	142	142	142
81–90	121	140	139	140
91–100	117	138	138	138
Mean	125	142	142	141

Note: Density given in number of cells/mm in successive 10% segments of the cochlea beginning at the apex.

in CBA and B6 mice. Hair cell density in CBA and B6 mice shows a small decline in the basal portion of the cochlea, from 60 to 100% of the distance from the apex. Second, hair cell density is greater in DBA/2 and BALB/cJ mice than in CBA and B6 mice. Third, OHC density is generally greater than IHC density. These differences illustrate the importance of having appropriate hair cell norms for each strain of mouse being studied and for quantitative comparison across strains.

A fundamental characteristic of the mammalian auditory system is the transfer of frequency onto a specific site of mechanical vibration along the cochlear partition. In humans, the full range of hearing, approximately 20 kHz, is transposed onto a cochlea that is approximately 34 mm long. The mouse cochlea, by contrast, has a hearing range of roughly 100 kHz; however, its cochlea is only about 6 mm in length. Mapping frequency onto place requires knowledge of the length of each strain's cochlea and its upper and lower frequency range of hearing (Greenwood, 1990). Table 13.5 shows the average length of the cochlea in the four inbred strains mentioned above.

TABLE 13.5
Mean Length (± SD) of Basilar Membrane

Strain	N	Mean ± SD
CBA/Ca	10	5.88 ± 0.29
B6	10	6.20 ± 0.20
DBA/2	6	6.32 ± 0.11
BALB/cJ	6	6.16 ± 0.27
B10	5	6.10 ± 0.19

Note: All mice approximately 1 month old.

TABLE 13.6
Total Number of Hair Cells/Cochlea

Strain	IHC	OHC1	OHC2	OHC3	OHC123
CBA	725	760	757	773	2291
C57BL/6	723	799	799	820	2420
DBA/2	806	899	897	898	2695
BALB/cJ	771	875	874	874	2624

Among the four strains shown here, the CBA has the shortest cochlea (5.88 mm on average), and the DBA/2 has the longest cochlea (6.32 mm). The length of the cochlea, together with knowledge of hair cell density, allow one to estimate the total number of IHCs and OHCs for each strain. As shown in Table 13.6, CBA mice have the fewest total IHCs and OHCs, while DBA/2 have the most hair cells. Such information can be especially useful when studying the effects of genes and growth factors that influence the length of the cochlea, the density and number of hair cells, and the arrangement of IHCs and OHCs with respect to supporting cells and neurons (W.-Q. Gao et al., 1999; Kelley et al., 1994; Represa et al., 1990).

HAIR CELL LOSS AND AGING

The cochleogram, a plot showing the percentage of missing IHCs and OHCs as a function of percent total distance from the apex of the cochlea, is a standard method of describing the location and size of sensory cell lesions resulting from various types of trauma, such as acoustic overstimulation and ototoxic drugs. However, hair cell lesions can develop in normal mice as they age, and certain strains of mice show a strong genetic predisposition to age-related hair cell loss and presbycusis. Thus, anyone planning a research study with mice that extends over a few months to a year should give careful consideration to the choice of strain because of potential confounding effects of age-related hair cell death.

Figures 13.1 through 13.4 show hair cell loss as a function of age for five strains of mice. For all strains except C57BL/10J (B10), hair cell loss is referenced to the total number of hair cells present in a normal cochlea of that strain. Hair cell losses for the B10 mice are relative to the norms for B6 mice. (*Note:* B6 and B10 are two of the seven major substrains of C57BL, separated prior to 1937. According to The Jackson Laboratory [www.informatics.jax.org/external/festing/mouse/docs/C57BL.shtml], the B6 and B10 substrains appear to be quite similar, although they differ at multiple loci on chromosome 4).

Among the common strains of laboratory mice, the CBA is one of the most resistant to age-related hair cell loss, showing minimal loss out to 8 months of age (Figure 13.1). Nevertheless,

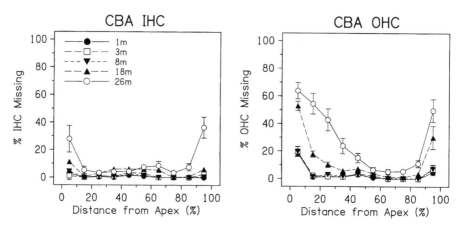

FIGURE 13.1 Average hair cell loss in successive 10% segments of the cochlea for CBA mice of various ages. Percent hair cells missing was determined relative to normal cochleae of the CBA strain. Left panel, IHC loss; right panel, OHC loss; bars show SEMs. There were ten mice in each age group except 8 month (n = 5). (Data from Spongr et al., 1997a.)

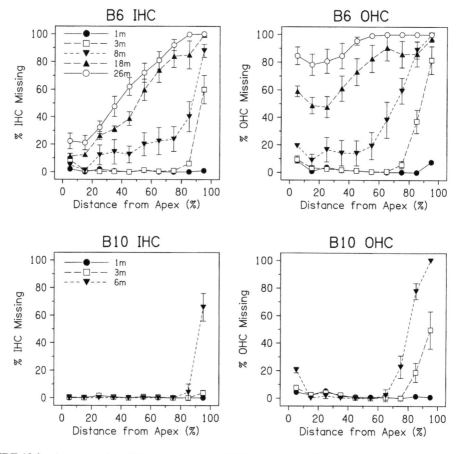

FIGURE 13.2 Average hair cell loss in successive 10% segments of the cochlea for B6 mice (top panels) and B10 mice (bottom panels) of various ages. Percent hair cells missing was determined relative to normal cochleae of the B6 strain. Left panels, IHC loss; right panels, OHC loss; bars show SEMs. There were ten mice in each B6 age group, and 4 to 5 mice in each B10 age group. (B6 data from Spongr et al., 1997a; B10 data not previously published.)

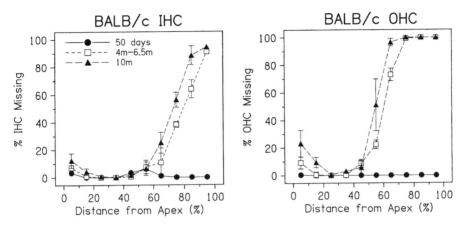

FIGURE 13.3 Average hair cell loss in successive 10% segments of the cochlea for BALB/cJ mice of various ages. Percent hair cells missing was determined relative to normal cochleae of the BALB/cJ strain. Left panel, IHC loss; right panel, OHC loss; bars show SEMs. There were three mice in each age group (50 days, 4 months, 6.5 months, and 10 months). Data for 4- and 6.5-month-old mice are combined. (See Willott et al., 1998 for hair cell counts of the same BALB/cJ mice.)

small to moderate OHC lesions appear at the high-frequency basal end of the cochlea and the low-frequency apical region around 18 months of age. By 26 months of age, the apical and basal OHC lesions have expanded toward the middle of the cochlea, and IHC lesions appear at the extreme base and apex. Thus, as long as the measurements do not extend much beyond 8 to 12 months of age, the confounding effects of age-related hair cell loss should be minimal in CBA mice.

On the other hand, if one wishes to study the effects of age-related hair cell loss, then the C57BL strains would be a highly desirable model. B6 mice develop large IHC and OHC lesions that spread from the base to apex with advancing age (Figure 13.2, top row). Most hair cells are present at 1 month of age; but by 3 months, clear evidence of OHC loss, and to a lesser extent IHC loss, are evident near the base of the cochlea. At 26 months of age, nearly all the OHCs are missing except for a small percentage in the apical third of the cochlea; IHC loss decreases from 100% in the base to roughly 25% at the extreme apex. Estimates of age-related hair cell loss in B10 mice are currently underway in our laboratory and preliminary data (Figure 13.2, bottom row) suggest that the growth of the lesion with age will be similar to that in the B6 substrain.

The BALB/cJ mouse is another inbred strain that exhibits early onset age-related IHC and OHC loss that progresses along a base to apex gradient (Figure 13.3). Most hair cells are present at 50 days of age; but by 10 months of age, most of the OHCs are missing over the basal third of the cochlea, and roughly 20% of the OHCs are missing in the extreme apex. Likewise, IHC loss declines from nearly 100% at the extreme base to less than 10% in the middle of the cochlea. While B6 and BALB/cJ exhibit a similar pattern and time course of age-related hair cell loss, inspection of the data suggests that the loss may develop a bit more rapidly in the BALB/cJ.

TECHNIQUES FOR ASSESSING MOUSE INNER-EAR PATHOLOGY

Because of its small size, the mouse inner ear presents special challenges for dissection and staining. Some methods for evaluating the mouse temporal bone (e.g., electron microscopy) require careful attention to embedding and sectioning of the tissue. Excellent techniques for preparing the mouse temporal bone through resin embedding are described by Bohne et al. in this volume. However, when the aim of histology is simple evaluation of hair cell loss or determination of gross histopathology, less time-consuming techniques that do not involve tissue embedding may be appropriate. Here, we describe several relatively simple methods that we have used successfully for preparing

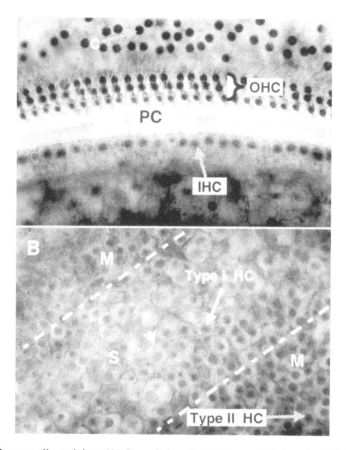

FIGURE 13.4 Hematoxylin staining. (A) Inner hair cells (IHC), outer hair cells (OHCs), and nuclei of supporting cells (Claudius cells, c) in the cochlea are strongly stained. Pillar cells (PC) separate IHC and OHC. (B) Nuclei of vestibular hair cells (HC) are strongly stained by hematoxylin. Type I hair cells can be distinguished from type II hair cells by the presence of the afferent chalice (arrowhead) surrounding the cell. Type I cells are more numerous in the striolar region (S), whereas type II cells are more numerous in the marginal region (M).

and staining the mouse inner ear for light microscopic examination of hair cells, ganglion cells, nerve fibers, and red blood cells (see also Chapter 12). Because many degenerative changes in the inner ear progress along a base-to-apex gradient (i.e., from high to low frequencies), it is generally necessary to assess the magnitude of sensory cell loss over the entire length of the cochlea. One of the most convenient methods of assessing the longitudinal extent of damage is to carefully dissect out the organ of Corti as a flat-surface preparation. It is quite common to dissect the entire organ of Corti in consecutive half-turn segments that are arranged in order on a glass slide. The specimens can be stained by several different methods, depending on the specific cell type or feature that one is interested in evaluating. Afterward, the specimen is cover-slipped and examined with a compound microscope (usually 200 to 400X) along its entire length.

To visualize hair cells and other inner-ear tissues with a light microscope, it is usually necessary to impart color to the tissue. This can be accomplished by three primary methods: (1) staining the tissue with dyes (e.g., eosin), (2) impregnating the tissue with metallic salts (e.g., silver nitrate), or (3) initiating chemical reactions that form either true dyes or colored chemical compounds that are not dyes (e.g., hematoxylin staining and succinate dehydrogenase histochemistry). The dye method employs compounds that possess the dual properties of color and the ability to bind to tissues. Dye uptake can be modified by fixatives and mordants (agents that act as a "bridge" between a dye and a particular tissue). For example, formalin fixation promotes the staining of proteins and nucleic acids. The second method, metallic salt impregnation, usually employs silver nitrate. There are three general reactions involving silver: *arygrophil* reactions, in which silver nitrate binds to structural elements with natural affinity for it (arygrophilia) and is subsequently reduced to form an opaque (usually black or brownish-black) silver compound; *argentaffin* reactions, in which substances (often phenols) present in structures directly reduce the silver salts; and *aldehyde* reactions, in which certain carbohydrate-containing tissues are oxidized to aldehydes that, in turn, reduce hexamine-silver nitrate compounds to a black product. Staining by metallic impregnation can be a one-step technique in tissues with powerful reducing agents such as myelin. The third method, formation of colored compounds by means of a chemical reaction, is a very old technique, dating back to a histochemical technique for demonstration of tyrosine devised by Millon in 1849 (Bancroft and Cook, 1984). Since Gomori introduced the use of the chemical reaction method for the demonstration of enzymes in 1939, this technique has become indispensable for enzyme histochemistry. One advantage of histochemical techniques is that they involve clearly understood, highly specific chemical reactions. In enzyme reactions, the enzymes do not combine with a chemical substrate to form a colored end-product. Rather, the enzymes react upon a substrate, and this either changes the substrate into a colored product at the site of enzyme activity, or it produces a colorless compound that can be turned into a colored compound in a subsequent reaction. A second advantage to using histochemical techniques is the ability to quantify results, because the intensity of the reaction is proportional to the quantity of the active reagent in the tissues (D.L. Ding et al., 1999). An obvious disadvantage to histochemical techniques is that staining must be accomplished rapidly to avoid the loss of labile substances following the removal of the inner ear.

We routinely use each of the three general staining methods for evaluating the mouse inner ear. For hair cell counting, our preferred staining methods are hematoxylin for fixed tissue and SDH histochemistry for fresh, unfixed tissue. Other stains we use routinely are eosin for red blood cells, acetylcholinesterase (AChE) histochemistry for efferent fibers, and osmium tetroxide for myelin in fresh or formalin-fixed tissue. Myelin is a complex substance containing protein, cholesterol, phospholipids, and cerebrosides. The lipids in myelin reduce osmium tetroxide to a black compound that is easily visualized. Nerve fibers can also be demonstrated using silver nitrate or mordant-hematoxylin solutions that attach to the phospholipid component of myelin.

Hematoxylin

Hematoxylin, a substance extracted from the bark of a small tree found in Mexico and Jamaica, was one of the first "dyes" used for histological purposes, and it is probably the most important early dye still in use today. Technically, hematoxylin is not a dye, because it lacks tissue-binding properties and has little inherent color; color appears only after hematoxylin is oxidized to hematein, a weakly anionic purple dye. To accelerate the oxidation of hematoxylin to hematein, an oxidizing agent (e.g., mercuric oxide, sodium iodate, or iodine) is added to the staining solution. Because hematein is anionic, it has no affinity for anionic structures such as chromatin. Therefore, the hematoxylin must be combined with a metallic salt mordant to produce a cationic dye–metal complex. The particular mordant used depends on the desired demonstration; for example, aluminum ammonium sulfate for chromatin staining, potassium dichromate for phospholipids, or iron alum for normal myelin.

We typically use Harris' hematoxylin solution (Humason, 1972), which uses mercuric oxide as the oxidizing agent and aluminum ammonium sulfate as the mordant. This is an inexpensive, reliable, and convenient stain for hair cells and certain supporting cells in fixed tissue. Harris' hematoxylin is a powerful and selective stain that sharply delineates the nucleus of hair cells and supporting cells in the cochlear and vestibular sensory epithelium. Figure 13.4A shows the orderly pattern of staining seen in a flat surface preparation of the mouse inner ear. The nuclei of the three rows of OHCs and single row of IHCs are distinctly labeled and separated by a clear region formed

TABLE 13.7
Essential Steps for Harris' Hematoxylin Staining

1. Anesthetize animal; remove cochlea and vestibular system.
2. Open round window and oval window, make hole in apex, and then gently perfuse 10% formalin through openings. Store specimen in fixative for a minimum of 4 h.
3. Immerse sample in Harris' hematoxylin solution[a] for 5 min.
4. Dip tissue into 0.3% hydrochloric acid to remove excess color (approximately 5 s).
5. Place tissue in aluminum ammonium sulfate solution for several seconds until the tissue turns blue.
6. Mount tissue on slide as surface preparation.

[a] Harris' hematoxylin staining solution:
- Dissolve 0.9 g hematoxylin in 10 cc of 100% alcohol using gentle heat.
- Dissolve 20 g aluminum ammonium sulfate in 200 cc distilled water using heat with frequent stirring.
- Mix the hematoxylin-alcohol and hot aluminum ammonium sulfate solutions and bring to a boil, stirring frequently.
- Remove from heat and add 0.5 g red mercuric oxide.
- Return to heat and bring to a boil; remove immediately; solution should be dark purple.
- Filter the hematoxylin solution before use.

by the inner and outer pillar cells. The nuclei of the Claudius cells are seen as sharp, intensely labeled spots lateral to OHCs. Figure 13.4B shows a flat surface preparation of the crista of a semicircular canal stained by hematoxylin. The striola, or central region of the crista, is populated mainly by type I hair cells that are surrounded by large chalice-like nerve endings of the afferent vestibular neurons (dashed lines show approximate boundaries of striola). The nuclei of the type I hair cells are stained darkly by hematoxylin, whereas the surrounding afferent terminals, largely devoid of chromatin, form a clear circular envelope around the type I hair cells. Hematoxylin also stains the nuclei of type II hair cells, which are mainly found outside the striolar region. In a surface preparation view, type II hair cells appear closely packed together because they lack large, clear chalice-like afferent terminals. Thus, type II hair cells can be distinguished from type I hair cells based on the absence of a large, clear space surrounding the hair cell. The general procedures for Harris' hematoxylin staining are presented in Table 13.7 (Humason, 1972).

SUCCINATE DEHYDROGENASE (SDH) HISTOCHEMISTRY

One of the most reliable and convenient methods for evaluating the presence or absence of IHCs and OHCs utilizes SDH histochemistry. The histochemical procedures for visualizing the activities of SDH and other dehydrogenases are based on the fact that colorless tetrazolium salts are reduced to distinct colored formazans in the presence of hydrogen donors (Altman, 1974; Altman, 1976). When succinate is included in the incubation medium, SDH will catalyze its oxidation to fumarate (Clarke et al., 1989; Spector, 1975; Vosteen, 1960), and the liberated hydrogen ion will reduce the electron-accepting tetrazolium salt to an insoluble, blue formazan (Koide et al., 1964; Spoendlin and Balogh, 1963; Yang et al., 1990).

Because SDH and other mitochondrial enzymes involved in aerobic metabolism are expressed at much higher levels in IHCs and OHCs than in supporting cells, the SDH-labeled hair cells stain dark blue with little background staining (Figure 13.5A). SDH labeling is absent in regions where the hair cells are missing or is greatly reduced in hair cells that are metabolically compromised. For example, C57 mice, which exhibit early onset hair cell loss and hearing loss, show much lower levels of SDH labeling than CBA mice of any age (D.L. Ding et al., 1999). SDH also distinctly labels the hair cells in the vestibular sensory epithelium, as shown in Figure 13.5B. The hair cells in the crista of the posterior semicircular canal are intensely labeled. The hair cells in the posterior semicircular canal are separated into two distinct regions separated by a "bar," a region devoid of

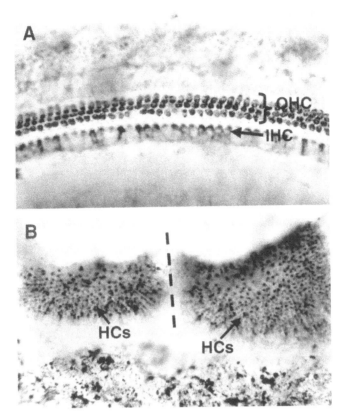

FIGURE 13.5 SDH histochemistry. (A) Inner hair cells (IHC) and outer hair cells (OHC) in the cochlea are strongly labeled. (B) Hair cells (HC) of the posterior semicircular canal are strongly labeled. Note the presence of a bar (indicated by dashed line) in the central portion of the crista. The bar is a region devoid of hair cells that effectively separates nerve fibers into two prominent bundles (see Figure 13.8). The bar is found in all three semicircular canals of birds and in the posterior and superior semicircular canals of mice, but not in semicircular canals of humans.

hair cells. The bar is found in all three semicircular canals of birds and in the posterior and superior semicircular canals of mice, but not in semicircular canals of humans. The essential steps involved in SDH staining of the cochlear and vestibular sensory epithelia are shown in Table 13.8 (Humason, 1972). Because the SDH staining solution labels dehydrogenase enzymes involved in aerobic metabolism, it must be perfused into the cochlea and vestibular system prior to fixation.

TABLE 13.8
Essential Steps in Succinate Dehydrogenase Histochemistry

1. Anesthetize animal; remove cochlea and vestibular system.
2. Open round window and oval window, make hole in apex, and then gently perfuse SDH staining solution[a] through openings. Immerse specimen in SDH solution for 45 min at 37° C.
3. Fix specimens in 10% formalin for 4 h.
4. Microdissect out sensory epithelium and mount on glass slide as a surface preparation.

[a] SDH Staining Solution:
- 0.2 M sodium succinate (2.5 mL)
- 0.2 M phosphate buffered saline (pH 7.6) (2.5 mL)
- 0.2 M nitro-BT (tetranitro blue tetrazolium) (5.0 mL)

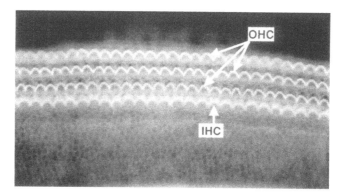

FIGURE 13.6　Staining for filamentous actin (F-actin) protein using rhodamine-conjugated phalloidin. Surface preparation view of the organ of Corti showing stereocilia bundles on inner hair cells (IHC) and three rows of outer hair cells (OHC).

TABLE 13.9
Essential Steps for Phalloidin Staining

1. Anesthetize animal; remove cochlea and vestibular system.
2. Open round window and oval window; make hole in apex.
3. Perfuse cochlea and vestibular systems with 4% paraformaldehyde in 0.1 M phosphate buffer (pH 7.2) for 2 h.
4. Immerse sample in 0.25% Triton-X 100 for 5 min.
5. Immerse sample in rhodamine-labeled phalloidin (dilution 1:200) in phosphate buffered saline for 30 min.
6. Rinse sample with phosphate buffered saline.
7. Mount on slide in 50% glycerol with 100 mg/mL of 1,4-diazobicyclo-octane, an anti-fade compound.
8. View with a microscope equipped with epi-fluorescent illumination with excitation and emission filters appropriate to the fluorescent probe that is conjugated to phalloidin.

PHALLOIDIN STAINING

A useful method for identifying hair cells is to use fluorescently labeled phalloidin, a toxin that binds selectively to filamentous actin (F-actin), a structural protein that is abundant in the stereocilia bundles in hair cells (Raphael, 1991). When phalloidin is conjugated to a fluorescent probe such as rhodamine, it can be visualized with a microscope equipped with epi-fluorescence illumination and the appropriate excitation and emission filters for visualizing the fluorochrome (for more detailed information, see Molecular Probes at www.probes.com). Figure 13.6 shows a surface preparation of the mouse organ of Corti that was maintained as an organ culture from postnatal day 3 to 5. The blunt V-shaped stereocilia bundles can be clearly seen on the three rows of OHCs. The stereocilia on the IHCs tend to form more gently curving arcs. Much higher resolution of the stereocilia bundles and other actin-containing structures can be obtained with a confocal microscope that reduces stray fluorescence from structures outside the plane of focus (Attanasio et al., 1994). The F-actin staining technique is particularly useful for assessing the general status of stereocilia bundles in developing or regenerating hair cells and the actin along the lateral wall of OHCs. In mature animals, intense F-actin labeling is also seen in pillar cells and Deiters' cells (Attanasio et al., 1994). The general protocol for phalloidin labeling is presented in Table 13.9 (Attanasio et al., 1994).

SILVER NITRATE

Silver nitrate provides auditory researchers with a convenient and useful method for labeling the stereocilia on IHCs and OHCs, as illustrated in Figure 13.7A. The stereocilia bundles, labeled

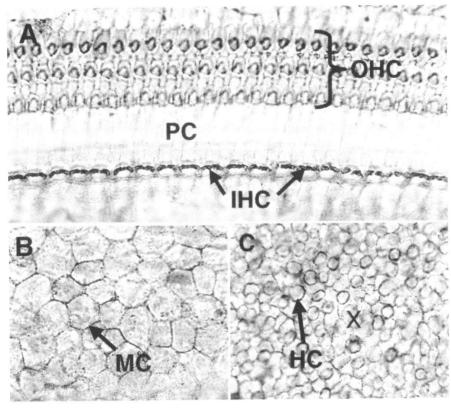

FIGURE 13.7   Silver nitrate staining. (A) Surface preparation of the organ of Corti, showing silver nitrate deposits on surfaces of inner hair cell (IHC) and outer hair cell (OHC) stereocilia and cell borders on the cuticular plate. Pillar cells (PC) separate the single row of IHC from three rows of OHC. (B) Stria vascularis, showing outlines of marginal cells (MC). (C) Surface preparation of the macula of the utricle, showing outlines of vestibular hair cells (HC). X indicates missing HC.

brownish-black, form a distinct blunt V-shape on the three rows of OHCs, while those on IHCs form gently curving arcs. Light staining is also seen on the cuticular plate of some OHCs. The heads of the pillar cells form a clear boundary between the OHCs and IHCs. Figure 13.7B shows a surface view of the stria vascularis with the plane of focus at the outermost marginal cell layer. The junctions between adjacent marginal cells are labeled brown-black by silver nitrate, allowing the outline of each marginal cell to be visualized. Silver nitrate also labels the perimeter of the vestibular hair cells as illustrated in Figure 13.7C, which shows a surface preparation view of the macula of the utricle. The cylindrical boundary of each hair cell is labeled brownish-black. The absence of these brown cylindrical boundaries from a small portion of this sensory epithelium is indicative of hair cell loss. An overview of the methods for silver nitrate staining of the inner ear is presented in Table 13.10 (Humason, 1972).

Osmium Tetroxide

Osmium tetroxide preserves the nuclei and cytoplasm of cells; but because of poor tissue penetration, it often leaves the tissue soft and difficult to section (Humason, 1972). For this reason, osmium tetroxide is often used together with glutaraldehyde to obtain better tissue preservation. Osmium tetroxide forms cross-links with proteins, and is reduced by most lipids, resulting in the formation of a dark black stain around the myelinated portions of the auditory and vestibular nerves that

TABLE 13.10
Essential Steps in Silver Nitrate Staining

1. Anesthetize animal; remove cochlea and vestibular system.
2. Open round window and oval window; make hole in apex, remove bone and open up vestibular epithelium.
3. Perfuse 0.5% silver nitrate solution[a] through the cochlear and vestibular sensory epithelium three times.
4. Fix specimens in 10% formalin for 2 h.
5. Microdissect out sensory epithelium and mount on glass slide as a surface preparation.
6. Expose slides to sunlight for approximately 1 h to enhance the silver stain.

[a] Silver nitrate staining solution: 0.5% silver nitrate in phosphate buffered saline (5–10 mL).

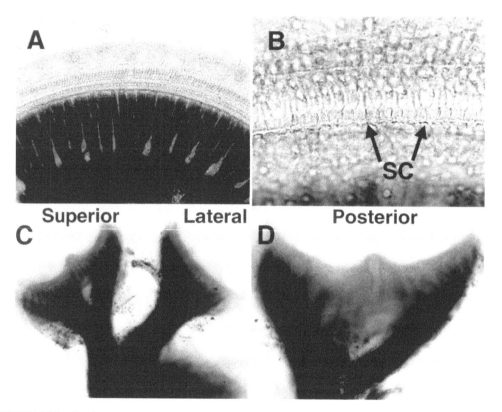

FIGURE 13.8 Osmium tetroxide stain. (A) Strongly stained myelinated nerve fibers (NF) are seen entering the habenula perforatae in the osseous spiral lamina of the cochlea. The nerve fibers lose their myelin sheath as they enter the organ of Corti, and are therefore poorly stained in the region of the hair cells. (B) Higher magnification of hair cell region shown in (A), showing poor definition of non-myelinated structures such as hair cell stereocilia (SC). (C) Myelinated nerve fibers (NF) innervating hair cells in the superior semicircular canal (note bar), lateral semicircular canal (no bar), and macula of utricle are strongly stained. (D) Myelinated nerve fibers (NF) of the posterior semicircular canal are strongly stained. (Note the presence of a bar separating nerve fibers into two bundles.)

innervate the sensory epithelium. Figure 13.8A shows a surface preparation view of the organ of Corti stained with osmium tetroxide. Large fascicles of darkly stained myelinated nerve fibers can be seen emerging from the spiral ganglion. The bundles of fibers proceed toward the habenular openings in the osseous spiral lamina and, as they pass through this region, they lose their myelin sheath and dark osmium staining. Structures within the organ of Corti proper are only very lightly

TABLE 13.11
Essential Steps in Osmium Tetroxide Staining

1. Anesthetize animal; remove cochlea and vestibular system.
2. Open round window and oval window; make hole in apex, remove bone, and open up vestibular epithelium.
3. Perfuse cochlear and vestibular cavities with 2% glutaraldehyde in 0.1 M phosphate buffer (pH 7.2) for 4 h at 4°C.
4. Rinse with phosphate buffered saline.
5. Immerse sample in 2% osmium tetroxide solution for 2 h at 4°C.
6. Microdissect out sensory epithelium and mount on glass slide as a surface preparation.

Note: Osmium tetroxide fumes from crystals and solution are dangerous. Mix and use this stain under a fume hood, and handle with care.

stained by osmium tetroxide. Figure 13.8B shows a higher magnification view of the IHCs; the stereocilia are faintly labeled with this method. Figures 13.8C and 13.8D show the intense staining of the branches of the vestibular nerve as the fibers enter the superior and lateral semicircular canals and the posterior semicircular canal, respectively. The essential procedures for osmium tetroxide staining of the inner ear are listed in Table 13.11. It should be noted that the fumes from osmium tetroxide crystals and solutions are dangerous; thus, this stain should be handled carefully and prepared and used only under a fumehood.

Acetylcholinesterase Histochemistry

The inner ear is innervated by both afferent and efferent neurons, and myelin stains such as osmium tetroxide do not distinguish between these classes of neurons. In cases where it is desirable to identify the efferent innervation of the cochlea, investigators can take advantage of the fact that the major neurotransmitter of the efferent system is acetylcholine. Most of the acetylcholine released into the synaptic cleft is rapidly hydrolyzed by acetylcholinesterase (AChE), which limits the duration of acetylcholine action on the post-synaptic neuron. Because the cochlear efferent neurons contain high levels of AChE, they can be precisely identified with stains directed against AChE. Figure 13.9 shows the pattern of efferent innervation in a surface preparation view of the organ of Corti as revealed by AChE staining. The AChE-containing neurons running within the inner and outer spiral bundles, and those crossing the tunnel of Corti in the upper tunnel region, take on a dark-brown label. The terminal swellings of the efferent neurons can also be seen near the base of the OHCs. This method has proved extremely effective in our hands for identifying the degree of efferent damage caused by surgical section of the efferent axons entering the cochlea (X.Y. Zheng et al., 1997; X.Y. Zheng et al., 1999). A brief overview of the AChE staining procedure is found in Table 13.12.

Eosin Staining

In some cases, it is desirable to stain the vascular structures within the cochlear and vestibular labyrinth; and this can easily be achieved by eosin, a xanthene dye derived from fluorescein that stains connective tissue (Drury and Wallington, 1980). Eosin is available in two main forms: (1) eosin B, a bluish-red dye, and (2) the more commonly used eosin Y, a yellowish-red dye that is readily soluble in water. Figure 13.10A shows a surface preparation view of the organ of Corti stained with eosin. The inner spiral vessel, which runs beneath the basilar membrane near the lip of the osseous spiral lamina, can be seen as a pinkish-red beaded structure. The outline of a blood vessel within the spiral ganglion is also visible. Figure 13.10B presents an eosin-stained flat surface preparation of the stria vascularis. The extensive vascular bed with extensive radiating arterioles

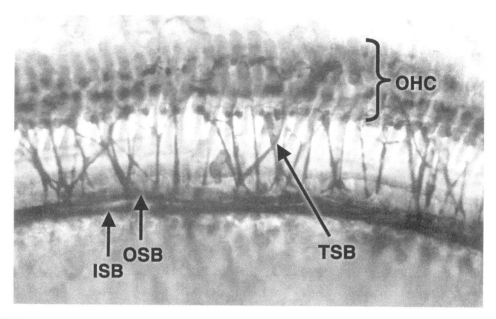

FIGURE 13.9 Acetylcholinesterase (AChE) stain for efferent nerve fibers. Dark staining is seen in the inner spiral bundle (ISB), outer spiral bundle (OSB), the tunnel crossing fibers (TSB), and beneath the outer hair cells (OHC). Efferent fibers within the ISB innervate afferent nerve fibers beneath the inner hair cells, whereas efferent fibers crossing through the upper portion of the tunnel of Corti terminate directly on the OHCs.

TABLE 13.12
Essential Steps in Acetylcholinesterase Staining

1. Anesthetize animal; remove cochlea and vestibular system.
2. Open round window and oval window, and make hole in apex.
3. Perfuse 4% paraformaldehyde in 0.1 M phosphate buffer (pH 7.2) through the inner ear and immerse specimen in fixative for 2 h.
4. Microdissect out the organ of Corti in 0.1 M phosphate buffer.
5. Incubate specimen in 0.1 M acetate buffer (pH 6.0) for 30 min.
6. Incubate in AChE staining solution[a] for 30 min.
7. Wash specimens 3 times in 0.1 M acetate buffer.
8. Immerse tissue in 1% ammonium sulfide for 1 min.
9. Wash tissue in 0.1 M sodium nitrate 5 times.
10. Immerse tissue in 0.1% silver nitrate for 1 min.
11. Wash tissue in 0.1 M sodium nitrate and mount in glycerin on slides.

[a] AChE staining solution: dissolve 5 mg acetylthiocholine iodide (substrate) in 6.5 mL of 0.1 M acetate buffer (pH 6.0). Add 0.5 mL of 0.1 M sodium citrate, 1 mL of 30 mM copper sulfate, 1 mL distilled water, and 1 mL of 5 mM potassium ferricyanide.

and collecting venules stain bright red. Figure 13.10C shows a surface preparation view of an eosin-stained crista of the posterior semicircular canal. In contrast to the organ of Corti, the crista shows a rather diffuse staining pattern. Figure 13.10D shows a low magnification view of an eosin-stained membranous duct of the semicircular canal. The large blood vessels surrounding the duct are labeled bright red. The essential procedures for staining the vascular bed of the cochlear and vestibular systems with eosin are presented in Table 13.13.

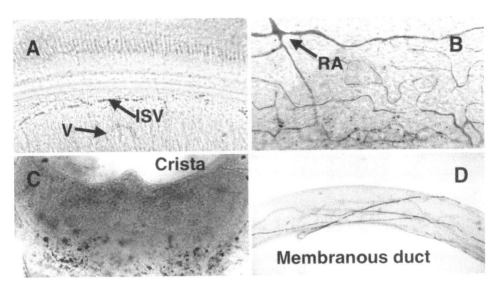

FIGURE 13.10   Eosin stain highlights: (A) the inner spiral vessels (ISV) and other vessels (V) of the basilar membrane; (B) the radiating arterioles (RA) and collecting venules in the stria vascularis; (C) the crista in the vestibular system; and (D) the vessels running along the surface of the membranous duct of the semicircular canal.

TABLE 13.13
Essential Steps in Eosin Staining

1. Anesthetize animal; remove cochlea and vestibular system.
2. Open round window and oval window, make hole in apex, remove bone, and open up vestibular epithelium.
3. Perfuse 10% formalin through the cochlear and vestibular sensory epithelium and immerse in fixative for 4 h or more.
4. Microdissect out sensory epithelium and mount on glass slide as a surface preparation.
5. Immerse samples in 0.5% eosin-alcohol solution for 5 min.
6. Rinse samples with distilled water.
7. Mount specimens in glycerin as surface preparation on glass slides.

[a] Eosin-alcohol staining solution:
   * Dissolve 0.5 to 1 g of eosin Y or eosin B in 6 mL of distilled water.
   * Add acetic acid drop by drop into eosin solution until an eosin deposit appears.
   * Continue adding distilled water (~2–3 mL) until the eosin deposit does not change in size.
   * Filter the solution to extract the eosin deposit.
   * Dry the eosin deposit by heating.
   * Make a solution of 0.5% eosin in 95% alcohol.

SUMMARY

This chapter has provided normative data on hair cell density in several strains of mice, along with an overview of relatively simple staining techniques for assessing the mouse inner ear. The information provided is not meant to be exhaustive, by any means. Instead, we have presented several procedures that we have found to be convenient and reliable for evaluating the mouse cochlea and vestibular system for gross histopathology. As more auditory researchers turn to the mouse as the model of choice for understanding various types of hearing disorders, they will need to develop techniques for rapidly and accurately assessing the inner ear.

14 Effects of Exposure to an Augmented Acoustic Environment on the Mouse Auditory System

James F. Willott, Victoria Sundin, and Jennifer Jeskey

INTRODUCTION

Millions of people of all ages suffer from sensorineural hearing loss. The majority of sensorineural disorders involve progressive sensorineural cochlear pathology, most notably in the basal end of the cochlea and resulting in loss of high-frequency hearing (Dublin, 1976; Northern and Downs, 1991; Schuknecht, 1974; Willott, 1991). At this time, little if anything can be done to effectively slow or ameliorate the progression of sensorineural cochlear degeneration. Similarly, little can be done to improve "central" correlates of sensorineural hearing loss, a collection of problems including difficulty hearing speech and other stimuli in acoustically degraded or noisy conditions (Schuknecht, 1974; Willott, 1991a). Recent studies have investigated a simple yet intriguing phenomenon that holds promise as a means of altering the severity and time course of progressive sensorineural hearing loss: exposure to augmented levels of controlled acoustic stimulation, an *augmented acoustic environment* (AAE) (Turner and Willott, 1998). The essential notion is that appropriate stimulation of the degenerating cochlea and the central auditory system by an appropriate AAE may have ameliorative effects, similar to the effects of "exercise" or increased neural activity in other neural systems (e.g., Cotman and Neeper, 1996).

A number of inbred strains of mice have been employed thus far, including C57BL/6J (C57), DBA/2J (DBA), several BXD recombinant inbred strains, BALB/cJ, and CBA/CaJ (CBA). With the exception of CBA mice, these possess recessive genes that inevitably result in degeneration of outer hair cells (OHCs) beginning in the basal end of the cochlea, accompanied by loss of sensitivity for high-frequency sounds; this is followed by degeneration of other cochlear structures (Erway et al., 1993a; Henry and Chole, 1980; Hunter and Willott, 1987; Li and Borg, 1991; Mikaelian, 1979; Parham and Willott, 1988; Parham et al., 1997; Ralls, 1967; Willott, 1981; 1986; Willott and Bross, 1996; Willott et al., 1984; 1995).

Our experimental strategy has been to expose mice to a moderate-intensity broadband noise AAE prior to the onset of significant hearing loss, beginning at age 25 days, just after weaning. Mice of the same ages are used as non-exposed controls. The auditory brainstem response (ABR) was used as a measure of auditory sensitivity; the acoustic startle response was used as a measure of responsiveness to intense sounds; and prepulse inhibition (PPI) was used as a response to moderately intense suprathreshold tones. As discussed in Chapter 5, PPI is a phenomenon in which a "prepulse" tone (S1) (e.g., a 70-dB SPL tone burst), presented 10 to 200 ms before an intense startle-evoking stimulus (S2), results in a smaller ("inhibited") startle response. The magnitude of PPI produced by a tone defines its behavioral salience (e.g., Hoffman and Ison, 1980). PPI is generally viewed as a measure of central auditory processing because the inferior colliculus (IC) and other higher-order structures comprise the pathway(s) by which the prepulse modulates the startle response (Carlson and Willott, 1998; M. Davis, 1984; Fox, 1979; Hoffman and Ison, 1980; Leitner and Cohen, 1985; L. Li et al., 1998a; b; Parham and Willott, 1990; Swerdlow and Geyer, 1993).

A complete description of vivarium conditions, equipment, and procedures are found in earlier papers (Turner and Willott, 1998; Willott and Turner, 1999). These are outlined here.

Mice were placed in plastic cages (12 × 13 × 30 cm) with a wire lid, where they received consecutive 12-h nights of AAE. The AAE was a broadband noise (rise/fall = 10 ms, duration = 200 ms, rate = 2/s) of 70 dB SPL (re: 20 µPa). SPLs measured within third-octave bands between 4 and 25 kHz rolled off above and below this range. Like-aged control animals (usually littermates) received no AAE exposure, and were reared in the vivarium.

For all strains, AAE was initiated at 25 days of age, and auditory testing was performed for various durations up to 1 year or more. Age-matched controls were tested at the same time.

Auditory sensitivity was assessed with ABR thresholds for tone bursts (1-ms rise/fall, 3-ms duration, rate 21 Hz) of 4, 8, 12, 16, and 24 kHz, using Tucker-Davis hardware and software (*AeP* and *Siggen* packages).

The startle stimulus (S2) was a 100-dB (re: 20 µPa) 4-kHz tone burst (10-ms duration, 1-ms rise/fall time). Prepulse stimuli (S1s) were tone bursts (1-ms rise/fall, 10-ms duration) of 4, 8, 12, 16, and 24 kHz at 70 dB SPL. They were presented with a Radio Shack super tweeter in a startle chamber that transduced the animals' movements into voltage units displayed on a digital storage oscilloscope. The acoustic startle response caused a spike-like voltage change; amplitude was defined as the largest peak-to-peak voltage deflection in the first 30 ms following startle stimulus onset.

AAE EFFECTS ON ABR THRESHOLDS IN INBRED STRAINS OF MICE EXHIBITING PROGRESSIVE HEARING LOSS

Exposure to the AAE has been shown to ameliorate hearing loss in strains of mice that exhibit progressive sensorineural cochlear pathology including C57, DBA, BALB/cJ, and BXD recombinant inbred strains BXD-12, BXD-22, and BXD-16. We focus here on data from C57 and DBA mice, the two strains that have been most thoroughly evaluated.

Figure 14.1 shows mean ABR thresholds from a study by Willott and Turner (1999) in which C57 mice were exposed to the AAE from age 25 days to 14 months. The exposed mice and a control (non-exposed) cohort group were longitudinally tested during the AAE exposure period. It is clear that exposure to the AAE had striking effects on progressive elevation of ABR thresholds for high-frequency tones. The drastic, progressive elevation of high-frequency thresholds (which becomes quite evident by 6 months of age) is substantially ameliorated in exposed mice.

DBA mice exhibit much more rapid progressive hearing loss. As seen in Figure 14.2 (also from Willott and Turner, 1999), progressive elevation of ABR thresholds was diminished in AAE-exposed DBA mice. However, the AAE was not effective on ABR thresholds for 24 kHz, and only minimally effective at 16 kHz; by 5 months of age, both exposed and control mice failed to respond to these frequencies, although some savings are evident in 2-month-olds. By 7 to 9 months of age, the only remaining benefits of AAE exposure for DBA mice were observed for 4-kHz tones.

Interestingly, the longitudinal data for both strains suggest some degree of *improvement* of ABR thresholds for lower frequency tones in AAE-exposed mice (Figures 14.1 and 14.2). Longitudinal reductions in ABR thresholds were evident in exposed 8-month-old C57 mice and 2-month-old DBA mice. After these ages, progressive threshold elevations commenced.

AAE EFFECTS ON PREPULSE INHIBITION IN INBRED STRAINS OF MICE EXHIBITING PROGRESSIVE HEARING LOSS

The broadband AAE resulted in stronger PPI for the same inbred strains whose ABR thresholds benefitted: C57, DBA, BALB/cJ, and BXD recombinant strains. AAE effects on PPI are nicely

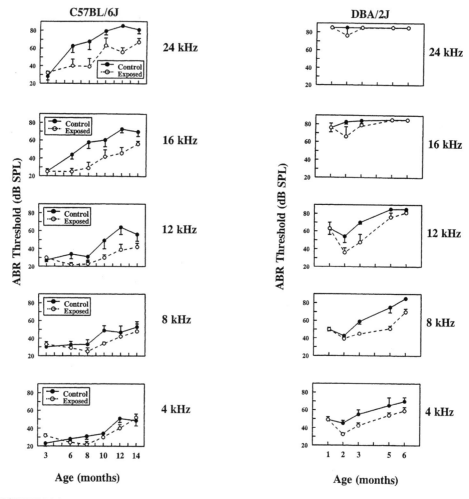

FIGURE 14.1 Longitudinal changes in ABR thresholds for C57 mice. Threshold elevations in mice exposed to the AAE (open circles) are not as severe as those of non-exposed controls. Error bars = standard errors of the mean. (From Willott, J. F. and Turner, J. G. 1999. *Hearing Res.*, 135, 78–88. With permission.)

FIGURE 14.2 Longitudinal changes in ABR thresholds for DBA mice. Threshold elevations in mice exposed to the AAE (open circles) are not as severe as those of non-exposed controls. Error bars = standard errors of the mean. (From Willott, J. F. and Turner, J. G. 1999. *Hearing Res.*, 135, 78–88. With permission.)

demonstrated in C57 mice, as shown in Figure 14.3, which summarizes the longitudinal changes in PPI for the same mice used in the ABR experiments (Figure 14.1). PPI is expressed as startle amplitude when the prepulse is present relative to the S2-only amplitude. Thus, lower % values indicate stronger PPI. It is clear from Figure 14.3 that exposure to the AAE resulted in superior PPI for all S1 frequencies. Even in 3-month-old C57 mice (exposed to the AAE since age 25 days), PPI was superior in the AAE-exposed mice, and this effect was still present when the mice were 14 months old.

It can also be seen from Figure 14.3 that PPI improved somewhat in control C57 mice, for S1s of 4, 8, and 12 kHz. For example, S1s of 4 to 12 kHz produced PPI in the range of 55 to 70% in 3-month-old control mice, compared to 35 to 40% in 12-month-olds. This is the typical hearing-loss-induced (HLI) plasticity effect, whereby high-frequency hearing loss is accompanied by stronger PPI for low-middle-frequency S1s (as well as stronger central auditory responses to these frequencies; see Chapter 24). Thus, the improvement in PPI in the AAE-exposed mice occurs on top of improved PPI from HLI plasticity.

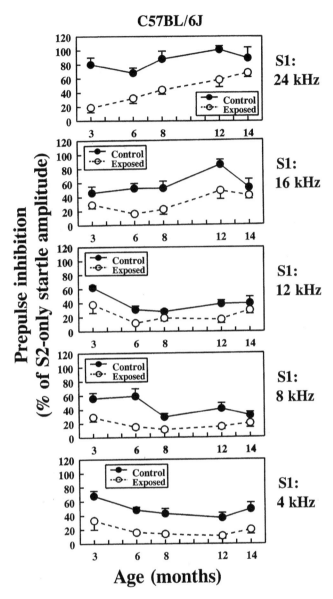

FIGURE 14.3 Longitudinal changes in PPI for C57 mice. PPI is superior in mice exposed to the AAE (open circles), compared to non-exposed controls. Error bars = standard errors of the mean.

AAE EFFECTS ON BASELINE STARTLE AMPLITUDE IN INBRED STRAINS OF MICE EXHIBITING PROGRESSIVE HEARING LOSS

In DBA mice, startle amplitudes become smaller as hearing loss progresses, and by 5 months of age, startle responses are unreliably evoked and amplitudes are quite small. By contrast, startle amplitudes became increasingly large in AAE-exposed mice, and were twice as large as occurred when the mice were 1 to 2 months old. Increased baseline startle amplitudes were also observed in C57 and BXD-12 mice, but AAE-exposed BALB/c mice and the other hearing-impaired BXD strains did not exhibit increased baseline startle amplitude. Thus, the effect of the AAE on baseline startle is the least robust and consistent of the AAE effects.

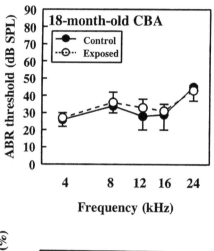

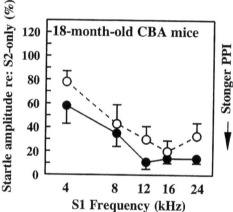

FIGURE 14.4 ABR thresholds (upper panel) and PPI (lower panel) in 18-month-old CBA/CaJ mice. ABR thresholds remain near normal at this age. Differences between exposed and control groups were not significant for either measure. Error bars = standard errors of the mean.

THE ABSENCE OF AAE EFFECTS IN NORMAL-HEARING MICE

Willott, Turner, and Sundin (2000) found that the only effect of 9 months of AAE exposure observed in normal-hearing CBA mice was *slightly worse* PPI in exposed mice with the 4-kHz S1. Figure 14.4 presents more recent data from the same cohort, now 18 months of age. The control and exposed groups did not differ significantly (ANOVAs) with respect to ABR thresholds, PPI, or baseline startle amplitude. Indeed, the trend for PPI continues to be slightly stronger PPI in control mice — the opposite of the ameliorative AAE effects observed in hearing-impaired strains.

The absence of AAE effects (particularly on ABR thresholds) is also observed in C57, BALB/c, and BXD-14 mice prior to the development of hearing loss. For example, 55-day-old BXD-14 mice exhibit normal ABR thresholds from 4 to 16 kHz and slightly elevated thresholds for 24-kHz tones; and mice exposed from day 25 did not differ significantly from controls for ABR thresholds, PPI, or baseline startle amplitude at this age (Willott et al., 2000).

TIME COURSE FOR THE ACQUISITION OF AAE EFFECTS

It appears that AAE effects on ABR thresholds and PPI occur irrespective of whether the onset of hearing loss occurs during the age ranges of preweaning (e.g., the BXD-16 strain), postwean-

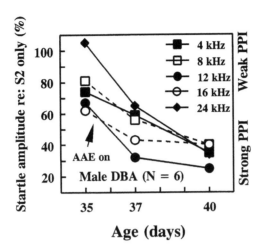

FIGURE 14.5 Acquisition of improved PPI with nightly AAE exposure in DBA mice. Significant improvements occurred after 5 days of exposure.

ing/adolescence (BXD-22; BXD-12; DBA/2J strains), or adulthood (BALB/cJ; C57 strains). An essential variable seems to be progressive high-frequency hearing loss, irrespective of age (Willott et al., 2000). The emergence of AAE effects is in part dictated by the time course of high-frequency hearing loss. Thus, AAE effects can be observed in 35-day-old DBA mice exposed from age 25 days (Turner and Willott, 1998). In contrast to DBA mice, the loss of hearing progresses gradually in BALB/c mice, as do the benefits of AAE exposure (e.g., after 3 months of age) (Willott et al., 2000).

We have recently performed experiments on DBA mice to determine how rapidly AAE treatment can bring about changes in PPI. Figure 14.5 presents data obtained from male mice (females were more variable, and a clear picture could not be obtained in this time frame). AAE treatment was initiated at age 35 days in DBA mice (already exhibiting high-frequency hearing loss). After 2 nights of treatment, PPI had begun to show improvement, and by 5 days of treatment the changes were statistically significant. An earlier study on DBA mice had shown that both PPI and ABR thresholds (but not baseline startle amplitude) could be significantly affected after 10 days of AAE treatment (Turner and Willott, 1998).

LIMITATIONS OF AAE EFFECTS

The ameliorative effects of AAE exposure are limited under two conditions. First, the effects are attenuated by delaying AAE treatment until after hearing loss has already progressed too far. Second, even when AAE exposure has greatly slowed progressive hearing loss, the negative effects of the *ahl* and other genes are eventually expressed.

DELAYING AAE TREATMENT

In a study by Sundin, Turner, and Willott (2000), initiation of AAE treatment in C57 mice was delayed until either 3 months of age (shortly after hearing loss begins to develop) or 5 months (when high-frequency hearing loss had become significant). The results are depicted in Figure 14.6 for ABR thresholds (upper row) and PPI (lower row). Control mice (solid circles) exhibited the strain-typical progressive elevations of ABR thresholds, which are most severe at high frequencies. Mice exposed to the AAE nightly beginning at age 25 days (unfilled circles; from Willott and Turner, 1999) had substantially less severe threshold elevations. Delaying AAE treatment until 3 months of age (unfilled squares) or 5 months (gray squares) had little effect, as ABR thresholds were similar to those of control mice.

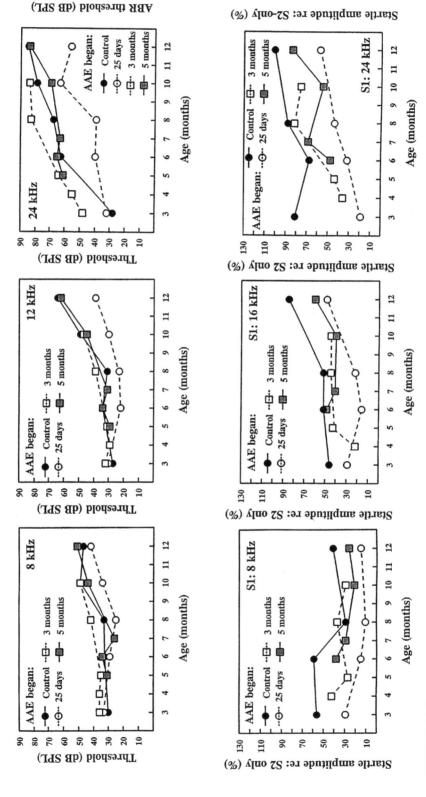

FIGURE 14.6 Longitudinal changes in ABR thresholds (upper row) and PPI (lower row) in C57 mice. AAE treatment was initiated at 25 days, 3 months, or 5 months of age.

The PPI data in Figure 14.6 demonstrate the typical AAE effect: mice exposed to the AAE beginning at 25 days (unfilled circles) maintained PPI (lower %) that was superior to that of non-exposed controls (filled circles). When treatment was delayed until 3 or 5 months of age, PPI tended to be intermediate between the latter two conditions.

From the ABR thresholds of this study, it can be concluded that the benefits of exposure to an AAE are greatly reduced when treatment is implemented after significant hearing loss has already occurred. In contrast, PPI can still benefit from delayed AAE treatment, albeit to a lesser extent than what occurs when treatment is initiated early. Other studies from our laboratory have found similar results in the DBA/2J and BXD-22 strains, which exhibit more rapid hearing loss. In these strains, withholding AAE treatment until age 4 to 5 weeks also diminishes AAE effects, especially for ABR thresholds. Moreover, in BXD-16 mice, which exhibit severe high-frequency hearing loss even at 3 weeks of age (Willott and Erway, 1998), benefits of AAE exposure do not accrue for ABR thresholds for tones of 16 and 24 kHz. In BXD-16 mice, ABRs could not be obtained at 55 days of age in either control mice or mice exposed to the AAE from 25 days of age. The only significant AAE effects were for ABR thresholds at 4 to 12 kHz, where thresholds were 10 to 15 dB lower than controls in 55-day-olds (Willott et al., 2000).

THE BENEFICIAL AAE EFFECTS ARE ULTIMATELY LOST

There are also limitations to how long the beneficial effects of AAE treatment can last in the face of genetically determined mechanisms that cause severe sensorineural pathology. Eventually, the ameliorative effects of AAE exposure are "overcome." For example, in 3-month-old BXD-22 mice, ABR thresholds for 16- and 24-kHz tones no longer differed from those of controls, although AAE effects were present earlier, at 55 days of age. And, in both DBA and C57 mice, high-frequency ABR thresholds ultimately become elevated in AAE-exposed mice, albeit at a much older age than in non-exposed controls (Figures 14.1 and 14.2).

DURATION OF AAE EFFECTS ON PPI

Jeskey and Willott (2000) performed a study to determine how long the improved PPI would persist after AAE treatment was terminated. The strategy was to establish the behavioral AAE effects by exposing DBA mice to the AAE from age 25 days to 12 weeks, with control mice maintained in the vivarium. After this, mice were kept in normal acoustic conditions and tested weekly for 4 weeks, as were age-matched controls.

Jeskey and Willott found that the PPI of exposed 12-week-olds (60 nights of AAE treatment) was generally stronger than that of controls, the typical AAE effect on PPI. One to two weeks after removal from the AAE, PPI had become weaker for all S1 frequencies, whereas PPI in controls did not change significantly in this age range. The clearest effects were observed for the 8- and 12-kHz S1s, where mean values of PPI for exposed mice converged with those of controls over a 1 to 2 week period. More recently, we evaluated changes in PPI on a shorter time scale. As seen in Figure 14.7, the AAE effect for high-frequency S1s had begun to fade after 3 days without AAE treatment; however, changes at 4- to 12-kHz S1s were minimal. Thus, it would appear that it takes about a week (±, depending on the S1) for the AAE effects on PPI to fade in DBA mice.

POSSIBLE MECHANISMS FOR THE AAE EFFECTS: ONE, TWO, OR MORE?

Exposure to the broadband noise AAE slows the progressive decline of auditory performance for three rather different paradigms: ABR thresholds (i.e., tones that were not very intense), the salience of moderately intense (70 dB SPL) tones in PPI, and amplitude of the startle response to a very intense (100 dB SPL) tone. The generality of AAE effects might suggest that a single mechanism

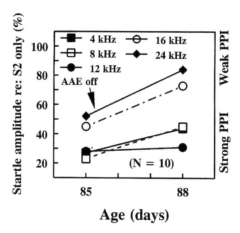

FIGURE 14.7   Changes in PPI after termination of AAE treatment in DBA mice.

is responsible for all three types of changes. On the other hand, AAE effects also exhibited important differences across the three measures, suggesting that more than one mechanism may be involved. For example, AAE exposure can produce improved PPI under some conditions where ABRs are not altered. When exposed to the AAE, PPI tends to improve for all S1 frequencies, whereas the occurrence of AAE effects on ABR thresholds is more closely related to the pattern and magnitude of threshold elevations observed in control mice. Moreover, the effects of the AAE on PPI generally occur at an earlier age than the effects on ABR thresholds, and in some cases remain evident at an older age. Possible mechanisms for the AAE effects have been discussed elsewhere (Jeskey and Willott, 2000; Turner and Willott, 1998; Willott and Turner, 1999; 2000), with the following points being made.

It should first be noted that several other phenomena may have relevance for the AAE effects. In the "toughening" phenomenon, exposure to noise (albeit substantially more intense than 70 dB SPL used for AAE) can protect the ear from subsequent noise-induced trauma (e.g., Canlon, 1996; Henderson et al., 1996b; Subramaniam et al., 1996). Also potentially relevant are studies of electrical stimulation of the auditory system via cochlear implants, which can be beneficial to spiral ganglion cells and central auditory neurons (e.g., Leake et al., 1991; Miller et al., 1996). In addition, a large body of literature has shown that "enriched" environments and neural activity *per se* can alter neural structure and physiology (e.g., Cotman and Neeper, 1996).

While the relationships between AAE and these other phenomena remain to be determined, both peripheral and central mechanisms need to be considered. One hypothesis is that cochlear function is maintained longer in exposed mice and even improved with continued exposure to the AAE. This would also result in augmented peripheral tone-evoked input to the central auditory system, accounting for the beneficial effects on PPI and startle. Presumably, the AAE might benefit cochlear function by affecting the condition and/or performance of the still-intact hair cells and/or their synapses (*cf.* Willott and Turner, 1999), spiral ganglion cells and/or their central synapses (*cf.* Leake et al., 1991; Lousteau, 1987; Miller et al., 1996), and/or efferent influences.

Alternatively, central auditory function is likely to become altered in AAE-exposed mice. It is well-established in C57 mice and in other species that the loss of high-frequency sensitivity in the cochlea produces hearing-loss-induced (HLI) plasticity in the IC, auditory cortex, and elsewhere, whereby responses evoked by still-audible middle-frequencies become stronger (Calford et al., 1993; Popelár et al., 1994; Rajan et al., 1993; Robertson and Irvine, 1989; Schwaber et al., 1993; Willott, 1984; 1996a; Willott et al., 1993). In the absence of AAE exposure, HLI plasticity is accompanied by improved PPI for middle-frequency prepulse tones between 1 and 2 months of age in DBA mice (Willott et al., 1994b) and in middle-aged C57 mice (Carlson and Willott, 1996; Willott and Carlson, 1995). This is presumably due to the fact that PPI is mediated by descending circuits from the upper auditory system (including the IC) which inhibit the startle circuit (Davis, 1984; Fox, 1979; Hoffman and Ison, 1980; Leitner and Cohen, 1985; L. Li et al., 1998a; b; Parham and Willott, 1990; Swerdlow and Geyer, 1993). As HLI plasticity occurs, low- and middle-frequency prepulses activate the descending inhibitory circuit(s) more effectively, and PPI improves. We have hypothesized that the AAE facilitates HLI plasticity. Indeed, neurophysiological evidence suggests that the "over-representation" of middle frequencies in the IC is exaggerated in AAE-exposed mice (Turner and Willott, 1999; see also Chapter 24). Enhanced inhibitory modulation by the IC would be consistent with the improvement in PPI in exposed mice.

To shed additional light on the hypothesis that AAE effects on PPI represent a form of central neural plasticity, the Jeskey and Willott (2000) study also reintroduced nightly AAE exposure in DBA mice 4 weeks after removal from the AAE, when the original AAE effect had faded. The mice were tested weekly for baseline startle amplitude and PPI (testing was always during the day in quiet). A general improvement in PPI was observed over 3 weeks of reinstated AAE treatment (except for 24 kHz). Thus, the evidence indicates that AAE exposure modulated PPI up and down in DBA mice, much like the introduction and removal of stimuli modulate behavior in other forms of centrally mediated behavioral plasticity.

SUMMARY AND CONCLUSIONS

Chronic exposure to a broadband AAE has significant effects on the progressive changes in auditory function in various inbred strains that exhibit progressive sensorineural hearing loss. AAE exposure results in improved auditory performance: PPI is enhanced, ABR thresholds are lower, and baseline startle amplitudes are (for some strains) increased. The effects are not observed in the absence of hearing loss, but they occur in all hearing-impaired mouse strains thus far studied. The effects occur irrespective of a mouse's age at the onset of hearing loss, as long as initiation of AAE treatment precedes the occurrence of severe hearing loss. If AAE treatment is delayed beyond such a point, loss of threshold sensitivity progresses as usual, although PPI may still benefit. AAE treatment can slow, but not prevent, the occurrence of severe genetically determined hearing loss.

The AAE effect is particularly interesting because it appears to involve two interacting processes: (1) neural changes induced (or set in motion) by the partial loss of sensory input (HLI plasticity); and (2) changes induced by the augmentation of sensory input (the AAE). Moreover, the fact that progressive high-frequency sensorineural hearing loss is, by far, the most prevalent form of hearing impairment in humans adds a compelling clinical dimension as well. It opens up the possibility of modulating auditory functions in hearing-impaired individuals by manipulation of auditory stimulation.

ACKNOWLEDGMENTS

This research was supported by NIH grant R01 AG07554 to J.F.W. Preliminary findings were presented at the Association for Research in Otolaryngology.

15 Cochlear Blood Flow

Alfred L. Nuttall

INTRODUCTION

The homeostatic mechanisms of the cochlea include those that regulate energy supply, fluid volume and ionic balance, and removal of metabolic waste products. The blood circulation of the inner ear is the major system providing some aspects of these specific functions. The control of the circulation is critical to normal function. However, there is much that needs to be learned about basic patho-physiological questions on inner-ear blood flow and specifically about microcirculation of the inner ear. Does sound influence cochlear blood flow in ways that have important physiological consequences to hearing? Is vascular permeability (and the pathology of permeability) a determinant of ear lymphatic volume or pressure or ionic content? What percentage of sudden hearing loss in the human population is due to vascular insufficiencies? Clearly, the answers to such questions require unique studies of inner-ear circulation. It is not sufficient to generalize the findings from other organ systems to the inner ear because considerable heterogeneity occurs in different vascular beds. For example, in the choroid arterioles of the guinea pig, four different neurotransmitters/neuro-modulators (norepinephrine, ATP, acetylcholine, and nitric oxide) are found to be active (Hashitani et al., 1998). In the cochlea, neuropeptides are also likely to be important for vasoregulation (e.g., Carlisle et al., 1990a).

The physiological study of cochlear blood flow (CBF) is now about a half century old and considerable advances have been made. It is a technically challenging research area because of the measurement problems. Although most cochlear physiological studies face measurement difficulties, blood flow-related studies are particularly hampered by instrumentation limitations and the shortcomings of miniature sensors. Translating these problems to the mouse, it is not surprising that few investigators have attempted mouse cochlear blood flow studies. A MEDLINE literature search (April, 2000) reveals only six peer-reviewed articles.

This chapter has three goals: (1) to outline the measurement problems so that a scientist interested in applying known technologies will have a starting point; (2) to review this small body of investigative work; and (3) to briefly introduce some useful aspects of mouse mutants for the future study of inner-ear blood flow. The focus of this chapter is restricted to issues related to cochlear blood flow (CBF), as there is no literature on the vestibular component of inner-ear blood flow from the mouse.

THE MEASUREMENT PROBLEM

MICROELECTRODE SENSORS

All of the studies conducted on mice have utilized laser Doppler flowmetry (LDF) as a solution to the measurement problem. Thus, LDF merits the more comprehensive discussion given below. There are, however, a number of other approaches that could be used, depending on the purpose of the study. The main limiting factor, of course, is the size of the cochlea and its relatively hidden position in the medial wall of the auditory bulla. Unlike the gerbil, chinchilla, and guinea pig cochleae, the rat, hamster, and mouse cochleae are a less visible, flattened feature of the medial wall of the temporal bone. All turns of the cochlea are not as clearly demarked. The size and the lack of clear landmarks make the placement of access holes into the perilymphatic and endolymphatic spaces extremely difficult. Such holes would be necessary to place probes which serve as primary (e.g., hydrogen clearance; Maass and Kellner, 1984) or secondary sensors (e.g., oxygen tension; Haupt et al., 1991; Lawrence and Nuttall, 1972; Misrahy et al., 1958; Morgenstern and Kessler, 1978; Nuttall and Lawrence, 1980) of CBF. Nonetheless, the fact that the endocochlear potential has been measured in mice (e.g., Carlisle et al., 1990b; Sadanaga and Morimitsu, 1995) is evidence that microelectrode approaches to fluid oxygen, pH, and ionic concentrations are possible.

INTRAVITAL MICROSCOPY

The oldest of the blood flow techniques used in the cochlea is termed "intravital microscopy" (IVM) (Lawrence, 1971; Nuttall, 1986; Seymour, 1954; Weille et al., 1954). IVM is nothing more than the adaptation of a compound microscope for *in vivo* observations of blood circulation (Nuttall, 1986; Prazma et al., 1989; Slaaf et al., 1981; Wayland, 1975). Bright field, transilluminated or fluorescent observations can be accomplished for many tissues. The most practical and useful application in the cochlea is fluorescent vertical illumination, in which the objective lens also serves as the condenser lens for the illumination (Slaaf et al., 1982; Wayland, 1975), or contrast-enhancing bright-field microscopy (e.g., using light polarization manipulations) (Ren et al., 1993a). Typically, these microscopes use long working distance objectives, because water immersion objectives do not generally have the physical profile dimensions to access the surface of the cochlea. However, a custom-made lens, such as that designed by Maier et al. (1997), might prove a good choice.

IVM is used when it is important to measure rheological parameters such as red blood cell velocity, leukocyte adherence to the endothelium, vessel vasomotion, vessel diameters, or hydromechanical properties such as vessel permeability and hydraulic conductivity. Of course, the vessels of interest must be visible in the microscope, and this raises the technical question of preparation of the mouse cochlea for such visualization. Thus far, no studies have described the physical opening of the mouse cochlear lateral wall, as can be done for the guinea pig (Nuttall, 1986; Prazma et al., 1989), to observe the microcirculation of the spiral ligament and stria vascularis. It should be noted that observations of cochlear circulation are generally limited to the microcirculation, with arterioles, venuoles, and the supplying arteries and veins of the cochlea being deeper and relatively inaccessible. Should the physical opening of an observation hole be impractical in the mouse, two approaches could be explored that might still yield IVM data. The first approach takes advantage of the fact that the mouse otic capsule is thin. In the case of thin bone (which might be thinned further by shaving with a small knife), a contrast-enhancing fluorescent dye, of different fluorescent emission character than the auto-fluorescence of bone, could render some "transparency" to the bone.

The other "route" to observe the circulation would be via the round window (RW). Although there are vessels of the RW itself (as there are vessels in otic capsule) that could interfere with observations, capillaries of the osseous spiral lamina and the spiral capillary of the basilar membrane could be studied.

It would also be possible to dissect the spiral modiolar artery (the central artery of the cochlea) from the cochlea and study it as an *in vitro* preparation. The isolated vessel approach has been quite productive using the gerbil and guinea pig (Jiang et al., 1999; Wangemann and Gruber, 1998). Mutant mouse models will eventually serve to define the cellular characteristics of endothelial cells and smooth muscle cells in pathophysiological experiments.

MICROSPHERE, INDICATOR DILUTION METHODS, AND 2-DEOXYGLUCOSE

The use of microspheres, either radioactive (e.g., Angelborg et al., 1977; Hillerdal, 1987) or nonradioactive (e.g., Prazma et al., 1984), is a well-established method to obtain absolute blood flow to organs. Using grouped data, microspheres can be used to compare the control flow state to the stimulated flow state. It has not been applied in studies of mouse CBF but has been used in a number of auditory studies in other animals. The main advantage of the method is determination of the actual flow (e.g., in microliters per minute), while the main disadvantage is the small number of measurements in time (typically one or two). To accomplish microsphere determinations of blood flow, a bolus injection of a large quantity of spheres (approximately 3 million for the guinea pig) about 10 to 15 μm in diameter is given into the left ventricle of the heart. For absolute measurements of organ flow, a known sample of arterial blood is drawn over the minute that the spheres become trapped in tissues. The microsphere method has theoretical limitations that set both the number of sequential measurements and accuracy of the measurement (Hillerdal, 1987). The size of the spheres must be correctly chosen to permit them all to be captured in arterioles and capillaries and not pass through the capillary beds. If they are too large, they will stop flow in larger arteries, leading to a significant vascular peripheral resistance increase. The accuracy is, in part, a function of the number of spheres captured in an organ and the variability of the number of captured spheres. It is likely the mouse would present a special challenge to the microsphere technique, due to the small size of the cochlea (the size and number of blood vessels) and the small size of the heart, which must accept the injection of spheres. Therefore, it is not clear that the microsphere technique would work for the mouse cochlea, although there is a good rationale for using this technique; that is, the microsphere method would allow direct comparison of CBF in different mouse strains and genetic variants.

Another approach to the direct measurement of CBF would be via the use of "indicator" molecules that distribute in an organ according to blood flow. Typically, these are radioactive compounds, an example of which is ^{14}C-labeled iodoantipyrine that was used to measure gerbil CBF (Ryan et al., 1988). This radiopharmaceutical is given as a bolus injection and tissues are then processed for autoradiography.

When 2-deoxyglucose (2-DG) has been used to study mouse CBF, interesting results have been obtained. Sound caused an increase in 2-DG uptake in a number of auditory tissues, reaching a peak uptake value at about 80 dB SPL (Canlon and Schacht, 1983). An important technical issue, however, is just how closely the level of 2-DG represents actual blood flow. The molecule is transported into tissues according to rate processes that depend on cellular metabolism as well as the availability of substrate. Possibly the most powerful approach would be to combine the 2-DG method with an indicator dilution molecule and measure the resulting radioactivity from two different labels, one giving energy metabolism information and one giving blood flow information.

Laser Doppler Flowmetry (LDF)

The LDF method is arguably the most useful approach for the study of CBF in any animal model. It is a simple, real-time method and one that is noninvasive to the cochlea because it is only necessary to open the bulla to gain access to the cochlea. Thus far, there are no published reports of chronic CBF determinations in any animal model. Typically, the experiment is done as an acute study, with the animal under deep anesthesia. The use of LDF is restricted to those studies where there is a stimulus causing CBF change. The absolute level of CBF cannot be determined using LDF. This is an important limitation, as many questions that might be addressed using specific mouse genetic variants would require absolute flow measurements. For example, the age-dependent investigation of CBF in the C57 mouse, which undergoes premature (early in age onset) loss of hearing acuity, has not been addressed in a straightforward way. Instead, what has been studied is the age dependence of blood pressure autoregulation, a parameter that can be manipulated in acute experiments.

LDF is "simple" to use, but the mouse presents certain technical problems leading to errors in flow measurement. The reader may wish to consult a text on LDF to become conversant with the technology and the relevant measurement issues (e.g., Shepherd and Oberg, 1990); the chapter by

Miller and Nuttall (1990) covers the use of LDF for the cochlea in greater detail. The LDF instrument contains complex electronics to analyze the backscattered laser light from tissue when the probe emitting the laser light is put in approximation to the tissue surface or within the bulk of the tissue. The instrument reads out in units of arbitrary blood flux (the product of the number of red blood cells [RBC] and their mean velocity). An assumption is that the hematocrit in the analyzed volume of tissue does not change* so the readout can be interpreted as changing mean RBC velocity. An initial stable value is determined during a control time period; then the stimulus is given. Some manufacturers "calibrate" their instruments in units of absolute flow, but generally this calibration is only useful for well-characterized tissues such as skin.

To properly use LDF, it is important to control the quality of the interface between the probe and the tissue:

1. The probe must not move with respect to the tissue, as the instrument will see this movement as RBC velocity.
2. Extraneous particles (such as RBCs) must be excluded from between the probe tip and the tissue, as movement of these will affect the reading.
3. The number of capillaries in the tissue analyzed should dominate over large vessels to get an accurate mean flow value.
4. It is best if the tissue is homogeneous, but the cochlea is not.
5. The measurement volume should be understood; however, it has not been well-characterized for the cochlea.

Regarding point 4, the inhomogeneity of the cochlea means the laser light can penetrate to different depths as it spreads out. The optically clear lymph of the inner ear makes it possible for forward-scattered photons from interactions with RBCs to travel to deep areas of the cochlea before being backscattered. Possibly, those photons will interact with secondary RBCs, from the modiolar vessels for example, and certainly from any flow in the otic capsule. A determination of lateral wall blood flow might thus be contaminated by modiolar blood flow. The small size of the mouse cochlea will promote this form of error.

The related issue of measurement volume causes more obvious errors. It has been said that the typical LDF probe measures a radius of about 1 mm diameter (Bonner and Nossal, 1981; Nilsson et al., 1980). A direct study of the measurement depth revealed that the depth can be greater (Johansson et al., 1987). Clearly, this is important in the mouse, where the cochlea is of such small size. Not only will the large extent of the measurement volume defeat attempts to measure tonotopic (regional) flow, but it will also mix lateral wall and modiolar flow together. Because the mouse cochlea is not as separated from the bulla wall as it is in the guinea pig, gerbil, and chinchilla, it is not possible to direct the laser illumination to avoid even deeper tissues. The laser light could reach the brain, for example.

There are optical design methods for controlling the depth of measurement, the principal one being the design of the probe. One important factor governing depth of measurement is the size and distance between the optical fibers from which the probe is constructed (Johansson et al., 1991). For mouse CBF measurements, a probe of 0.4 mm diameter (e.g., from the Perimed Company) has been used successfully (T. Suzuki et al., 1998). The residual CBF that is found in the mouse when the supplying arterial system to the cochlea is clamped (the anterior inferior cerebellar artery)

---

* The assumption of constant number of measured cells is not a trivial point and the status of the capillary microhematocrit is a topic of research (Duling and Desjardins, 1987; Sarelius and Duling, 1982). Most CBF studies ignore this parameter but the stability of the population of cells in capillaries is generally unknown. Some LDF instruments output derived signals that approximate the moving mass of RBCs and the RBC mean velocity, but these parameters have not been systematically studied for the cochlea.

is about 37% (T. Suzuki et al., 1998), a number similar to the guinea pig (Ren et al., 1993b). This residual flow is attributed to collateral circulation to the labyrinthine artery. Suzuki et al. (2000) have found that, in the rat, about 20 to 30% of the residual LDF measured flow is due to the otic capsule. This would leave 7 to 17% for collateral flow and noncochlear flow if the mouse were to have otic capsule flow of the same proportion as the rat.

COCHLEAR BLOOD FLOW STUDIES IN THE MOUSE

Thus far, there have been no studies of CBF in the mouse using chemical microsensors (e.g., oxygen tension measuring electrodes), IVM, microspheres, or indicator compounds. Those studies that comprise the small body of literature can be divided into those indirectly concerned with (and measuring) CBF and those directly measuring CBF. In the first category can be placed histological and morphological approaches to the study of cochlear circulation and the 2-DG work.

Nakae and Tachibana (1986) studied a spontaneously diabetic mouse using transmission electron microscopy to characterize the morphological changes of various tissue types within the cochlea. Although the morphology of the stria vascularis was abnormal, including swollen intermediate cells and abnormal marginal cells, they noted that no obvious changes were visible for capillaries. Of course, the latter finding says nothing about the state of cochlear blood flow, but it must be noted that there are a number of morphological papers in other animal models where observations on strial capillaries can lead to the conclusion that blood flow must be altered. For example, Hawkins (1971) found swollen endothelial cells of the guinea pig spiral vessel of the basilar membrane following loud sound exposures in the guinea pig. Also, Vertes and Axelsson (1981) quantified many parameters of the circulation such as RBC packing density and plasma gaps to conclude that loud sound did reduce CBF in the guinea pig.

The 2-DG studies, as mentioned above, are an indirect measure of CBF because the uptake of 2-DG is metabolically driven. One can definitely say the increased 2-DG levels in tissue represent increased metabolism, but one cannot conclude that the blood flow was increased. Nonetheless, the results of the mouse 2-DG studies using sound stimuli are very important because they provide support for the hypothesis of a metabolically driven range of CBF. The nonsensory portions of the cochlea, the stria vascularis and spiral ligament, all respond with an increase in parallel to the neurosensory tissues (organ of Corti, VIII nerve, and inferior colliculus) (Canlon and Schacht, 1981; 1983) (Figure 15.1). High sound levels (>100 dBA SPL of broadband noise) resulted in a reduced deoxyglucose uptake compared to the peak produced by 85 dBA SPL noise. The metabolically driven change in CBF is still a matter needing further study, as the control mechanisms for such a cochlear blood flow increase are not known. Ryan et al. (1982) showed actual CBF increase in the gerbil using ^{14}C-iodoantipyrine and autoradiography, while Scheibe et al. (1993) found increased CBF in guinea pigs using LDF. These two studies are to be contrasted to the many reports that show loud sound (>100 to 115 dB SPL) decreases CBF (e.g., Scheibe et al., 1990; Thorne and Nuttall, 1987). The pathological mechanisms contributing to reduced CBF with loud sound are also not known. However, they could be related to the production of ROS because loud sound reduction in blood flow has an analogy to ischemia/reperfusion injury (Nuttall, 1999).

Ohlemiller et al. (1999b) used the mouse to demonstrate the production of ROS in the cochlea by sound stimulation and by compression of the anterior inferior cerebellar arterial network to the cochlea (Ohlemiller and Dugan, 1999). These were elegant studies that sampled the inner-ear chemical state by perfusion of the perilymphatic space with artificial perilymph and then analyzed the perfusate using high-performance liquid chromatography.

The direct studies of mouse CBF (using LDF) have been concerned with three issues: autoregulation and its strength dependence on age, vasoactive agents, and the age-dependent reactivity of mouse CBF to vasoactive agents. As mentioned, it is essential to have some stimulus to CBF that allows the assessment of blood flow change in relation to the initial baseline flow. The first

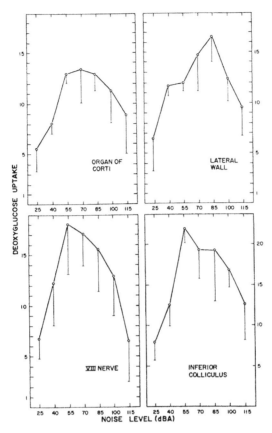

FIGURE 15.1 Response of deoxyglucose uptake to noise exposure. Animals received a pulse of 5 mCi [^{3}H]-deoxygluscose/kg body wt and were killed after 60 min of exposure to the noise levels indicated. Values are means ±S.D. from 3 to 8 animals each. Differences between 25 dBA and 85 dBA and between 85 dBA and 115 dBA are significant at $p < 0.001$ for all tissues. (From Canlon, B. and Schacht, J. 1983. *Hear. Res.,* 10, 217–226. With permission.)

study on mouse autoregulation of CBF was done in CBA mice by Nakashima et al. (1994). It used the agent angiotensin II to increase systemic blood pressure and the systematic withdrawal of whole blood from the femoral artery to reduce systemic mean blood pressure. They found that young, 2-month-old mice had significantly reduced ability to regulate a flow when blood pressure was slowly changed by angiotensin or blood withdrawal.

A more advanced method to examine autoregulation was applied to the mouse by T. Suzuki et al. (1998). The method was based on the occlusion of supplying arteries to the cochlea (e.g., Randolf et al., 1990 in the guinea pig), refined for repeated vessel occlusions and analysis of the LDF-measured dynamic flow waveform (see Ren et al., 1993b; Ren et al., 1995, for more on the method). Figure 15.2 shows the change in the LDF-measured CBF signal caused by clamping the AICA (anterior inferior cerebellar artery) in the young CBA mouse. The key feature of this waveform is the adaptation that occurs between timepoints O and O′. With the vessel clamped, the blood pressure driving blood into the cochlea may be considered constant and reduced in value from normal, yet the flow returns to normal over 60 seconds. This example is therefore representative of perfect or complete autoregulation. The vascular system of the cochlea and its supply vessels downstream of the clamp must dilate to achieve the flow increase. Figure 15.3 shows the striking effect of age on the waveform. The 21-month-old mouse has nearly lost the ability to adjust flow in the presence of abnormal conditions. Also seen in Figure 15.3 is the larger amount of CBF

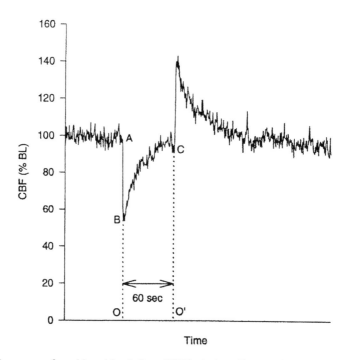

FIGURE 15.2 Response of cochlear blood flow (CBF) during 60-second occlusion of anterior interior cerebellar artery (AICA) in young mouse. To calculate AICA contribution and change in vascular conductance (vascular responsiveness), the following measurements are made: A — baseline (BL) of CBF; B — CBF at onset of acute occlusion; C — CBF prior to clamp release. Percent AICA contribution to CBF is indicated by AB. Vascular responsiveness was calculated as follows: Vascular responsiveness = CO'. (From Suzuki, T., Ren, T., Nuttall, A.L., and Miller, J.M. 1998. *Ann. Otol. Rhinol. Laryngol.*, 107, 648–653. With permission.)

change induced by the clamp. This indicates that the amount of collateral blood supply to the cochlea decreased with age in the CBA mouse.

In other studies, it has been possible to assess the actions of vasoactive agents on cochlear circulation using LDF. The most straightforward approach to applying drugs is the topical delivery of the agent to the RW membrane. This approach was explored initially by Ohlsen et al. (1989) and has been used primarily in the guinea pig in a number of other studies (e.g., Ohlsen et al., 1990; 1992; 1993). In the mouse, Nakashima et al. (1994) showed that RW application of the vasodilators sodium nitroprusside and hydralazine could elevate CBF. Sodium nitroprusside was decidedly the more powerful agent and there did not seem to be any difference in the vasodilation response across CBA mice ranging in age to 18 months. In contrast, Brown et al. (1995) showed that the inherent cochlear vessel dilation capacity of C57BL/6 mice, which had early onset hearing loss, was deficient in comparison to age-matched, normal-hearing CBA mice. The old (20 to 21 months) CBA mice exhibited similar deficient vasodilative capability in response to the sodium nitroprusside agent applied to the RW. These studies, which use different mouse strains and creative approaches to test the status and reactivity of the CBF, demonstrate the potential for mouse models to provide information about the mechanisms of blood flow control and homeostatic condition. It should also be noted that the pharmacological manipulation of CBF in the mouse, while difficult, is not limited to the RW approach. Yet clearly, the topical application of drugs to the ear is to be preferred over systemic applications when those systemic treatments involve changes in systemic blood pressure, for example. While it is possible to inject agents into the AICA in the rat and guinea pig (e.g., Coleman et al., 1998; McLaren et al., 1993; Quirk et al., 1994), this has not yet been accomplished in the mouse. The topical approach can be improved by perfusion of agents directly into the perilymph and one way to achieve this is via a catheter such as that described by Prieskorn and Miller (2000).

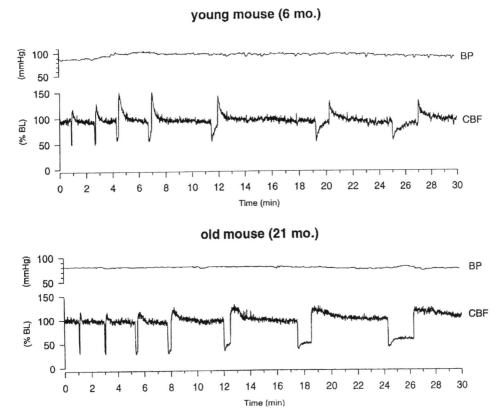

FIGURE 15.3   Response of blood pressure (BP) and CBF to 3-, 5-, 10-, 15-, 30-, 60-, and 120-second AICA clampings in young and aged mice. Abrupt decline in CBF is observed with clamp initiation followed by gradual recovery toward BL during 30-, 60-, and 120-second occlusions in both animals. Decreased amplitude is larger and recovery amplitude is smaller in the aged mouse. (From Suzuki, T., Ren, T., Nuttall, A.L., and Miller, J.M. 1998. *Ann. Otol. Rhinol. Laryngol.,* 107, 648–653. With permission.)

FUTURE DIRECTIONS

Of course, the value of the mouse model for CBF will be the availability of genetic variants that make the physiological or pathophysiological mechanisms of the cochlea understandable. Five areas of human hearing loss have potential components related to the circulation: Ménière's disease, autoimmune hearing loss, sound-induced hearing loss, age-related hearing loss, and sudden hearing loss. In each situation, there is a suspected pathology of the vasculature. In animal models (usually guinea pig), the vascular deficiencies are permeability change, decline in vascular density, altered vascular reactivity, and/or decreased blood flow. Mice having altered expression of proteins that specifically influence these and other vascular parameters will aid in sorting out the relative role of CBF in hearing loss.

As an example, consider the problem of how loud sound causes loss of sensory function. As mentioned, a medium level of sound (i.e., approximately 70 to 80 dBA SPL) is a driving force for increased energy metabolism (e.g., Canlon and Schacht, 1983) in the auditory system and for increased blood flow (Scheibe et al., 1993). Most studies show abnormal vascular-related parameters that point to decreased CBF above about 100 dB SPL. It has been proposed that this decreased flow could be the functional equivalent of ischemic stroke. Stroke damage in the brain generates two zones of damage: the peri-infarct zone, where complete hypoxia and stopped flow leads to necrotic cell death; and the penumbra, where ischemia is followed by reperfusion leading to various outcomes from the cellular point of view and activation of the apoptotic cell death pathway.

In the cochlea, it is not known if a critical ischemic level is reached prior to sensory cell damage and death. It is also not known how to divide the cause of ischemia into the portion related to vascular insufficiency and the portion due to excess metabolic demand. It is the combination of these two factors that probably makes the relatively mild CBF changes (compared to stroke) functionally important. The two factors could compound to become the equivalent of an ischemic stroke. Indeed, the hallmarks of ischemia and reperfusion injury — energy failure and excitotoxicity, an excess of ROS, inflammation, and apoptotic cell death — now have a significant literature in relation to loud sound damage in the cochlea.

Certain mouse mutants have already been used to begin to clarify ototoxic mechanisms. For example, homozygous 129/CD-1 mice with no measurable Cu/Zn superoxide dismutase (SOD) activity develop a more pronounced age-related auditory sensitivity loss than age-matched controls (McFadden et al., 1999b; Chapter 32 in this book). The targeted deletion of the *Sod1* gene causes an increased susceptibility to noise. Homozygous mice develop additional permanent threshold shifts relative to wild-type controls (Ohlemiller et al., 1999a). Studies such as these lend support to the role of ROS in the aging process and in noise-induced damage. Of course, it is possible that the age-dependent factor includes a component from the life long exposure to sound and other unknown parameters (such as diet) that influence the metabolic state of the cochlea. The pathological role of superoxide (which is regulated by Cu/Zn SOD) that occurs in direct correlation with sound exposure, as found by Ohlemiller et al. (1999a), appears to confer importance to the direct observation of superoxide generated by the stria vascularis (of the guinea pig) following loud sound exposure (Yamane et al., 1995a,b).

Again, it must be remembered that studies such as those on SOD do not speak strictly to the question of the role of CBF. Blood flow is one aspect of the metabolic equation, and it is difficult to sort out metabolic shortfall (caused by ischemia) from deficiencies of the tissue antioxidant mechanisms. With loud sound, it is likely that the antioxidant defense mechanisms of the cochlea will be important. For example, Jacono et al. (1998) showed sound-related up-regulation of glutathione-related enzymes; Yamasoba et al. (1998) showed that the pharmacological depletion of glutathione enhances loud sound damage; and Ohinata et al. (1999) showed the protective effect of glutathione supplementation.

There are many relevant mouse knockout/knockin models that will be useful in defining the CBF-related pathology. Examples would be the mutants for nitric oxide synthase (NOS). There are now specific knockouts available for the three isoforms of NOS. These have not yet been investigated to determine the role of the significant amount of NOS in the cochlea distributed across a wide number of cell types (e.g., Fessenden et al., 1994; Franz et al., 1996; Gosepath et al., 1997; Ruan et al., 1997; Zdanski et al., 1994). Endothelial NOS (eNOS or NOS III) produces NO that is locally vasodilative to smooth muscle of arteries and arterioles. A basal level of NO is shown to contribute about 10% of the baseline CBF in the guinea pig (Brechtelsbauer et al., 1994). Will the eNOS-deficient mouse have increased susceptibility to noise because of the expected compromised CBF? This is the type of experiment that speaks fairly closely to the question of ischemia and can be done in mouse models at this time.

We have been using NOS knockout mice to study the production of NO in the cochlea and its physiological roles. NO is produced by a number of different cell types in the cochlea including inner and outer hair cells (Shi et al., 2000). The function of the endogenically produced NO is largely unknown, but we have shown that in nNOS, –/– mice have significant protection against noise-induced permanent threshold shift (Omelchenko et al., 2001).

Ischemia is known to result in delayed damage to cells via apoptotic cell death pathways, so interventions to prevent cell death due to ischemia are possible. For example, brain stroke leads to caspase-mediated neuronal death, and caspase-1 knockout mice are resistant, suggesting a role for inflammation (Schielke et al., 1998). Generally, the cell death mechanism is identified by terminal-deoxynucleotidyl-transferase-mediated dUTP nick end (TUNEL) labeling. While the TUNEL method is currently controversial for the cochlea (Nishizaki et al., 1999; Orita et al., 1999) (i.e., apoptotic vs. necrotic cell death), it is important to continue to understand the apoptotic pathways, which are the final common route from which cells may be rescued. Indeed, a general caspase inhibitor has been found to protect cultured rat spiral ganglion cells from hypoxic injury (Cheng et al., 1999). Of course, there are other calcium-dependent proteases, gene products, and neurotrophic factors involved in ischemia-induced cell death that will benefit from future mouse mutant models.

One must not overlook the usefulness of examining the direct susceptibility of the cochlea to ischemia using traditional whole-organ approaches. Different organ systems have different susceptibilities to injury. While the pathophysiological mechanisms of sound, autoimmune disease, Ménière's disease, aging, and sudden hearing loss will be complex and diverse, the ischemic hypoxia model, by arterial clamp, offers a direct test-bed for the acute study of short-term cell damage mechanisms. T. Suzuki et al. (1998) showed the feasibility of clamping the arterial supply to the mouse cochlea. Previously, the vascular clamp approach was limited to rats (e.g., Seidman et al., 1991), guinea pigs (e.g., Randolf et al., 1990), and gerbils (e.g., Ren et al., 1995; Mom et al., 1997). Its use for the mouse opens up the possibility of using knockout mice in well-defined ischemia experiments, where physiological parameters such as otoacoustic emissions can be measured. Such studies not only can serve to clarify ischemic damage mechanisms, but can also clarify the role of certain genes in the normal physiology of the cochlea, where energy metabolism is a parameter of interest.

ACKNOWLEDGMENTS

This work was supported by NIH grants NIDCD R01 DC 00105, DC00105-25S1, DC00141, and DC00141-22S1.

16 Development of the Endbulbs of Held

Charles J. Limb and David K. Ryugo

INTRODUCTION

The cochlear nucleus of the brainstem receives direct input from the inner ear and is therefore the first synaptic station of the central auditory system. The resident neurons of the cochlear nucleus in turn give rise to all ascending pathways. Consequently, the organization between incoming auditory nerve fibers and second-order neurons plays a key role in the central processing of sound. A corollary is that abnormalities in the cochlear nucleus are likely to have downstream effects throughout the system. The cochlear nucleus contains a variety of different cell types (see Chapters 18 and 19), each of which exhibits different somatic and dendritic properties (Osen, 1969; Brawer et al., 1974), associates with a particular constellation of afferent endings (Lorente de Nó, 1981; Cant, 1982; Smith and Rhode, 1989), projects to different targets (Van Noort, 1969; Warr, 1982a; Schofield and Cant, 1996a), and expresses different response properties to sound (Pfeiffer, 1966a; Evans and Nelson, 1973; Rhode et al., 1983a; b). The particular combinations of these various properties are thought to underlie separate functions in hearing. Within the anteroventral cochlear nucleus (AVCN), myelinated auditory nerve fibers produce one or several large axosomatic endings known as endbulbs of Held (Held, 1893; Ramón y Cajal, 1909). The endbulb is one of the largest synaptic endings in the brain (Lenn and Reese, 1966), exhibits an elaborately branched appearance in adult animals (Ryugo and Fekete, 1982), expresses an estimated 500 to 2000 synaptic active zones (Ryugo et al., 1996), and contacts a population of second-order neurons called spherical bushy cells (Brawer and Morest, 1975; Cant and Morest, 1979a; Ryugo and Fekete, 1982). These features reflect a highly secure synaptic interface, consistent with the suggestion that every pre-synaptic discharge produces a postsynaptic spike (Pfeiffer, 1966b). The postsynaptic spherical bushy cell exhibits rapid depolarizations and repolarizations, thereby maintaining the temporal fidelity of incoming signals (Romand, 1978; Oertel, 1983; Manis and Marx, 1991). In addition, spherical bushy cells project to the superior olivary complex (Cant and Casseday, 1986) where they form a circuit implicated in the processing of interaural timing differences (Yin and Chan, 1990; Fitzpatrick et al., 1997). Thus, this component of the auditory pathway faithfully preserves the temporal changes and transients of acoustic streams necessary for the localization of sound sources in space and for the comprehension of speech (Moiseff and Konishi, 1981; Takahashi et al., 1984; Blackburn and Sachs, 1990).

The structure of endbulbs exhibits several activity-related features. Endbulb branching patterns and the ultrastructure of their synapses in cats with normal hearing have been shown to vary system-atically with respect to average levels of spike discharges (Ryugo et al., 1996). The endbulbs of auditory nerve fibers having relatively low levels of spike discharges exhibit smaller swellings in their arborization and are associated with larger postsynaptic densities compared to endbulbs of relatively active fibers. Activity-related features of synaptic structure were further documented by using deafness as an extreme form of activity reduction (Ryugo et al., 1997; 1998). The endbulbs of adult congenitally deaf white cats, where auditory nerve activity is almost entirely abolished, exhibit reduced branching and hypertrophied synaptic structures when compared to hearing littermates. It is clear that endbulb morphology is strongly influenced by levels of activity, and most likely impacts on signal transmission from nerve to brain.

These observations have clinical implications for intervention strategies in cases of deafness. Strategies for hearing restoration have progressed from simple sound amplification to digital speech encoding and direct neuronal stimulation. The most widely used of the latter modalities is the cochlear implant, which uses an external speech processor to control an electrode array implanted within the cochlea (Marangos and Laszig, 1996; Cheng and Niparko, 1999). This array directly stimulates spiral ganglion cells, thus initiating neuronal transmission from these first-order sensory neurons to cochlear nucleus neurons of the brainstem. Thus, the physiological condition of primary neurons and their synapses is a major determinant in the success of the implant. Post-lingually deafened patients appear to benefit more from cochlear implants than pre-lingually deafened patients, and younger children benefit more than older children (Nikolopoulos et al., 1999; Waltzman et al., 1994; Gantz et al., 1994). These clinical data indicate that time windows during maturation define "critical periods" that are important factors in the normal development of the central auditory system. The endbulbs of Held may be especially relevant to the acquisition of language because speech comprehension relies on accurate temporal coding of acoustic input. It is plausible that deafness-induced abnormalities in endbulb structure and function are mostly limited to cases of congenital deafness, and that such kinds of early developmental changes are responsible for the differential effects of hearing loss in young vs. old populations. The efficacy of treatments for deafness might be improved with a better understanding of the exact nature of the changes that occur during the earliest periods of development in the auditory system.

NORMAL AND MUTANT MICE

We demonstrated in the congenitally deaf white cat that synaptic changes occur in the endbulbs of Held, where abnormal endbulb synapses appear in animals that have been deaf for 6 months or longer. One of our concerns regarding these observations, however, was whether the abnormalities of endbulb structure in congenitally deaf white cats were simply part of the genetic syndrome or whether they were due to deafness (e.g., lack of auditory nerve activity). In this regard, a different animal model was sought in order to test hypotheses developed from cat data. The mouse provides a compelling model with which to begin because of its relatively rapid development, its genetic homogeneity that limits interanimal variability, the presence of well-defined mutant strains, some with point mutations causing deafness, and the potential for single gene manipulations using transgenic techniques. A first step was to study the development of endbulbs of Held in normal-hearing mice. The next step was to compare the effects of deafness on endbulb development. The goal was to provide insight into the significance of specific time periods for proper development and the nature of activity-related features of synaptic structure. In this chapter, we report on endbulb development in normal-hearing CBA/J mice, and compare the adult endbulb morphology to that of deaf adult *shaker-2* mice ($Myo15^{sh2/sh2}$) and normal-hearing heterozygous littermates ($Myo15^{+/sh2}$).

The *shaker-2* mouse has a mutation on the MYO15 gene, causing an amino acid substitution from cysteine to tyrosine within the motor domain of the unconventional myosin 15 protein (Probst et al., 1998; see also Chapter 27). Myosin 15 appears to be involved in the maintenance of the actin organization in the hair cells of the organ of Corti and vestibular sensory epithelia. As a result of this mutation, stereocilia of homozygous mutants appear short and stubby, and the mice display phenotypic deafness and circling behavior (Deol, 1954; Probst et al., 1998). There are early pathologic alterations in the organ of Corti, but cell loss in the spiral ganglion is undetectable until after 100 days postnatal (Deol, 1954). The identified point mutation found in *shaker-2* mice has also been found in humans with DFNB3, a nonsyndromic form of recessive deafness (Wang et al., 1998). This condition emphasizes the potential of *shaker-2* mice as a model for understanding human deafness and for studying the effects of a natural form of deafness on brain development.

AUDITORY BRAIN STEM RECORDINGS (ABRS)

The bulk of the data reported in this chapter was generated from normal-hearing CBA/J mice of either sex and aged 1 day, 1 week, 2 weeks, 4 weeks, 8 to 10 weeks, and >6 months (Limb and Ryugo, 2000). The CBA/J strain of mouse was selected because it retains good hearing across most of its life span (e.g., Henry, 1983), and we needed normal baseline data with which to compare mutants. The ages of the homozygous *shaker-2* mice ($Myo15^{sh2/sh2}$) and heterozygous, hearing littermates ($Myo15^{+/sh2}$) ranged between 8 and 11 weeks. Mice were obtained from a licensed vendor (Jackson Laboratories, Bar Harbor, ME), and appeared healthy, with normal respiratory activity, normal tympanic membranes, and no evidence of external- or middle-ear infection.

Studying development in mice is not a trivial task because newborn mice are small, their peripheral auditory systems are immature (e.g., the external ear canal is closed), and they are difficult to anesthetize. Consequently, ABRs were obtained for all CBA/J mice 4 weeks of age or older. The day of birth is defined as postnatal day 1, and each successive day is numbered consecutively. All mice older than 2 weeks of age were tested for behavioral responses to free-field auditory stimuli (loud handclap from behind). CBA/J and $Myo15^{+/sh2}$ mice exhibited startle responses, but the *shaker-2* mice were unresponsive. For all mice 4 weeks of age and older, ABRs were recorded in response to clicks as a function of intensity. Mice were anesthetized using intraperitoneal injections of 3.5% chloral hydrate (0.008 mL/kg) and xylazine hydrochloride (0.006 mg/kg). ABRs were recorded with a vertex electrode and an electrode inserted behind the pinna ipsilateral to the stimulated ear. Click levels were determined in dB peak equivalent SPL (dB peSPL) referenced to 1 kHz by recording levels just inside the tip of a hollow ear bar using a calibrated microphone (Burkard, 1984). The ear bar, coupled to an electrostatic speaker (Sokolich, 1977), was then placed into the external ear canal. Clicks (n = 1000) of 100-μs duration and alternating polarity were presented monaurally in 5-dB increments, starting at 0 dB and progressing to 95 dB peSPL.

Representative ABR tracings from one 4-week-old animal and one 7-month-old animal are shown in Figure 16.1. The mean threshold for hearing in all CBA/J mice used in this study was 41.7 ± 7.1 dB peSPL, similar to previously reported values (Wenngren and Anniko, 1988; Mikaelian and Ruben, 1965; Hunter and Willott, 1987; X.Y. Zheng et al., 1999). At 4 weeks of age (n = 8), the mean threshold for hearing was 45.4 ± 9.0 dB peSPL. At 8 to 10 weeks of age (n = 6), the mean threshold was 40.2 ± 5.8 dB peSPL. At 7 months of age (n = 9), the mean threshold was 39.3 ± 5.0 dB peSPL. These differences were not statistically significant (ANOVA, $p > 0.1$), indicating that ABR thresholds are stable by 4 weeks of age and remain relatively constant for the next 6 months.

ENDBULB DEVELOPMENT

POSTNATAL DAY 1

The newborn mouse weighed 1.33 ± 0.1 g, with a cochlear nucleus less than 0.8 mm in length. The histologic appearance of the ventral division was characterized by tightly packed cell bodies. Each cell body contained scant cytoplasm but housed a prominent nucleus. The ventral division was separated from the dorsal division by a lamina of granule cells, and the dorsal division already exhibits its characteristic layering of neuropil and cell bodies. Auditory nerve fibers were labeled by neurobiotin injections into the cochlea, and labeled fibers were observed to enter from the ventrolateral aspect, travel dorsally a short distance, and bifurcate into ascending and descending branches. At this age, individual fibers were thin (<0.5 μm in diameter) and relatively unbranched. At the rostral end of each fiber, a small terminal swelling (1 to 3 μm in diameter) could be located (Figure 16.1). Typically, the swellings appeared as rounded boutons, but the contour of the swelling

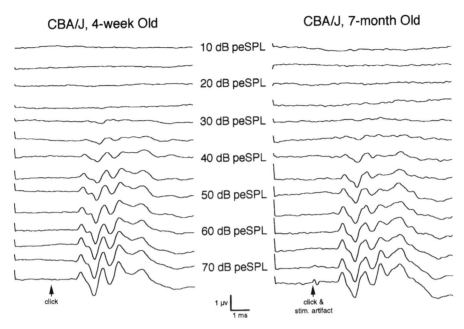

CBA/J, 4-week Old   CBA/J, 7-month Old

10 dB peSPL
20 dB peSPL
30 dB peSPL
40 dB peSPL
50 dB peSPL
60 dB peSPL
70 dB peSPL

click   1 μv   click &
                               1 ms   stim. artifact

FIGURE 16.1 Representative auditory brainstem response (ABR) recordings of normal CBA/J mice, aged 4 weeks (left) and 7 months (right) in response to click stimuli. The gray arrows indicate the presentation of each click. The mean threshold of CBA/J mice (n = 23) was 41.7 ± 7.1 dB peSPL. Thresholds do not show any significant change between 4 weeks and 7 months. (Adapted from Limb and Ryugo, 2000.)

could also be elongated or triangular in shape. These terminal swellings did not resemble the mature endbulbs of Held, but we inferred their identify by virtue of their origin in the auditory nerve and their axosomatic contacts in the rostral anteroventral cochlear nucleus (AVCN).

Postnatal Week 1

During the first week, the light microscopic appearance of the swellings of auditory nerve fiber did not undergo much change. By the end of the week, the mouse weighed 3.2 ± 0.3 g, but swellings still appeared as small buds (Figure 16.2). Some of the endings were bouton-like in shape and, occasionally, two buds emanated from one fiber to form a doublet onto the same cell body. The buds themselves did not exhibit filopodia or branches.

Neurons in the rostral AVCN could not be separated into morphological groups on the basis of Nissl patterns or somatic shapes at this early age. In adults, neurons in this location are called spherical bushy cells and are described as having a round cell body, a centrally placed round nucleus surrounded by a cytoplasmic "necklace" of Nissl bodies, and a perinuclear Nissl cap (Osen, 1969; Cant and Morest, 1979a; Webster and Trune, 1982). In the neonatal mouse, the cell bodies are angular in shape and their surface is invaginated, often more than once, producing a jagged appearance. In addition, the nuclear envelope is pleated, and perinuclear Nissl caps are not observed. The mean somatic silhouette area at this age is 62.9 ± 13.8 μm^2.

Although the nuclear and cytoplasmic characteristics of cells in the rostral AVCN did not change during the first week, cell body size doubled to a mean silhouette area of 114.0 ± 14.7 μm^2. The cell outline still has frequent irregularities, but the overall impression was that they were less pronounced and that cell shape was less angular. The nuclear envelope appeared rippled, the chromatin generally dispersed, and there was no cap of perinuclear Nissl substance. In many cases, cresyl violet staining revealed the proximal portions of large dendrites.

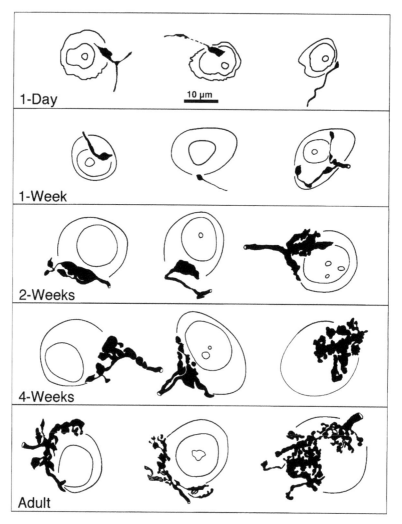

FIGURE 16.2 Representative examples of neurobiotin-labeled, axosomatic, terminal swellings in the rostral AVCN of an age-graded series of CBA/J mice, spanning from 1 day postnatal to adulthood. The endings begin as small, sometimes irregularly shaped boutons, and grow in size during the first week (Stage 0). At 2 weeks, the endings appear large, club-shaped with occasional branches (Stage 1). By 4 weeks of age, endbulbs have a central trunk that usually gives rise to two or three short branches, each of which has *en passant* swellings and bouton-like terminations (Stage 2). Adult status is reached by 9 weeks of age, and no changes in endbulb morphology can be detected out to 7 months (Stage 3). A central trunk can usually be identified that gives rise to branches that are longer and more varied in arrangement than at 4 weeks of age. The branches themselves give rise to other small branches with *en passant* swellings and complex terminations. (Adapted from Limb and Ryugo, 2000.)

POSTNATAL WEEK 2

By the end of the second postnatal week, mice weighed 5.0 ± 0.8 g and exhibited a startle response to sudden loud sounds (Mikaelian and Ruben, 1965; Ehret, 1976a; Shnerson and Pujol, 1983). The parent axon ranged from 1 to 3 μm in diameter as it ascended through the AVCN. As each axon approached one pole of the target cell, it gave rise to a large terminal swelling having a variety of shapes (Figure 16.2). The simplest endings at this age were bouton-like, but they were 10- to 15-fold larger compared to those of 1-day-old mice. A few filopodia could be seen arising from this main swelling. In some cases, there was a coarse pattern of branches, where the parent branch gave rise to several smaller and irregular branchlets (Figure 16.2). The branchlets formed a cluster of endings that was generally confined to the same pole of the cell and did not appose much of the cell surface.

The cells of the rostral AVCN increased in mean silhouette area to 163.9 ± 18.5 μm^2. A perinuclear cap could be seen in stained, light microscopic preparations, revealing a defining feature of the spherical bushy cells. The contour of the cell was more regular compared to that at 1 week of age, with fewer and smaller somatic invaginations. The overall shape of the cells was oval-to-round. The nuclear envelope appeared more regular in contour and nucleoli became clearly visible.

POSTNATAL WEEK 4

At this age, CBA/J mice were approximately half their final body weight (17.4 ± 2.9 g) and terminal swellings have been replaced by endings with definite branches (Figure 16.2). These endings were identifiable as nascent endbulbs, where a central trunk (2 to 4 μm in diameter) often gave rise to more branches with *en passant* swellings and irregular terminal swellings. The main branch usually divided into two or three additional branches, each of which was nearly the same in caliber as the parent axon. The branches were separable from each other and did not extend far from the main trunk.

The cell body of the spherical bushy cell reached its adult size. The mean cross-sectional area was 204.0 ± 36.7 μm^2, which is significantly greater than that at 2 weeks of age ($p < 0.05$). The spherical bushy cell itself appeared similar to previous descriptions of neurons in the AVCN of cats and mice (Osen, 1969; Cant and Morest, 1979a; Webster and Trune, 1982). The cell surface lost most of its irregular contour, and now had an oval-to-round shape. The population of spherical bushy cells was generally homogeneous. The nucleus was pale and round, occupying a slightly eccentric position. Nucleoli were prominent, and a perinuclear Nissl cap had become a definable feature by light microscopic examination.

ADULT MICE

Nine weeks is the mean age for initial fertile matings in mice (Crispens, 1975). At this age, the mouse weighed 30.9 ± 4.3 g and the terminal arborization of auditory nerve fibers was clearly definable as an endbulb (Figure 16.6). The main axon formed branches of approximately equal caliber, ranging from 1 to 3 μm in thickness. A central trunk with a variety of lumpy branches extended to cover up to half the somatic surface. The branches themselves gave rise to more branches with *en passant* swellings and irregular terminations, yielding an elaborate three-dimensional arrangement that encircled the cell body. Spherical bushy cells exhibited a prominent perinuclear Nissl cap and had a mean cross-sectional area of 189.8 ± 26.4 μm^2.

Growth continued but at a slower pace, until at least 7 months of age. On average, these old mice weighed 34.36 ± 2.9 g, and the complex pattern of endbulb arborizations persisted (Figure 16.2). The mature spherical bushy cell was characterized by a centrally located nucleus with a distinct perinuclear Nissl cap and a prominent nucleolus (Figure 16.7b). The mean cross-sectional area of spherical bushy cells in 7-month-old animals was 219.10 ± 50.2 μm^2.

DEAF MOUSE OBSERVATIONS

ABR DATA, SHAKER-2 MICE

Myo15$^{sh2/sh2}$ mice, 2 to 3 months of age, exhibited nearly constant circling behavior and were noticeably smaller (19.25 ± 0.6 g) than CBA/J mice of comparable age. At 6 months, *Myo15$^{sh2/sh2}$* mice weighed 25.71 ± 1.3 g, approximately 75% of the weight of age-matched CBA/J mice. They exhibited no evoked potentials in response to clicks up to 95 dB peSPL (Figure 16.3), and were therefore considered deaf. Although heterozygous *Myo15$^{+/sh2}$* littermates were also small (23.19 ± 0.6 g), they exhibited

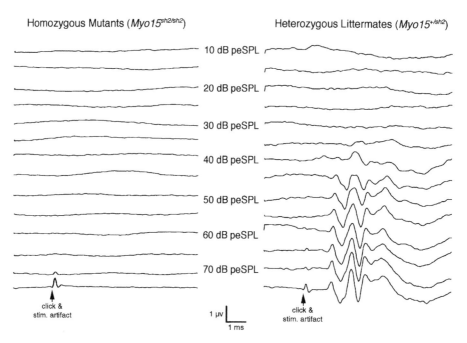

Homozygous Mutants ($Myo15^{sh2/sh2}$)   Heterozygous Littermates ($Myo15^{+/sh2}$)

10 dB peSPL

20 dB peSPL

30 dB peSPL

40 dB peSPL

50 dB peSPL

60 dB peSPL

70 dB peSPL

click & stim. artifact

1 μV

1 ms

click & stim. artifact

FIGURE 16.3 Representative auditory brainstem response (ABR) recordings from deaf $Myo15^{sh2/sh2}$ mice (left) and $Myo15^{+/sh2}$ littermates (right). No evoked responses were observed for $Myo15^{sh2/sh2}$ mice even after presentation of clicks up to 95 dB peSPL. On the right, $Myo15^{+/sh2}$ littermates are shown to have normal hearing in response to click stimuli, with a mean threshold of 38.5 ± 3.5 dB peSPL. The gray arrows indicate the presentation of the click stimulus. (Adapted from Limb and Ryugo, 2000.)

similar ABR thresholds (38.5 ± 3.5 dB peSPL) as those recorded in normal CBA/J mice of the same age (Figure 16.3).

Cochlear Morphology

The histologic appearance of the cochleae of CBA/J and $Myo15^{+/sh2}$ mice was normal, although the sample size for $Myo15^{+/sh2}$ was small. In contrast, the cochleae of $Myo15^{sh2/sh2}$ mice were distinctly abnormal. A general histopathologic description for the cochleae of $Myo15^{sh2/sh2}$ mice has been previously published (Deol, 1954), and our data are generally consistent with this earlier report. Briefly, the tectorial membrane is swollen in the apical turn of the cochlear duct and becomes thinner by the middle half-turn. It remained thin to the basal end. Throughout, however, the tectorial membrane failed to extend over the region of outer hair cells (OHCs). Typically, all inner hair cells were present in the apex although their intermittent absence was noted in the middle half-turn and they were mostly missing in the base. OHCs were more seriously affected. In the apex, OHCs of row 3 were often missing. Progressively more OHCs were absent throughout the rows in the middle half turn of the cochlear duct, and there were few if any OHCs in the base. The tunnel of Corti was consistently intact in the apex, but outer pillar cells were sometimes missing in the lower middle turn of the cochlear duct, and the tunnel was often difficult to discern in the base. Irrespective of the appearance of the organ of Corti, spiral ganglion cells were present throughout Rosenthal's canal for all cochleae of $Myo15^{sh2/sh2}$ mice. There were occasional empty spaces, 20 to 25 μm in diameter, scattered throughout Rosenthal's canal, but mostly in the basal half-turn; these spaces seemed to represent sites of ganglion cell loss. In the cochlear base, some sections exhibited up to 30% ganglion cell loss as estimated by reductions in cell density. Throughout the rest of Rosenthal's canal, however, the full complement of ganglion cells was present and appeared normal.

Shaker-2 Mutant   Heterozygous Littermate

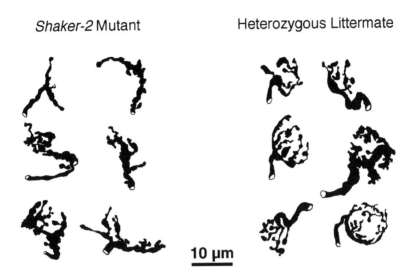

10 µm

FIGURE 16.4 Drawing tube reconstructions of neurobiotin-labeled endbulbs from deaf, adult $Myo15^{sh2/sh2}$ mice (left) and hearing, adult $Myo15^{+/sh2}$ mice (right). Endbulbs exhibit variable morphology, but overall there is a decrease in complexity of endbulb morphology in the *shaker-2* mutant mice. Many of the endbulbs of the deaf mice appear stunted in shape, without many branches or filopodia. It is particularly interesting that the endbulbs of *shaker-2* mice do not resemble those of normal mice at younger ages, suggesting that deafness does not simply arrest endbulb development. (Adapted from Limb and Ryugo, 2000.)

Endbulb Morphology

The diameter of auditory nerve fibers from 2-month-old deaf (2.88 ± 0.4 µm) and hearing (2.9 ± 0.4 µm) mice were comparable (ANOVA, $p > 0.3$). The appearance of endbulbs from normal hearing CBA/J mice of the same age. Adult hearing mice exhibited endbulbs with elaborate arborizations (Figures 16.2 and 16.4). Most striking for the deaf $Myo15^{sh2/sh2}$ mice was a decrease in the amount of endbulb branching (Figure 16.4). The main trunk was thick with irregular bumps, yet without interconnecting filaments or higher levels of branching. Endbulbs from deaf mice could exhibit more extensive branching and present a near normal appearance, but such occurrences were rare.

Fractal Analysis of Endbulb Complexity

Fractal geometry provides a means of quantifying the complexity of natural structures (Mandelbrot, 1982), and has been used to assess endbulb complexity (Ryugo et al., 1997). We applied the box counting technique (Fractal Dimension Calculator v1.5), in which a grid of squares having 11 different sizes is placed over the outline of an endbulb; and for each size (s), the number of squares N(s) that contain any portion of the endbulb is counted. As the size of the squares on a grid became progressively smaller, the number of intersections increased, and this increase is faster for more complicated structures. The fractal dimension D is given by the slope of the linear portion of the line when log [N(s)] is plotted against log (1/s), derived from the relationship log [N(s)] = D log (1/s). As a result, the greater the slope of the line, the greater the structural complexity. Fractal values range between 1 and 2, and each increase of 0.1 in the fractal dimension represents a doubling of structural complexity (Porter et al., 1991).

We calculated the fractal index of CBA/J endbulb silhouettes with respect to age to quantify developmental features (Figure 16.5). The mean fractal index of endbulbs progressively increases with age, beginning at 1.02 ± 0.02 in 1-day-old mice and stabilizing at 1.29 ± 0.05 at 10 weeks. The data demonstrate statistically significant changes in endbulb complexity with respect to age up to 10 weeks, but no change in complexity between the 10-week-old and the 6- to 7-month-old

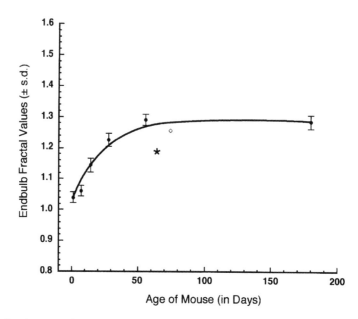

FIGURE 16.5 Graph comparing quantitative data for endbulbs of normal hearing, adult CBA/J (●) and $Myo15^{+/sh2}$ mice (○) to data from deaf adult $Myo15^{sh2/sh2}$ mice (*). This graph shows a change in fractal index with age in CBA/J mice, indicative of the increased complexity in endbulb structure. Fractal index undergoes a marked increase during the first 4 to 6 weeks of life, at which time the adult endbulb structure is reached and stabilizes throughout adulthood. Endbulb complexity is similar for hearing heterozygous $Myo15^{+/sh2}$ mice but seriously reduced in littermate deaf $Myo15^{sh2/sh2}$ mice. This graph stresses the idea that the first 2 months of life in the mouse represent a period during which significant growth, change, and structural refinement occur, and that endbulb elaboration is compromised by congenital deafness. (Adapted from Limb and Ryugo, 2000.)

mice (ANOVA, $p < 0.05$). As already stated, the fractal index (1.25 ± 0.03) of endbulbs from $Myo15^{+/sh2}$ mice with normal ABR thresholds was not statistically different from that of normal-hearing, adult CBA/J mice (1.29 ± 0.05). The endbulbs of deaf *shaker-2* mice, however, were less structurally complex (1.19 ± 0.04), revealing a twofold reduction in structural complexity ($p < 0.01$) and implying that endbulb structure is dependent on hearing.

SPHERICAL BUSHY CELL SIZE

There was a rapid, statistically significant, age-related increase in the average size of spherical bushy cells in the first month of life. Cell body size at birth was 62.9 ± 13.8 μm^2, increased to 204 ± 36.7 μm^2 at 4 weeks ($p < 0.05$), and remained constant out to 7 months of age ($p > 0.45$). The body weight of $Myo15^{sh2/sh2}$ and $Myo15^{+/sh2}$ mice was consistently less than those of age-matched CBA/J mice. Likewise, the size of their spherical bushy cells was smaller than that of adult CBA/J mice. Deaf $Myo15^{sh2/sh2}$ mice exhibited somatic silhouette areas of 147.68 ± 26.9 μm^2, whereas hearing $Myo15^{+/sh2}$ littermates exhibited a mean of 150.59 ± 32.8 μm^2. A comparison of cell body size between the three groups of mice demonstrated no difference between $Myo15^{sh2/sh2}$ and $Myo15^{+/sh2}$ mice ($p > 0.40$), but a significant difference when compared to CBA/J mice (ANOVA, $p < 0.01$). These observations suggest that cell body size is related to strain differences rather than deafness.

DISCUSSION

Endbulbs of Held represent a class of large, axosomatic synaptic endings that arise from myelinated auditory nerve fibers and terminate in the AVCN. One or several endbulbs are found on every

Mouse

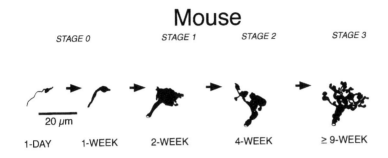

STAGE 0   STAGE 1   STAGE 2   STAGE 3

1-DAY   1-WEEK   2-WEEK   4-WEEK   ≥ 9-WEEK

Cat

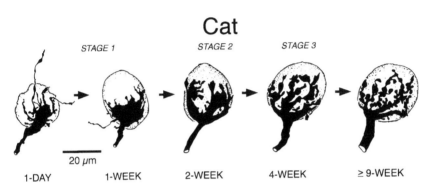

STAGE 1   STAGE 2   STAGE 3

1-DAY   1-WEEK   2-WEEK   4-WEEK   ≥ 9-WEEK

FIGURE 16.6 Developmental comparison of endbulbs of mice and cats. (Top) Schematic diagram showing developmental changes in the endbulb of Held in normal hearing CBA/J mice. The endbulb begins as a small bouton (Stage 0), grows rapidly in size to a large club-shaped ending by 2 weeks of age (Stage 1), forms definite branches by 4 weeks of age (Stage 2), and reaches its mature shape by 9 weeks of age (Stage 3). After this age, the appearance of the endbulb does not undergo significant change. (Adapted from Limb and Ryugo, 2000.) (Bottom) Schematic diagram showing the developmental appearance of endbulb of Held from cats. (Adapted from Ryugo and Fekete, 1982.) Note that the endbulbs of both species progress through essentially the same developmental stages. Reprinted by permission of Wiley-Liss, Inc., a subsidiary of John Wiley & Sons, Inc.

auditory nerve fiber, spanning the entire audible frequency range, and endbulbs are clearly identifiable throughout vertebrates (reviewed by Szpir et al., 1990). The characteristic endbulb arborization embraces the somata of spherical bushy cells, and together they form part of the circuit involved in processing of acoustic timing information. Endbulbs begin as small axosomatic swellings evident just after birth, develop gradually into larger club-shaped endings, and finally blossom into an intricate network of branches interconnected by fine filaments. This sequence of development is inferred from findings in the mouse, as well as from observations in cats (Ryugo and Fekete, 1982). Keep in mind, however, that there are differences in the duration of each developmental stage, and that the mouse auditory system seems relatively less mature at birth (Figure 16.6).

ENDBULB STAGING

The terminal swellings of auditory nerve fibers in the AVCN exhibit a range of appearances, but with a predominant form at each age (Figure 16.6). At the earliest ages, the presumptive endbulb appears as a simple, small bouton. During the next 2 weeks, this bud continues to enlarge, forming the classic club-shaped ending with filopodial extensions (Held, 1893; Ramón y Cajal, 1909; Lorente de Nó, 1981). This large, club-like form of the endbulb is defined as a Stage 1 endbulb in the newborn cat (Ryugo and Fekete, 1982). It appears that endbulbs of newborn mice have not yet reached this first developmental stage, while endbulbs of newborn cats have already passed through the small bouton stage. Thus, bouton endings of the auditory nerve in the just-born mouse are defined as Stage 0 endbulbs, a stage not observed in neonatal kittens. Mice do not exhibit Stage 1 endbulbs until about 2 weeks of age. By the 4th week, the endbulb has sprouted several branches and become somewhat irregular in form. This form of the endbulb is equivalent to the Stage 2 endbulb in cats. At 9 weeks postnatal, endbulbs have become more complex in arrangement, with extensive secondary and tertiary branching that covers a large portion of the postsynaptic cell. By this age, the endbulb is considered to be adult-like and is called Stage 3. Beyond this age, endbulbs do not change in branching complexity, but become slightly finer in caliber. Thus, the endbulbs of postnatal mice begin at an earlier stage than in cats, but eventually pass through the same sequential stages of development. The qualitative descriptions of endbulbs and their staging are confirmed quantitatively by the results of fractal analysis because each stage is statistically more complex than the previous one.

Branching of Endbulbs

Development of the endbulb is likely dependent on the interaction between both pre- and postsynaptic mechanisms. The exact participants involved (whether neurotransmitters, trophic factors, action potentials, etc.) remain unidentified, but it is probable that two-way communication between endbulbs and spherical bushy cells occurs. Presynaptic activity appears to be a necessary requirement for endbulb integrity. Previous work has suggested that synapses of spherical bushy cells undergo a compensatory hypertrophy in response to sensory deprivation (Ryugo et al., 1997; 1998). What mechanisms might be responsible for such changes? Depolarization or electrical field potentials are known to influence the branching of axons and formation of lamellipodia in cultured cortical neurons (Ranmakers et al., 1998; Stewart et al., 1995; Erskine et al., 1995). Although the mechanisms underlying this branching phenomenon remain to be determined, voltage-dependent calcium channels are likely responsible for activity-dependent growth. Reduction of calcium activity has been found to block the effect of electrical current on branching (Erskine et al., 1995; Stewart et al., 1995; Graf and Cooke, 1994). Normal development of endbulbs with an intact peripheral auditory system might serve to maintain a certain minimum level of electrical activity in auditory nerve fibers, which, through a calcium-mediated process, could promote terminal branching. With deafness, however, the reduction in auditory nerve activity and presumably calcium influx might diminish terminal branching in endbulbs. Although this idea is quite speculative, the proposed mechanism is consistent with the observations in endbulb morphology associated with deafness.

Deafness and the Development of Hearing

The mouse is a useful model for study because of its homogenous genetic background, its potential for gene manipulation with transgenic techniques, and its relative immaturity at birth. The central auditory system is not functional at birth and its maturation may be dependent on that of peripheral structures. The onset of hearing in the mouse occurs around postnatal day 11, but thresholds at this age are roughly 70 dB above those of adults (Mikaelian and Ruben, 1965; Ehret, 1976a). Preyer's reflex, the acoustic startle response, is present by 9 to 14 days of age, approximately around the time that sound-evoked cochlear potentials first appear (Alford and Ruben, 1963). The organ of Corti exhibits a nearly mature appearance by the end of the second week, but continues to undergo morphologic changes until the end of the second month (Kraus and Aulbach-Kraus, 1981). Mesenchyme clears from the middle-ear space by postnatal days 14 to 16 (Mikaelian and Ruben, 1965), but the ear canal itself is not patent along its entire length until the end of the third week (unpublished observations). These findings reveal an orchestrated pattern of structural and functional development. Hearing is not only contingent on the central and peripheral maturation of auditory structures, but also on our technical and analytic abilities to detect and identify critical events.

An important distinction should be made between onset of hearing and functional hearing. By 4 weeks of age, the mice exhibited stable ABR thresholds and waveforms, despite the continued maturation of the endbulbs of Held. It is this period between hearing readiness (around the second week) and cochlea and cochlear nucleus maturation (around the eighth week; Kraus and Aulbach-Kraus, 1981) that is crucial to the interplay between sensory input and proper development. Given that normal mice have extremely high auditory thresholds until the second postnatal week, hearing does not appear to influence early brain development. Nevertheless, the demonstration that deafness produces highly abnormal endbulbs of Held emphasizes the role of sound on development. Environmental sounds presumably enable the expression of a predetermined genetic program of development at those crucial ages.

Homozygous mutants ($Myo15^{sh2/sh2}$) and heterozygous littermates ($Myo15^{+/sh2}$) were smaller in size and body weight than CBA/J mice. These mice also had smaller spherical bushy cells. There was, however, no difference in body weight or spherical bushy cell size between these two groups of littermates. In contrast, there was a significant difference in endbulb morphology between the $Myo15^{sh2/sh2}$ and $Myo15^{+/sh2}$ mice. In the deaf $Myo15^{sh2/sh2}$ mouse, mature endbulbs exhibited relative structural simplicity, as evidenced by a smaller fractal index. There was no difference in endbulb complexity between $Myo15^{+/sh2}$ and CBA/J mice, both of which have normal hearing. These findings on endbulbs in the deaf mouse are consistent with observations in the congenitally deaf white cat (Ryugo et al., 1997; 1998) and demonstrate the effects of auditory deprivation on synaptic structure.

Endbulbs of deaf $Myo15^{sh2/sh2}$ mice have a similar appearance to those of congenitally deaf white cats (Ryugo et al., 1997; 1998). In deaf white cats, there is a reduction of endbulb branching complexity and a corresponding hypertrophy of postsynaptic densities (Ryugo et al., 1997). Due to the unknown genetic background of the deaf white cat, it was not known whether endbulb changes were due to the consequences of deafness or whether they were part of the constellation of abnormalities seen in the genetic syndrome. The genetic differences between deaf white cats and $Myo15^{sh2/sh2}$ mice in contrast to the similarities in endbulb structure, however, imply that the manifestations in endbulb abnormalities are attributable to deafness. This interpretation, while still tentative, is also the most parsimonious. Collectively, the data suggest that the endbulb synapse is responsive to both normal variations in activity (Ryugo et al., 1996) and to the pathologic absence of sound. Furthermore, the structure of these abnormal endbulbs does not resemble a state of arrested development. That is, endbulbs of normal-hearing mice and cats do not seem to pass through a stage where they resemble those of congenitally deaf animals.

The most common cause of sensorineural deafness in humans is hair cell loss within the cochlea (Kveton and Pensak, 1995). The disparate results achieved by the surgical restoration of hearing disorders, however, suggest that providing acoustic information to the brain via cochlear implantation is not by itself always sufficient to restore functionally useful hearing (Waltzman et al., 1995; Tyler and Summerfield, 1996). The endbulbs of Held, necessary for the temporal processing of sound, may be especially relevant to the acquisition of language because speech comprehension relies on accurate temporal coding of acoustic streams. Our data reveal that maturation of the endbulb and spherical bushy cell in the mouse proceeds rapidly during the first month of life and continues steadily through the second. It is plausible, then, that sound and early developmental events are responsible for the differential effects of hearing loss on young vs. old populations. The efficacy of treatments for deafness might be improved with a better understanding of the exact nature of the changes that occur at the earliest periods of auditory development. By comparing the changes seen in deafness with those seen in normal cases, we might also derive insight into the significance of particular time periods for proper development of synaptic structure.

ACKNOWLEDGMENTS

Support was provided by NIH/NIDCD research grant DC00232, NIH/NIDCD training grant DC00027, and a resident research grant from the American Academy of Otolaryngology-Head and Neck Surgery.

Section III

The Central Auditory System

The mouse has not been one of the traditional favorites of neurophysiologists and neuroanatomists who have studied the central auditory system. A proliferation of single-unit recording studies of the central auditory system in the 1960s tended to focus on cats and other species, with little attention paid to mice. Similarly, studies of connectivity, cytoarchitecture, neurochemistry, and other aspects of central auditory system anatomy made little use of mice prior to the 1980s. This is understandable because the majority of earlier neurophysiological and anatomical studies were primarily interested in how the normal auditory system worked. This required "typical" young adult animals with hearing somewhat similar to that of humans. With their high-frequency hearing range, small size, and sparse history in neurophysiology, mice did not fit this conceptual mold the way cats, primates, chinchillas, and other species did. However, as the body of knowledge and understanding of "normal" central auditory systems grew, questions could be asked about variations and abnormalities in auditory systems. It is here that interest in the mouse central auditory system began to grow, due to the availability of inbred strains and mutants with hearing loss or other interesting phenotypes and the attractiveness of mice as subjects for gerontological studies.

As is always the case, practical and economical forces also elevated the value of mice as research subjects. Because complete serial sections of the mouse auditory brainstem can be mounted on a manageable number of microscope slides, techniques such as immuno-labeling of neurons could be performed extraordinarily quickly and cheaply, as could morphometric analyses. Moreover, mice proved to be outstanding for *in vitro* slice preparations to unravel the physiological and histological details of the cochlear nucleus.

The chapters in this section provide ample evidence that the auditory research community has been exploiting these advantages. Chapter 18, by Frisina and Walton, building on the earlier review by Willard and Ryugo (1983), reveals that the current state-of-the-art of mouse central auditory anatomy is quite impressive. The anatomical literature becomes even more noteworthy with the addition of a new cytoarchitectionic map of the CN developed by Trettel and Morest, presented in Chapter 19. The cochlear nucleus is, indeed, the primary focus of this section, with the elegant work on *in vitro* slices reviewed by Ferragamo and Oertel in Chapter 20, followed by additional details on inhibitory neurotransmitters (Chapter 21; Caspary) and calcium binding proteins (Chapter 22, Idrizbegovic, Bogdanovic, and Canlon). We are, however, reminded by Carlson in Chapter 23 that neurons outside of the primary auditory system also respond to sounds to accomplish certain functions. Finally, the unique advantages of mice in presbycusis research is made quite evident by Frisina, Walton, Ison, and O'Neill in Chapters 24 and 25.

17 Focus: Diversity of the Mouse Central Auditory System

James F. Willott

INTRODUCTION

A number of *in vivo* single- and multiple-unit neurophysiological studies of auditory processing in the mouse central auditory system have examined the cochlear nucleus (CN) (e.g., Ehret and Moffat, 1984; Willott, Parham, and Hunter, 1991); inferior colliculus (IC) (e.g., Ehret and Moffat, 1985a; b; Ehret and Romand, 1992; Romand and Ehret, 1990; 1992; Walton et al., 1997; Willott, 1981; 1984; 1986; Willott and Demuth, 1986; Willott et al., 1988b; c); and auditory cortex (Stiebler and Ehret, 1985; Stiebler, Neulist, Fichtel, and Ehret, 1997; Willott, Aitkin, and McFadden, 1993). In general, response properties of central neurons in mice are similar to those of other mammals. However, the considerable differences among strains of laboratory mice with respect to peripheral sensitivity and myriad other traits, coupled with the capacity of the central auditory system to exhibit plasticity, make it problematic to talk about response properties in neurons of "the" mouse, as is typically done for other species.

For example, in normal-hearing mice, the general tonotopic organization of the CN and IC follows the basic mammalian scheme in normal-hearing mice: a dorsoventral progression of high- to low frequencies in CN subdivisions and low-to-high frequencies in the IC, an orderly representation in cortex. However, the commonly used inbred strain, DBA/2J exhibits high-frequency hearing loss at an early age (Chapters 14, 28, and 29), and its tonotopic organization is far from typical. As shown in Figure 17.1, tonotopic organization in the CN progresses dorsoventrally from high to low frequencies, as expected in young C57BL/6J mice (which hear well at this age). By contrast, in DBA mice with high-frequency hearing loss, tonotopic variation is virtually nonexistent. Given that a number of the most commonly used inbred strains exhibit high-frequency hearing loss at some stage of life (Chapters 24, 27–29), it is wise to avoid referring to tonotopic organization or frequency representation typical of "the mouse."

This, of course, is not a weakness but a strength of using mice in research on the central auditory system. Individuals of our own and other species differ from one another with respect to genotype and hearing ability. It seems likely that their central auditory systems likewise vary, as is the case for inbred strains of mice. Thus, mice may provide an avenue for investigating the interesting *differences* among individuals that are much more germane than some abstract "standard" for a species.

The differences in the central auditory systems of inbred mice also spawn valuable animal models. Staying with the example of DBA/2J mice, they have excellent frequency difference limens at 12 and 16 kHz (Kulig and Willott, 1984). This suggests that normal tonotopic organization is not necessary for good frequency discrimination. Mice such as this provide unique ways to correlate neural and behavioral phenotypes.

Whereas high-frequency hearing loss and abnormal tonotopic organization are present in DBA/2J mice at or around the onset of hearing, a different scenario is seen in C57BL/6J mice, as discussed in detail in Chapter 24. They start out with normal hearing and tonotopic organization (Figure 17.1), but exhibit progressive hearing loss, with profound deafness by 15 to 18 months of

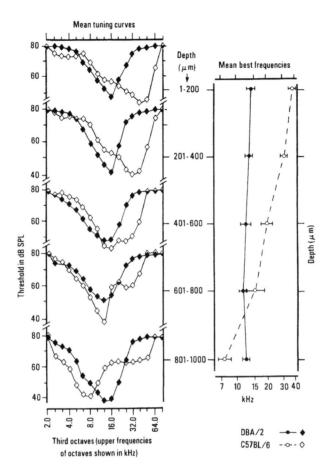

FIGURE 17.1   Tonotopic organization in the ventral CN divisions of 1-month-old C57BL/6J and DBA/2J mice. (From Willott, J.F., Demuth, R.M., Lu, S.M., Van Bergem, P., 1982. *Neurosci. Lett.,* 34, 13–17. With permission.

age. Situations such as this also allow interesting questions to be posed with respect to the central correlates of hearing loss. For example, as the functional representation of sounds changes and is ultimately lost, what happens to various metabolic properties of the IC? Micrographs presented in Figures 17.2 and 17.3 provide interesting insight into this question. The tissue sections, from C57BL/6J mice, were stained for cytochrome oxidase, an enzyme involved in oxidative metabolism. The central nucleus of the IC stains intensely, and this persists in the 25-month-old mouse, despite its chronic deafness. It appears that the pattern of activity in the 25-month-old C57 mouse is generally similar to that of the 1.5-month-old (as was that for a 6-month-old, not shown). By this indicator, metabolic activity seems to continue unabated in the IC, irrespective of the ability to hear. A similar conclusion was arrived at from a study using radioactive 2-deoxy-D-glucose as a measure of metabolic activity (Willott, Hunter, and Coleman, 1988a).

These examples show how mice can be used to move from questions about the "typical" or "normal" central auditory system to questions about genetic and phenotypic variance, plasticity, abnormality, and deafness.

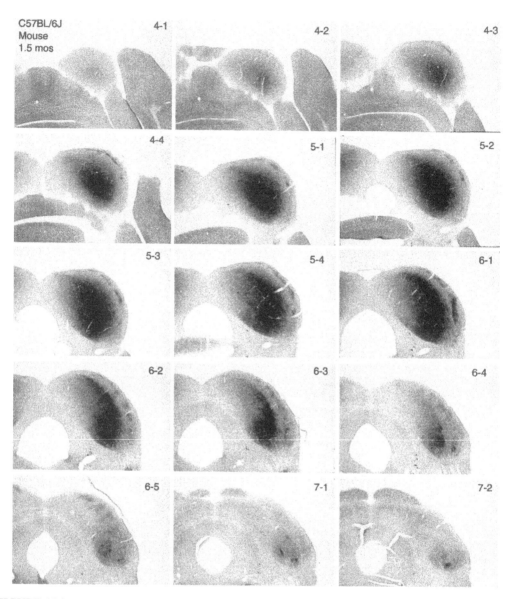

FIGURE 17.2 Frontal sections of the IC of a 1.5-month-old C57BL/6J mouse stained with cytochrome oxidase. The central nucleus is clearly labeled by intense staining. Sections progress from the caudal pole of the IC (4.1) through the rostral pole (7-2). (Courtesy of Dr. Nell Cant who prepared the sections. Lori Bross provided additional technical assistance.)

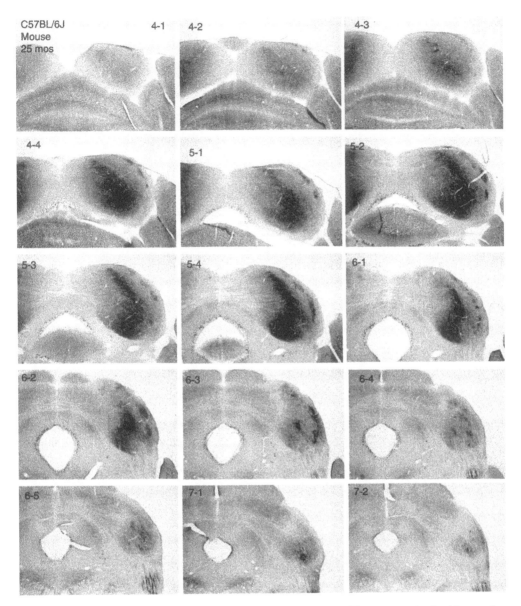

FIGURE 17.3 Frontal sections of the IC of a 25-month-old C57BL/6J mouse stained with cytochrome oxidase. Despite the fact that the mouse was chronically and profoundly deaf, intense staining is still observed. (Courtesy of Dr. Nell Cant who prepared the sections. Lori Bross provided additional technical assistance.)

18 Neuroanatomy of the Central Auditory System

Robert D. Frisina and Joseph P. Walton

INTRODUCTION

One advantage of using mammals such as the mouse to study the neural bases of human hearing and deafness is that the phylogenetic similarities of the central auditory systems of mammals far outweigh their evolutionary differences. For this reason, rodents, relative to other mammalian orders, have provided the most information about the functional anatomy of the auditory portions of the brain relevant to the human condition. Of all mammals, cats, mice, and rats are the most popular species for neuroscientific investigations of neural mechanisms for the coding of biologically relevant acoustic signals containing speech-like characteristics. In fact, more species of rodents have been utilized for investigations of the central auditory system than any other mammalian order. Mice, gerbils, rats, guinea pigs, and chinchillas are some of the most popular rodents to have been used thus far. It is for reasons like these that handbooks and this chapter in particular are quite useful to those interested in the general workings of the mammalian auditory system.

This chapter follows a systems analysis path for exploring the anatomy of the mouse central auditory system, as diagrammed in Figure 18.1. So we begin in the most peripheral portion of the system, at the level of the cochlear nucleus, and proceed in an ascending manner through the superior olivary complex (SOC), the lateral lemniscus (LL), the inferior colliculus (IC), the medial geniculate body (MGB), and conclude in the auditory cortex. Portions of the descending auditory system that have significant influence on the ascending system will be described where the two systems interact significantly, with possible functional implications pointed out. A general organizational scheme will be given for each level of the system, with important mouse studies highlighted. We will also point out differences in the structure, connections or cell types regarding the mouse and other mammals, or different strains of mice, and discuss clear phylogenetic trends. In some cases, the outputs of a region may be presented in a section on the inputs to another region. For example, many of the connections between the IC and other brainstem nuclei, including the cochlear nucleus, will be examined in the IC connections segment of this chapter.

MEDULLA/PONS: COCHLEAR NUCLEUS

BASIC ORGANIZATION AND CYTOARCHITECTONICS

Information about sound is conducted from the cochlea, the auditory portion of the inner ear, to the brain via the auditory division of the eighth cranial nerve. The axons of all auditory nerve fibers terminate in the cochlear nucleus. The mammalian cochlear nucleus (CN), including mice, has three major divisions: anteroventral (AVCN), posteroventral (PVCN), and dorsal (DCN) (rat: Harrison and Irving, 1965; 1966; cat: Osen, 1969; Brawer et al., 1974; mouse: Willott et al., 1994a). Each division is topographically organized with regard to incoming auditory nerve fibers. In general, apical regions of the cochlea are connected to ventral portions of each division, auditory nerve fibers from the middle turns of the cochlea terminate in central regions, and nerve fibers originating

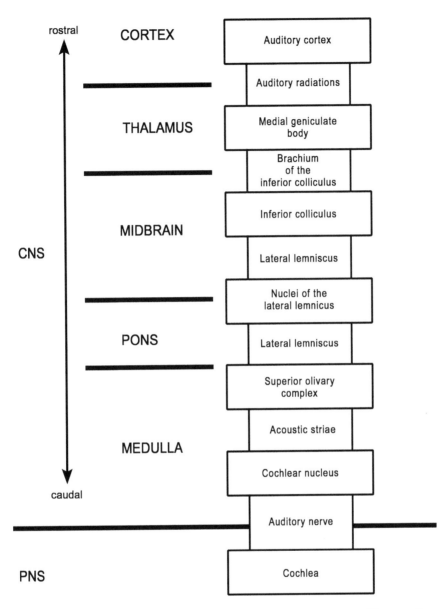

FIGURE 18.1   A simplified block diagram of the mouse central auditory system. The overall organization of the mouse central auditory system portrayed here is the same as exists in other mammals. Wide rectangles designate auditory nuclei, and thin rectangles indicate interconnecting fiber pathways. (From Willard, F.H. and Ryugo, D.K., *The Auditory Psychobiology of the Mouse,* 1983, p. 203. Courtesy of Charles C. Thomas, Publisher, Ltd., Springfield, Illinois.)

in the basal turn of the cochlea send information to dorsal portions of the cochlear nucleus divisions. This topographic or cochleotopic organization underlies the tonotopic organization of the cochlear nucleus: high-frequency information lies dorsally, middle-frequency coding takes place in interme-diate regions of each division, and low-frequency processing takes place in the ventral areas. This principle of cochleotopic or tonotopic organization is important because it manifests itself in significant ways at each level of the central auditory system.

A cytoarchitectonic atlas of the mouse cochlear nucleus is presented in Chapter 19, where the reader can find much information in addition to what is presented here. In the light microscope at low magnification, the boundaries of the three divisions are typically apparent. In Nissl-stained sections (cell body stain), when viewed with a bright-field microscope, a thinning of the density of perikarya occurs in the middle (anterior-posterior axis) of the ventral cochlear nucleus (VCN). The posterior border of this region of less dense cell-bodies where auditory nerve fibers are entering the brainstem (sometimes referred to as the interstitial nucleus) marks the boundary between the AVCN and PVCN. Broadly speaking, the VCN is separated from the DCN by a cap of small cells, or portions of a granule cell layer, particularly in the anterior areas. Some overall differences have been reported for the AVCN in different strains of mice. Specifically, Willott et al. (1987) found that in young adult mice, C57s have a greater volume and number of neurons than CBA/J mice.

In terms of cytoarchitectonics, the DCN has a laminar appearance when viewed at low magnification, whereas the VCN lacks a stratified appearance. The DCN laminar structure in many ways resembles that of the nearby cerebellar cortex (Mugnaini et al., 1980a; b). In the DCN, the dorsal-most zone is called the molecular layer, superficial layer, or Layer I (Chapter 19; and Willard and Ryugo, 1983). Moving in a ventral direction, the next layer is referred to as the fusiform cell layer, intermediate layer, the granule cell layer, or Layer II. The most ventral regions of the DCN are generally called the deep layers, of which there are two in the mouse. Layer III is also called the polymorphic layer. Layer IV, sometimes called the strial layer, primarily contains efferent fibers making up the dorsal acoustic stria. As generally occurs with immunocytochemical labeling techniques for specific neural proteins, the DCN laminae can become more prominent when mouse sections are treated with antibodies for molecules such as calcium-binding proteins, including calbindin and calretinin. For example, calbindin labeling is quite prominent in and around the fusiform cell layer (Frisina et al., 1995).

ANTEROVENTRAL DIVISION: CELL TYPES

In general, cell types of the central auditory system are classified either with Nissl staining, which preferentially labels RNA in the cell bodies, or with Golgi stains, which randomly impregnate the cell body and dendrites of certain cells. Representative cochlear nucleus cell types, and their relations to the major subdivisions of the mouse cochlear nucleus, are given in Figure 18.2 (see also Chapter 19). In the Nissl stain nomenclature, three major neuronal types are found in the AVCN. Spherical cells have relatively smooth, round cell bodies, and are associated with the incoming end bulbs of Held from auditory nerve fibers. Globular cells are like spherical cells, except that they have a more oblong cell body, have a few more smaller end bulbs of Held, and are found primarily in the posterior AVCN where the auditory nerve fibers first penetrate the cochlear nucleus. Multipolar neurons have a more irregular perikaryon, due to the presence of a significant number of major, primary dendrites emanating from the cell body, and are associated with many punctate inputs from auditory nerve fibers.

In the Golgi classification scheme, the two major cell types include the bushy cells, with one or two primary dendrites that branch and ramify from the cell body to resemble a bush. In contrast, stellate cells display more typical primary dendrites that protrude in a star-shaped pattern from the perikaryon, and are rarely found in the anterior AVCN. There is a rough correspondence between the spherical/globular neurons and bushy cells, and the multipolar cells and stellate neurons, respectively.

ANTEROVENTRAL DIVISION: CONNECTIONS

The inputs to spherical or globular bushy cells, via end bulbs of Held, functionally induce a secure synaptic connection (see also Chapter 16). Therefore, it is usually the case that an incoming spike dominates the post-synaptic cell so that a one-to-one relationship holds for incoming and outgoing action potentials. Spherical or globular bushy neurons also receive many small synaptic inputs, which can modify this "relay cell" under certain conditions that are not known with certainty. In contrast, multipolar/stellate cells, which receive distributed, small synaptic inputs from many auditory nerve fibers, carry on a more considerable amount of distributed neural processing.

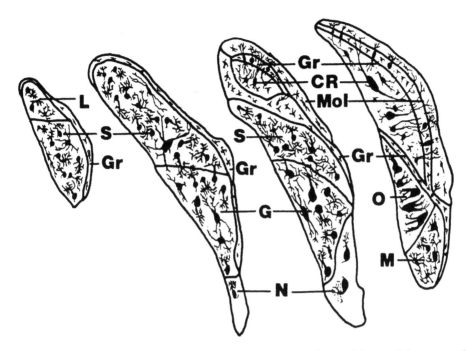

FIGURE 18.2   Camera lucida drawings of CBA/J mouse cochlear nucleus serial coronal (transverse, frontal) sections stained with luxol fast blue-cresyl violet Nissl stain. Cytoarchitectonic boundaries between the cochlear nucleus divisions were determined with the luxol fast blue-cresyl violet staining, and the morphology of the representative cells in each area was derived from Golgi preparations. The left-most section is most anterior, and the right-most is the most posterior. CR — central region or deep layers of the DCN; G — globular cell area of the posterior AVCN; GR — granule cell layer of the VCN and DCN; L — large spherical cell area of the anterior AVCN; M — multipolar cell area of PVCN; N — interstitial nucleus of the posterior AVCN where the auditory nerve enters the cochlear nucleus; O — octopus cell area of posterodorsal PVCN; S — small spherical cell area of the AVCN. (From Webster and Trune (1982, Fig. 3b, p. 108). With permission.)

The trapezoid body is the major output fiber tract of the VCN. It has been generally found that spherical/bushy cells of the anterior AVCN, which carry primarily low-frequency acoustic information, project bilaterally to the medial superior olivary nucleus (MSO). This excitatory neural pathway is somewhat small in the mouse, a species that does not have good low-frequency hearing. For example, Webster and Trune (1982) report on the relatively small size of the large spherical cell region in the CBA/J mouse strain. The large spherical cell region of the anterior AVCN lies ventrally and receives inputs from the cochlear apex — low-frequency coding.

Spherical/bushy neurons also project ipsilaterally to the lateral superior olive (LSO) in an excitatory fashion. Globular/bushy cells of the posterior AVCN send a prominent projection to the contralateral medial nucleus of the trapezoid body (MNTB), which in turn provides inhibitory inputs to the LSO on the same side of the brainstem. The specificity of multipolar/stellate afferent pathways is less well-known, but typically they project to certain regions of the SOC, LL, and IC. For example, Willott et al. (1985) for C57 mice, and Frisina et al. (1998) for CBA mice, have demonstrated direct connections from the AVCN to the contralateral central nucleus of the IC that involve stellate cells.

POSTEROVENTRAL DIVISION: NEURON TYPES

The predominant cell of the PVCN is the multipolar/stellate cell, which may have certain morphological subtypes based upon proximity of auditory nerve inputs to the cell body. In addition, in the

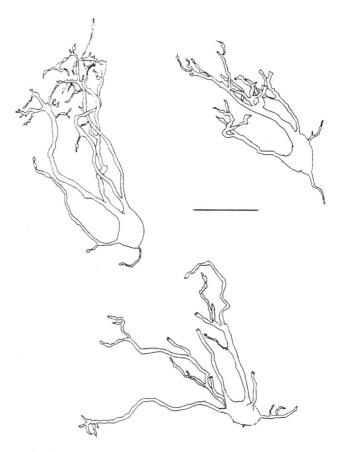

FIGURE 18.3 Camera lucida reconstructions of three different octopus neurons from 2-month-old C57 mice. Scale bar = 50 micron. Upper right: frontal plane, dorsal third of octopus cell area (OCA); upper left: frontal plane, middle of OCA; lower: horizontal plane (anterior is to the left), middle OCA. (From Willott and Bross (1990, Fig. 12, p. 73). With permission.)

most posterior/dorsal area of the PVCN, a homogenous pocket of octopus cells exists (mouse: Webster and Trune, 1982). Octopus cells are so named because they have large cell bodies that send out a group of thick, long, tentacle-like dendrites from one pole of their perikaryon. Willott and Bross (1990) present basic morphology of octopus cells as displayed here in Figure 18.3. It is noteworthy that, unlike other cochlear nucleus cell types, the long, prominent octopus cell dendrites project *across* isofrequency laminae, imparting to the octopus cells a broad frequency response, rather than a narrow one like most cochlear nucleus units.

POSTEROVENTRAL DIVISION: CONNECTIVITY

Berglund and Brown (1994) utilized the mouse (CD-1) to elegantly investigate the central trajectories of type II spiral ganglion cells. These auditory nerve fibers receive their inputs from outer hair cells, in contrast to type I auditory nerve fibers that are more numerous and synapse with inner hair cells. Utilizing extracellular horseradish peroxidase (HRP) injections in the spiral ganglion, they demonstrated that type II fibers displayed predominantly *en passant* synaptic swellings in the cochlear nucleus (mean = 95) and only a few *boutons terminaux* (mean = 6), with fibers from the cochlear base having more swellings than those from the apex. Type II fibers traveled with type I fibers in a cochleotopic manner, and formed ascending and descending branches in the VCN;

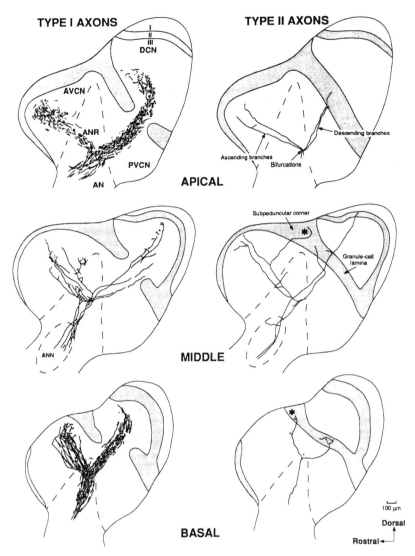

FIGURE 18.4 Camera lucida reconstructions (parasagittal plane) of the cochlear nucleus of three individual mice. HRP injections were made in the apical (top), middle (center), and basal (bottom) cochlear turns. Left: type I spiral ganglion cell central projections that were large enough to be drawn at low magnification. Right: individually reconstructions of type II fibers and terminals originally drawn at high magnification and then reduced for illustration. Shading indicates mouse granule cell regions. These regions differ on the left and right because type I fibers pass medial to the granule cell lamina on their way to the DCN, whereas type II processes travel directly into the lamina without proceeding to the DCN. Stars indicate terminations of ascending branches. I, II, III are DCN layers; AVCN — anteroventral cochlear nucleus; AN — auditory nerve; ANR — auditory nerve root; DCN — dorsal cochlear nucleus; PVCN — posteroventral cochlear nucleus. (From Berglund and Brown (1994, Fig. 1, p. 123). With permission.)

however, they differed from type I fibers in that type II axons, particularly those from the base, sent many more branches into the granule cell regions (poorly innervated by type I fibers), especially those separating the VCN and DCN. These differing projection patterns are displayed in Figure 18.4.

Berglund et al. (1996) pursued this line of investigation and examined type II fiber synapses in the cochlear nucleus at the ultrastructural, electron micrsocopic (EM) level. Focusing on swellings in the PVCN and AVCN near the granule cell regions, and in the auditory nerve root region, they observed that the synapses were asymmetric, containing clear round vesicles, indicating that type II inputs are excitatory. Relative to type I fibers, there were fewer and smaller presynaptic vesicles. These had a greater proportion of membrane apposition with postsynaptic density, and had more discontinuous or perforated densities. In all cochlear nucleus regions examined, the postsynaptic targets of type II synapses were dendrites, the majority of which were granule cells.

DORSAL DIVISION: CELL CLASSIFICATION

The molecular layer of the DCN is relatively devoid of cell bodies, except for its ventral areas that contain some cartwheel and stellate cells, small neurons, and granule cells (see also Chapter 19). In the next layer down, the fusiform or granule cell layer, fusiform (pyramidal) cells are the major cell type. These have large, elongated cell bodies tending to have their long axes oriented in a dorsal/ventral direction. Large tufts of primary dendrites extend from each end of the fusiform cell body, one bunch heading dorsally and the other coursing ventrally, as shown in Figure 18.5. Small, round granule cells also populate the fusiform cell layer of the DCN profusely. In the more apical portion of this layer, other prominent cell types can be found, such as the cartwheel cells. Another prominent cell type in the mouse fusiform-cell layer is sometimes referred to as the Purkinje-like neuron due to its similarity to cerebellar Purkinje cells, and differs from fusiform cells in having smaller perikarya, rounder cell bodies, no basal dendrites, a sagittal dendritic orientation, more elaborate dendritic arborizations, and abundant dendritic spines (Webster and Trune, 1982; Willott et al., 1992). In the deeper layers of the DCN, different varieties of stellate neurons abound, such as giant cells (examples given in Figure 18.6). In the CBA/J mouse, vertical, elongate, and radial types of stellates can be found (Webster and Trune, 1982).

DORSAL DIVISION: CONNECTIONS

Many cells of the DCN receive some form of excitatory input from auditory nerve fibers. For example, the basal dendrites of fusiform cells receive many punctate inputs from the auditory nerve, and preserve tonotopicity. The local interconnections of the DCN, however, are much more complicated than the VCN and have not yet been elucidated in a comprehensive way in the mouse. It is known that granule cells provide excitatory inputs to the apical dendrites of fusiform cells and molecular layer stellate cells, via their axons that comprise the parallel fiber network of the DCN molecular layer (Mugnaini et al., 1980a; b).

Fusiform and giant cells are the main output neurons of the DCN (Golgi type I cells). They both send a significant contralateral projection, via the dorsal acoustic stria, to the central nucleus of the IC in a tonotopic fashion, and also to the external nucleus (Willard and Ryugo, 1983; Ryugo and Willard, 1985), as illustrated in Figure 18.7. Available evidence suggests that these crossed inputs to the IC are excitatory in nature.

COCHLEAR NUCLEUS: DEVELOPMENT

Mice have been used effectively to track the ontogenetic development of the cochlear nucleus (see Chapter 16). For example, Ivanova and Yuasa (1998), examined neuronal migration in the mouse (ICR strain) DCN utilizing immunohistochemical bromodeoxyuridine labeling. They found that granule cells were generated later in development, and traveled a different migratory pathway than large multipolar neurons. It was only later in development (at the time of perinatal maturation) that they become mixed again to form the fusiform-granule cell layer (Layer II) of the DCN. The homology of this sequence of developmental events is quite similar to that of the Purkinje and granule neurons of the cerebellar cortex, supporting analogies in structure and function of these areas.

Developmental studies involving the cochlear nucleus often take the form of measuring the effects of cochlear ablation (or some other form of cochlear deafening) on the structure and function of the central auditory system. Generally, it has been found that disruption of the peripheral inputs

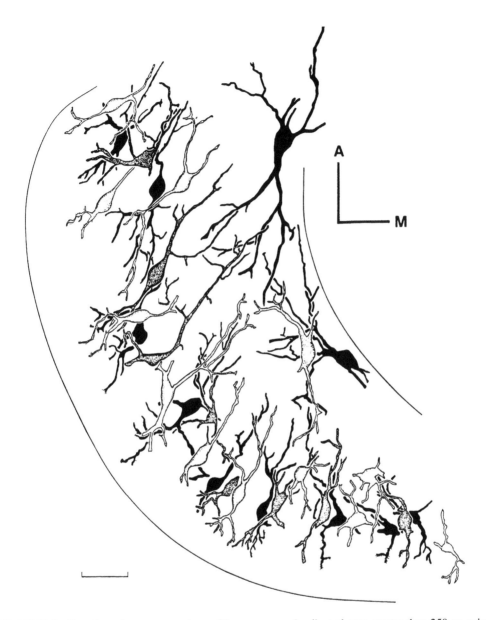

FIGURE 18.5 Drawing tube representations of large neurons (perikaryal area greater than 250 sq. micron) found in a single 100-micron-thick horizontal section of the mouse DCN. Notice that pyramidal cells, when viewed edgewise, have compressed dendritic fields. The dendritic fields of the giant cells, lying deep in the DCN along the medial border, contact a larger proportion of the DCN, and a significant number of their distal dendrites are aligned with pyramidal cell basal dendrites. Golgi-Kopsch, 60-day-old mouse. Scale bar = 50 micron. (From Ryugo and Willard (1985, Fig. 13, p. 393). With permission.)

to the cochlear nucleus during development will cause declines in the number of auditory nerve synaptic contacts on cochlear nucleus cells, and cochlear nucleus neuron size reductions. This vast field cannot be reviewed here in a comprehensive manner, but a representative mouse study will be presented (see also Chapter 16). Trune and Morgan (1988) examined the neuronal ultrastructure in the CBA/J AVCN following unilateral sound deprivation. The deprivation was achieved by removal of the blastemas of the right external auditory meatus on postnatal day 3. This prevented normal meatal opening on day 8, resulting in complete meatal occlusion throughout hearing

ICM-77

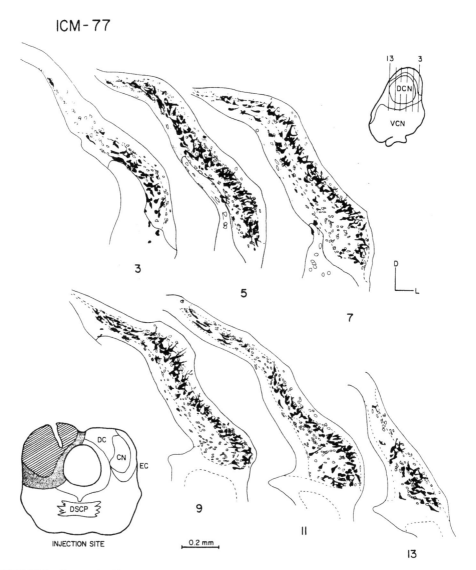

FIGURE 18.6 Camera lucida reconstructions showing all labeled and unlabeled neurons in alternate sections of the contralateral DCN after a large HRP injection into the IC (bottom inset indicates the injection site; top inset shows the planes of the sections). Notice that the labeled cells tend to be the largest neurons in the DCN, and are concentrated in Layer II. CN — central nucleus of IC; DC — dorsal cortex of IC; DSCP — decussation of superior cerebellar peduncle; EC — external cortex of IC. (From Ryugo and Willard (1985, Fig. 8, p. 389). With permission.)

development (days 8–45). These experimental mice and controls were sacrificed on day 45, and the AVCN was examined using electron microscopy. Analyses yielded quantitative reductions in auditory nerve synaptic contacts, AVCN cell body cytoplasmic volume, and declines in mitochondrial activity and wellness pre- and post-synaptically.

COCHLEAR NUCLEUS: COMPARATIVE DIFFERENCES

Although homologies abound between the mouse central auditory system and that of higher mammals such as the human, some important differences do exist (see also Chapter 19). As mentioned, the low-frequency neural networks between the cochlear nucleus and the SOC are

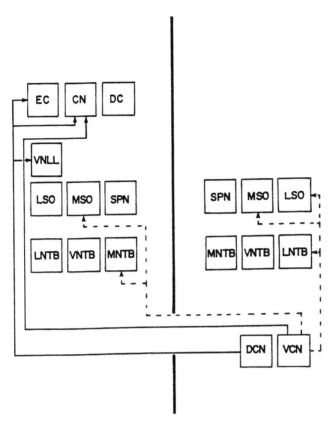

FIGURE 18.7   Schematic summary diagram of the outputs of the cochlear nucleus to other auditory brain-stem centers. Thick vertical line is the midline. Solid lines are pathways demonstrated in mouse. Dashed lines were originally demonstrated in rat, and later confirmed in mice. CN — central nucleus of IC; DC — dorsal cortex of IC; DCN — dorsal cochlear nucleus; EC — external cortex of IC; IC — inferior colliculus; LSO — lateral superior olive; LNTB — lateral nucleus of TB; MNTB — medial nucleus of TB; MSO — medial superior olive; SOC — superior olivary complex; SPN — superior paraolivary nucleus; TB — trapezoid body; VCN — ventral cochlear nucleus; VNLL — ventral nucleus of the lateral lemniscus; VNTB — ventral nucleus of TB. (From Willard, F.H. and Ryugo, D.K., *The Auditory Psychobiology of the Mouse,* 1983, p. 221. Courtesy of Charles C. Thomas, Publisher, Ltd., Springfield, Illinois.)

attenuated in the mouse because of its poor low-frequency hearing. In addition, there is a phylogenetic trend for the DCN to become less differentiated as one moves from rodents to primates to man (Moore and Osen, 1979). Specifically, the cytoarchitectonic laminae, and therefore the layout and circuitry of the cell types within these laminae, become significantly less organized in higher mammals (Moore, 1980; Frisina et al., 1982). It is hypothesized that this is due to the encephalization of DCN functionality to higher levels of the auditory system as one proceeds up the phylogenetic scale from rodents, through the felines and primates, and finally to *homo sapiens.*

Mugnaini and co-workers (1980a; b) have investigated the morphological analogies between the laminar structure of the DCN and that of the adjacent cerebellar cortex in mice and other mammals. In particular, they note the similarity of the structure and connections of granule cells. For example, in both the DCN and cerebellum, the axons of granule cells, whose perikarya are in the granule cell layer (Layer II), comprise the parallel fibers of the molecular layer (Layer I). These axons possess excitatory synaptic specializations that contact the apical dendrites of fusiform cells. Additional evidence for the homology between the DCN and cerebellar cortex neuronal circuitries come from investigators such as Dumesnil-Bousez and Sotelo (1993). They grafted embryonic cerebellar Purkinje cells onto the surface of the adult Lurcher mouse DCN. They found, using anti-calbindin antibodies, that Purkinje cells migrated into the molecular layer (Layer I) of the host DCN, and developed dendritic trees that were isoplanar. This dendritic development suggested synaptic interactions with DCN parallel fibers, similar to those occurring normally.

COCHLEAR NUCLEUS: FUNCTIONAL IMPLICATIONS

What are the functional implications of the morphological organization of the cochlear nucleus? Different cell types of the cochlear nucleus abstract different features of the incoming information from the auditory nerve at the expense of other acoustic features. In the next section, some neural mechanisms based on differing morphologies of cochlear nucleus neurons and their inputs are put forth as a neural basis of rudimentary acoustic feature abstraction. The reader is also referred to Chapter 20 for a more detailed discussion of this topic.

COCHLEAR NUCLEUS: ABSTRACTION OF ACOUSTIC INFORMATION

One aspect is that as one proceeds posteriorly from the AVCN through the PVCN and up to the DCN, the morphology of the cochlear nucleus principal cells (output neurons) becomes more complex. This is also true of the inputs that these neurons receive from the auditory nerve, as noted for the CBA/J mouse by Webster and Trune (1982). For example, spherical bushy cells, with their simple dendritic structure, are most prominent in the anterior AVCN. Physiologically, these neurons function as relay cells, and are referred to as "primary-like" because their responses strongly resemble those of the auditory nerve fibers providing their inputs (Pfeiffer, 1966b). As one moves caudally through the posterior AVCN, one encounters the globular bushy cells that receive several, smaller end bulbs as inputs. Physiologically, these neurons are associated with the "primary-like-with-notch" physiological response category, which exhibits a slightly different response than the typical auditory nerve fiber. The multipolar stellate cells are associated with physiological responses that significantly differ from auditory nerve fibers. For example, responses to pure tones are more transient than in the auditory nerve, and have been dubbed "chopper" or "onset," with subcategories within these broad unit types. Pure tone response patterns become even more complex in the DCN, with some units even showing true inhibition to pure tones. They have been given names such as "pauser," "buildup," and "inhibitory." Using more complex acoustic stimuli such as amplitude modulated sounds, physiologists have noted an increased ability to encode temporal acoustic features, as one proceeds from the AVCN through the PVCN and into the DCN. This hierarchy of enhancement for coding of sound envelope timing features beyond that of the auditory nerve is consistent with the increased morphological complexity and responses to simple sounds just described for the cochlear nucleus (Frisina et al., 1985; 1990a; b; 1994; 1996).

COCHLEAR NUCLEUS: ORIGIN OF PARALLEL PROCESSING PATHWAYS

To the extent that the various cell types of the cochlear nucleus project to different regions of the brainstem, parallel processing pathways are established at the level of the cochlear nucleus. For example, as will be described later in this chapter, low-frequency inputs from the AVCN travel along the trapezoid body pathway bilaterally to the MSO for processing of interaural time differences. The projections from the AVCN to the LSO (contralaterally via the MNTB) comprise a separate pathway more concerned with high-frequency sound localization. Outputs of the intermediate acoustic stria comprise another parallel processing tract, possibly involved in acoustic reflexes such as the auditory startle response. Fibers of the dorsal acoustic stria project directly to the contralateral IC and serve a different function.

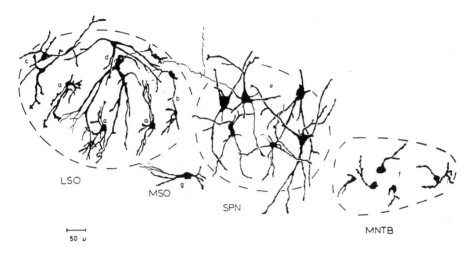

FIGURE 18.8 Golgi-Cox composite drawings from coronal (frontal) sections of the SOC, presenting the relative locations of cells from many different C57 mouse brains. (a) Principal neurons of LSO; (b) LSO spindle-shaped cells; (c) LSO marginal cells; (d) LSO marginal cells in the dorsal hilus region; (e) SPN principal cells; (f) MNTB principal cells; (g) a caudal MSO principal neuron. LSO — lateral superior olive; MNTB — medial nucleus of the trapezoid body; MSO — medial superior olive; SOC — superior olivary complex; SPN — superior paraolivary nucleus. (From Ollo and Schwartz (1979, Fig. 3, p. 355). With permission.)

PONS: SUPERIOR OLIVARY COMPLEX (SOC)

General Topography

The SOC is a multinuclear cluster at the level of the pons. Generally, the two most prominent nuclei are the medial and lateral superior olives, although the former in the mouse is relatively small. However, certain other regions are more prominent in the mouse than in higher mammals as mentioned below.

LATERAL SUPERIOR OLIVE

In most mammals, the lateral superior olive (LSO) takes on an S-shaped appearance. Examples of the primary LSO cell types of the mouse are given in Figure 18.8. Principal neurons have oblong perikarya that are aligned along the long axis of the S, with the major axis of their cell body orthogonal to the S axis (neurons labeled with "a"). These neurons are bitufted, with one branch of dendrites extending approximately in the medial direction and the other branch in the opposite direction. The laterally oriented dendrites receive inputs from spherical/bushy cells of the ipsilateral AVCN via their axons that comprise the trapezoid body. Evidence suggests that these inputs are primarily excitatory in nature. The medially oriented dendritic tufts receive inputs from the ipsi-lateral MNTB, and are inhibitory in nature. Principal cells of the MNTB receive inputs via large end bulbs of Held from globular/bushy cells of the contralateral posterior AVCN. Thus, LSO principal cells receive excitatory inputs from the ipsilateral ear and inhibitory inputs from the contralateral ear. LSO neurons in mice project bilaterally to IC (Willard and Ryugo, 1983).

MEDIAL SUPERIOR OLIVE

Principal cells of the medial superior olive (MSO) are in many ways similar to those of the LSO: they have elongated cell bodies with a tuft of dendrites on each end, an example of which is shown in Figure 18.8. The medial bunch of dendrites receives excitatory inputs from spherical/bushy cells of the contralateral AVCN. The lateral group of dendrites receives excitatory inputs from spherical/bushy

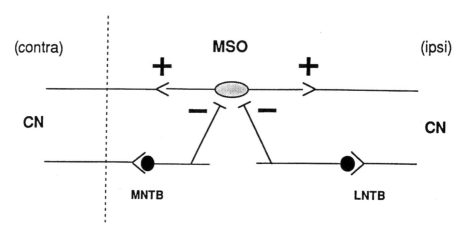

FIGURE 18.9 Schematic diagram summarizing the ascending inputs to principal cells of MSO. Direct excitatory inputs to the MSO arise bilaterally from CN, and inhibitory inputs come from the contralateral CN via principal cells of MNTB. In addition, inhibitory projections also came from the ipsilateral CN via elongate neurons of LNTB. CN — cochlear nucleus; LNTB — lateral NTB; MNTB — medial NTB; MSO — medial superior olive; NTB — nucleus of the trapezoid body. (From Kuwabara and Zook (1992, Fig. 9, p. 533). With permission.)

neurons of the ipsilateral AVCN. In both cases, these inputs tend to come from the anteroventral AVCN, an area specialized for processing low-frequency sound information, and are excitatory in nature. In rodents such as mice, these excitatory inputs are modulated by bilateral inhibitory inputs from the cochlear nucleus via the ipsilateral MNTB and lateral nucleus of the trapezoid body (LNTB) (Kuwabara and Zook, 1992), as diagrammed in Figure 18.9. In mice, the MSO projects ipsilaterally to the IC central nucleus and bilaterally to the IC dorsal cortex (Willard and Ryugo, 1983; Gonzalez-Hernandez et al., 1987; Frisina et al., 1998).

NUCLEI OF THE TRAPEZOID BODY

The fibers of the trapezoid body (TB) are axons originating primarily from the VCN on both sides. The TB lies medial and ventral to the MSO, and ventral and lateral to the LSO. There are several noticeable neuron groups clustered within the TB, including the MNTB, ventral nucleus of the TB (VNTB), and LNTB.

NUCLEI OF THE TRAPEZOID BODY: MEDIAL NUCLEUS

The MNTB serves an important neural processing role in the SOC. As in cat (Morest, 1968a; b), there are three main cell types in the mouse MNTB: principal, stellate, and elongate cells (Kuwabara and Zook, 1991). Principal cells, examples of which are given in Figure 18.8, have spherical or oval perikarya with an eccentrically placed nucleus and one or two thick primary dendrites that terminate in a spray of secondary branches. Spines are sparse on primary dendrites, but frequently seen on distal dendritic branches. Different subclasses of principal cells may subserve different functions. For example, one subclass had dendrites that spread beyond the borders of the MNTB. Axonal projections were utilized to distinguish additional subgroups. All principal cells projected to the ipsilateral LSO; however, one subclass had axonal collaterals that entered the LL, and another had recurrent collaterals. Stellate cells had a large, elongate soma, a radial dendritic pattern usually extending beyond the MNTB boundaries, a centrally placed nucleus, and abundant cytoplasm. Elongate neurons were sparse in number and characterized by the presence of five or six small-diameter long dendrites, small round or oval perikarya, and axons that branched within the MNTB. Examples of morphology and connections of MNTB cell types are given in Figure 18.10.

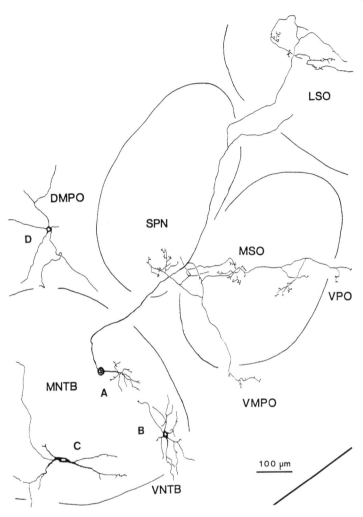

FIGURE 18.10 A composite reconstruction of the three MNTB main cell types. (A) A typical principal neuron with bushy dendrites and a single axon that projects to the ipsilateral LSO. Axon collaterals send branches to the MSO, SPN, VPO and VMPO. Other principal cells also send axon collateral to the VNTB (not shown). (B) An MNTB elongate cell with dendritic ramifications in a characteristic dorsoventral orientation and invading the VNTB. (C) An MNTB stellate neuron with dendrites extending beyond the MNTB borders. (D) A typical radiate cell in DMPO, sending an axon collateral into MNTB. DMPO — dorsomedial periolivary nucleus; LSO — lateral superior olive; MNTB — medial nucleus of the TB; MSO — medial superior olive; SPN — superior paraolivary nucleus; TB — trapezoid body; VMPO — ventromedial periolivary nucleus; VNTB — ventral nucleus of TB; VPO — ventral periolivary nucleus. (From Kuwabara and Zook (1991, Fig. 2, p. 710). With permission.)

Principal cells of the MNTB receive inputs from globular/bushy cells of the contralateral AVCN via very large terminal endings of the globular/bushy cell axons, the end bulbs of Held referred to earlier. Functionally, the MNTB principal cells serve primarily as relay cells. The excitatory transmitter release from the presynaptic end bulb of Held dominates the response of the MNTB post-synaptic cell body that is partially encapsulated by the end bulb. The MNTB, in turn, provides inhibitory inputs to the medial tuft of dendrites for the principal cells of the ipsilateral LSO and to somata of principal neurons in the MSO central cell column (rodents, including mouse, as shown in Figure 18.9, Kuwabara and Zook, 1992).

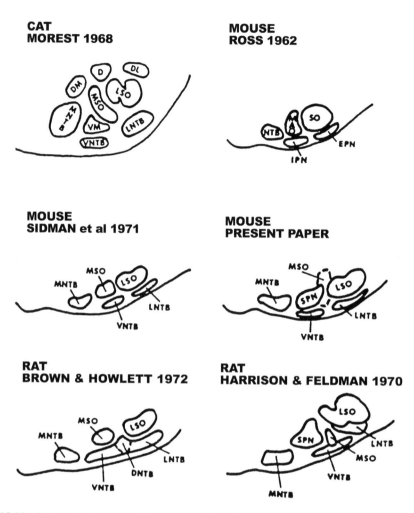

FIGURE 18.11 Schematic diagrams of transverse (frontal, coronal) sections through a middle level of the SOC in mouse, rat, and cat, showing locations of the main nuclei and periolivary cell groups. D — dorsal periolivary group; DL — dorsal lateral periolivary group; DM — dorsal medial periolivary group; DNTB — dorsal nucleus of TB; EPN — external paraolivary nucleus; IPN — internal paraolivary nucleus; LSO — lateral superior olive; MAO — medial accessory olive; MNTB or NTB — medial nucleus of TB; MSO — medial superior olive; SO — superior olive; SOC — superior olivary complex; SPN — superior paraolivary nucleus; VM — ventromedial periolivary nucleus; VNTB or VTB — ventral nucleus of TB; TB — trapezoid body. (From Ollo and Schwartz (1979, Fig. 1, p. 352). With permission.)

NUCLEI OF THE TRAPEZOID BODY: VENTRAL AND LATERAL NUCLEI

Four different smaller cell groups have been identified embedded in the fibers of TB ventral to the MNTB, MSO, and LSO: the VNTB and LNTB, and the ventral (VPO) and ventromedial (VMPO) periolivary nuclei. The VNTB is situated ventral to MNTB; the VMPO is situated ventromedial to MSO; the VPO is ventrolateral to MSO; and the LNTB is ventrolateral to LSO, as indicated in Figures 18.10 and 18.11. Little is known of the function and connections of these cell groups, although in mice they do receive some collateral inputs from MNTB principal cell axons (Kuwabara and Zook, 1991). LNTB principal neurons project bilaterally to IC, whereas VNTB cells send axons ipsilaterally to IC (Willard and Ryugo, 1983; Frisina et al., 1998). LNTB principal cells project to ipsilateral MSO and LSO principal cells in an inhibitory fashion, and these perisomatic bouton contacts have been demonstrated in rodents such as mice and gerbils (Kuwabara and Zook, 1992). This MSO projection is shown schematically in Figure 18.9.

SOC: Para- and Periolivary Nuclei

In most mammals, cell bodies comprising the olivocochlear auditory efferent system reside in regions of the SOC medial and dorsal to the MSO and LSO. This efferent system sends projections back to the cochlea and cochlear nucleus. In the mouse, the prominent components of this system are the superior paraolivary nucleus (SPN), a small dorsomedial periolivary nucleus (DMPO), and the dorsolateral periolivary nucleus (DLPO).

SOC: Superior Paraolivary Nucleus

The SPN is a prominent nucleus medial and dorsal to the MSO in the mouse. The major SPN cell type is the large multipolar cell (shown in Figure 18.8). Some of these cells send axons bilaterally to the outer hair cells of the cochlea and to neurons of the cochlear nucleus (Ollo and Schwartz, 1979; Willard and Ryugo, 1983). The SPN neurons that contribute to the auditory descending system are sometimes referred to as the medial olivocochlear system (MOC). Some SPN multipolar cells of the CBA mouse also send ascending projections to the ipsilateral IC (Frisina et al., 1998). For mice, this projection is topographic, in that lateral SPN neurons project to dorsolateral IC, and medial SPN cells send outputs to the ventromedial IC (Willard and Ryugo, 1983).

SOC: Dorsolateral Periolivary Nucleus

The DLPO is a small, scattered group of neurons, situated dorsally and dorsolaterally to the LSO. In the general mammalian plan, these neurons contribute axonal fibers that make the lateral efferent system that projects bilaterally to the outer hair cells of the cochlea and to neurons of the cochlear nucleus. The principal cells, which are elongate in shape, not only participate in the lateral efferent system, but some also send ascending projections to the ipsilateral IC in the mouse (Frisina et al., 1998).

SOC: Anterolateral Periolivary Nucleus

In contrast to the rest of the SOC, particularly the small MSO, the anterolateral periolivary nucleus (ALPO) is quite large in mice. In small mammals, this nucleus is situated rostral and lateral to the LSO, borders upon the ventromedial boundary of the ventral nucleus of the LL, and contains an abundance of multipolar cells (Frisina et al., 1989; Kelley et al., 1992). In young adult CBA mice, there is a strong afferent, topographic projection to the ipsilateral IC (Frisina et al., 1998).

SOC: Structure and Function

The SOC is the first level of the central auditory system where sounds from the two ears are compared in a systematic manner. In addition, it is thought that SPN and DLPO cell groups participate in the medial and lateral auditory efferent systems, respectively.

SOC: Sound Localization

In the LSO, high-frequency signals are processed such that contralateral sounds induce inhibition in LSO principal cells and ipsilateral cells produce excitation. In the LSO, this processing occurs for sound intensity differences at the two ears. Depending on the strength and timing of the binaural inputs, each LSO principal cell has a specific sound source location in space that yields a maximum firing rate response. Somewhat analogously, each MSO principal cell has a maximal firing rate for an optimal interaural time or phase difference associated with a particular location in space. LSO neurons could participate in the processing of interaural time differences, in the sense that they receive inputs that carry information on the temporal properties of high-frequency sounds. For example, if an amplitude-modulated sound were present, depending on its location in space, a particular LSO principal cell would fire maximally when the interaural stimulus envelope features display a particular time difference, as suggested in a study by Joris and Yin (1995). In any of these three cases, this sound-source information is projected out of the LSO and MSO to the IC where it is further processed.

SOC: Descending Pathways

The descending systems modulate cochlear transduction and cochlear nucleus processing. Physiological evidence suggests that these systems may be involved in reducing the deleterious effects of background noise, thus increasing the signal-to-noise ratio for biologically relevant signals and operating as a type of gain control mechanism. Psychoacoustic and otoacoustic emissions studies implicate the auditory efferents in masking-level difference phenomena and certain types of release from masking.

Mice have been utilized in investigations of the projection patterns of the efferent system. For example, Benson and Brown (1990) made injections of HRP into the spiral ganglion area basal turn of the CD-1 mouse cochlea to examine cochlear nucleus efferent inputs, as shown in Figure 18.12. They found that MOC neuron axonal branches often terminated in or near the VCN granule cell regions, as diagrammed in Figure 18.13. The MOC axons displayed both *en passant* and terminal boutons containing round vesicles and exhibiting asymmetric axodendritic synapses. This suggests that they are excitatory in nature. The morphological features of reconstructed MOC postsynaptic dendrites suggest that they belong to VCN multipolar/stellate cells. Based on these findings, Benson and Brown (1990) hypothesize that MOC excitatory inputs to VCN multipolar/stellate cells could help boost their responses to counterbalance reduced cochlear outputs due to MOC feedback in the presence of loud sounds, as diagrammed in Figure 18.14. Using similar tracing techniques involving cochlear injections, M.C. Brown (1993) subsequently demonstrated in mice that collaterals of both the MOC and lateral olivocochlear systems send inputs into various vestibular nuclei, thus providing a basis for auditory/vestibular system interaction mechanisms.

In a subsequent investigation, Benson et al. (1996) examined the targets of HRP-stained MOC collaterals into the CD-1 mouse cochlear nucleus in greater detail. Using serial reconstructions, they found that the dendritic targets of these collaterals were either "large" or "varicose" (Figure 18.15). This allowed them to examine other, non-HRP-labeled synapses onto these dendrites. On large dendrites, the predominant non-HRP synapses had small round vesicles, suggesting that they are excitatory. In contrast, varicose dendrites had many synaptic specializations with pleomorphic vesicles. This suggests inhibitory inputs, possibly arising from more rostral centers of the auditory system or brain. These results suggest a convergence, in and near cochlear nucleus granule cell regions, of type II auditory nerve fiber inputs from outer hair cells and descending inputs from MOC fibers — constituting part of the basis for a cochlea/cochlear nucleus/SOC feedback loop.

SOC: Monaural vs. Binaural Pathways

The MSO and LSO are exemplary with respect to how sounds from the two ears can be processed to yield information on sound localization. Descending projection neurons from the SPN and DLPO are also bilateral in nature, in that portions of the medial and lateral efferent systems are both crossed and uncrossed. Other portions of the SOC are unilateral or monaural in nature. ALPO, for example, has a major ipsilateral projection to the IC; and the SPN, VNTB, and DLPO have minor ones to the ipsilateral IC of mice (Frisina et al., 1998).

SOC: Comparisons with Other Species

The mouse has SOC nuclear complex features that are similar to other mammals except that the medial superior olive is relatively underdeveloped, like other small mammals relative to bigger

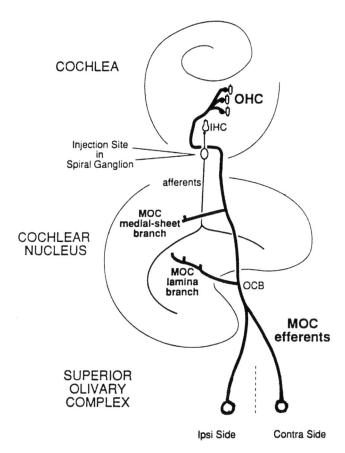

FIGURE 18.12 Diagrammatic cartoon of the results of an HRP injection made in the MOC and identified projections of MOC axons. MOC cell bodies of origin are displayed bilaterally in SPN of SOC. Branches to the cochlear nucleus primary areas of termination, and terminals to OHCs are shown. Note that in this experiment, the HRP reaction product generally faded before it reached the MOC cell bodies shown here. Consequently, axons were identified as efferent by their pathways. One type I afferent innervating an IHC is also shown. IHC — cochlear inner hair cell; MOC — medial olivocochlear system; OCB — olivocochlear bundle; OHC — cochlear outer hair cell; SOC — superior olivary complex; SPN — superior paraolivary nucleus. (From Benson and Brown (1990, Fig. 1, p. 53). With permission.)

mammals, as shown in Figures 18.8 and 18.11. This goes with the notion that mammals with larger heads can make use of greater interaural time differences than mammals with small heads such as mice. Thus, large mammals tend to have better low-frequency hearing. In addition, in mice, except for ALPO, the quantity of SOC ascending projections to certain regions of the IC may be attenuated relative to other brainstem regions, including the contralateral cochlear nucleus and the ipsilateral nucleus of the LL (Frisina et al., 1998).

PONS/MIDBRAIN: NUCLEI OF THE LATERAL LEMNISCUS (LL)

Overall Organization

For most mammals, there are three prominent nuclei making up the nuclei of LL (NLL): the dorsal NLL (DNLL), the intermediate NLL (INLL), and the ventral NLL (VNLL). The commissure of Probst is a fiber tract connecting the two DNLL with each other and with the contralateral inferior

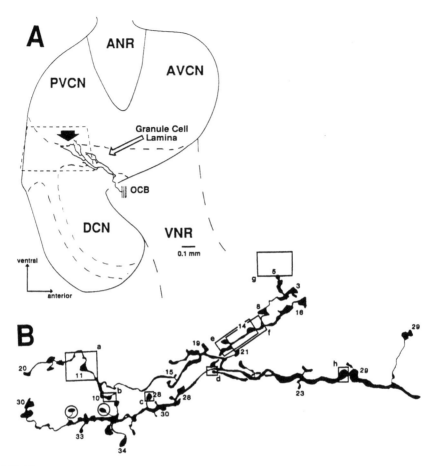

FIGURE 18.13 (A) Camera-lucida assisted reconstruction of an HRP-labeled OCB collateral, from its parent axon of the OCB in the VNR. This sketch was generated from nine parasagittal sections, each 50 microns thick, and was projected on a representation of the single 50-micron section utilized for EM. In this two-dimensional representation, the positions of the three anterior-most "terminal areas" relative to the GCL are not accurately portrayed. Each actually ended at the boundary of the GCL, not in it. The "terminal areas" designated by the tip of the solid arrow is magnified in (B). Notice that the GCL separating the VCN and the DCN, melds with the GCL of the DCN. The dashed trapezoid designates the region investigated with EM. (B). The circled swellings were not part of the original camera lucida drawing. They were added based upon EM observations. ANR — auditory nerve root; AVCN — anteroventral CN; CN — cochlear nucleus; DCN — dorsal CN; EM — electron microscopy; GCL — granule cell lamina; OCB — olivocochlear bundle; PVCN — posteroventral CN; VCN — ventral CN; VNR — vestibular nerve root. (From Benson and Brown (1990, Fig. 2, p. 54). With permission.)

colliculus. These areas, at the level of the LL, have received little attention in mice, and therefore will not be emphasized in this chapter.

LL: Dorsal Nucleus

The DNLL is situated just ventral to the ventral portions of the central nucleus of the IC. Major bundles of LL fibers course through it, organizing the DNLL cells into columns. Most DNLL cells have a striking dendritic arrangement, where the dendritic domains are essentially two-dimensional, flattened in the horizontal plane, with the ascending LL fibers penetrating through these stacks (mouse: Willard and Ryugo, 1983). The DNLL is bounded ventrally by the INLL, and in most mammals laterally by the sagulum. The sagulum, due to differential connections, is thought to be

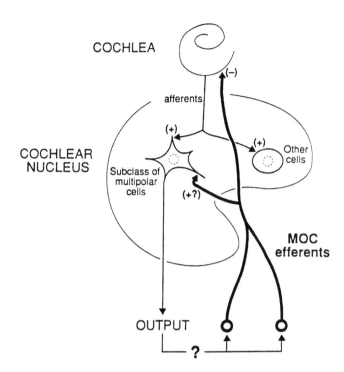

FIGURE 18.14 Hypothesis stating that a subclass of VCN multipolar/stellate neurons have outputs that are somewhat independent of MOC cochlear negative feedback in the presence of loud sounds. Primary afferents (auditory nerve fibers) are known to excite VCN neurons (+). MOC efferents provide feedback to the cochlea (–), thus indirectly decreasing excitatory input to VCN cells. MOC collaterals to the VCN are postulated to be excitatory (+?) and provide excitation enough to keep the VCN cells' outputs somewhat independent of the MOC cochlear negative feedback, thus keeping loud auditory signals within the functional operating range of the VCN neurons. MOC — medial olivocochlear bundle; VCN — ventral cochlear nucleus. (From Benson and Brown (1990, Fig. 14, p. 69). With permission.)

an auditory nucleus separate from DNLL. In contradistinction to VNLL, DNLL is referred to as a "binaural" nucleus in that its inputs from lower auditory centers and its outputs to the IC tend to be bilateral, and no doubt play some critical roles in sound localization.

LL: Intermediate Nucleus

The INLL is positioned between the DNLL lying dorsally and the dorsal division of VNLL (VNLLd) situated ventrally, when viewed in a coronal (frontal) plane of section. The primary cell type arrangement and cytoarchitectonic organization of the mouse INLL are similar to that of DNLL, except that with cresyl violet stains (for Nissl substance), the INLL principal cells stain intensely, in contrast to the more lightly stained DNLL neurons (Willard and Ryugo, 1983).

A main distinguishing feature of the INLL vs. the adjacent VNLLd cell groups is its differential projections. For example, outputs of the INLL tend to be bilateral in nature, whereas those of the VNLL tend to be ipsilateral. In the CBA mouse, INLL principal cells project to the IC (Frisina et al., 1998). In a single plane of section, this projection appears to be organized in a complex fashion topographically, but probably represents a concentric ring of tonotopic laminae in INLL.

LL: Ventral Nucleus

The VNLL has a dorsal (VNLLd) and a ventral division (VNLLv), and in the mouse is the largest of the three NLL. VNLLd principal cells are large (15 to 20 µm) multipolar neurons that are loosely

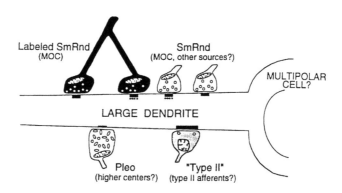

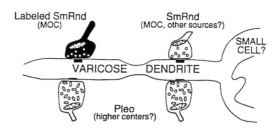

FIGURE 18.15 Cartoon summary of synaptic terminal types (their origins in parentheses) onto two classes of MOC target dendrites. Large dendrites likely arise from multipolar cells and varicose dendrites probably come from small cells. HRP-labeled terminals emanate from MOC axon branches and have small round synaptic vesicles. Many unlabeled terminals also have small round vesicles. Other unlabeled terminals have pleomorphic vesicles. Synaptic terminals showing some signs of neuronal degeneration are termed "type II" and probably originate from damaged primary afferent auditory nerve fibers from outer hair cells. MOC — medial olivocochlear bundle. (From Benson et al. (1996, Fig. 9, p. 38). With permission.)

scattered among the LL fibers. They project ipsilaterally to the IC (Frisina et al., 1998), including the central nucleus and external cortex (Willard and Ryugo, 1983). These cells exhibit long, relatively unbranched dendrites oriented orthogonal to the LL axons.

A signature of VNLLv is its striking columnar organization. This appears in both Nissl-stained material and when HRP injections are made in the IC. In the latter case, tonotopic columns of retrogradely labeled neurons are visible in the mouse (Frisina et al., 1998), along with a band of lightly labeled neurons orthogonal to the vertical columns. Mouse principal cells have small (10 to 15 μm) round somata and long, relatively thin dendrites that tend to be oriented parallel to the trajectory of the surrounding LL fibers as shown by Willard and Ryugo (1983). These investigators demonstrated in protargol preparations that these VNLLv principal neurons receive large, axosomatic calycine endings, similar in form but slightly smaller than the calyx of Held endings in the MNTB. Inputs to the mouse VNLL have not been well worked out, but some come from the contralateral DCN, and outputs are similar to VNLLd.

MIDBRAIN: INFERIOR COLLICULUS (IC)

ORGANIZATIONAL OVERVIEW OF THE AUDITORY MIDBRAIN

The largest portion of the auditory midbrain is the central nucleus of IC (ICC). Dorsal and caudal to the ICC lies a strip commonly referred to as the dorsal cortex (DC). Ventrolateral and rostral to ICC lies the external nucleus. A region anterior to ICC and external nucleus, including the deepest layers

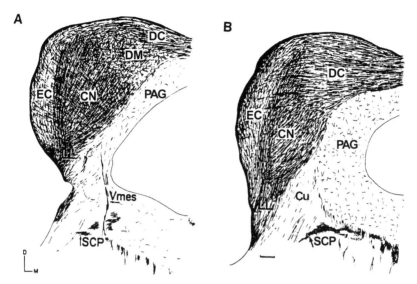

FIGURE 18.16   Camera lucida drawing of protargol-stained sections illustrating the fibroarchitecture of the mouse IC. The CN is characterized by dense neuropil, with a major component coming from the ascending fibers of LL. The CN also has output fibers that course dorsolaterally to penetrate EC prior to their entry into the brachium of IC (which then projects to the medial geniculate body, not shown). The DC is characterized by the presence of horizontally directed fascicles of axons from the commissure of IC. The DM portion of the central nucleus exhibits a criss-cross neuropil pattern (A). Scale bar = 0.2 mm. Section A is more caudal than section B. CN — central nucleus of IC; CU — cuneiform nucleus; DC — dorsal cortex of IC; EC — external cortex of IC; IC — inferior colliculus; LL — lateral lemniscus; PAG — periaqueductal gray; SCP — superior cerebellar peduncle; Vmes — trigeminal mesencephalic nucleus. (From Willard, F.H. and Ryugo, D.K., *The Auditory Psychobiology of the Mouse*, 1983, p. 251. Courtesy of Charles C. Thomas, Publisher, Ltd., Springfield, Illinois.)

of the superior colliculus (SC), is involved in multimodality (auditory, visual) processing of spatial maps. One of the most striking procedures for visualizing the divisions of the IC is with fiber stains. Willard and Ryugo (1983) made elegant use of the protargol stain for just this application (Figure 18.16).

IC: CENTRAL NUCLEUS

Much of the general mammalian plan for the organization and cytoarchitectonics of ICC have been worked out in cat by Morest, Oliver, and colleagues (Oliver and Morest, 1984; Oliver and Huerta, 1992). Many similarities exist between this basic organization in cat and the ICC of the mouse and other rodents (Meininger et al., 1986; Willott et al., 1994a). There are two main principal cell types in the ICC: disc-shaped neurons, with elongate somata and flattened dendritic fields, and stellate neurons whose dendritic arborizations extend across the ICC laminae. The presence and organization of these ICC cell types is shown for the mouse in Figure 18.17.

Central Nucleus: Watershed of Ascending Information and Diverse Inputs

Virtually all of the processing in lower centers of the auditory brainstem project onto the neurons of ICC, as shown in Figure 18.18. Primary projections in the mouse originate from the contralateral cochlear nucleus, the ipsilateral SOC, the ipsilateral VNLL, and the IC bilaterally. Lesser inputs come from the DNLL and INLL bilaterally, the contralateral DC and external nucleus, the ipsilateral central gray (reticular formation), and all three divisions of the ipsilateral MGB in the thalamus. Major inputs, such as those from the contralateral cochlear nucleus and NLL, are tonotopically organized, as exemplified in Figure 18.19. In the albino mouse, Ryugo et al. (1981) demonstrated that axonal projections from the contralateral cochlear nucleus were tonotopic in nature, and that

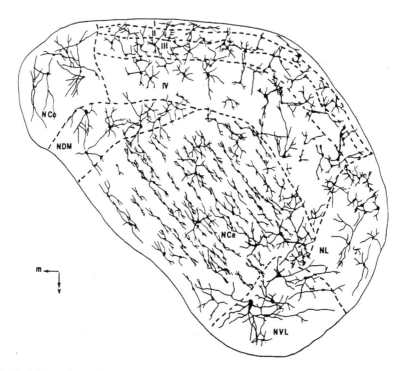

FIGURE 18.17 Mid-section of the mouse IC in the frontal (coronal) plane of section of Golgi-impregnated material. In the NCe, two principal cell types are evident: disc-shaped (bipolar) neurons constituting the NCe laminae and multipolar/stellate cells whose dendritic fields cut across the laminae. These principal cell types become larger in NDM and NVL. The dorsal cortex of IC is composed of four layers, with Layer I being the most superficial and dorsal, and Layer IV making up the deepest most ventral region. IC — inferior colliculus; NCe — central nucleus of IC; NCo — nucleus of the commissure of IC; NDM — dorsomedial nucleus of IC; NL — lateral or external nucleus of IC; NVL — ventrolateral IC. (From Meininger et al. (1986, Fig. 8, p. 1173). With permission.)

the DCN projected not only to ICC, but also to the external nucleus. No connections were observed from the cochlear nucleus to DC.

Reetz and Ehret (1999) conducted an elegant and technically challenging investigation of inputs to the mouse IC. They made intracellular recordings from mouse ICC neurons while being able to electrically stimulate LL, the commissure of IC, or the commissure of Probst (CP), and followed this by intracellular injection of biocytin to examine the morphology of the cell studied. They found that ICC neurons investigated, including disc-shaped and stellate cells, had axon collaterals that provided inputs to several adjacent iso-frequency laminae, as well as projecting to the external nucleus, the brachium of IC, LL, CP, or the commissure of IC. An example of one of the ICC neurons studied is given in Figure 18.20.

Central Nucleus: Laminar Structure

The ICC has a striking fibrodendritic laminar organization. The laminae are composed of the somata and dendrites of the main principal cells: the disc-shaped neurons. These neurons have oval-to-fusiform shaped perikarya and flattened dendritic fields parallel to the ICC laminae, as displayed in Figure 18.17. These characteristics of the ICC principal neurons, together with the incoming LL fibers that project onto these cells and their dendrites, make up the ICC laminae (Figure 18.16). The laminae in most mammals, such as cat and mouse, are oriented like a stack of pancakes, with the main surface of the each pancake approximately in the horizontal plane, with a tilt in the dorsomedial/ventrolateral direction. Therefore, as one moves from dorsal to ventral through the

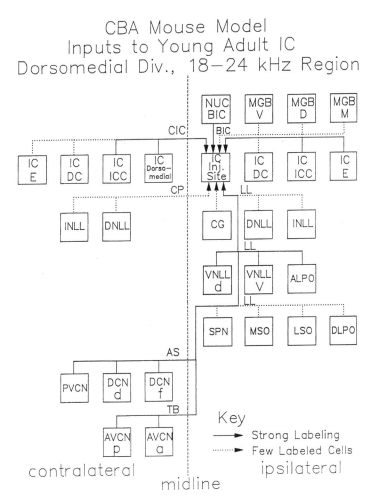

FIGURE 18.18 Schematic flow diagram of inputs to the CBA mouse IC dorsomedial region, determined with focal HRP injections. Certain inputs would be emphasized or attenuated when HRP injections are made in other regions of the IC, or if they cover a larger area. Inputs are exclusively contralateral at the level of the cochlear nucleus, ipsilateral for the SOC and MGB, and bilateral for the NLL and auditory midbrain. ALPO — anterolateral periolivary nucleus; AVCNa — anteroventral CN, anterior region; AVCNp — anteroventral CN, posterior region; BIC — brachium of IC; CG — central gray, reticular formation; CN — cochlear nucleus; DC — dorsal cortex of IC; DCNd — dorsal CN, deep layers; DCNf — dorsal CN, fusiform cell layer; DLPO — dorsolateral periolivary nucleus; DNLL — dorsal NLL; E — external nucleus of IC; IC — inferior colliculus; ICC — central nucleus of IC; INLL — intermediate NLL; LSO — lateral superior olive; MGB — medial geniculate body of the thalamus; MGBd — dorsal MGB; MGBm — medial MGB; MGBv — ventral MGB; MNTB — medial nucleus of the trapezoid body; MSO — medial superior olive; NLL — nuclei of the lateral lemniscus; PVCN — posteroventral CN; SOC — superior olivary complex; SPN — superior paraolivary nucleus; VNLLd — ventral NLL, dorsal division VNLLv — ventral NLL, ventral division. (From Frisina et al. (1998, Fig. 15, p. 76). With permission.)

ICC, one proceeds through the stack of laminae. In terms of tonotopic organization, the dorsal laminae encode low frequencies, and the ventral laminae are for the processing of high frequencies. Thus, although the frequency organization of inputs to the ICC is preserved, topographic organization is sometimes altered in nuclei of the brainstem auditory system. For example, the tonotopic progression in the VCN is reversed from that in the ICC. In the former, low frequencies are processed ventrally, and in the latter, they are encoded dorsally.

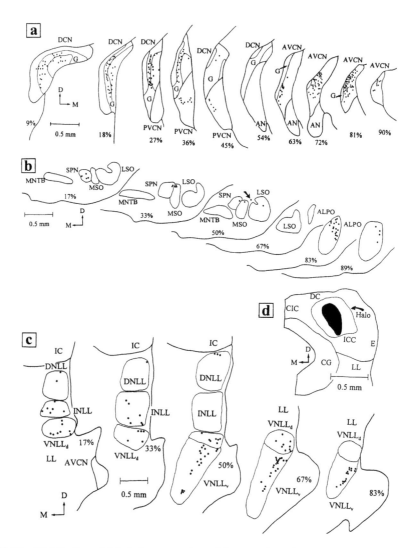

FIGURE 18.19 Distribution of labeled neurons in serial coronal sections of contralateral CN, ipsilateral SOC, and ipsilateral NLL. These are major inputs to the CBA mouse IC dorsomedial region, determined with focal HRP injections. Certain inputs would be emphasized or attenuated when HRP injections are made in other regions of the IC, or if they cover a larger area. (a) Cochlear nucleus inputs derive contralaterally; (b) ipsilateral SOC inputs, with the arrow designating a labeled neuron in DLPO; (c) labeled neurons of ipsilateral NLL; (d) camera lucida reconstruction showing spatial extent of an injection site in the CBA mouse dorsal IC. Percentages indicate the distances from the caudal boundary of each region. ALPO — anterolateral periolivary nucleus; AN — auditory nerve; AVCN — anteroventral CN; BIC — brachium of IC; CG — central gray, reticular formation; CIC — commissure of IC; CN — cochlear nucleus; DC — dorsal cortex of IC; DCN — dorsal CN; DLPO — dorsolateral periolivary nucleus; DNLL — dorsal NLL; E — external nucleus of IC; G — granule cell layer of CN; IC — inferior colliculus; ICC — central nucleus of IC; INLL — intermediate NLL; LSO — lateral superior olive; MNTB — medial nucleus of the trapezoid body; MSO — medial superior olive; NLL — nuclei of the lateral lemniscus; PVCN — posteroventral CN; SOC — superior olivary complex; SPN — superior paraolivary nucleus; VNLLd — ventral NLL, dorsal division; VNLLv — ventral NLL, ventral division. (From Frisina et al. (1998, Fig. 14, p. 75). With permission.)

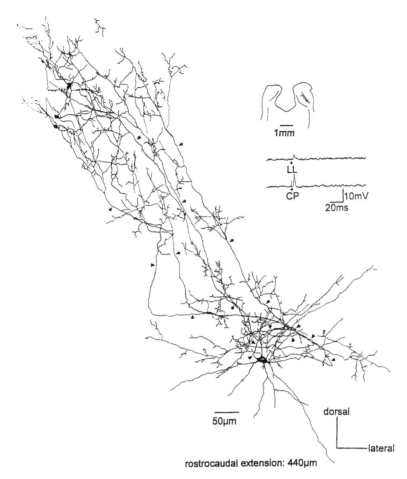

FIGURE 18.20 Drawing of a large multipolar cell in ventral ICC, with multiple axon collaterals (arrowheads) projecting dorsomedially and parallel to the ICC laminae. This neuron received excitatory inputs from LL and from CP. Note the three labeled, small bipolar neurons in the upper-left portion of the dendritic tree. These were apparently dye-coupled, possibly via electrical gap junctions, to the stained neuron, and had dendritic fields that overlapped with the axonal arborizations of the large multipolar cell. Location of this cell in the ICC is given in the inset. CP — commissure of Probst; IC — inferior colliculus; ICC — central nucleus of IC; LL — lateral lemniscus. (From Reetz and Ehret (1999, Fig. 6, p. 533). With permission.)

Central Nucleus: Output Pathways

The major output pathway of the IC is the brachium of the IC (BIC). Primarily, the BIC projects to all three divisions of the ipsilateral MGB, although there is a small contralateral projection in some cases. In the CBA mouse, additional smaller output pathways have been demonstrated. For example, auditory information is relayed to the visual system via ipsilateral inputs to the superior colliculus, and to the reticular formation through a bilateral pathway to the central gray region. Axonal processes also terminate in the other regions of the ipsilateral IC away from the area of the HRP injection sites used to determine these connections. A summary of the output regions for the ICC of the CBA mouse is presented in Figure 18.21.

Central Nucleus: Commissure

The commissure of the IC (CIC) is a prominent decussation at the level of the auditory midbrain, providing a major transfer of information between the IC on both sides of the brain. The most

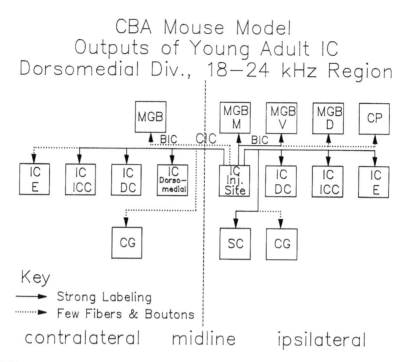

FIGURE 18.21   Schematic diagram of the outputs of the CBA mouse dorsomedial IC, as determined by focal iontophoretic injections of HRP. BIC — brachium of IC; CG — central gray, reticular formation; CIC — commissure of IC; CP — cerebral peduncle; DC — dorsal cortex of IC; E — external nucleus of IC; IC — inferior colliculus; ICC — central nucleus of IC; MGB — medial geniculate body of the thalamus; MGBd — dorsal MGB; MGBm — medial MGB; MGBv — ventral MGB; SC — superior colliculus. (From Frisina et al. (1997, Fig. 6, p. 2752). With permission.)

significant connections are between homologous regions of the ICC, as exemplified in Figure 18.22, from a CBA mouse. Other crossed connections exist between the ICC and the other IC regions such as the dorsal cortex and external nucleus, shown schematically in Figure 18.21 (Frisina et al., 1997). There are also scattered neurons whose cell bodies reside within the CIC, exhibiting a simple dendritic branching pattern that is parallel or orthogonal to the CIC axons. These neurons receive synaptic specializations from collaterals of some of the CIC fibers.

IC: Dorsal Cortex

The principal cells of DC are the stellate and pyramidal neurons, examples of which are presented in Figure 18.17. The DC has been distinguished from ICC and the external nucleus based on considerations such as ontological development and orientation of neuronal perikarya and dendritic fields (Meininger et al., 1986). Gonzales-Hernandez et al. (1987) note that ICC can also be distinguished from DC based on afferent inputs. In the albino mouse, they report that the ICC receives more non-auditory inputs than the DC, such as from substantia nigra, deep layers of the superior colliculus, and the hypothalamic nuclei. However, from a functional point of view, it may be that DC is actually an extension of the dorsomedial IC. For example, in the mouse it has been found that the tonotopic map of single-unit best frequencies flows smoothly from the DC to the dorsomedial IC (Stiebler and Ehret, 1985; Willott, 1986; Walton et al., 1997). The presence of a continuous tonotopic map for the mouse DC and ICC suggests that the functions of these two regions may coincide.

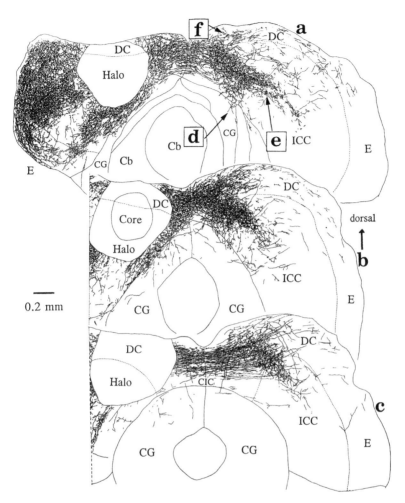

FIGURE 18.22 Camera lucida reconstruction of IC connections identified with injections of HRP in the IC. Injections in dorsomedial IC sent labeled processes to all major divisions of the contralateral IC, as well as bilaterally to CG. Dashed lines indicate that boundaries between ICC, DC, and E should be considered approximate, because they are based on Nissl-stained material (not Golgi). Coronal sections extend from caudal (a) to rostral (c), and are 180 micron apart. Section thickness: 60 micron; Cb — cerebellum; CG — central gray, reticular formation; CIC — commissure of IC; DC — dorsal cortex of IC; E — external nucleus of IC; IC — inferior colliculus; ICC — central nucleus of IC. (From Frisina et al. (1997, Figure 4, p 2749). With permission.)

IC: EXTERNAL NUCLEUS

The external nucleus (also called external cortex) lies lateral, ventral, and rostral to the ICC in most mammals. It has been divided into a superficial layer composed of densely packed small stellate cells, and a deep region containing more loosely packed large pyramidal cells with thick primary dendrites that taper distally. In terms of the functional organization of its laminae, the external nucleus can also be differentiated from the neighboring ICC and DC (Stiebler and Ehret, 1985). Specifically, defined in terms of both anatomy and physiology, its isofrequency laminae are oriented differently from those of the adjacent ICC and DC, being separated by a laminar discontinuity. The connectional patterns of the external nucleus also differ from those of ICC, including participation in more multimodality interactions. For example, the superficial layer receives inputs from the contralateral spinal tract of the trigeminal nerve (Gonzales-Hernandez et al., 1987) and the somatic sensory system dorsal column nuclei (Willard and Ryugo, 1983). In contrast, the deep layer receives significant input from the DCN. Auditory projections to the external cortex are similar to those going to the ICC, except that the VCN contributes little input to the external nucleus.

IC: CONNECTIONS WITH SUPERIOR COLLICULUS: MULTIMODALITY PROCESSING

The deep layers of the superior colliculus (SC) functionally merge with rostral portions of the IC external nucleus to form a multimodality spatial location processing area, with maps of visual space that coincide with auditory maps. Thus, these regions contain spatially coincident visual and auditory inputs. The anatomical and physiological details of these relationships, and what the ontogenetic development sequence of these maps is, has been worked out by Knudsen and colleagues in birds (Cohen and Knudsen, 1999; Knudsen, 1999; Gold and Knudsen, 2000). These types of maps may exist to a less-developed extent in mammals such as mice, depending on the neuroethological importance of spatial maps for the survival (as predator or prey) of a particular mammalian species.

IC: STRUCTURE/FUNCTION RELATIONSHIPS

A wealth of information exists on the functional organization of IC that has been derived primarily from species other than mice. This body of information cannot be covered in this anatomy chapter, but may be gleaned from other chapters of this handbook. One of several general principles concerning structure/function relationships in the IC is that specific functional maps or organizations are superimposed on the tonotopic laminae of the ICC. For example, Langner and Schreiner have demonstrated neurophysiologically the presence of maps for single-unit best-amplitude-modulation frequencies within ICC laminae (Langner, 1992).

THALAMUS: MEDIAL GENICULATE BODY (MGB)

BASIC ORGANIZATION OF THE AUDITORY THALAMUS

The MGB lies on the posterolateral surface of the mouse thalamus as a rounded protrusion, delineating the rostral termination of the BIC. It has been divided into several areas in mammals (cat: Morest, 1964; tree shrew: Oliver and Hall, 1978; rat: Winer et al., 1999), usually including these major divisions: ventral (MGBv), dorsal (MGBd), and medial (MGBm). Considering all centers of the central auditory system, in mice the MGB is probably the least studied, and will not be an area of emphasis in this chapter.

MGB: VENTRAL DIVISION

The MGBv is the only auditory diencephalic structure with a prominent laminar, tonotopic cytoarchitectonic typography, and in mice is the largest MGB division. It contains densely packed, small- and medium-sized neurons, examples of which are displayed in Figure 18.23. The small cells are probably homologous to Golgi II cells of cat swirls (Willard and Ryugo, 1983). The larger neurons are characterized by three to five stout primary dendrites, and most likely correspond to the thalamocortical relay cells in cat MGBv. Nissl-stained analysis of MGBv reveals that the perikarya of most neurons are arranged in curved rows, forming a pattern of tonotopic organization, which is superimposed on the trajectory of BIC axons providing ICC inputs to MGBv.

MGB: DORSAL DIVISION

The MGBd caps MGBv on its dorsal and caudal borders. It possesses small round cells, with dichotomously radiating dendrites that ultimately form a spherical dendritic field (Willard and

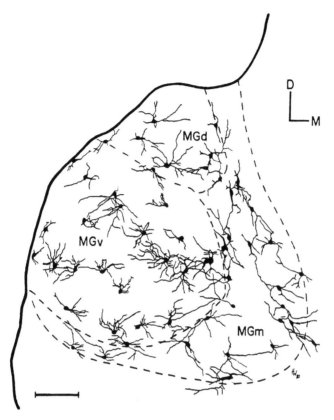

FIGURE 18.23 Neuronal cytoarchitecture of the major subdivisions of the mouse MGB as drawn with a camera lucida from a Golgi-stained section (Golgi-Kopsch, Stensaas modification, juvenile age). Scale bar = 100 micron. D — dorsal; M — medial; MGB — medial geniculate body of the thalamus; MGd — dorsal division of MGB; MGm — medial division of MGB; MGv — ventral division of MGB. (From Willard, F.H. and Ryugo, D.K., *The Auditory Psychobiology of the Mouse*, 1983, p. 265. Courtesy of Charles C. Thomas, Publisher, Ltd., Springfield, Illinois.)

Ryugo, 1983), some of which are drawn in Figure 18.23. The mammalian MGBd also contains a circumscribed region of large multipolar neurons, often called the suprageniculate region, which lies dorsally in MGBd. The MGBd receives significant auditory inputs from dorsal cortex of IC, and sends a small projection back to the ipsilateral external nucleus of IC.

MGB: Medial Division

The MGBm bounds MGBv medially and rostrally. Large multipolar neurons, as shown in Figure 18.23, characterize this region, along with some smaller cells with round or elongate perikarya that are fewer in number. Myelinated fibers are also prominent, running rostrocaudally (Willard and Ryugo, 1983). Besides receiving auditory inputs from the IC external nucleus, MGBm receives somatosensory information from the dorsal column nuclei. The MGBd has an output pathway back to the ipsilateral IC external nucleus, with which it has reciprocal connections.

MGB: Reciprocity with Auditory Cortex

A fundamental property of the connections of MGB is the reciprocal feedback loops it has with primary and secondary auditory cortices. Specifically in the mouse (Caviness and Frost, 1980; Frost and Caviness, 1980), Class I axons of the acoustic radiation (AR, connects MGB with cortex) project mainly to auditory cortex Layers III and IV, with some collaterals penetrating Layers I and VI. Class I fibers originating in MGBv project primarily to primary auditory cortex (area 41), whereas those coming from MGBd terminate in secondary cortical fields (areas 36 and 36a). In contrast, AR Class II axons are small-caliber and more diffusely distributed in the cortical layers, with their heaviest concentration in Layers I and VI. Class II axons derive mostly from MGBm to cortical areas 41, 22, 36, and 36a (Willard and Ryugo, 1983). Overall, the connectivity of the MGB is similar to what is known for rat.

MGB: FUNCTIONAL IMPLICATIONS

Of the major central auditory nuclei, the functionality of the MGB is probably least understood. It certainly plays some role in multimodality processing, especially MGBd and MGBm. The MGBv is an important relay center to the auditory cortex. Specific modulation of auditory cortical activity also takes place within the many feedback loops with the cortex, and to a lesser extent with IC. In addition, much of the specificity of cortical physiological responses and receptive fields is set up and initiated in MGB neurons of its three divisions that probably subserve different sensory processing functions.

CEREBRUM: AUDITORY CORTEX

GENERAL TOPOGRAPHY AND LOCATIONS OF CORTICAL FIELDS

In all mammals, cortical area 41 corresponds to the primary auditory cortex (AI), and is located on the dorsal surface of the temporal lobe, just dorsal to the rhinal fissure (Caviness, 1975). However, its exact location, topography, and the positions, functions, and sizes of the secondary auditory cortical fields vary to a great extent across different mammalian species. In mice, AI is bounded rostrally and dorsally by area 22, and caudally and ventrally by area 36 (Willard and Ryugo, 1983). The major auditory cortical areas for the mouse are laid out in Figure 18.24, as defined by Stiebler (1987) and Hofstetter and Ehret (1992). Unlike the auditory centers of the brainstem where, in general, homologies exceed species differences, phylogenetic diversity is a theme at the level of the cerebral cortex.

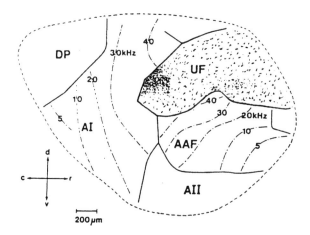

FIGURE 18.24 Example of the field topography of the mouse auditory cortical fields. Note that some fields, such as AI and AAF, have tonotopic organizations. Other fields, such as UF (gray shading), DP, and AII, lack regular tonotopy in their physiological responses. AI — primary auditory cortex; AII — secondary auditory cortex; AAF — anterior auditory field; DP — dorsoposterior field of auditory cortex; UF — ultrasonic field. c — caudal; d — dorsal; r — rostral; v — ventral. (From Hofstetter and Ehret (1992, Fig. 1, p. 371). With permission.)

CORTEX: PRIMARY AUDITORY CORTEX

Primary auditory cortex, like most areas of the cerebral cortex, has a columnar and laminar structure overlaid orthogonally to the basic tonotopic organization received from the lower auditory centers. The mouse cortical laminar structure is composed of six layers, with Layer I lying most superficially and Layer VI positioned most deeply (see Willard and Ryugo, 1983, for Nissl analyses of these laminae in areas 41, 22, and 36; and Willott et al., 1993, for tonotopic organization). Area 41 has the greatest dorsal/ventral thickness, primarily due to an expanded Layer V, which receives many incoming axons from the auditory brainstem and other cortical areas. Layer I is thin, composed of mainly fibers and a few scattered somata. Layer II consists of small pyramidal cells, and a slightly greater cell density than Layer III, which also contains small pyramidal neurons. Layer IV is made of granule cells at high density. Layer V, consisting of large pyramidal cells, has three sublayers: Va has a decreased cell density, Vb is the broadest of the sublayers with the densest cell packing, and Vc has a markedly diminished neural density. AI is sometimes referred to as koniocortex, receiving this name due to the dense population of granule cells in Layer IV, and receives the strongest input from MGBv.

Inputs to auditory cortex come from the MGB, with an ipsilateral bias, from other areas of cortex, and from the contralateral cortex via the corpus callosum, primarily the auditory areas (Willard and Ryugo, 1983). The laminar distribution of inputs to mouse area 41 is given in Figure 18.25. The cells of origin of these callosal connections are primarily the medium-to-large cells of cortical Layers III and V, and a few from Layer VI (Yorke and Caviness, 1975).

A significant descending pathway projects from cortical pyramidal cells of Layer Vb bilaterally, with an ipsilateral emphasis, to the IC central nucleus, and ipsilaterally to the dorsal cortex of IC, as displayed in Figure 18.26 (Gonzalez-Hernandez et al., 1987). Additional descending projections provide heavy inputs to MGBv, and sparser ones to MGBm and MGBd, as presented in Figure 18.27 (Willard and Ryugo, 1983).

CORTEX: SECONDARY CORTICES

As presented in Figure 18.24, three cortical fields lie rostral to AI in mice. The ultrasonic field (UF) lies most dorsally, the secondary auditory cortex (AII) is most ventral, and the anterior auditory field (AAF) is situated between the two. The dorsoposterior field (DP) is located dorsocaudal to AI in mice.

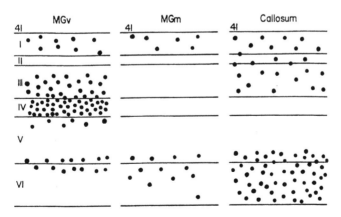

FIGURE 18.25 Diagram illustrating area 41 laminar distribution, density, and source of axon terminals. Thalamocortical inputs arise from MGv and MGm, whereas the contralateral cerebral hemisphere contributes projections through the corpus callosum. (Based on Yorke and Caviness (1975), Caviness and Frost (1980), and Frost and Caviness (1980).) MGm — medial division of medial geniculate body; MGv — ventral division of medial geniculate body. (From Willard, F.H. and Ryugo, D.K., *The Auditory Psychobiology of the Mouse,* 1983, p. 274. Courtesy of Charles C. Thomas, Publisher, Ltd., Springfield, Illinois.)

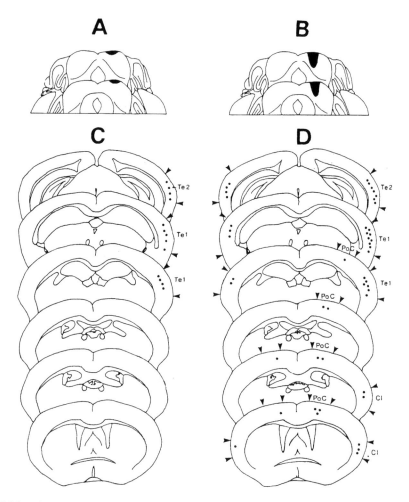

FIGURE 18.26 (A, B) Diagrams showing location of injection sites in dorsal cortex (A) and dorsomedial central nucleus (B) of IC. The distribution of labeled somata following injections of HRP into the dorsal cortex (C) and the dorsomedial central nucleus (D) of IC in the albino mouse. Cl — claustrocortex; IC — inferior colliculus; PoC — postcentral cortex. (From Gonzalez-Hernandez et al. (1987, Fig. 1, p. 317). With permission.)

Hofstetter and Ehret (1992), utilizing focal HRP injections into the superficial (Layers I–IV) and deep (Layers IV–VI) of UF, delineated some of the connections of the secondary auditory cortices. Superficial injections led to reciprocal (stained somata and terminals) in ipsilateral AI, AII, DP, dorsal association area, MGBv, MGBd, MGBm, caudal posterior nucleus, and secondary somatosensory cortex. Contralaterally, reciprocal connections were observed in homotopic UF. Deep injections showed the same results and, in addition, labeled terminals were observed ipsilaterally in caudal caudatoputamen, nucleus limitans, nucleus reticularis of the thalamus, dorsomedial ICC, external nucleus of IC, stratum griseum intermediale of the superior colliculus, and in ALPO. This connectivity pattern of UF, due to its similarities with the connections of AI and AAF, suggest that UF may be an extension of one of these other auditory cortical fields.

Area 22 has inputs from the contralateral cerebral hemisphere that are similar to those of area 41, as depicted in Figure 18.25. Area 36's contralateral hemisphere inputs are a bit different, with terminals mainly found in Layers I and II, Layer VI, and the most ventral portion of Layer V. Areas 22 and 36 pyramidal neurons send a few output projections to the dorsal cortex of IC, as summarized in Figure 18.27 (Willard and Ryugo, 1983).

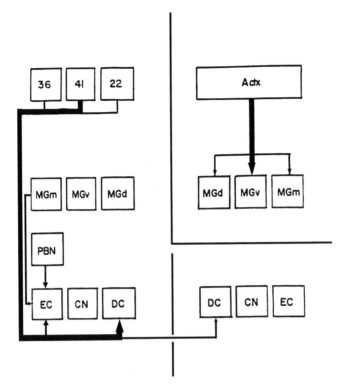

FIGURE 18.27 Flow diagram illustrating the known descending, efferent pathways originating in the mouse auditory cortex and MG. Relative innervation density is indicated by line thickness. Actx — auditory cortex; CN — central nucleus of IC; DC — dorsal cortex of IC; EC — external nucleus of IC; IC — inferior colliculus; MG — medial geniculate body of the thalamus; MGd — dorsal MG; MGm — medial MG; MGv — ventral MG; PBN — parabrachial nucleus (near the brachium of the IC). (From Willard, F.H. and Ryugo, D.K., *The Auditory Psychobiology of the Mouse*, 1983, p. 279. Courtesy of Charles C. Thomas, Publisher, Ltd., Springfield, Illinois.)

CORTEX: COMPARATIVE ANALYSES

The comparative organization of the auditory cortex (Figure 18.28), regarding layouts for macaque monkey, cat, gerbil, and mouse, are presented clearly in a diagram from Stiebler et al. (1997). Notice that all these mammals have an AI and AAF that are tonotopically organized (isofrequency laminae are given), and an AII region that fails to show tonotopy. As indicated in the figure, additional tonotopic areas have been mapped in cat (PAF, VPAF by Reale and Imig, 1980) and gerbil (DP, VP by Thomas et al., 1993).

In regard to UF's location in the mouse cortex and its connections to the posterior nucleus complex of the thalamus, the dorsal area may correspond functionally to the suprasylvian association area of cat auditory cortex, which has connections with thalamic nuclei processing acoustical, somatosensory, and visual information. Consistent with this pattern of connectivity, neurons in this region respond to stimuli from all three of these sensory modalities (Hofstetter and Ehret, 1992). Reciprocal connections of UF with AI, DP, and AII are also reported for cat and monkey. Contralateral connections of UF seen in mice have also been observed in rat and cat.

CORTEX: COLUMNAR ORGANIZATION AND FUNCTIONAL IMPLICATIONS

Columns in mouse auditory cortex, whose major axes run in a dorsoventral direction like those of the somatosensory (Mountcastle, 1957) and visual (Hubel and Wiesel, 1963) systems, share similar physiological properties such as firing patterns, best frequencies, minimum thresholds, sharpness

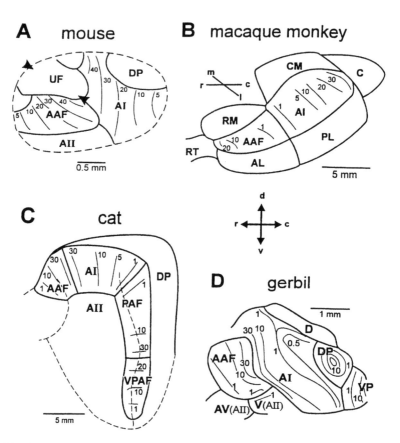

FIGURE 18.28 Comparative organizations of auditory cortex in (A) mouse; (B) monkey; (C) cat; and (D) gerbil. The left auditory cortex is shown in each case. Arrowheads in UF show a line dividing UF into rostral and caudal parts, whereby the latter may be an extension of AI. Auditory cortex fields: AI — primary; AII — secondary; AAF — anterior auditory field; AL — anterior lateral; AV — anteroventral; C — caudal; CM — caudomedial; D — dorsal; DP — dorsoposterior; PAF — posterior; PL — posterior lateral; RM — rostro-medial; RT — rostrotemporal; UF — ultrasonic field; V — ventral; VP, VPAF — ventroposterior. c — caudal; d — dorsal; l — lateral; m — medial; r — rostral; v — ventral. (From Stiebler et al. (1997, Fig. 5, p. 567). With permission.)

of frequency tuning, and onset latency (Shen et al., 1999). Moreover, a number of cortical columns display ear dominance properties, similar to the ocular dominance columns discovered in the visual cortex. Ear dominance refers to the physiological properties of cortical cells being preferentially responsive to one ear vs. the other.

Functional differences from one auditory field to the next relate to some specializations for subserving certain auditory perceptual phenomena preferentially over others. Little is known about the functionality of the mouse auditory cortical fields. Hofstetter and Ehret (1992) speculate that UF, due to its lack of tonotopy and sensitivity to ultrasonic signals from 45 to 70 kHz, may be specialized for encoding ultrasonic vocalizations and communication signals for juvenile and adult mice. Stiebler et al. (1997) report that the left auditory cortex of the house mouse is larger than the right, by a factor of 1.3, whereas the relative sizes of the five main cortical fields were the same on both sides.

ACKNOWLEDGMENTS

Work supported by the National Institute on Aging NIH Grant P01 AG09524, and the International Center for Hearing and Speech Research, Rochester, New York.

19 Cytoarchitectonic Atlas of the Cochlear Nucleus of the Mouse

Joseph Trettel and D. Kent Morest

INTRODUCTION

The central auditory system has received increasing attention in the field of comparative neurobiology. One reason for this is that it presents the opportunity to correlate specific sensory and behavioral adaptations to structural features of the neurons and their connections. For example, owls and echolocating bats present obvious specializations that can be exploited in establishing structure/function relationships. Because a number of methods and approaches are being used in the field, it is often necessary to refer experimental findings to specific groups of neurons, because these are known to have different connections and to support different functions. Studies, based on distantly related species, can be more effectively compared when there is a common architectural plan that can be referenced.

In the case of the mouse, the current interest stems largely from the availability of detailed genetic information concerning hearing and hearing deficits. As is evident from other chapters in this book, much of hearing research on mice has focused on the cochlea, where the normal anatomical structure is better known than in the central auditory system. Meanwhile, there is growing interest in the mouse central auditory system as a suitable substrate for analyzing the role of aging and neurodegeneration in hearing loss, as well as normal hearing. The small size of the brain provides several strategic advantages in facilitating anatomical and physiological studies of the central auditory system, for example, in the use of brain slices for morphological and electrophysiological experiments (e.g., see Chapter 20).

The cochlear nucleus (CN) has received considerable attention in structure/function relationships. A major topic in this research has been the correlation of signal processing operations with specific types of neurons. This line of research provides the opportunity to relate synaptic organization and the circuits of cell types to auditory response properties. It leads directly to hypotheses about the cellular and molecular mechanisms and the network properties responsible for signal coding (see Morest, 1993, for a review). Progress in this effort requires the availability of an architectural plan of sufficient detail to support such hypotheses. The cytoarchitecture of the CN has been the subject of a number of comparative light microscopic investigations on cats (e.g., Lorente de Nó, 1981; Osen, 1969; Brawer et al., 1974; Brawer and Morest, 1975; Cant and Morest, 1979a); primates (Strominger and Strominger, 1971; Moore and Osen, 1979); rabbits (Disterhoft et al., 1980); and various rodents (e.g., Harrison and Irvine, 1966, in the rat; Webster et al., 1968; Martin, 1981; and Webster and Trune, 1982, in the mouse; Morest et al., 1990, in the chinchilla). One purpose of the present effort is to provide an adequate guide to the neuroanatomical structure of the CN, sufficient to allow significant observations of the perturbations provided by genetic engineering and multidisciplinary approaches to normal function of the mouse. While generally useful guides for the mouse exist (e.g., Webster and Webster, 1977; Martin, 1981; Webster and

Trune, 1982; Chapter 18), there is still a need to provide a more detailed analysis, to permit unambiguous comparisons with the schemes available for the cat and the chinchilla, where a good deal of neuroanatomical, electrophysiological, and neurochemical data have already been collected. We believe that the level of sophistication in the experimental study of the central auditory pathways is necessarily limited by the detailed information available on specific neuroanatomical structures.

In mammals, the axons constituting the cochlear nerve terminate in the CN. Cochlear nerve fibers synapse on the principal neurons of the CN in a tonotopic array over the rostrocaudal extent of the nucleus. The principal cells send collateral fibers within the CN, and also project out of the CN to initiate the parallel ascending pathways of the auditory brainstem, each of which encodes and processes different features of acoustic stimuli. The CN also contains populations of intrinsic neurons whose connectivity does not extend beyond the anatomical boundaries of the CN. Anatomically, the CN is generally divided into the dorsal cochlear nucleus (DCN) and the ventral cochlear nucleus (VCN). The cochlear nerve enters the VCN on the ventral surface and bifurcates in the rostrocaudal plane into ascending and descending branches. Ascending fibers enter the anteroventral CN (AVCN), and the descending branch enters the posteroventral CN (PVCN), while heading dorsally to innervate the DCN. Each of these primary regions can be further divided, as defined by cell types and standard cytoarchitectonic criteria.

This chapter presents a detailed cytoarchitectonic atlas of the mouse cochlear nucleus based on the topographic scheme of Brawer et al. (1974) and Morest et al. (1990). This atlas could serve as a reference tool for future studies on the mouse auditory system, and this should facilitate more general comparisons with the other species. Anatomical or physiological analyses, in which the resolution of specific cell populations is desired, require atlases useful for navigating and identifying common structures within and between orders of animals. The atlas should provide this tool for those wishing to employ the mouse as their model system in studies of the central auditory system.

MATERIALS AND METHODS

Fifteen female mice (C57BL/CBA; Jackson Laboratories) between 6 and 12 weeks old and weighing between 16.8 and 21 g were used. All procedures were done in accordance with the guidelines established by the Internal Animal Care Committee of the University of Connecticut Health Center; and in all circumstances, an effort was made to minimize pain and discomfort to the animals. All reagents used were of the highest grade commercially available, unless otherwise specified.

HISTOLOGY

The cytoarchitectonic atlas was based on the brains of five mice (average age of 7.25 weeks), sectioned and stained with either a modified buffered thionin or cresyl violet. Fibers were visualized in two mice by staining myelin with Luxol fast Blue, or lipids with the Sudan black method of Rasmussen (1961). All animals were deeply anesthetized with 0.1 mL sodium pentobarbital IP and perfused intracardially with 25 mL of 0.15 M phosphate-buffered saline (PBS, pH 7.4) at 38°C, followed by 35 mL of 10% formol-saline (Fisher, Scientific, Pittsburgh, PA) at 9 mL · min^{-1}. The vestibulocochlear nerve was cut at the opening of the internal auditory meatus, and the brain was quickly removed, immersed in the same fixative for 5 days, and transferred successively to 10%, 20%, and 30% sucrose in formol-saline for 24 h each. The tissue was then trimmed, frozen on dry ice, and sectioned in the anatomical transverse plane at 20 or 24 μm. Sections were collected serially on poly-L-lysine coated slides and air-dried for 24 h. For thionin staining, the tissue was dehydrated through 100% EtOH, defatted in ether-chloroform, rehydrated, and stained with a 0.1% buffered thionin stain (pH 3.7). Following differentiation in acidic 70% EtOH, the tissue was dehydrated, cleared in xylene, and coverslipped with Permount (Fisher). The procedures for the cresyl violet stain were identical to that of the thionin stain with the exception of the delipidation step in chloroform, which was replaced by a 24-h wash in 95% EtOH. Sudan black staining was done on hydrated sections with a saturated solution of Sudan black B in 70% EtOH. Sections were preserved in the aqueous state and mounted in glycerin for microscopic examination.

SHRINKAGE FACTOR CALCULATION

To determine the tissue shrinkage factor for the formalin fixation and histological processing, we developed an ink track/injection method. Briefly, one mouse (MS01-061899; 19.2 g) was anesthetized with 0.12 mg xylazine and 0.1 mg ketamine, and placed in a stereotaxic apparatus. Glass pipettes (World Precision Instruments, 1.0 mm) were pulled to 4 to 8 μm I.D. and filled with black indigo ink. Two holes (radius = 0.25 mm), spaced 2.5 mm apart on the rostrocaudal axis, were made on the superior surface of the right temporal bone. An ink-filled micropipette was then connected to a Pico-spritzer (General Valve) and inserted into the parietal cortex to a depth of 1.5 mm below the surface of the cortex; the pipette was slowly retracted with 15-ms pulses of ink at a pressure of 1.8 bar at each 0.25-mm interval. Upon completion of the injections, the animal was given a lethal dose of sodium pentobarbital (0.15 ml) and perfused as outlined above. The tissue was processed identically to that of the brains used for histology, and stained with buffered thionin. The distance between the pipette marks was recorded and the shrinkage factor was determined to be 9.2%.

PHOTOMICROGRAPHY

The Nissl-stained sections were photographed with a 4X Zeiss objective lens (planapochromat, NA0.13) on a Zeiss Photomicroscope III, using TechPan 100 (Kodak), and printed at X7.5. The subdivisions of the CN were observed in the microscope and outlined on the photographic prints of every other section in a complete series. The prints were then scanned into Adobe Photoshop. Following adjustments to equalize contrast and brightness uniformly throughout the series, the images, with the outlines superimposed, were printed at the same magnification illustrated in the atlas section of the "Results." The cytoarchitectonic terminology in the CN was based on Brawer et al. (1974) and Morest et al. (1990).

RESULTS

GENERAL ANATOMY OF THE MOUSE COCHLEAR NUCLEUS
(See Abbreviations, Table 19.1)

The CN of the mice used in this study is similar to that of other strains of mice as reported in previous studies (Webster and Trune, 1982; Willard and Ryugo, 1983). The CN lies on the lateral surface of the medulla, bounded dorsally by the lateral recess of the fourth ventricle, medially by the spinal trigeminal tract, and dorsomedially by the restiform body (inferior cerebellar peduncle). The CN is covered by the ependymal cells of the fourth ventricle on its dorsal aspect, and by pia mater from the taenia choroidea ventrally. The nucleus is divided into the dorsal, posteroventral, and anteroventral divisions (DCN, PVCN, and AVCN, respectively). The DCN is located dorsally with respect to the VCN, and the PVCN and AVCN are partitioned by the caudal aspect the cochlear nerve root, which enters on the ventral side of the CN. The somata of the cell types found in the mouse CN ranged in size from 4 μm in diameter (granule cells) to 25 μm (giant cells); neurons are divided into granule (4 to 7 μm), small (8 to 13 μm), and large (14 to 25 μm) cells, based on the diameter of the soma in the transverse plane (adopted from Morest et al., 1990).

DORSAL COCHLEAR NUCLEUS (DCN)

In the transverse plane, the mouse DCN is displaced somewhat caudodorsally with respect to the VCN. It appears slightly elongated along its anteroposterior axis, and its rostral end overlaps the

TABLE 19.1
Abbreviations in Figures

Brainstem Insets

6	Abducens nuc	mlf	Medial longitudinal fasciculus
7	Facial nuc	Mo5	Motor trigemninal nuc
7n	Facial nerve root	MVe	Medial vestibular nuc
8v	Vestibular nerve root	PB	Parabrachial nuc
8c	Cochlear nerve root	PCRt	Parvocellular reticular nuc
CGPn	Central gray pons	PF	Paraflocculus
CxIC	Caudal cortex inferior colliculus	Pn	Pontine reticular nuc
DCN	Dorsal cochlear nuc	Pr5	Principal sensory trigeminal nuc
DMTg	Dorsomedial tegmental area	PrH	Prepositus hypoglossal nuc
Fl	Flocculus	pyr	Pyramidal tract
g7	Genu facial nerve root	R	Raphe nuc
Gi	Gigantocellular reticular nuc	scp	Superior cerebellar peduncle
Int	Interposed cerebellar nuc	SOC	Superior olivary complex
icp	Inferior cerebellar peduncle	sol	Solitary nuc
Lat	Lateral cerebellar nuc	Sp5	Spinal trigeminal tract
LC	Locus coeruleus	Sp5O	Spinal trigeminal nuc, oral
LVe	Lateral vestibular nuc	SVe	Superior vestibular nuc
mcp	Middle cerebellar peduncle	Tg	Dorsal tegmental nuc
ml	Medial lemniscus		

Cochlear Nucleus (CN)

AS	Dorsal + intermediate acoustic striae	ML	Molecular layer
AVCNP	Anteroventral CN, posterior	FL	Fusiform layer
PV	Ventral part	PL	Polymorphic layer
PD	Dorsal part	PVCN	Posteroventral CN
AVCNA	Anteroventral CN, anterior	A	Anterior part
AA	Anterior part	AD	Anterodorsal part AV anteroventral part
AP	Posterior part	V	Ventral part
APD	Posterodorsal part	C	Central part
DAP	Dorsal part	D	Dorsal part
VAP	Ventral part	S	Small cell shell
bv	Blood vessel	TC	Taenia choroidea
DCN	Dorsal CN		

AVCN. In gross conformation, the DCN appears to be rotated slightly toward the lateral aspect of the CN, compared to other rodents. The DCN is bounded medially by the restiform body and laterodorsally by the lateral recess of the fourth ventricle and overlying flocculus rostrally and paraflocculus caudally. The superficial ependyma is continuous with the rest of the lateral recess of the fourth ventricle, extending to the taenia choroidea at the level of the internal lamella of the small cell shell, which separates the DCN and VCN. Beyond that point, the pia mater covers the VCN. The DCN is somewhat smaller in size than the VCN, but extends farther in the caudal plane, sometimes seeming to separate from the brainstem in the initial 20 to 30 μm of its caudal extent. The output tract for DCN, the dorsal acoustic stria (DAS), exits dorsomedially and runs in the medial direction above the vestibular complex. Neuronal elements are interspersed through the DAS — especially small and elongate neurons. As in other mammals, the mouse DCN is a laminated structure, and this pattern is evident throughout the anteroposterior axis. The mouse DCN can be divided into (1) the cell-poor superficial (molecular) layer, (2) the intermediate or fusiform cell layer, and (3) the deep or polymorphic layer.

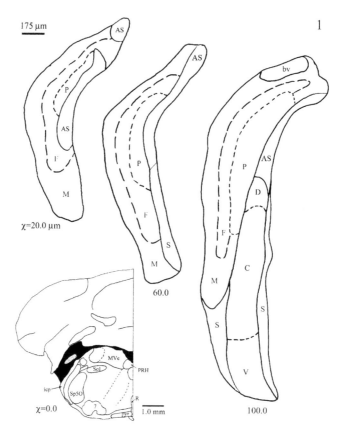

FIGURES 19.1 to 19.10 Cytoarchitectonic atlas of the mouse cochlear nucleus in the transverse plane. Figures are arranged with Nissl sections on one page and the parcellations of each section drawn on the preceding page. Nissl plates are ordered with the caudal section to the left; the numerals below each photomicrograph indicate the rostral distance from the caudal pole of the DCN (0.0 μm). Solid lines represent boundaries of the primary divisions, and dashed lines represent subdivisions. The axis at the bottom left of Figure 19.2 indicates the lateral (L) and dorsal (D) directions. Gray shading indicates the cochlear nucleus; black shows the fourth ventricle. Scale = 175 μm for the Cochlear Nucleus; scale = 1.0 mm for Brain Stem Insets. For abbreviations see Table 19.1.

Molecular Layer (ML; Figures 19.1 to 19.8)

The molecular layer (ML) appears as a half-shell, covering the deeper layers of the DCN. It is characterized by a low density of cellular elements and dense neuropil. Granule cells and small, oval neurons are scattered diffusely throughout this layer; some of the small cells exhibit circular profiles, containing a homogenous, lightly stained Nissl substance. The packing density of cartwheel cells, small to large or intermediate in size, is greatest at the margin of the fusiform and molecular layers. Some (~10%) small oval and small spherical cells possessed a "halo" of Nissl substance around the nucleus. Elongate neurons could also be found in this area just beneath the ependyma. The ML continues for the entire anteroposterior length of the DCN and wraps around the deeper layers at the rostral and caudal poles. It is bound ventromedially and dorsomedially by the small cell shell.

Fusiform (Intermediate) Layer (FL; Figures 19.1 to 19.6)

The fusiform layer (FL) (intermediate zone), otherwise known as the granular layer, of the DCN is a highly cellular region with a distinct band of tightly packed granule cells. The FL contains

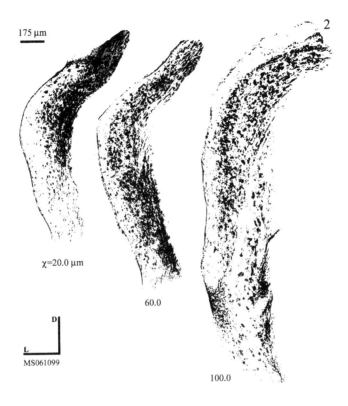

175 μm

χ=20.0 μm

60.0

D

L

MS061099

100.0

2

FIGURE 19.2

neurons of all size classes. The small cells of the FL are similar in appearance to those of the ML, with the exception of being more numerous and more variable in shape. The large cells are of two types. The first type is the characteristic principal cell of the FL, that is, the fusiform cell (also called the pyramidal cell), with an obvious large, spindle-shaped soma that ranges from 18 to 22 μm in diameter. The fusiform cells in the mouse are not consistently oriented and do not form a linear band. Many, but not all, fusiform cells are orientated with their long axis perpendicular to the ependymal surface. The Nissl substance of the fusiform cell is deeply stained, granular, and distributed through the entire cell body, occasionally forming dense aggregates that tend to be located in the apical portion of the cell. The apical dendrites of the fusiform cells extend into the ML and the basal dendrites, into the polymorphic layer. The nucleus is eccentric. Cartwheel cells also have a large, eccentric nucleus, but the smaller perikaryon is more lightly stained. Despite their multipolarity, one of the thick dendritic trunks is filled with Nissl-stained material and projects vertically into the ML. The FL is contiguous with the small cell shell at the lateral margin of the DCN/VCN boundary just medial to the taenia choroidea.

Polymorphic (Deep) Layer (PL; Figures 19.1 to 19.8)

This is the deepest cell layer of the DCN. It possesses several cell types, ranging in size from 4 μm (granule cells) to 25 μm (giant cells), with varying morphologies. The overall cell packing density is lower than that of the FL; however, the prevalence of small and large neurons is greater. The region flanking the DAS has a moderate density of elongate neurons with deeply stained Nissl substance and somata that are aligned between the tightly packed fibers coursing dorsomedially. Dendritic trunks well-stained for Nissl material give these cells a similar appearance to bipolar neurons, only with a more compressed cell body. An occasional small cell can be found in the DAS. The shape of these cells often seem to comply with the tight fiber bundles surrounding the cell; indeed, most small cells are slightly compressed and elongated. The granule cells of the PL

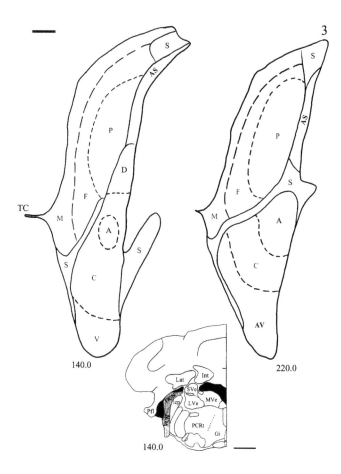

FIGURE 19.3

are evenly distributed and similar to those in other areas of the CN, with scant cytoplasm, and no dendrites evident in Nissl preparations. Small cells, including small stellate cells, are scattered about the PL and tend to form small aggregates, or cell clusters. This is especially true on the dorsal side of the small cell shell of the VCN. Morphologically, the small cells are either oval with intensely stained Nissl bodies, or spherical, with more lightly stained Nissl substance and, infrequently, a perinuclear rim. The large cells in the PL are diverse in morphology and size. The giant cell, the largest cellular element in the CN, ranges in size from 22 to 25 μm and is located in the central regions of the PL. The morphology of the giant cell body is saddle-like, with two to four dendritic appendages that tend to originate from polar ends of the cell, and the Nissl substance is evenly distributed. The nucleus is large, centrally placed, has a prominent nucleolus, and is frequently surrounded by a "cap" of Nissl bodies half-way around its circumference. Besides giant cells, the deep layer contains numerous vertical elongate neurons (corn cells). There are also a number of displaced fusiform cells. As reported by Martin (1981), these cells often occur in clusters of two to four cells, especially in the dorsomedial regions of the PL and at more rostral levels. A variety of large neurons occur, multipolar or spherical, more or less well-stained. These may represent varieties of giant cells, which have been described in the cat (Brawer et al., 1974; Kane, 1974), but we did not attempt to characerized them systematically.

Posteroventral Cochlear Nucleus (PVCN)

The PVCN is a heterogenous collection of cells of variable size and mixed packing density. It lies ventral to the DCN and posterior to the primary bifurcations of the cochlear nerve root. The primary

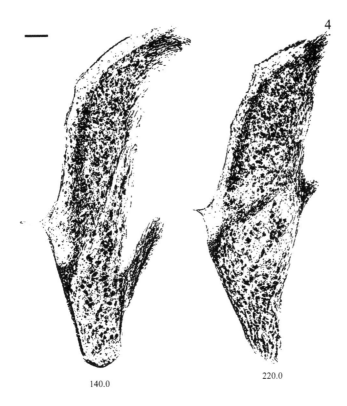

FIGURE 19.4

cytoarchitectonic regions include the ventral, dorsal, central, anterior, anteroventral, and anterodorsal parts. PVCN is surrounded more or less completely by the small cell shell.

Dorsal Part (D; Figures 19.1 to 19.4)

The dorsal part is marked by a high prevalance of large elongate neurons and other cells of small and large profile. Elongate cells found in D are among the largest cells with this geometric profile in the mouse CN. They are typically surrounded by fibers of the acoustic stria, and contain densely stained Nissl substance. The frequency of elongate cells decreases from the dorsal to the ventral areas. Small cells and some bushy neurons are found; the packing arrangement is consistent and relatively loose.

Central Part (C; Figures 19.1 to 19.4)

The central part is the octopus cell region of Osen (1969), so named because the primary neuronal type is represented by the octopus cell (Brawer et al., 1974). The octopus cell is large (15 to 18 μm) with heterogeneously stained Nissl substance and an eccentric nucleus. Thick dendritic trunks, when stained in Nissl preparations, often branch from the cell on each end of the soma, forming a crescent shape. In myelin preparations, many fibers course between each cell. Octopus cells do not appear in clusters; rather, they bask in solitary splendor amid a veritable sea of myelin. Other cells of C include small stellate neurons and occasional granule cells. Globular bushy cells begin to intermingle with the octopus cells more rostrally, marking the appearance of the anterior part of PVCN.

Ventral Part (V; Figures 19.1 to 19.4)

The ventral part in the mouse is small. It forms the ventral boundary of PVCN and is flanked rostrally by AV. The neurons of V are smaller than those of C. There are various types, including stellate, bushy, and granule cells. Granule cells are most conspicuous in the ventromedial region

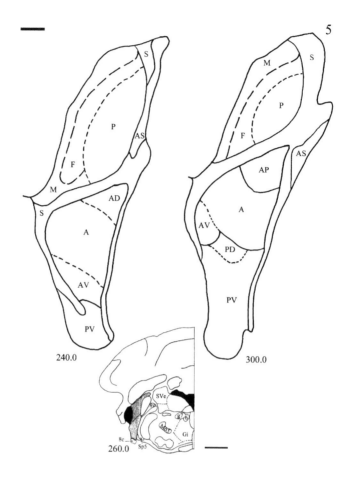

FIGURE 19.5

of V, where outcroppings of the small cell shell show up in more rostral sections. The cell packing density of V is similar to C, but again, neuronal size is significantly reduced.

Anteroventral Part (AV; Figures 19.3 to 19.6)

The anteroventral region has not been previously reported in other species. In the mouse, AV is characterized by small, ovoid cells of high packing density and irregular-to-intense Nissl staining. This group of cells appears to be predominantly small stellate and granule cells, with few bushy cells in the rostral region of AV. The small cells of AV become apparent 190 μm rostral to the caudal pole of DCN, and they continue to the posterior boundary of AVCN. On the lateral margin of AV, the cells of the small cell shell are interspersed so as to give the impression of a merger with this cell group (Figure 19.6, left). At its rostral tip, AV is displaced laterally against the shell and is bounded medially and ventrally by AVCN. An occasional small globular bushy cell can be found throughout AV, as well as octopus cells on the caudodorsal border of AV and C.

Anterior Part (A; Figures 19.3 to 19.6)

The anterior part is the largest subdivision in mouse PVCN and is characterized by a mixed population of cells ranging in size from small stellate cells (~8 μm) to displaced giant cells (~22 μm). Globular bushy cells are found in this region and tend to be arranged in clusters with smaller stellate neurons. Elongate neurons are common along the medial boarder of A, where this subdivision merges with fibers of the intermediate acoustic stria. The packing density of cells in

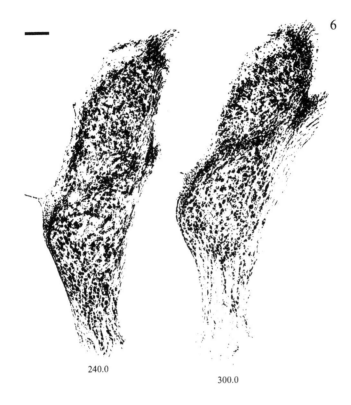

240.0

300.0

FIGURE 19.6

A is uniform through its central core, but increases slightly in lateral and rostral areas, where this division meets the shell and AVCN, respectively. As described in the chinchilla (Morest et al., 1990) and cat (Brawer et al., 1974), the myelinated fibers of A have the classic "whirling" appearance in Luxol fast blue and Sudan black preparations. These fibers constitute the majority of those in the descending branch of the auditory nerve, projecting to caudal cell groups.

Anterodorsal Part (AD; Figures 19.5 and 19.6)

This cell group is small and was not observed in all mice, but it had a very characteristic appearance when it was found. Overall, the neurons tend to have a greater packing density than is seen in *A* or *AP*. Some of the cells in AD are notably larger than those of A. AD is bounded laterally and dorsally by the small cell shell and medially by fibers of the acoustic stria.

Anteroventral Cochlear Nucleus (AVCN)

AVCN begins in the cochlear nerve root, includes the zone of bifurcations, and continues as the rostral-most division of the CN, associated with the ascending branch of the cochlear nerve. Its border with PVCN is formed by the caudal aspect of the cochlear nerve root. AVCN can be dichotomously parcellated into the posterior and anterior subdivisions, which contain the globular and spherical bushy neurons, respectively. The posterior division contains the posteroventral, posterodorsal parts. We did not identify the ventromedial part previously observed in the chinchilla (Morest et al., 1990). The anterior division contains the posterior, posterodorsal, and anterior parts.

Posterior Division (P; Figures 19.5 to 19.10)

The posterior division of AVCN, designated P, is comprised of globular bushy cells and stellate cells. In the ventral part of P, fibers of the cochlear nerve enter the CN and create a characteristic

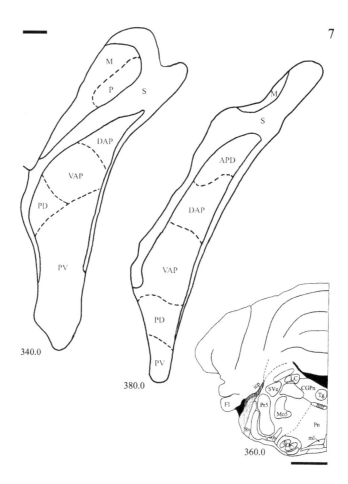

FIGURE 19.7

fascicular pattern of globular cell arrangement. The globular cells in the mouse are smaller than those in cat and chinchilla, have heterogeneously distributed Nissl substance, an eccentric nucleus, and a number of dendrites that can be seen in Nissl preparations as rising from many areas on the soma. These dendrites give the bushy cell a classic multipolar appearance. Stellate cells are frequently found in association with globular cells, although this is not a distinguishing characteristic of the posterior division. The stellate neurons are similar to those found in PVCN, but in AVCN their Nissl substance forms small aggregates; a prominent nucleolous is common in posterior division stellate cells. They also have a multipolar appearance, but differ from the bushy cells in having a more oval, even rectangular-shaped body. We did not examine the accessory nucleus of the cochlear nerve root (auditory nerve nucleus), because that requires a special dissection. This nucleus has already been nicely described in the mouse by the Spanish neuroanatomists (Lorente de Nó, 1926; López et al., 1993).

Ventral Part (PV; Figures 19.5 to 19.8)

This part of AVCN was formerly referred to as the interstitial nucleus of Lorente de Nó (1933) because of its characteristic fasciculated arrangement within the cochlear nerve root and the zone of bifurcations. Globular cells in PV are arranged in columns aligned with the fibers of the cochlear nerve. The cell columns contain between 3 and 15 cells; globular cells in the columns are smaller than those in the dorsal part of the posterior division. Stellate neurons are also encountered in the columns. The orientation of the cell bodies within the groups of cells is typically dorsoventral, but

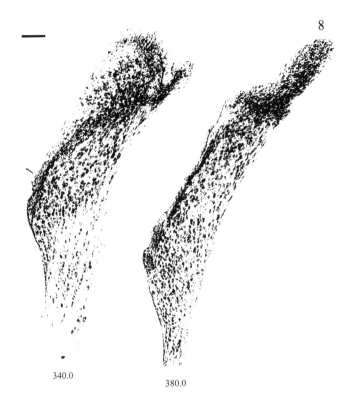

340.0

380.0

FIGURE 19.8

occasionally a neuron is tilted laterally and positioned in line with the fibers exiting the CN and projecting to the trapezoid body. Elongate cells are usually aligned with the exiting fibers to the trapezoid body. Occasional clusters of small cells (Hurd et al., 1999) are seen in this area, suggesting some continuity of the shell through the nerve root region (Figures 19.6, right; 19.8, left).

Dorsal Part (PD; Figures 19.5 to 19.10)

The dorsal part is easily recognized by a higher packing density of neurons than that seen in PV, and by the orientation of many cells in the centrifugal fibers streaming toward the trapezoid body. Stellate neurons are common components of this subdivision; they are evenly distributed throughout its rostrocaudal extent. Giant cells in the PD were not as clearly distinguished from other large cells on the basis of perikaryal size, unlike those in both cat and chinchilla.

Anterior Division (Figures 19.7 to 19.10)

The anterior division of AVCN consists of anterior and posterior parts. The anterior part (AA) in the mouse contains the spherical bushy cells, and a large contingent of medium and large stellate cells. The appearance and number of mouse AA spherical bushy cells in thionin sections differ from what has been reported for other mammals (Brawer et al., 1974; Moore and Osen, 1979; Disterhoft et al., 1980; Morest et al., 1990). Mouse spherical cells are fewer in number, smaller in size, less clearly spherical, and lack a perinuclear rim of Nissl substance. The pattern of Nissl staining is heterogeneous, with some cells staining more intensely than others. In fact, some spherical cells have very little stained Nissl material, making their delineation difficult. The spherical cells extend into the core of the anterior division, but not to the anterior pole. Unlike the cat and chinchilla, the stellate cells in the anterior division of the mouse are more common than bushy

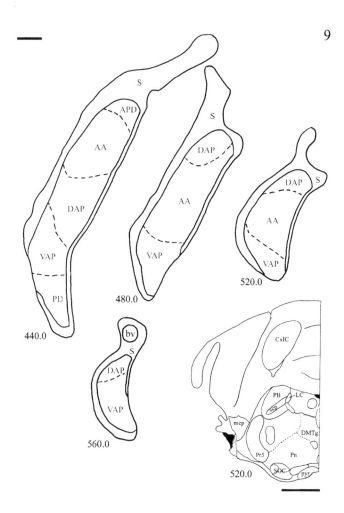

FIGURE 19.9

cells. The anterior division also has an extensive elaboration of the small cell shell along the dorsal regions where the DCN was located at more caudal levels. This part (subpeduncular corner of Mugnaini et al., 1980a) spreads in some areas up to 400 μm in the dorsomedial plane, forming a finger-like extension of the AVCN extending toward the vestibular nuclei.

Posterior Part (AP; Figures 19.5 to 19.10)

This part of AVCN has a moderate packing density of stellate neurons and spherical bushy cells. Of the three parts, AP comprises the greatest volume of AVCN. The cytoarchitecture of AP is dichotomous: the dorsal region (DAP) is comprised of larger stellate and spherical neurons with a homogeneous packing density. The staining pattern in DAP also tends to be more intense than the ventral region (i.e., VAP). In VAP, the stellate and spherical cells are smaller and more clustered in their distribution. The neurons in the ventral region of VAP are slightly smaller than in the dorsal area of VAP; however, the overall cell size is still less than in DAP. There is a cell-size continuum in AP, which was noted in all animals studied. This consisted of an increased somatic size in the areas central to the rostro-caudal axis, flanked by a decrease in the anterior and posterior extremities. Similar observations have been reported for the spherical cells in the chinchilla AVCN (Morest et al., 1990).

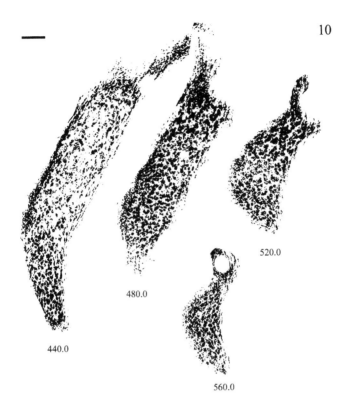

10

520.0

480.0

440.0

560.0

FIGURE 19.10

Posterodorsal Part (APD; Figures 19.7 to 19.10)

A small cluster of small stellate cells sits beneath the dorsal margin between the anterior part and the small cell shell; it has a very high packing density of cells with intensely stained Nissl substance. The frequency of spherical bushy cells is very low, and in some cases, cells were not readily identified as spherical cells. On the dorsal boundary of DAP, there were some granule cells, which may be slightly displaced from the overlying small cell shell.

Anterior Part (AA; Figures 19.9 and 19.10)

This region is the classic spherical cell domain. The principal neurons are the spherical bushy cells, and it is in AA that their morphological standard would usually be established. AA spherical cells are the largest in the entire AVCN and possess clumps of Nissl substance heterogeneously stained with thionin. No perinuclear cap is observed in the mouse spherical cells, as observed in the cat. A few stellate cells can also be found in this region, many of which possess a somewhat irregular shape. On the lateral margin, where AA meets the shell, some small neurons are evident, most likely representing small stellate cells and perhaps a few granule cells. It is noteworthy that AA in the mouse does not extend to the anterior pole and that the somatic shape of the spherical cells is not nearly as robust as it is in chinchilla, rat, and guinea pig. Nonetheless, the resident cell population is clearly analogous to AA in other mammals.

SMALL CELL SHELL

The small cell shell (Figures 19.1 to 19.10), including the so-called granular cell domain, is a large and complex component of the CN. The shell separates the DCN and VCN and essentially surrounds the VCN. In its lateral lamella, the shell appears to be stratified into three distinct layers. Accordingly, these layers have been described in the cat (Brawer et al., 1974) and chinchilla (Morest et al., 1990). A superficial plexiform layer, an intermediate granular layer with many more glial cells and granule cells than small stellate cells, and an inner stellate cell layer that contains small stellate neurons as well as some granule cells.

The shell forms a cap surrounding the VCN, albeit with some gaps in the medial lamella. A discontinuity exists where the cochlear nerve root enters the CN and physically displaces the small cells of the shell. However, the small cell clusters described by Hurd et al. (1999) can be found in this region. The small cells of the clusters are similar to those found in the stellate cell layer of the shell.

ATLAS OF THE MOUSE COCHLEAR NUCLEUS

A cytoarchitectonic atlas of the mouse cochlear nucleus was prepared from Nissl-stained mouse medulla (Figures 19.1 to 19.10). The figure plates are arranged as follows. The transverse thionin-stained sections (Figures 19.2, 19.4, 19.6, 19.8, 19.10), with the distance from the caudal pole indicated below each section, are faced on the opposite page by a cross-section of the brainstem at the rostro-caudal level indicated below the drawing (Figures 19.1, 19.3, 19.5, 19.7, 19.9). Major landmarks are outlined and labeled for orientation. All figures are drawn to the scale indicated by the scale bar on each page. Scales are noted in the figure legends.

DISCUSSION

The cytoarchitectonic atlas of the mouse cochlear nucleus was prepared from Nissl-stained material in the transverse plane. Cytoarchitectonic criteria included somatic size and shape, cell packing density, and the appearance of Nissl staining in the cytoplasm. The Nissl observations were supplemented with myelin-stained sections (Sudan black). The cytoarchitectonic subdivisions were readily compared to those previously described in the cat (Brawer et al., 1974) and chinchilla (Morest et al., 1990).

The CN is divided into the dorsal, posteroventral, and anteroventral regions. The DCN consists of a deep, or pleiomorphic layer, the fusiform cell layer, and an external neuropil, or molecular layer. PVCN is subdivided into ventral, dorsal, central, anteroventral, and anterior parts, while the AVCN is parcellated into posterior and anterior divisions. The posterior division contains the ventral and dorsal parts, and the anterior division is comprised of the posterior, posterodorsal, and anterior parts. Each subdivision was considered analogous to those described in the cat and chinchilla, based on cytoarchitectonic criteria.

The present scheme proposed for the mouse compares with previous architectural schemes in general use. Osen (1969) developed a system of nomenclature derived from categorizing Nissl-stained cell types that dominated a given region. This parcellation scheme is relatively simple, but it has a disadvantage in that it lumps together a number of different types of neurons which actually are spatially distinct. Taking advantage of this circumstance, subsequent, more detailed descriptions of cytoarchitecture and morphology were possible, using a variety of neurohistological techniques, including Golgi, Nissl, reduced silver methods, as well as immunohistochemstry and electron microscopy (for a review, see Morest, 1993). The nomenclature was developed based on topography. The resulting architectural schemes have provided a finer resolution of more coherent cell popuations useful for anatomical and physiological analyses which address the roles of specific types of neurons in studies of structure/function relations. The higher resolution and greater homogenity is also useful for navigating and identifying common structures within and between orders of animals.

The first descriptions of the mouse CN were provided by Ramón y Cajal (1909) and Lorente de Nó (1933). However, their observations were amalgamated with those of other rodents. Ross (1965), Taber-Pierce (1967), and Sidman et al. (1971) have reported on the mouse CN in Nissl-stained material, but they did not provide a systematic mapping. Martin described the anatomy of the mouse CN and applied Osen's cytoarchitectonic terminology to Luxol Fast Blue-cresyl violet stained tissue, as well as some of the patterns of histogenesis in the mouse CN (Martin and Rickets, 1981). While investigating neonatal development and noise deprivation, Webster and Webster (1977) have also provided a parcellation of the mouse CN based on Osen's nomenclature, as did Browner and Baruch (1982) in the DCN. To date, the most comprehensive anatomical description of the mouse CN has come from Webster and Trune (1982), based on Nissl-stained and Golgi-impregnated material. Their work summarized a number of the cell types found in the mouse CN, including a description of "Purkinje-like" cells in the DCN. As with the preceding studies on mouse CN, Webster and Trune (1982) utilized the cytoarchitectonic nomenclature of Osen. Nevertheless, there are no cytoarchitectonic atlases available for the mouse that have employed the detailed parcellation scheme and nomenclature of Brawer et al. (1974).

A number of anatomical observations made in the mouse deviate considerably from those reported in other rodents and mammals. The gross conformation of the CN is variable among rodents. Most notably, the DCN of the mouse sits relatively dorsal, and not so much dorsomedial with respect to the VCN, as is the case, for example, in the guinea pig (personal observations). In other words, it is displaced dorsorostrally with respect to the VCN, and rotated slightly laterally on its longitudinal axis, compared to other rodents The chinchilla DCN also sits more dorsomedial with respect to the VCN. In the cat and the human, on the other hand, the DCN occupies a more caudal location with respect to the VCN. These differences may result from anatomical variations in the structure of the cranium, or they may reflect functional and structural demands that the DCN requires in its own ontogenic and phyletic development.

The lamination of the DCN in the guinea pig is much more clear than that in the mouse. The DCN is somewhat more laminated in the chinchilla than in the mouse. In the cat, the lamination of DCN is very well developed. However, in the human, it is hardly even apparent. This may reflect species differences in the underlying synaptic organization of the neuronal components. But, in any case, the prevalence of displaced fusiform cells reflects a less well coordinated migration of these neurons during development in the mouse and the human. It is tempting to argue that lamination is correlated with structural evolution, but the directionality of such evolutionary changes could only be surmised. Cortical structures may provide a basis for synaptic organization of different exogenous inputs in relation to the local circuitry. For example, cochlear inputs to the basal dendrites and soma of the fusiform cells are situated so that they might interact with the inhibitory synapses formed by local interneurons, such as the projections from cartwheel cells and the recurrent collaterals of corn cells (Brawer et al., 1974; Kane, 1974). However, a more complex brain system does not necessarily equate with stratification of the individual components.

Perhaps the most striking morphological feature of the mouse CN is the overall size of the neurons themselves. Not only are the neuronal somata of the mouse much smaller than those previously described in common rodents, but their size range is much more compressed, making size a less useful criterion for defining different cell types. For example, the giant cells as a category were not readily discriminated from large projection neurons, such as stellate and globular cells throughout the CN. Another example is especially apparent in PVCN. In PVCN-V, the neurons are generally somewhat smaller than those found in the same subdivision of other rodents. However, in regions just rostral to PVCN-V (see Figure 19.4), the cell size decreases dramatically, and the packing density increases. This region, which we called the anteroventral (AV) part of PVCN, contains the smallest population of cells in this subdivision, except for granule cells. This is quite surprising in view of the tonotopic organization of the CN. Descending fibers from the mouse cochlear nerve enter the PVCN and synapse with bushy cells and stellate cells in a frequency-mapped fashion: high-frequency fibers remain in the dorsal regions and low-frequency fibers synapse in more ventral areas (Willott, 1983). Correlations between a cell's size and its best frequency suggested that high-frequency-sensitive cells tend to have smaller diameters compared to lower frequency-sensitive cells (e.g., Willard and Ryugo, 1983). The hearing range of the mouse is shifted to a higher frequency range compared to some other rodents (Ehret, 1983b). It may be that this frequency shift is responsible for the small cell size in the typical low-frequency regions of PVCN. Could there be subdivisions analogous to AV in chinchilla and cat? This remains to be determined. However, if these other species have an AV, it is unlikely to be as well developed as in the mouse. On the other hand, we did not find the posterior part of PVCN in the mouse, as previously described in cat and chinchilla. Because this cell group consists of only a few cells in these larger species, it may be that its representation in the mouse was so tiny as to escape notice. Perhaps for the same reason, we failed to find the ventromedial part of AVCN, previously described in the chinchilla (Morest et al., 1990). After all, size is perhaps the most impressive difference between the CN of these species. This applies not only to the overall volume of the CN and the volumes of the subdivisions, but also to the sizes of the constituent neurons, all being much smaller in the mouse.

The small cell shell is well developed in the mouse. The PVCN is fully bounded dorsally, dorsomedially, and laterally to the shell. This is typical for terrestrial mammals (Glendenning and Masterton, 1998). There is evidence that the shell may have been, either phyletically or developmentally, continuous around the ventral portions of PVCN as well. In the mouse CN, the shell continues some distance ventromedially into parts of the VCN, and medial to this there are small cell clusters. The small cell clusters in AVCN-PV, like those in the chinchilla (Hurd et al., 1999), are formed by the interrupting fascicles of the cochlear nerve, leaving only "islands" of very small stellate neurons similar to those in the rest of the shell. Presumably, the small cell clusters are a categorical continuation of the lateral and medial lamellae of the small cell shell.

The anterior portions of AVCN are sometimes referred to as the spherical cell region (Hackney et al., 1990), so named because the principal neuron in cats and guinea pigs have spherical cell bodies. These cells correspond to the spherical bushy cell in the cat (Brawer and Morest, 1975) and presumably in the mouse (Webster and Trune, 1982; D.K. Morest, unpublished). In the mouse, as in other species, the spherical bushy cells receive large end-bulb synapses from cochlear nerve fibers and presumably project to a poorly developed medial superior olivary complex, where they might participate in the computation of interaural time differences that are potentially useful in localization of low-frequency sounds in some mammals. In the mouse, however, as we and others (Webster and Trune, 1982) have observed, the spherical bushy cells in AVCN, and more especially those in the presumed low-frequency region of AA, do not display the quintessential features that characterize the more stereotypical spherical bushy cells of the cat and chinchilla. They tend to be smaller, less numerous, and often not very spherical. The Nissl method stains the cytoplasm only faintly and no perinuclear cap stands out. No doubt, all of these features reflect the murine deficiencies in low-frequency hearing and localization (e.g., see Ehret, 1983b). Be that as it may, it is only to challenge future studies to show what adaptive functions are expressed by the bushy cells of the mouse.

In this study, we provide a detailed cytoarchitectonic atlas of the mouse CN in the transverse plane. The comparative similarities and differences that have been noted should be verified by other anatomical analysis, including impregnation for the visualization of neuronal dendritic and axonal arborizations. Furthermore, it wll be of interest to compare the cytoarchitecture of the CN in different strains of mice, including mutants and transgenics, to determine what differences there are and how these may relate to phenotype. Based on previous experience (see, e.g., Morest and Winer, 1986), we are encouraged to believe that analogous, and presumably homologous, cell types and cell groups can be identified and compared between strains and species. Knowledge of the specific connections and physiological properties of well-characterized cell types and cell groups in mice should lead to new insights into structure and function and their contributions to hearing disorders.

SUMMARY

A cytoarchitectonic atlas of the mouse cochlear nucleus (CN) was constructed by identifying cell populations analogous to those described previously in the cat, chinchilla, and guinea pig. The atlas is based on Nissl-stained, serial sections in the transverse plane. The overall cell size in the CN is quite small compared to that of other mammals, but the main nuclear groups can be readily discerned. The dorsal CN (DCN), anteroventral CN (AVCN), and posteroventral CN (PVCN) divisions have about the same relative sizes as in other rodents. Although the DCN is clearly laminated, it is displaced dorsorostrally with respect to the VCN, and rotated slightly laterally on its longitudinal axis, compared to other rodents. The VCN is surrounded by a well-developed small cell shell, which contains a high concentration of granule cells and numerous small stellate neurons. Most of the neuronal cell types previously described in other species could be identified in the DCN and VCN of the mouse. However, some of them (e.g., spherical bushy cells) may be less distinctly differentiated than in the cat or chinchilla. There appears to be a less well-developed population of projection neurons in the low-frequency region of the AVCN. This correlates with the relative lack of low-frequency hearing in the mouse. This atlas is intended to serve as a reference to facilitate pursuit of modern studies on the structure, function, and biochemistry of specific cell populations and cell types in the mouse CN. It should also provide the basis for comparisons between the mouse and other species.

ACKNOWLEDGMENTS

Supported by NIH grants R01DC00127 (DKM) and T32DC00025 (JT). We thank Drs. Susan Muly and Eleanor Josephson for advice.

20 Functional Circuitry of the Cochlear Nucleus: *In Vitro* Studies in Slices

Michael J. Ferragamo and Donata Oertel

INTRODUCTION

The mouse, like all vertebrates, critically examines acoustic patterns that reveal where events arise in the environment and what they represent. A central question concerns what are the important features of sounds for the detection, localization, and interpretation of external events and how those features are detected by the nervous system. Incoming sound is transformed by the sensory epithelium of the cochlea into temporal firing patterns across the tonotopic array of auditory nerve fibers. The cochlear nucleus, the obligate terminal for auditory nerve fibers, serves as the initial platform to begin deciphering this code, a duplex of time and frequency, and rebuilding its elements into a coherent image of the external world. Whereas much is known about auditory behaviors and abilities in mice (e.g., Chapters 1 through 7), we can also look to behavioral/psychophysical studies in other mammals to help interpret results obtained with *in vitro* methods in the mouse auditory system. For example, bats with a similar head size and audiogram to the mouse, can precisely localize and orient toward prey during flight; and in discriminating among prey, they rely on patterns of frequency and amplitude modulations, similar to those measured in natural speech signals (reviewed in Moss and Schnitzler, 1996). These behaviors suggest that mammals have evolved sophisticated mechanisms for examining spatiotemporal firing patterns to interpret sounds before choosing an appropriate response. The circuitry of the cochlear nuclei described in this chapter is the foundation of those mechanisms.

A series of electrophysiological and anatomical studies done in mice over the past two decades has revealed some patterns in biophysical properties and anatomical connections that are common to all mammals. Much of the work in this chapter describes intracellular recordings from specific cell types in slices of the cochlear nucleus from the mouse (see Appendix at the end of this chapter). This technique enables a well-controlled approach for studying intrinsic conductances and for elucidating functional circuitry that obviates the associated technical problems of intracellular recording *in vivo*. One commissural and six ascending pathways emerge in parallel from specific cell types in the cochlear nucleus (Figure 20.1). Each can be typified by its association with incoming auditory nerve fibers and by its interconnection with other groups of cells within the cochlear nucleus and by its projections, and in some cases, by specialized anatomical and biophysical characteristics that customize it for performing a specific function. The morphology, intrinsic responses, and synaptic responses of most of the cell types described in this chapter are summarized in Figures 20.2, 20.3, and 20.4, respectively.

The mammalian cochlear nuclear complex is divided into two subdivisions, a ventral cochlear nucleus (VCN) with anteroventral and posteroventral divisions (see Chapters 18 and 19) and a dorsal cochlear nucleus (DCN). The VCN comprises pathways specialized for preserving the temporal firing patterns from the auditory nerve and for faithful transmission of those patterns to other nuclei in the brainstem and midbrain. Auditory nerve fibers in mammals can discharge action potentials at

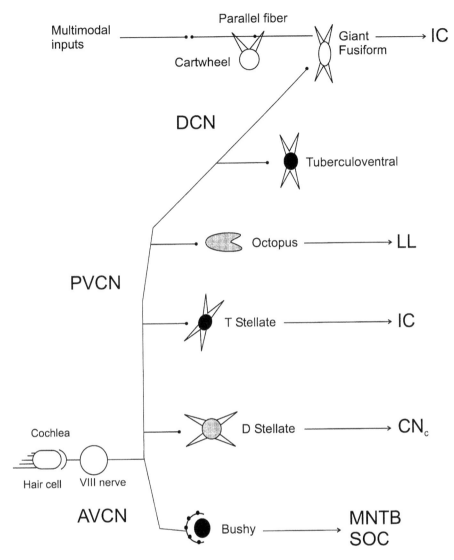

FIGURE 20.1 A schematic representation of different cell types of the cochlear nucleus showing the excitatory inputs and the auditory areas to which they project. The shading of the filled cells indicates tuning width: the black cells are narrowly tuned and the gray cells are widely tuned. Auditory nerve fibers bifurcate, the ascending branch innervates bushy cells (calyceal terminal indicated by arc) and T stellate cells located in the anterior ventral cochlear nucleus (AVCN). The descending branch innervates T stellate and octopus cells in the posteroventral cochear nucleus (PVCN), and continues into the deep layer of the dorsal cochlear nucleus (DCN) where its terminals contact dendrites of tuberculoventral and giant fusiform cells. D stellate cells are distributed throughout the VCN. Parallel fibers, the axons of granule cells, innervate the dendrites of DCN interneurons, cartwheel cells, and its projection neurons, giant and fusiform cells. Projections are to inferior colliculus (IC), lateral lemniscus (LL), contralateral cochlear nucleus (CN$_c$), medial nucleus of the trapezoid body (MNTB) and the superior olivary complex (SOC). (From Gardner, S.M., Trussell, L.O., and Oertel, D., *J. Neurosci.*, 19, 8721-8729, With permission. Copyright 1999 by The Society for Neuroscience.)

the same phase of a waveform up to about 4000 Hz. The time-of-occurrences in the sequence of action potentials can be transformed into an estimate of sound source location, or alternatively, be transformed to the frequency domain by accumulating a count of the intervals between discharges. There is much similarity in the organization and properties of these timing pathways across birds,

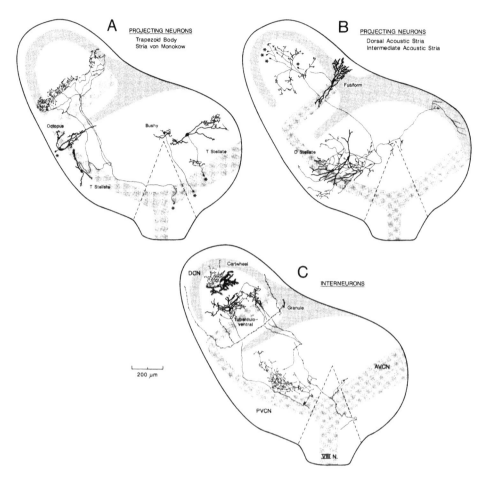

FIGURE 20.2 Reconstructions of cochlear nuclear neurons intracellularly labeled with HRP and positioned in an idealized parasaggital slice. Dendrites are shown with thick lines, axons are shown with thin lines, and the point where the axon was cut is indicated by an *. An idealized isofrequency laminae of auditory nerve fibers is indicated with fine stippling, and the areas that contain many granule cells, the granule regions and the fusiform layer, are indicated with coarse stippling. (From Oertel, D., Wickesberg, R.E., 1996. In Ainsworth, W.A., Evans, E.F., Hackney, C.M. (Eds.) *Advances in Speech, Hearing and Language Processing*, JAI, London, 293-321. With permission.)

reptiles, and mammals (Oertel, 1999). The dorsal cochlear nucleus (DCN) has many features in common with cerebellum, and molecular and electrophysiological evidence suggests a shared lineage between the two structures (Berrebi et al., 1990; Berrebi and Mugnaini, 1991; Manis et al., 1994; Zhang and Oertel, 1993a; Golding and Oertel, 1996; 1997). The eclectic mix of inputs to the DCN foreshadows its place in integrating audition with cues from other sensory modalities, and subsequently referring that information to the midbrain. Correlation of multisensory spatial information would enhance accuracy in orienting the body and in directing visual attention to acoustic signals.

INTRINSIC CIRCUITRY OF THE VCN

TIMING PATHWAYS: OCTOPUS CELLS

Octopus cells form a circuit that signals synchronous discharges of auditory nerve fibers to targets in the superior paraolivary nucleus and to the ventral nucleus of the lateral lemniscus. While the

Neurons Vary in their Electrical Properties

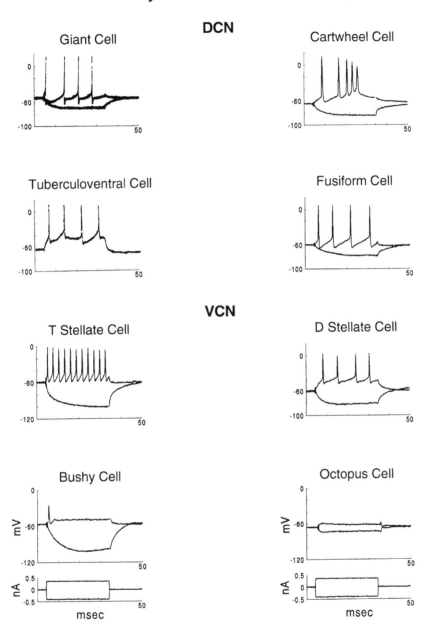

FIGURE 20.3 Voltage changes produced by symmetrical depolarizing and hyperpolarizing current pulses (stimuli plotted at bottom) in intracellularly labeled cells in the mouse cochlear nucleus. Giant, tuberculoventral, and fusiform cells of the DCN and D stellate cells of the VCN fire large action potentials followed by a fast and a slower undershoot. Cartwheel cells fire complex action potentials with a regenerative, slow calcium current that triggers a burst of action potentials generated by an inward sodium current. T stellate cells fire action potentials with a single, brief undershoot. Bushy and octopus cells fire one action potential when they are depolarized and remain steadily depolarized by a few millivolts. In contrast, the large hyperpolarization to a hyperpolarizing current of equal magnitude is indicative of a strong rectification (see Figure 20.5).

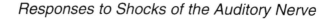

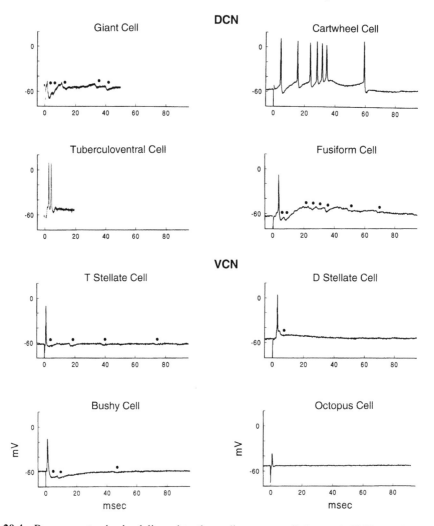

FIGURE 20.4 Responses to shocks delivered to the auditory nerve. Polysnaptic IPSPs are indicated by a filled circle. Late glycinergic IPSPs in giant and fusiform cells mirror the firing pattern of cartwheel cells. Giant cells are dominated by early inhibition, presumably from tuberculoventral cells. Disynaptic inhibition in T stellate and bushy cells arises from tuberculoventral cells that are probably tuned to similar frequencies. D stellate cells are the source of late glycinergic inhibition to both VCN and DCN cells.

integrative role of this pathway is not completely understood, it has been suggested that the ventral nuclei of the lateral lemniscus may play a role in pattern recognition (Covey and Casseday, 1991). The octopus cell area has a sharply defined border that can be visualized by the absence of glycine-positive puncta (Wickesberg et al., 1991; 1994). Aptly named, thick dendrites always emanate from the rostral pole of the soma and spread anteriorly in mice (Figure 20.2) (Willard and Ryugo, 1983; Oertel et al., 1990; Willott and Bross, 1990; Golding et al., 1995; 1999). Willott and Bross (1990) have estimated that there are about 200 octopus cells in each ventral cochlear nucleus in mice. Fascicles carrying the descending branches of myelinated type I auditory nerve fibers are bundled tightly as they travel through the octopus cell area on their way to the DCN. Dendrites of octopus cells are arranged orthogonal to the tonotopic axis. Without exception in mice, dendrites of octopus cells are oriented proximally across low-frequency fibers and distally across high frequency fibers (Willard and Ryugo, 1983; Oertel et al., 1990; Willott and Bross, 1990; Golding et al., 1995; 1999). *In vitro*, recruitment of auditory nerve inputs is apparent in the graded appearance of excitatory postsynaptic potentials (EPSPs) in response to electrical stimuli at the auditory nerve that vary incrementally in strength (Golding et al., 1995). Octopus cells fire action potentials only when multiple small increments sum. In cats, in which recordings from octopus cells have been made *in vivo*, the requirement of convergent input from many auditory nerve fibers is reflected in the responses of octopus cells to sounds (Godfrey et al., 1975; Britt and Starr, 1976; Rhode et al., 1983a; Rhode and Smith, 1986a). Octopus cells are broadly tuned, have a high threshold to pure tone-bursts, respond robustly to clicks, and prefer frequency-modulated signals sweeping in the direction from low to high frequency (Godfrey et al., 1975; Rhode and Smith, 1986a; Joris et al., 1992).

Forming a major ascending pathway from the VCN, the axons of octopus cells course through the intermediate acoustic stria, terminating in endbulbs at the contralateral ventral nucleus of the lateral lemniscus (VNLL) (Vater and Feng, 1990; Smith et al., 1993b; Adams, 1997; Schofield and Cant, 1997; Vater et al., 1997). Octopus cells also ascend to the superior paraolivary complex, primarily contralaterally (Schofield, 1995). Terminals from intrinsic collaterals are observed among granule cells and other octopus cells, and less commonly among cells in the deep layers of the DCN (Golding et al., 1995). The presence of endbulb synapses in the VNLL suggests a circuit involved in maintaining temporal patterns of electrical signals. Accordingly, the responses to acoustic signals *in vivo* or electrical stimulation *in vitro* are strikingly similar between octopus cells and cells of the VNLL (Golding et al., 1995; Adams, 1997; Covey and Casseday, 1991; Wu, 1999). Octopus cells and their targets in the VNLL respond preferentially to transients and broadband sounds, and do so by firing a single precisely time action potential at the onset of the stimulus, a temporal response pattern classified as Onset-i (Godfrey et al., 1975; Rhode, 1998; Feng et al., 1994). A short integration time enables octopus cells to entrain to clicks or tones at every cycle at frequencies up to almost 1 kHz while maintaining a constant latency (Rhode and Smith, 1986a; Smith et al., 1993b; Joris et al., 1992). Functionally, the hypertrophy of the VNLL in both bats and humans suggests that this brainstem pathway plays a role in the analysis of temporal features, presumably for the recognition of acoustic patterns such as speech and echolocation signals (Covey and Casseday, 1991; Adams, 1997; Vater et al., 1997). In cats, it has been demonstrated that octopus cells show the most robust synchronization to the fundamental of single formant speech sounds among all of the cell types of the VCN (Rhode, 1998).

The intrinsic properties of octopus cells embody features specialized for fast and precise signal transmission (Golding et al., 1995; 1999). In slices of cochlear nuclei of mice, stimulation of the auditory nerve evokes suprathreshold EPSPs that are rapid and can entrain with a constant latency to shocks delivered at a rate that exceeds the range of naturally occurring auditory nerve discharges (Figure 20.5). The jitter in the timing of such discharges has a standard deviation of between 20 and 40 µs (Golding et al., 1995). Octopus cells discharge a single action potential in response to steps of injected current. Their input resistance and membrane time constant are on average about 6 MΩ and 200 µs, respectively, perhaps making octopus cells the fastest in the brain (Golding et al., 1995; 1999; Bal and Oertel, 2000). The low input resistance is traced to a hyperpolarization-activated, mixed cationic conductance, g_h, and a low-threshold, depolarization-activated potassium conductance, g_{KLT}. The currents through these two conductances, the inward I_h and outward I_{KLT}, are balanced at rest. Like other cells of the VCN, the receptors that detect firing of auditory nerve fibers have rapid rates of activation and deactivation, producing rapidly rising and falling excitatory synaptic currents (Gardner et al., 1999). Large synaptic currents, boosted only slightly by sodium and calcium conductances, are necessary to counteract the large membrane conductances to generate action potentials. The high resting conductance attenuates action potentials as they spread from the point where they are generated, presumably at the axon hillock, to the soma where they are recorded. The small size at the soma insures that the timing of the peak of synaptic activation is not distorted.

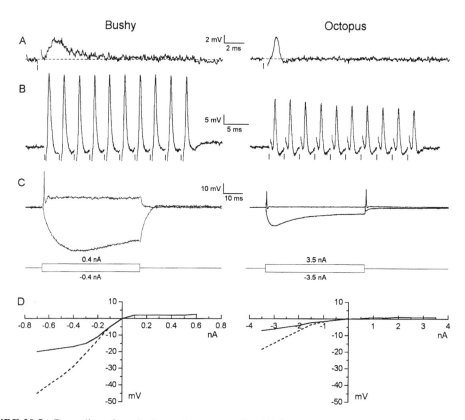

FIGURE 20.5 Recordings from bushy and octopus cells. (A) Synaptic responses to auditory nerve stimulation are brief. (B) Well-timed responses to a 300-Hz train of shocks. (C) Asymmetrical responses to depolarizing and hyperpolarizing current pulses. A low-threshold K⁺ conductance is activated in the depolarizing range, making responses brief and preventing repetitive firing. (D) Plot of voltage change at steady state (solid line) as a function of injected current. The flat appearance in the depolarizing voltage range is where input resistances are low. Peak hyperpolarizations are indicated with broken lines, and the levels at the end of 50 ms are shown with solid lines. (From Oertel, D., 1997, *Neuron*, 19, 959-962. With permission.)

A functional property of strong outward rectification is that octopus cells fire within a narrow temporal window when depolarized rapidly, but fail to fire when depolarized slowly. This sensitivity has been examined by systematically changing the rate of depolarization by injecting ramps of current at varying speeds (Ferragamo and Oertel, 1998a). Action potential initiation depends on the rate of change of membrane potential, and as a consequence, even large currents fail to be suprathreshold when increased slowly. The activation of the potassium rectifying conductance, $g_{KLT,}$ under slow conditions, prevents the sodium conductance from becoming regenerative. Computational modeling supports the idea that g_{KLT} is primarily responsible for the onset response, and that its behavior cannot be described by a static membrane conductance (Cai et al., 2000).

The low input resistance of octopus cells guarantees that synaptic responses to activation of individual auditory nerve fibers will be brief and small. To activate octopus cells, inputs distributed throughout the extensive dendritic tree must deliver especially large currents to the spike initiation zone. Because many, small, subthreshold inputs are required to drive action potentials, octopus cells serve as coincidence detectors for convergent activity from auditory nerve fibers. Octopus cells are well designed to detect common interspike intervals among a population of incoming auditory nerve fibers, and therefore may be an initial temporal processor in encoding the periodicity of complex sounds (Golding et al., 1995).

Timing Pathways: Bushy Cells

A well-studied timing specialist is the mammalian bushy cell of the anterior ventral cochlear nucleus (AVCN). Bushy cells are anatomically distinctive in that they are the targets of calyceal terminals from one to a few auditory nerve fibers. Calyceal endings, also known as endbulbs, blanket the bushy cell body, and present multiple release sites to ensure the release and detection of the release of large amounts of neurotransmitter. As a consequence, bushy cells transmit faithfully the signaling of their auditory nerve inputs, avoiding the slowing that dendritic transmission would impose. In all mammals, bushy cells generally have one or a few primary dendrites that branch profusely and are only sparsely innervated (Figure 20.2) (Brawer et al., 1974; Cant and Morest, 1979b; Wu and Oertel, 1984). These morphological features are shared with principal cells in the medial nucleus of the trapezoid body (MNTB) and the VNLL, and in nonmammalian homologues in reptiles and birds.

Mammals have three types of bushy cells that are distinguished by their targets in the superior olivary complex. Large, spherical bushy cells are found in the anterior AVCN. They are engulfed by large endbulbs from a few auditory nerve fibers and project to the medial superior olivary nucleus (Smith et al., 1993a). Those found in the posterior division appear globular, receive inputs through smaller endbulbs, and project to the medial nucleus of the trapezoid body (Cant and Morest, 1979b; Tolbert and Morest, 1982; Smith et al., 1991; Spirou et al., 1990; Vater and Feng, 1990). This group provides excitation to the ispilateral lateral superior olivary nucleus (Cant and Casseday, 1986). The range of frequency tuning represented by large spherical and globular bushy cells overlap, but is skewed to low frequencies in large spherical bushy cells and to high frequencies in globular bushy cells (Liberman, 1991; Smith et al., 1991; 1993a). Small spherical bushy cells, like globuluar bushy cells, are presumably skewed to higher frequencies as are their targets in the lateral superior olive.

In mice, the distinction between these types of bushy cells is not very clear. No detectable differences have been observed in intracellularly labeled bushy cells. In Nissl-stained tissue, some spherical and globular bushy cells can be identified with considerable confidence but others cannot unambiguously be distinguished from one another or from multipolar cells. At the anterior pole of the nucleus, auditory nerve fibers form larger calyceal endings than more posteriorly. Presumably, the bushy cells that are the targets of these terminals correspond to the large spherical cells but they are not as distinctive in Nissl-stained tissue as in cats (Cant and Morest, 1979b; Willard and Ryugo, 1983). In mice, the number of large spherical cells seems to be small, in accordance with the small size of the medial superior olive. More posteriorly, some bushy cells have the typical oval cell bodies and eccentric nuclei. Small spherical bushy cells have not specifically been identified in mice, but they are presumably intermingled among the globular bushy cells. The mouse audiogram spans well into the ultrasonic range, thus one would expect that globular and small spherical bushy cells are more common than large spherical bushy cells, but anatomically they are not sufficiently distinct in mice for reliable estimates to be made of their relative proportions.

Shocks to the auditory nerve evoke large EPSPs with well-timed peaks (Figure 20.5). It has been estimated that roughly four to seven inputs converge on one bushy cell, with some being subthreshold (Oertel, 1983; 1985; Wu and Oertel, 1984). The peaks of EPSPs are precisely timed, with the standard deviation of the latency from the beginning of a train of identical shocks being between 20 and 40 µs.

Synaptic excitation is mediated through glutamate receptors with uniquely rapid kinetics. The α-amino-3-hydroxy-5-methyl-4-isoxazoleproprionic acid (AMPA) class of glutamate receptor mediates fast excitatory transmission in mammalian bushy cells (Isaacson and Walmsley, 1995; Gardner et al., 1999) as well as in their avian homologues, neurons of nucleus magnocellularis (nMAG) (Zhang and Trussell, 1994). AMPA receptors studied in the cells of the nMAG restrict excitatory postsynaptic currents (EPSCs) to a short duration by opening briefly, and desensitizing at a rate that is rapid in comparison to non-auditory regions (Raman et al., 1994; reviewed in

Trussell, 1997; 1999). Auditory nerve stimulation evokes brief EPSCs in bushy cells and octopus cells in the mouse cochlear nucleus (Gardner et al., 1999).

Bushy cells have intrinsic electrical properties well suited to preserving and conveying the timing of their inputs from the auditory nerve. The intrinsic conductances of bushy cells have properties similar to octopus cells, and are part of a recurring motif among vertebrate auditory neurons considered as timing specialists (reviewed in Oertel, 1997; 1999; Trussell, 1999). Bushy cells typically fire one action potential when depolarized with injected current (Figures 20.4 and 20.5) (Oertel, 1983; 1985; Manis and Marx, 1991). The current-voltage relationship reveals a low input resistance resulting from an outwardly rectifying current in the physiological voltage range in mouse bushy cells (Figure 20.5) (Oertel, 1983) and in nMAG (Reyes et al., 1994; Zhang and Trussel, 1994; Trussell, 1999). Intrinsic outward currents reduce the ensuing voltage changes from synaptic currents and prevent repetitive firing. The consequences of a low input resistance mandate that a large current be delivered to the synapse to bring the cell to threshold and place a constraint on the variability in threshold crossing to a minimum, functionally narrowing the jitter in latency. Voltage-clamp has revealed the presence of at least two potassium currents underlying outward rectification in rat bushy cells (Manis and Marx, 1991) and in chick nMAG (Rathouz and Trussell, 1998). The characteristic single discharge is transformed into repetitive firing subsequent to application of blockers specific for the low threshold, voltage-activated potassium current, K_{LT} (Manis and Marx, 1991; Rathouz and Trussell, 1998).

The firing patterns of bushy cells *in vivo* in response to sound have not been recorded in mice, but in all species in which such recordings have been made, their firing reflects their input from the auditory nerve and their firing is referred to as "primary-like." Their firing mirrors that of their auditory nerve input in their sharp tuning to frequency. Their ability to encode timing and periodicity has been observed to be enhanced over that of their inputs through a convergence of auditory nerve fibers upon individual bushy cells (Spirou et al., 1990; Smith et al., 1991; Joris et al., 1994a; b).

In departure from merely relaying auditory nerve activity, bushy cells in mice have been shown *in vitro* to be influenced by inhibition (Figure 20.4) (Oertel, 1983; Wu and Oertel, 1984, 1986; Wickesberg and Oertel, 1990). At least some of this inhibition arises through tuberculoventral cells, glycinergic interneurons that are probably tuned to similar frequencies (Wickesberg and Oertel, 1988; 1990). Tuberculoventral cells have axon collaterals in the vicinity of bushy cell bodies (Figure 20.2) (Zhang and Oertel, 1993c). In guinea pigs, inhibition tuned to the same frequency as excitation in bushy cells has been documented in *in vivo* studies (Winter and Palmer, 1990). The suggestion has been made that such inhibition could serve to suppress echoes in localization of sound (Wickesberg and Oertel, 1990). Spherical and globular bushy cells participate in circuitry important for localizing sounds in the horizontal plane.

T STELLATE CELLS

T stellate cells are the most numerous cell type in the magnocellular regions of the VCN. Stellate cells are distinguished from bushy cells by their multiple dendrites that radiate from the cell body (Figure 20.2). (In Nissl-stained material, these cells have been termed "multipolar".) T stellate cells are named for the trajectory of their axon through the *t*rapezoid body (Oertel et al., 1990). They presumably form a pathway that conveys information from the auditory nerve to the contralateral inferior colliculus. (mice: Oertel et al., 1990; Ryugo et al., 1981; cats: Adams, 1979; 1983; Cant, 1982; Osen, 1972; Oliver, 1987; Roth et al., 1978). Collaterals are found locally in the VCN, and in the DCN they are restricted to a narrow band of tissue parallel to the entire rostral-caudal extent of the tonotopic axis of the fusiform cell layer (Oertel et al., 1990; Ferragamo et al., 1998b; Doucet and Ryugo, 1997).

T stellate cells lie intermingled with bushy cells in the caudal AVCN and rostral PVCN, becoming more frequent caudally where bushy cells are least frequent. T stellate cells comprise the bulk of the rostral PVCN. The most striking anatomical attribute of T stellate cells is the elongate architecture of their dendritic field, which lies parallel to the plane of incoming auditory nerve fibers (Figure 20.2) (Oertel et al., 1990; Ferragamo et al., 1998b; rat: Doucet and Ryugo, 1997; Brawer et al., 1974). In mice, the tips of the elaborate and curly dendrites of T stellate cells consistently lie in the vicinity of granule cells.

At least four sources of synaptic input to T stellate cells have been identified by delivering shocks to the auditory nerve in slices from mice.

1. Auditory nerve fibers excite T stellate cells with large EPSPs (Oertel, 1983; Wu and Oertel, 1984; Oertel et al., 1990; Ferragamo et al., 1998b). Approximately five myelinated auditory nerve fibers innervate a single T stellate cell (Ferragamo et al., 1998b). The peak of excitation after shocks to the auditory nerve occurs with little temporal jitter. Peaks occur about 1 ms after the shock, with standard deviations between 20 and 40 μs.
2. T stellate cells receive glycinergic inhibition through tuberculoventral cells of the DCN (Figure 20.4). Tuberculoventral cells receive acoustic input from roughly the same group of auditory nerve fibers as their T stellate cell targets; inhibition from tuberculoventral cells must therefore be tuned to roughly the same frequency as excitation through the auditory nerve (Wickesberg and Oertel, 1988; 1990). Tuberculoventral cells terminate in isofrequency laminae of the AVCN and PVCN (Figure 20.2) (Zhang and Oertel, 1993c).
3. T stellate cells receive a second source of glycinergic inhibition that is present even when the DCN is cut away. The glycinergic interneurons that remain in slices of only the VCN are likely to correspond to D stellate cells (Ferragamo et al., 1998b). Not only does the morphology of these neurons match the location of the inhibition, but the temporal patterns of the timing of discharges recorded from D stellate cells match those of inhibitory postsynaptic potentials (IPSPs) (Figure 20.4) (Ferragamo et al., 1998b).
4. Slower, less sharply timed excitation arises through neurons of the cochlear nucleus. This excitation, which has a slow component, arises through AMPA and also N-methyl-d-aspartate (NMDA) receptors (Ferragamo et al., 1998b). The excitation probably arises from local collaterals from the axons of other T stellate cells. T stellate cells have collaterals within the same isofrequency lamina as the parent soma in the rostral PVCN (Oertel et al., 1990). Because the majority of cells in the vicinity are other T stellate cells, these are likely to be the targets of those collaterals. The morphology of synaptic terminals of the corresponding cells in other species suggests that T stellate cells are likely to be excitatory (Oliver, 1984; Smith and Rhode, 1989).

Although extracellular recordings have not been made in mice, the arrangement of dendrites with respect to tonotopy suggests that T stellate cells are tuned narrowly. Smith and Rhode (1989) labeled multipolar cells in cats that projected through the trapezoid body and responded as "choppers." Choppers are characterized by a sharp, well-timed onset spike, followed by a pattern of steady firing at regular intervals independent of the phase of a tone-burst at best frequency. Choppers of cats, rats, and chinchillas are tuned narrowly with the excitatory regions flanked by inhibitory bands (Rhode and Smith, 1986a; Wickesberg, 1996). Individual choppers are more sensitive to signal envelope than their auditory nerve inputs (Blackburn and Sachs, 1989; Frisina et al., 1990b; Rhode and Greenberg, 1994; Wang and Sachs, 1994); and as a population, choppers can provide a rate-representation of speech sounds (Keilson et al., 1997).

D Stellate Cells

D stellate cells in mice are so named because they send their axons *d*orsalward through the intermediate acoustic stria (Oertel et al., 1990). These presumably correspond to commissural stellate cells in cats, which have been shown to project to the contralateral cochlear nucleus (cats: Cant and Gaston, 1982; Wenthold, 1987; Smith and Rhode, 1989; guinea pigs: Schofield and Cant,

1996). Sparse in number, with a relatively large cell body that tends to lie just underneath the granule cell regions, D stellate cells violate tonotopy by radiating extensive dendrites across the orderly trajectory of auditory nerve fibers (Figure 20.2). Their axons, too, extend over broad regions of the VCN and DCN (Oertel et al., 1990). Local collaterals are found in the neighborhood of T stellate cells in the VCN and also in the overlying granule cell region (Smith and Rhode, 1989; Oertel et al., 1990; Doucet and Ryugo, 1997; Ferragamo et al., 1998b). Axons of D stellate cells also project to the tuberculoventral cells of the DCN (Oertel et al., 1990; Oertel and Wickesberg, 1996).

Because they are relatively rare, D stellate cells have been less well studied than other types of cells in the VCN of mice. They receive both monosynaptic excitation and disynaptic inhibition through the auditory nerve (Figure 20.3) (Oertel et al., 1990; Ferragamo et al., 1998b). Because at least some of the excitation is of short latency, some of the excitation is presumably through myelinated, type I auditory nerve fibers. The dendrites of D stellate cells are, however, located in the vicinity of the unmyelinated, type II auditory nerve terminations (Brown and Ledwith, 1990). Type II fibers specifically terminate on the proximal dendrites of unidentified multipolar cells (Benson et al., 1996). Indirect evidence indicates that at least part of the inhibition arises through Golgi cells and is mediated through γ-aminobutyric acid (GABA). Removal of inhibition with picrotoxin, a $GABA_A$ receptor antagonist, augments the frequency and duration of firing in D stellate cells (Ferragamo et al., 1998b).

Several lines of evidence suggest that D stellate cells are inhibitory and glycinergic. First, T stellate cells receive inhibition through the VCN (Ferragamo et al., 1998b). D stellate cells are the only group of cells that are candidates for being inhibitory interneurons through their local collaterals. Second, in the VCN, neurons labeled with antibodies to glycine conjugates match the location where D stellate cells are found (Wickesberg et al., 1994). Third, stellate cells have been shown to be of two types, one excitatory and the other inhibitory, in many studies in other species. In cats, two types of stellate cells are distinguished on the basis of somatic innervation (Cant, 1981). One type is labeled with antibodies to glycine conjugates and projects to the contralateral cochlear nucleus (Wenthold, 1987). This type has terminals with pleomorphic vesicles, the morphology usually associated with inhibitory neurons (Smith and Rhode, 1989). Commissural cells with a morphology similar to D stellate cells were shown to project to all major cell types located in the contralateral cochlear nucleus of guinea pigs, including those that project to the inferior colliculus (Schofield and Cant, 1996). In rats, also, two types of stellate cells have been identified (Doucet and Ryugo, 1997).

Responses to sound have been recorded from neurons in cats that are likely to correspond to D stellate cells. Those neurons have wide dynamic ranges and respond with a burst of action potentials at the onset of a tone, the "onset-chopper" pattern (Smith and Rhode, 1989). These cells encode the precise timing of the onset of a response, sacrificing a representation of signal spectrum (Rhode and Smith, 1986a; Jiang et al., 1996; Palmer et al., 1996). It has been proposed that D stellate cells participate as a "wide-band inhibitor" in a circuit of the DCN to detect peaks and notches in the spectrum of a sound source (see below; Nelken and Young, 1994).

Golgi Cells

Recent results from mice have raised the intriguing possibility that type II auditory nerve fibers could influence the activity of cells in the magnocellular regions of the ventral cochlear nucleus. This influence may be exerted through an interneuron found intermingled in the granule cell domains within and around the cochlear nuclei, the Golgi cell. A recent study (Ferragamo et al., 1998c) in slices from the mouse revealed that the morphology of these previously elusive cells resembled Golgi cells associated with the granule cells of the cerebellum (Alvarez-Otero and Anadón, 1992; Midtgaard, 1992). Labeling single Golgi cells overlying the VCN in mice revealed a remarkable axonal arbor that uniformly pervades a patch of approximately 0.5 mm diameter within the plane of the superficial granules overlying the VCN. Terminal beads are laced throughout the dense and far-reaching network of fibers, and are found in close apposition to granule cells. The mycelium-like pattern makes it difficult to distinguish whether there is more than one axon emanating from the same cell. Golgi cells exert inhibition on their targets, and are labeled with antibodies to glycine and GABA (Kolston et al., 1992) and glutamic acid decarboxylase (GAD), an enzyme involved in the synthesis of GABA (Mugnaini, 1985). Several indirect lines of evidence imply that Golgi cells are GABAergic (Ferragamo et al., 1998c), but the possibility that they are glycinergic cannot be eliminated. The granule cells in a patch innervated by a Golgi cell, on the order of hundreds of granule cells, share a common inhibitory input that could functionally serve to coordinate extensive portions of the granule cell region overlying the VCN.

In slices, shocks delivered to the auditory nerve activate Golgi cells (Ferragamo et al., 1998c). Synaptic responses include three components: an initial EPSP, a late EPSP, and late inhibition. Shocks evoked an initial EPSP at a latency that was on average 0.6 ms longer than monosynaptic responses in nearby octopus and stellate cells whose input is known to arise from myelinated, type I auditory nerve fibers. This observation raises the question of what the source is of this comparatively slow excitatory input. The possibility of an additional synaptic delay within a disynaptic pathway is unlikely (Ferragamo et al., 1998c) simply because there are no known excitatory neurons with terminals in the area where Golgi cells were recorded which could serve as interneurons. It is more likely that excitation is provided through unmyelinated, type II auditory nerve fibers. Type II auditory nerve fibers end in the superficial granule cell domain of mice (Brown and Ledwith, 1990) and specifically terminate on the proximal dendrites of unidentified multipolar cells near the Golgi cells (Benson et al., 1996).

Trains of shocks mimicking trains of action potentials from auditory nerve inputs also elicit late EPSPs that last for up to hundreds of milliseconds in slices (Ferragamo et al., 1998c). Because the cut end of an axon fires only a single action potential, the late excitation observed in Golgi cells reflects the presence of excitatory interneurons. Manipulations that affected the function of NMDA receptors affected the frequency of late EPSPs. Granule cells, and another interneuron associated with granule cells (i.e., unipolar brush cells) are excitatory, and each contacts Golgi cells (Mugnaini et al., 1994; 1997) and possesses NMDA receptors (Rossi et al., 1995). Unipolar brush cells in cerebellum fire at regular temporal intervals, suggesting that they are an unlikely source of the irregularly occurring late EPSPs in Golgi cells. A similar pattern of late excitation is traced to parallel fiber-Golgi synapses in the cerebellum (Dieudonné, 1998).

Golgi cells receive glycinergic inhibition (Ferragamo et al., 1998c). This input could reflect a functional connection between the cells of the magnocellular regions of the VCN and the superficial granule layer. D stellate cells with collaterals that penetrate the overlying granule cell region are a likely source of this glycinergic inhibition (Oertel et al., 1990; Ferragamo et al., 1998b).

Functional Implications

The ventral cochlear nuclei contribute to the processing of acoustic information in at least two ways. One is that the auditory pathway is split into several parallel ascending pathways (Figure 20.1). The second is that, within the cochlear nuclei, some processing takes place (Figure 20.6).

Processing of acoustic information along parallel ascending pathways allows that processing to be rapid and to accommodate rapid, ongoing sound stimuli to be localized and understood. The auditory pathway at the level of the auditory nerve can be considered as a single tonotopic pathway. In the ventral cochlear nucleus, each auditory nerve fiber contacts several different types of cells with separate targets in the brainstem and midbrain. In doing so, the auditory pathway is split into several parallel ascending pathways, with each of the groups of principal cells of the ventral cochlear nucleus, bushy, T stellate, and octopus cells, forming a separate ascending pathway. Such an arrangement allows acoustic information to be processed simultaneously in several different ways. Pathways through the bushy cells and their targets in the medial and lateral superior olivary nuclei

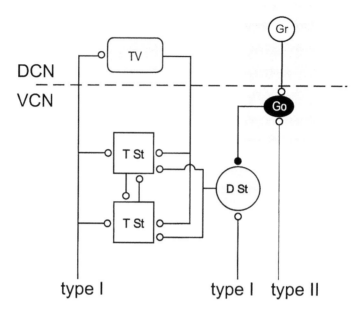

type I   type I   type II

FIGURE 20.6 Proposed connections of T stellate cells (T St). A few type I auditory nerve fibers excite T stellate monosynaptically, and proceed to contact tuberculoventral cells in the DCN. A larger group of type I fibers excite D stellate (D St) cells. Both D stellate and tuberculoventral (TV) cells inhibit T stellate cells. T stellate cells excite one another. Golgi (Go) cells are excited by type II auditory nerve fibers and granule (Gr) cells, and act to inhibit D stellate cells. (clear symbol, glutamergic input; stippled symbol, glycinergic; black symbol, GABAergic; background stippling, granule cell region). (Adapted from Ferragamo, M.J., Golding, N.L., Oertel, D., 1998, *J. Neurophysiol.,* 79, 51-63. With permission.)

contribute to the localization of sound sources in the horizontal plane (Smith et al., 1993a; Joris and Yin, 1995; Joris, 1996; 1998). Pathways through the octopus cells and ventral nuclei of the lateral lemniscus may be involved in the recognition of patterns including synchronicity, periodicity, directionality of frequency sweeps, and duration (Covey and Casseday, 1999). It has been suggested that the homologues of T stellate cells in birds are involved in the localization of sound in elevation (Takahashi et al., 1984). In mammals, the function of this pathway is not well understood.

It is not easy to assign a function to the integrative neuronal circuits in the cochlear nuclei. The circuitry described in this section is summarized diagrammatically in Figure 20.6. T stellate cells are innervated by a small number of auditory nerve fibers, as well as by collaterals contributing late EPSPs from other T stellate cells. An interconnected network of T stellate cells in an isofrequency lamina could account for the transformation of the primary-like input from auditory nerve fibers into the chopper pattern observed in T stellate cells. Auditory nerve fibers stimulate choppers with an initial transient at the onset of a tone-burst, but choppers presumably tuned to similar frequencies fill in subsequent excitation so that choppers fire more tonically in response to tones than their auditory nerve inputs. The existence of feed-forward excitation raises the issue of how the chopping response is terminated after the offset of a sound stimulus. It seems likely that inhibition from either tuberculoventral or D stellate cells contributes to cessation of excitation. In that regard, it is interesting that D stellate cells provide trains of IPSPs to T stellate cells after responses to strong, single shocks and after trains of shocks to the auditory nerve (Ferragamo et al., 1998b). What that transformation accomplishes in terms of the representation of the acoustic stimulus is not well established.

Although responses from individual cells have not been recorded from mice, in cats inhibition from neurons that correspond to D stellate cells in mice has been linked to the inhibitory side bands in neurons that correspond to T stellate cells (Smith and Rhode, 1989). If a chopper is driven by tone-bursts in the vicinity of the characteristic frequency, the inhibition contributed by onset-choppers can be overcome, but this model predicts that excitation from the auditory nerve would be cut short at the edges of the response area. As predicted, the regularity of the chopping responses is transformed into a transient response as the stimulating frequency is moved away from the characteristic frequency (W.S. Rhode, personal communication).

The suggestion has been made that inhibition through the deep layer of the DCN can contribute to the suppression of echoes. Roughly the same group of auditory nerve fibers that innervate T stellate cells, proceed to contact tuberculoventral cells in the deep DCN, which, in turn, provide delayed feedback inhibition to T stellate and bushy cells (Wickesberg and Oertel, 1988; 1990). That delayed inhibition can serve to suppress monaurally excitation evoked by the detection of echoes. The timing of inhibition through the DCN in an *in vitro* preparation corresponds to the timing of echo suppression measured in psychoacoustic experiments in humans (Wickesberg and Oertel, 1990).

Golgi cells of the granule cell domain are a likely source of $GABA_A$ergic inhibition to both D and T stellate cells. If Golgi cells are activated by type II auditory nerve fibers, stellate cells are poised to integrate auditory information conveyed through both rapidly and slowly conducting pathways. GABAergic inhibition from Golgi cells may sculpt the onset pattern characteristic of D stellate cells. Application of bicuculline, a $GABA_A$ receptor antagonist, transforms a phasic to a tonic discharge pattern and increases the jitter in the initial spike in response to pure tone-bursts in the PVCN (Palombi and Caspary, 1992). T stellate cells respond with slow, subtle GABAergic IPSPs (Ferragamo et al., 1998b) and have distal dendrites that receive contacts from terminals containing pleiomorphic vesicles (Josephson and Morest, 1999). Extracellular recordings revealed neurons, presumably Golgi cells, with a wide dynamic range in the granule cell region of cats (Ghoshal and Kim, 1997). A source of inhibition delivered over a wide dynamic range would modulate the membrane potential and input conductance of T stellate cells over a broad range of stimulus intensity. A similar explanation for the role of GABA in both divisions of the cochlear nuclei has been proposed (Evans and Zhao, 1993; Caspary et al., 1994). One action of type II auditory nerve fibers may be to regulate the gain of circuits in the magnocellular regions of the cochlear nuclei through Golgi cells.

INTRINSIC CIRCUITRY OF THE DCN

ORGANIZATION

The primary feature that distinguishes the DCN from the VCN is that the DCN is layered while the VCN is not. The DCN is a three-layered structure with auditory nerve fibers terminating along a rostro-caudal band in the deep layer. Isofrequency sheets in the deep layer are stacked dorsoventrally, with higher frequencies represented dorsally and lower frequencies represented ventrally. Parallel fibers, the axons of granule cells, form beams of excitation in the outermost molecular layer, perpendicularly to the isofrequency laminae, along the dorso-ventral axis. Each system of excitation, both superficial and deep, is associated with a glycinergic system of inhibition that shapes the output of the two principal output pathways that originate mainly from the intermediate layer, the fusiform cell layer. The DCN serves as the initial site of multimodal integration along the ascending auditory pathways. Much of the recent work using intracellular recording in murine slices has focused on how the complex integration occurring in the superficial layer influences its principal cells. A summary of the connections among DCN cells and their synaptic pharmacology is shown diagrammatically in Figure 20.7. Additional descriptions of DCN anatomy are found in Chapters 18 and 19.

Granule cells lie in sheets and clusters around the VCN and also within the DCN (Muganini et al., 1980a). They convey to the principal cells of the DCN not only auditory input from many levels of the auditory system, but also inputs from other sensory modalities. Granule cells are the

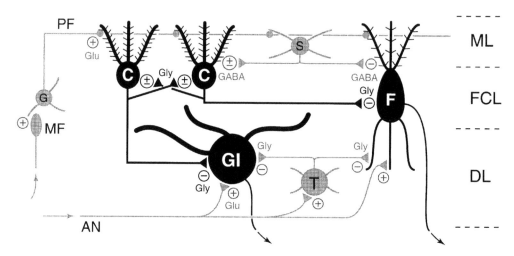

FIGURE 20.7 Connections and synaptic pharmacology of cells in the DCN. Granule cells (G) receive excitation from mossy fibers (MF) and convey that excitation via their axons, called parallel fibers (PF), through glutamatergic synapses to cartwheel cells (C), superficial stellate cells (S), and fusiform cells (F). Tuberculoventral, fusiform and giant cells are excited by auditory nerve fibers through glutamatergic synapses. Cartwheel cells inhibit fusiform and giant cells, and can either suppress or excite firing in other cartwheel cells through glycinergic synapses. (ML, molecular layer; FCL, fusiform cell layer; DL, deep layer). (From Oertel, D., Golding, N.L., 1997. In Syka, J. (Ed.), *Acoustic Signal Processing in the Central Auditory System.* Plenum, New York, 127-138. With permission.)

target of ascending projections from unmyelinated type II auditory nerve fibers and octopus cells of the VCN, as well as descending inputs from the superior olivary complex, inferior colliculus, and auditory cortex (M.C. Brown et al., 1988a; b; Brown and Ledwith, 1990; Caicedo and Herbert, 1993; Feliciano et al., 1995; Berglund et al., 1996; Golding et al., 1995). Non-auditory afferents arise from the vestibular nuclei (Burian and Gestoettner, 1988) and from the spinal trigeminal and cuneate nuclei of the somatosensory system (Itoh et al., 1987; Weinberg and Rustioni, 1987; Kevetter and Perachio, 1989; Wright and Ryugo, 1996; Weedman and Ryugo, 1996). The mossy fiber inputs from octopus cells of the VCN (Golding et al., 1995), auditory cortex (Feliciano et al., 1995; Weedman and Ryugo, 1996) and the cuneate nucleus (Wright and Ryugo, 1996) form the core of synaptic glomeruli, that not only include contacts to granule cells, but also to Golgi and unipolar brush cells (Mugnaini et al., 1997). The axons of granule cells, the parallel fibers, are the major source of excitation to the molecular layer (Kane, 1974; Mugnaini et al., 1980a; Wouterlood and Mugnaini, 1984; Wouterlood et al., 1984; Manis 1989). Few recordings have been made from granule cells because the currents associated with their activity are small. Their activity is, however, reflected in their targets: Golgi, stellate, cartwheel, and fusiform cells. In slices from mice, shocks that activate granule cells evoke slow, glutamatergic excitation that is AMPA and NMDA receptor mediated (Zhang and Oertel, 1993a; b; 1994; Golding and Oertel, 1996; 1997; Ferragamo et al., 1998c).

A striking feature of the outer layers of the DCN is the similarity with the cerebellum (Mugnaini et al., 1980a; Mugnaini, 1985; Berrebi and Mugnaini, 1991). Lying just beneath the cerebellar flocculus, the granule cells of the DCN form a continuous sheet with those of the overlying cerebellum. Similar to the cerebellum, the axons of granule cells form a molecular layer that impinges on smooth dendrites of stellate cells (Zhang and Oertel, 1993a). As in the cerebellum, granule cells are contacted through mossy fibers (Dunn et al., 1996). Golgi cells associated with granule cells of the cochlear nuclei resemble Golgi cells of the cerebellum (Alvarez-Otero and Anadón, 1992; Midtgaard, 1992; Ferragamo et al., 1998c). Parallel fibers in the molecular layer of the DCN contact the spiny dendrites of cartwheel cells, cells that are homologous to cerebellar

Purkinje cells in their labeling for immunocytochemical markers, GAD, GABA, and PEP 19 (Mugnaini, 1985; Berrebi and Mugnaini, 1991). Cartwheel cells fire simple and complex action potentials, as do Purkinje cells (Manis et al., 1994; Zhang and Oertel, 1993a; Golding and Oertel, 1997). Unlike cerebellar Purkinje cells, cartwheel cells contact other cartwheel cells and neurons that are also targets of parallel fibers. Cartwheel cells are glycinergic, whereas Purkinje cells are GABAergic (Golding and Oertel, 1996; 1997).

CARTWHEEL CELLS

Cartwheel cells transform excitatory input from parallel fibers into inhibition that is in turn conveyed to principal cells (Hirsch and Oertel, 1988; Zhang and Oertel, 1993a; Manis et al., 1994; Golding and Oertel, 1996). Cartwheel cells located at the border between the molecular and fusiform cell layers are numerous in mice (Figure 20.2). They have several thick, branched, spiny dendrites that reach up into the molecular layer to sample activity from parallel fibers (Brawer et al., 1974; Wouterlood and Mugnaini, 1984; Zhang and Oertel, 1993a). Their axonal arbor is largely restricted to the molecular and fusiform layer, where they contact fusiform, giant, and other cartwheel cells (Berrebi and Mugnaini, 1991; Zhang and Oertel, 1993a; Manis et al., 1994; Golding and Oertel, 1997).

Cartwheel cells, unlike any other cell recorded in the cochlear nucleus *in vitro*, fire complex action potentials — a slow action potential formed from a regenerative calcium current that triggers a burst of rapid action potentials that are generated by inward sodium current (Figures 20.3 and 20.4) (Zhang and Oertel, 1993a; Golding and Oertel, 1997). In response to shocks of their inputs, cartwheel cells fire in variable patterns for up to hundreds of milliseconds beyond the stimulus (Manis et al., 1994; Golding and Oertel, 1996; 1997).

The characteristic bursty firing can be used as a physiological tag to identify the targets of cartwheel cells. The targets of cartwheel cells include other cartwheel, fusiform, and giant cells, but not superficial stellate or tuberculoventral cells (Golding and Oertel, 1997). Although labeled by antibodies to GAD, unexpectedly in slices from mice, no GABA$_A$ergic PSPs have been recorded in their targets (Zhang and Oertel, 1994; Golding and Oertel, 1996; 1997). Instead, all spontaneous and evoked postsynaptic potentials that mirror the burst pattern of complex spikes are glycinergic.

Cartwheel cells have an unusually elevated intracellular chloride concentration that causes glycinergic and GABAergic synaptic responses to be depolarizing and excitatory (Golding and Oertel, 1996; 1997). Conventional GABA$_A$ and glycine receptors in cartwheel cells mediate synaptic potentials whose reversal potentials are more depolarized than the threshold of firing, whereas it lies below threshold, and indeed below the resting potential, in all other cells of the cochlear nuclei. Therefore, the action of GABAergic and glycinergic PSPs is context dependent — suppressing firing when cartwheel cells are strongly depolarized and promoting activation from the resting potential (Golding and Oertel, 1996; Oertel and Golding, 1997). The interaction of these synaptic inputs with the voltage-dependent conductances can be predicted to limit the dynamic range of the firing frequency of cartwheel cells. Because primary auditory afferents do not invade the molecular layer, the response of cartwheel cells to sounds *in vivo* would be expected to be weak. As predicted, in cat and gerbil, a majority of complex-spiking units, presumed to be cartwheel cells, are only weakly driven and sluggish in responding to pure tone-bursts and broadband noise (Parham and Kim, 1995; Davis et al., 1996; Ding and Voigt, 1997; J. Ding et al., 1999).

PRINCIPAL CELLS: FUSIFORM AND GIANT

The major output pathway of the DCN originates with the fusiform cells underlying the molecular layer. Spiny, apical dendrites extend from the cell body into the molecular layer and basal dendrites radiate narrowly in parallel to isofrequency sheets of the deep layer (Figure 20.2). Fusiform cells are poised to integrate excitation from the parallel fiber system with excitation from the auditory nerve (Figure 20.7) (Zhang and Oertel, 1994; Golding and Oertel, 1997). Fusiform cells also receive inhibition from two powerful systems, one associated with each of the excitatory systems. The outcome of this complex processing is delivered to the contralateral inferior colliculus through the dorsal acoustic stria. A second output pathway to the inferior colliculus originates from the giant cells in the deep layer. The basal dendrites of giant cells are not restricted to the isofrequency plane but extend widely, and in contrast to fusiform cells, apical dendrites are sparse in the molecular layer (Zhang and Oertel, 1993b; Golding and Oertel, 1997). Their responses to shocks to the auditory nerve reflect these differences (Figure 20.4). Long duration, evoked, and spontaneous glutamatergic excitation arising from parallel fiber inputs is more prominent in fusiform cells than in giant cells. In addition to the glycinergic inhibiton arising from cartwheel cells, both cell types receive short-latency, glycinergic input that most likely emanates from tuberculoventral cells and D stellate cells in the VCN (Zhang and Oertel, 1993b; Oertel and Golding, 1997). Fusiform cells balance excitation from the molecular and deep layers with intrinsic inhibition, while giant cells, with greater access to the deeper lying terminals of tuberculoventral and D stellate cells, are dominated by inhibition. Early glycinergic inhibition masks early excitation in giant cells (Figure 20.4).

The interplay between these excitatory and inhibitory influences is apparent in intracellular recordings of responses to sounds in giant and fusiform cells in cats (Rhode et al., 1983b; Rhode and Smith, 1986b; Joris, 1998) and gerbils (J. Ding et al., 1999). Poststimulus-time histograms recorded from principal cells clearly show that the timing of auditory nerve inputs is degraded by robust inhibition in the DCN (Rhode and Smith, 1985; 1986b).

TUBERCULOVENTRAL CELLS

Tuberculoventral cells, also known as corn or vertical cells, have cell bodies that share the deep layer of the DCN with giant cells. Unlike giant cells, their dendrites are aligned along the isofrequency sheet of auditory nerve fibers, and their axons do not project out of the cochlear nuclear complex. Tuberculoventral cells deliver feedback inhibition to bushy and stellate cells that lie in the corresponding isofrequency region along the ascending branch of the auditory nerve in the VCN (Wickesberg and Oertel, 1988; Wickesberg et al., 1991; Zhang and Oertel, 1993c). In addition, local collaterals innervate an isofrequency lamina near the dendrites, which presumably contact giant and fusiform cells. Shocks to the root of the auditory nerve elicit a monosynaptic EPSP, late EPSPs that may be mediated through T stellate cells, and late glycinergic IPSPs that presumably originate from D stellate cells (Zhang and Oertel, 1993c).

On the basis of measurements in cats, tuberculoventral cells presumably respond with one, or few, poorly timed action potentials at the onset of a tone-burst. They have sharp tuning and fail to respond to broadband noise (Young and Brownell, 1976; E.D. Young, 1980; Voigt and Young, 1980; 1990; Rhode, 1999).

FUNCTIONAL CONSIDERATIONS

The function of the DCN has not been studied in the mouse, and while studies in the cat provide some insights, its role remains enigmatic. The pioneering work of Young and colleagues suggests that the DCN is involved in integrating multimodal cues in interpreting the spectral profile imposed by the passive filtering properties of the convolutions of the pinna. Notches and peaks are created by the external ear at specific frequencies that are elevation dependent (Musicant et al., 1990; Rice et al., 1992). These features are available as cues in localizing sounds in space (humans: Wightman and Kistler, 1989; bat: Wotton et al., 1996). Projection cells show complex response patterns, so-called type IV response patterns, that are sensitive to notches introduced into broadband sounds (Spirou and Young, 1991; Nelken and Young, 1994; Joris, 1998). With narrow-band stimuli, type IV responses are dominated by inhibition at best frequency that presumably arises from type II inputs from tuberculoventral cells. A second source of inhibition, putatively from D stellate cells in the

VCN, emerges under broadband conditions, and can suppress excitation to type IV units when a narrow band centered at best frequency is notched out of noise. DCN circuitry activated by sound is strongly affected by electrical activation of somatosensory inputs originating from the dorsal column and vestibular nuclei, or by tactile somatosensory stimuli at the pinna (Young et al., 1995; Davis et al., 1996; Davis and Young, 1997). Presumably, the principal cells of the DCN combine information regarding head and pinna position with information describing the signal spectrum to direct attention to an acoustic signal in space. However, behavioral experiments have not been able to demonstrate salient deficits in sound localization subsequent to lesion of the dorsal acoustic stria (Sutherland, 1991).

CONCLUSIONS

The cochlear nucleus serves to segregate information from auditory nerve inputs into functional streams, yet the role of its intrinsic circuitry in transforming that information into a format that is recognizable as a basis for complex psychological attributes precludes it from being considered a simple relay nucleus. A significant investment in precise and faithful encoding of the timing of electrical signals is manifested in the anatomical and electrophysiological features of the VCN. Bushy cells and octopus cells have converged upon a similar palette of intrinsic conductances to maintain brevity in EPSPs. Bushy cells extract and convey temporal information to other sites in the brainstem to assist in localizing in the horizontal plane. Octopus cells are ideally suited to precisely detect common intervals in complex sounds such as speech formants, but this hypothesis must be further investigated *in vivo*. T stellate cells can capably detect energy within a narrow band of frequencies and as a population represent signal spectrum. Their association with two different classes of inhibitory systems, glycinergic from the magnocellular region and GABAaergic from the overlying granule cell layer, appears to be important in encoding transients through mechanisms that enhance spectral and temporal contrast. Transients appear to be essential in understanding speech sounds by humans. The DCN, a structure with a lineage shared with the cerebellum, integrates excitation from two major systems along with the intrinsic inhibition that each source uniquely activates. Evidence is accumulating that suggests that the DCN is involved in evaluation of elevation-dependent acoustic cues and combines that with information about head and pinna orientation from the somatosensory and vesibular systems. Yet disruption of this site results in only subtle behavioral deficits. Electrophysiological studies of behaving animals may refine our understanding of the function of the DCN.

ACKNOWLEDGMENTS

We are grateful to Janine Wotton for her thoughtful comments on the manuscript.

APPENDIX: INTRACELLULAR RECORDING FROM MOUSE BRAIN SLICES

TISSUE PREPARATION

A mouse between the ages of 17 and 28 days was decapitated with a pair of scissors, and the head was immersed in carbogen-infused saline (in mM: 130 NaCl, 3 KCl, 1.2 K_2HPO_4, 2.4 $CaCl_2 \cdot H_2O$, 1.3 $MgSO_4$, 3 HEPES, 20 $NaHCO_3$, 10 glucose; pH 7.4) warmed to 31°C. After removing the brain from the skull, a cut was made through the midline at the approximate angle parallel to which the cut for the slice will be made, and the cut surface of one-half of the tissue was affixed with cyanoacrylate (Crazy Glue) to a teflon stage. The cochlear nucleus was removed from the brainstem with a single parasagittal cut with a tissue slicer (Frederick Haer, New Brunswick, Maine).

Slices, estimated between 250 and 400 μm at the thickest point, were immersed in saline in a custom-built tissue chamber. The tissue chamber is described in detail in Oertel (1985); briefly, it was constructed of magnetic rubber affixed to a glass slide with dental wax, and the shape of the chamber was hollowed out of the rubber to an approximate volume of 0.3 mL. A slice was visualized with dark-field illumination from below. The tissue was placed on a nylon gauze base that was glued over a plastic spacer, and was maintained in place with an overlaying piece of nylon gauze that was held down by metal clips. Saline was gravity fed, and continuously replaced at a rate of 10 to 12 mL per minute. Saline was aspirated through a glass capillary from a canal that adjoins the chamber. Pharmacological agents were introduced into the chamber without a break in the flow. A thermoregulator (UW-Madison Medical Electronic Shop), with feedback supplied by a temperature probe (Physitemp, Clifton, New Jersey) placed close to the slice, maintained the temperature of the saline at 34°C. Slices were allowed to "rest" in the chamber for between 60 and 90 min before electrophysiological recording.

ELECTROPHYSIOLOGICAL RECORDING

Intracellular recordings were made with sharp microelectrodes filled with 1% biocytin (Sigma, Inc.) in 2 M K$^+$-acetate, pH 7.0. Electrode impedances ranged from 120 to 250 MΩ. Voltages were amplified, and low-pass filtered at 10 kHz (ICX2-700; Dagan, Inc., Minneapolis, Minnesota). Membrane potential was monitored audiovisually, recorded on chartpaper (Gould, Inc., Valley View, Ohio), and individual traces were recorded digitally at a sampling rate of 25 kHz. Data acquisition, current injection, and shock triggering were performed with a Digidata 1200A computer interface in conjunction with pCLAMP software (Axon Instruments, Inc., Foster City, California). Shocks were delivered to the auditory nerve root, to the surface of the VCN, or to the dorsal tip of the DCN through a pair of insulated tungsten, each with a 50-μm exposed tip. Stimulation voltage (0.1 to 100 V; 100-μs duration) was delivered through an optical stimulus isolator (S-100; Winston Electronics Co., Millbrae, California) under the control of a digitally triggered timer (A-65; Winston Electronics Co.).

HISTOLOGY

Recorded cells were routinely labeled by iontophoretic injection of biocytin with depolarizing current steps (0.5 to 2.0 nA; 150 to 200 ms) at a rate of two per second for 1 to 2 min. At the end of the experiment, slices were fixed in 4% paraformaldehyde, 0.1 M phosphate buffer, pH 7.4, and stored overnight at 4°C. Individual slices were embedded in a mixture of gelatin and albumin cross-linked with glutaraldehyde, and sectioned at 60 μm on a vibratome. Sections were reacted with avidin conjugated to horseradish peroxidase (Vector ABC kit, Vector Laboratories, Burlingame, California), intensified with Co^{2+} and Ni^{2+}, and conterstained with cresyl violet.

21 Focus: GABA and Glycine Neurotransmission in Mouse Auditory Brainstem Structures

Donald M. Caspary

INTRODUCTION

The inhibitory amino acids, gamma-aminobutyric acid (GABA) and glycine, play a critical role in the coding of acoustic information in auditory brainstem structures. The cochlear nucleus, superior olivary complex, or nuclei of the lateral lemniscus and inferior colliculus contain numerous extrinsic and intrinsic circuits that utilize GABA and/or glycine in the detection of signals in noise, echo suppression, and the localization of sound in space. This chapter focuses on what is known about GABA and glycine from studies conducted in mouse auditory brainstem.

GENERAL INHIBITORY AMINO ACID FINDINGS IN THE AUDITORY BRAINSTEM OF OTHER MAMMALS

The inhibitory amino acid neurotransmitters, GABA and glycine, play a major role in shaping responses to acoustic stimuli in the major brainstem auditory nuclei of most mammals. Functional and anatomical studies on the chinchilla, guinea pig, rat, cat, and bats that examine possible roles for these inhibitory amino acids are mentioned for comparison only when necessary. In general, those studies identify important glycinergic circuits in the cochlear nucleus which may adjust dynamic range, function in echo suppression (see Chapter 20), and shape responses to both transient and complex stimuli (see Young, 1998, for a review).

In the first binaural complex of the auditory brainstem, the superior olivary complex (SOC), glycine has been shown to mediate binaural inhibition in the lateral superior olivary nucleus (LSO) through a projection from the glycinergic medial nucleus of the trapezoid body (MNTB) (Finlayson and Caspary, 1991; Moore and Caspary, 1983). In the pathways that lead to the midbrain lie the nuclei of the lateral lemniscus. In bats and other mammals, the ventral nucleus of the lateral lemniscus (VNLL) has been found to be a glycinergic structure (Saint Marie et al., 1997). In other mammals, the dorsal nucleus of the lateral lemniscus (DNLL) neurons are primarily GABAergic. Cells in the VNLL are thought to project glycinergic inputs onto the more ventral portions of the inferior colliculus.

Extrinsic GABA inputs and intrinsic GABA connections play a role in shaping cochlear nucleus (CN) response properties. Superior olivary complex circuits involved with binaural processing utilize either/or both glycine and GABA in the medial superior olivary nucleus (MSO) and other subnuclei within the SOC. The DNLL, as noted, contains primarily GABAergic neurons while the midbrain auditory relay station, the inferior colliculus (IC), receives both glycinergic and GABAergic inputs from a number of ascending and descending pathways. In addition, the IC contains a large number of GABAergic neurons that form numerous intrinsic GABAergic connections within the IC. Although the number of inhibitory neurotransmitter studies in the mouse auditory system is modest, findings from studies reviewed below are generally in agreement with findings in other mammals.

As detailed below, brainstem inhibitory neurotransmitter systems in mouse strains with no significant peripheral anomalies or neurotransmitter knockouts appear similar to the same neurotransmitter systems in other mammals. In their recent comparative morphometric review of brainstem auditory systems across 53 mammals, Glendenning and Masterton (1998) found that the mouse CN, MNTB, LSO and MSO, DNLL, VNLL, and IC are not categorically different from the same structures in other small mammals.

GABA AND GLYCINE IN THE BRAINSTEM AUDITORY SYSTEM OF THE MOUSE

GLYCINE NEUROTRANSMISSION IN MOUSE COCHLEAR NUCLEUS

The CN has been extensively studied in perinatal, adult, and aged mouse, as described elsewhere in this handbook (Chapters 16, 18 to 20, and 24). As in other mammals, there is a significant intrinsic inhibitory circuitry in the dorsal and ventral CN as well as extrinsic descending pathways, primarily from the SOC (Golding and Oertel, 1996; Wickesberg et al., 1994; Wu and Oertel, 1986; Wu and Kelly, 1993; 1995). The work of Oertel and colleagues (Hirsch and Oertel, 1988; Wickesberg et al., 1994; Wu and Oertel, 1986; Zhang and Oertel, 1993a; b; c) as well as Willott et al. (1997) has suggested that the vertical cells (tuberculoventral cells) in the dorsal cochlear nucleus (DCN) represent a major source of an intrinsic glycinergic backbone in CN (Hirsch and Oertel, 1988; Wickesberg et al., 1994; Wu and Oertel, 1986). These cells project onto and shape the output of the pyramidal/fusiform cells, which comprise the major output neurons from the DCN (Hirsch and Oertel, 1988; Wickesberg et al., 1994; Wu and Oertel, 1986). Vertical cells also provide a significant inhibitory input onto two major cell types in the anteroventral cochlear nucleus (AVCN), bushy and stellate neurons (Wickesberg et al., 1994). Oertel and colleagues provide an elegant argument for a role of this pathway in echo suppression, and their findings are consistent with studies in other mammals that suggest that these glycinergic neurons function in dynamic range adjustment, forward masking, and detection of signals in noise (Wickesberg et al., 1994; Wu and Oertel, 1986; Zhang and Oertel, 1993a; b; c).

Further support for glycinergic input onto neurons in the CN has been presented in a number of strychnine binding studies. These studies map the presence of inhibitory glycine receptors in the different regions of the CN using quantitative receptor binding autoradiography, with strychnine as the ligand for glycine receptors (Frostholm and Rotter, 1986; Willott et al., 1997). Kakehata et al. (1992) described the presence of both strychnine-sensitive and strychnine-insensitive glycine receptors within the DCN. These studies in mouse are consistent with binding studies in other species and are suggestive of extrinsic as well as intrinsic glycinergic inputs onto the cells of both the DCN and VCN. Several studies have described age-related changes in the glycine system of the mouse CN (Willott et al., 1992; 1997) similar to those observed in the rat (Milbrandt and Caspary, 1995; Krenning et al., 1998).

GABA NEUROTRANSMISSION IN MOUSE COCHLEAR NUCLEUS

There is evidence of GABAergic neurons in the superficial layers of the DCN (Hirsch and Oertel, 1988) and significant binding of muscimol (a selective GABA ligand) within all the layers of the DCN (Frostholm and Rotter, 1985; 1986). Depending on the physiologic state of the cartwheel cells, their GABAergic output may be either excitatory or inhibitory (Golding and Oertel, 1996).

Frostholm and Rotter (1986) used quantitative receptor binding autoradiography to map both glycine and $GABA_A$ receptors in mouse DCN and posteroventral cochlear nucleus (PVCN). The selective ligands, strychnine (glycine receptor), flunitrazepan, and muscimol ($GABA_A$ receptor), were used to map glycine and $GABA_A$ receptors. Frostholm and Rotter (1986) describe strychnine binding clustered around fusiform cells of the DCN as well as several other cell types in the granular and deep layers of DCN. A different pattern was observed using muscimol. Except for the area immediately surrounding fusiform cells, most cells in all three layers of the mouse DCN showed significant muscimol binding. The subunit makeup of the $GABA_A$ receptor in mouse appears similar to observations from other species. These findings suggest that $GABA_A$ receptor subunit makeup in DCN differs from the wild-type subunit composition most commonly found in other mammalian brain regions (McKernan and Whiting, 1996). Bahn et al. (1997) suggested that DCN $GABA_A$ receptors express the alpha 6 subunit type, a subunit generally found only in cerebellum. Binding studies by Varecka et al. (1994) were the first to describe the presence of the alpha 6 subunit within the granule cell domain of the CN and within the cerebellum in both developing and adult mice.

GABA AND GLYCINE NEUROTRANSMISSION IN MOUSE SUPERIOR OLIVARY COMPLEX

The inhibitory neurotransmitters GABA and glycine are critically involved in the processing of binaural acoustic information in the subnuclei of the SOC. Observations by Wu and Kelly (1994; 1995) in mouse SOC support previous findings, from other species, of a large glycinergic input onto LSO neurons from the glycinergic neurons of the MNTB. Electrical stimulation of the contralateral fibers of the trapezoid body (ventral acoustic stria) evokes robust strychnine-sensitive inhibitory postsynaptic currents (IPSCs) during intracellular recordings from LSO neurons (Wu and Kelly, 1993; 1995). Strychnine binding studies indicated the presence of glycine receptors on the somata and dendrites of LSO neurons (Frostholm and Rotter, 1985). Both glycinergic and GABAergic inputs/receptors were found to be present on MNTB neurons, and LSO neurons exhibited $GABA_A$ receptors in a relatively low number (Wu and Kelly, 1993, 1994; 1995). Most neurons in the major SOC nuclei were sensitive to bath-applied GABA and glycine.

GABA AND GLYCINE NEUROTRANSMISSION IN MOUSE NUCLEI
OF THE LATERAL LEMNISCUS

The somatic and axonal properties of DNLL neurons of the mouse have been described in Golgi preparation, with an appearance similar to those found in other rodent species (Iwahori, 1986). In slice studies in mouse by Reetz and Ehret (1999) and in rat by L. Chen et al. (1999), stimulation of the lateral lemniscus fibers or commissure of Probst projecting to IC evoked both IPSCs and excitatory postsynaptic currents (EPSCs). Based on immunocytochemical data from other mammalian species and blockade of electrically evoked IPSCs following lemniscal stimulation, these slice studies suggest that cells in the mouse DNLL are GABAergic (Reetz and Ehret, 1999; Wagner, 1996).

GABA AND GLYCINE NEUROTRANSMISSION IN MOUSE INFERIOR COLLICULUS

Frisina et al. (1998b) recently mapped inputs to the mouse IC and found them to be similar to projections in other mammals. Contreras and Bachelard (1979) found high levels of GABA and its synthetic enzyme, glutamic acid decarboxylase (GAD), in the IC relative to other auditory structures. More recently, Wagner (1996) recorded from 34 neurons in the central nucleus of the IC in mouse brain slices. He was able to back-fill neurons for identification as multipolar cells (Wagner, 1996). Late IPSCs induced by electrical stimulation of the lateral lemniscus were blocked by the GABA antagonist bicuculline (Wagner, 1996). Wagner (1996) concluded that GABA plays an important role as an inhibitory neurotransmitter in the IC. Studies by Reetz and Ehret (1999) recorded from and labeled different neuronal types within the IC. They were able to evoke IPSCs from nonoriented neurons more readily than from oriented (bipolar) neurons (Reetz and Ehret, 1999). Peris et al. (1989) described relatively high levels of binding of a picrotoxin analog (GABA antagonist) in the IC of seizure-susceptible mice. Altogether, these findings are in agreement with numerous studies in rat, guinea pig, chinchilla, and bat that find an important role for GABA in shaping the responses of IC neurons to simple and complex monaural as well as binaural stimuli.

ACKNOWLEDGMENTS

Judy Bryan helped with the preparation of the manuscript and Dr. R. Helfert provided useful comments. The author is supported by NIH grant DC 00151.

22 Calcium Binding Proteins in the Central Auditory System: Modulation by Noise Exposure and Aging

Esma Idrizbegovic, Nenad Bogdanovic, and Barbara Canlon

INTRODUCTION

In recent years, an effort has been made to understand the role of altered calcium homeostasis in different neurodegenerative conditions such as noise-induced hearing loss, ototoxicity, and aging. Calcium plays a crucially important role as an intracellular mediator in activating and regulating various physiological processes in neurons, including fast axonal transport, membrane excitability, cell motility, differentiation, synthesis and release of neurotransmitters, long-term potentiation, secretion, apoptosis, and synaptic plasticity (Ghosh and Greenberg, 1995). All of these processes must be tightly controlled, because neuronal activity can lead to marked increases in the concentration of cytosolic calcium. With concentrations of below 10^{-6} M, intracellular calcium levels are kept at a level that is about four orders of magnitude below the extracellular calcium concentration of 2 to 5 mM. Because an elevated concentration of intracellular calcium is toxic for the cell, control of cytosolic Ca^{2+} is of fundamental significance (Orrenius and Nicotera, 1994). As a result of Ca^{2+} overload, there is an activation of biochemical processes leading to enzymatic breakdown of proteins and lipids, malfunctioning of mitochondria, energy failure, and finally cell death (reviewed by Heizmann and Braun, 1995). Thus, Ca^{2+} homeostasis is essential for the appropriate functioning of neurons and may be very important with respect to the operation and maintenance of the auditory system.

CALCIUM BINDING PROTEINS

A crucial step toward understanding calcium-evoked responses is the identification and characterization of calcium binding proteins. Calcium binding proteins have been found to regulate intracellular calcium concentrations, and an increase in intracellular Ca^{2+} triggers activity of calcium binding proteins. They restrict the Ca^{2+}-mediated signals in the cytoplasm and buffer the calcium concentration (Chard et al., 1993). Different strategies have led to the identification of a number of calcium binding proteins that may be involved in regulating intracellular calcium. Two of these are parvalbumin and calbindin-D_{28k}, cytosolic calcium binding proteins. They are of particular interest in neuroanatomical, neurophysiological, and neuropathological studies because the immunocytochemistry for parvalbumin and calbindin has been useful for the morphological and chemical analysis of subpopulations of neurons in the central nervous system. These proteins are also of special interest because of their suggested protective role in neurons and their associations with several diseases of the brain. Therefore, they have been used to study the alterations of neuronal circuits in several diseases in the human brain and in experimental models (reviewed by Celio, 1990; Baimbridge et al., 1992; Heizmann and Braun, 1992; 1995; Andressen et al., 1993).

PARVALBUMIN

In the brain, parvalbumin exhibits a neuron-specific distribution and is frequently localized in fast firing nerve cells, especially in a subpopulation of mammalian neurons containing the inhibitory neurotransmitter, γ-aminobutyric acid (GABA) (Celio et al., 1996). Parvalbumin is expressed both in the central and peripheral nervous system, and has proven to be an excellent neuronal marker in the nervous system (Celio, 1990). It is also expressed in non-neuronal tissue such as muscle, seminal vesicles, the prostate, adipose tissue, testis, ovary, and kidney (Celio et al., 1996; Heizmann and Berchtold, 1987). Parvalbumin is present in high levels in fast anaerobic muscle fibers that are found most frequently in fast contracting/relaxing muscles. In muscle, parvalbumin is believed to facilitate the transfer of Ca^{2+} from the myofibrils to the sarcoplasmic reticulum (Gailly et al., 1993).

Parvalbumin is a Ca^{2+} and Mg^{2+} binding protein (Eberhard and Erne, 1994). Parvalbumin is known to be a slower buffer than calbindin because Mg^{2+} (bound to the protein in the resting state) must first dissociate before Ca^{2+} binding can occur (Heizmann, 1984; Hou et al., 1991). It has been hypothesized that parvalbumin could act in neurons as a Ca^{2+} buffer and modulator of free calcium levels, thereby protecting cells from Ca^{2+} overload (Sloviter, 1989). The differential distribution of parvalbumin in neuronal compartments suggests that this protein might act as a mobile buffer of Ca^{2+} transport within neurons, as suggested for skeletal muscles (Hou et al., 1993). It is believed that alterations in Ca^{2+} homeostasis due to an altered expression of calcium binding proteins, modification in Ca^{2+} and Mg^{2+} binding sites, or intra- or extracellular interactions might be involved in some neurodegenerative disorders. Parvalbumin is highly expressed in the auditory system of all species studied thus far (Lohmann and Friauf, 1996; Caicedo et al., 1996; Vater and Braun, 1994). In the highly active auditory neurons, parvalbumin may function primarily as a stabilizer of the intracellular calcium concentration.

CALBINDIN-D_{28k}

Calbindin-D_{28k} is present in all vertebrate species and in a wide range of different cells (Heizmann and Braun, 1995). Calbindin was first discovered by Wasserman and Taylor (1966) in chick intestinal mucosa and is common in intestines. In mammals, calbindin-D_{28k} is found in subpopulations of nerve cells in the nervous system, kidney, and pancreas. Furthermore, calbindin-D_{28k} has been localized in specific sensory pathways, including cones and horizontal cells in the retina (Pasteels et al., 1987), and cochlear and vestibular hair cells of the inner ear (Rabie et al., 1983). Antibodies against calbindin-D_{28k} are commonly used as neuroanatomical markers (Celio, 1990). The highest concentration of brain calbindin-D_{28k} is found in the Purkinje cells in the cerebellum. Other central nervous system regions that contain significantly high levels of calbindin-D_{28k} include the auditory system, limbic system, visual system, basal ganglia, and pathways concerned with the integration of movement (Christakos et al., 1989).

Calbindin-D_{28k} has a very high-affinity Ca^{2+}-binding site. It functions as a pure Ca^{2+} buffer in order to hold the cytoplasmic Ca^{2+} below toxic levels. Increased calbindin-D_{28k} immunoreactivity has also been associated with neurodegenerative diseases such as Alzheimer's and Parkinson's disease (Heizmann and Braun, 1992). It was reported that calbindin-D_{28k} is up-regulated in the kidney and the pancreas by 1,25-dihydroxyvitamin D_3, the active metabolite of vitamin D (reviewed by Celio et al., 1996). Although a vitamin D-dependent response has been reported in the intestinal and renal calbindins, brain calbindin-D_{28k} is unresponsive to vitamin D or to any of its metabolites (Schneeberger et al., 1985). In neurons, calbindin-D_{28k} is distributed throughout the cytoplasm, and this cytoplasmic localization allows it to function as a buffering system that can protect nerve cells against excess calcium concentrations (Heizmann and Braun, 1992). Calbindin is also localized within the nucleus of nerve cells in the rodent brain, suggesting its role in regulating nuclear calcium signals (German et al., 1997).

In the central auditory system, the neuronal circuitry involved in sound localization contains very high levels of calbindin-D_{28k} and this expression is conserved across species. Thus, the potential functional implications of calbindin-D_{28k} in the auditory brainstem are its possible role in the mechanisms underlying rapid transmission of temporal information in auditory neurons by maintaining physiological levels of intracellular calcium (Caicedo et al., 1996). However, the predominance of calbindin-D_{28k} in these neurons suggests functions in addition to buffering intracellular calcium transients. For example, a role of calbindin-D_{28k} in synapse stabilization during development was suggested because of its transient expression in neurons of certain auditory nuclei (Friauf, 1994).

CALBINDIN-D_{28K} AND PARVALBUMIN IMMUNOREACTIVITY IN RELATION TO INJURY AND NEURODEGENERATIVE DISORDERS

A prominent feature of acute central nervous system injury is disturbed calcium homeostasis. Changes at the level of gene expression related to cellular homeostasis are becoming an increasingly apparent aspect of the neuronal response to injury. It was shown that mRNA for calbindin-D_{28k} increased in the rat hippocampus following acute CNS injury by global ischemia. This suggests a potential role of calbindin-D_{28k} in buffering intracellular calcium as a cellular response to disturbed calcium homeostasis in acute CNS injury (Lowenstein et al., 1994). It was also reported that neuronal excitation via the perforant path leads to an increased expression of calbindin-D_{28k} mRNA in the rat hippocampus, suggesting that the neuronal activation is associated with elevated cytosolic Ca^{2+}, including a system of feedback control at the level of gene expression (Lowenstein et al., 1991). The expression of calbindin-D_{28k} and parvalbumin was observed in the immature rat hippocampus following anoxia, with modifications in calbindin immunoreactive neurons and a transitory effect on parvalbumin immunoreactivity (Dell Anna et al., 1996). In the lateral geniculate nucleus of adult monkeys, it was shown that parvalbumin and calbindin-D_{28k} fibers were depleted 1 to 7 months after monocular enucleation (Gutierrez and Cusick, 1994). Increased expression of calbindin-D_{28k} in deafferented neurons of the lateral geniculate nucleus was observed in the same study. A substantial increase in the number of calbindin immunoreactive fibers and boutons in the ventral subdivisions of the ipsilateral cochlear nucleus, following unilateral cochleotomy in mature rats, was demonstrated; and, at the same time, calbindin positive astrocytes in the dorsal and ventral cochlear nucleus emerged (Förster and Illing, 2000). It is clear that there is altered expression of calcium binding proteins during development or after injury, but the functional basis for the different responses of calbindin and parvalbumin containing neurons and the relation to neuronal impair are poorly understood.

Calbindin and parvalbumin are of particular interest in relation to neurodegenerative diseases such as Alzheimers's, Huntington's, and Parkinson's. Expression of these calcium binding proteins may be one of the determinants of selective vulnerability in neurodegenerative diseases. For example, impaired Ca^{2+} homeostasis with elevated calcium concentrations may play a role in neuronal degeneration in Alzheimer's disease. Loss of calbindin immunoreactive neurons from the cortex in Alzheimer-type dementia has been found (Ichimiya et al., 1988), but not in the visual cortex of normal and Alzheimer brains (Leuba et al., 1998). Regional variability in the expression of parvalbumin and calbindin has been reported in many studies relevant to dementia. However, the findings have ranged from no notable changes to significant reductions in immunoreactivity in different types of dementia (reviewed by Heizmann and Braun, 1995). Moreover, calbindin-D_{28k} and parvalbumin may have a protective capacity (reviewed by Heizmann and Braun, 1992; Andressen et al., 1993), because cells containing one or the other of these proteins appear to be more resistant to cell death. The reasons for the contradictory findings are not clear, but one possibility is that so many different methods have been used.

EFFECT OF NOISE EXPOSURE ON CALCIUM BINDING PROTEIN IMMUNOREACTIVITY

It is important to know if calcium homeostasis is altered in the central auditory nervous system after noise exposure. For example, if prolonged sound over-stimulation affected intracellular neuronal calcium concentration, the result could be dysfunction of neuronal activity. However, if the activity of calcium binding proteins were simultaneously increased, protection from damage might be afforded. To determine the activity of calbindin and parvalbumin after noise exposure, Idrizbegovic, Bogdanovic, and Canlon (1998) exposed young CBA mice to a broadband noise (6 to 12 kHz) at an intensity of either 80 dB SPL or 103 dB SPL for 2 hours. The lower level sound stimulation did not alter auditory brainstem thresholds compared to pre-exposure values when measured immediately post-exposure, while the 103-dB exposure caused between a 36- and 52-dB threshold shift. Quantitative immunocytochemistry was performed on the dorsal- and posteroventral cochlear nucleus (DCN, PVCN) and the inferior colliculus (IC) to determine the effects of noise exposure on calbindin and parvalbumin.

CALBINDIN-D_{28k} IMMUNOREACTIVITY

Noise exposure caused statistically significant increases in calbindin immunoreactivity in the DCN (Idrizbegovic et al., 1998). Calbindin-D_{28k} immunoreactivity was more notable in the DCN in the group of mice exposed to 103-dB broadband noise than in the group exposed to 80 dB (Figure 22.1A). Qualitatively, increased calbindin immunoreactivity was observed both in the neurons and the surrounding neuropil in the deep layers of the DCN. The unexposed group was characterized by the least calbindin immunoreactivity. In the PVCN, the apparent trend toward a graded increase in calbindin immunoreactivity with increasing sound stimulation was not statistically significant.

Calbindin immunoreactivity in the IC showed statistically significant differences in the noise-exposed groups, compared to the control group, but not between the 80 and 103 dB exposed groups (Figure 22.1B). Qualitatively, calbindin-positive neurons in the control group were observed in the neuronal soma and neuropil of the dorsal cortex (DC) and the external cortex (EC) superficial layers, as well as the commissural nucleus (NCO). After noise exposure, an increase of calbindin-positive neurons was observed in the superficial and deep layers of the EC and the DC (Idrizbegovic et al., 1999). In general, calbindin immunoreactivity in the IC was much weaker, both in the noise-exposed and control groups, compared to the calbindin immunoreactivity in the DCN and PVCN. The same pattern of weak calbindin immunoreactivity has been shown in the IC of CBA/CaJ mice (Zettel et al., 1997).

PARVALBUMIN IMMUNOREACTIVITY

Parvalbumin immunoreactivity in the DCN was more prominent in the group of mice exposed to 103-dB broadband noise than in the group exposed to 80 dB (Figure 22.2). Qualitatively, both the neurons and the neuropil in the deep layers in the DCN were more intensely stained for parvalbumin with increasing sound stimulation. The least intense parvalbumin staining was noted in the unexposed group. In the PVCN, parvalbumin immunoreactivity was also more pronounced in the group of mice exposed to 103-dB and 80-dB broadband noise compared to the control group, and in the 103-dB compared to the 80-dB exposed group (Figure 22.2). An increase of parvalbumin-stained neurons was observed in the octopus cell area with increasing sound stimulation (Figure 22.3A).

In the IC, parvalbumin immunoreactivity was more prominent in the mice exposed to 103 dB compared to either the 80 dB group or the control group. Parvalbumin displays an intensive staining pattern in the neuronal soma and surrounding neuropil of the ICC, the deeper layer of the EC, and to a lesser extent in the DC, but not in the NCO. After sound stimulation, more parvalbumin immunopositive neuronal profiles were obtained in these regions of the IC (Figure 22.3B).

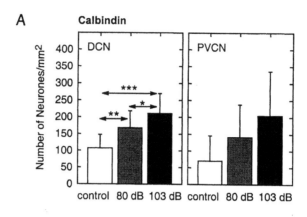

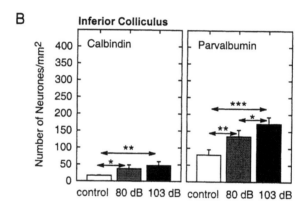

FIGURE 22.1 (A) The number of calbindin immmunopositive neurons per square millimeter in the DCN (left) and in the PVCN (right) for the three different groups (control, 80 dB SPL, and 103 dB SPL), showing a graded increase in immunoreactivity with increasing sound stimulation. (Reprinted from *Brain Res.,* 800, 86-96, 1998. With permission from Elsevier Science.) (B) The number of calbindin (left) and parvalbumin (right) immmunopositive neurons per square millimeter in the inferior colliculus (IC) for the three different groups (control, 80 dB SPL, and 103 dB SPL), showing a graded increase in immunoreactivity with increasing sound stimulation. (Reprinted from *Neuroscience Lett.,* 259, 49-52, 1999. With permission from Elsevier Science.)

SIGNIFICANCE OF AN ALTERED CALBINDIN AND PARVALBUMIN IMMUNOREACTIVITY AFTER NOISE EXPOSURE

The results of the study by Idrizbegovic et al. (1998) showed that increasing sound stimulation caused a graded increase in the expression of calbindin and parvalbumin immunoreactivity in the DCN, PVCN, and the IC (with a non-significant trend for calbindin immunoreactivity in the PVCN). These findings may indicate a possible protective role of the calcium binding proteins in the cochlear nucleus and IC associated with noise exposure and the resulting increased neuronal activity or physiological stress (see Batini et al., 1993; Celio et al., 1986). Alternatively, the increase in calbindin and parvalbumin immunoreactivity in these central nervous auditory structures might be in response to higher (non-stressful) auditory evoked metabolic activity connected with sound stimulation.

The expression of parvalbumin in the neurons and neuropil of the DCN, PVCN, and IC, was statistically greater than the calbindin immunoreactivity. This pattern of a stronger immunoreactivity of parvalbumin in the DCN, PVCN, and IC has also been found in a variety of other species,

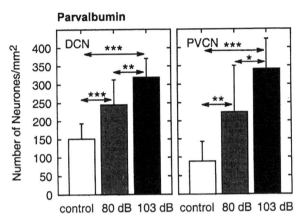

FIGURE 22.2 The number of parvalbumin immmunopositive neurons per square millimeter in the DCN (left) and PVCN (right) for the three different groups (control, 80 dB SPL, and 103 dB SPL), showing a graded increase in immunoreactivity with increasing sound stimulation. (Reprinted from *Brain Res.*, 800, 86-96, 1998. With permission from Elsevier Science.)

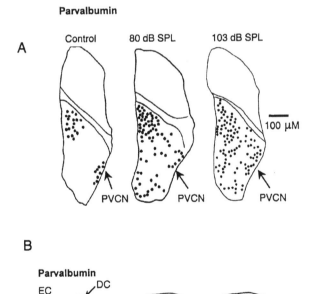

FIGURE 22.3 (A) Camera lucida tracings showing a graded increase in parvalbumin labeling with increasing sound stimulation in the PVCN in control, 80 DB SPL and 103 dB SPL. Scale bar: 100 μm. (Reprinted from *Brain Res.*, 800, 86-96, 1998. With permission from Elsevier Science.) (B) Camera lucida tracings illustrating the graded increase in parvalbumin labeling with increasing sound stimulation (in control, 80 dB SPL, and 103 dB SPL), in the inferior colliculus (IC). Scale bar: 100 μm. (Reprinted from *Neuroscience Lett.*, 259, 49-52, 1999. With permission from Elsevier Science.)

including the rat, guinea pig, and bat (Lohmann and Friauf, 1996; Caicedo et al., 1997; Vater and Braun, 1994). It has also been shown that parvalbumin has been localized in neuronal pathways characterized with high spike rates and high levels of metabolic activity and that parvalbumin staining is in the more highly active neurons (Kawaguchi et al., 1987; Braun et al., 1985). These results suggest that parvalbumin plays a more dominant role in buffering calcium in response to highly active neurons in the central auditory pathways.

AGING, CA²⁺, AND CALCIUM BINDING PROTEINS

Whereas there are a number of theories of aging, changes in calcium homeostasis are likely to play a key role (Khachaturian, 1989). Age-dependent alterations in the cellular mechanisms of Ca^{2+} homeostasis result in sustained changes in the regulation of intracellular Ca^{2+} concentration, which contribute to neuronal degeneration that often accompany aging. Khachaturian (1989) suggested that a small disturbances in Ca^{2+} homeostasis, with increased Ca^{2+} over a long period, can have similar cell-injuring consequences to those produced by a large increase in Ca^{2+} over a shorter period. Whereas there are indeed a number of alterations in calcium homeostasis and calcium-related neuronal processes, they tend to be complex and difficult to understand (see Verkhratsky and Toescu, 1998). For example, age-related decreases in the number of calbindin and parvalbumin neurons were found in the hippocampus of the rat (Krzywkowski et al., 1996). It has also been shown that the number of hippocampal interneurons expressing these calcium binding proteins decrease with aging in rats (Shetty and Turner, 1998). In different regions of the hamster brain, however, parvalbumin and calretinin mRNA expression was unchanged, while calbindin-D_{28k} mRNA expression decreased (Kishimoto et al., 1998).

AGING AND CALBINDIN AND PARVALBUMIN IMMUNOREACTIVITY IN THE AUDITORY SYSTEM OF CBA MICE

The complexity of age-related changes in calcium binding proteins is clearly revealed by studies on the CBA mouse central auditory system. As discussed elsewhere (e.g., Chapters 5, 13, 24, and 28), CBA mice maintain good hearing well into old age, and there is little age-related neuronal loss in the cochlear nucleus or IC. Thus, quantifying the number of calbindin-D_{28k} and parvalbumin neurons may give insight into the fate of calcium binding proteins in the central auditory system during aging.

We estimated the total number of calbindin-D_{28k} and parvalbumin immunopositive neurons in the DCN and PVCN of CBA/CaJ mice (1 to 24 months of age) using the optical fractionator procedure, an unbiased quantitative stereological method. This technique involves counting immunopositive neurons with optical disectors in a uniform and systematic sample that constitutes a known fraction of the region to be analyzed. The estimation is not affected by tissue shrinkage (West et al., 1991).

Parvalbumin immunoreactivity was distributed evenly throughout all layers of the DCN, both in the neurons and the neuropil. Most parvalbumin immunopositive neurons appeared to be stellate, large multipolar, fusiform, and granule cells. Quantitative analysis in the DCN showed a statistically significant increase of parvalbumin immunopositive neurons with increasing age (Figure 22.4A). Parvalbumin immunoreactivity was also found in neurons and surrounding neuropil throughout the PVCN, and this also showed a statistically significant increase with age (Figure 22.4A). Parvalbumin immunopositive neurons were mainly octopus and globular cells. Calbindin immunoreactivity in the DCN was predominantly found in the superficial layer, both in the neurons and surrounding neuropil. Most calbindin-stained neurons appeared to be cartwheel and stellate cells. On the cellular level, calbindin-positive staining was detected both in the cytoplasm and in the nucleus. Quantitative analysis in the DCN showed a statistically significant increase of calbindin immunopositive neurons with increasing age (Figure 22.4B). In the PVCN, calbindin immunoreactivity was found mostly

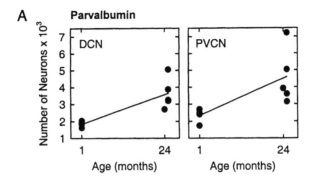

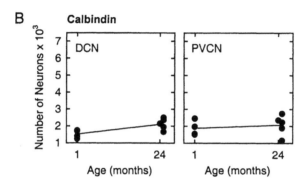

FIGURE 22.4   (A) Quantitative analysis showing statistically significant increases in the total number of parvalbumin immunopositive neurons in the DCN (left) and in the PVCN (right) with increasing age (1 and 24 months). (B) Quantitative analysis showing statistically significant increases in the total number of calbindin immunopositive neurons in the DCN (left) with increasing age (1 and 24 months). In the PVCN (right), statistically significant differences between 1- and 24-month-old mice were not found.

in the globular cells in the ventral part of the PVCN, and in the surrounding neuropil. Statistically significant differences were not found for calbindin positive neurons in the PVCN with increasing age (Figure 22.4B).

For other regions of the central auditory system, the picture may be more complicated, however. Other studies have shown a decrease in calbindin immunoreactivity in the CBA mouse IC, whereas calretinin immunoreactivity increased (Zettel et al., 1997). In the medial nucleus of the trapezoid body (MNTB), no change in calbindin immunoreactivity was found between young and old CBA mice (O'Neill et al., 1997).

SUMMARY

Calbindin-D$_{28k}$ and parvalbumin immunoreactivity is modulated in neurons of the cochlear nucleus and IC after noise exposure and during aging in CBA mice. The effect of noise exposure on calbindin and parvalbumin immunoreactivity in the DCN, PVCN, and IC was studied using two-dimensional quantification. Sound stimulation (80 dB SPL and 103 dB SPL) caused a graded increase in the appearance of calbindin and parvalbumin immunoreactivity in the DCN and IC, and parvalbumin immunoreactivity in the PVCN. The up-regulation of these calcium binding proteins may be associated with a protective role against over-stimulation and/or their response to a higher auditory-evoked metabolic activity.

Studies on aging CBA mice found an increase in the total number of parvalbumin immunopositive neurons in the DCN and PVCN, and increases in the total number of the calbindin immunopositive neurons in the DCN. An increase of parvalbumin and calbindin immunopositive neurons during aging may reflect a functional protective role of these calcium binding proteins in the cochlear nucleus. However, the results of several studies demonstrate the complexity of age-related changes in calcium binding proteins: an increase in the number of parvalbumin immunopositive neurons increases with age in both DCN and PVCN; an increase in calbindin immunopositive neurons in the DCN, a decrease in the IC, and no change in the PVCN or MNTB.

ACKNOWLEDGMENTS

Supported by The Swedish Council for Work Life Research (96-0509), The Swedish Medical Research Council (9476), Stiftelsen Tysta Skolan, Kapten Arthur Erikssons Stiftelse, AMF Trygghetsförsäkring, Svenska Sällskapet för Medicinsk Forskning, Gun and Bertil Stohne Stiftelse, NIH grant AGO7554, and Karolinska Institute.

23 Auditory Neurons in the Reticular Formation of C57BL/6J Mice

Stephanie Carlson

INTRODUCTION

Most physiological studies investigating auditory response properties of neurons have focused on neurons within the auditory system, from cochlear nucleus to auditory cortex. However, auditory stimuli are also processed in other regions of the central nervous system, such as the reticular formation of the brainstem. This chapter discusses one such region, the caudal pontine reticular nucleus (PnC), a structure thought to be the sensorimotor interface of the acoustic startle reflex circuit.

THE ROLE OF THE PNC IN STARTLE

Numerous studies have investigated the role of the PnC in startle. Leitner, Powers, and Hoffman (1980) made selective lesions of the PnC in rats and assessed the impact of these lesions on startle elicited by acoustic as well as footshock stimuli. Startle amplitudes in response to both types of stimuli were significantly reduced. Davis, Gendelman, Tischler, and Gendelman (1982) lesioned specific regions (dorsal and ventral) of the PnC in rats and found that only ventral PnC lesions reduced startle to a significant degree. Davis and colleagues (1982) also stimulated these nuclei electrically and observed startle-like behavior in response to ventral PnC stimulation, but not in response to dorsal PnC stimulation.

Wu, Suzuki, and Siegel (1988) began to characterize the response properties of startle-related neurons within the reticular formation. They measured startle electromyographically from the neck and simultaneously sampled the activity of 396 single units in the pontomedullary reticular formation of awake cats. Startle-inducing stimuli elicited action potentials in 26.5% of the cells. Wu and co-workers found a strong correlation between unit response magnitudes and motor response magnitudes, strengthening the evidence for a role of these neurons in the acoustic startle responses.

Yeomans and Cochrane (1993) used the collision technique to determine if the neural response to intense acoustic signals in the startle circuit could be affected by antidromic action potentials originating in the PnC. They implanted an electrode in the caudal PnC and stimulated cells with electric pulses that were time-locked to an acoustic signal. They found sharp increases in the current threshold for electrical startle when the electrical pulse followed the acoustic stimulus by 1.5 to 4.6 ms, but not when the electric pulse occurred during or before the acoustic stimulation. These findings were presumably due to collisions between acoustically evoked action potentials and antidromic electrically evoked AP. This indicates that both types of stimuli caused the activation of a common pool of axons and supports the role of the PnC in startle. More recent studies (Koch, Lingenhöhl, and Pilz, 1992; Lingenhöhl and Friauf, 1992; 1994) have investigated a specific subpopulation of PnC neurons (giant cells) that are likely to mediate the startle response. These giant cells receive auditory input from the cochlear nucleus, superior olivary complex, and the inferior colliculus and project to the ventral horn of the spinal cord (Lingenhöhl and Friauf, 1992), which contains spinal motoneurons capable of eliciting the startle response.

PREPULSE INHIBITION

The behavioral startle response is subject to modification by prepulse stimuli. When a low-intensity prepulse (S1) precedes the startle stimulus (S2), by an interval of 5 to 200 milliseconds, the amplitude of the startle reflex is reduced (prepulse inhibition, or PPI; see Chapter 5). The degree to which the startle is reduced is an indicator of the behavioral salience of the prepulse. Previous studies using C57 mice have investigated prepulse inhibition and how it is affected by hearing loss, and these are reviewed in Chapters 5 and 14. Briefly, C57 mice mature into young adulthood (1 to 2 months) with normal hearing but exhibit progressive high-frequency hearing loss beginning at 2 to 3 months of age. By 5 to 6 months of age, high-frequency (>20 kHz) hearing loss is substantial. Concurrent with the cochlear pathology, functional changes are observed in central auditory structures such as the inferior colliculus, thought to be involved in prepulse inhibition of the startle response: as high frequency sensitivity is lost, neurons in the formerly high-frequency regions of the primary auditory cortex and inferior colliculus become more sensitive to middle-frequency tones (4 to 16 kHz) (Willott, 1984; 1986; Willott, Aitkin, and McFadden, 1993). This increased sensitivity to middle-frequency tones is reflected behaviorally in the prepulse inhibition paradigm. Middle-frequency prepulses inhibit the startle reflex to a greater degree in 6-month-old mice than in 1-month-old mice (Willott, Carlson, and Chen, 1994b; Carlson and Willott, 1996). Thus, the middle frequencies that become "over-represented" in the 6-month-old mice become more behaviorally salient as well.

RESPONSES OF PNC NEURONS IN C57 MICE

With all of the above in mind, Carlson and Willott (1998) assessed extracellular response properties of PnC neurons in 1- and 6-month-old C57 mice. Because this seems to be the only published study investigating PnC responses in mice, it is described here in some detail. The mice had been behaviorally pretested and demonstrated the typical pattern of PPI: Prepulse frequencies of both 4 and 12 kHz provided superior inhibition in the 6-month-old animals, whereas 24-kHz prepulses became less effective.

Extracellular recordings were obtained with tungsten microelectrodes from PnC neurons in mice anesthetized with sodium pentobarbital and chlorprothixene. In contrast to the situation in typical auditory nuclei, it was necessary to employ 90 dB SPL noise bursts as "search stimuli" (i.e., an intensity capable of eliciting startle responses in awake animals). It was also necessary to present search stimuli at a rate of 0.1 Hz because PnC neurons readily habituate when a faster presentation rate is employed. Neural responses were measured using stimuli similar to those used in the behavioral tests: S2-only (4 kHz tone pip, 90 dB SPL, 10 ms duration, 1 ms rise-fall) and various S1-S2 combinations (S1 = 70 dB SPL, either 4, 12, or 24 kHz tones, 10 ms duration, 1 ms rise-fall).

Latency

Figure 23.1 is a frequency distribution, plotting latency of the response of each neuron evoked by an S2-only stimulus for each age group. It is evident that a greater number of neurons demonstrated short-latency (<6 ms) responses in the 1-month-old C57 mice, when compared to the responses of neurons in 6-month-old mice (20 vs. 3 neurons demonstrating short latencies). Many PnC neuron response latencies in the 6-month-old mice were clustered around 8 ms, whereas the responses in the younger mice were distributed more evenly across the shorter latencies. The latency of these responses would allow sufficient time for the completion of the startle circuit before behavioral startle is initiated. In a previous experiment using 1- and 6-month-old C57 mice, Parham and Willott

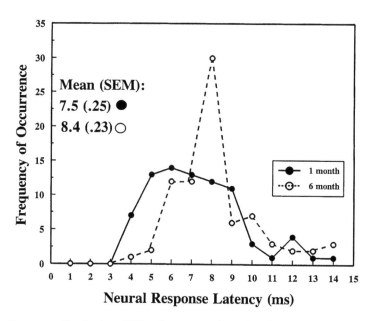

FIGURE 23.1 Frequency distribution of S2-only response latencies of all PnC neurons in 1- and 6-month-old mice (n = 81 and 80 neurons, respectively). Fewer PnC neurons responded with short latencies in 6-month-olds. (Reprinted with permission from The American Physiological Society from Carlson, S.C., Willott, J.F., 1998. Caudal pontine reticular formation of C57BL/6J mice: responses to startle stimuli, inhibition by tones, plasticity. *J. Neurophysiol.*, 79, 2603-2614.)

(1988) found that mean startle latencies of 1-month-old C57's were 9 ms and those of 6-month-olds were 10 ms. The latencies of S2-evoked PnC responses in the present study should allow 1 to 2 ms for the completion of the startle circuit and reflect the 1-ms age difference seen in C57 mice as well.

THRESHOLD

PnC neurons generally had high thresholds for excitation by auditory stimuli. Many neurons gave no response when S1 stimuli of 4, 12, and 24 kHz were presented at a level of 70 dB SPL. For 1-month-old animals, 74% of neurons had no response to 4-kHz stimuli (the same frequency as all S2 stimuli used in this experiment). Stimuli of 12 and 24 kHz elicited no response in 5% and 40% of neurons, respectively. For 6-month-old animals, 63% of neurons had no response to 4 kHz stimuli presented at 70 dB SPL. Stimuli of 12 and 24 kHz elicited no response in 6% and 96% of neurons, respectively. The mean thresholds were 63 and 57 dB SPL for 1- and 6-month old mice, respectively. These values are 30 to 40 dB higher than thresholds of inferior colliculus neurons in C57 mice at the respective ages (Willott, 1986).

The acoustic startle response is evoked exclusively by abrupt, high-intensity stimuli (Davis, 1984). Thresholds for startle were determined in 1- and 6-month-old C57 mice by Parham and Willott (1988). Thresholds were similar for both age groups; between 85 and 90 dB SPL for a 4-kHz S2. The absolute threshold sensitivity (i.e., the minimal SPLs a mouse can detect) measured electrophysiologically in both ages of C57 mice were between 55 and 60 dB SPL. Startle thresholds are "high" when compared to the absolute threshold sensitivity for these mice.

SENSITIVITY TO STIMULUS PRESENTATION RATE

PnC units exhibited sensitivity to the stimulus presentation rate, specifically a reduction in the number of responses elicited by rapidly presented stimuli when compared to those elicited by stimuli presented at a slower rate. All neurons responded well to the relatively slow rate of

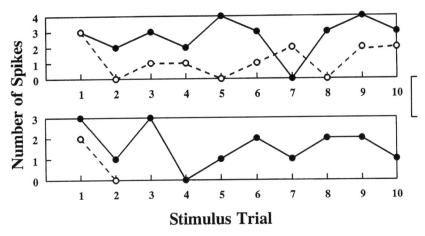

Stimulus Trial

FIGURE 23.2   Effects of stimulus presentation rate. Responses of two representative neurons to slow (0.1/s) and fast (1/s) S2 presentation rates. Top panel: this neuron responded to the S2 with 2 to 4 action potentials on most trials, when the S2 was presented at 1/s; at the faster rate, the unit continued to respond across 10 trials, but with fewer action potentials. Bottom panel: this unit responded well for 10 stimulus trials at the slower rate, but stopped responding after the first stimulus when the rate was 0.1/s. Whereas the top panel is from unit SC5C (1-month-old mouse), and the bottom panel is from unit SC9D (6-month-old mouse), these response patterns were common in both age groups. (Reprinted with permission from The American Physiological Society from Carlson, S.C., Willott, J.F., 1998. Caudal pontine reticular formation of C57BL/6J mice: responses to startle stimuli, inhibition by tones, plasticity. *J. Neurophysiol.*, 79, 2603-2614.)

presentation (0.1 Hz) used in the recording protocols. However, they typically did not respond well when a more rapid rate (1 Hz) was employed. The vast majority of neurons tended to respond to the first of a train of rapidly presented startle stimuli. Subsequent stimuli elicited fewer action potentials or no responses at all. Figure 23.2 shows potentials for each stimulus presentation elicited by rapidly or slowly presented stimuli in two representative neurons. In both neurons, action potentials were evoked by nine out of ten S2 stimuli presented at the slow rate. The neuron represented in the upper panel responded to the first stimulus presented at the rapid rate, and subsequent responses to the stimuli were diminished (fewer action potentials were evoked). The neuron represented in the lower panel responded to the first stimulus presented at the rapid rate and ceased to respond to subsequent S2s in the stimulus train.

The relationship between presentation rate and the number of action potentials evoked by ten S2 stimuli is shown in Figure 23.3. The number of action potentials evoked by S2 only stimuli was measured using fast and slow stimulus presentation rates. The fast presentation rate produced fewer action potentials, regardless of the age of the animals.

These response properties are also similar to those of behavioral startle. Previous studies examining the startle response in C57 mice have demonstrated sharp decrements in startle amplitude in response to rapidly presented stimuli. For example, Willott, Shnerson, and Urban (1979) elicited startle responses in C57 mice using a fast rate of 1 Hz or a slower, variable rate. For the fast presentation rate, startle amplitude elicited by the second stimulus was approximately 30% of the response elicited by the first stimulus. Subsequent responses to stimuli presented at the fast rate were reduced as well. Startles elicited by the stimuli presented at a slower rate were robust, and their amplitudes did not decrement with repeated stimulation.

PPI DEMONSTRATED IN PNC NEURONS

To evaluate PnC responses to moderately intense tones, a "neural PPI" paradigm was employed (this also helps to establish a relationship between PPI and PnC responses). Neural PPI was defined as the number of action potentials evoked by the S2 when the S1 was present, divided by the

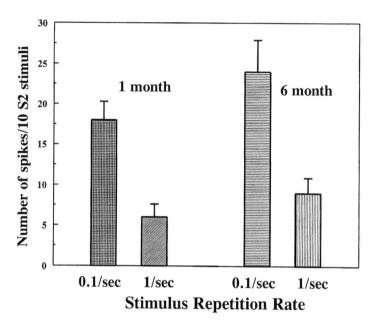

FIGURE 23.3 Bar graph depicting the number of action potentials evoked by slow (0.1/s) and fast (1/s) S2 presentation rates for 1- and 6-month-old mice. Error bars indicate 1 standard error of the mean; number of neurons = 13 (1-month-olds) and 15 (6-month-olds). Irrespective of age, the faster repetition rate was much less effective in evoking action potentials in PnC neurons. (Reprinted with permission from The American Physiological Society from Carlson, S.C., Willott, J.F., 1998. Caudal pontine reticular formation of C57BL/6J mice: responses to startle stimuli, inhibition by tones, plasticity. *J. Neurophysiol.*, 79, 2603-2614.)

number of action potentials evoked by S2-only (S1-S2/S2-only), expressed as a percentage. PnC neurons in both age groups of mice demonstrated neural PPI. In each unit examined, at least one of the three S1 frequencies employed produced neural PPI in that fewer discharges were evoked by S2 when S1 was present. These findings would be expected if PPI were mediated by a reduction in evoked discharges in PnC neurons that trigger the startle response.

Post-stimulus time histograms (PSTHs) from two representative neurons demonstrating the typical response characteristics of PnC neurons to S1 and S2 stimuli are shown in Figures 23.4 (1-month-old) and 23.5 (6-month-old). Unit SC12e (Figure 23.4) showed substantial PPI when each S1 was employed. Thirty responses were initiated by the S2 stimulus alone. This was decreased to 10 responses when the 4-kHz S1 was present (PPI = 33%), 1 response when the 12-kHz S1 was present (PPI = 3%), and 9 responses when the 24-kHz S1 was present (PPI = 30%). Note that all of the S1 frequencies were capable of eliciting action potentials in this unit, although responses to the 12-kHz S1 were the most robust. The response of this neuron to S2 when a 4- or 12-kHz S1 was employed showed a latency shift when compared to the S2-only response. Figure 23.5 shows a substantial reduction in the response of unit SC9d when S1 stimuli preceded the S2 stimuli. Twenty-seven responses were initiated by the S2 stimulus alone. This was decreased to 14 responses when the 4-kHz S1 was present (PPI = 52%), 1 response when the 12-kHz S1 was present (PPI = 4%), and 16 responses when the 24-kHz S1 was present (PPI = 59%). Note that the only S1 that was capable of eliciting a response in this unit was 12 kHz. Substantial PPI occurred when the S1 did not evoke a response (4- and 24-kHz S1s). The response of this neuron to S2 when a 12-kHz S1 was employed showed a 5-ms latency shift when compared to the S2-only response.

Neural PPI was apparent for all S1 frequencies in both age groups, with the exception of 24 kHz in the 6-month-old mice. Several studies (Carlson and Willott, 1996; Willott and Carlson, 1995; Willott et al., 1994b) have demonstrated better behavioral PPI for low- and middle-frequency S1s in 6-month-old C57 mice when compared to PPI in 1-month-old C57 mice, whereas poor PPI is

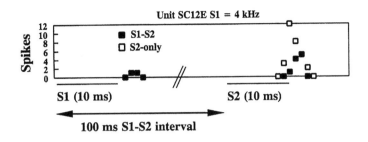

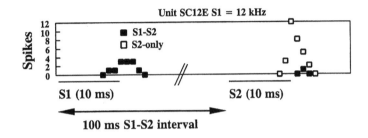

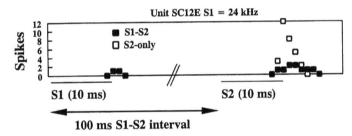

FIGURE 23.4 Representative post-stimulus time histograms showing responses of PnC unit SC12E (1-month-old mouse) to S1 and S2 stimuli for each frequency of S1. PSTH bin width = 1 ms. The horizontal lines under each PSTH show the occurrence of the S1 and S2, separated by 100 ms. The open squares show the number of action potentials in each 1-ms time bin evoked by the S2-only; filled squares show the number of action potentials when S1 preceded S2 by 100 ms. For each S1 frequency, the number of responses evoked by S2 was reduced when S1 preceded S2. This unit also responded to the S1 (especially 12 kHz). (Reprinted with permission from The American Physiological Society from Carlson, S.C., Willott, J.F., 1998. Caudal pontine reticular formation of C57BL/6J mice: responses to startle stimuli, inhibition by tones, plasticity. *J. Neurophysiol.*, 79, 2603-2614.)

obtained with 24-kHz S1s in the older mice. The reduction of S2-evoked action potentials in startle-related PnC neurons by 4-kHz S1s was greater for 6-month-old C57 mice than for 1-month-old C57 mice.

S1–S2 Intervals

Neural PPI data obtained using different S1–S2 intervals provided further evidence that PnC responses have parallels with behavioral PPI. A 2-ms S2 interval is too short to produce behavioral PPI (Willott and Carlson, 1995). Similarly, neural PPI was not evident with a 2-ms S1–S2 interval. Behaviorally, intervals of 5 to 500 ms do result in PPI in C57 mice, with optimal intervals of 50 to 100 ms (Willott and Carlson, 1995). As seen in Figure 23.6, similar PPI was observed in PnC neurons in the present study. A study by Willott and Carlson (1995) showed that long S1–S2 intervals (200 and 500 ms) provided good PPI in 6-month-old C57 mice, but not in 1-month-old

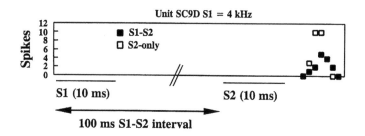

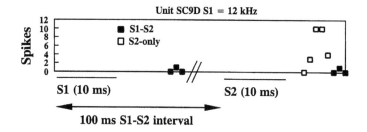

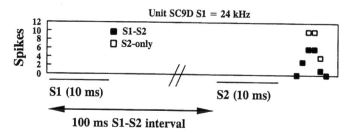

FIGURE 23.5 Representative post-stimulus time histograms showing responses of PnC unit SC9D (6-month-old mouse) to S1 and S2 stimuli for each frequency of Sl. The open squares show the number of action potentials in each 1-ms time bin evoked by the S2-only; filled squares show the number of action potentials when S1 preceded S2 by 100 ms. For the 4-kHz, and especially the 12-kHz S1, the number of responses evoked by S2 was reduced when S1 preceded S2. The latency of the response to S2 was prolonged when the 12-kHz S1 was present. When the S1 was 24 kHz, inhibition of the S2 response was minimal. This unit did not respond to the S1. (Reprinted with permission from The American Physiological Society from Carlson, S.C., Willott, J.F., 1998. Caudal pontine reticular formation of C57BL/6J mice: responses to startle stimuli, inhibition by tones, plasticity. *J. Neurophysiol.*, 79, 2603-2614.)

C57 mice. The reduction of S2-evoked action potentials by middle-frequency (12 kHz) S1s lasted for a longer duration in 6-month-old C57 mice than in 1-month-old C57 mice.

Spontaneously Active Neurons

Some spontaneously active neurons were present in the PnC (although none of the PnC units used for startle-PPI recordings exhibited spontaneous activity). Some of these units were inhibited for a brief time (about 100 ms) after the presentation of S1 or S2 stimuli. Others showed no change in response rate or a small increase in discharge rate after the presentation of an S2 stimulus.

Anatomical Considerations

A variable that influenced the PPI data was the anatomical location of PnC neurons. There appeared to be a crude "tonotopic organization" *with respect to S1 efficacy.* In young mice, PPI with the

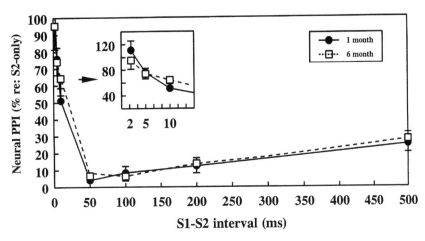

FIGURE 23.6 Neural PPI as a function of S1–S2 interval and age group; S1 = 12 kHz. Error bars indicate 1 standard error of the mean. In both age groups, S1–S2 intervals of 2 ms produced no neural PPI; intervals of 5 and 10 ms produced a moderate degree of PPI; 50 to 100 ms intervals were optimal; PPI remained strong with 200- and 500-ms S1–S2 intervals. (Reprinted with permission from The American Physiological Society from Carlson, S.C., Willott, J.F., 1998. Caudal pontine reticular formation of C57BL/6J mice: responses to startle stimuli, inhibition by tones, plasticity. *J. Neurophysiol.*, 79, 2603-2614.)

4-kHz S1 tended to be better in the lateral PnC than in the medial PnC. By contrast, the 24-kHz S1 was more effective in the medial PnC. This organization did seem important with respect to the neural manifestation of stronger PPI using 4-kHz S1 stimuli. The age difference was quite clear in the lateral PnC but absent in the medial PnC. Perhaps the descending inputs to the PnC that were affected by hearing loss-induced plasticity (for 4 kHz stimuli) project primarily to the lateral PnC causing enhanced behavioral PPI through their influence on cells in this region.

SUMMARY

Responses of PnC neurons are quite different from those in most nuclei of the auditory system. For reliable responses to be evoked, acoustic stimuli must be very intense and presented at a relatively slow rate. Moreover, PnC neurons exhibit very strong neural PPI: excitatory responses evoked by intense (startle) stimuli are modulated (inhibited) by moderately intense tones, although those tones cannot evoke excitatory responses in PnC neurons. Responses of PnC neurons clearly parallel the startle response with respect to latency, threshold, responses to repetitive stimuli, spontaneous activity, and PPI. In 6-month-old C57 mice, the modulation of PnC responses by 4-kHz S1s is enhanced, as is the case for behavioral PPI. This suggests that plasticity in pathways that modulate startle (e.g., the inferior colliculus) influence neural PPI in PnC neurons.

24 Aging of the Mouse Central Auditory System

Robert D. Frisina and Joseph P. Walton

INTRODUCTION

Aside from investigations that directly measure aging changes of the human central auditory system, as summarized comprehensively by Willott (1991a), a strong case can be made that the most productive animal model for understanding the neural bases of presbycusis — age-related hearing loss — is the mouse. Mice have afforded many advantages along these lines. Different strains of mice lose their hearing at different rates. For example, CBA strains (e.g., CBA/J, CBA/CaJ) have a slow, relatively flat, progressive hearing loss with a time frame similar to that of humans, if one corrects for the different absolute lifespans of mice and men. In contrast, the DBA/2J (DBA) and C57BL/6J (C57) mouse strains have very rapid, high-frequency hearing losses. Comparing neural changes with age in these different strains allows for determination of peripheral vs. central etiologies. For example, a 6-month-old C57 mouse has a young brain, but an "old" ear; whereas, a 2-year-old CBA mouse has both an old ear and old brain. Last, breakthroughs in molecular biology, including mapping of the human and mouse genomes, make the mouse especially relevant for utilization of genetically engineered mice and development of gene therapies that eventually may cure or prevent age-related sensory disorders.

One of the challenges to sensory neuroscientists interested in discovering the neural bases of presbycusis is determining the contributions of various structural and functional changes that accompany aging. For example, changes in the central auditory system can result from "biological aging" — changes linked to free radical damage, somatic mutations, or other putative "causes" of aging that affect tissue throughout the body. Alternatively, plasticity of the central auditory system can result from age-related reductions in inputs from the peripheral auditory system (i.e., secondary effects of aging of the ear). Declines in hair cells and spiral ganglion neurons, starting in the high-frequency turn of the cochlea, disrupt high-frequency channels to the brain. Lack of these inputs to brainstem and cortical portions of the auditory system can induce reorganization that is overlaid on other age-related changes in the brain. The distinctions between these three different aging effects are presented diagrammatically in Figure 24.1.

This chapter is organized following the logic of Figure 24.1. First, articles focusing on direct age effects on the central auditory system are reviewed. Next, investigations primarily aimed at uncovering peripherally induced central effects are presented. At the end of this chapter, comparative information is highlighted, along with future research directions and implications of mouse research for understanding human age-related hearing loss.

AGE-RELATED CHANGES IN THE CENTRAL AUDITORY SYSTEM

COCHLEAR NUCLEUS

The outputs of the auditory portion of the inner ear project to and terminate in the cochlear nucleus, a lateral bulge on the brainstem, near the junction of the pons and medulla. The cochlear nucleus

0-8493-2328-2/01/$0.00+$.50
© 2001 by CRC Press LLC

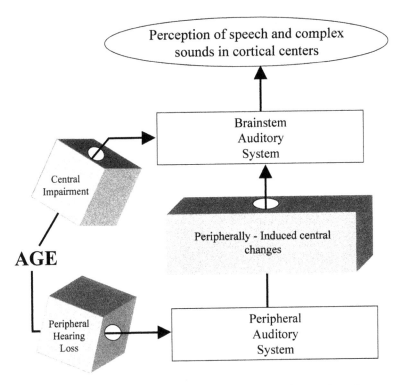

FIGURE 24.1 Schematic diagram indicating the possible neural sites of deleterious changes associated with aging on the auditory system. Changes in the central auditory system can result from biological aging, or age-related insults can induce changes in the central auditory system due to reduction or distortion of neural inputs from the aging ear. Here, we have termed this indirect influence of age on the auditory central nervous system as "peripherally induced central changes." (From Frisina et al. (2001, Fig. 1, p. 566). With permission.)

(CN) consists of three main divisions: anteroventral cochlear nucleus (AVCN), posteroventral cochlear nucleus (PVCN), and dorsal cochlear nucleus (DCN). Functionally, the cochlear nucleus sets up parallel processing pathways that ascend through the auditory brainstem, eventually proceeding to the auditory cortex and beyond for the purposes of complex sound analysis and perception. Because all auditory information is processed in the cochlear nucleus, age-related anatomical, neurochemical, or physiological changes here will affect many aspects of hearing.

Modest Changes in Gross Anatomy and Neuron Properties with Age

Willott and colleagues have examined aging changes in the cochlear nucleus in both CBA and C57 strains, and found that gross anatomical changes are relatively minor, and that in some cases hearing loss has little effect. Willott and Bross (1990) investigated the structure of the octopus cell area (OCA) of PVCN in CBA mice and C57 mice, using light microscopy staining, including Golgi sections. They found that aging was associated with declines in OCA volume, neuron number, neuron size, number of primary dendritic branches, and increased packing density of glial cells. The most significant changes took place in extreme old age; and in the OCA region of PVCN, age-related changes were not exacerbated by hearing loss (C57 data). These investigators observed great variations with aging in individual octopus cells in the older animals.

In similar studies, Willott et al. (1992; 1994a) made light microscopy investigations of other parts of the cochlear nucleus in CBA mice. They found only minor declines in cell numbers and volumes of the cochlear nucleus divisions primarily in the second year of life, even in cases where age and noise exposure were commingled. Lambert and Schwartz (1982) and Willott et al. (1987)

specifically reported small declines in the perikaryal size of AVCN bushy and multipolar cells. Nuclear volume and neuron cell body reductions were more apparent in the VCN, which receives relatively more inputs from the auditory nerve, vs. the DCN which receives ascending inputs from the auditory nerve along with significant descending inputs from other parts of the brain.

No Change in 2-DG Patterns with Age

Willott et al. (1988a) utilized [2-^{14}C]deoxy-D-glucose (2-DG) autoradiography in the auditory brainstem of young and old CBA and C57 mice to determine functional changes with age. Animals were injected with 2-DG and placed in quiet for 45 minutes before being sacrificed. The presence of 2-DG in the AVCN, the inferior colliculus (IC), and the trigeminal nerve (TN) were quantified using densitometry. In young adult animals, the degree of labeling was maximal in the IC, followed in order by the AVCN and TN. No age effects were observed, indicating that basic metabolic activity in these areas remained stable with age, with or without peripheral hearing loss.

INFERIOR COLLICULUS

The IC is the watershed for virtually all ascending acoustic information from the brainstem auditory centers. The majority of information reaching the IC comes from the ear on the opposite side of the head. Virtually all basic auditory perceptual phenomena and capabilities are formulated at the level of the IC, and then passed onto the thalamus and cortex for further refinements and final perceptions. The central nucleus of the IC (ICC) has a striking laminar appearance, reflecting a strong tonotopic (cochleotopic) organization. Overlaid upon this tonotopic map are other functional organizations such as spatial receptive field maps based on excitatory and inhibitory interactions, temporal processing capabilities for amplitude modulation (AM), and reflex arcs within the auditory system and between the auditory system and other sensorimotor systems. Age-related changes in the IC will no doubt have an effect on most auditory functions due to the IC's pivotal processing position in the central auditory nervous system, including the coding of complex sounds in quiet and background noise (Frisina and Frisina, 1997).

Stability of Nuclear Volume, Neuron Size, Numbers, and Basic Response Properties

Willott et al. (1994a) evaluated basic anatomical features of the CBA and C57 IC as a function of age utilizing light microscopy methodologies. For both strains, they found that age-related changes were minimal with respect to IC volume and regional areas, the size of IC principal neurons, the number of neurons, or their packing density. They noted that old CBA mice developed spongiform lesions similar to those originally discovered to be plentiful in certain portions of gerbil auditory brainstem nuclei as a function of age and metabolic activity. The absence of noteworthy declines in neuron numbers and dimensions in the C57 strain suggest that the chronic, high-frequency sensorineural age-related hearing loss of this strain does not manifest itself at the light microscope level in the IC, and that the basic anatomy of the IC is fairly stable in the face of aging (Willott et al., 1994a).

Kazee and West (1999) did a similar cross-sectional aging study for CBA mice, but studied features of ICC principal cells at the electron microscopy (EM) level. Like Willott and colleagues' light microscopy investigation, they reported that no changes occurred in the sizes of principal neurons with age. In terms of ultrastructure, synapses on the somata showed no change in the number, type, length, or size of the terminal area, confirming the notion that anatomical features of the CBA IC are undaunted with age.

Consistent with stability of basic anatomical features of the IC and its principal cells, response properties of IC cells as a function age in CBA mice show little change in the old mice. Willott et al. (1988b) surveyed the extracellular responses of IC cells to simple tones and noise bursts in

CBA mice and measured small declines in hearing thresholds and the number of spiral ganglion cells in the cochlear modiolus. Their main finding was the discovery that most IC units in old animals were indistinguishable from their young counterparts in terms of response patterns, response areas, and rate-level functions. An exception to the lack of an age effect was that there were more units that were sluggish in the old animals: 3% in young and 22% in old. They defined sluggish units as those responsive to acoustic stimulation but responding with very low driven spike rates. In addition, they reported a trend toward increasing spontaneous activity rates in the ventral (high-frequency) region of IC, and the opposite effect in the dorsal (low-frequency) IC.

Changes in Temporal Processing: Behavioral and Neural Declines

Interestingly, in contrast to the basic anatomical and physiological properties of CBA mice that show little change with age, Walton and co-workers have demonstrated in a multidisciplinary manner that there are declines in processing of complex sounds with age for CBA mice in regard to the brainstem auditory system. Walton et al. (1997), for the first time in the mammalian auditory system, demonstrated possible neural correlates at the level of the IC for a behavioral temporal processing task. Gap detection is commonly used by psychoacousticians and hearing scientists to assess auditory temporal acuity, and Walton et al. measured behavioral gap detection thresholds utilizing an inhibition of startle response paradigm (see Chapters 5 and 25 for more on this). With this methodology, the more perceptible the gap in a wideband noise, the greater the inhibition of the acoustic startle response, which is measured quantitatively. Results of this behavioral portion of the study are presented in Figure 24.2A for a suprathreshold intensity level. At short gap durations, lengthening the gap results in dramatic increases in detection; whereas at longer gap durations, greater than 3 ms, responses tend toward an asymptote.

In the neurophysiological part of this investigation, single-unit responses to suprathreshold gaps in a wideband noise burst were recorded in awake CBA mice, examples of which are given in Figures 24.3 and 24.4. Figure 24.3 displays the typical gap encoding responses of an IC unit that had a sustained response to tones. For these units, gap encoding consists of a *decrease* in spike firing rate in response to the gap (arrows), followed by an *increase* in firing in response to the end of the gap (asterisks). Units with transient (onset) responses encode gaps a bit differently. Their main coding mechanism consists of an *increase* in neuronal firing rate in response to the end of the gap (arrows in Figure 24.4). Walton et al. (1997) plotted the behavioral results on the same axes as the representative neural findings, as shown in Figure 24.2B, demonstrating the correspondence between the behavioral measures of CBA gap encoding and the single-unit responses in the IC of the awake CBA.

Having established a correspondence between temporal processing behavior and single-neuron electrophysiology at the auditory midbrain level, Walton et al. (1998) went on to examine changes in processing of gaps as a function of age for CBA mice. They repeated the single-unit experiments just described in young and old unanesthetized CBA mice. Single-unit recordings revealed that the proportion of units with very good (short duration) gap thresholds significantly declined in the old animals relative to the young adults (Figure 24.5). In addition, the strength of the response for encoding gaps was diminished in the old animals (Figure 24.6). The neural recovery functions here demonstrate that in young animals, neural firing rates increase faster with increases in gap duration, relative to units in old animals. In addition, there are many units from young animals whose gap responses exceed their initial responses to the wideband noise bursts. This "facilitation" was rarely observed in units from old animals.

Decreased Inputs from the Cochlear Nucleus and Olivary Complex

Frisina, Walton, and colleagues obtained data on the possible neural bases of these age-related declines in auditory temporal processing by making horseradish peroxidase (HRP) injections into the IC region studied in the gap encoding experiments just described (Walton et al., 1997; 1998).

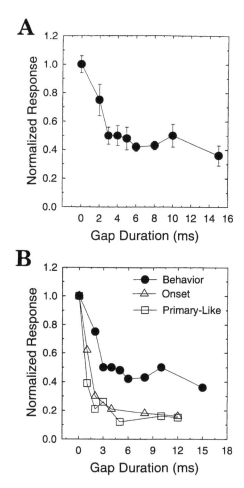

FIGURE 24.2 (A) Increases in the duration of a silent gap embedded in noise result in rapid improvements in perception. Mean acoustic startle response amplitude for five young adult CBA mice plotted as a function of gap duration. Amplitudes are normalized to the average of three startle responses in the absence of any pre-startle inhibiting gap. Gaps in a 70-dB continuous white noise were placed 60 ms in front of the startle stimulus. Error bars indicate the standard error of the mean (SEM). (B) Functional similarities of IC single-unit responses to behavioral data suggest that IC units are part of the neural basis for the auditory temporal processing of gaps. Filled data points are the mean acoustic startle responses replotted from(A). Open data points are average single-unit normalized gap coding functions for onset (N = 13) and primary-like (N = 3) units measured from the IC of the same mice as used in the behavioral experiment. These physiological recordings were made in awake animals. The single-unit data were normalized to the spike counts in response to a noise burst with no gap. For onset units, *increases* in firing rate in response to gaps were measured; and for primary-like units, *decreases* in firing rate in response to the gaps were calculated. (From Walton et al. (1997, A: Fig. 1, p. 164; and B: Fig. 12, p. 173). With permission.)

HRP injections provide information about where the single-unit recordings are made, in this case the dorsomedial region of the CBA mouse IC, and the connections of this region (Frisina et al., 1997; 1998). The inputs to this region for young adult CBA mice are given in the schematic flow diagram of Figure 24.7. Frisina (2001) and Frisina et al. (2001) reported on how the ascending inputs change with age in the CBA mice. Major projections from the AVCN (Figure 24.8), PVCN, and DCN (Figure 24.9) of the contralateral cochlear nucleus show statistically significant declines with age, as presented in Figure 24.10. Note that the largest decline in inputs occurs in the middle age group. Functionally, the middle age mice have minimal peripheral sensitivity changes or

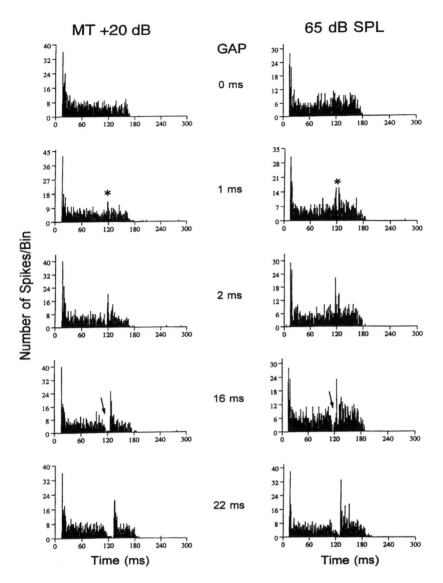

FIGURE 24.3 Sustained units of the unanesthetized mouse IC encode gaps with a *decrease* in response to the gap, and an *increase* in firing rate at the end of the gap. Representative responses in post-stimulus-time histogram (PSTH) format for a CBA mouse IC primary-like unit to gaps of varying widths are presented here at an intensity level of 20 dB above threshold (left column) and at 65 dB SPL (right column). Gap widths are listed in the center column (ms = milliseconds). Asterisks denote an increase in firing at the end of the gap, and while the arrows delineate the reduction in spike rate time-locked to the offset of the first wideband noise-burst. Unit BF = 39.6 kHz, threshold (MT) = 19 dB SPL. (From Walton et al. (1997, Fig. 5, p. 166). With permission.)

cochlear sensory cell loss (Spongr et al., 1997a; b), yet behaviorally they show temporal processing declines that are correlated with the diminution of inputs seen here. Statistically significant reductions in inputs from the ipsilateral anterolateral periolivary nucleus (ALPO, Figure 24.11) also occur with age, but inputs from the rest of the superior olivary complex (Figure 24.12) do not change as a function of normal aging. Bilateral inputs from the dorsal nuclei of the lateral lemniscus (Figure 24.13), bilateral projections from the intermediate nuclei of the lateral lemniscus (Figure 24.14), and ipsilateral inputs from the ventral nucleus of the lateral lemniscus (Figure 24.15) remain constant as a function of the lifespan, as tabulated in Figure 24.16 (Frisina, 2000; Frisina et al., 2000).

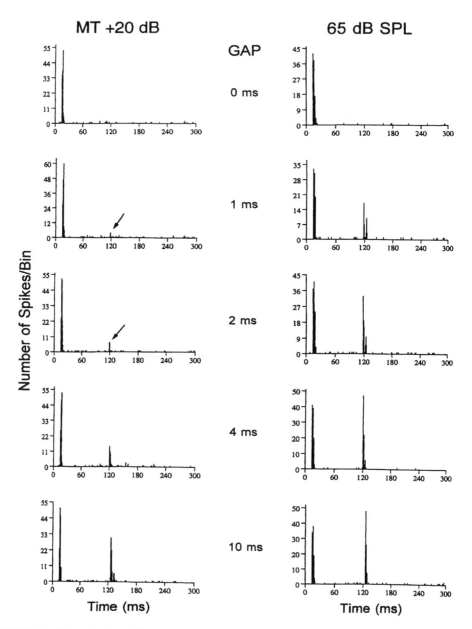

FIGURE 24.4 The majority of IC units in the unanesthetized mouse respond transiently to noise and tone-bursts. They encode gaps in a wideband noise-burst by *increasing* their firing rate in response to the gap. PSTH responses of a representative onset unit are given here for gaps of varying widths. Format same as Figure 24.3. Arrows denote the gap response, which in this unit is time-locked to the onset of the post-gap wideband noise burst. Unit BF = 20.3 kHz, threshold (MT) = 25 dB SPL. (From Walton et al. (1997, Fig. 6, p. 168). With permission.)

Up-regulation of Calretinin, Declines in Calbindin

To further investigate the possible neural bases for the age-related behavioral and single-unit temporal processing deficits of CBA mice discovered by Walton et al. (1998), age-correlated alterations in the presence of calcium binding proteins were investigated in the dorsomedial region of IC, where Walton and colleagues made their single-unit recordings (Zettel et al., 1997). It was

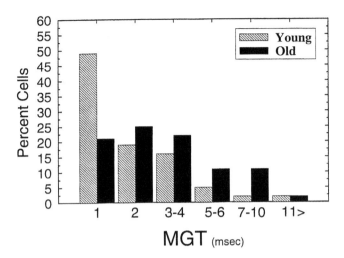

FIGURE 24.5   The proportion of single-units in the unanesthetized CBA mouse IC with short gap thresholds *declines* in old animals. This histogram tabulates the percentage of units in young and old CBA mice having minimum gap thresholds (MGT) ranging from 1 to >11 ms for young adults (hatched, N = 78) and for old mice (solid, N = 108). Notice that the distribution is skewed toward longer gap thresholds for the units from old animals. (From Walton et al. (1998, Fig. 8, p. 2771). With permission.)

found that in both CBA and C57 mice, that calbindin immunoreactivity diminished with age. However, in CBA mice only, the degree of antibody labeling for calretinin *increased* with age. Quantitative data for the down-regulation of calbindin and the up-regulation of calretinin are given in Figure 24.17. Because age-linked intracellular calcium excitotoxicity or misregulation can adversely affect neural functioning, these changes in the presence of calcium-regulatory proteins may result in neural impairment, or may play a role in protecting these neurons from age-related calcium toxicity. More needs to be known concerning the exact functional role of these calcium binding proteins in neuron development and aging (see also Chapter 22).

PERIPHERALLY INDUCED EFFECTS ON THE AUDITORY CENTRAL NERVOUS SYSTEM: INTERACTIONS OF AGE AND PERIPHERAL HEARING LOSS

As portrayed in Figure 24.1, age can be associated with deleterious biological changes in the ear and brain, as well as secondary effects of changes in the cochlea, which in turn alter normal inputs to the brain. Because current neuroscientific evidence suggests that even the adult brain has a certain amount of structure/function plasticity, the brains of aging animals can alter their organization based upon changing or diminished inputs from the auditory periphery. We now examine studies where these changes have been demonstrated, particularly in terms of advancing our understanding of the neurological bases of presbycusis.

Cochlear Nucleus

As the brainstem region receives the terminations of auditory nerve fibers carrying information from the inner ear to the brain, age-related changes in the outputs of the cochlea would likely manifest themselves most dramatically here. Subdivisions such as the AVCN and PVCN receive more auditory nerve inputs than the DCN, in relative terms. This is because the DCN, in addition to its ascending inputs from the cochlea, receives a significant number of inputs from other brain regions, including descending inputs from higher auditory centers.

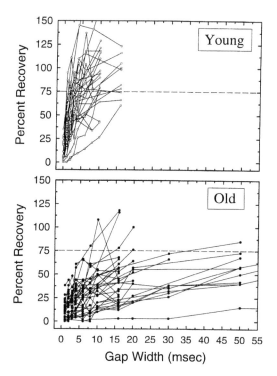

FIGURE 24.6 IC units in young adult CBA mice encode gaps with higher firing rates than IC units in old animals. Neural recovery functions are plotted for 30 phasic units in young (top) and old (bottom) animals. Neural recovery was measured by computing the number of spikes elicited by the noise-burst following the gap, divided by the spike count in response to the noise-burst preceding the gap, X 100. This calculation was performed for every gap duration in the gap series for each unit. A recovery value of 100% represents equal discharges to the first and second noise-bursts. Recovery of the gap response (response to the post-gap noise-burst) to 75% is complete by <10 to 15 ms for almost every young neuron, whereas most units from old animals do not reach this criterion for even the longest gap widths tested (horizontal dashed line in each graph). Notice also that many young units show "facilitation," that is, the response to the gap exceeds the response to the initial (pre gap) noise-burst, while this is rarely seen in the old units. (From Walton et al. (1998, Fig. 9, p. 2772). With permission.)

Volume Stability and Reduction of Neuron Number

The loss of sensory cells in the basal turn of the cochlea in C57 mice, approximately 6 months of age and older, results in a significant progressive high-frequency hearing loss, eventually resulting in profound deafness for old C57 mice. One consequence of this is that auditory nerve fibers providing input to high-frequency areas of the cochlear nucleus stop sending neural signals into these regions with age, with the eventual outcome being the death and disappearance of many of these auditory nerve fibers in middle-aged and old C57 mice. Willott and colleagues have conducted a series of inquiries into the effects of these aging changes on the functional anatomy of the cochlear nucleus.

Willott et al. (1987) performed a morphometric study of the AVCN in C57 and CBA mice, including measurements of AVCN dimensions, volume, neuron density, perikaryal size, and neuron number. The CBA results were mentioned in detail above, and in both strains no significant changes in AVCN dimensions or volume occurred with age. In C57 mice, cell number and packing density decrease up to 7 months of age and remain stable thereafter, despite continued declines in hearing sensitivity through 2 years of age. In addition, in C57 mice, the sizes of spherical and globular bushy cells increase slightly with age, whereas multipolar cells shrink. These age-related C57 changes are

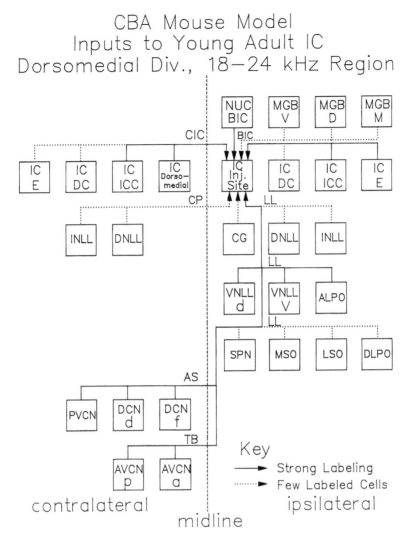

CBA Mouse Model
Inputs to Young Adult IC
Dorsomedial Div., 18—24 kHz Region

FIGURE 24.7 Schematic flow diagram of inputs to the young adult CBA mouse IC dorsomedial region, determined with focal HRP injections following single-unit recordings in unanesthetized animals (Walton et al., 1997; 1998). Certain inputs would be emphasized or attenuated when HRP injections are made in other regions of the IC, or if they cover a smaller or larger area. Inputs are exclusively contralateral at the level of the cochlear nucleus, ipsilateral for the SOC and MGB, and bilateral for the NLL and auditory midbrain. ALPO — anterolateral periolivary nucleus; AVCNa — anteroventral CN, anterior region; AVCNp — anteroventral CN, posterior region; BIC — brachium of IC; CG — central gray, reticular formation; CN — cochlear nucleus; DC — dorsal cortex of IC; DCNd — dorsal CN, deep layers; DCNf — dorsal CN, fusiform cell layer; DLPO — dorsolateral periolivary nucleus; DNLL — dorsal NLL; E — external nucleus of IC; IC — inferior colliculus; ICC — central nucleus of IC; INLL — intermediate NLL; LSO — lateral superior olive; MGB — medial geniculate body of the thalamus; MGBd — dorsal MGB; MGBm — medial MGB; MGBv — ventral MGB; MNTB — medial nucleus of the trapezoid body; MSO — medial superior olive; NLL — nuclei of the lateral lemniscus; PVCN — posteroventral CN; SOC — superior olivary complex; SPN — superior paraolivary nucleus; VNLLd — ventral NLL, dorsal division VNLLv — ventral NLL, ventral division. (From Frisina et al. (1998, Fig. 15, p. 76). With permission.)

most apparent in dorsal regions of the AVCN, where cochlear inputs are diminishing with age (cochlear basal turn, high frequencies). Willott and colleagues also report a strain difference in that the AVCN volume and neuron number are significantly greater in the C57 mice relative to CBA.

Willott and Bross (1996) expanded on this theme by comparing AVCN light microscopy age-related changes in DBA mice to those of C57. The DBA strain loses its hearing at an even faster rate than C57 mice. The anatomical changes discovered in the DBA AVCN as a function of age were, for the most part, what one would expect given the more rapid peripheral hearing loss of this strain. For example, AVCN volume and neuron number reductions were more rapid in the DBA mice relative to the CBA mice. It was interesting to note that these rapid changes in the DBA slowed with age (negatively accelerated), and the eventual total relative volume and neuron number declines in the old DBA mice were similar to the old C57 mice. In another comparative strain investigation, Willott et al. (1998) examined age-related gross anatomical changes in the BALB/c mouse AVCN. This strain loses its hearing very rapidly, at a rate between that of the DBA and the C57. AVCN volume reductions were what would be expected based on the previous findings in the DBA and C57; however, no cell loss occurred as was reported for the DBA and C57. In this latter regard, the BALB/C is like the CBA (no significant AVCN neuron loss with age).

Utilizing Golgi impregnations, Browner and Baruch (1982) investigated neuron morphology changes in the DCN of young and old C57 mice. They found that some fusiform and cartwheel neurons of Layers I and II had more dendritic abnormalities, such as blunted and sparser dendritic spines relative to young adult mice. Willott et al. (1992) performed a light microscopy study of the DCN in C57 and CBA strains using Nissl and fiber stains. In C57 mice, DCN volume decreased rapidly with age, particularly in Layer III, as presented in Figure 24.18. In CBA mice, DCN volume *increased* in the first year of life and declined at very old ages. In C57 mice, neuron size diminished with age, starting in young adulthood, as shown in Figure 24.19, whereas only a small trend toward shrinking neurons was seen in CBA mice, starting in the second year of life. In the three DCN layers, it was only in Layer III of C57 mice that an age-related loss in neurons was seen, as shown in Figure 24.20. Taken as a whole, the neurons in Layer III of the C57 appear to be most susceptible to age-related pathology and death in the DCN, no doubt induced by the peripheral hearing loss since similar deficits are not seen in Layer III of the CBA mice.

Ultrastructural Changes Due to Progressive Hearing Loss

In a study complementary to Willott and colleagues' light microscopy investigations, Briner and Willott (1989) examined the ultrastructural changes in bushy and multipolar neurons of the C57 AVCN as a function of subject age. Two features changed with age in both cell types, irrespective of the location within the AVCN: the incidence of neurons with heterochromatic nuclei increased and the percent of the perikaryon occupied by lipofuscin increased with age. For multipolar neurons, there was a decrease in the roundness of nuclei and a rise in the number of nuclear invaginations. Features that changed much more for bushy cells in the dorsal regions of the AVCN, the areas that lose their inputs from the basal turns of the cochlea dramatically with age, included: *declines* in the terminal ending lengths making contact with the perikaryon and in the percentage of soma surface opposed by terminals, and *increases* in the incidence of neurons contacted by myelinated axons and in mean synaptic vesicle densities.

Reductions in Glycine Neurons Due to Peripheral Loss

Willott et al. (1997) investigated glycine immunoreactivity and receptor binding in the cochlear nucleus of C57 and CBA mice. In old C57 mice, they discovered a significant decline in the density of glycine immunoreactive neurons, as presented in Figure 24.21. Moreover, in the old C57 DCN, the number of strychnine-sensitive glycine receptors decreased relative to young and middle-age animals of both strains, and relative to old CBA mice. CBA mice showed no significant decreases with age. These age and hearing-loss dependent reductions in glycine, the predominant cochlear nucleus inhibitory neurotransmitter important for complex sound encoding, would presumably contribute to deficits in neural processing of biologically relevant sounds in the old C57 mice.

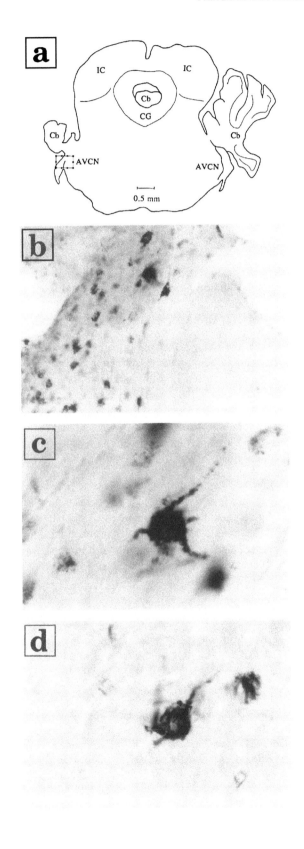

Consistent with this mouse study, Milbrandt and Caspary (1995) showed that strychnine, a glycine antagonist, binding to glycine receptor sites significantly declined in the anteroventral and dorsal cochlear nucleus of old Fisher 344 rats, with no significant change in affinity.

SUPERIOR OLIVARY COMPLEX

The superior olivary complex (SOC) is the first level of the central auditory system where information from the two ears is systematically compared and analyzed to enable the precise localization of sounds in the azimuthal plane. Low-frequency information, for analysis of interaural time differences, is preferentially encoded by the medial superior olive (MSO). High-frequency information, processed in the form of interaural intensity differences, takes place in the lateral superior olive (LSO). Information from the contralateral cochlear nucleus reaches the LSO via the ipsilateral medial nucleus of the trapezoid body (MNTB). Functionally, the MNTB performs a sign change on the acoustic information passing through it. Specifically, the MNTB receives *excitatory* inputs from the contralateral dorsal AVCN, but sends *inhibitory* information to the medial dendrites of principal cells of the ipsilateral LSO (see Chapter 18 for more details on this circuitry). Age-related structural or neurochemical changes in this circuitry should have an impact on sound localization coding.

Reduction in Calbindin in MNTB Due to Peripheral Hearing Loss

O'Neill et al. (1997) examined age-related changes in calbindin immunoreactivity in the MNTB of C57 and CBA mice. They reported significant declines in the number of calbindin immunoreactive neural somata in middle-age and old C57 mice, relative to young mice. There were no age-dependent changes in cell counts in the CBA mice. Only a portion of the calbindin declines in C57 mice could be accounted for by overall reductions in cell numbers, as displayed in Figure 24.22. The difference between the C57 and CBA mice found by O'Neill and colleagues mirrors the greater age-related cell losses in the C57 cochlear nucleus, which provides inputs to the MNTB, relative to CBA mice, as described previously in this chapter.

INFERIOR COLLICULUS

A major contribution to our understanding of neuronal plasticity due to declines in peripheral inputs for the adult auditory central nervous system, comes from an initial discovery by Willott (1984). He and co-workers then followed up the original finding with more rigorous characterizations and explorations of the possible neural bases and consequences of this activity-driven reorganizational plasticity in the central auditory system.

Reorganization of Best Frequencies with Age and Peripheral Loss

In response to declining inputs from the high-frequency region of the C57 cochlea with age, the tonotopic organization of the IC is reorganized such that ventral regions of the IC, previously most

---

FIGURE 24.8 Following HRP injections into the dorsomedial IC of an unanesthetized young adult CBA mouse, numerous retrogradely labeled neuronal somata were found in anterior regions of the contralateral AVCN. (a) Schematic diagram of a coronal section at the level of the anterior AVCN. The box indicates the location of the photomicrograph of Figure 24.8b. Animal #: 23, chromagen: TMB, counterstain: safranin-O. (b) Micrograph displaying labeled neurons in the dorsal region of anterior AVCN (20X obj.) (c) High-magnification view of a stained spherical bushy cell of Figure 24.8b, 60X obj. (d) High-magnification photomicrograph of a darkly labeled bushy neuron from the anterior AVCN of another animal. Animal #: 27, chromagen: TMB, counterstain: safranin-O, 60X obj. AVCN — anteroventral cochlear nucleus, IC — inferior colliculus, TMB — tetramethylbenzidine.

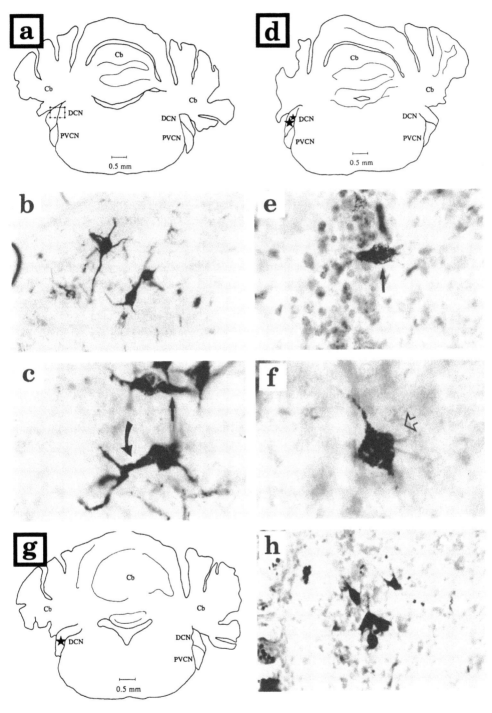

FIGURE 24.9 After an HRP injection into the dorsomedial IC of an unanesthetized young adult CBA mouse, many darkly stained neurons were observed in the fusiform cell layer and some in the deep layers of the contralateral DCN. (a) Schematic diagram of a coronal section through the DCN. The box indicates the location of the photomicrograph of Figure 24.9b. Animal #: 24, chromagen: TMB, counterstain: safranin-O. (b) Micrograph showing strong labeling of cells in the fusiform-cell layer with prominent dendritic staining, and a few darkly stained cells in the deeper layers (20X obj.) (c) Higher power micrograph of more stained

sensitive to high frequencies, is rewired so that neurons in this region become maximally sensitive to middle and low frequencies (Willott, 1984; 1986). Willott discovered this by recording from single units at different depths in the ICC of C57 and CBA mice of different ages. Representative threshold tuning curves from C57 mice of various ages and recorded at different depths in the ICC are presented in Figure 24.23. Notice that in the young adult animals, the mean tuning curve data at the lowest depths have tips at 25 kHz, whereas in the older animals at the same depths, the mean data have tips in the 10 to 12 kHz range.

Willott (1991b) and Willott et al. (1988c; 1991) followed up the initial discovery of the tonotopic reorganization to determine if other response properties change in the IC due to the peripheral hearing loss present in middle age C57 mice. By recording extracellularly from single units in different sectors of the IC, they found that some response properties were resistant to age/hearing impairment changes, and others were modified in the middle age animals relative to the young adults. For example, there was an increase in the number of sluggish units (2% to 11%) with age, as they had reported for the CBA IC. They also observed an increase in the percentage of neurons that were spontaneously active with age in the ICC. The parameters of unit response areas were altered in the ventromedial region of ICC, as one would expect from the changes in tonotopic organization there, whereas these parameters were unchanged in the dorsal ICC. Finally, the proportion of neurons with non-monotonic rate-level functions declined with age, especially in the dorsal cortex of IC. In contrast, the types of PSTH response patterns and their relative incidence in the unit populations were similar for young adult and middle-age C57 mice.

To gain some understanding of the neural mechanisms responsible for the IC tonotopic reorganization in middle-age C57 mice, Willott et al. (1991) compared single- and multi-unit neural response properties in the IC of aging C57 and CBA mice to those in the VCN and DCN for mice of the same ages. One main finding was that as C57 mice age, ventral regions of the ICC shift their neural tuning curve tips to lower frequencies, but yet maintain relatively good sensitivity. This maintenance of good sensitivity was not found in the VCN when inputs to the high-frequency regions declined with age, whereas it was observed in the DCN to a degree similar to the IC, as portrayed in Figure 24.24. In CBA mice, little change was seen for the sensitivities of units in the VCN, DCN, or IC with age.

Pathway Input Reorganization: High-Frequency Region of the VCN that Projects to the IC

Willott et al. (1985), utilizing retrograde tracing of HRP-labeled cell bodies from dorsal, middle, and ventral regions of the IC, examined connections between the contralateral AVCN and the IC as a function of the age of C57 mice. They found that dorsal regions of the AVCN (high-frequency place in young adult animals) were still connected to ventral regions of the IC (high-frequency

---

FIGURE 24.9 (continued)   cells in and near DCN Layer II, from a section 180 microns caudal to that of Figure 24.9b. A darkly stained fusiform cell (curved arrow) with prominent primary and secondary apical dendrites, and another nearby with a basal dendrite (straight arrow) are portrayed (40X obj.) (d) Schematic drawing of a coronal section from another animal at the level of the DCN. The large star designates the location of the micrograph displayed in Figure 24.9e, and the small star that of Figure 24.9f. Animal #: 20, chromagen: TMB, counterstain: safranin-O. (e) Numerous lightly stained neurons, and a darkly labeled fusiform cell with the classic long-axis orientation orthogonal to the DCN surface (arrow), located in the fusiform cell layer (40X obj.). (f) Example of a darkly stained giant cell in the deep layers of DCN (arrow). (60X obj.) (g) Schematic diagram of a coronal section through the DCN. The star indicates the location of the photomicrograph of Figure 24.9h. Animal #: 24, chromagen: DAB, counterstain: safranin-O. (h) HRP-labeled neurons in middle layers of the DCN. Notice the lack of label in the DCN superficial layers (40X obj.). CN — cochlear nucleus, DAB — diaminobenzidine, DCN — dorsal CN, IC — inferior colliculus, PVCN — posteroventral CN, TMB — tetramethylbenzidine.

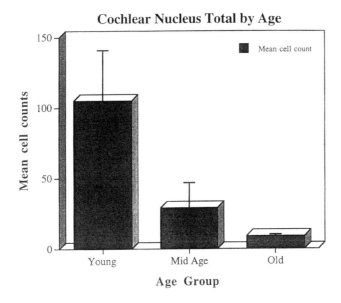

FIGURE 24.10 Significant age-related declines occurred for the inputs to the dorsomedial IC from the contralateral cochlear nucleus in the middle-age and old CBA mice relative to the young animals. (Top) Large declines occurred for the total number of labeled neurons from all three divisions of the cochlear nucleus. The most dramatic decline was from the young to the middle-age group. (Bottom) Breakdown of mean cell counts for each division of the contralateral cochlear nucleus. As with the total number of cells (top), the most noticeable decline occurred in middle age. The relative declines were similar for all three divisions; that is, the DCN always had the most labeled neurons, and the PVCN the least. AVCN — anteroventral cochlear nucleus; DCN — dorsal cochlear nucleus; PVCN — posteroventral cochlear nucleus. (From Frisina et al. (2001, Fig. 13, p. 577). With permission.)

place in young adult animals) in old animals, despite the fact that the ventral IC in old C57 mice becomes sensitive to middle sound frequencies (Figure 24.25). Because this investigation demonstrates that the locations of anatomical pathways between the AVCN and the IC are stable with age, it may be that the middle- and low-frequency inputs to the AVCN are modified such that they

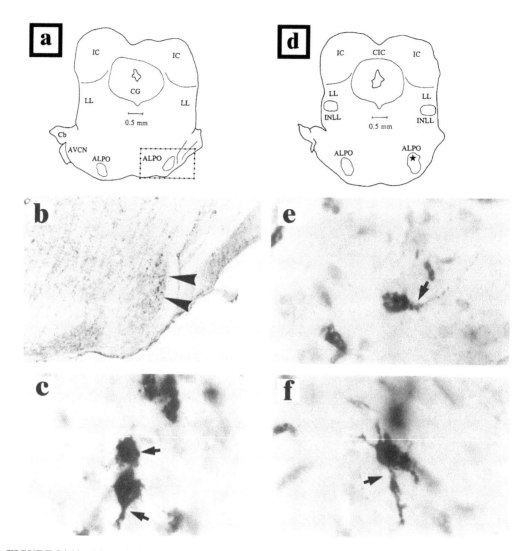

FIGURE 24.11 Many darkly labeled cells were observed in the ipsilateral ALPO when HRP was injected into the dorsomedial IC following extracellular mapping experiments in young adult mice. (a) Schematic diagram of a coronal section at the level of the ALPO. The box shows where the micrograph of Figure 24.11b is located. Animal#: 20, chromagen: TMB, counterstain: safranin-O. (b) Micrograph of many darkly stained of ALPO (arrowheads). The lower arrowhead designates two darkly stained of Figure 24.11c (arrows). (4X obj.) (c) Close-up view of darkly stained ALPO cells of Figure 24.11b (60X obj.) (d) Schematic diagram of a coronal section including ALPO from another animal. The star indicates the location of the neurons of Figure 24.11e. Animal #: 19, chromagen: TMB, counterstain: safranin-O. (e) Intensely stained ALPO soma with prominent, long process (arrow). (20X obj.) (f) Another example of a darkly stained multipolar neuron with prominently labeled dendrites (arrow) from a section adjacent to that of Figure 24.11d-e. Animal #: 19, chromagen: DAB, counterstain: cresyl violet, 60X obj. ALPO — anterolateral periolivary nucleus, AVCN — anteroventral cochlear nucleus, Cb — cerebellum, CG — central gray, DAB — diaminobenzidine, IC — inferior colliculus, INLL — intermediate nucleus of LL, LL — lateral lemniscus, TMB — tetramethylbenzidine.

provide inputs to the dorsal regions of the AVCN, which in turn convey the information to the ventral IC. This could occur through sprouting of new terminal endings by middle- and low-frequency fibers of the ascending branch of the auditory nerve, strengthening of previously weak connections of these fibers with dorsal AVCN regions, or other possible neuronal plasticity mechanisms in other divisions of the cochlear nucleus or IC.

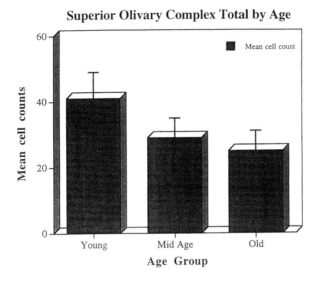

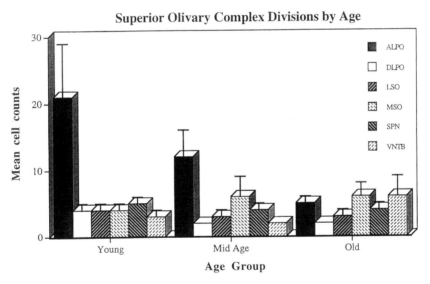

FIGURE 24.12 Significant declines occurred for the inputs from the ipsilateral SOC in the middle-age and old CBA mice relative to the young animals, based on HRP injections in the dorsomedial IC. (Top) Large declines occurred for the total number of labeled neurons summed over all the divisions of the SOC. (Bottom) However, examination of the SOC nuclei that contained HRP-labeled neurons indicates that only in ALPO, which contains most of the stained cells in young animals, is there a significant age-related decline. ALPO — anterolateral periolivary nucleus; DLPO — dorsolateral periolivary nucleus; LSO — lateral superior olivary nucleus; MSO — medial superior olivary nucleus; SOC — superior olivary complex, SPN — superior paraolivary nucleus; VNTB — ventral nucleus of the trapezoid body. (From Frisina et al. (2001, Fig. 14, p. 577). With permission.)

Changes in Synaptic Contacts from Ascending Input Pathways

In the IC, Kazee et al. (1995) demonstrated with EM techniques using young adult, middle-age, and old C57 mice, that there was a significant reduction in the number and size of synaptic contact areas on principal nerve cells of the ICC, and that the size of the principal cells declined with age. Surprisingly, there was no difference in the extent of these age effects in different quadrants of the

IC. Thus, the same synaptic reductions were observed in ventral (high-frequency) regions of the IC, that receive middle- and low-frequency information in old C57 mice, as occur in the dorsal (low-frequency) areas. A follow-up investigation, using the same quantitative EM procedures, found that no age-related reductions occur in the IC of the CBA mouse (Kazee and West, 1999). Taken together, these studies suggest that reductions in synaptic efficacy in the auditory midbrain are a result of, or are in response to, synaptic reorganization or degradation caused by reductions in peripheral inputs, not to the aging brain itself. It may be that to preserve the number and size of synaptic inputs to IC neurons, relatively normal input from the auditory periphery is required.

Neurophysiological Declines in Binaural Processing

McFadden and Willott (1994a) examined binaural properties of IC single units in C57 mice of different ages by measuring azimuth functions: discharge rates evoked by tone-bursts as a function of stimulus azimuth. Like other mammals, nearly all ICC single units were sensitive to azimuth for best-frequency (BF) tones as revealed by greater than a 50% firing rate change from maximum to minimum as a function of stimulus location. Some response properties remained stable with age, such as azimuth function shapes and the proportion of units having functions meeting the criteria for directional sensitivity. However, relative to young adults, in 7- and 12-month-old C57 mice, the proportion of IC neurons in which the strongest excitation was evoked by ipsilateral stimuli was significantly larger, azimuth function borders were more likely to be reversed (high rates evoked by a more ipsilateral angle), and direction sensitivity was reduced. These findings suggest deficits in binaural excitation/inhibition interactions in the IC of the middle-age C57 relative to young adults.

In a companion study, McFadden and Willott (1994b) again recorded responses to BF tones from young adult and middle-age C57 mice, but this time in the presence of a wideband masking noise at different azimuthal locations. The major finding was that changing the location of the masker for the 2-month-old mice significantly reduced the masking effects, whereas movement of the masker in the azimuthal plane had no effect on the coding of BF tones in middle-age animals. An example of these findings is given in Figure 24.26, indicating that the 6-month-old mice did not benefit from movement of the noise source; and that for a given masking stimulus configuration, the amount of masking was greater in the older animals. Another indicator of a binaural processing deficit in the middle-age C57 mice was that movement of the background noise away from the signal source in the azimuthal plane often enhanced the response to the signal in young mice, but rarely did so in old mice, as presented in Figure 24.27. Because sound localization deficits have been implicated as part of the presbycusic speech processing problem (i.e., inability to discriminate a speaker in one location from background noise in another spatial location), the results of McFadden and Willott's studies suggest that part of the neural etiology resides at the level of the auditory midbrain.

Physiological Temporal Processing Deficits

Walton et al. (1995) used auditory brainstem response (ABR) neurophysiological techniques to investigate the possibility of temporal processing deficits in C57 mice that might be correlated with, or produced by, the anatomical and neurochemical changes with age described thus far for aging C57 mice. Walton and colleagues measured ABR waves 1 (P1) and 5 (P5) in young adult C57 and CBA mice and in middle-age C57 mice. P1 represents the output of the cochlea in mice and other mammals. P5 in mice probably corresponds to responses from the lateral lemniscus or its nuclei, and may have some contribution from IC neurons with short latencies (see Chapter 4). Temporal processing recovery functions were measured using masking and probe tone-bursts, with a variable time delay between the bursts, and a carrier frequency of 12 kHz. For each time delay, which ranged from 2 to 64 ms, the intensity of the masker required to reduce the probe to 50% of

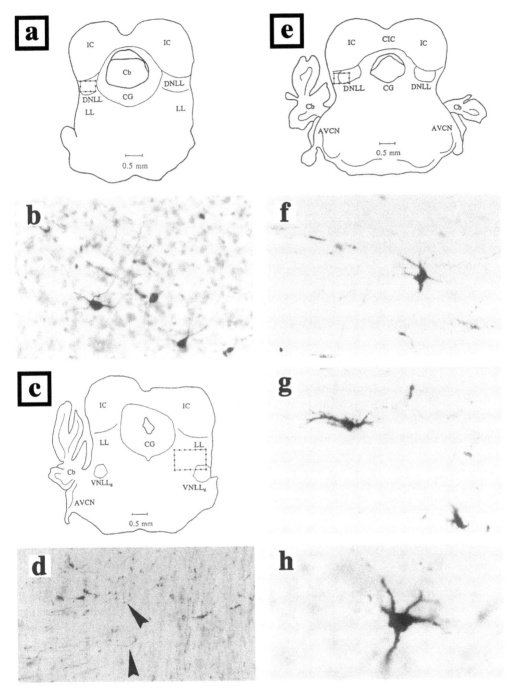

FIGURE 24.13 Darkly stained neurons were found in the contralateral DNLL, resulting from HRP injections into dorsomedial IC of young adult CBA mice. (a) Schematic diagram of a coronal section that includes DNLL. The box indicates the location of the section of Figure 24.13b. Animal#: 32, chromagen: DAB, counterstain: cresyl violet. (b) Intensely stained multipolar neuron cell somata with prominently labeled, long tapering dendrites are displayed in this micrograph (20X obj.) (c) A drawing of a coronal section at the level of LL. The box indicates where the micrograph of Figure 24.13d is. (d) Micrograph showing the branching off of the commissure of Probst fibers from the labeled ipsilateral LL. These commissure fibers are most likely axons of the labeled neurons of the contralateral DNLL and INLL (Figures 24.13 and 24.14). (e) Schematic diagram of a coronal section at the DNLL level. The box designates the location of Figure 24.13f's neuron.

its control value was determined by altering the masker level in 2-dB steps. Examples of ABR waveforms for a middle-age C57 mouse are given in Figure 24.28. ABR recovery functions for P5 from a young adult C57 are presented in Figure 24.29, along with time constants computed from these functions. Mean time constants for P1 and P5 were then compared for the young adult mice of both strains, relative to the middle-age, hearing-impaired C57 mice: young adult CBA — 90 ms; 1 month C57s — 82 ms; 8 month C57s — 198 ms. The mean latency shifts of P1 and P5 for the 50% reduction of the probe tone are given in Figure 24.30. It is elucidating to note that except for the 3-ms time delay point, temporal processing at the level of the auditory nerve is unaltered with aging and hearing loss, and therefore cannot account for the significant shift of the P5 function over all time delays tested. This suggests a temporal processing deficit has occurred in the auditory brainstem that cannot be accounted for by shifts in the cochlear portion of the ABR.

AUDITORY CORTEX

Ultimately, perception of biologically relevant sounds such as speech and animal vocalizations take place in the auditory cortex and related cerebral cortex areas. Unfortunately, from an aging neuroscience perspective, little is known about how the functional anatomy and organization of the auditory cortex in any mammal changes with age. A noteworthy study has been conducted in the C57 mouse that is now presented.

Reorganization of Best Frequencies (BFs) with Age and Peripheral Loss

Willott et al. (1993) made multi-unit recordings for the primary auditory cortex (AI) in C57 and CBA mice of different ages. In young adult mice of either strain, as presented in Figure 24.31, BFs comprise a tonotopic organization with high frequencies located dorsally and low frequencies residing ventrally, but with variability from animal to animal. The major effect of the age-related peripheral high-frequency hearing loss for C57 mice is a significant *over-representation of frequencies in the middle of the mouse audiogram*, as depicted here in Figures 24.32 and 24.33. Note the absence of units with high BFs that reside in the dorsal region of young adult animals. This middle-frequency over-representation has good sensitivity, and therefore was not simply a consequence of Willott and colleagues' recording the tails of tuning curves that had lost their high-frequency tips. This middle-frequency reorganization was not seen in the CBA strain as a function of age.

COMPARATIVE ANALYSES

BINAURAL PROCESSING IN THE LSO

Only one study has investigated age-related changes in single-unit responses to binaural stimuli in the LSO (Finlayson and Caspary, 1993). These authors hypothesized that the alteration in neurochemistry of GABA and glycine found in the auditory brainstem nuclei might lead to deficits in the ability of neurons to encode binaural signals, because neural processing of inputs from the two ears in the LSO is shaped by the interplay of excitatory (E) and inhibitory (I) circuits arising binaurally. To test this hypothesis, they recorded from single neurons in the LSO of young and old

---

FIGURE 24.13 (continued)   Animal #: 35, chromagen: TMB, counterstain: none. (f) Photomicrograph of a darkly-stained neuron of contralateral DNLL (20X obj.) (g) Another intensely labeled neuron with prominently labeled dendrites in contralateral DNLL. This section is 180 microns rostral to that of Figure 24.13f (20X obj.) (h) A heavily stained multipolar cell of contralateral DNLL. Animal #: 35, chromagen: DAB, counterstain: cresyl violet, 40X obj. AVCN — anteroventral cochlear nucleus, Cb — cerebellum, CG — central gray, CIC — commissure of IC, DNLL — dorsal nucleus of LL, IC — inferior colliculus, LL — lateral lemniscus, VNLLd — dorsal division of ventral nucleus of LL.

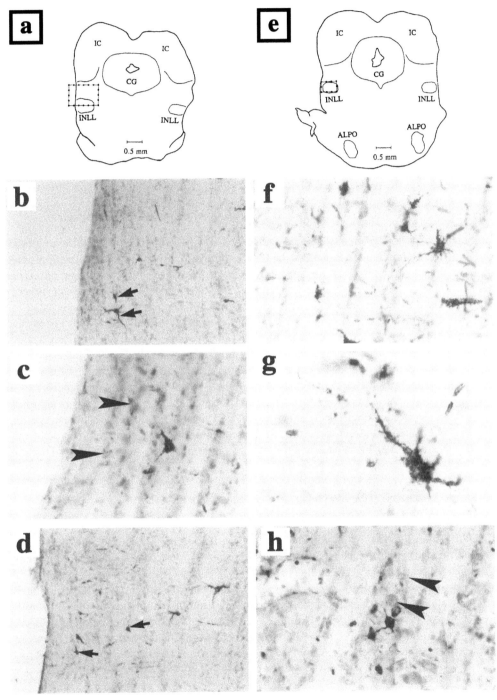

FIGURE 24.14   For HRP injections into dorsomedial IC of young adult mice, retrogradely stained neurons were observed in the contralateral INLL. (a) Line drawing of a coronal section including the INLL. The box designates the boundaries of the photomicrograph of Figure 24.14b. Animal #: 32, chromagen: TMB, counterstain: safranin-O. (b) Micrograph highlighting darkly labeled INLL neurons (arrows) (10X obj.) (c) More darkly and lightly stained (arrowheads) INLL neurons from a section 180 microns caudal to those of Figure 24.14b. (20X obj.) (d) Additional examples of darkly-stained INLL neurons from another animal (arrows). Animal #: 35, chromagen: TMB, counterstain: safranin-O, 10X obj. (e) Line drawing of a coronal

Fisher 344 rats. Except for the characteristic age-related threshold shift that is a reflection of the peripheral hearing loss, nearly all other parameters studied remained stable with age. They did find that a greater proportion of neurons from old rats exhibited lower inhibitory drive when the contralateral ear was stimulated. This result, although not statistically significant, is supportive of the idea that a decline in inhibition may reduce the contrast in binaural signals. Palombi and Caspary (1996a) measured binaural response properties for IC neurons in young and old rats. Because binaural responses are shaped by the summation of excitatory and inhibitory inputs, Palombi and Caspary hypothesized that if there were an age-related alteration in inhibitory neurotransmitters, binaural processing would be affected. Surprisingly, they found no statistically significant differences in any of the binaural responses properties, for units from young and old rats. The authors did report a trend toward encountering fewer E/I units in the aged rat IC as compared to the young rat IC.

Responses to Simple Sounds in the Rat IC: Minimal Age Effects as in Mouse

Palombi and Caspary (1996b) also studied age-related changes in monaural response properties to simple sinusoidal stimuli in the Fisher 344 rat IC. The temporal response patterns of neurons located in the central nucleus and external nucleus of the IC were classified into four groups: onset, pause, sustained, and inhibitory. They found that in the central nucleus there was a decline in the proportion of units with onset type patterns with advancing age, and this appeared to be compensated for by a slight increase in pause and sustained patterns. In the external nucleus, aging was not associated with changes in the proportion of the different types of temporal response patterns. They also found no change in the spontaneous rates or the mean absolute first spike latency of IC neurons from old rats when compared to young rats. Neurons of old rats did appear to be affected in the manner in which stimulus intensity was encoded. Specifically, there was a decline in the percentage of units displaying nonmonotonic rate-level functions. The mean maximum discharge was significantly lower in neurons of old animals, decreasing over 11%. The authors conclude that these age-related changes reflect a subtle, but real, deficit in the dynamic range of many neurons recorded from old rats. They postulate that the alteration in dynamic range might be due to a loss of inhibition, especially at higher intensities.

Declines in Inhibitory Transmitter in the Inferior Colliculus?

Caspary, Helfert, and colleagues have uncovered evidence suggesting that there are significant declines in inhibitory synaptic circuitry in the aged rat IC (Caspary et al., 1995). GABA (gamma-aminobutyric acid) is a primary inhibitory neurotransmitter in the brainstem auditory system that is particularly prominent in nerve endings and nerve cells in the IC, especially its central nucleus. It is likely that this inhibitory transmitter plays a crucial role in several aspects of auditory functioning such as spatial coding, temporal processing, and discrimination of signals from background noise. Caspary et al. (1990) examined IC nerve cell immunolabeling against GABA in young (2 to 7 month) and old (18 to 29 month) Fischer 344 rats. Quantitative analyses showed that in the ventrolateral ICC (high-frequency region), the number of labeled neurons decreased by 36%

FIGURE 24.14 (continued)   section including INLL. The box shows the location of the micrograph of Figure 24.14f. Animal #: 19, chromagen: TMB, counterstain: safranin-O. (f) Darkly stained principal neurons of contralateral INLL (20X obj.) (g) Another darkly-stained elongate neuron of contralateral INLL from a section adjacent to that of Figure 24.14e and f. Animal #: 19, chromagen: TMB, counterstain: none, 40X obj. (h) A group of darkly and lightly stained (arrowheads) neurons from the contralateral INLL of another animal. Animal #: 24, chromagen: DAB, counterstain: cresyl violet, 20X obj. ALPO — anterolateral periolivary nucleus, CG — central gray, IC — inferior colliculus, INLL — intermediate nucleus of LL, LL — lateral lemniscus.

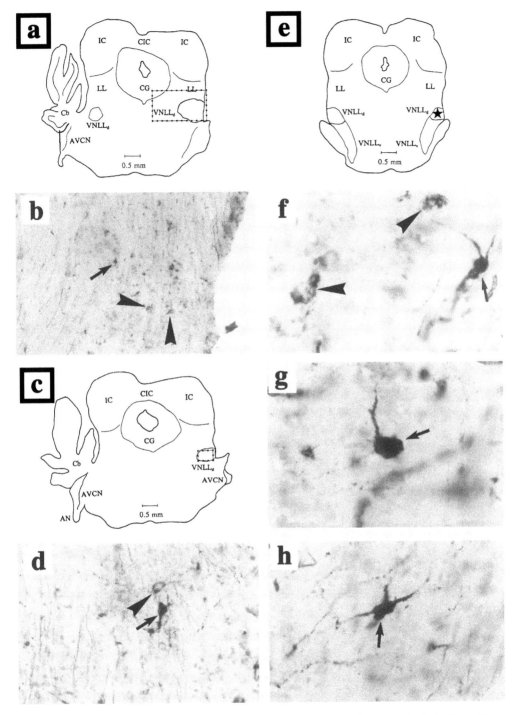

FIGURE 24.15 A large number of darkly and lightly stained cells were discovered in the ipsilateral VNLLd for young adult CBA mice, as a consequence of placing an HRP injection in dorsomedial IC. (a) Schematic drawing of a coronal section at the level of the VNLLd. The box designates the location of the micrograph of Figure 24.15b. Animal #: 20, chromagen: TMB, counterstain: safranin-O. (b) Low-magnification micrograph showing pattern of HRP-labeling in ipsilateral VNLLd, including lightly (arrowheads) and darkly stained (arrow) somata. Notice the lack of labeled cells in adjacent, non-auditory areas of the brainstem. (10X obj.) (c) Schematic drawing of a coronal section at the level of the VNLLd, at a level 180 microns caudal to that

in the old rats. Neurochemical experiments measured the basal (resting) and K^+-evoked (potassium-evoked) efflux of GABA. ICC tissue from old animals showed statistically significant reductions in both basal and K^+-evoked release of GABA relative to young adults. As a control, release of excitatory neurotransmitters such as glutamate and aspartate, as well as other endogenous amino acids and the inhibitory neurotransmitter acetylcholine, were measured and found to be stable with age.

Caspary's group went on to demonstrate an age-related decline in GABAb receptor binding in the rat IC (Milbrandt et al., 1994). Using quantitative receptor autoradiography, reductions were demonstrated in the ICC, the dorsal cortex, and external nucleus, whereas no age-related deficits were observed in nearby cerebellar tissue. The IC effects were observed despite no change in the cross-sectional area of the rat IC with age. Milbrandt et al. (1994) went on to demonstrate that GABAb receptor binding decreased in old rats. In contrast, the number of GABAa receptors increased with age, perhaps as a partial compensation for the GABAb declines (Milbrandt et al., 1996).

Using immunogold EM methodologies, Helfert et al. (1999) quantitatively compared changes in the organization of GABA(+) and GABA(–) terminals and synapses in the rat IC. They found that the density of both types of terminals and synapses declined with age by 24 to 33% in old rats relative to young adults, with the range reduced by 9% if the densities were corrected for overall shrinkage of the IC with age. Because the age-related declines were similar for GABA(+) and GABA(–) synapses, the results of this study suggest that excitatory and inhibitory inputs decline proportionately with age, avoiding an age-related imbalance. Following the Helfert et al. study, Milbrandt et al. (1997) examined the GABAa receptor subunit composition, and found that this changes with age in the rat IC such that enhanced responses to GABA can occur. Specifically, as the rats age, the gamma1 protein subunit *increased*, and the alpha1 subunit *decreased* (Caspary et al., 1999). They also demonstrated an age-related increase in GABA-mediated chloride influx, which is functionally consistent with these changes in subunit composition. If similar redistributions occur for excitatory synapses which enhance their responsiveness, then the relative balance and strength of excitation and inhibition could be maintained with age to help preserve normal functioning of the IC in the face of other age-related structural and neurochemical declines, such as those involving GABAb receptors. An informative summary of Caspary and Helfert's line of investigation is given by Caspary et al. (1995). The conclusion is that — at least in rats — there are reductions in most aspects of GABA biochemistry in the IC, including the presence of GABA, its receptors, and its activity levels.

FUTURE RESEARCH DIRECTIONS

Research reviewed here for age-related changes in the mouse auditory system, taken with information gained from other mammalian studies of neural substrates for presbycusis, including those

---

FIGURE 24.15 (continued) of Figures 24.15a,b. The box designates the location of the micrograph of Figure 24.15d. (d) A darkly stained oval multipolar neuron of VNLLd (arrow), and lightly labeled perikarya (arrowhead) surrounded by prominently stained ascending fibers of LL. Some labeled neurons displayed significant dendritic staining. (20X obj.) (e) Another line drawing of a coronal section at the VNLL level. The star indicates the location of the cell in Figure 24.15f. Animal #: 19, chromagen: TMB, counterstain: safranin-O. (f) Higher-power view of lightly (arrowheads) and darkly labeled neuron (arrow) of VNLLd. (40X obj.) (g) High-magnification micrograph of an intensely stained multipolar cell with round soma (arrow) and prominently labeled processes. (60X obj.) (h) Darkly impregnated neuron of VNLLd with relatively thick proximal dendrites (arrow). Animal #: 35, chromagen: TMB, counterstain: safranin-O, 60X obj. AVCN — anteroventral cochlear nucleus, Cb — cerebellum, CG — central gray, CIC — commissure of IC, IC — inferior colliculus, LL — lateral lemniscus, VNLLd — dorsal division of ventral nucleus of LL, VNLLv — ventral division of ventral nucleus of LL.

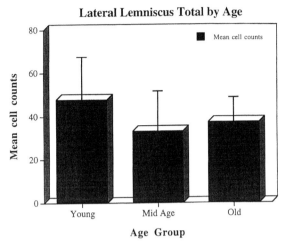

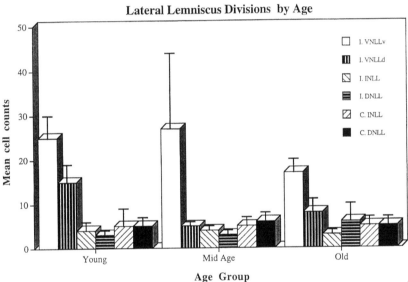

FIGURE 24.16 In contrast to the cochlear nucleus and SOC, only modest age-related declines (not statistically significant) were observed from the ipsilateral nuclei of the lateral lemniscus (NLL), following HRP injections into the dorsomedial IC of young adult, middle age, and old CBA mice. (Top) Overall declines in labeled neurons from NLL were small. (Bottom) Ipsilateral VNLLv had the most labeled cells and showed a small decline in the old animals. Ipsilateral VNLLd showed a modest decline in middle-age mice. The rest of the nuclei had small numbers of stained neurons that showed no age trends. C. — contralateral; DNLL — dorsal nucleus of LL; I. — ipsilateral; INLL — intermediate nucleus LL; LL — lateral lemniscus; VNLLd — ventral nucleus of LL, dorsal division; VNLLv — ventral nucleus of LL, ventral division. (From Frisina et al. (2001, Fig. 15, p. 578). With permission.)

of humans reviewed in Willott (1991a), gives much information needed to initiate interventional research. For example, age-related declines in cochlear hair cells or spiral ganglion neurons may be preventable with applications of proteins that nourish or protect inner ear sensory cells from age-linked insults such as fever, noise, or ototoxic agents. The latter includes strong antibiotics such as kanamycin, or chemotherapeutic agents such as cisplatin. Walsh and Webster (1994) conducted an investigation along these lines concerning occurrence and prevention of conductive hearing loss and its damaging effects in the VCN in CBA mice. They examined the cochlea and VCN in neonatal animals with atresia of the external auditory meatus. They found that relative to

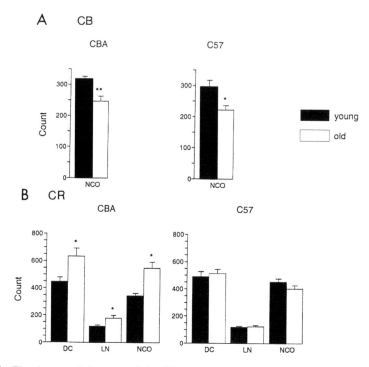

FIGURE 24.17 The dorsomedial region of the CBA mouse IC shows a reduction in calbindin immunore-activity with age, but an *up-regulation* of calretinin immunostaining as a function of age. (A) The mean number of CB+ cells in the NCO of young (filled) vs. old (unfilled) CBA and C57 mice. CB+ counts declined significantly (*) in old mice of either strain. (B) The average number of CR+ neurons in DC, LN, and NCO of young vs. old CBA and C57 mice. CR+ neurons increased significantly (*) in all three regions for old CBA mice, but not for C57. Error bars designate the standard error of the mean (SEM). *: $p < 0.05$, **: $p < 0.01$. CB+ — neurons staining positively for calbindin, CR+ — neurons staining positively for calretinin, DC — dorsal cortex of IC, IC — inferior colliculus, LN – lateral nucleus of IC, NCO – nucleus of the commissure of IC. (From Zettel et al. (1997, Fig. 12, p. 109). With permission.)

controls, the cochlea had a reduction in spiral ganglion cells, and the VCN had a somewhat smaller volume and reduction in neuron number for these atresia subjects. They then repeated the experiment, but made post-surgical daily subcutaneous injections of GM1 ganglioside. The application of the ganglioside significantly cut down on spiral ganglion cell loss and VCN volume and neuron number reductions, presumably due to the ganglioside's ability to potentiate or stimulate growth factor production. This, in turn, helped sustain spiral ganglion cells in the face of the conductive hearing loss. As knowledge becomes more comprehensive concerning age-related central auditory deficits, such as those presented in this chapter, biochemical, pharmacological, or molecular genetic interventions targeted at aging changes in the brain will come forth from interdisciplinary neuro-scientific research groups.

CONCLUSIONS AND IMPLICATIONS FOR UNDERSTANDING PRESBYCUSIS

Where direct comparisons can be made, mouse findings appear to shed light and expand on the human presbycusic condition. For example, as presented above, in terms of neuron numbers and volumes of the cochlear nucleus divisions, age effects are minimal, even when combined with peripheral hearing loss due to age or noise damage. Post-mortem investigations of the human cochlear nucleus in old subjects confirm the resiliency of the cochlear nucleus with age. Konigsmark

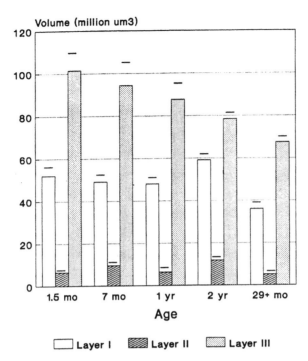

FIGURE 24.18 Age-related declines in the volume of the dorsal cochlear nucleus (DCN) occur throughout the lifespan in the C57 strain. This histogram delineates the DCN volume as a function of age and DCN layer. Note that the more superficial layers, Layers I and II, have relatively constant volumes, whereas Layer III has a monotonic decline in volume throughout life. Horizontal lines = standard error of the mean (SEM). (From Willott et al. (1992, Fig. 2, p. 669). With permission.)

and Murphy (1970; 1972) and Crace (1970) found no significant loss of cochlear nucleus neurons in autopsy tissue from old humans. Modest reductions in VCN volume and neuron size were seen (Seldon and Clark, 1991). On the functional side, it is the case that older listeners who experience speech perception problems in background noise also tend to have auditory temporal processing deficits (Snell and Frisina, 2000), a portion of whose etiologies reside in the brainstem auditory system (Frisina and Frisina, 1997). As presented above for CBA mice, Walton, Frisina, Ison, and their colleagues have demonstrated that a functional age-related temporal coding deficit develops for neurons in the auditory midbrain. These neurons are likely part of the mammalian auditory brainstem circuitry whose temporal analysis abilities decline with age. These age-related changes for responses to complex stimuli in humans and mice, are in contrast to small or nonexistent age effects in mice and men for perception, behavior, and physiology experiments involving simple stimuli or non-complex listening situations. Finally, as genetically engineered mice become more plentiful and molecular biology studies continue to utilize the mouse as the mammalian species of choice, we will push closer to a knowledge base necessary for understanding, preventing, and curing presbycusis in humans.

ACKNOWLEDGMENTS

We thank Martha Erhardt, Martha Zettel, and Jonathan Byrd for technical anatomical assistance, and Patricia Bardeen for analysis support. Work supported by the National Institute on Aging NIH grant P01 AG09524, and the International Center for Hearing and Speech Research, Rochester, New York.

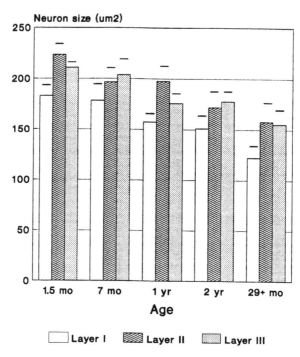

FIGURE 24.19 Age-related declines in neural soma size occur in all three DCN layers for C57 mice. This histogram displays the mean cross-sectional area for perikarya as a function of age and DCN layer. Horizontal lines = standard errors of the mean (SEM). (From Willott et al. (1992, Fig. 8, p. 675). With permission.)

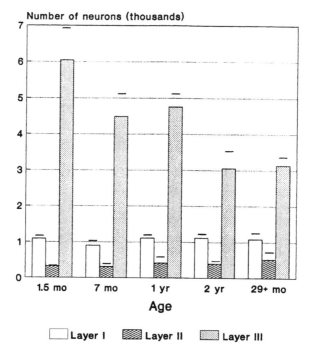

FIGURE 24.20 Age-related declines in neuron number occur only in Layer III of the DCN for C57 mice. This histogram displays the mean number of neural cell bodies as a function of age and DCN layer. Horizontal lines = standard errors of the mean (SEM). (From Willott et al. (1992, Fig. 12, p. 676). With permission.)

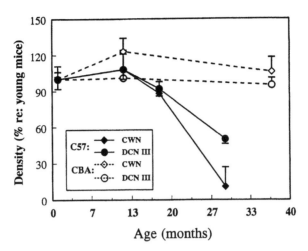

FIGURE 24.21   In the cochlear nucleus, a significant age-related decline in glycine immunoreactivity occurs in the second year of life of C57 mice, but the presence of glycine is constant throughout the CBA mouse lifespan. The functions plotted here display the density of glycine immunoreactive DCN neurons in C57 and CBA mice. Specifically, these functions show the relative changes in packing density of glycine+ neurons as a function of age, where 100% = the density of glycine immunoreactive neurons in a 1-month-old mouse. CWN — DCN Layer I, DCN III — Layer III. (From Willott et al. (1997, Fig. 2, p. 410). With permission.)

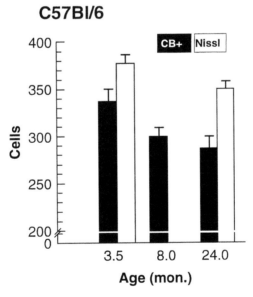

FIGURE 24.22   An age-related decline in calbindin immunoreactivity occurs in the medial nucleus of the trapezoid body (MNTB) of C57 mice, but not in CBA mice. An overall reduction in the number of cells in MNTB occurs with age, but this reduction is not nearly enough to account for the decline in calbindin+ (CB+) neurons. This histogram displays cell counts (means ± standard error of the mean [SEM]) of calbindin+ cells (filled bars) and Nissl-stained neurons (open bars) in the MNTB of young, middle age, and old C57 mice. Relative to young adults, there is a statistically significant ($p < 0.05$) decline in CB+ cells of 11% in middle-age and 14.8% in old C57 mice; whereas there is only a 7.1% reduction in total cells (Nissl-stained) from young to old age in C57 mice. (From O'Neill et al. (1997, Fig. 4, p. 162). With permission.)

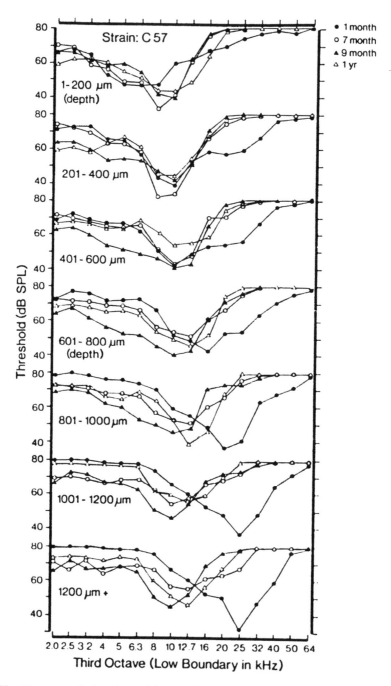

FIGURE 24.23 The tonotopic (cochleotopic) map of best frequencies (BFs) in the C57 inferior colliculus (IC) undergoes a reorganization due to the age-related decline in inputs from the high-frequency (basal turn) region of the cochlea. This graph shows mean frequency-threshold tuning curves (MTCs) for units from C57 mice as a function of age and dorsoventral depth within the IC central nucleus. There is a statistically significant shift of the MTCs' BFs from high frequencies (25 kHz) to middle frequencies (10 to 12 kHz) at the three lowest depths for the 7- to 12-month-old mice relative to the young adults. The number of single-unit tuning curves comprising each of the MTCs is a follows: 1 month, N = 90; 7 month, N = 74; 9 month, N = 50; 12 month, N = 56. (From Willott (1986, Fig. 2, p. 395). With permission.)

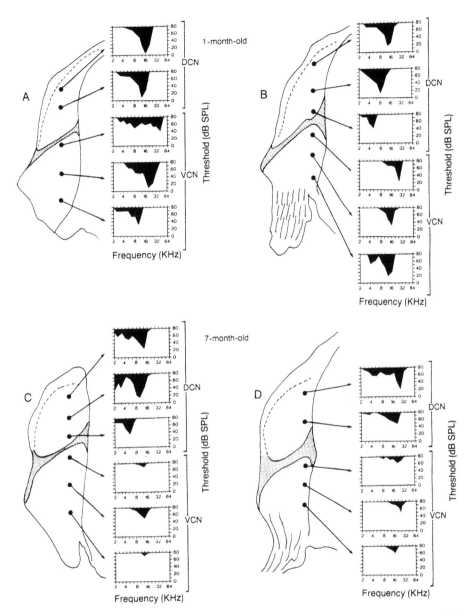

FIGURE 24.24 Drastic elevations in the sensitivities of AVCN units occur with age, but relatively good sensitivity is maintained in the DCN of middle-age C57 mice. Representative individual frequency-threshold tuning curves (TCs) recorded from electrode penetrations through the C57 CN. (A, B) 1-month old. (C, D) 7-month old. The camera lucida drawings were traced from frontal sections. The stippled region is the granule cell border between the DCN and AVCN. The dashed line denotes the DCN molecular layer boundary. The filled circles indicate the recording locations of the TCs. AVCN — anteroventral CN, CN — cochlear nucleus, DCN — dorsal CN. (From Willott et al. (1991, Fig. 5, p. 84). With permission.)

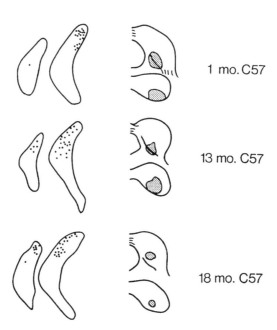

1 mo. C57

13 mo. C57

18 mo. C57

FIGURE 24.25 Anatomical pathway connections between the AVCN and the IC remain in the same location with age in the C57 strain. These projections from the *dorsal AVCN* subserve *high-frequency* coding in young adult animals. The anatomical stability of this projection pathway occurs despite the fact that the high-frequency sensitivity of the ventral IC is re-wired to a *middle-frequency* sensitivity. This frequency range is normally coded in *middle regions of the AVCN* in young adult mice. This figure displays camera lucida drawings of WGA-HRP injections restricted to ventral IC regions in C57 mice of different ages (right column). Left column shows locations of retrogradely labeled soma located in dorsal regions of the AVCN. Scale bar = 500 microns. Each upper IC section is more rostral, and each AVCN section on the left is more rostral. AVCN — anteroventral cochlear nucleus, IC — inferior colliculus, WGA-HRP – wheat germ agglutinin-horseradish peroxidase. (From Willott et al. (1985, Fig. 3, p. 549). With permission.)

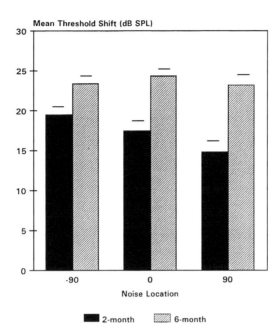

FIGURE 24.26   In the IC of aging C57 mice, movement of a background noise source away from a sound signal does *not* give the perceptual benefit that occurs from this separation of signal and noise in young adult mice. In addition, the amount of background noise masking at a given masker location was always greater in the older mice (greater threshold shifts). The histogram presented here tabulates the mean threshold shifts of a BF tone in the presence of a 20 dB SL wideband masking noise as a function of the location of the masker (–90, 0, or 90 degrees), for 2- and 6-month-old C57 mice. The threshold shift represents the tone threshold in the presence of the noise, minus the threshold in quiet. The tone signal source was always placed contralateral to the IC being recorded from (tone source at –90 degrees). Although the standard errors of the mean (SEM, horizontal bars) were fairly small (1.53 to 1.88 dB), threshold shifts as large as 70 dB sometimes occurred in the presence of the masking noise for individual units. BF — best frequency of a unit, IC — inferior colliculus, SL — sensation level. (From McFadden and Willott (1994b, Fig. 3, p. 135). With permission.)

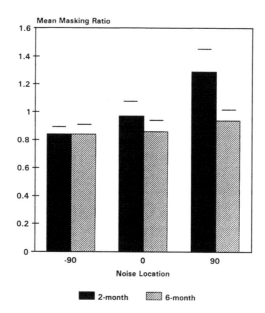

FIGURE 24.27 IC neural responsiveness to a tonal signal (spike firing rates) improved when the background noise source moved away from the signal source in young animals, but not in the middle-age C57 mice. This histogram plots mean masking ratios for BF tones in 20 dB SL wideband noise for 2- and 6-month-olds. Masking ratios increase with signal/masker separation in 2-month-olds, exceeding 1.0 at 90 degrees. The masking ratio is defined as the ratio between the maximum spike count obtained in the presence of the noise and the maximum count obtained in response to the tone alone. A masking ratio <1.0 indicates that the presence of the noise reduced the discharge rate of the unit; a ratio >1.0 shows that the noise enhanced the response to the tone; and a ratio equal to 1.0 indicates that the background noise had no effect on the tonal response over the intensity range tested. The standard errors of the mean (SEM, horizontal bars) were small, except for the 90-degree noise location. BF — best frequency of a unit, IC — inferior colliculus, SL — sensation level. (From McFadden and Willott (1994b, Fig. 5, p. 136). With permission.)

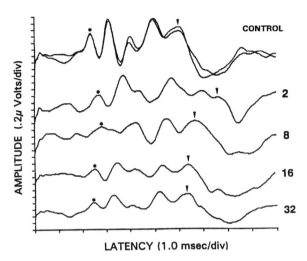

FIGURE 24.28   In the mammalian auditory system, temporal processing can be measured utilizing auditory brainstem response recordings (ABRs). In mice and other mammals, Wave I (P1) reflects the neurophysio-logical response of the cochlea and auditory nerve. Wave V (P5) in the mouse and most mammals reflects the neural activity of the lateral lemniscus, its nuclei, and possibly some short-latency neurons of the inferior colliculus. Examples are given here of some ABR waveforms elicited by a 20 dB SL, 12 kHz probe tone (masking tone of the same frequency). The forward masking series consisted of masker/probe gaps ranging from 0 (no gap) to 32 ms. Recordings shown here were obtained from an 8-month-old, hearing-impaired C57 mouse with a 12-kHz threshold of 48 dB SPL, or approximately a 28-dB threshold shift from the normal mean threshold of a young adult mouse. The P1 wave is designated by asterisks and the P5 with arrowheads. Note the decrease in latency of both waves as the masking/tone gap increases, and the increase in the amplitude of P5 as the gap increases. SL — sensation level. (From Walton et al. (1995, Fig. 4, p. 22). With permission.)

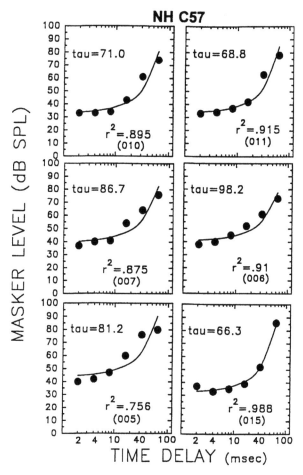

FIGURE 24.29 In a forward masking experiment, such as that in Figure 24.28, as the intensity (masker level) of a masking tone increases, the amplitude of the probe tone declines. If one plots the intensity of the masker required for a 50% reduction in the probe response amplitude, as a function of the time delay (gap) between the masking tone and the probe, a neural recovery function is obtained. Recovery functions for six 1-month-old C57 mice are displayed here. Tau (τ) gives the time constant of the functions fitted to the data points, and r^2 gives the least-squares goodness of fit. The time constants ranged from 66 to 98 ms, and the r^2 values were all greater than 0.75. The young adult C57 recovery functions, such as those shown here, are similar to those obtained in this study for young adult CBA mice up to 6 months of age. However, for hearing-impaired, middle-age C57 mice, the time constants were significantly longer: 119 to 350 ms (graphs not shown). (From Walton et al. (1995, Fig. 6, p. 23). With permission.)

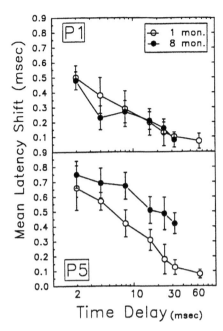

FIGURE 24.30 P5 of the ABR shows an age-related temporal processing deficit that cannot be accounted for by latency shifts at the level of the auditory nerve. In a forward masking experiment, such as that in Figure 24.29, as the intensity (masker level) of a masking tone increases, the amplitude of the probe tone declines. If one plots the probe *latency shift* resulting from the presence of a fixed-intensity masker vs. the gap between the masker and probe, one obtains latency-shift functions such as those given here. P1 (top) and P5 (bottom) group data are plotted for young adult and middle-age C57 mice. A 0-ms mean latency shift signifies that the masker had no effect on the latency of the probe tone. With the exception of the 3-ms gap, age had no effect on the P1 latencies; but for the P5 waves, age resulted in a significant shift toward longer latencies (temporal slowing). (From Walton et al. (1995, Fig. 8, p. 24). With permission.)

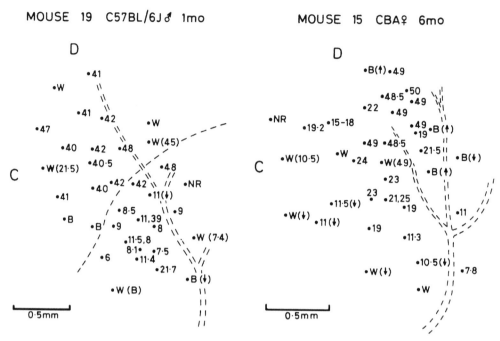

FIGURE 24.31 Tonotopic (cochleotopic) maps of the young adult mouse auditory cortex (AI) cover the full range of mouse hearing, with physiological BFs ranging from those in the ultrasonic bands (50-kHz range) dorsally, to those with low BFs (below 10 kHz) in the ventral areas. Maps here are given for a typical 1-month-old C57 (left) and a 6-month-old CBA (right). Each number designates the BF (frequency in kHz for which the unit gives a threshold response) of a unit or unit cluster measured 0.2 to 0.4 mm below the pia mater. Dashed lines indicate major blood vessels. BF — unit best frequency; C — caudal; D — dorsal; NR — no response; W — weak response, BF in parentheses if measurable; arrow — frequency range extends upward or downward. (From Willott et al. (1993, Fig. 4, p. 406). With permission.)

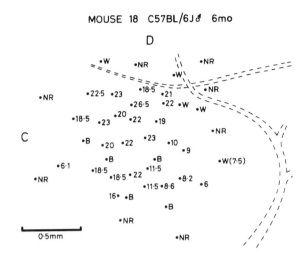

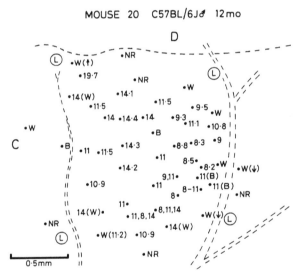

FIGURE 24.32   The reduction in units with BFs above 25 kHz (top) and higher than 20 kHz (bottom) is the main age-related change in the cortical tonotopic (cochleotopic) organization in the middle-age and old C57 auditory cortex, respectively. The format of this figure is the same as that of Figure 24.31. Top map is from a 6-month animal and the bottom from a 1-year old mouse. (From Willott et al. (1993, Fig. 6, p. 407; Fig. 7, p. 408). With permission.)

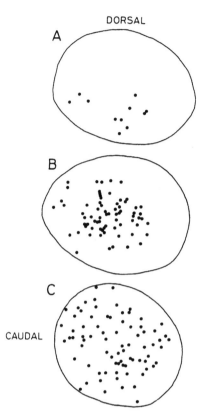

FIGURE 24.33 Schematic summary of the major age-related invasion of auditory cortex tonotopic maps by units with BFs in the middle of the mouse audiogram, at the expense of those with higher BFs in young animals. The drawings here were obtained by superimposition of the most detailed individual maps, with the centers of the maps aligned as accurately as possible. The boundaries of these three fields are each an average of the superimposed maps of that group. The points represents units or small clusters of units with BFs ranging from 10 to 13 kHz. (A) Map obtained from data of 1-month C57s and 6-month CBA mice. (B) Summary map for 2-month-old C57 mice. (C) Unit map for 6- and 12-month C57 mice. (From Willott et al. (1993, Fig. 8, p. 409). With permission.)

25 Focus: Elicitation and Inhibition of the Startle Reflex by Acoustic Transients: Studies of Age-Related Changes in Temporal Processing

James R. Ison, Joseph P. Walton, Robert D. Frisina, and William E. O'Neill

There is a growing literature on the anatomical changes in the central auditory system that accompany the aging process in the CBA/CaJ mouse, which, as described in Chapter 24, helps us understand in some measure age-related changes in auditory function, particularly the important changes in temporal acuity seen in the physiological studies that they summarize. Here we examine temporal processing in the behavioral correlates of aging, referring back where possible to certain of these anatomical and physiological effects. The subjects are CBA/CaJ mice, and also F1 hybrid mice from a C57BL/6J x CBA/CaJ cross. Both strains retain their threshold sensitivity across the spectrum until well into their second year of life, and thus provide a picture of the relatively pure effects of age on behaviors that depend on auditory processing. The history and rationale for the reflex methods used in these experiments and the procedures common to this work are given in Chapter 5. All experiments measured the acoustic startle response (ASR), as elicited by relatively intense stimuli and modified by relatively weak preliminary stimuli. This chapter addresses the question of how age affects behaviors that depend on the ability to resolve brief perturbations in the acoustic environment.

Figure 25.1 provides fundamental data on the effects of age on ASR amplitude over a wide age span, 6 weeks to 29 months, in CBA and F1 hybrid mice. The ASR was elicited by 115 dB SPL wide-band noise, 20-ms duration, ~0 ms rise and decay times, presented against a 70-dB noise background. The data come from different experiments, but all include this same baseline condition. The shape of the ASR amplitude by age function for both strains consists of an early increase in ASR vigor that reaches a peak between 3 and 6 months of age, followed then by a gradual but continuous decline. A similar decrement in the ASR with age has been seen in both rats (Krauter et al., 1981) and in humans (Ford et al., 1995). Our data agree with those provided by Krauter et al. in showing that the effect of age on this form of auditory behavior begins in middle age. The early increase in the ASR can be understood at least in part as a reflection of an increasing muscle strength in young mice up to 4 to 6 months old. The later decrement has a parallel with the changes in connectivity of the cochlear nucleus (CN) with higher centers summarized in Chapter 24, which also first appear in middle age. It may, however, have multiple causes located at both central and peripheral sites. Thus, for example, skeletal muscle changes with age to include a greater ratio of slow twitch fibers (Einsiedel and Luff, 1992), compared to the fast twitch fibers important in the fast and vigorous ASR. It is also possible that neural transmission from sensory to motor control

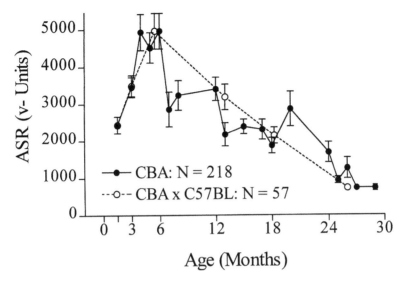

FIGURE 25.1 Mean amplitude of the ASR (±SEM) as a function of age in CBA mice and in the F1 hybrid offspring of a CBA/CaJ sire and a C57BL/6J dam. The startle stimulus was a 115 dB SPL noise burst (20 ms in duration) and a 70 dB noise was always present. The ABR is measured as the integrated output (100 ms) of an accelerometer under the floor of a test cage. See, for example, Ison et al. 1998 for procedural details. Note the increase in ASR amplitude in both strains up to about 4 to 6 months of age, and then the terminal linear decline.

neurons may be less effective in aging mice, and certainly age affects the integrity of the octopus cells of the posterior ventral CN (Willott and Bross, 1990). Their role in the ASR is not certain, but they have desirable structural and physiological characteristics that would usefully contribute to its rapidity and its vigor. Three major variables that affect the ASR are the level and the duration of the eliciting stimulus and the presence of background noise. Hogan and Ison (2000) examined these variables in hybrid mice aged 3, 12, and 30 months, with stimuli of 1, 2, 4, 8, and 16 ms in duration, and levels of 105, 115, and 125 dB SPL. These stimuli were presented in quiet and in 70-dB wide-band noise. Figure 25.2 suggests that the age-related changes shown in Figure 25.1 depend in detail on both the level of the startle stimulus chosen in those experiments and on the presence of background noise. Young and middle-age mice show the usual substantial facilitation of the ASR by noise, especially at the higher stimulus levels (note especially the 3 to 1 increase in 12-month-old mice, which required a change in the scale along the y-axis, and the increase of about 2 to 1 in 3-month-old mice). In contrast, the ASR for the oldest mice was depressed by noise at the lower levels and shorter durations of startle stimulus input, and was not enhanced by noise at the highest stimulus level. Evidently, noise loses its normal positive "arousal" effect in old mice, and also more seriously suppresses the ASR to weak startle inputs. This is an intriguing finding, but the major rationale for the experiment had been to examine age effects on temporal integration. In this regard, while some age differences in ASR growth rate with increased duration can be seen in the data, they primarily occur at lower stimulus values and seem to mostly relate to increases in noise-produced masking and to changes in ASR thresholds with age. The fact that the overall shapes of the functions obtained with 125-dB stimuli are very similar at the three ages suggests that there is no intrinsic age-related change in temporal integration for the ASR.

Turning now to reflex modification, the offset of a noise just prior to the onset of the startle stimulus has a substantial inhibitory effect on the ASR: how might this effect vary with age? Ison et al. (1998) examined the effects of noise decrements of 10 to 40 dB in a 70-dB background on the relative ASR to 115-dB startle stimuli in CBA/CaJ mice (Figure 25.3). Overall the effect of the decrement was greater with larger decrements up to asymptotic values of about 30 to 40 dB, and

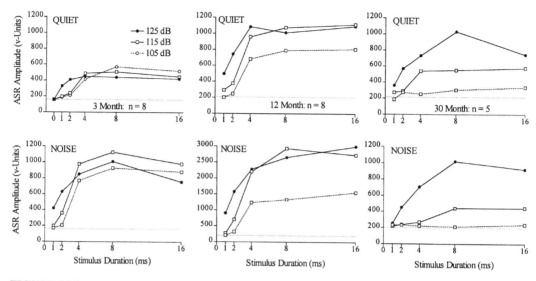

FIGURE 25.2 Mean amplitude of the ASR as a function of age in F1 hybrid mice when the eliciting noise burst stimuli were varied in duration (1, 2, 4, 8, and 16 ms) and level (105, 115, and 125, dB SPL), and these stimuli were presented in quiet (in the upper graphs) or in noise (in the lower graphs). Note the increase in the ASR with background noise in young and middle-aged mice, but not old mice; and note that in quiet, the age effects in the ASR are relatively small, especially with the higher startle level. It is hypothesized that the longer high-intensity startle stimuli evoke a self-limiting recurrent inhibitory process in younger mice. The dotted lines provide a "no-stimulus" activity level.

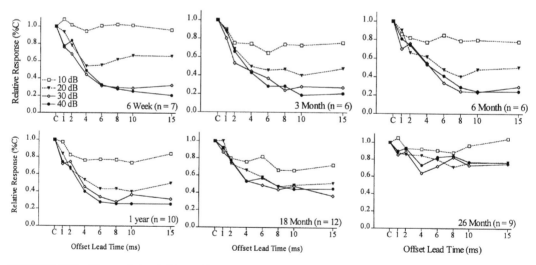

FIGURE 25.3 Mean relative ASR amplitude (percent of control responding) when the startle stimulus was preceded at different lead times by a decrement (of 10, 20, 30, or 40 dB) in a 70 dB noise background, as a function of age in CBA mice. Note especially that ASR inhibition is stronger the greater the decrement in the noise background, develops very rapidly, and reaches an asymptote between about 6 and 10 ms across conditions. The major age effect age is reduced asymptotic inhibition.

also with an increase in its lead time up to asymptotes reached at about 6 to 10 ms. Time constants generally were lower for the smaller decrements, and the youngest mice showed no inhibition for the decrement of 10 dB, suggesting a relative insensitivity to small decrements. However, there was otherwise little sign of age-related effects on the shapes of the four functions in the first year

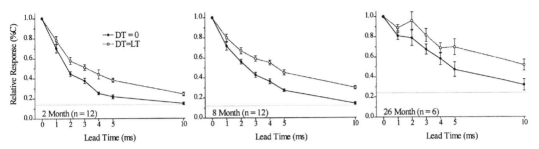

FIGURE 25.4 Mean relative ASR amplitude (±SEM) when the startle stimulus was preceded by noise offset at different lead times (LT) in hybrid mice as a function of age. Noise offset was either abrupt (Decay Time = 0) or had a decay time that equaled the lead time (DT = LT). Inhibition developed very rapidly, and the difference between abrupt offset and the more gradual offset was apparent for a 1-ms decay time, regardless of age. Old age was associated with reduced asymptotic inhibition.

of life. At 18 months, the mice remained sensitive to the 10-ms decrement, but decrements of 30 and 40 dB were less effective in producing inhibition. This tendency was then exaggerated in very old mice, which showed reliable but reduced inhibition for the larger decrements. There were clear and significant differences in asymptotic levels of inhibition beyond the age of 12 months, but no indication of any age-related change in the time constant for ASR inhibition with increasing lead time. The overall effect is similar to that of Figure 25.2, where there is no age effect on the time course of integration of excitatory input on ASR elicitation but the asymptotic ASR is reduced. These data sets both show that transient stimuli generally lose their effectiveness with age. In addition, we can conclude that the decline in ASR inhibition must be greater than that for excitation because inhibition is measured against the weakened excitatory impulse produced by eliciting stimuli: if age effects were equal for both inhibitory and excitatory processes, then relative inhibition would be stable across age.

Because the inhibitory effects of noise offset on the ASR are evident with lead times of just 1 ms, it seems certain that the neural processing for this form of inhibition must involve a minimal number of stages that are probably confined to the CN. While onset cells of the CN are constructed and sited so as to integrate across frequency, their special membrane characteristics minimize temporal integration for continued excitatory input (Golding et al., 1999) and thus the fact that the time constants for the growth of excitation do not vary with age should not be surprising. However, the stability of time constants for inhibition seems more remarkable, and one particularly compelling example of stability in temporal processing across age is given in the next set of data (see Figure 25.4, taken from Ison et al., 1999). Here, hybrid mice at three ages (2, 8, and 26 months) were presented with noise offsets under two conditions: one in which offset decay time was abrupt (DT = 0), and the other in which the decay time equaled the lead time (LT) by which the beginning of the offset preceded the startle stimulus. Quite obviously, ASR inhibition increased with offset lead time and was greater for DT = 0 than DT = LT; and further, younger mice showed more inhibition. However, a more subtle finding emerges from these data. The procedure was taken from von Bekesy (1960/1930) and Miller (1948) to track the hypothetical decay of sensation at noise offset in young mice, and to determine if this function changed with age. Their idea was that if the sensory effect of abrupt decay is equal to that of a non-zero decay time, then the internal decay of excitation for that abrupt offset can be no faster than the objective non-zero decay time. Conversely, if the abrupt decay yields a bigger sensory effect, then the internal rate of decay must be faster than the objective non-zero decay rate. Two important features of Figure 25.4: (1) abrupt offsets with a 1-ms lead time were more inhibitory than the equivalent 1-ms decay time, indicating that the internal rate of decay was very fast; and (2) this difference did not vary with age. This very sophisticated measure of one form of temporal acuity showed absolutely no trace of an age

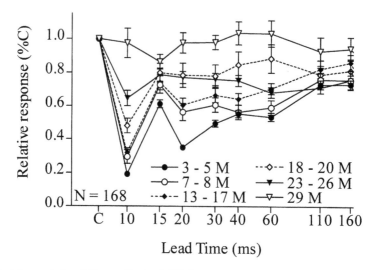

FIGURE 25.5 Mean relative ASR amplitude (±SEM) when the startle stimulus was preceded by a 10-ms gap in a background noise, the gap beginning 10 ms to 160 ms prior to startle onset, as a function of age in CBA/CaJ mice. In young mice, two phases of inhibition occur in rapid succession, just 10 ms apart. With increased age, the overall levels of inhibition are reduced and the second phase of inhibition is delayed.

effect; thus, in all of the data described thus far, age seems to diminish the asymptotic excitatory and inhibitory effects of transient stimuli without affecting their intrinsic rate of growth.

All of the behaviors described to this point can be attributed to neural processing at early brainstem levels; and it might be expected that as this information ascends to more rostral sites, the effects of the reduced output of the caudal brainstem would branch out and reduce central response speed and possibly also temporal acuity. Evidence for this hypothesis is presented in Figure 25.5, taken from an experiment in which a 10-ms gap in a 70-dB background noise was presented at various lead times before the startle stimulus, and the CBA mice (N = 167) ranged in age from 3 to 29 months. The youngest group of mice showed the usual W-shape in the relative response, with strong inhibition at the 10-ms lead time, a substantial recovery at 15 ms, and then a second inhibitory phase beginning at 20 ms. (In rats, this second inhibitory phase is sensitive to decortication, while the first is not: Ison et al., 1991). Note how this second phase occurred progressively later with age, although the first phase was at 10 ms in all but very old mice. The lead time of maximal inhibition beyond that occurring at 10 ms was calculated for each mouse, with results seen in Figure 25.6. The means ranged from just over 20 ms in young mice to about 60 ms in old mice, and the linear increase in this function with age was very striking.

What are the behavioral changes with age on gap detection at these later lead times? At the level of the inferior colliculus, relatively few cells in the old mouse have the same high temporal acuity of those in the young mouse; also, these old cells are much slower to recover their normal level of reactivity following the gap (see Chapter 24, Figures 24.5 and 24.6). A clear age-related behavioral effect of gaps presented at lead times of 60 ms in these same CBA mice is shown in Figure 25.7, with the older mice showing reliable inhibition but with a much reduced asymptotic strength (data from Barsz et al., 2000). A threshold for gap detection was calculated for each mouse, as the shortest gap duration at which inhibition was 50% of its asymptotic. The means for each age group are given in Figure 25.8. A linear regression function provides a reasonable fit to these data, but strong evidence for an age-related loss of temporal acuity as measured by gap-detection thresholds is only apparent beyond about 18 months of age. These data are also interesting in the fact that although there were large age effects seen in ABR thresholds for tone pips, the ABR did not correlate with gap detection (O'Neill and Ison, 2000).

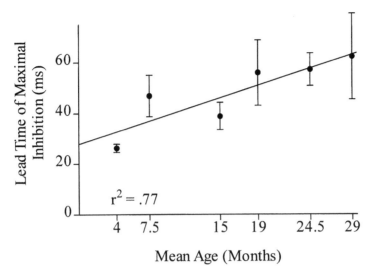

FIGURE 25.6   The mean lead time (±SEM) at which maximal ASR inhibition occurred, not counting the inhibition present at the 10-ms lead time, as a function of age in CBA/CaJ mice (taken from the data displayed in Figure 25.5, the values being calculated for each individual mouse).

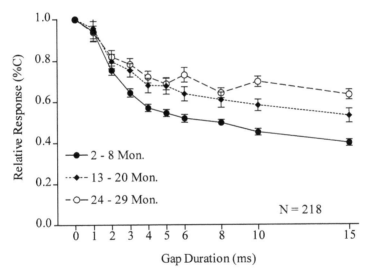

FIGURE 25.7   Mean relative ASR amplitude (±SEM) when the startle stimulus was preceded by gaps of various durations at an interval of 60 ms (offset of gap to onset of startle), as a function of age in CBA/CaJ mice. Inhibition developed less rapidly here with increased gap duration than it does in a noise offset condition, but the major effect of age is still to reduce the asymptotic level of inhibition.

CONCLUSIONS

The neural process that provides temporal integration of the acoustic transient that elicits the ASR must be different from that responsible for ASR inhibition by noise offset at short lead times. In turn, it is likely that noise-offset inhibition is different from inhibition by complete gaps at long lead times. Despite these differences, common outcomes do appear at each level to support the hypothesis that peripheral and brainstem mechanisms retain their threshold sensitivity to small

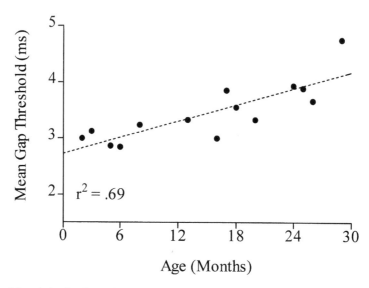

FIGURE 25.8 Mean behavioral gap thresholds as a function of age in CBA/CaJ mice, derived from the data for individual mice for which grouped age means for inhibition are presented in Figure 25.7. These threshold values were calculated for each mouse, and were defined as the minimal gap duration at which the level of inhibition was at least 50% of the maximal level of inhibition found for that mouse at any gap duration. It might be noted that a threshold of about 3 ms is very close to that obtained in young humans, and the age-related increase of about 1 ms is again close to that reported (Snell, 1997) in old human listeners.

variations in the acoustic envelope in aged mice. Moreover, the major consequence of old age appears in the lower asymptotic effect of transient input, either positive or negative. These behavioral data suggest that very brief acoustic transients are detected but are less able to generate a significant neural response, a conclusion that is consistent with the physiological data showing that there are fewer high-acuity cells in older mice. Age-related shifts in the timing of the second phase of gap inhibition and increased gap thresholds may result because the diminished neural output achieved in the early stages of neural processing spreads out through more rostral sites. This would result in delays in the time course and increases in the jitter in the input to higher processing stations. This effect must be further exacerbated by the age-related loss of transmission links from the CN to more rostral sites. There is also strong evidence for intrinsic changes at those rostral sites, for example, in the delayed recovery of aged gap-sensitive neurons in the inferior colliculus, as summarized in Chapter 24.

It has been hypothesized that the older human listeners suffer from two auditory deficits, one being a loss of audibility for certain spectral frequencies, and the second being some degree of distortion in the perception of the acoustic event. Age-related changes in sensitivity at the auditory periphery are certainly responsible for the loss of audibility. However, deficits in the neural responses to acoustic transients, which we believe are responsible for the behavioral and physiological evidence for age-related decrements in temporal acuity, seem likely to contribute to a distorted perceptual representation of the complex acoustic events that we know as speech.

ACKNOWLEDGMENT

The research described herein was supported by the USPHS, by way of Research Grant AG09524 and Center Support Grant EY01319. Correspondence should be addressed to James R. Ison, Department of Brain and Cognitive Sciences, University of Rochester, Rochester, New York 14627. Electronic mail may be sent to Ison@bcs.rochester.edu.

Section IV

Genetics and the Mouse Auditory System

Mouse genetics is one of the hottest and most fruitful topics in current science, and many auditory scientists are part of the research scene. With the arsenal of behavioral, anatomical, physiological, and other biological tools discussed in earlier sections, the stage is set for many exciting findings. Indeed, exciting findings are already accruing in impressive numbers, as shown in this section.

The topic is introduced in Chapter 26 by Dr. James Battey. In his role as director of the National Institute of Deafness and other Communicative Disorders, he has championed the use of mouse models in auditory research, and his efforts are paying off. Johnson, Zheng, and Letts, scientstists working out of the world's premier mouse research facility, The Jackson Laboratory, review the incredibly impressive body of research that is being produced from studies of auditory mutations in mice. The range of research approaches and empirical findings is further elaborated upon in Chapter 28 (Erway, Zheng, and Johnson).

In Chapter 29, Hitzemann, Bell, Rasmussen, and McCaughran review the use of quantitative trait loci analysis to map genes that modulate the acoustic startle response and prepulse inhibition the BXD recombinant inbred strains.

Finally, the production and use of transgenic mice in auditory research is the topic of Chapter 30 (Mullen and Ryan).

26 Human Hereditary Hearing Impairment: Research Progress Fueled by the Human Genome Project and Mouse Models

James F. Battey, Jr.

INTRODUCTION

Roughly one child in a thousand is afflicted with hearing impairment severe enough to potentially compromise the development of normal spoken communication skills. In over one half of these children, an alteration in one or more genes is the primary cause of hearing impairment. The Human Genome Project has provided a rich bounty of resources, including genetic markers, databases of expressed human sequences, comprehensive libraries of clones spanning the human genome, and sequencing of the human genome. These resources make it possible to determine the location of the genes and identify with precision the genetic changes that underly hereditary hearing impairment. Given this unprecedented opportunity to understand the fundamental basis for hereditary hearing impairment, the National Institute on Deafness and Other Communication Disorders gives high priority to research that elucidates the structure, function, and regulation of genes responsible for hereditary hearing impairment.

WHAT HAS BEEN LEARNED

In contrast to many other disorders that are genetically complex (e.g., diabetes, hypertension, autism, stuttering), hereditary hearing impairment in children often involves one or more mutations in a single gene that is inherited in a predictable Mendelian fashion. Several hundred different genetic loci have been identified that harbor one or more genes where mutations cause hearing impairment, and the list is growing by the day. Approximately 70% of individuals with hereditary hearing impairment have no other obvious clinical manifestation; this type of hearing impairment is called nonsyndromic hereditary hearing impairment. The remaining 30% have hearing impairment, together with other associated clinical findings that constitute a syndrome; these individuals are referred to as having syndromic hearing impairment.

Initial efforts to map and clone genes causing hereditary hearing impairment were focused on syndromic hereditary hearing impairment because genetic material from affected individuals in many different families could be used in the analysis when mutations in the same gene cause the syndrome, as is the case in Pendred syndrome (Everett et al., 1997). However, molecular genetic analysis of other syndromes such as Usher syndrome, where deafness is one of the clinical features, has shown that mutations in more than one gene can result in the same clinical syndrome. Attention has shifted back to identifying genes involved in the more common nonsyndromic hereditary hearing impairment. About 50 genetic loci have been shown to contain one or more genes, and a standard nomenclature has been adopted (reviewed in Griffith and Friedman, 1999). All loci inherited in an autosomal dominant fashion (about 20% of cases) are named DFNAz, where z is the numerical order in which the locus was discovered. Similarly, autosomal recessive loci (close to 80% of cases) are named DFNBz, and the relatively rare X-linked loci are named DFNz. The relevant gene has been identified and cloned in about twenty of these nonsyndromic loci.

MAPPING AND CLONING GENES WHERE MUTATIONS CAUSE NONSYNDROMIC HEREDITARY HEARING IMPAIRMENT

The quest to identify a gene for hereditary hearing impairment usually begins with the identification of a large, multigeneration (or multiplex) family in which hearing impairment is inherited in a clear-cut Mendelian fashion. It is even better to pool the gene mapping data from two or more large multiplex families where it is likely that the same gene is involved. This simplifies identifying the correct candidate gene and provides confirmation that the right gene has been found. The advantages of studying multiple families underscore the critical need for collaboration among laboratories around the world. These collaborations will undoubtedly play an increasingly important role in accelerating the pace of gene discovery.

The next step is to map the gene, or determine its location in relation to genetic markers whose location in the genome is known (reviewed in Green, 1999). Thousands of markers particularly useful for this purpose have been developed. Many are called Short Tandem Repeats (STRs). These consist of short nucleotide repeats (such as CACACACACAÀ) flanked by unique sequences. The length of the short nucleotide repeat is quite variable (or highly polymorphic) within the human population, making it likely that two unrelated individuals will have different genotypes. The length of STRs is easy to determine by using polymerase chain reaction (PCR) to amplify the STR repeat and the flanking unique sequences, followed by gel electrophoresis to determine the length of the product (Figure 26.1).

The procedure for mapping a gene is predicated on two principles of genetics: (1) genes (or markers) that are close to each other on the same chromosome tend to be inherited together, or are linked; (2) however, during the meiotic cell division process that creates germ cells, there is frequently crossing-over, or homologous recombination, creating new recombinant chromosomes each containing portions of the starting homologous chromosome. Because crossing-over is essentially a random event, the chance that recombination will occur between two genetic loci is a function of the distance separating them. The higher the frequency of recombination between the gene and the marker, the greater the genetic (and usually physical) distance between the gene and marker. A 1% frequency of recombination between two genetic loci or markers is referred to as a centiMorgan (cM), and, on average, corresponds to about 1 million bases of the human genome, or a megabase. Gene mapping is simply the process of determining the likelihood that the gene of interest and one or more known genetic markers remain together and are not separated by a crossing-over event.

A panel of STR markers evenly spaced throughout the genome is used to study members of a multiplex family, or families, that are affected or not affected. If one or several contiguous genetic markers (called a haplotype) is invariably associated with the affected status, these markers are assumed to be linked to the hearing impairment gene in that family. The likelihood that the presumptive linkage is real — and not just a chance event — increases with the number of affected and unaffected individuals studied. In a given multiplex family, or families, the probability that association between a marker and hereditary hearing impairment is happening by chance rather than physical linkage can be calculated using powerful computer algorithms. Gene linkage to a given locus (defined by the location of STR markers) is established when: (1) the likelihood of

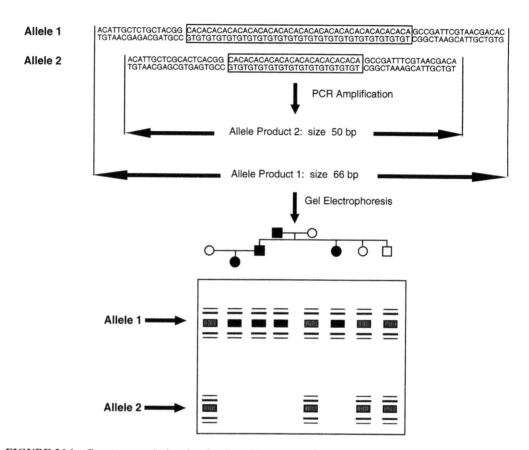

FIGURE 26.1 Genotype analysis of a family with autosomal recessive hereditary hearing impairment, showing a short tandem repeat (STR) marker linked to the gene where mutations cause the disorder. Two alleles, or forms, of the STR (allele 1 [66 base pairs] and 2 [50 base pairs]), which differ in length due to a difference in the number of "CA" dinucleotide repeats, are shown. After PCR amplification using primers corresponding to unique sequences that flank the repeat, the two STR alleles are resolved by gel electrophoresis. All individuals in the multiplex pedigree (circles, indicating females, and squares indicated by males, joined by lines) who are hearing impaired (filled symbols) carry two copies of allele 1, the form of this STR that is linked to the mutant hearing impairment gene. All individuals that are not affected (open symbols) carry one copy of allele 1 and one copy of allele 2.

random association between gene and marker becomes very small compared to the number of markers used to "cover" the human genome, and (2) only one region of the genome has a marker, or markers, that invariably associate with the disorder.

Once the location of a gene is determined, the next step is to identify the gene by positional cloning (reviewed in Green, 1999) (Figure 26.2). A set of overlapping recombinant DNA clones spanning the gene locus is isolated. The initial clones of human genomic DNA clones are usually yeast artificial chromosomes (YACs), consisting of millions of bases of human genome sequence. However, YAC inserts are often unstable, and thus it is desirable to use the YACs to identify overlapping collections, or contigs, of BACs (bacterial artificial chromosomes). BACs contain inserts that range from 80,000 to 150,000 bases of contiguous human genome sequence, and are both stable and relatively easy to isolate.

After a complete BAC contig covering the region of interest is established, it is necessary to identify all the genes within that "interval" of the genome. The most comprehensive technique for gene identification is partial sequence analysis of the BACs, an activity facilitated by the Human Genome Project. A draft genome sequence in the interval known to contain candidate genes is

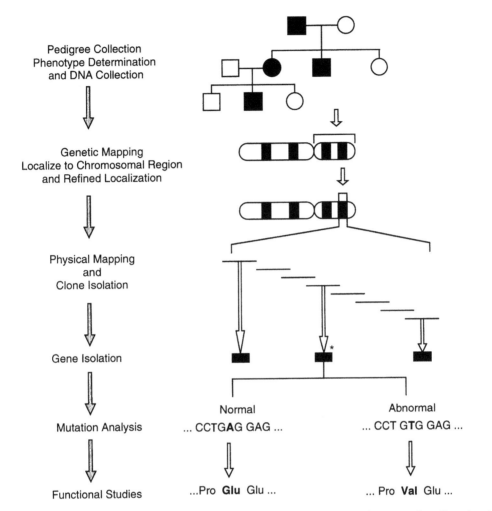

Pedigree Collection
Phenotype Determination
and DNA Collection

Genetic Mapping
Localize to Chromosomal Region
and Refined Localization

Physical Mapping
and
Clone Isolation

Gene Isolation

Mutation Analysis

Functional Studies

Normal
... CCTGAG GAG ...

...Pro **Glu** Glu ...

Abnormal
... CCT GTG GAG ...

... Pro **Val** Glu ...

FIGURE 26.2 Flowchart showing the steps taken to identify a gene where mutations cause hereditary hearing impairment. The location of the gene is determined by performing gene linkage analysis on a multiplex family with hereditary hearing impairment (circles and squares, connected by lines). The location is refined by combining data from other multiplex families with mutations in the same gene. A collection of clones (YAC and BAC) that form an overlapping contig and span the locus containing the gene (horizontal lines) are isolated, and DNA sequence analysis is used to find candidate genes (filled rectanges depicted with arrows). DNA sequence comparison between the gene sequence from affected and unaffected individuals is used to identify which candidate gene carries a mutation, a DNA sequence change that is invariably associated with hearing impairment in this family. If an *in vitro* assay for the gene product is available, functional studies of the protein encoded by the gene can be used to determine the effect of the mutation. Alternatively, the mutation can be recreated in the mouse genome to create an animal model of the human disorder, which can be tested for auditory function using auditory brainstem responses or other physiologic procedures to assess auditory function.

compared to computerized databases of cDNA sequences expressed as messenger RNA. These databases contain sequence information (called "expressed sequence tags," or ESTs) from the majority of genes expressed in the human genome. In addition to searching for ESTs to identify candidate genes, there are computer programs that analyze genomic sequence and predict the identity and location of expressed segments of human genes, called exons. For each gene identified within an interval harboring a hearing impairment gene (called a positional candidate gene), a complete cDNA is isolated and sequenced to determine the normal sequence of the coding region. In most cases, the larger the interval, the more candidate genes are likely to be found. While it is clear that there are relatively gene-rich and gene-poor regions of the human genome, the average spacing of genes is estimated to be about one every 100,000 bases, or about every 10 million bases (or megabase).

To determine which gene from among the candidates harbors the mutation causing hearing impairment, the candidates are searched for evidence of a mutation in the DNA from affected individuals. This search can be a daunting task if the interval is large with many candidates, as is often the case when only a single human pedigree is available for study. When a mutation is found that modifies the predicted protein structure, tentative gene identification is established. In some cases, a sequence change completely disrupts the protein-coding sequence (e.g., by creating a premature termination codon, or a shift in the protein reading frame). These mutations are readily distinguishable from a benign single nucleotide polymorphism, or variation between human individuals, that has little or no consequence for protein function. However, some gene sequence changes are subtle, and the distinction between a deleterious mutation and a benign sequence variation can be more difficult. In these instances, data from one or more independent families implicating the same gene are very helpful in confirming the identity of a hearing impairment gene. However, even in these cases, the physiological consequences of the DNA change can only be inferred. Alternatively, a mouse model, where the same genetic change is introduced into the mouse genome resulting in hereditary hearing impairment, can provide confirmation of the mutation identity, as well as a model for performing functional analyses of the gene product.

A PIVOTAL ROLE FOR MOUSE MODELS

For decades, mouse geneticists have identified strains with heritable auditory and vestibular abnormalities. These strains often display circling or head-bobbing behavior not observed in normal mice, or fail to show a Preyer, or startle, reflex in response to a loud sound. More recently, more subtle forms of hearing impairment have been measured in mice using auditory brainstem responses. In some mouse strains, the mutant gene has been mapped to a region of the mouse genome that shows evolutionary homology to a region of the human genome where linkage studies map a human hearing impairment locus. When this fortuitous convergence of research findings occurs, it is very likely that hearing impairment in both species is a result of mutations in the same gene. The availability of a mouse model where mutations in a given gene cause hereditary hearing impairment can be very helpful both in gene identification and in understanding why a mutation causes hearing impairment.

Using the mouse, thousands of individual animals can be generated by carefully planned matings. These animals can then be checked for hearing impairment and their genotype determined using STR markers, which allows the interval containing the hearing impairment gene to be narrowed to as little as 100,000 bases, the size of a single BAC. Comparable multiplex families with thousands of members simply do not exist in the human population; and as a consequence, the interval containing a human hearing impairment gene is often megabases in size. The increased precision in mapping that is possible in the mouse reduces the number of candidates that need to be searched for mutations that segregate with hearing impairment to a manageable collection for analysis. For example, the *shaker 1* mouse model was critical in the studies that showed that mutations in *myo7a* cause deafness, and lead directly to the identification of the homologous gene in humans (*MYO7A*), where mutations cause Usher syndrome type 1B (Weil et al., 1995). Once the *MYO7A* gene was cloned, studies of families where nonsyndromic hereditary hearing impairment mapped close to *MYO7A* revealed that other mutations in this gene cause both autosomal dominant (Li et al., 1998) and recessive (Weil et al., 1997; Liu et al., 1997a) nonsyndromic hearing impairment.

The study of genetically engineered mouse models can provide important clues about candidate genes for human hereditary hearing impairment. One example is provided by the identification of the gene underlying the autosomal dominant hearing impairment in the DFNA15 locus. Gene linkage studies on a multiplex Israeli Jewish family placed this gene in a 25-centiMorgan interval of human chromosome 5q31 (Vahava et al., 1998). A genetic interval of this size is predicted to correspond to a physical interval of tens of megabases, a region much too large for a systematic search for all candidate genes, and no other families were available for any attempt to narrow the interval. However, mice with a targeted *pou4f3* gene encoding a POU domain transcription factor were known to become progressively deaf immediately after birth, and the gene was shown to be selectively expressed in hair cells (Erkman et al., 1996). When it was noted that the human *POU4F3* mapped to chromosome 5q31, within the DFNA15 region, it became an obvious candidate. Nucleotide sequence analysis of DNA derived from affected members of the Israeli Jewish family revealed an 8-base deletion in the coding region that resulted in a truncated protein, providing compelling evidence that this mutation in *POU4F3* was the cause of deafness in this family (Vahava et al., 1998). Clearly, clues from the gene-targeted mouse model greatly accelerated the discovery of this gene. However, one interesting paradox remains: deafness in the Israeli Jewish family is inherited in an autosomal dominant fashion, while deafness in the gene-targeted mouse is inherited in an autosomal recessive fashion with heterozygote animals unaffected. The authors speculate that when the truncated POU4F3 protein is expressed in humans, it may function as a dominant negative protein by forming dimers with normal POU4F3 protein expressed from the normal allele, thereby explaining the autosomal dominant mode of expression.

An additional benefit to working with mouse models is that the use of inbred mouse lines reduces the problem of confounding benign sequence variations often found in outbred human populations. With a mouse model in hand, an investigator can obtain proof that the mutation in a gene causes hearing impairment by using transgenic technology to introduce a normal version of the gene into the mouse genome and restore auditory function. This functional approach was used to identify the *shaker 2* gene, whose human counterpart is the autosomal recessive hearing impairment gene, DFNB3 (Probst et al., 1998; Wang et al., 1988).

To fully exploit the advantages of mouse models, the National Institutes of Health is supporting efforts to generate many more mouse models for human diseases and disorders, through systematic mutagenesis of the mouse genome. In an ideal scenario, one or more mouse models for most, if not all, human hereditary hearing impairment genes will be found in this ambitious project. These mouse models will greatly accelerate the pace of gene discovery, and will allow a thorough analysis of the abnormal anatomy and pathophysiology of the auditory system that underlies hereditary hearing impairment. Indeed, when a human hearing impairment gene is discovered in the absence of a mouse model, the first step in understanding the functional basis for hearing impairment is often the creation of a mouse model using gene targeting technology. Given the wealth of spontaneous mutants and genetically engineered animals that are currently available and will be available in the future, the mouse has clearly become the mammalian animal model of choice for auditory research. To take full advantage of this resource, every effort should be made to adapt powerful and informative assays of auditory function developed in other mammalian models for use in the mouse.

THE NATURE OF GENES UNDERLYING NONSYNDROMIC HUMAN HEREDITARY HEARING IMPAIRMENT

Remarkable progress has been made in determining the identity of genes where mutations cause nonsyndromic hereditary hearing impairment. A list of some of these genes is presented in Table 26.1. Although the field has just begun to identify these interesting genes, several generalities are already emerging, including:

1. There are examples in which different mutations in the same gene can cause either syndromic or nonsyndromic hearing impairment (PDS; DFNB4 or Pendred Syndrome; or MYO7A; Usher Syndrome Type 1b, or DFNA11, or DFNB2). This observation underscores the fact that different mutations can have relatively more or less drastic

TABLE 26.1
Genes Where Mutations Cause Nonsyndromic Hereditary Hearing Impairment

Locus	Gene Symbol	Name of Protein	Affected Auditory Structure	Ref.
DFNA1	*DIAPHII*	Diaphonous 1	Hair cell cytoskeleton?	Lynch et al., 1997
DFNA2	*KCNQ4*	Potasssium channel subunit	Outer hair cell	Kubisch et al., 1999
DFNA3 and DFNB1	*GJB2 (Cx26)*	Connexin 26	Support cell stria vascularis	Kelsell et al., 1997
DFNA5	*DFNA5*	DFNA5 V	—	Van Laer et al., 1998
DFNA9	*COCH*	Coch	—	Robertson et al., 1997
DFNA8 and DFNA12	*TECTA*	α-Tectorin	Tectorial membrane	Verhoeven et al., 1998
DFNA1 1, DFNB2, and USH1B	*MY07A (Myo7A; shaker-1 in mouse)*	Unconventional myosin-7A	Hair cell (?)	Liu et al., 1997a; b
				Weil et al., 1997
DFNA15	*POU4F3 (Brn 3.1)*	—	Hair cell (m) Support cell (?)	Vahava et al., 1998
DFNB3	*MY015 (Myo-15; shaker-2 in mouse)*	Unconventional myosin-15	Inner and outer hair cells have short stereocilia (m)	Wang et al., 1998
				Probst et al., 1998
DFNB4 and PDS	PDS	Pendrin	Chloride and iodide transporter	Everett et al., 1997 Li et al., 1998

effects on protein function. Further, different mutations in the same protein can result in either an autosomal dominant or recessive pattern of inheritance, as is observed for MYO7A where mutations underlie both DFNA11 or DFNB2 in different families. Presumably, the mutations in DFNB2 are traditional loss-of-function mutations, whereas the mutations found in DFNA11 prevent the myosin 7A protein from forming functional dimers with other normal myosin 7A proteins, functioning as a dominant negative allele.

2. Some of the genes (DFNA9, *COCH*, DFNA8, *TECTA*) are expressed selectively in the inner ear, with the gene TECTA encoding the protein alpha-tectorin (Verhoeven et al., 1998), an integral protein within the tectoral membrane; and *COCH* encoding a protein called Coch5B2 whose function in the inner ear is unknown (Robertson et al., 1997). Both genes were initially identified based on the property of selective expression in the inner ear. These examples underscore the potential value of identifying genes selectively expressed in the inner ear as potential candidates for genes where mutations cause nonsyndromic hereditary hearing impairment. This strategy, initially pursued by Dr. Cynthia Morton and collaborators (Robertson et al., 1994), shows great promise for identifying good candidate genes in a genetic interval known to harbor a hereditary hearing impairment gene.

3. Unconventional myosins are a prominent and unexpected class of genes where mutations cause hearing impairment in humans (*MYO7a, MYO15*) (Weil et al., 1995; 1997; Liu et al., 1997a; 1997b; Wang et al., 1998) and mice (*myo7a, myo6, myo15*) (Weil et al., 1995, Avraham et al., 1995; Probst et al., 1998). All three genes are expressed in inner ear hair cells. In the mouse, hair cell damage is a prominent feature accompanying mutations that alter the structure of all three proteins. Unconventional myosins are thought to play a role in moving molecular "cargo" from one intracellular location to another. The function of unconventional myosins, which are clearly essential for normal hair cell structure and development, is currently unknown and is an important area for future research.

4. Auditory scientists have known for years that the extracellular endolymph fluid in the cochlea has a remarkably high potassium concentration, and that this high concentration is needed for normal auditory function. It is not unexpected that mutations in a potassium channel expressed in hair cells might lead to hearing impairment. Recently, scientists have shown that mutations in the potassium channel gene *KCNQ4* are the cause of the autosomal dominant hearing impairment mapped to the DFNA2 locus (Kubisch et al., 1999). In fact, certain mutations in two other potassium channel genes (*KCNQ1, KCNE1*) are known to cause Jervell and Lang-Nielsen syndromes, which combine a long QT segment in the individual's electrocardiogram and accompanying cardiac arrhythmias with congenital hearing impairment (Neyroud et al., 1997; Schultze-Bahr et al., 1997). Given these fascinating discoveries, it seems likely that other genes whose proteins are critical for potassium metabolism in the inner ear will be targets for mutations that cause hearing impairment.

5. Mutations in one gene (*GJB2*, which encodes the gap junction subunit protein connexin 26 [Kelsell et al., 1997]) are a particularly frequent cause of deafness within certain population groups. Mutations that alter the structure of the connexin 26 protein are known to cause both autosomal dominant (DFNA3) and recessive (DFNB1) hereditary hearing impairment. A study of nonsyndromic deafness in Italy and Spain concluded that 49% of individuals with recessive deafness had mutations in *GJB2*, with a carrier frequency for the mutated allele of about 3% in the general population (Estivill et al., 1998). In a study of the genetic epidemiology of hereditary deafness among Ashkenazi Jews, Morell et al. (1998) concluded that the majority of cases of nonsyndromic deafness were a result of mutations in *GJB2*, although the predominant mutation in the Ashkenazi Jewish population (a deletion of a thymidine nucleotide at position 167 in the gene sequence [167delT]) is different from the most common mutation in the Italian and Spanish population (a deletion of a guanine nucleotide at position 35 in the gene sequence [35delG]). These studies underscore the observation that the genetic epidemiology of hereditary hearing impairment will differ between defined human population groups.

Cohn et al. (1999) have studied the clinical features of the hearing loss attributable to mutations in *GJB2* gene. Although all persons had hearing impairment, no consistent audiologic phenotype was observed, even within individual families. Hearing loss varied from mild-moderate (about 1/3 of cases) to profound (about 2/3 of cases), even within the group of families with the same mutation in the gene. In about 1/3 of the individuals where serial audiograms were available, the hearing loss was observed to be progressive. Similar findings were reported in a study correlating clinical findings with mutations in *GJB2* in Europe (Denoyelle et al., 1999). This heterogeneity in the phenotype associated with the same mutation in *GJB2* indicates that other factors (presumably mutations or allelic variation in other genes) play an important role in determining the clinical outcome. Identifying the nature of these "modifier" genes will be an important research goal for future studies. In any case, these modifying factors will need to be better understood before any accurate prediction of clinical outcome based on the result of a genetic test for mutations in *GJB2* can be unambiguously communicated to parents and relatives of children carrying a mutant *GJB2* allele.

CLINICAL IMPLICATIONS

As the genetic basis for hereditary hearing impairment is unraveled, the possibility of timely diagnosis based on genotype of this genetically diverse disorder will become a reality for most individuals. These advances will allow clinical studies that correlate the efficacy of different intervention strategies with the genetic basis for hearing impairment, with the promise of improving the communication skills of individuals with hereditary hearing impairment. In many cases of autosomal dominant nonsyndromic hereditary hearing impairment, the hearing loss is progressive. Genetic diagnosis will help determine which individuals in families carrying the dominant allele need careful follow-up and intervention to try to prevent or delay progressive hearing loss.

There is increasing evidence that susceptibility to noise-induced hearing loss and presbycusis has a genetic basis. It is not unreasonable to speculate that different mutations in the genes that cause profound hearing impairment in children may predispose individuals to noise-induced hearing loss and/or presbycusis. In the future, genetic testing may allow individuals at risk for progressive hearing loss to be identified at a young age, so that their career and lifestyle choices can be modified to help preserve their hearing. In any case, understanding the structure, function, and regulation of the genes that underlie hereditary hearing impairment will teach us a great deal about hitherto unknown physiologic processes essential for normal auditory function. In other organ systems, this basic understanding has often been the first step in developing intervention strategies in the future that cannot even be imagined at this time. There is no question that mouse model systems will play a pivotal role in furthering this basic understanding.

ACKNOWLEDGMENTS

The author thanks Eduardo Sainz and Lisa Blumenthal for expert assistance in preparing the figures and table. In addition, the author thanks Drs. Donald Luecke, Bob Wenthold, Thomas Friedman, Andrew Griffith, Rob Morell, and Amy Donahue, as well as Lori Hampton and Eduardo Sainz, for a critical review of the manuscript.

27 Genetic Analyses of Non-Transgenic Mouse Mutations Affecting Ear Morphology or Function

Kenneth R. Johnson, Qing Yin Zheng, and Verity A. Letts

INTRODUCTION

THE MOUSE AS A MODEL FOR HUMAN HEARING IMPAIRMENT

The mouse is an excellent animal model for the study of human deafness or hearing impairment (Steel, 1991; Steel and Brown, 1996). The mouse inner ear is anatomically similar to that of humans and hereditary pathologies have been shown to be similar in humans and mice (Brown and Steel, 1994; Steel and Bock, 1983). Because of these similarities, identification of the genes causing hearing impairment or deafness in mice may also identify homologous human genes and genetic disorders. Defined regions of chromosomes are highly conserved for gene content and gene linkages between these two mammalian species. Major efforts are well underway to sequence the entire genomes of both species that, when completed, will provide highly increased resolution of homologies.

The genetic analysis of mouse mutations has helped to identify several human deafness genes (Probst and Camper, 1999), including *PAX3* (responsible for WS1 and WS3), *MITF* (responsible for WS2), *MYO7A* (responsible for DFNB2, DFNA11, and USH1B), *MYO15* (responsible for DFNB3), and *POU4F3* (responsible for DFNA15). For example, the spontaneous mouse mutations shaker 1 (*sh1*) and shaker 2 (*sh2*) were instrumental in identifying two human genes responsible for four deafness syndromes. Both *sh1* and *sh2* are characterized by hyperactivity, head-shaking, and circling behaviors, and also are deaf due to neuroepithelial defects of the cochlea. *sh1* was shown by positional cloning to be a mutation of the *Myo7a* gene, which encodes an unconventional myosin-type protein (Gibson et al., 1995). Subsequently, the homologous *MYO7A* gene in humans was shown to be responsible for both dominant (DFNA11) and recessive (DFNB2) forms of nonsyndromic deafness (Liu et al., 1997a; 1997b), as well as for Usher syndrome type1B (Weil et al., 1995). *sh2* was shown to be a mutation of the *Myo15* gene (Probst et al., 1998), which encodes a different unconventional myosin. Aided by this information, the homologous *MYO15* gene in humans was shown to be responsible for *DFNB3* (Wang et al., 1998).

There are nearly 100 genes in the mouse with mutations that have been reported to cause hearing impairment, some of which may serve as models for human deafness (MGD, 2000; Steel, 1995). A major focus of this chapter is to provide an updated list of these mutations, their effects on hearing and balance, their chromosomal map positions, their pathological classifications, and their underlying genes, if known. This chapter covers naturally occurring or spontaneous mutations and those that have been randomly induced by irradiation or chemical treatments. The study of such non-directed mutations is a phenotype-driven approach that can be used to identify new genes as opposed to the targeted mutational analysis of already-known genes by genetic engineering techniques, a subject dealt with in Chapter 30. These two approaches to the study of mouse mutations are complementary, and both have made important contributions to hearing research.

Additional mouse mutations with hearing impairment or deafness continue to be discovered, and the pace of their discovery is likely to increase as the mouse becomes a greater focus of biomedical research. Molecular characterization of these mutations is necessary to identify the affected genes, to establish or confirm human–mouse gene homologies and, ultimately, to permit the study of the underlying pathophysiological mechanisms that result in deafness. This chapter also describes positional cloning approaches that are now being used for molecular gene identification of non-targeted mouse mutations.

EARLY STUDIES OF MOUSE DEAFNESS MUTATIONS

Early studies of deaf or hearing-impaired mutant mice were restricted to those occurring spontaneously or those resulting from irradiation. Most of these mutations were identified on the basis of more obvious non-auditory symptoms. Nearly all early studies of mouse deafness mutations were limited to the two phenotypes most commonly associated with hearing impairment — balance disorders and pigmentation anomalies. Many pigmentation mutants have impaired hearing, often caused by the absence of melanocytes in the stria vascularis of the cochlea, as discussed later in this chapter.

If ever you have seen a hyperactive circling mouse in action, you will understand why these creatures have fascinated mouse fanciers (and scientists) for centuries. There are references to them in China as far back as 80 BC (Keeler, 1931). Mice with this characteristic head-shaking and circling behavior are also known as waltzers, spinners, whirlers, twirlers, shakers, and dancers. The abnormal behavior of these mutant mice is caused by defects of the vestibular organs of the inner ear. Many of the mutations causing this vestibular dysfunction also affect the cochlea, resulting in deafness or hearing loss. Ear infections may also cause mice to circle; however, most ear infections involve only a single ear and therefore usually cause unilateral rather than bidirectional circling.

To assess hearing in mice, early investigators observed their startle response to a loud sound, such as a whole-body jump or the backward flick of the pinna (Preyer reflex). The acoustic startle response (ASR) test detects supra-threshold responses and thus can identify only mice that are deaf or profoundly hearing-impaired. However, the simplicity of this test makes it useful for screening very large numbers of mice. Other behavioral and physiological methods have been developed to more accurately assess hearing in mice, including prepulse inhibition (PPI), auditory-evoked brain-stem response (ABR), distortion product otoacoustic emissions (DPOAE), and recordings of endo-cochlear potential (EP). Methods for examining inner-ear anatomy and pathology include whole mount preparations for stereoscopic examination of gross anatomy (with staining or paint-filling to enhance features) and cross-sections or surface preparations for light or electron microscopic examination of fine anatomy. All of these methods for hearing and anatomical assessment are described in detail in other chapters of this handbook.

During the past decade, the mouse has become the premier mammalian model for biomedical research (Malakoff, 2000). Consequently, many new investigators are entering the field of mouse genetics and making important contributions. These new discoveries have built upon the solid foundation provided by earlier investigators. It is important to acknowledge the many contributions that early studies of mouse mutations have made to hearing research. These contributions include the discovery and genetic characterization of a large number of mouse deafness mutations (which laid the groundwork for later gene discovery efforts), and the anatomical characterization of the inner ears from these mutant mice (which has provided insight into pathological mechanisms of hearing and balance dysfunction). Three prominent researchers who pioneered the study of mouse mutations in deafness research are H. Gruneberg (University College, London, U.K.), M.S. Deol (University College, London, and The Jackson Laboratory, Bar Harbor, ME, USA), and K.P. Steel (Medical Research Council, Nottingham, U.K.). Other researchers who made important early contributions include M.M. Dickie, M.C. Green, and P.W. Lane of The Jackson Laboratory, and M.F. Lyon of the Medical Research Council, Harwell, U.K.

Gruneberg was one of the first geneticists to study shaker-waltzer type mice and wrote the first review article describing this class of mutations (Gruneberg, 1956). Many contradictions occurred in the early reports of these mutants because investigators did not realize that the generic waltzer phenotype can be caused by mutations of many different genes. Gruneberg helped clarify that the Japanese waltzing mice imported from Japan into Europe and the United States around 1890 were probably the original source of the waltzer (*v*) mutation, but that many of the other shaker-waltzer type mice then being studied were caused by mutations of different genes (Gruneberg, 1952). M.S. Deol, the premier mouse ear pathologist of his time, contributed to more than 20 papers between 1954 and 1983 that described the anatomy and development of inner ears from more than 15 different mutants. Deol also wrote about the relationship of deafness with abnormalities of pigmentation (1970), neural tube formation (1966), and hypothyroidism (1973a; b), and was one of the first to espouse the importance of mouse mutations as models for human hearing defects (1968). Since 1980, K. Steel has contributed to more than 40 papers describing hearing and deafness in mice; and her authorship of more than ten review articles attests to her prominence in the field today. The comprehensive review published in 1995 (Steel, 1995) was a major source of information and a model for this chapter.

MOUSE MUTATIONS CAUSING EAR MALFORMATIONS OR DYSFUNCTION

LIST AND DESCRIPTION OF MUTATIONS

Many recent review articles have listed and described human and mouse genes and mutations that are involved in hearing and deafness (Brown and Steel, 1994; Cremers et al., 1995; Fekete, 1999; Fritzsch and Beisel, 1998; Holme and Steel, 1999; Kalatzis and Petit, 1998; Keats and Berlin, 1999; Probst and Camper, 1999; Steel, 1995; Steel and Brown, 1994; 1996; Steel and Bussoli, 1999; Van Camp et al., 1997). This chapter presents a comprehensive list of non-transgenic mouse mutations with ear malformations or dysfunction (Table 27.1) and a very brief overview of the pathologies associated with these mutations. The primary literature should be consulted for details on particular genes and mutations. The references listed in Table 27.1 are by no means exhaustive; they are limited to the first reports of the functional or morphological ear defects associated with the mutations and a few of the most important subsequent papers, with a maximum of three entries. Searches of PubMed (http://www.ncbi.nlm.nih.gov/entrez/query.fcgi?db = PubMed) and the Mouse Genome Informatics (MGI) Web site at The Jackson Laboratory (http://www.informatics.jax.org/) can be used to obtain additional references for each of these mutations. For example, using the search terms "mouse AND shaker-1 OR Myo7a" retrieves 49 references from PubMed, with the oldest reference dated 1967. The MGI entry for "Myo7a" includes 36 references, including the original 1929 reference that first described the shaker-1 mutation (Lord and Gates, 1929).

Symbols for non-targeted mouse mutations beginning with a capital letter indicate dominant inheritance, and those beginning with a lower case letter indicate recessive inheritance. When the mutated gene is identified at the molecular level, the original mutation symbol becomes a superscript for the new gene symbol. All mouse gene symbols begin with a capital letter and are italicized. To simplify presentations in Figures 27.1 to 27.5 and Table 27.1, mutant allele symbols are given separately from their gene symbols.

In Figures 27.1 through 27.5, chromosomal map positions are shown for all mouse mutations (including transgene-induced mutations) and strain polymorphisms that have been reported to be associated with hearing and balance defects or with malformations of the outer, middle, or inner ear. These include 76 spontaneous mutations (sp), 14 random transgene insertions (tg), 19 radiation-induced mutations (ra), 12 chemically induced mutations (ch), 33 targeted mutations (tm), and

TABLE 27.1
Mouse Mutations Reported to Cause Ear Malformations or Dysfunction

Symbol	Mutation Name	Gene[a]	Chr	Ear Pathology	Hearing[b]	Balance	Ref[/c]
adr	Arrested development of righting	Clcn1	6	Unknown	Impaired, ABR *	Retarded righting response; myotonia	1
av	Ames waltzer		10	Hair cell defects	Deaf, ABR *	Circling, head tossing	2–4
bor	Branchio-oto-renal syndrome	Eya1	1	Inner ear development	Deaf, ABR *	Circling, head tossing	5; tm 6
bs	Blind-sterile		2	Unknown	Impaired, ABR *	Normal	7
Bst	Belly spot and tail		16	Unknown	Impaired, ABR *	Normal	8
bv	Bronx waltzer		5	Hair cell defects	Deaf	Circling, head tossing	9–11
Cm	Coloboma		2	Unknown	Impaired, ABR *	Circling, head tossing	12
cmd	Cartilage matrix deficiency	Agc	7	Cartilage abnormality	Impaired	Unknown	13
cn	Achondroplasia		4	Unknown	Impaired, ABR *	Normal	14
co	Cocked		11	Otolith defect	Unknown	Head tilting	15
cog	Congenital goiter	Tgn	15	Thyroid hormone	Impaired, ABR *	Normal	16
cpk	Congenital polycystic kidneys		12	Unknown	Normal, ABR	Normal	17
Dc	Dancer		19	Vestibular defects	Not deaf	Circling, head tossing	18; 19
ddl	Dreidel	Pou4f3	18	Hair cell defects	Deaf, ABR *	Circling, head tossing	20; tm 21
de	Droopy ear		3	Malformed pinna	Unknown	Normal	22
df	Ames dwarf	Prop1	11	Thyroid hormone	Impaired, ABR *	Normal	23
dfw	Deaf waddler	Atp2b2	6	Calcium transport	Deaf, ABR *	Wobbly gait, head tossing	24–26; tm 27
Dmm	Disproportionate micromelia	Col2a1	15	Inner ear malformation	Unknown	Normal	28–30
dn	Deafness		19	Hair cell defects	Deaf	Slight head tossing	31; 32
Dom	Dominant megacolon	Sox10	15	Melanocyte development	Unknown	Normal	33; 34
dr	Dreher	Lmx1a	1	Inner ear development	Deaf	Circling, head tossing	35–37
Dre	Dominant reduced ear		4	Malformed pinna	Unknown	Normal	38
dt	Dystonia musculorum	Dst	1	Unknown	Unknown	Uncoordinated movement	39
dw	Dwarf	Pit1	16	Thyroid hormone	Impaired, ABR *	Normal	40
dwg	Dwarf grey		10	Unknown	Deaf, ABR *	Circle when old	41
Eh	Hairy ears		15	Malformed pinna	Normal, ABR	Normal	42
fi	Fidget		2	Inner ear development	Impaired, ABR *	Circling, head tossing	43–45
fsn	Flaky skin		17	Autoimmune?	Impaired, ABR *	Normal	46
ft	Flaky tail		3	Malformed pinna	Unknown	Normal	47
Fu	Fused	Axin	17	Inner ear development	Impaired, ABR *	Circling	48; 49
Gy	Gyro	? Phex	X	Hair cell defects	Impaired, ABR *	Circling	50–52

Symbol	Name	Gene	Chromosome	Defect	Hearing	Behavior	References
het	Head tilt		17	Otolith defect	Normal, ABR	Head tilting	53–55
hyh	Hydrocephaly with hop gait		7	Unknown	Impaired ABR *	Hop gait	56
hyt	Hypothyroid	*Tshr*	12	Thyroid hormone	Impaired, ABR *	Normal	57
le	Eye-ear reduction		X	Malformed pinna	Unknown	Normal	58
jc	Jackson circler		10	Hair cell defects	Impaired/deaf, ABR *	Circling, head tossing	59
je	Jerker		4	Hair cell defects	Deaf, ABR *	Circling, head tossing	60–62
js	Jackson shaker		11	Hair cell defects	Deaf, ABR *	Circling, head tossing	63; 64
jv	Jackson waltzer	*Otx1*	11	Inner ear development	Normal, ABR	Circling, head tossing	65; our unpublished results
kr	Kreisler	*Mafb*	2	Inner ear development	Unknown	Circling, head tossing	66–68
lm	Lethal milk	*Slc30a4*	2	Otolith defect	Unknown	Delayed righting	69; 70
Lp	Loop-tail		1	Neural tube defect	Normal, ABR	Head wobbling	71–73
lpr	Lymphoproliferation	*Fas*	19	Autoimmune	Impaired	Normal	74–76
ls	Lethal spotting	*Edn3*	2	Melanocyte development	Unknown	Normal	77–79
Lse	Low set ears		U	Malformed pinna	Unknown	Normal	80
mdx	X-Linked muscular dystrophy	*Dmd*	X	Unknown	Normal, ABR	Normal	81; 82
mes	Mesenchymal dysplasia		13	Unknown	Impaired, ABR *	Normal	83
mh	Mocha	*Ap3d*	10	Otolith defect and cochlear degeneration	Impaired, ABR *	Head tilting	84–86
mi	Microphthalmia	*Mitf*	6	Melanocyte development	Impaired, ABR *	Normal	87–89
mps	Mucopolysaccharidosis	*Gus*	5	Lysosome storage defect	Impaired	Normal	90; 91
mu	Muted		13	Otolith defect	Unknown	Head tilting	92; 93
nr	Nervous		8	Central nervous system	Normal, ABR	Wobbly gait	94
nv	Nijmegen waltzer		7	Unknown	Not deaf	Circling, head tossing	95
oc	Osteosclerotic		19	Unknown	Impaired	Circling	96; 97
ocd	Osteochondrodystrophy		19	Unknown	Impaired, ABR *	Normal	98
oto	Otocephaly		1	Craniofacial	Unknown	Unknown	99
pa	Pallid		2	Otolith defect	Unknown	Head tilting	100–102
pcd	Purkinje cell degeneration		13	Central nervous system	Normal, ABR	Ataxia	103
pi	Pirouette		5	Hair cell defects	Deaf, ABR *	Circling, head tossing	104–106
pkr	Punk rocker	*Kcne1*	16	K± transport	Deaf, ABR *	Circling, head tossing	107; tm 108
pr	Porcine tail		U	Inner ear development	Unknown	Circling	109
Q	Quinky		8	Unknown	Unknown	Circling, head tossing	110
qk	Quaking	*qk*	17	Myelin deficiency	Impaired, ABR **	Tremor	111; 112
qv	Quivering		7	Central nervous system	Impaired, ABR **	Quivering	113; 114
rg	Rotating		U	Inner ear development	Not deaf	Circling, head tossing	115
rl	Reeler	*Reln*	5	Central nervous system	Unknown	Ataxia	116–118

TABLE 27.1 (continued)
Mouse Mutations Reported to Cause Ear Malformations or Dysfunction

Symbol	Mutation Name	Gene[a]	Chr	Ear Pathology	Hearing[b]	Balance	Ref[c]
s	Piebald	Ednrb	14	Melanocyte development	Unknown	Normal	119; 120
se	Short ear	Bmp5	9	Malformed pinna	Normal, ABR	Normal	121
sh1	Shaker 1	Myo7a	7	Hair cell defects	Deaf, ABR *	Circling, head tossing	104; 122; 123
sh2	Shaker 2	Myo15	11	Hair cell defects	Deaf, ABR *	Circling, head tossing	60; 124; 125
shi	Shiverer	Mbp	18	Myelin deficiency	Impaired, ABR **	Tremor	126
Sig	Sightless		6	Inner ear development	Normal, ABR	Unknown	127
Sl	Steel	Mgf	10	Melanocyte development	Impaired	Normal	87; 128; 129
slf	Sex-linked fidget (also KO)	Pou3f4	X	Inner ear development	Deaf, ABR *	Head tossing	130; tm 131; 132
Sp	Splotch	Pax3	1	Melanocyte development	Normal, ABR	Normal	133
sr	Spinner		9	Hair cell defects	Deaf, ABR *	Circling, head tossing	134
stg	Stargazer	Cacng2	15	Central nervous system	Normal, ABR	Ataxia, head tossing	135; 136
sv	Snell's waltzer	Myo6	9	Hair cell defects	Deaf, ABR *	Circling, head tossing	137–139
swe	Slow-wave epilepsy	Slc9a1	4	Central nervous system	Impaired, ABR **	Ataxia	140
syj,syjns	Shaker with syndactylism	Slc12a2	18	K± transport	Deaf, ABR *	Circling, head tossing	141–143; tm 144
thd	Tilted head		1	Otolith defect	Unknown	Head tilting	100; 145
Tim	Translocation-induced mutation		4	Unknown	Normal, ABR	Circling, head tossing	146
tlt	Tilted		5	Otolith defect	Normal, ABR	Head tilting	147–149
Tr	Trembler	Pmp22	11	Myelin deficiency	Impaired	Tremor	150–152
Ts	Tail-short		11	Unknown	Impaired, ABR *	Normal	153–155
Tsk	Tight-skin	Fbn1	2	Extracellular matrix	Impaired, ABR *	Normal	156; 157
tub	Tubby	tub	7	Hair cell defects	Impaired, ABR *	Normal	158–160
Tw	Twirler		18	Inner ear development	Not deaf	Circling, head tossing	161–163
twt	Twister		7	Unknown	Unknown	Circling, head tossing	164
v	Waltzer		10	Hair cell defects	Deaf, ABR *	Circling, head tossing	104; 165; 166
Va	Varitint-waddler		3	Inner ear degeneration	Impaired/deaf, ABR *	Circling, head tossing	60; 167; 168
W	Dominant spotting	Kit	5	Melanocyte development	Impaired, ABR *	Normal	169–171
Whl	Wheels		4	Inner ear development	Unknown	Circling	172
wi	Whirler		4	Hair cell defects	Deaf	Circling, head tossing	173–175
Wt	Waltzer type		U	Inner ear development	Not deaf	Circling	176
Xt	Extra-toes	Gli3	13	Inner ear development	Normal, ABR *	Normal	177; 178

(Transgene-induced and targeted mutations are not included.)

[a] Gene symbols are given for those mutations whose underlying genes have been cloned and molecularly characterized.

[b] Hearing: ABR indicates that hearing was assessed as part of The Jackson Laboratory's auditory screening program supported by NIH grant DC62108 (our unpublished data). A single asterisk indicates elevated ABR thresholds; two asterisks indicate an abnormal ABR wave pattern. Mice homozygous for the semi-dominant mutations *Bst, Cm, Dc, Eh, Lp, Sp, Ts, Tsk* and *Xt* die before or at birth; in these cases, only heterozygous mice could be tested. Both homozygous and heterozygous mice were tested for all other mutations.

[c] References: Limited to first reports or most important papers; maximum of three. References for targeted mutations are indicated by "tm."

1. Steinmeyer, K., Klocke, R., Ortland, C., Gronemeier, M., Jockusch, H., Grunder, S., and Jentsch, T.J., 1991. Inactivation of muscle chloride channel by transposon insertion in myotonic mice. *Nature*, 354, 304-308.

2. Schaible, R.H., 1961. Ames waltzer, *av. Mouse News Lett.*, 24, 38.

3. Zobeley, E., Sufalko, D.K., Adkins, S., and Burmeister, M., 1998. Fine genetic and comparative mapping of the deafness mutation Ames waltzer on mouse chromosome 10. *Genomics*, 50, 260-266.

4. Alagramam, K.N., Kwon, H.Y., Cacheiro, N.L., Stubbs, L., Wright, C.G., Erway, L.C., and Woychik, R.P., 1999. A new mouse insertional mutation that causes sensorineural deafness and vestibular defects. *Genetics*, 152, 1691-1699.

5. Johnson, K.R., Cook, S.A., Erway, L.C., Matthews, A.N., Sanford, L.P., Paradies, N.E., and Friedman, R.A., 1999. Inner ear and kidney anomalies caused by IAP insertion in an intron of the *Eya1* gene in a mouse model of BOR syndrome. *Hum. Mol. Genet.*, 8, 645-653.

6. Xu, P.X., Adams, J., Peters, H., Brown, M.C., Heaney, S., and Maas, R., 1999. Eya1-deficient mice lack ears and kidneys and show abnormal apoptosis of organ primordia. *Nat. Genet.*, 23, 113-117.

7. Varnum, D.S., 1983. Blind-sterile: a new mutation on chromosome 2 of the house mouse. *J. Hered.*, 74, 206-207.

8. Rice, D.S., Williams, R.W., Ward-Bailey, P., Johnson, K.R., Harris, B.S., Davisson, M.T., and Goldowitz, D., 1995. Mapping the Bst mutation on mouse chromosome 16: a model for human optic atrophy. *Mamm. Genome*, 6, 546-548.

9. Bussoli, T.J., Kelly, A., and Steel, K.P., 1997. Localization of the bronx waltzer (bv) deafness gene to mouse chromosome 5. *Mamm. Genome*, 8, 714-717.

10. Deol, M.S. and Gluecksohn-Waelsch, S., 1979. The role of inner hair cells in hearing. *Nature*, 278, 250-252.

11. Deol, M.S., 1981. The inner ear in Bronx waltzer mice. *Acta Otolaryngol.*, 92, 331-336.

12. Hess, E.J., Collins, K.A., Copeland, N.G., Jenkins, N.A., and Wilson, M.C., 1994. Deletion map of the coloboma (Cm) locus on mouse chromosome 2. *Genomics*, 21, 257-261.

13. Yoo, T.J., Cho, H., and Yamada, Y., 1991. Hearing impairment in mice with the cmd/cmd (cartilage matrix deficiency) mutant gene. *Ann. N.Y. Acad. Sci.*, 630, 265-267.

14. Lane, P.W. and Dickie, M.M., 1968. Three recessive mutations producing disproportionate dwarfing in mice: achondroplasia, brachymorphic, and stubby. *J. Hered.*, 59, 300-308.

15. Peterson, A.C., 1970. The genetics of cocked, a new behavioural mutant in the house mouse. *Can. J. Genet. Cytol.*, 12, 391-392.

16. Beamer, W.G., Maltais, L.J., DeBaets, M.H., and Eicher, E.M., 1987. Inherited congenital goiter in mice. *Endocrinology*, 120, 838-840.

17. Cho, H., Buchanan, J., Strong, D., Yamada, Y., and Yoo, T.J., 1991. The molecular and structural basis of hearing impairment in mice with the cpk mutant gene. *Ann. N.Y. Acad. Sci.*, 630, 262-264.

18. Deol, M.S. and Lane, P.W., 1966. A new gene affecting the morphogenesis of the vestibular part of the inner ear in the mouse. *J. Embryol. Exp. Morphol.*, 16, 543-558.

19. Wenngren, B.I. and Anniko, M., 1988. Age-related auditory brainstem response (ABR) threshold changes in the dancer mouse mutant. *Acta Otolaryngol.*, 106, 386-392.

20. Frankel, W., Mahaffey, C., and Bartlett, F.N., 1999. The mutant mouse dreidel (ddl) contains a mutation in the Pou4f3 gene. Personal communication, MGI Electronic submission.

21. Erkman, L., McEvilly, R.J., Luo, L., Ryan, A.K., Hooshmand, F., O'Connell, S.M., Keithley, E.M., Rapaport, D.H., Ryan, A.F., and Rosenfeld, M.G., 1996. Role of transcription factors Brn-3.1 and Brn-3.2 in auditory and visual system development. *Nature*, 381, 603-606.

TABLE 27.1 (continued)
Mouse Mutations Reported to Cause Ear Malformations or Dysfunction

22. Curry, G.A., 1959. Genetical and developmental studies on droopy-eared mice. *J. Embryol. Exp. Morphol.*, 7, 39-65.

23. Sornson, M.W., Wu, W., Dasen, J.S., Flynn, S.E., Norman, D.J., O'Connell, S.M., Gukovsky, I., Carriere, C., Ryan, A.K., Miller, A.P., Zuo, L., Gleiberman, A.S., Andersen, B., Beamer, W.G., and Rosenfeld, M.G., 1996. Pituitary lineage determination by the Prophet of Pit-1 homeodomain factor defective in Ames dwarfism. *Nature*, 384, 327-333.

24. Lane, P.W., 1987. Deaf waddler (dfw). *Mouse News Lett.*, 77, 129.

25. Noben-Trauth, K., Zheng, Q.Y., Johnson, K.R., and Nishina, P.M., 1997. mdfw: a deafness susceptibility locus that interacts with deaf waddler (*dfw*). *Genomics*, 44, 266-272.

26. Street, V.A., McKee-Johnson, J.W., Fonseca, R.C., Tempel, B.L., and Noben-Trauth, K., 1998. Mutations in a plasma membrane Ca²⁺-ATPase gene cause deafness in deafwaddler mice. *Nat. Genet.*, 19, 390-394.

27. Kozel, P.J., Friedman, R.A., Erway, L.C., Yamoah, E.N., Liu, L.H., Riddle, T., Duffy, J.J., Doetschman, T., Miller, M.L., Cardell, E.L., and Shull, G.E., 1998. Balance and hearing deficits in mice with a null mutation in the gene encoding plasma membrane Ca²⁺-ATPase isoform 2. *J. Biol. Chem.*, 273, 18693-18696.

28. Berggren, D., Frenz, D., Galinovic-Schwartz, V., and Van de Water, T.R., 1997. Fine structure of extracellular matrix and basal laminae in two types of abnormal collagen production: L-proline analog-treated otocyst cultures and disproportionate micromelia (Dmm/Dmm) mutants. *Hear. Res.*, 107, 125-135.

29. Brown, K.S., Cranley, R.E., Greene, R., Kleinman, H.K., and Pennypacker, J.P., 1981. Disproportionate micromelia (Dmm): an incomplete dominant mouse dwarfism with abnormal cartilage matrix. *J. Embryol. Exp. Morphol.*, 62, 165-182.

30. Pace, J.M., Li, Y., Seegmiller, R.E., Teuscher, C., Taylor, B.A., and Olsen, B.R., 1997. Disproportionate micromelia (Dmm) in mice caused by a mutation in the C-propeptide coding region of Col2a1. *Dev. Dyn.*, 208, 25-33.

31. Deol, M. and Kocher, W., 1958. A new gene for deafness in the mouse. *Heredity*, 12, 463-466.

32. Keats, B.J., Nouri, N., Huang, J.M., Money, M., Webster, D.B., and Berlin, C.I., 1995. The deafness locus (dn) maps to mouse chromosome 19. *Mamm. Genome*, 6, 8-10.

33. Herbarth, B., Pingault, V., Bondurand, N., Kuhlbrodt, K., Hermans-Borgmeyer, I., Puliti, A., Lemort, N., Goossens, M., and Wegner, M., 1998. Mutation of the Sry-related Sox10 gene in Dominant megacolon, a mouse model for human Hirschsprung disease. *Proc. Natl. Acad. Sci. U.S.A.*, 95, 5161-5165.

34. Southard-Smith, E.M., Kos, L., and Pavan, W.J., 1998. Sox10 mutation disrupts neural crest development in Dom Hirschsprung mouse model. *Nat. Genet.*, 18, 60-64.

35. Deol, M.S., 1964. The origin of the abnormalities of the inner ear in dreher mice. *J. Embryol. Exp. Morphol.*, 12, 727-733.

36. Lyon, M.F., 1961. Linkage relations and some pleiotropic effects of the dreher mutant of the house mouse. *Genet. Res.*, 2, 92-95.

37. Millonig, J.H., Millen, K.J., and Hatten, M.E., 2000. The mouse Dreher gene Lmx1a controls formation of the roof plate in the vertebrate CNS [see comments]. *Nature*, 403, 764-769.

38. Kelly, E.M., 1968. Dominant reduced ear, E (orB<e>). *Mouse News Lett.*, 38, 31.

39. Brown, A., Bernier, G., Mathieu, M., Rossant, J., and Kothary, R., 1995. The mouse dystonia musculorum gene is a neural isoform of bullous pemphigoid antigen 1. *Nat. Genet.*, 10, 301-306.

40. Li, S., Crenshaw, E.B.R., Rawson, E.J., Simmons, D.M., Swanson, L.W., and Rosenfeld, M.G., 1990. Dwarf locus mutants lacking three pituitary cell types result from mutations in the POU-domain gene Pit-1. *Nature*, 347, 528-533.

41. Harris, B. and Davisson, M.T., 1990. Dwarf grey (dwg). *Mouse Genome*, 86, 238.

42. Bangham, J.W., 1965. Hairy ears, Eh. *Mouse News Lett.*, 33, 68.

43. Cox, G.A., Mahaffey, C.L., Nystuen, A., Letts, V.A., and Frankel, W.N., 2000. The mouse fidget gene defines a new role for AAA family proteins in mammalian development. *Nat. Genet.*, 26, 198-202.

44. Gruneberg, H., 1943. Two new mutant genes in the house mouse. *J. Genet.*, 45, 22-28.

45. Truslove, G.M., 1956. The anatomy and development of the fidget mouse. *J. Genet.*, 54, 64-86.

46. Pelsue, S.C., Schweitzer, P.A., Beamer, W.G., and Shultz, L.D., 1995. Mapping of the flaky skin (fsn) mutation on distal mouse chromosome 17. *Mamm. Genome*, 6, 758.

47. Lane, P.W., 1972. Two new mutations in linkage group XVI of the house mouse. Flaky tail and varitint-waddler-J. *J. Hered.*, 63, 135-140.

48. Deol, M.S., 1966. The probable mode of gene action in the circling mutants of the mouse. *Genet. Res.*, 7, 363-371.

49. Zeng, L., Fagotto, F., Zhang, T., Hsu, W., Vasicek, T.J., Perry, W.L., 3rd, Lee, J.J., Tilghman, S.M., Gumbiner, B.M., and Costantini, F., 1997. The mouse fused locus encodes axin, an inhibitor of the Wnt signaling pathway that regulates embryonic axis formation. *Cell*, 90, 181-192.

50. Lyon, M.F., Scriver, C.R., Baker, L.R., Tenenhouse, H.S., Kronick, J., and Mandla, S., 1986. The Gy mutation: another cause of X-linked hypophosphatemia in mouse. *Proc. Natl. Acad. Sci. U.S.A.*, 83, 4899-4903.

51. Meisler, M., 1997. Mutation watch: PEX PLUS? Gene(s) for X-linked hypophosphatemia and deafness. *Mamm. Genome*, 8, 543-544.

52. Strom, T.M., Francis, F., Lorenz, B., Boddrich, A., Econs, M.J., Lehrach, H., and Meitinger, T., 1997. Pex gene deletions in Gy and Hyp mice provide mouse models for X-linked hypophosphatemia. *Hum. Mol. Genet.*, 6, 165-171.

53. Bergstrom, R.A., You, Y., Erway, L.C., Lyon, M.F., Schimenti, J.C., 1998. Deletion mapping of the head tilt (het) gene in mice: a vestibular mutation causing specific absence of otoliths. *Genetics*, 150, 815-822.

54. Jones, S.M., Erway, L.C., Bergstrom, R.A., and Schimenti, J.C., and Jones, T.A., 1999. Vestibular responses to linear acceleration are absent in otoconia- deficient C57BL/6JEi-het mice. *Hear. Res.*, 135, 56-60.

55. Sweet, H.O., 1980. Head tilt (het). *Mouse News Lett.*, 63, 19.

56. Bronson, R.T. and Lane, P.W., 1990. Hydrocephalus with hop gait (hyh): a new mutation on chromosome 7 in the mouse. *Brain Res. Dev. Brain Res.*, 54, 131-136.

57. O'Malley, B.W., Jr., Li, D., and Turner, D.S., 1995. Hearing loss and cochlear abnormalities in the congenital hypothyroid (hyt/hyt) mouse. *Hear. Res.*, 88, 181-189.

58. Hunsicker, P., 1974. [le = eye-ear reduction X linked]. *Mouse News Lett.*, 50, 51-52.

59. Southard, J.L., 1970. Jackson circler, jc. *Mouse News Lett.*, 42, 30.

60. Deol, M.S., 1954. The anomalies of the labyrinth of the mutants varitint-waddler, shaker-2 and jerker in the mouse. *J. Genet.*, 52, 562-588.

61. Gruneberg, H., Burnett, J.B., and Snell, G.D., 1941. The origin of jerker, a new gene mutation of the house mouse, and linkage studies made with it. *Proc. Natl. Acad. Sci. U.S.A.*, 27, 562-565.

62. Steel, K.P. and Bock, G.R., 1983. Cochlear dysfunction in the jerker mouse. *Behav. Neurosci.*, 97, 381-391.

63. Dickie, M.M. and Deol, M.S., 1967. Jackson shaker, *js. Mouse News Lett.*, 36, 39.

64. Kitamura, K., Kakoi, H., Yoshikawa, Y., and Ochikubo, F., 1992. Ultrastructural findings in the inner ear of Jackson shaker mice. *Acta Otolaryngol.*, 112, 622-627.

65. Dickie, M.M. and Deol, M.S., 1966. Jackson waltzer, jv. *Mouse News Lett.*, 35, 31.

66. Cordes, S.P. and Barsh, G.S., 1994. The mouse segmentation gene *kr* encodes a novel basic domain-leucine zipper transcription factor. *Cell*, 79, 1025-1034.

67. Deol, M.S., 1964. The abnormalities of the inner ear in Kreisler mice. *J. Embryol. Exp. Morphol.*, 12, 475-490.

68. Hertwig, P., 1942. Neue Mutationen und Koppelungsgruppen bei der Hausmaus. *Z. Indukt. Abstamm. Vererbungsl.*, 80, 220-246.

69. Erway, L.C. and Grider, A., Jr., 1984. Zinc metabolism in lethal-milk mice. Otolith, lactation, and aging effects. *J. Hered.*, 75, 480-484.

70. Huang, L. and Gitschier, J., 1997. A novel gene involved in zinc transport is deficient in the lethal milk mouse. *Nat. Genet.*, 17, 292-297.

71. Deol, M.S., 1966. Influence of the neural tube on the differentiation of the inner ear in the mammalian embryo. *Nature*, 209, 219-220.

72. Strong, L.C. and Hollander, W.F., 1949. Hereditary loop-tail in the house mouse accompanied by inperforate vagina and craniorachischisis when homozygous. *J. Hered.*, 40, 329-334.

73. Wilson, D.B., 1985. An ultrastructural analysis of abnormal otic development in exencephalic mutant mice. *Arch. Otorhinolaryngol.*, 241, 203-208.

74. Kusakari, C., Hozawa, K., Koike, S., Kyogoku, M., and Takasaka, T., 1992. MRL/MP-1pr/1pr mouse as a model of immune-induced sensorineural hearing loss. *Ann. Otol. Rhinol. Laryngol. Suppl.*, 157, 82-86.

75. Ruckenstein, M.J., Mount, R.J., and Harrison, R.V., 1993. The MRL-lpr/lpr mouse: a potential model of autoimmune inner ear disease. *Acta Otolaryngol.*, 113, 160-165.

TABLE 27.1 (continued)
Mouse Mutations Reported to Cause Ear Malformations or Dysfunction

76. Trune, D.R., Craven, J.P., Morton, J.I., and Mitchell, C., 1989. Autoimmune disease and cochlear pathology in the C3H/lpr strain mouse. *Hear. Res.*, 38, 57-66.

77. Baynash, A.G., Hosoda, K., Giaid, A., Richardson, J.A., Emoto, N., Hammer, R.E., and Yanagisawa, M., 1994. Interaction of endothelin-3 with endothelin-B receptor is essential for development of epidermal melanocytes and enteric neurons. *Cell*, 79, 1277-1285.

78. Edery, P., Attie, T., Amiel, J., Pelet, A., Eng, C., Hofstra, R.M., Martelli, H., Bidaud, C., Munnich, A., and Lyonnet, S., 1996. Mutation of the endothelin-3 gene in the Waardenburg-Hirschsprung disease (Shah-Waardenburg syndrome). *Nat. Genet.*, 12, 442-444.

79. Pavan, W.J., Liddell, R.A., Wright, A., Thibaudeau, G., Matteson, P.G., McHugh, K.M., and Siracusa, L.D. 1995. A high-resolution linkage map of the lethal spotting locus: a mouse model for Hirschsprung disease. *Mamm. Genome*, 6, 1-7.

80. Theiler, K. and Sweet, H.O. 1986. Low set ears (Lse), a new mutation of the house mouse. *Anat. Embryol.*, 175, 241-246.

81. Raynor, E.M. and Mulroy, M.J. 1997. Sensorineural hearing loss in the mdx mouse: a model of Duchenne muscular dystrophy. *Laryngoscope*, 107, 1053-1056.

82. Pillers, D.A., Duncan, N.M., Dwinnell, S.J., Rash, S.M., Kempton, J.B., and Trune, D.R., 1999. Normal cochlear function in mdx and mdx(Cv3) Duchenne muscular dystrophy mouse models. *Laryngoscope*, 109, 1310-1312.

83. Sweet, H.O. and Bronson, R.T. 1988. Mesenchymal dysplasia (mes). *Mouse News Lett.*, 81, 70.

84. Lane, P.W. and Deol, M.S., 1974. Mocha, a new coat color and behavior mutation on chromosome 10 of the mouse. *J. Hered.*, 65, 362-364.

85. Rolfsen, R.M. and Erway, L.C., 1984. Trace metals and otolith defects in mocha mice. *J. Hered.*, 75, 159-162.

86. Kantheti, P., Qiao, X., Diaz, M.E., Peden, A.A., Meyer, G.E., Carskadon, S.L., Kapfhamer, D., Sufalko, D., Robinson, M.S., Noebels, J.L., and Burmeister, M., 1998. Mutation in AP-3 delta in the mocha mouse links endosomal transport to storage deficiency in platelets, melanosomes, and synaptic vesicles. *Neuron*, 21, 111-122.

87. Deol, M.S., 1970. The relationship between abnormalities of pigmentation and of the inner ear. *Proc. R. Soc. Lond., B. Biol. Sci.*, 175, 201-217.

88. Hodgkinson, C.A., Moore, K.J., Nakayama, A., Steingrimsson, E., Copeland, N.G., Jenkins, N.A., and Arnheiter, H., 1993. Mutations at the mouse microphthalmia locus are associated with defects in a gene encoding a novel basic-helix-loop-helix-zipper protein. *Cell*, 74, 395-404.

89. Tassabehji, M., Newton, V.E., and Read, A.P., 1994. Waardenburg syndrome type 2 caused by mutations in the human microphthalmia (MITF) gene [see comments]. *Nat. Genet.*, 8, 251-255.

90. O'Connor, L.H., Erway, L.C., Vogler, C.A., Sly, W.S., Nicholes, A., Grubb, J., Holmberg, S.W., Levy, B., and Sands, M.S., 1998. Enzyme replacement therapy for murine mucopolysaccharidosis type VII leads to improvements in behavior and auditory function. *J. Clin. Invest.*, 101, 1394-1400.

91. Sands, M.S., Erway, L.C., Vogler, C., Sly, W.S., and Birkenmeier, E.H., 1995. Syngeneic bone marrow transplantation reduces the hearing loss associated with murine mucopolysaccharidosis type VII. *Blood*, 86, 2033-2040.

92. Lyon, M.F. and Meredith, R., 1969. Muted, a new mutant affecting coat colour and otoliths of the mouse, and its position in linkage group XIV. *Genet. Res.*, 14, 163-166.

93. Swank, R.T., Reddington, M., Howlett, O., and Novak, E.K., 1991. Platelet storage pool deficiency associated with inherited abnormalities of the inner ear in the mouse pigment mutants muted and mocha. *Blood*, 78, 2036-2044.

94. Berrebi, A.S. and Mugnaini, E., 1988. Effects of the murine mutation 'nervous' on neurons in cerebellum and dorsal cochlear nucleus. *J. Neurocytol.*, 17, 465-484.

95. Abeelen, J.H.V. and Kroon, P.H.v.d., 1967. Nijmegen waltzer—a new neurological mutant in the mouse. *Genet. Res.*, 10, 117-118.

96. Dickie, M.M., 1967. Osteosclerotic (oc). *Mouse News Lett.*, 36, 39.

97. Marks, S.C., Jr., Seifert, M.F., and Lane, P.W., 1985. Osteosclerosis, a recessive skeletal mutation on chromosome 19 in the mouse. *J. Hered.*, 76, 171-176.

98. Sweet, H.O. and Bronson, R.T., 1991. Osteochondrodystrophy (ocd): a new autosomal recessive mutation in the mouse. *J. Hered.*, 82, 140-144.

99. Juriloff, D.M., Sulik, K.K., Roderick, T.H., and Hogan, B.K., 1985. Genetic and developmental studies of a new mouse mutation that produces otocephaly. *J. Craniofac. Genet. Dev. Biol.*, 5, 121-145.

100. Erway, L.C., Fraser, A.S., and Hurley, L.S., 1971. Prevention of congenital otolith defect in pallid mutant mice by manganese supplementation. *Genetics*, 67, 97-108.

101. Huang, L., Kuo, Y.M., and Gitschier, J., 1999. The pallid gene encodes a novel, syntaxin 13-interacting protein involved in platelet storage pool deficiency. *Nat. Genet.*, 23, 329-332.

102. Lyon, M.F., 1953. Absence of otoliths in the mouse: An effect of the pallid mutant. *J. Genet.*, 51, 638-650.

103. Berrebi, A.S., Morgan, J.I., and Mugnaini, E., 1990. The Purkinje cell class may extend beyond the cerebellum. *J. Neurocytol.*, 19, 643-654.

104. Deol, M.S., 1956. The anatomy and development of the mutants pirouette, shaker-1 and waltzer in the mouse. *Proc. R. Soc. Lond., B. Biol. Sci.*, 145, 206-213.

105. Kocher, W., 1960. Untersuchungen zur Genetik und Pathologie der Entrwicklung von 8 Labyrinthmutanten (deaf-waltzer- shaker-Mutanten) der Maus. *Z. Vererbungsl.*, 91, 114-140.

106. Woolley, G.W. and Dickie, M.M. 1945. Pirouetting mice. *J. Hered.*, 36, 281-284.

107. Letts, V.A., Valenzuela, A., Dunbar, C., Zheng, Q.Y., Johnson, K.R., and Frankel, W.N., 2000. A new spontaneous mouse mutation in the Kcne1 gene. *Mamm. Genome*, 11, 831-835.

108. Vetter, D.E., Mann, J.R., Wangemann, P., Liu, J., McLaughlin, K.J., Lesage, F., Marcus, D.C., Lazdunski, M., Heinemann, S.F., and Barhanin, J., 1996. Inner ear defects induced by null mutation of the *Isk* gene. *Neuron*, 17, 1251-1264.

109. McNutt, W., 1968. Abnormalities of the inner ear in choreic porcine tail (pr) mice. *Anat. Rec.*, 160, 392-393.

110. Schaible, R.H., 1961. "Quinky". *Mouse News Lett.*, 24, 38-39.

111. Shah, S.N. and Salamy, A., 1980. Auditory-evoked far-field potentials in myelin deficient mutant quaking mice. *Neuroscience*, 5, 2321-2323.

112. Sidman, R.L., Dickie, M.M., and Appel, S.H., 1964. Mutant mice (quaking and jumpy) with deficient myelination in the central nervous system. *Science*, 144, 309-311.

113. Bock, G.R., Frank, M.P., Steel, K.P., and Deol, M.S., 1983. The quivering mutant mouse: hereditary deafness of central origin. *Acta Otolaryngol.*, 96, 371-377.

114. Deol, M.S., Frank, M.P., Steel, K.P., and Bock, G.R., 1983. Genetic deafness of central origin. *Brain Res.*, 258, 177-179.

115. Deol, M.S. and Dickie, M.M., 1967. Rotating, a new gene affecting behavior and the inner ear in the mouse. *J. Hered.*, 58, 69-72.

116. D'Arcangelo, G., Miao, G.G., Chen, S.C., Soares, H.D., Morgan, J.I., and Curran, T., 1995. A protein related to extracellular matrix proteins deleted in the mouse mutant reeler [see comments]. *Nature*, 374, 719-723.

117. Kanzaki, J., Mikoshiba, K., and Tsukada, Y., 1985. Auditory brainstem response in neuropathological mutant mice (shiverer and reeler). ORL. *J. Otorhinolaryngol. Relat. Spec.*, 47, 294-298.

118. Martin, M.R., 1981. Morphology of the cochlear nucleus of the normal and reeler mutant mouse. *J. Comp. Neurol.*, 197, 141-152.

119. Deol, M.S., 1967. The neural crest and the acoustic ganglion. *J. Embryol. Exp. Morphol.*, 17, 533-541.

120. Hosoda, K., Hammer, R.E., Richardson, J.A., Baynash, A.G., Cheung, J.C., Giaid, A., and Yanagisawa, M., 1994. Targeted and natural (piebald-lethal) mutations of endothelin-B receptor gene produce megacolon associated with spotted coat color in mice. *Cell*, 79, 1267-1276.

121. King, J.A., Marker, P.C., Seung, K.J., and Kingsley, D.M., 1994. BMP5 and the molecular, skeletal, and soft-tissue alterations in short ear mice. *Dev. Biol.*, 166, 112-122.

122. Gibson, F., Walsh, J., Mburu, P., Varela, A., Brown, K.A., Antonio, M., Beisel, K.W., Steel, K.P., and Brown, S.D., 1995. A type VII myosin encoded by the mouse deafness gene shaker-1. *Nature*, 374, 62-64.

123. Lord, E.M. and Gates, W.H., 1929. Shaker, a new mutation of the house mouse (Mus musculus). *Am. Naturalist*, 63, 435-442.

124. Probst, F.J., Fridell, R.A., Raphael, Y., Saunders, T.L., Wang, A., Liang, Y., Morell, R.J., Touchman, J.W., Lyons, R.H., Noben-Trauth, K., Friedman, T.B., and Camper, S.A., 1998. Correction of deafness in shaker-2 mice by an unconventional myosin in a BAC transgene [see comments]. *Science*, 280, 1444-1447.

125. Wang, A., Liang, Y., Fridell, R.A., Probst, F.J., Wilcox, E.R., Touchman, J.W., Morton, C.C., Morell, R.J., Noben-Trauth, K., Camper, S.A., and Friedman, T.B., 1998. Association of unconventional myosin MYO15 mutations with human nonsyndromic deafness DFNB3 [see comments]. *Science*, 280, 1447-1451.

126. Fujiyoshi, T., Hood, L., and Yoo, T.J., 1994. Restoration of brainstem auditory-evoked potentials by gene transfer in shiverer mice. *Ann. Otol. Rhinol. Laryngol.*, 103, 449-456.

TABLE 27.1 (continued)
Mouse Mutations Reported to Cause Ear Malformations or Dysfunction

127. Deol, M.S., 1980. Genetic malformations of the inner ear in the mouse and in man. *Birth Defects Orig. Artic. Ser.*, 16, 243-261.

128. Copeland, N.G., Gilbert, D.J., Cho, B.C., Donovan, P.J., Jenkins, N.A., Cosman, D., Anderson, D., Lyman, S.D., and Williams, D.E., 1990. Mast cell growth factor maps near the steel locus on mouse chromosome 10 and is deleted in a number of steel alleles. *Cell*, 63, 175-183.

129. Schrott, A., Melichar, I., Popelar, J., and Syka, J., 1990. Deterioration of hearing function in mice with neural crest defect. *Hear. Res.*, 46, 1-7.

130. Phippard, D., Boyd, Y., Reed, V., Fisher, G., Masson, W.K., Evans, E.P., Saunders, J.C., and Crenshaw, E.B., 3rd., 2000. The sex-linked fidget mutation abolishes Brn4/Pou3f4 gene expression in the embryonic inner ear. *Hum. Mol. Genet.*, 9, 79-85.

131. Minowa, O., Ikeda, K., Sugitani, Y., Oshima, T., Nakai, S., Katori, Y., Suzuki, M., Furukawa, M., Kawase, T., Zheng, Y., Ogura, M., Asada, Y., Watanabe, K., Yamanaka, H., Gotoh, S., Nishi-Takeshima, M., Sugimoto, T., Kikuchi, T., Takasaka, T., and Noda, T., 1999. Altered cochlear fibrocytes in a mouse model of DFN3 nonsyndromic deafness [see comments]. *Science*, 285, 1408-1411.

132. Phippard, D., Lu, L., Lee, D., Saunders, J.C., and Crenshaw, E.B., 3rd., 1999. Targeted mutagenesis of the POU-domain gene Brn4/Pou3f4 causes developmental defects in the inner ear. *J. Neurosci.*, 19, 5980-5989.

133. Steel, K.P. and Smith, R.J., 1992. Normal hearing in Splotch (Sp/±), the mouse homologue of Waardenburg syndrome type 1. *Nat. Genet.*, 2, 75-79.

134. Deol, M.S., Robins, M.W., 1962. The spinner mouse. *J. Hered.*, 53, 133-136.

135. Letts, V.A., Felix, R., Biddlecome, G.H., Arikkath, J., Mahaffey, C.L., Valenzuela, A., Bartlett II, F.S., Mori, Y., Campbell, K.P., and Frankel, W.N., 1998. The mouse stargazer gene encodes a neuronal Ca^{2+}-channel γ subunit. *Nat. Genet.*, 19, 340-347.

136. Noebels, J.L., Qiao, X., Bronson, R.T., Spencer, C., and Davisson, M.T., 1990. Stargazer: a new neurological mutant on chromosome 15 in the mouse with prolonged cortical seizures [published erratum appears in *Epilepsy Res.*, 11(1), 72, 1992. *Epilepsy Res.*, 7, 1291-35.

137. Avraham, K.B., Hasson, T., Steel, K.P., Kingsley, D.M., Russell, L.B., Mooseker, M.S., Copeland, N.G., and Jenkins, N.A., 1995. The mouse Snell's waltzer deafness gene encodes an unconventional myosin required for structural integrity of inner ear hair cells. *Nat. Genet.*, 11, 369-75.

138. Deol, M.S. and Green, M.C., 1966. Snell's waltzer, a new mutation affecting behaviour and the inner ear in the mouse. *Genet. Res.*, 8, 339-345.

139. Green, M.C., 1960. New mutant — Snell's waltzer — sv. *Mouse News Lett.*, 23, 34.

140. Cox, G.A., Lutz, C.M., Yang, C.L., Biemesderfer, D., Bronson, R.T., Fu, A., Aronson, P.S., Noebels, J.L., and Frankel, W.N., 1997. Sodium/hydrogen exchanger gene defect in slow-wave epilepsy mutant mice [published erratum appears in *Cell*, 91(6), 861, 1997. *Cell*, 91, 139-148.

141. Deol, M.S., 1963. The development of the inner ear in mice homozygous for shaker-with-syndactylism. *J. Embryol. Exp. Morphol.*, 11, 493-512.

142. Dixon, M.J., Gazzard, J., Chaudhry, S.S., Sampson, N., Schulte, B.A., and Steel, K.P., 1999. Mutation of the Na-K-Cl co-transporter gene Slc12a2 results in deafness in mice. *Hum. Mol. Genet.*, 8, 1579-1584.

143. Johnson, K.R., Cook, S.A., and Zheng, Q.Y., 1998. The original shaker-with-syndactylism mutation (sy) is a contiguous gene deletion syndrome. *Mamm. Genome*, 9, 889-892.

144. Delpire, E., Lu, J., England, R., Dull, C., and Thorne, T., 1999. Deafness and imbalance associated with inactivation of the secretory Na-K-2Cl co-transporter. *Nat. Genet.*, 22, 192-195.

145. Kelly, E.M. and Hartman., 1958. Tilted head. th. *Mouse News Lett.*, 19, 37.

146. Lewis, S.E., Barnett, L.B., Akeson, E.C., and Davisson, M.T., 1990. A new dominant neurological mutant induced in the mouse by ethylene oxide. *Mutat. Res.*, 229, 135-139.

147. Lane, P.W., 1986. Tilted (tlt). *Mouse News Lett.*, 75, 28.

148. Ornitz, D.M., Bohne, B.A., Thalmann, I., Harding, G.W., and Thalmann, R., 1998. Otoconial agenesis in tilted mutant mice. *Hear. Res.*, 122, 60-70.

149. Ying, H.C., Hurle, B., Wang, Y., Bohne, B.A., Wuerffel, M.K., and Ornitz, D.M., 1999. High-resolution mapping of tlt, a mouse mutant lacking otoconia. *Mamm. Genome*, 10, 544-548.

150. Falconer, D.S., 1951. Two new mutants, "trembler" and "reeler," with neurological actions in the house mouse. *J. Genet.*, 50, 192-201.

151. Suter, U., Welcher, A.A., Ozcelik, T., Snipes, G.J., Kosaras, B., Francke, U., Billings-Gagliardi, S., Sidman, R.L., Shooter, E.M., 1992. Trembler mouse carries a point mutation in a myelin gene. *Nature*, 356, 241-244.

152. Zhou, R., Assouline, J.G., Abbas, P.J., Messing, A., and Gantz, B.J., 1995. Anatomical and physiological measures of auditory system in mice with peripheral myelin deficiency. *Hear. Res.*, 88, 87-97.

153. Deol, M.S., 1961. Genetical studies on the skeleton of the mouse. XXVIII. Tail-short. *Proc. R. Soc. Lond., B. Biol. Sci.*, 155, 78-95.

154. Morgan, W.C., 1950. A new tail-short mutation in the mouse — Whose lethal effects are conditioned by the residual genotypes. *J. Hered.*, 41, 208-215.

155. Paterson, H.F., 1980. *In vivo* and *in vitro* studies on the early embryonic lethal tail-short. *J. Exp. Zool.*, 211, 247-256.

156. Green, M.C., Sweet, H.O., and Bunker, L.E., 1976. Tight-skin, a new mutation of the mouse causing excessive growth of connective tissue and skeleton. *Am. J. Pathol.*, 82, 493-512.

157. Siracusa, L.D., McGrath, R., Ma, Q., Moskow, J.J., Manne, J., Christner, P.J., Buchberg, A.M., and Jimenez, S.A., 1996. A tandem duplication within the fibrillin 1 gene is associated with the mouse tight skin mutation. *Genome Res.*, 6, 300-313.

158. Ikeda, A., Zheng, Q.Y., Rosenstiel, P., Maddatu, T., Zuberi, A.R., Roopenian, D.C., North, M.A., Naggert, J.K. Johnson, K.R., and Nishina, P.M., 1999. Genetic modification of hearing in tubby mice: evidence for the existence of a major gene (moth1) which protects tubby mice from hearing loss. *Hum. Mol. Genet.*, 8, 1761-1767.

159. Noben-Trauth, K., Naggert, J.K., North, M.A., and Nishina, P.M., 1996. A candidate gene for the mouse mutation tubby. *Nature*, 380, 534-538.

160. Ohlemiller, K.K., Hughes, R.M. Lett, J.M., Ogilvie, J.M., Speck, J.D., Wright, J.S., and Faddis, B.T., 1997. Progression of cochlear and retinal degeneration in the tubby (rd5) mouse. *Audiol. Neurootol.*, 2, 175-185.

161. Griffith, A.J., Radice, G.L., Burgess, D.L., Kohrman, D.C., Hansen, G.M., Justice, M.J., Johnson, K.R., Davisson, M.T., and Meisler, M.H., 1996. Location of the 9257 and ataxia mutations on mouse chromosome 18. *Mamm. Genome*, 7, 417-419.

162. Lyon, M.F, 1958. Twirler: a mutant affecting the inner ear of the house mouse. *J. Embryol. Exp. Morphol.*, 6, 105-116.

163. Ting, C.N., Kohrman, D., Burgess, D.L., Boyle, A., Altschuler, R.A., Gholizadeh, G., Samuelson, L.C., Jang, W., and Meisler, M.H., 1994. Insertional mutation on mouse chromosome 18 with vestibular and craniofacial abnormalities. *Genetics*, 136, 247-254.

164. Lane, P.W., 1981. [Twister (twt)]. *Mouse News Lett.*, 64, 59.

165. Deol, M.S., 1956. A gene for uncomplicated deafness in the mouse. *J. Embryol. Exp. Morphol.*, 4, 190-195.

166. Bryda, E.C., Ling, H., and Flaherty, L., 1997. A high-resolution genetic map around waltzer on mouse Chromosome 10 and identification of a new allele of waltzer. *Mamm. Genome*, 8, 1-4.

167. Cable, J. and Steel, K.P., 1998. Combined cochleo-saccular and neuroepithelial abnormalities in the Varitint-waddler-J (VaJ) mouse. *Hear. Res.*, 123, 125-136.

168. Cloudman, A.M. and Bunker, L.E., 1945. The varitint-waddler mouse. *J. Hered.*, 36, 258-263.

169. Deol, M.S., 1970. The origin of the acoustic ganglion and effects of the gene dominant spotting (Wv) in the mouse. *J. Embryol. Exp. Morphol.*, 23, 773-784.

170. Geissler, E.N., Ryan, M.A., and Housman, D.E, 1988. The dominant-white spotting (W) locus of the mouse encodes the c-kit proto-oncogene. *Cell*, 55, 185-192.

171. Steel, K.P., Barkway, C., and Bock, G.R., 1987. Strial dysfunction in mice with cochleo-saccular abnormalities. *Hear. Res.*, 27, 11-26.

172. Nolan, P.M., Sollars, P.J., Bohne, B.A., Ewens, W.J., Pickard, G.E, and Bucan, M., 1995. Heterozygosity mapping of partially congenic lines: mapping of a semidominant neurological mutation, Wheels (Whl), on mouse chromosome 4. *Genetics*, 140, 245-254.

173. Lane, P.W., 1963. Whirler mice, a recessive behavior mutation in linkage group VIII. *J. Hered.*, 54, 163-166.

174. Fleming, J., Rogers, M.J., Brown, S.D., and Steel, K.P., 1994. Linkage analysis of the whirler deafness gene on mouse chromosome 4. *Genomics*, 21, 42-48.

175. Rogers, M.J., Fleming, J., Kiernan, B.W., Mburu, P., Varela, A., Brown, S.D., and Steel, K.P., 1999. Genetic mapping of the whirler mutation. *Mamm. Genome*, 10, 513-519.

176. Stein, K.F. and Huber, S.A., 1960. Morphology and behavior of waltzer-type mice. *J. Morphol.*, 106, 197-203.

177. Hui, C. and Joyner, A.L., 1993. A mouse model of Greig cephalo-polysyndactyly syndrome: the extra-toesJ mutation contains an intragenic deletion of the Gli3 gene. *Nat. Genet.*, 3, 241-246.

178. Johnson, D.R., 1967. Extra-toes: anew mutant gene causing multiple abnormalities in the mouse. *J. Embryol. Exp. Morphol.*, 17, 543-581.

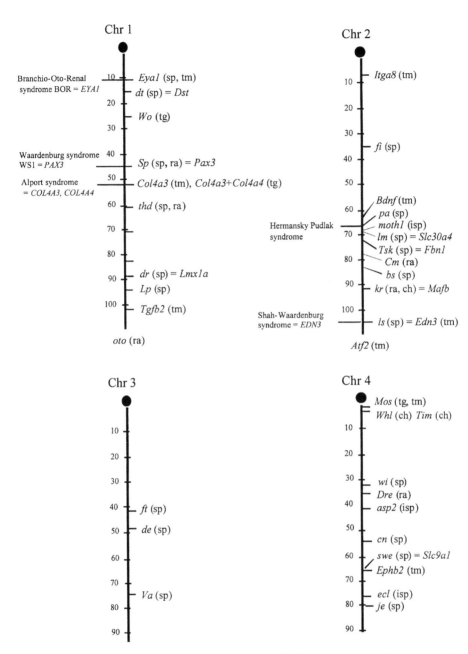

FIGURE 27.1 Chromosomal map positions (chromosomes 1–4) for loci reported to be associated with hearing and balance defects or with malformations of the outer, middle, or inner ear. For this and Figure 27.2, loci are identified as spontaneous mutations (sp), random transgene insertions (tg), radiation-induced mutations (ra), chemically induced mutations (ch), targeted mutations (tm), and inbred strain polymorphisms (isp). When known, gene symbols are given for loci originally identified as mutations. Human hearing disorders that are proven homologs of mouse gene mutations are shown to the left of each chromosome representation.

7 inbred strain polymorphisms (isp). Altogether, these mutations and polymorphisms identify a total of 126 gene loci. Human hearing disorders that are proven homologs of mouse gene mutations are shown to the left of each chromosome representation. Other homologies between human hearing disorders and mouse mutations probably exist but cannot be proven until their responsible genes are identified.

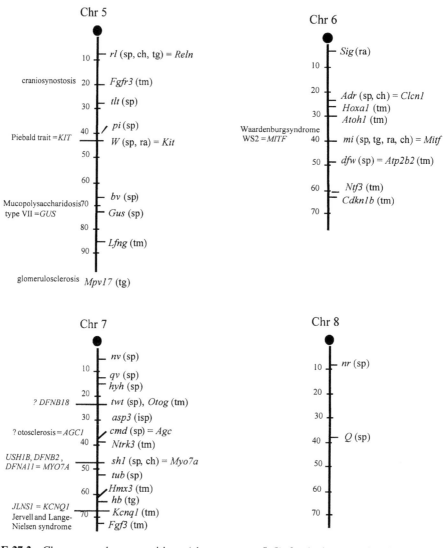

FIGURE 27.2 Chromosomal map positions (chromosomes 5–8) for loci reported to be associated with hearing and balance defects or with malformations of the outer, middle, or inner ear. See caption for Figure 27.1 for explanation of symbols.

Table 27.1 includes only spontaneous mutations and those induced by chemical or radiation treatments; it does not include targeted and transgenic mutations and inbred strain polymorphisms, which are the subjects of other book chapters. In Table 27.1, a total of 95 mutations are listed alphabetically by their mutant allele symbols (column 1) followed by their full names (column 2). The genes responsible for 43 of the mutations have been identified at the molecular level, and these gene symbols are shown in column 3. Also shown in Table 27.1 are the chromosomes to which the mutations have been mapped (column 4), the types of ear pathology they cause (column 5), the effects they have on hearing and balance (columns 6 and 7), and a few pertinent references (column 8).

A large-scale, auditory screening project is in progress at The Jackson Laboratory (Bar Harbor, Maine) to identify genes that contribute to hearing loss in both inbred and mutant strains of mice. This project is supported by the National Institutes of Health (contract DC62108). The screening project uses ABR thresholds to assess hearing, systematically testing representative mice from the nearly 2000 available strains. The first phase of the project concentrated on screening standard

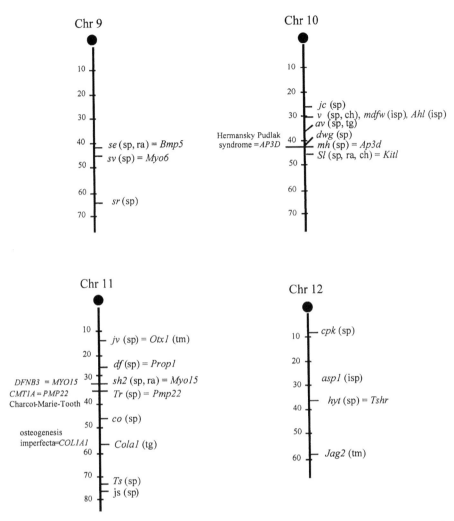

FIGURE 27.3 Chromosomal map positions (chromosomes 9–12) for loci reported to be associated with hearing and balance defects or with malformations of the outer, middle, or inner ear. See caption for Figure 27.1 for explanation of symbols.

inbred strains of mice (Q.Y. Zheng et al., 1999), but the emphasis has now shifted to examining mutant mice. The mutations that so far have been screened as part of this program are indicated by "ABR" in column 5 of Table 27.1. In some cases, these results represent the first report of a hearing loss associated with a mutation. Many mutant mice discovered on the basis of other phenotypic abnormalities also have an associated hearing loss that has gone undetected. For example, the $Pit1^{dw}$ mutation was originally discovered because it causes dwarfing, but ABR testing revealed that homozygosity for this mutation also causes deafness. Similarly, hearing impairments associated with the mutations *adr, bs, Bst, Cm, cn, cog, df, dt, dwg, fsn, hyh, mes, ocd, swe, Ts,* and *Tsk* were first discovered by the ABR screening program. Updated results from this screening program and other information related to the mouse as a model for human inherited hearing disorders is accessible at the following URL: http://www.jax.org/research/hhim/.

In the following brief overview, some of the mutations listed in Table 27.1 are grouped into categories according to their associated ear pathologies, expanding on those described by Holme and Steel (1999). These mutant categories are more thoroughly discussed in a recent review article by Steel et al. (2001). Until their underlying genes have been identified and characterized, the

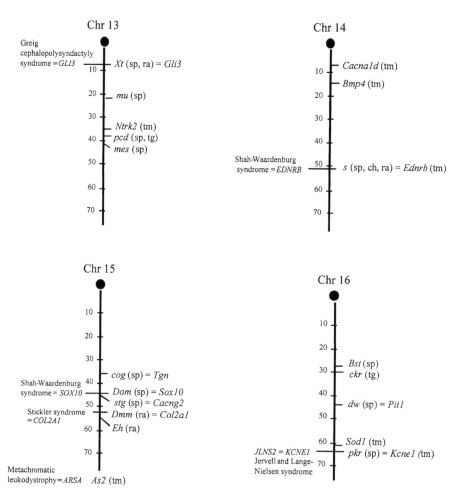

FIGURE 27.4   Chromosomal map positions (chromosomes 13–16) for loci reported to be associated with hearing and balance defects or with malformations of the outer, middle, or inner ear. See caption for Figure 27.1 for explanation of symbols.

assignment of mutations to primary pathological categories is often difficult. No classification scheme in biology is without exceptions; and in some cases, the categories we have chosen partially overlap. For example, morphogenetic defects can include malformations of the outer and middle ear as well as the inner ear. Defects of melanocyte development can cause dysfunction of the stria vascularis, thereby affecting endolymph homeostasis. Secondary effects of disrupted ion transport often include degeneration of hair cells and spiral ganglia. Yet, assembling the mutations into these categories helps to illustrate our growing knowledge of the pathological mechanisms and gene pathways involved in the intricate processes of hearing and balance. Much of this knowledge came about through the study of these mouse mutations.

OUTER AND MIDDLE EAR DEFECTS

Mice with the mutations *de, Dre, Eh, ft, Ie, Lse,* and *se* have malformations of the external ears or pinna. Only two of these mutations, *Eh* and *se*, have been assessed for their effects on hearing by ABR analysis, and neither exhibited a detectable impairment. The malformed pinna may decrease the ability to discern the correct direction of a sound source, but such tests have not been reported for these mutant mice. Genetic hearing impairment attributable to the middle ear is usually the result of ossicle malformations or fusions. Mice with such conductive hearing loss probably would

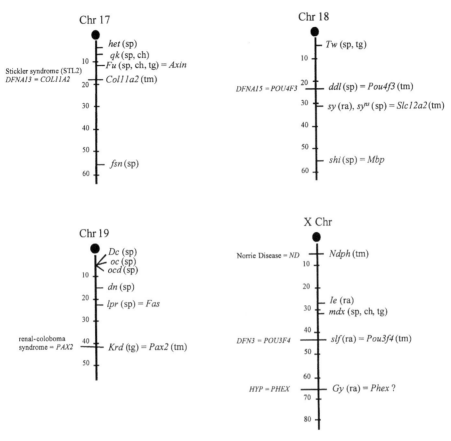

FIGURE 27.5 Chromosomal map positions (chromosomes 17–X) for loci reported to be associated with hearing and balance defects or with malformations of the outer, middle, or inner ear. See caption for Figure 27.1 for explanation of symbols.

go undetected without a specific auditory screening program, and this may explain why so few mouse mutations have been identified with middle-ear defects. The middle-ear defects that have been identified in mice are usually part of a larger syndrome, sometimes associated with craniofacial and outer or inner ear developmental abnormalities.

OTOLITH DEFECTS

Otoliths (or otoconia) are minute calcium carbonate crystals embedded in a gelatinous material overlying the maculae (or sensory epithelia) of the utricle and saccule. Their deficiency or malformation causes balance defects, resulting in a head-tilting behavior and/or an inability to swim. Mouse pigmentation mutations with otolith defects include *mh*, *mu*, and *pa*; the *mh* mutation also causes cochlear degeneration. The *mh* gene has been identified as *Ap3d* and its product has been shown to mediate intracellular vesicle transport, including melanosomes; however, the precise mechanism causing hearing loss has not yet been determined. The *mh*, *mu*, and *pa* mutations also cause plate storage pool deficiencies and are models for human Hermansky Pudlak syndrome. Other mouse mutations with otolith defects include *co*, *het*, *lm*, *thd*, and *tlt*.

MORPHOGENETIC DEFECTS

The mutations *Eya1^bor*, *Dc*, *Lmx1a^dr*, *fi*, *Axin^Fu*, *jv*, *Mafb^kr*, *pr*, *rg*, *Sig*, *Pou3f4^slf*, *Tw*, *Whl*, and *Wt* alter normal otic development, causing malformations of the inner ear. Mice with *Dc*, *Sig*, *Tw*, *jv*, and *rg* mutations exhibit balance defects but can hear; thus, these mutations primarily affect development of the vestibular end-organs. Mice with $Eya1^{bor}$, $Lmx1a^{dr}$, $Pou3f4^{slf}$, *fi*, and $Axin^{Fu}$ mutations have both balance and hearing deficits, because they alter the normal development of both the cochlea and the vestibular organs. The semidominant mutations *Sp* and *Xt* affect inner-ear development only when homozygous; however, homozygosity for these mutations also causes pre- or perinatal death. The genes responsible for inner-ear malformations are often transcription factors important in controlling early otic development.

ENDOLYMPH HOMEOSTASIS

The hearing impairment in some pigmentation mutants is caused by the absence of melanocytes in the stria vascularis of the cochlea. Melanocytes (or pigment cells) form an integral part of the stria vascularis, the highly vascularized granular cells on the outer wall of the cochlear duct that regulate the ionic composition of the enclosed endolymph. Absence of melanocytes in the stria results in loss of endocochlear potential and hearing impairment. Examples of pigmentation mutants affecting melanocyte development and survival include splotch (*Sp*), dominant spotting (*W*), piebald (*s*), lethal spotting (*ls*), microphthalmia (*mi*), and dominant megacolon (*Dom*). The homologous genes responsible for these mutations (that is, *Pax3*, *c-Kit*, *Ednrb*, *Edn3*, *Mitf*, and *Sox10*, respectively) underly the multiple forms of human Waardenburg syndrome. Mutations of the *c-Kit* and *Mitf* genes are known to cause hearing impairment in mice. The *Mgf* gene altered by the steel mutation (*Sl*) also affects pigmentation and hearing in mice.

Other mouse mutations without pigmentation defects have been shown to disrupt the ionic balance of the endolymph. Compared with the surrounding perilymph, the endolymph has a high concentration of K^+ ions and a low concentration of Na^+ ions. This ionic balance is actively maintained by marginal cells of the stria vascularis in the cochlea and by the dark cells of the vestibular organs. The targeted and *pkr* mutations of *Kcne1* and the targeted and *sy* and sy^{ns} mutations of *Slc12a2* disrupt potassium transport and recycling to the endolymph, thereby causing both hearing and balance defects.

SENSORY HAIR CELL DEFECTS

Mouse mutations that affect the sensory hair cells of the cochlea and vestibular organs cause both deafness and the classic shaker-waltzer phenotype. This group includes mutations of genes encoding important structural components of hair cells, such as the unconventional myosins *Myo7a*, *Myo6*, and *Myo15* that are disrupted by the *sh1*, *sv*, and *sh2* mutations, respectively. The group also includes mutations affecting hair cell development, such as the targeted and *ddl* mutations of the *Pou4f3* gene. The targeted and deaf waddler (*dfw*) mutations of the *Atp2b2* gene disrupt the normal regulation of intracellular calcium in hair cells. Other mouse mutations that affect hair cells but that are less well understood at the molecular level include *av*, *bv*, *dn*, *jc*, *je*, *js*, *pi*, *sr*, *v*, *Va*, and *wi*. Efforts are underway to identify the underlying genes for these mutations.

MYELIN AND CENTRAL NERVOUS SYSTEM DEFECTS

Myelin forms a membranous sheath that insulates axons and facilitates transmission of the nerve impulse. Myelin deficiencies can affect axons of both the peripheral and central nervous systems. Myelin mutations in mice usually cause an overt shivering or shaking behavior. Hearing can also be impaired in these mutants because of obstructed neurotransmission along the auditory pathway. Examples of myelin mutations with associated hearing deficits include quaking (*qk*), shiverer (Mbp^{shi}), and trembler (Pmp^{Tr}). Mouse mutations affecting the cerebellum, brainstem, or other parts of the CNS may impair hearing. ABR screening has identified a hearing loss associated with the quivering (*qv*) and slow-wave epilepsy ($Slc9a1^{swe}$) mutations, but not with the neurological mutants *nr*, *pcd*, and *stg*. Mice with myelin or central nervous system defects display abnormal ABR wave patterns, with increased latencies and reduced peak amplitudes following the initial auditory nerve response.

OTHER TYPES OF MUTATIONS

Abnormalities of extracellular matrix proteins, such as collagens, tectorin, and otogelin, can cause anomalies of membranes and other inner-ear structures that result in impaired hearing. ABR threshold analysis has shown an association between hearing impairment and several mouse mutations that affect thyroid hormone levels, including cog^{Tgn}, $Prop1^{df}$, $Pit1^{dw}$, and $Tshr^{hyt}$. Some mutations affecting immune responses, such as Fas^{lpr} or fsn, may also affect hearing. The pathophysiological mechanisms of hearing loss are not well understood for many mutations, but as their underlying genes are identified by the molecular cloning approach described below, many new insights into the hearing process will be revealed.

GENETIC APPROACHES TO ANALYZE MOUSE MUTATIONS

The extensive list of mouse mutants with hearing and vestibular defects illustrates the considerable research that has taken place in this field. With constantly improving reagents, it is now feasible to progress from first observing a mutation to finding the exact DNA change within a couple of years. Below, we outline the steps that are presently followed in characterizing a new mutation. Most mice with hearing defects are first noticed because of an irregular gait or coat color abnormality; subsequent testing then reveals that they are also deaf or hearing impaired. There are many mouse mutations that cause only vestibular problems, such as dancer (*Dc*), head tilt (*het*), and Jackson waltzer (*jv*); however, at present there is only one example of an existing mouse mutation causing uncomplicated deafness without vestibular defects (the deafness mutation, *dn*). Mutagenesis programs may generate and allow the identification of additional mutations causing non-syndromic deafness (see "Future Directions").

Genetic analyses of a new phenotypic deviant mouse include determining its heritability and mode of inheritance, its chromosomal map location, and its allelic relationships with known mutations (if any) that map to the same location and cause similar phenotypes. Ultimately, positional cloning approaches can be used to identify and characterize the mutated gene by molecular screening of candidate genes. The book *Mouse Genetics* (Silver, 1995) provides detailed background information on basic strategies and methods used in mouse genetics. In the following, we briefly describe the essential features of the approaches we have used to map and clone mouse mutations.

DETERMINING INHERITANCE

On observing a mouse with a defect, the first priority is to determine if it is a genetically inherited trait. Do the parents continue to throw affected pups? And if the pup is mated to one of its parents, are the offspring also affected? Upon establishing that the mutation has a genetic basis, can it be clearly defined as a single gene mutation? Problems with defining traits can occur if the phenotype cannot be accurately measured due to incomplete penetrance (when not all mice with mutant genotypes show a mutant phenotype) or variable expressivity (when not all mutant mice are equally affected). In both situations, one may have to consider that modifier genes or epigenetic factors are playing a significant role, as discussed further at the end of this chapter.

Single gene mutations, either spontaneous or induced, are characterized as dominant or recessive and are inherited following Mendel's laws. Dominant mutations express in every generation. A further refinement of the description of dominance is the semi-dominant phenotype, wherein the heterozygous phenotype is intermediate between the normal and homozygous. Conversely, a recessive mutation can skip generations, and both parents must be carriers (heterozygous) to give rise to an affected offspring. To determine mode of inheritance, a new mutant mouse is mated to a mouse from an unrelated strain producing F1 hybrid progeny. If the deviant dies at a young age or is infertile, the breeding test is done with the parents or siblings.

For a dominant or semi-dominant mutation, the abnormal phenotype is expected to appear in about 50% of the F1 progeny. If the abnormal phenotype does not appear among the F1 progeny, then F1 progeny are intercrossed to determine if the aberrant phenotype reappears in F2 offspring. A recessively inherited gene will reappear in about one-fourth of the F2 progeny. A semi-dominant gene will produce an intermediate phenotype in F1 progeny, and both the intermediate and original phenotypes will be recovered in the F2 generation. Deviations from expected Mendelian ratios are usually due to a deficiency of mutants. This deficiency can be caused by partial pre- or perinatal lethality of mutant homozygotes, or by incomplete penetrance of the mutant phenotype (not uncommon in mice heterozygous for semi-dominant mutations).

MAPPING MUTATIONS

The next step in analyzing a single gene mutation is to map the mutation to one of the 20 mouse chromosomes. X- and Y-linked mutations are ascertained by their sex-linked mode of inheritance. Because each new mutation is a unique event, a new linkage cross must be produced to genetically map each one. First, mutation-carrying F1 hybrids must be produced from mating mutant mice with mice from a different inbred strain. If homozygous mutant mice cannot breed, heterozygotes must be used to produce F1 hybrids, but the F1 hybrids must be tested to determine if they carry the mutant allele.

The choice of inbred strain utilized to produce F1 hybrids is important. The strain should be genetically distinct from the strain on which the mutation arose, so that enough polymorphic DNA markers are available for linkage analysis. Most of the standard laboratory strains of mice were derived from admixtures of *Mus mus musculus* and *M. m. domesticus*. Examples of genetically divergent strains include those derived from wild populations of *M. mus castaneus, M. m. molossinus*, and *M. spretus* (however, F1 hybrid males from the *M. spretus* cross are infertile, restricting linkage analysis to backcrossing). One of the most popular strains for linkage crosses is the *M. m. castaneus*-derived inbred strain CAST/Ei, which is genetically well characterized and distinct from all of the common laboratory strains. It usually breeds well to give sufficient F1s for either interbreeding to produce the F2 generation, or for backcrossing to the affected strain. Occasionally, a mutant phenotype may fail to appear in linkage crosses involving the CAST/Ei strain, and an alternative strain must then be chosen by evaluation of breeding performance and numbers of known inter-strain marker polymorphisms. Approximately 50% of all SSLP markers are polymorphic between standard inbred strains, offering a variety of strain choices for mapping crosses.

To best explain linkage mapping, let us assume that a recessive mutation affecting hearing arose on the C57BL/6J (B6) inbred strain, and that the affected mouse (genotype m/m) is capable of breeding (Figure 27.6). If the affected mouse is crossed to a normal hearing male mouse of a different inbred strain background (e.g., BALB/c, Figure 27.6), the F1 generation will carry both parental strain alleles, and none of the mice will be affected (but all will be carriers). If an F1 hybrid is backcrossed to an affected mouse, about one half of the N2 generation will be affected (homozygous for the mutant allele) and one half will be normal (heterozygous for the two parental alleles). If F1 hybrids are intercrossed, approximately one fourth of the F2 progeny will be affected. For recessive mutations, F1 hybrids are usually intercrossed to produce F2 progeny. The use of F2 progeny for genetic mapping is efficient because each mouse analyzed represents two potentially recombinant chromosomes — one from each F1 parent. For dominant mutations, F1 hybrids are usually backcrossed to the non-mutant strain because heterozygous and homozygous mutants cannot be distinguished.

Several procedures are available for mapping mutations to specific chromosomes, but probably the easiest and most efficient is the "pooling" method (Taylor et al., 1994). For backcrosses, DNAs (extracted from tail-tips or blood) from about 20 affected N2 mice are pooled and a second pool of DNA from an equal number of unaffected N2 mice is prepared for comparison. For intercrosses,

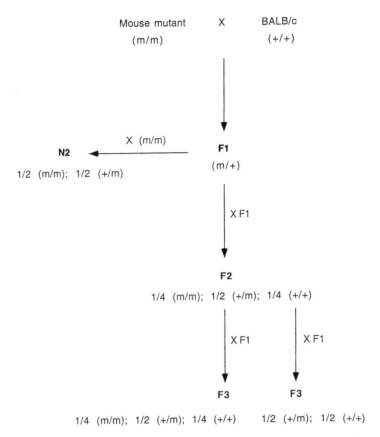

FIGURE 27.6   Mating schemes for the analysis of recessive mutations with geneotypes shown in parenthesis.

a single DNA pool is prepared from about 20 affected F2 mice for comparison with DNA from F1 hybrids. MIT microsatellite markers are selected that roughly map to the top, middle, and bottom of each chromosome (Dietrich et al., 1992). The polymerase chain reaction (PCR) products for the selected markers should be at least two, and preferably more than ten, base pairs different in size between the parental strains. PCR products for each set of primers with each template DNA to be compared (DNA pools and F1 hybrid DNA) are individually separated on high percentage agarose gels to resolve the different allele sizes (Figure 27.7).

Linkage of a marker with the mutation increases the proportion of the mutant strain allele relative to the non-mutant strain allele. In the case of complete linkage, only the mutant strain allele would be amplified from the DNA pool of mutant mice. In the case of backcrosses, the ratios of strain-specific PCR products are compared between the mutant and non-mutant DNA pools. For intercross linkage analysis, the ratio of strain-specific PCR products from the DNA pool of affected F2 progeny is compared with that from the F1 hybrid, whose 1:1 ratio of parental alleles is the same as that expected for no linkage. To confirm suspected linkage, DNAs from individual mice are typed for additional markers in the region.

TESTING ALLELISM WITH PREVIOUSLY DESCRIBED MUTATIONS

Once the position of the mutation has been initially determined, databases containing previously mapped mouse mutations, such as the one maintained by The Jackson Laboratory (http://www.informatics.jax.org), should be consulted to determine if the new mutation maps close to a previously identified hearing-deficient mutation or otherwise potentially allelic mutation. From the preliminary analysis of the new mutation and its map position, it might become evident that this mutation

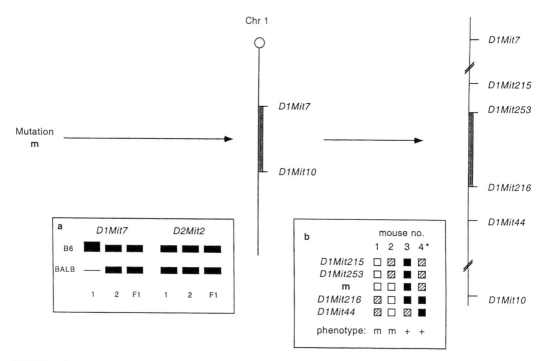

FIGURE 27.7 Pooling strategy for efficient genetic mapping of mutations and recombinant haplotype analysis for high-resolution mapping. Mutation m is mapped to mouse chromosome 1 within the shaded area using the pooling method shown in (a). The B6 runs above the BALB allele and pool 1, containing only mutant DNA, has a stronger B6 and reduced BALB band for *D1Mit7*. Pool 2 is unaffected DNAs and F1 is the heterozygous control. (b) illustrates the haplotype of four recombinant F2 DNAs with crossovers close to the mutation, m, thus refining the area covering the mutation. Open box represents homozygous B6; hatched box, heterozygous B6/CAST; black box, homozygous CAST. Phenotype: m is affected mouse; +, unaffected mouse. 4*, this F2 mouse was progeny-tested to determine its genotype at the mutation locus.

resembles a particular, previously identified mutant. More refined mapping of the new mutation with reference to markers used to map the previously identified mutation can sometimes eliminate the possibility of allelism by crossover exclusion.

For recessive mutations, functional allelism can be determined by testing for complementation by making direct crosses between mice carrying the two mutations. If mice inheriting mutant alleles from both mutations have a mutant phenotype (do not functionally complement), then the mutations are considered allelic (alterations of the same gene). If a mutant phenotype is not observed in these test crosses, then the two mutations are considered to be in different genes. For dominant mutations or semidominant mutations with homozygous lethality, allelism cannot be tested by functional complementation. In these cases, high-resolution genetic mapping can sometimes distinguish separate genes. If, however, the two dominant mutations cannot be separated by genetic recombination, then ultimate proof of allelism will depend on molecular gene identification.

As more mutations are found, the chances of a new mutation being a "remutation" increase. How do the phenotypes of the new and old mutants compare? Even if the new mutation turns out to be a remutation, subtle differences between the new and old mutants may make the new mutation interesting to pursue further. Furthermore, if the gene altered by the old mutation remains to be identified, the new allele will help in this endeavor, as described below. If the affected gene has been identified, the researcher must carefully weigh whether or not the new mutation is worthy of further study to find the actual gene defect in the new mutant. Characterization of different mutations of the same gene can sometimes provide insight into gene function; for example, multiple *Myo7a* gene mutations result in differing severity of the shaker-1 phenotype, corresponding to functional domains of the protein (Mburu et al., 1997). At the very least, DNA and RNA from the new mutant should be prepared and frozen for possible future studies.

IDENTIFYING CANDIDATE GENES

Once the new mutation has been shown to identify a new gene by its genetic map location and allelism tests (if needed), mouse and human gene databases should be consulted to determine potential candidate genes that are present within the same or homologous chromosomal location. Useful Internet Web sites include The Jackson Laboratory (http://www.informatics.jax.org), The Whitehead Institute (http://www.genome.wi.mit.edu), Baylor College of Medicine (www.hgsc.bcm.tmc.edu), and the National Center for Biotechnology Information (NCBI; http://www.ncbi.nlm.nih.gov). The NCBI Web site for Mouse Genome Resources (http://www.ncbi.nlm.nih.gov/genome/guide/M_musculus.html) includes sequence, mapping, and clone information. The NCBI Web site for Human/Mouse Homology Relationships (http://www3.ncbi.nlm.nih.gov/Homology/) is valuable for determining the human chromosomal region that corresponds to the map position of a new mouse mutation. This information allows the identification of human genes whose homologs may be potential candidate genes for a mouse mutation. To evaluate candidate genes on the basis of their expression profiles, reference should be made to the MRC Institute of Hearing Research Web site (http://www.ihr.mrc.ac.uk/hereditary/genetable/index.html), which lists known genes expressed in the developing ear in different animal species. The Morton fetal cochlear cDNA library Web site (http://hearing.bwh.harvard.edu/cochlearcdnalibrary.htm) facilitates identification of genes and expressed sequence tags (ESTs) that are expressed in the human cochlea. A gene showing RNA expression in the inner ear would be a strong candidate for a hearing-deficient mutation, but there are also many examples of ubiquitously expressed genes where, surprisingly, mutations in these genes affect only specific tissues, as in slow-wave epilepsy (swe) (Cox et al., 1997). Pursuing candidate genes at this stage, when the map position of the mutation has not been well refined, may be justified only for particularly compelling cases in which gene function and expression closely match expectations gleaned from the mutant phenotype.

POSTIONAL CLONING OF NEW MUTATIONS

REFINING THE GENETIC MAP POSITION OF THE MUTATION

Once a mutation is localized to a specific region of a chromosome, further fine-mapping requires a considerable extension of the mapping cross to allow production of a large number of progeny (often more than 1000). For both F2 and N2 linkage analysis, the selection of markers flanking the mutation is critical. It is important to use markers that are certain to encompass the site of the mutation and that can easily and reliably be typed by PCR, such as MIT microsatellite markers. All offspring are typed with the two flanking markers, and those with crossovers between these markers are further genotyped with intervening markers (Figure 27.7).

We favor the F2 route for mapping recessive mutations because each F2 mouse is the product of two meiotic events, whereas each N2 backcross mouse represents only one meiotic event. In some cases, deducing the genotypes of non-mutant recombinant F2 progeny requires progeny testing to distinguish between heterozygotes and +/+ mice (Figure 27.6 and genotype illustrated in Figure 27.7b, mouse no. 4). If the normal-appearing test mouse produces any affected progeny when mated with a known homozygous mutant (or heterozygote in cases where homozygous mice cannot breed), then the F2 mouse must carry the mutant allele. If inheritance of the mutation is dominant, the backcross approach becomes more informative.

As more mice are genotyped, the site of the mutation is progressively narrowed to an interval between two closely linked markers. Genetic distance is calculated in cM units (number of recombinants multiplied by 100, divided by the total number of meiotic events). For example, one recombinant between the mutation and the closest marker in a total of 500 F2 mice (each F2 mouse is the product of two meiotic events) represents $(1 \times 100) \div (500 \times 2) = 0.1$ cM, a physical distance of approximately 200 kilobases (kb). This estimate assumes that recombination is equally distributed throughout the entire mouse genome (~1500 cM; 3 million kb). Assuming that each gene is roughly 30 kb in size, this distance encompasses about six genes; however, actual gene density varies throughout the genome. How many F1 mating pairs need to be set up to produce 500 F2 mice? If ten mating pairs are set up, and each produces one litter of eight pups every five to six weeks, it will take approximately a year to reach this number. Therefore, fine mapping a mutation does require a commitment of both time and mouse room space.

Testing Candidate Genes

With the narrowing of the genetic interval, the few candidate genes remaining in this region can be more vigorously pursued. Many of the genes associated with spontaneous and induced mutations causing ear defects have been identified by testing previously mapped candidate genes, without having to resort to physical mapping efforts (e.g., the *Eya1*, *Sox10*, *Dst*, and *Krm1* mutations).

PCR primers are designed from DNA sequences of candidate genes to amplify probes for Northern and Southern blot analyses and to amplify DNA and cDNA from mutant and control mice. Northern blot and RT-PCR analyses are used to compare RNA differences between mutants and controls, such as absences or changes in message level or alterations in the size of message. Southern blots can reveal DNA changes, including restriction fragment length polymorphisms and gross deletions and insertions. For finer molecular analysis of the gene, single-strand conformation polymorphism (SSCP) analysis (Brady et al., 1997) comparing the mutant and wild-type PCR products of up to 400 bp can reveal more subtle rearrangements, such as single base changes. Improvements in DNA sequencing methods now make it feasible to sequence large clones for direct mutation identification.

Ultimately, the mutation is identifed as a change in DNA sequence that results in an altered protein product or a change in its regulation. Specifically, these genetic rearrangements may be as little as a single base change affecting one amino acid codon (missense mutation) or introducing a stop codon resulting in premature termination of the protein product (nonsense mutation). More radical changes include deletions, insertions, inversions, and splice site mutations. The kinds of mutations induced by chemical or radiation treatment can often be predicted; for example, N-ethyl-N-nitrosourea (ENU) mutagenesis most often generates single base changes to small deletions, whereas X-ray radiation often produces large deletions. In contrast, spontaneous mutations are not so restricted and can include the entire range of exonic and intronic rearrangements. Most spontaneous mouse mutations do not produce gross DNA rearrangements unless they are the result of insertional disruptions by endogenous retroviruses.

Constructing Physical Maps and Identifying New Genes

If all the previously mapped candidate genes in the refined genetic interval have been exhausted, a physical map of the region can be prepared to identify additional genes. At this stage, the interval encompassing the mutation should be as small as possible; a walk of over 2 megabases (approximately 1 cM) is a daunting prospect. The tools available for the physical map include the YAC, BAC, and P1 libraries. Essentially, each library consists of large mouse clones ligated to yeast or bacterial vectors for propagation as artificial chromosomes. The yeast artificial chromosome (YAC) libraries contain mouse genomic inserts of an average size from 600 to 800 kb (Haldi et al., 1996; Hamilton et al., 1996), whereas the bacterial BAC and P1 libraries have smaller mouse inserts of 130 to 200 kb and 90 kb, respectively (deJong et al., 1999; Francis et al., 1994; Korenberg et al., 1999). The second Whitehead YAC library has been screened with numerous MIT markers, and the coordinates of the YACs containing these loci are available from The Whitehead Institute Web site (www.genome.wi.mit.edu).

For large physical distances, the general approach is to assemble an array of YACs covering the interval. However, YACs frequently harbor rearrangements such as chimerisms and internal deletions; and, for the critical region of the mutation, coverage by BACs (or P1s) is preferential. The ends of the mouse DNA clones are sequenced to generate sequence tag sites (STSs) for selecting further overlapping clones and, if they are polymorphic between the parental strains of the linkage cross, can be used to orientate the physical with the genetic map.

The BAC or BACs encompassing the mutation can then be sequenced directly to identify all their genes, as was done to positionally clone the *dr* mutation (Millonig et al., 2000). Alternatively, exons can be selected using the exon-trapping procedure or cDNA selection. Exon-trapping was successfully used to find the *Myo6^{sv}* and *Myo7a^{sh1}* mutations (Avraham et al., 1995; Gibson et al., 1995), and direct cDNA selection was employed for the isolation of the *Slc9a^{swe}*, *Cacng2^{stg}*, and *tub* mutations (Cox et al., 1997; Letts et al., 1998; Noben-Trauth et al., 1996). For both methods, specifically selecting the 3′ exons is advantageous because many identified ESTs in the BLAST database (www.ncbi.nlm.nih.gov/BLAST) are 3′ clones of genes. The full length cDNA sequence, if not present in the database, is then retrieved by screening cDNA libraries or by 5′ RACE (rapid amplification of cDNA ends). The entire sequence is submitted for a BLAST search to determine the identity of the gene or to find related DNA species, and each gene is pursued using the approaches described above for candidate genes.

Proving Causality

The direct comparison of the genomic DNA between mutant and control, where it is clear that the mutant arose on an inbred strain background, provides very strong evidence that the causative defect has been found. Additional evidence may also be provided by the severity of the mutation, if the DNA alteration would be expected to abolish or alter gene function. If the parental strain of the mutant is unknown, surveying a number of inbred strains can provide some confidence to show the DNA change is restricted to the mutant. More definitive proof also comes from finding changes within the same gene in other allelic mutants, as exemplified in the *Myo7a* mutation analysis (Gibson et al., 1995). Finally, transgenics and knockouts can be constructed to complement or reproduce the mutant phenotype. For example, the correction of mutant phenotypes by the introduction of wild-type genes contained in large transgenic clones, as was done for the *Myo15* gene and the *sh2* phenotype (Probst et al., 1998), would provide functional proof of causality.

FUTURE DIRECTIONS

This final section discusses probable future directions that genetic studies of mouse mutations will take to identify genes and molecular pathways important in the hearing process. Looming foremost in the not-too-distant future is the expansion of large-scale mutagenesis programs that will produce many new deafness mutations. The development of improved genotyping methods will enable the rapid and efficient genetic mapping of these new mutations and their modifying genes. Completion of both the human and mouse genome sequencing programs will greatly aid candidate gene identification, thereby reducing the effort needed to positionally clone mutations. The future contributions of mouse models to human hearing impairment are further addressed in Chapter 26.

Mutagenesis Programs

With the emerging prominence of the mouse in biomedical research and the new genome initiatives now underway (Battey et al., 1999), the study of mouse mutations will undoubtedly play an increasingly important role in unraveling the genetic basis of hearing and deafness. Large-scale mutagenesis programs will produce large numbers of mouse mutations with hearing deficits. The incidence of mutation can be greatly increased by treating mice with chemical mutagens. An optimal dose of N-ethyl-N-nitrosourea (ENU) generates a frequency of 1.5×10^{-3} mutations per locus (Russell and Russell, 1992) and thus makes screening for individual mice with specific defects more approachable, rather than picking the rare spontaneous mutant from a large breeding colony (Brown and Nolan, 1998). The high frequency of ENU-induced mutations allows for sensitive screening methods to identify subtle phenotypes that would not be feasible for spontaneous mutations. This phenotype-driven approach can generate mouse models for many human deafness traits that are not presently available. For example, mutagenized mice could be screened to identify models for non-syndromic deafness, completely devoid of associated non-auditory phenotypes.

Two major mouse mutagenesis programs have been established in Europe (in Neuherberg, Germany, and in Harwell, U.K.), both using ENU as a mutagen (Hunter et al., 2000). Male mice are injected intraperitoneally with ENU, allowed several weeks to recover their fertility, and then mated to normal females. The F1 offspring from these matings are examined for new dominant mutations. A simple hand-held auditory clickbox has been used for the primary screen to test mice for a startle response to a calibrated sound burst. Selected mice are then further characterized physiologically and anatomically for auditory deficits. In the United States, several funded mutagenesis programs are part of the Trans-NIH Mouse Initiative (http://www.nih.gov/science/models/mouse/). Strategies have been described for both whole-genome and targeted chromosomal regions, for the identification of both dominant and recessive mutations, for the use of different chemical mutagens and treatment regimes, and for the use of embryonic stem cells as well as spermatogonia (Munroe et al., 2000; Schimenti and Bucan, 1998).

IMPROVEMENTS IN METHODS FOR GENETIC ANALYSIS

Genetic mapping of these newly generated mutations will be aided by increases in the number of available genetic markers, such as single nucleotide polymorphisms (SNPs), and improvements in high-throughput genotyping efficiency, such as multiplexing reactions, high-density oligonucleotide arrays, and fluorescent detection (Lindblad-Toh et al., 2000; Sapolsky et al., 1999). Positional cloning of new mutations will be simplified by access to the completed DNA sequences of the human and mouse genomes. Candidate genes and potential human homologs will be readily identified by computer searches of these large databases. When all genes have been identified and mapped, the positional cloning approach will become a matter of genetically mapping the mutant phenotype to high resolution followed by molecular screening of candidate genes for causative mutations. Physical mapping efforts will no longer be required to identify candidate genes. Improved DNA sequencing and mutation-screening methods will simplify the molecular evaluation of candidate genes.

IDENTIFICATION OF MODIFYING GENES

A powerful approach to studying the function of a gene is to identify other loci that interact to modify the phenotype. The search for disease loci can be complemented by the search for such modifying loci. Identification of modifying loci can provide access to other genes/proteins in the disease pathway that may provide useful targets for therapeutic intervention. There are many instances of human and mouse genetic diseases that exhibit variable expressivity (when a given genotype exhibits a range of phenotypes) or incomplete penetrance (when some individuals inheriting a predisposing genotype do not manifest the trait). Many factors affect the phenotypic expression of a genetic disease. Environment (diet, infections, toxins, noise exposure), epigenetic factors (imprinting, somatic mutations, mitochondria), genetic background, and allelic heterogeneity can contribute to phenotypic variability. Mouse genetics provides means to distinguish among these alternative causes, which often cannot be distinguished in human genetic diseases.

Mice represent an attractive model system for the identification and characterization of modifying loci. The existence of inbred strains permits the generation of progeny in which the parental origin of alleles is defined. The great variety of inbred strains provides an increased likelihood of finding genetic differences in modifying genes. The development of dense genetic maps of highly polymorphic and easily typable genetic markers and computer programs for correlating genotype distribution with quantitative trait data has made the genetic localization of modifying loci feasible. Map positions for homologous human loci can be identified and tested for their potential modifying effects on human diseases.

Genetic background can have a profound effect on mouse mutations that affect hearing. Model systems have been described for two mouse mutations that affect hearing and that are influenced by modifying genes: the deaf waddler (*dfw*) — modifier of deaf waddler (*mdfw*) system (Noben-Trauth et al., 1997); and the tubby (*tub*) — modifier of tubby hearing (*moth*) system (Ikeda et al., 1999). Both of these systems represent examples of digenic epistasis, where the interaction of the two genes is not simply the sum of the individual gene effects. The *mdfw* and *moth* loci are examples of modifiers with large effects, but nearly all mutations are modified to some degree by strain background effects.

In future efforts to identify gene interactions and molecular pathways important to the hearing process, it will become practical to cross mutant mice with multiple inbred strains and efficiently screen for modifying genes that contribute to the phenotypic variability of mutant progeny. Individual modifying genes can then be isolated by rapid construction of congenic lines (Markel et al., 1997; Visscher, 1999; Wakeland et al., 1997), so that gene interactions can be evaluated and high-resolution map positions can be made in prelude to the positional cloning of the modifying genes.

28 Inbred Strains of Mice for Genetics of Hearing in Mammals: Searching for Genes for Hearing Loss

L.C. Erway, Q.Y. Zheng, and K.R. Johnson

INTRODUCTION

Early geneticists foresaw that mice could provide a useful model for the study of mammalian genetics. They generally started with "fancy" strains of mice available in pet stores. From 3 months of age, mice can generally produce litters of six or more pups in successive months; this is due to the short (18 to 21 days) gestation and possibility of post-partum matings. All of the early derived strains of mice were presumed to be from random matings, thus providing maximal genetic variability in the original populations. Selection of a few progenitors for any laboratory population progressively limited genetic variability within that breed or strain. Mouse geneticists have from the beginning deliberately inbred the stocks of mice, typically by brother-sister matings, maintained and pedigreed over successive generations. Given 20 consecutive generations of brother-sister matings, such an inbred strain is considered to be homozygous at virtually all of the estimated 30,000 genetic loci. Given such degree of inbreeding, all concurrent mice within each inbred strain are virtually as genetically identical as identical twins derived from the same zygote. Nearly 500 inbred strains of mice have been produced and listed. It is important to note, however, that inbreeding to genetic homozygosity for all genetic loci does not eliminate phenotypic variability. In fact, genetic homozygosity may make individuals more susceptible to certain environmental factors.

Surviving inbred strains of mice have obviously escaped early death, infertility, and most debilitating disorders. Laboratory conditions with cages, food, and care hardly resemble natural conditions to which mice were originally adapted in their natural habitats. The common laboratory mice, *Mus musculus domesticus*, mixed with *M. m. musculus*, were originally derived from some stocks naturally adapted to agrarian environment about the farm and home. In nature, genetic variability, not uniformity as produced by inbreeding, is the norm for well-adapted animal species. However, agricultural geneticists learned that despite the very many and undesirable traits of inbred strains, hybrid crosses between specific inbred strains actually produce the most uniform and desirable qualities in those plants and animals. The axiom is that hybrid vigor increases productivity and resistance to adverse conditions. Such F1 hybrid strains are reproduced in each generation from deliberate crosses among many inbred strains selected and proven for producing the most highly valued characters. All mice within the same F1 hybrid strain are also genetically homogeneous, that is, homozygous for many loci (e.g., AA; bb; CC) and heterozygous (Xx; Yy; Zz) for many other loci. Extensive heterozygosity at various loci contributes most to hybrid vigor (e.g., see discussion of noise-induced hearing loss below).

IMPORTANT EFFECTS OF INBRED STRAIN BACKGROUND

One way that geneticists can identify genes that may contribute to normal hearing is to identify mutant genes that impair hearing. In doing so, however, the genetic background of the mice must be taken into account. For example, a variety of hearing-impaired transgenic mice can be produced, as discussed in detail in Chapter 30. The basic technique for making transgenic mice, by means of embryonic stem cells, has been done with cells derived from the 129 substrains. Yet, some of these strains appear to possess a major gene on chromosome 10 that contributes to early hearing impairment, and this gene is expected to be segregating among progeny derived for a particular transgene. One must be aware of these possibilities before attributing differences in hearing to a particular transgene of interest. Furthermore, any two different inbred strains involved in producing and selecting for the transgenic genotypes will segregate for innumerable background genotypes. The only practical solution to this problem is to genetically backcross the transgene onto an acceptable, well-hearing inbred strain. This requires ten successive backcross generations to effectively make the transgene congenic on that particular inbred strain. The CBA/CaJ inbred strain is a recommended, well-hearing strain for making such congenic strains. An alternative may be the congenic B6.CAST^{+Ahl} without age-related hearing loss. The C57BL/6J and 19 other inbred strains with early hearing loss (Q.Y. Zheng et al., 1999b) are not recommended for producing strains congenic for any transgenes with potential effects on hearing.

FIRST GENETIC EVIDENCE FOR AGE-RELATED HEARING LOSS (AHL) AMONG FIVE INBRED STRAINS OF MICE

AHL has been identified in several inbred mouse strains (Henry, 1982a; Henry and Chole, 1980; Hunter and Willott, 1987; Li and Borg, 1991; Mikaelian, 1979; Parham and Willott, 1988; Willott et al., 1984; 1987). However, few genetic studies have been undertaken to determine its inheritance and to map responsible genes. In a study of genetic variability, dietary restriction, and longevity, Harrison and Archer (1983) chose five inbred strains of mice with a presumed greatest amount of genetic variability among those strains: CBA/H-T6J, C57BL/6J (B6), DBA/2J (D2), BALB/cByJ, and WB/ReJ. All ten F1 hybrid strains were included for genetic comparisons. Whereas the five inbred strains were originally selected without any knowledge regarding their hearing ability, the choice proved fortuitous when an AHL component was added to the study (Erway, Willott, Archer, and Harrison, 1993a). On the basis of auditory brainstem response (ABR) threshold testing at approximately 1, 2, and 3 years of age, the following conclusions were deduced: (1) the CBA/H-T6J mice exhibited essentially normal hearing throughout their life; (2) the D2 mice were deaf long before 1 year, as known from other studies; (3) the three other inbred strains exhibited AHL by 2 to 3 years of age; (4) all four F1 hybrids with the CBA strain exhibited the lowest normal ABR thresholds throughout their lifetime, which indicated that any gene(s) for AHL among these four strains were recessive to the CBA-wild-type gene(s). Being significantly lower than the CBA mice also suggested hybrid vigor; and (5) all three of the F1 hybrids with D2, exhibiting extensive AHL, indicated a common gene for hearing loss among these four strains.

The results were interpreted to indicate a major gene common to seven F1 strains [see (4) and (5)]. Nearly normal thresholds among the three F1 hybrid combinations of B6, BALB/cByJ, and WB/ReJ (parental strains that exhibit hearing loss) suggested the possibility of gene complementation among three different genes for AHL among these strains. However, the possibility cannot be ruled out that the observed differences for AHL among these three F1 strains may be attributable to a second locus.

RECOMBINANT INBRED STRAINS OF MICE

Several series of recombinant inbred strains have been produced. For example, Benjamin Taylor at The Jackson Laboratory crossed the C57BL/6J strain to the DBA/2J strain, thus producing F1 hybrids. Those F1 mice were mated among siblings, producing an effective F2 generation. With each successive generation of inbreeding among siblings, 25 or more recombinant inbred strains were established, all having been derived from the original F1 hybrid. From that first F1 generation, random recombinations occurred between different regions of the 20 pairs of chromosomes. The recombinant inbred strains between C57BL/6J and DBA/2J are designated BXD-1 to BXD-32, of which 26 are extant (see Chapter 29 for a discussion of the use of BXD strains in auditory behavioral genetics research).

Because hearing had been studied extensively in the B6 and D2 inbred strains, Willott and Erway (1998) evaluated ABR thresholds and cochlear pathology in the BXD strains. The parental D2 strain of mice loses hearing rapidly during the second month of life, whereas B6 has a more gradual loss beginning at about 2 months of age. It was not known at the time the study was done that C57BL/6J and DBA/2J have the same gene for AHL, so that all BXD strains would exhibit some degree of hearing loss (e.g., all are homozygous for the gene causing AHL). The severity ranged from being even worse than D2 to severity similar to B6. Seven more recently developed BXD strains of mice (Taylor et al., 1999) were screened for ABR thresholds at the Jackson Laboratory, and all of these BXD strains exhibited significant hearing loss as well (K.R. Johnson, unpublished data).

SPONTANEOUS MUTATIONS AMONG INBRED STRAINS AND GENETIC SEGREGATION FOR HEARING LOSS

Many spontaneous mutations have occurred within inbred strains (see Chapter 27), and genetic segregation has been the principal phenomenon for identifying and mapping genes to chromosomes. For example, in 1984, Dr. Priscilla Lane at The Jackson Laboratory observed a new mutant (nm808) within the C3H/HeJ inbred strain. These mice exhibited much circling behavior and head-shaking, and they were deaf. This mutant was named deaf-wadler (*dfw*), now known to code for the PMCA2 ATPase2 enzyme. The effects in the *dfw/dfw* mice could be readily identified by their behavior and complete deafness. Thereby, Lane collected 205 backcross progeny, of which 108 were normal (+/*dfw*) and 97 were circling and deaf (*dfw/dfw*). Such data were obviously not different from the expected 1:1 ratio. Furthermore, before chromosomal mapping was possible, Lane (1987) also published the linkage group: *Hd* 14 +/–2 cM *Mi^{wh}* 7+/–1 cM *dfw* (now part of chromosome 6).

Another new mutant (nm2187) was observed at TJL in 1996 with head-shaking and deafness. It was identified as allelic to *dfw*, and therefore a recurrent mutation designated *dwf*[2J] (Noben-Trauth et al., 1997). The original *dfw* gene has been cloned (Street et al., 1998), and it codes for the plasma membrane Ca^{2+}-ATPase2 enzyme (PMCA2). Kozel et al. (1998) have shown that mice homozygous for the disrupted PMCA2–/– transgene are deaf and exhibit extreme vestibular dysfunctions. The heterozygous PMCA2+/– transgenic mice exhibit hearing loss, depending on the strain background.

SEGREGATION FOR AHL GENE(S) FROM C57BL/6J AND DBA/2J PROGENIES

D2 mice exhibit very early onset hearing loss (severely impaired by 3 to 4 months of age); B6 mice exhibit later, slower onset AHL (beginning after 2 months); and CBA/J and CAST/Ei hear normally. Erway, Willott, Cook, Johnson, and Davisson (1993) made four crosses that exhibited segregation of progeny with normal vs. AHL. (1) CBA/J x C57BL/6J F2 progeny exhibited 9/41 (~¼) with AHL by 2 years; (2) CAST/Ei x B6-F1 backcrossed to B6 exhibited 22/47 (~½) AHL by 1 year; (3) CBA/J x DBA/2J F2 progeny exhibited 4/50 (~1/16) AHL by 4 months; (4) CBA/J x DBA/2J F1 backcrossed to DBA/2J exhibited 15/62 (~¼) AHL by 4 months. These results were consistent with one gene from the B6 strain segregating for AHL, among the F2 progeny (1) and among the backcross progeny (2). The earlier onset AHL among the D2 mice suggests possibility of two segregating genes: the observed $1/16$ of AHL F2 progeny (3) and $1/4$ AHL of backcross progeny (4) are consistent with segregation for two genes for AHL.

SEGREGATION FOR EARLY-ONSET OF HEARING LOSS AMONG 129XCAST/EI-F1-BACKCROSS PROGENY

As indicated earlier, the "129" designated inbred substrains of mice exhibit an early onset hearing loss. The 129/ReJ mice were outcrossed to the normally hearing CAST/Ei inbred mice, a subspecies for which thousands of Mit markers useful for mapping genes are known. There is no evidence that the CAST/Ei mice possess any genes contributing to AHL. Rather certainly, these mice would possess the wild-type alleles for any mutant gene(s) ascribed to the B6 and D2 inbred strains. CAST/Ei mice were crossed to the 129/ReJ mice, and those F1 hybrids were backcrossed to the 129/ReJ mice. The backcross mice were tested for segregation for the gene(s) that may contribute to the early onset hearing loss. By 2 months of age, many of the backcross mice exhibited very much elevated ABR thresholds of 80 to 100 dB. Out of 150 backcross mice tested, 54 (0.35) of the mice exhibited early-onset and profound hearing loss. The observed frequency is significantly less than would be expected (0.50) for equal segregation of one gene. The observed 0.35 frequency is also significantly more frequent than would be expected for independent assortment of two genes (0.25) contributing to such hearing loss. Alternatively, if two different genes were linked on the same chromosome and undergo 10 to 15% crossingover, that could explain these observed findings. Both of these deviations are significantly different by Chi-square test ($p < 0.005$). These unpublished results were obtained in collaboration with Q.Y. Zheng and K.R. Johnson at The Jackson Laboratory.

These preliminary attempts to detect segregation of a gene(s) for hearing loss illustrate the difficulties in detecting any clear-cut segregation for this complex trait with variable onset of hearing loss. More strains, more mice and additional methods were required for mapping any gene for age-related hearing loss.

MAPPING FIRST GENE FOR AGE-RELATED HEARING LOSS IN C57BL/6J MICE

Having obtained genetic evidence for AHL in B6 mice, K.R. Johnson et al. (1997) set up a CAST/Ei X C57BL/6J F1 hybrid backcrossed to C57BL/6J. This would afford possible detection of a gene for AHL, expecting $1/2$ heterozygous and $1/2$ homozygous genotypes among the backcross progeny. The very well-hearing CAST/Ei mice provided unlimited Mit markers across the mouse genome for mapping such a gene, if some bimodal distribution could be detected for normal vs. AHL mice among a small sample of 38 backcross mice. With onset of hearing loss from 10 to 18 months of age, a putative gene for Age-related Hearing Loss (*Ahl*) was mapped to the proximal end of chromosome 10, in proximity of D10Mit5/31 (K.R. Johnson et al., 1997).

PROVING THAT THE *AHL* REGION OF CHROMOSOME 10 AFFECTS AHL

When any new mutation has occurred within an inbred strain, that new mutation is assumed to be coisogenic with the wild-type allele already present in that inbred strain. To incorporate any gene from one strain into another strain requires at least ten generations of pedigreed backcrosses of the mutant gene, or region of chromosome, into the parent strain of interest. Thus, Johnson, Erway, Cook, Willott, and Zheng (1997) transferred the wild-type allele for AHL (*+Ahl*) (from the CAST/Ei strain) into the standard C57BL/6J strain of mice. Given the available Mit markers flanking *Ahl* on chromosome 10, that region of chromosome 10 was successively backcrossed for ten generations.

That congenic strain is designated B6.CAST^{+Ahl} and is available at The Jackson Laboratory. It is recommended as a control strain for comparison with any studies of hearing loss in the standard C57BL/6J mice or other inbred strains with this fairly common *Ahl* gene. Vazquez et al. (2000) have provided preliminary evidence that the B6.CAST^{+Ahl} mice homozygous for the +*Ahl* allele are more resistant to NIHL than are the standard B6-*Ahl/Ahl* mice.

SCREENING INBRED STRAINS OF MICE FOR EARLY ONSET HEARING IMPAIRMENT

By 1995, genetic studies of families had revealed the existence of some 45 different forms of non-syndromic hearing impairment among human populations. This was a great incentive for searching for genetic models among the inbred strains of mice. NIH funded such a project at The Jackson Laboratory, with its repository of inbred and mutant strains of mice. The procedure was to screen as many inbred strains of mice as possible by means of ABR thresholds, for at least five mice of each strain, over the first 3 months of age. This provided the possibility of detecting an early-onset hearing impairment in mice. All screened mice were tested at three or more ages for ABR thresholds for clicks and for pips (3-ms duration) at 8, 16, and 32 kHz. Given previous studies, cohorts of five to eight CBA/CaJ mice were repeatedly tested from 9 to 47 weeks of age as a standard for normal ABR thresholds. Each cohort was remarkably consistent over these tests with the following mean thresholds: clicks, 36 dB; 8 kHz, 24 dB; 6 kHz, 15 dB; 32 kHz, 39 dB, with a standard deviation of 3 to 5 (equivalent to error of judgment for threshold in 5-dB steps). Results for a number of strains are summarized in Tables 28.1, 28.2, and 28.3 and by (Q.Y. Zheng et al.,1999a,b).

Shown in Table 28.1 are 39 inbred strains exhibiting normal hearing when tested from 16 to 61 weeks of age. The grand means for ABR thresholds were: Clicks, 38 dB; 8 kHz 29 dB; 16 kHz, 18 dB; 32 kHz, 44dB, similar to CBA/CaJ. These means were used as criteria for judging whether other strains had significantly elevated ABR thresholds. Hearing loss was operationally defined as ABR thresholds equal to or greater than: clicks: 55 dB (+17); 8 kHz, 40 dB (+11); 16 kHz, 35 dB (+17); 32 kHz, 60 dB (+16).

TABLE 28.1
Normal Hearing Inbred Strains to Advanced Weeks of Age (Typically Tested as Retired Breeders)

A/HeJ	27	MOLF/Ei	28
AKR/J	26	MOLG/Dn	31
BALB/cBy J	34	NON/LtJ	29
BALB/cJ	34	NZB/B1NJ	18
BXSB/MpJ	34	NZO/NIJ	22
C3H/HeJ	21	PERA/camEi	45
C3HeB/FeJ	32	PL/J	30
C3H/HeOuJ	41	RBA/Dn	24
C57BL/10J	32	RBA/DnJ	27
C57BL/10SnJ	32	SENCARC/PtJ	43
CASA/RK	41	SF/CamEi	32
CAST/Ei	61	SHR/GnEi	22
CBA/J	28	SLJ/J	49
FVB/NJ	28	SM/J	58
HRS/J-hr/+	26	SPRET/Ei	19
MOLD/Rk	37	ST/bJ	30
		SWR/J	27

TABLE 28.2
Inbred Strains of Mice with Hearing
Impairment by 13 weeks of age[a]

	Stimuli:	Click	8K	16K	32K
Criteria (dB elevation):		55	40	35	60
Strain	Age (wks)				
129/J	9	52	*47*	33	69
129/J	13	*59*	*49*	*42*	*72*
129/ReJ	9	52	*45*	33	62
129/ReJ	12	*62*	*54*	*37*	*73*
129/SvJ	9	53	*55*	*41*	*68*
A/J	13	54	38	70	56
ALR/LtJ	26	*117*	*104*	*99*	*119*
ALS/LtJ	9	*60*	*55*	*55*	*70*
BUB/BnJ	3	*93*	*69*	*60*	*74*
BUB/BnJ	8	*102*	*83*	*79*	101
C57BLKS/J[a]	11	46	*41*	*36*	*61*
C57BR/cdJ[a]	7	48	48	23	*61*
C57L/J[a]	9	*69*	*73*	*47*	*83*
C57L/J	14	*85*	*77*	*53*	*93*
DBA/2J	5	*61*	*44*	*51*	*67*
DBA/2J	14	*68*	*52*	*60*	*72*
I/Ln/J	12	49	48	27	59
MA/MyJ	13	45	31	*52*	59
NOD.NON[b]	11	*64*	*66*	*79*	*88*
NOD/LtJ	3	*59*	*46*	*64*	*78*
NOD/LtJ	9	*83*	*86*	*88*	109
NOR/LtJ	9	*85*	*74*	*81*	100
SKH2/J-hr	10	*89*	*67*	*69*	*90*

[a] These three C57 strains share ancestry with C57BL/6J with later-onset hearing loss.
[b] Three congenic strains.

Using these criteria, a number of inbred strains, shown in Table 28.2, exhibited elevated thresholds by 13 weeks of age. Most of these strains were tested before, at, and after 13 weeks of age. For Table 28.2, the youngest age with significantly elevated ABR thresholds are shown as well as at 13 or older ages (thresholds significantly above normal are italicized). These may be viewed as strains of mice with early-onset hearing loss.

Among the inbred strains that were screened, 15 had normal hearing at 13 weeks of age; but between 19 weeks (~5 months) to 60 weeks of age, significant hearing loss emerged. These are shown in Table 28.3. The later onset of hearing loss in these strains suggests that they may be models for adult-onset hearing loss and/or presbycusis.

HOW MANY GENES CONTRIBUTE TO EARLY HEARING LOSS IN THESE INBRED INBRED STRAINS?

The standard test for allelism is to cross any two strains of mice that exhibit a similar phenotype, in this case the elevated ABR thresholds among strains exhibiting hearing loss (Table 28.1). To make

---

TABLE 28.3
Inbred Strains with Later Hearing
Loss after 19 Weeks of Age

Strain	Age Tested (weeks)[a]
129/SvEMS	35
A/WySnJ	34
C3H/HeSnJ	45
C58/J	30
CE/J	50
bDBA/1J	48
bDBA/1LacJ	33
KK/H1J	50
LG/J	48
LP/J	31, 49
MRL/MpJ	30
P/J	19
SENCARA/PtJ	44
SENCARB/PtJ	39
YBR/Ei	60

[a] Ages at which these mice happened to be available for testing. bDBA/1 strains shared ancestry with DBA/2 strains with very early hearing loss. No attempts have been made to identify the genetic bases for the later onset of hearing impairment in these inbred strains.

---

all possible reciprocal crosses would be impossible, but a few crosses were informative. If any two inbred strains with early hearing loss are crossed, producing F1 hybrids without hearing loss, then one can conclude that the two inbred strains do not possess the same mutant gene for hearing loss. They each presumably possess different genes for hearing loss, and the F1 hybrid is therefore heterozygous for two different genes, +/a; +/b. This is referred to as genetic complementation.

Reciprocal crosses (male vs. female of the two strains) between the DBA/2J and 129/ReJ did exhibit complementation; the progeny all exhibited normal ABR thresholds when tested to 31 weeks of age. Therefore, DBA/2J and 129/ReJ mice would appear to possess two different genes for hearing loss. The DBA/2J x A/J F1s appeared to complement to 14 weeks of age, but they did not complement to 29 weeks of age. The C57BR/cdJ and C57L/J strains crossed to the NOD.NON strains appear to complement to 13 weeks of age, but they were not tested at later ages. Four other crosses, including the NOD.NON strains to DBA/2J and to ALR/LtJ, do not exhibit any complementation from 13 to 31 weeks of age; this suggests that they both possess the same allele or different alleles for AHL. The genetic basis for these differences in onset of hearing loss depends on ultimately mapping any other genes which contribute to these differences.

SEGREGATION FOR EARLY-ONSET HEARING LOSS AMONG NINE BACKCROSS PROGENIES

Mapping genes for discrete phenotypes is relatively easy when the phenotypes occur in fixed ratios: for example, 3:1 among F2, or 1:1 among backcross (N2) progenies. Many phenotypes approach measurable, quantitative traits, as is the case for ABR thresholds. The earliest age of onset is one significant criterion, and those mice that have high ABR thresholds vs. those that do not, provides what approaches a qualitative segregation among N2 progeny of the backcross generation. The use of actual quantitative ABR threshold per mouse also affords a powerful statistical method by the so-called Quantitative Trait Loci (QTL), discussed in detail in Chapter 29. Both of these methods have been accomplished for the N2 backcross progeny from ten inbred strains. This was done first by mapping the *Ahl* gene in the C57BL/6J strain with only 38 N2 progeny, as presented above.

Nine of the 19 inbred strains with early-onset hearing loss were selected for mapping *Ahl* and/or any other contributing genetic factor(s). Crosses were made between the normal-hearing CAST/Ei (source of different microsatellite markers) and each of nine strains with early-onset hearing loss. Nine different sets of F1 hybrid mice were potentially heterozygous (e.g., +/*Ahl*). Each F1 hybrid was backcrossed to the parental strain with hearing loss, thus producing (N2) progeny with potentially normal ABR and with early onset hearing loss. (This same procedure allowed for the detection and mapping of one, two, or more genetic factors. As with all genetic crosses, the larger the number of N2 progeny, the more useful the results.) For each of the selected nine strains, 64 to 270 N2 progeny (a total of 1192) mice were tested and mapped.

All mice of each strain of N2 progenies were tested for ABR thresholds at approximately 1 to 6 months of age, with an attempt to distinguish the differences in age of onset and severity of hearing loss among these different N2 progenies. There were subtle differences among the nine N2 progenies. Nevertheless, all nine N2 progenies exhibited essentially normal hearing when young, but developed elevated ABR thresholds with increasing ages to about 6 months. Only the original C57BL/6J mice and the BALB/cByJ strain of mice included in this study exhibited later-onset hearing loss from 10 to 18 months of age. Regardless of these differences in the onset of hearing loss among these ten inbred strains, there is no evidence for other gene(s) contributing to these differences, because all of these strains clearly exhibited segregation for the *Ahl* allele.

The final genetic analysis conducted on the N2 progenies for ten inbred strains was the QTL analysis using all of the ABR thresholds obtained for each mouse as the measured parameter at each tested age. Based on the QTL analysis, each of these ten strains exhibited LOD (log of odds) scores of 4.7 for smallest sample size (64) to 72 for the largest sample (272). The original 38 N2 progeny for C57BL/6J had LOD scores of 13. All significant LOD scores are statistical probabilities that a major factor (supposed *Ahl* gene) may be located within a few centiMorgans (cM) of the known unique microsatellite markers along every chromosome.

A MAJOR GENETIC FACTOR FOR AHL AMONG TEN INBRED STRAINS OF MICE

K.R. Johnson et al. (1997) first demonstrated segregation of a gene for AHL among 38 backcross mice derived from the CAST/Ei x C57BL/6J cross. That *Ahl* gene affected a late-onset AHL about 18 months of age. We have demonstrated that some 19 other inbred strains of mice exhibit an early-onset AHL, as early as 2 months of age. To better define the genetics of early- vs. late-onset AHL, nine inbred strains of mice with early-onset AHL were selected for segregation and linkage analyses.

Each of the selected nine strains was out-crossed to the very normal-hearing CAST/Ei strain. Each of the nine F1 hybrid strains heard normally to advanced ages beyond when the parent AHL strain exhibited early-onset AHL. Each of the F1 hybrids was backcrossed to the parent strain characterized for early-onset AHL. Each of the backcross progenies (N2 generation) was tested at two or three ages to bracket the onset of AHL. Such N2 progenies would be expected to segregate +/*Ahl* (normal hearing) and *Ahl*/*Ahl* (early-onset AHL), if one major gene contributes to the early-onset AHL. However, if two genes contributed to AHL, then the N2 progenies might exhibit four categories, for example, (A_;B_: A_;bb: aa;B_: aa;bb), possibly with four different phenotype groups. However, the related AHL phenotypes for onset and severity of AHL could likely approximate a continuous or quantitative distribution.

Over a thousand backcross mice were produced and analyzed for the onset and severity of AHL. They were subsequently mapped for any potentially contributing gene(s) for early- to later-onset AHL. The results of this comprehensive study of AHL among these ten inbred strains (Johnson et al., 2000) indicate that of the nine strains with early-onset AHL yielded N2 progenies segregated for normal hearing (+/Ahl) vs. early-onset AHL (Ahl/Ahl). There were characteristic shifts in the age of onset of AHL among the different N2 progenies, reflecting the differences among the parental AHL strains. However, with increasing age of the N2 progenies, the segregation ratios approached the expected (normal hearing (+/Ahl) and with early-onset AHL (Ahl/Ahl). This general 1:1 segregation among each of the nine backcross progenies was tantamount to the segregation and expression of one gene (Ahl), as reported for the original 38 N2 progeny for the late-onset AHL from the C57BL/6J strain of mice.

Segregation for abstract genes does not by itself establish one vs. two or more different gene(s) contributing to AHL among the numerous inbred strains. Statistical analyses for variance of any measured quantitative traits have been used extensively for decades to identify heritable genetic contributions to measured traits in plants and animals. Comparisons of the analyses of variance among parental stocks, F1 hybrids, F2, and the N2 progenies help to distinguish between environmental vs. genetic factors for heritability of the measured trait(s). Such analyses of variances were done for the measured ABR thresholds in all mice within each of the above crosses. The analyses of variance among six strains with the earliest onset AHL yielded statistical heritabilities determined at 3 months of age (0.60 to 0.85), and the same analyses were (0.86 to 0.98) at 6 months of age. Such heritabilities (~1.0) are astronomically high compared to any standard quantitative traits. These statistical analyses effectively prove that a single, major genetic factor contributes most to AHL. It appears that an yet unknown "aging factor" moves the onset and severity of AHL toward deafness, but only among homozygotes (Ahl/Ahl).

Is there only one and the same mutant gene (Ahl), or are there different alleles among these ten strains (including CBA/CaJ, with late-onset AHL)? Ultimately, all genes must be mapped to their respective chromosomes. This is essential for eventually identifying the gene(s). Each of the nine N2 progenies was derived from the CAST/Ei x AHL strain, thus affording thousands of microsatelitte markers for mapping purposes. The late-onset AHL among the CAST/Ei x C57BL/6J N2 mice was mapped to chromosome 10 by this method. Each of the nine strains with early onset AHL was thus mapped for the Ahl-region on Chromosome 10.

Analyses QTL yield LOD scores such that LOD scores $\geq$ 3 are relatively equal to p values $\leq$ 0.001). The LOD scores reported for two strains with late-onset AHL and for eight strains with early-onset AHL ranged from LOD = 5 to 19 (six strains) and LOD = 29 to 72 (four strains). Those are astronomical probabilities for an Ahl gene being located near two markers (D10Mit130/299) on chromosome 10.

All nine strains with the early-onset AHL, plus C57BL/6J and BALB/cJ with late-onset AHL, appear to possess the same gene on chromosome 10, with either the same or different mutant allele(s). Different alleles of the D10Mit markers (varying for number of nucleotides) map in proximity to the Ahl gene: there is a dichotomy for the linked Mit alleles between four normally hearing strains vs. all ten of the AHL strains as shown in Table 28.4.

It is virtually certain that a gene for AHL is located on chromosome 10 in the region of the D10Mit299 marker. There is a complete dichotomy for the D10Mit299-185 allele in the four well-hearing strains vs. the 188 allele in the ten AHL strains. This dichotomy is consistent with close linkage between Ahl and D10Mit299. This suggests the possibility of one ancestral origin of the Ahl mutant allele. The D10Mit130 allele shows a similar dichotomy, albeit with two exceptions (*): these could be due to greater distance for crossingover between the Ahl gene and the D10Mit130. (Note that BUB mice with AHL have the same 158 allele as the normally hearing mice).

What contributes to the difference in onset of AHL? To approach this question, an F1 hybrid was produced between the NOD/LtJ strain with earliest-onset AHL and the C57BL/6J strain with

TABLE 28.4
Linkage Dichotomy Between *Ahl* and *D10Mit* Alleles Regarding:

	cM	CAST	C3H	AKR	NON	CBA				
				Normal Hearing Strains						
D10Mit130	24	170	158	158	158	158				
D10Mit299	24	192	185	185	185	185				

	cM	129	A/J	B6	DBA	BR	BALB	SKH	760	NOD	BUB
				Hearing-Impaired Strains							
D10Mit130	24	150	150	150	150	150	150	150	150	*154	*158
D10Mit299	24	188	188	188	188	188	188	188	188	188	188

late-onset AHL (~18 months). Those F1 hybrids were used to produce F2 progeny and N2 progeny for QTL analyses for linkages with different gene(s) for onset of AHL. No other genes were indicated from these crosses. Based on this long series of crosses and repeated tests for AHL in over a thousand mice, we must conclude that a "gene," yet without any known molecular function, must contribute to an extensive and varied onset AHL among these strains of mice. (Ten additional strains of mice were identified with early-onset AHL, but have not been mapped for *Ahl*.)

There are several homologies between mutant genes for hearing loss in mice and their syndromic mutations in humans. We suggest that the non-syndromic *Ahl* for AHL in mice may be a candidate for its homolog in humans that could contribute to the presbycusis (AHL) in the human population.

GENETIC AND NOISE-INDUCED INTERACTIONS FOR HEARING LOSS IN MICE

Erway et al. (1996) showed that two inbred strains of mice (CBA/CaJ and C57BL/6J) and two F1-hybrid strains of mice (CBxB6 and B6xD2) differed for susceptibility to hearing loss after noise exposure at 110 SPL dB for 1 hour. These differences were consistent with a major gene affecting NIHL. By contrast, the (CBAxB6)F1-progeny backcrossed to the B6 inbred strain, required an 8-hour exposure at 110 dB SPL to exhibit hearing loss comparable to that of the susceptible inbred and F1 hybrid strains (Davis et al., 1999). This difference in level of noise exposure ($2^3 = 8$-fold, or equivalent to +9 dB SPL) is consistent with heterozygosity for other genetic differences among the backcross that may ameliorate the damaging effects of noise exposure. Despite an altered genetic background for susceptibility to NIHL, segregation for the *Ahl/Ahl* genotypes exhibited a significantly greater susceptibility to NIHL than did the +/*Ahl* mice. Davis et al. (1999) also showed that the C57BL/6J mice are more susceptible to 1-hour exposures from 110 to 116 dB SPL, whereas the CBA/CaJ mice are more susceptible from 116 to 119 dB.

The evidence presented earlier indicates that a major genetic factor on chromosome 10 contributes to AHL. The noise-exposure studies indicate that the same genetic factor renders *Ahl/Ahl* mice more susceptible to NIHL. A lifetime of acoustic exposures, together with aging systems for adaptation and/or correction, may lead to loss of hearing acuity. All of the previous studies for AHL and NIHL in mice have been done on strains deduced to be *Ahl/Ahl* vs. +/*Ahl*, or +/+, but not including any mutant alleles at the *dfw*/PMCA2 locus on chromosome 6.

We have already indicated that two genes (products) interact and may contribute to AHL and to NIHL. A modifier gene (*mdfw*) on chromosome 10 affects the hearing ability of the heterozygous +/*dfw²ᴶ* mice (Noben-Trauth et al., 1997). The *mdfw/mdfw*; +/*dfw* mice have elevated ABR thresholds. Because the *mdfw* and *Ahl* genes map very closely to each other on chromosome 10, and both affect hearing thresholds, it is highly probable that *Ahl* and *mdfw* are one and the same gene, either the identical mutation or two different mutant alleles.

The original *dfw* mutation on chromosome 6 was cloned and identified as coding for the plasma membrane Ca-ATPase, isoform- 2 (PMCA2) (Street et al., 1998). The PMCA2 gene was disrupted and found to affect vestibular and hearing functions (Kozel et al., 1998). Homozygotes for the PMCA–/– were completely deaf. The PMCA+/– heterozygotes exhibited elevated ABR thresholds, dependent on the *mdfw*/*mdfw* genotype of chromosome 10. In the presence of a wild-type modifier (+*mdfw*) on chromosome 10, the PMCA+/– heterozygotes exhibit normal ABR thresholds. Exposure of these PMCA2+/– mice to 110 dB SPL for 8 hours causes significant levels of noise-induced hearing loss (NIHL) compared to their PMCA2+/+ littermates (P.J. Kozel et al., in preparation).

We propose that two major genes, *Ahl*/*mdfw* on chromosome 10 and *dfw*/PMCA2 on chromosome 6, contribute to AHL and to NIHL. There is no evidence for the product of the *Ahl*/*mdfw* gene, nor how it contributes to AHL or NIHL. However, the *mdfw*/*Ahl* locus appears to modify or regulate the *dfw*/PMCA2 locus.

The product of the *dfw* gene is the PMCA2 enzyme which pumps Ca^{2+} out of cells. Therefore, these mice may have insufficient ability to extrude Ca^{2+} from the outer hair cells. But what does Ca^{2+} have to do with acoustic over-stimulation? Fridberger et al. (1998) removed the temporal bones (with intact cochlea) from guinea pigs, incubated them *in vitro*, and then bombarded them for 30 minutes with acoustic over-stimulation. They assessed the accumulation of Ca^{2+}, by means of fluorescence, within the contractile outer hair cells of the cochlea. These data suggest the importance of PMCA2 for maintaining appropriate levels of Ca^{2+} in the ear, especially when the ear is acoustically over-stimulated. The PMCA2 function would likely be stressed during periods of intense acoustic stimulation. Their guinea pigs were presumably not prone to AHL; why should those ears have been susceptible to accumulation of Ca^{2+}? Those ears *in vitro* were obviously devoid of arterial circulation, hypoxic, and presumably unable to support the PMCA2-ATPase activity.

Data from Erway et al. (1996) show that C57BL/6J (*Ahl*/*Ahl*) mice exhibit NIHL, but that CBA/CaJ (+/+) mice are less susceptible to NIHL. Similarly, among F1 hybrids, B6xD2F1 mice (obligate *Ahl*/*Ahl*) also exhibit NIHL, but the CBxB6F1 mice (obligate +/*Ahl*) do not exhibit NIHL. Likewise, among the N2 progeny derived from the CBAxB6F1 backcross, the *Ahl*/*Ahl* progeny exhibit more NIHL than the +/*Ahl* progeny. The PMCA2 activity provides a reasonable role for maintaining normal auditory function. Might this mechanism also be contributing to AHL in the aging ear? Given the known modifier (*mdfw*/*mdfw*) of the (+/*dfw*) heterozygotes, the most important question is: what is the unknown product of (*Ahl*/*Ahl* ala *mdfw*/*mdfw*), and how does it modify PMCA2? It is possible that the (*Ahl*/*mdfw*) modifier may be a regulator for synthesis of mRNA for PMCA2. Then absence of the normal gene modifier would reduce PMCA2 activity, thus impairing the role of PMCA2 in maintaining normal intracellular Ca^{2+} within the contractile outer hair cells of the cochlea.

ACKNOWLEDGMENTS

We acknowledge the cooperation and analyses of the BXD data provided by Benjamin Taylor. The screening project was supported by the National Institute on Deafness and Other Communication Disorders, DC62108.

29 Mapping the Genes for the Acoustic Startle Response (ASR) and Prepulse Inhibition of the ASR in the BXD Recombinant Inbred Series: Effect of High-Frequency Hearing Loss and Cochlear Pathology

Robert Hitzemann, James Bell, Erik Rasmussen, and James McCaughran

BACKGROUND

The past decade has witnessed some remarkable advances in detecting and mapping the chromosomal position of genes associated with behavioral phenotypes. It is now clear that behavioral quantitative trait loci (QTLs) can be reproducibly mapped, with high log of odds (LOD) scores (Flint et al., 1995; Gershenfeld et al., 1997; Koyner et al., 2000), and that these QTL intervals can be reduced to 1 to 2 cM (Talbot et al., 1999; Demarest et al., 2000). Complimenting these advances, we now have a draft of the human genome and the mouse genome project should be completed soon. From these perspectives, QTL analyses will soon focus on selecting candidate genes within small QTL intervals and on determining which polymorphisms in the candidates selected are functionally relevant.

Although most preclinical behavioral phenotypes were developed and validated in the rat, genetic studies have largely focused on the mouse. Because of the availability of numerous inbred mouse strains, transgenic animals, and a well-described genome, the mouse has a clear advantage for genetic research. However, mice are not small rats. When rat paradigms are adapted to the mouse, especially paradigms involving higher order learning, mice tend to do poorly (Crawley et al., 1997). The question of whether or not this difference reflects a difference in "intelligence" or that new protocols need to be developed, specifically suited to the mouse's abilities and temperament, is unclear.

Another problem encountered when substituting mice for rats is that one frequently encounters marked sensory deficits. For example, the C3H/HeJ strain shows marked retinal degeneration at an early age. Obviously, such animals would be unsuitable for a task such as the Morris water maze, which requires the animal to remember spatial cues. More importantly (from the perspective of quantitative genetics), one would not use the C3H/HeJ strain as a part of a mapping intercross when the water maze is one of the phenotypes under investigation. This same argument would normally extend to phenotypes involving hearing acuity and the use of the DBA/2J (D2) and/or C57BL/6J (B6) inbred strains; as reviewed elsewhere in this volume and below, both strains exhibit high-frequency hearing loss (HFHL). However, there are significant gene mapping advantages to using intercrosses formed from the B6 and D2 strains or the BXD recombinant inbred (RI) strain series. The B6 and D2 strains are highly polymorphic (Dietrich et al., 1992; 1994), differ in a wide variety of behavioral phenotypes (Crawley et al., 1997), and have been widely used in QTL analysis (Crabbe et al., 1994; 1999). Importantly, the use of these strains and the associated crosses provides a cumulative record of information that allows one to compare results across studies. Because of this cumulative record, we have been able to address the following problem: does HFHL confound the QTL analysis of the acoustic startle response and prepulse inhibition of the acoustic startle response in the BXD RI series? The problem can be addressed since Willott and Erway (1998) have provided information on HFHL and cochlear pathology in 25 strains of the BXD RI series.

ACOUSTIC STARTLE RESPONSE AND PREPULSE INHIBITION OF THE ASR

There are several reasons for both the general and the genetic interest in the acoustic startle response (ASR) and prepulse inhibition (PPI) of the ASR (see also Chapter 5).

1. The circuits mediating both the ASR and PPI have been largely delineated (reviewed in Koch and Schnitzler, 1997); the PPI circuit is of special interest because the mesolimbic dopamine system (a target of numerous therapeutic agents and drugs of abuse) is an important regulatory component. Further, the circuits in man and laboratory animals appear to be largely identical, and the phenotypes can be measured in essentially isomorphic conditions.

2. PPI provides a measure of sensorimotor gating, which is known to be abnormal in a variety of psychiatric disorders including schizophrenia (Koch, 1996; Braff et al., 1978; 1992; Grillon et al., 1992; Swerdlow et al., 1993; Ornitz et al., 1992). The deficits of PPI observed in schizophrenic patients have been linked to the sensory overload and cognitive fragmentation seen in some patients (McGhie and Chapman, 1961; Braff et al., 1978).

3. Dopamine agonist-induced and naturally occurring deficits of PPI in laboratory animals are generally reversed by typical and atypical antipsychotics, suggesting that the PPI paradigm may be a useful model for drug development (Swerdlow et al., 1994; McCaughran et al., 1997).

4. Among both non-recombinant and recombinant inbred mouse strains, there are marked variations in both the ASR and PPI (Marks et al., 1989; Willott et al., 1994b; Logue et al., 1997; Paylor and Crawley, 1997). However, the two phenotypes appear to be genetically unrelated. For example, Logue et al. (1997) examined the ASR and PPI in 12 inbred mouse strains and 7 F_1 hybrids; the correlation between the ASR (to a 120-dB white noise stimulus) and the PPI (induced by a 90-dB prepulse stimulus) was 0.10. When a tactile-air puff was used for the startle stimulus, the correlation between PPI and the startle response was –0.33. Using 11 inbred strains, Paylor and Crawley (1997) were also unable to detect significant correlations between the strain distributions for startle response and PPI. Paralleling these genetic results, we have found that the phenotypic correlation between the ASR (110-dB pure tone) and PPI (80-dB white noise) for 500 B6D2 $F_{2 \, mice}$ is 0.03 (unpublished observation). Overall, these data suggest that the factors regulating the startle response and PPI are generally quite different.

5. Kline et al. (1998) have observed that in animals selectively bred for differences in haloperidol-induced catalepsy (the murine equivalent of neuroleptic-induced extrapyramidal symptoms) that there are marked differences in PPI. Animals resistant to the catalepsy response show both a poor ASR and PPI, which is reversed by moderate doses of haloperidol. These data suggest that some of the same genes that regulate the catalepsy response also regulate the ASR and PPI; importantly, four QTL for the catalepsy response have been identified (Kanes et al., 1996; Rasmussen and Hitzemann, 1999; Patel et al., 2000). One of these QTL is centered on *Drd2* (chromosome 9)(Kanes et al., 1996; Patel et al., 2000). B6.D2 congenic mice developed for this QTL not only show the appropriate change in catalepsy (decreased sensitivity) and dopamine D_2 receptor density (decrease), but also a reduction in the ASR (Rasmussen, 1999; see below).

HIGH-FREQUENCY HEARING LOSS IN THE B6 AND D2 INBRED STRAINS

Willott and colleagues (Willott et al., 1994b; Carlson and Willott, 1996) have followed the effects of HFHL on the ASR and PPI in the B6 and D2 strains. The ASR changes in a predictable fashion: the ASR amplitudes decline for high-frequency stimuli as expected from threshold elevations, but there is no change in the salience of the still audible frequencies (Parham and Willott, 1988; Carlson and Willott, 1996). The effect of HFHL on PPI differs from the effect on the ASR in that the salience of the still audible middle-frequency (12 to 16 kHz) tones to produce PPI increases (Carlson and Willott, 1996). This phenomenon appears to be an example of hearing-loss-induced plasticity of the central auditory system (Kaas, 1991; Salvi et al., 1996). Willott and colleagues have concluded this phenomenon (at least in the B6 strain) results from a tonotopic reorganization of the inferior colliculus such that middle-frequency portions of the inferior colliculus map expand as high-frequency portions are lost; thus, more vigorous suprathreshold responses are evoked by middle-frequency tones (see Chapters 23 and 24) .

The question addressed in the work described here concerns the extent to which HFHL contributes to differences in the ASR and PPI among individuals in genetically segregating populations formed from HFHL susceptible strains such as the B6 and D2. HFHL is a genetic defect that leads to cochlear pathology, including loss of hair cells and spiral ganglion cells (see Chapter 28). *A priori*, there is no reason to believe that these defects will parallel the genetic differences among individuals in the startle and prepulse circuits. Willott and Erway (1998) have provided the information necessary to test this assumption. These authors examined the cochlear pathology and the acoustic brainstem response in 25 strains of the BXD recombinant inbred series and the two parental strains. Both the cochlear pathology and the hearing loss were continuously distributed among the strains, indicating that these phenotypes were quantitative traits under the control of multiple genes. The B6 parental strain showed the least cochlear pathology and HFHL, but several RI strains showed significantly more pathology and HFHL than that observed in the D2 strain. Overall, these data made it possible to ask what, if any, association exists between HFHL and the ASR/PPI. (McCaughran et al., 1999).

BXD RECOMBINANT INBRED (RI) SERIES

The BXD RI series (26 strains) was developed by Taylor (1978; 1989) from the B6 and D2 strains. Because of recombination, each of the RI strains is genetically unique. However, at any given locus, the strains are homozygous for either the B6 or D2 allele. For a given phenotype, a strain distribution pattern is established; one tests sufficient individuals from each strain to accurately determine the strain mean. The reliability of this measurement is usually expressed as a split-halves reliability coefficient (Blizard, 1992). In the data reported here, 15 animals from each of 25 different RI

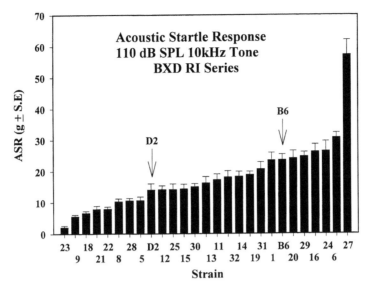

FIGURE 29.1 Distribution of strain means for the acoustic startle response in the BXD recombinant series (25 strains) and the C57BL/6 (B6) and DBA/2J (D2) parental lines. The ASR was measured as described in the text. Data is reported as mean grams of force above background + S.E. N = 9–15/animals/strain (see Table 29.1).

strains were tested; the reliability coefficients for the ASR and PPI (three different conditions) ranged from 0.78 to 0.97.

The ASR and PPI paradigm used was one that had been developed previously (McCaughran et al., 1997; Kline et al., 1998). A startle session consisted of 12 blocks of 5 trial types: startle stimulus (P) alone, prepulses of 56, 68, and 80 dB preceding P, and a null trial (no stimulus). In addition, within each test session, there were three trials of the 80-dB prepulse stimulus alone (not coupled to the startle stimulus); in no strain did these trials generate a startle response. Each trial type was presented in pseudo-random order and separated by an interval of 5 to 20 s (mean = 15 s). The startle stimulus alone (P-alone trials) consisted of a 60-ms 110-dB SPL 10-kHz tone. Each startle session was initiated by a 5-min habituation period, followed by an orientating P-alone trial. This trial was not included in the analysis. The prepulses were delivered as a 20-ms white noise burst, 100 ms prior to the startle stimulus. The ASR was defined as the difference in g of the peak response between the P-alone and null trial. Data were collected for 200 ms from the onset the startle stimulus; however, in all strains, the latency to the peak response was less than 100 ms and in general ranged from 50 to 70 ms after onset of the startle stimulus. PPI was defined as the percent change in the ASR.

The strain means for the ASR alone are illustrated in Figure 29.1. The means ranged from 2.7 g (RI#23) to 55 g (RI#27). The strain means for the D2 and B6 strains were 14 and 24 g, respectively. Neither of the parental strains were representative of the extreme phenotype (highest or lowest ASR), suggesting the presence of transgressive segregation in the RI strains and implying that the B6 strain has one or more alleles associated with low ASR while the D2 strain has one or more alleles associated with high ASR. From previous work (McCaughran et al., 1997), 3 g was established as the minimum ASR to test for PPI; thus, strain #23 was not included in subsequent analyses.

The PPI strain means (56-dB SPL prepulse stimulus) are shown in Figure 29.2. The means ranged from 3.4% (RI# 29) to 60% (RI# 8). For this phenotype, the D2 parental strain (PPI = 2.1%) was representative of the extreme poor PPI phenotype. However, there were numerous strains that showed greater PPI than the B6 strain (PPI = 27%). Apparently, the D2 strain is contributing one or more alleles that increase PPI. The floor effect does not allow any conclusions about whether or not the B6 strain is contributing alleles that decrease PPI.

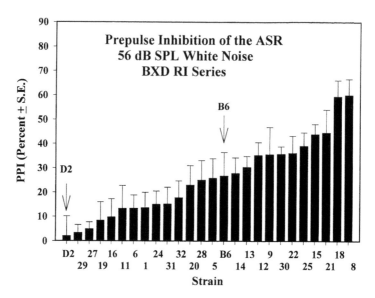

FIGURE 29.2 Distribution of strain means for prepulse inhibition (56 dB SPL) of the acoustic startle response (ASR) in the BXD recombinant series (24 strains) and the C57BL/6 (B6) and DBA/2J (D2) parental lines. PPI was measured as described in the text; background noise was approximately 50 dB. Data is reported as mean percent inhibition of the ASR + S.E. N = 9–15/animals/strain (see Table 29.1). Strain #23 was not included because of the low ASR (<3 gr).

The data for the 68-dB SPL prepulse stimulus are shown in Figure 29.3. Compared to the 56-dB prepulse, the average PPI at 68 dB increased from 26 to 34%. However, as with the 56-dB data, the D2 strain was representative of the extreme poor PPI phenotype while again numerous strains showed greater PPI than the B6 strain. The data for 80 dB SPL prepulse were also similar, except that there was a trend for RI #29 to have poorer PPI than the D2 strain (Figure 29.4). The RI average for PPI at 80 dB was 42%. Overall, the data in Figures 29.1 to 29.4 illustrate that both the ASR and PPI of the ASR were continuously distributed across the RI strains, indicating the likely involvement of multiple genes.

Willott and Erway (1998) obtained acoustic brainstem response data on 15 of the RI strains and the two parental strains and used these results to divide the RI strains into three groups: the B6 like (adult onset HFHL), the D2 like (juvenile onset HFHL), and an intermediate group. This classification provided the structural basis for the statistical analysis of the data in Figures 29.1 to 29.4. Additional RI strains were added to each of three categories on the basis of the age-related loss of spiral ganglion cells in the hook region of the cochlea; this maneuver to increase analysis power seemed reasonable given the strong relationship between cochlear pathology and the acoustic brainstem response. Table 29.1 summarizes the results. The ANOVA for the PPI data revealed that there was no significant effect for group ($F_{2,22}$ = 0.4, $p > 0.6$) or the group × intensity interaction ($F_{4,44}$ = 1.7, $p > 0.2$), but there was a significant intensity effect ($F_{2,44}$ = 37, $p > 0.00001$). Thus, there was no significant difference in PPI among the groups (e.g., adult onset HFHL vs. adolescent onset HFHL), and we conclude that under the experimental conditions used, the salience of the prepulse stimulus was not increased by HFHL. However, it should be noted that the animals used here were between 50 and 60 days old — sufficiently old to show HFHL but probably not old enough to show the tonotopic reorganization described by Willott and colleagues (see above).

MAPPING THE GENES FOR THE ASR AND PPI

The strain mean data illustrated in Figures 29.1 to 29.4 provide an entry for finding the genes associated with the variance in response. However, some background is needed on the use of the

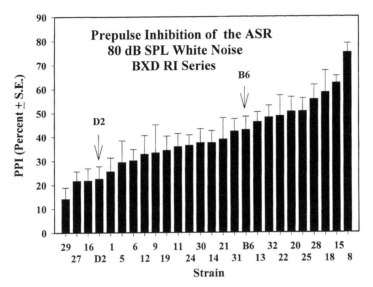

FIGURE 29.4 Distribution of strain means for prepulse inhibition (80 dB SPL) of the acoustic startle response (ASR) in the BXD recombinant series (24 strains) and the C57BL/6 (B6) and DBA/2J (D2) parental lines. PPI was measured as described in the text; background noise was approximately 50 dB. Data are reported as mean percent inhibition of the ASR + S.E. N = 9–15/animals/strain (see Table 29.1). Strain #23 was not included because of the low ASR (<3 gr).

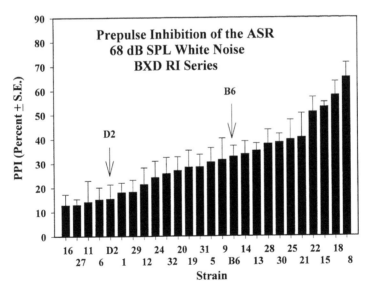

FIGURE 29.3 Distribution of strain means for prepulse inhibition (68 dB SPL) of the acoustic startle response (ASR) in the BXD recombinant series (24 strains) and the C57BL/6 (B6) and DBA/2J (D2) parental lines. PPI was measured as described in the text; background noise was approximately 50 dB. Data are reported as mean percent inhibition of the ASR + S.E. N = 9–15/animals/strain (see Table 29.1). Strain #23 was not included because of the low ASR (<3 gr).

BXD strains for finding genes or more precisely quantitative trait loci (QTLs) and on the limitations of the approach. The RI strains were originally developed to map dichotomous traits (e.g., dilute coat color), and for this purpose 26 strains have remarkable statistical power. The use of the RI

TABLE 29.1
Effect of Varying the Intensity of the Prepulse Stimulus (White Noise) on the Acoustic Startle Response to a 110 dB SPL 10 kHz Tone in the BXD RI Series Categorized According to Cochlear Pathology and Age-Related High-Frequency Hearing Loss

Strain (N)	Group	ASR-gr	PPI-80 dB (Mean Percent Inhibition ± SE)	PPI-68 dB	PPI-56 dB
RI#1 (15)	1	24 ± 2.4	62 ± 3.0	53 ± 2.1	44 ± 4.1
RI#25 (15)*	1	14 ± 1.8	51 ± 5.5	40 ± 8.0	39 ± 5.6
RI#28 (14)	1	11 ± 0.8	56 ± 6.0	38 ± 5.8	25 ± 8.0
RI#29 (15)	1	25 ± 1.4	14 ± 4.7	18 ± 4.9	3.4 ± 3.2
RI#30 (15)	1	15 ± 1.0	38 ± 5.9	38 ± 3.5	36 ± 3.1
RI#31 (15)	1	21 ± 2.2	42 ± 5.2	29 ± 5.2	15 ± 6.9
C57BL/6J (10)	1	24 ± 2.2	43 ± 5.5	33 ± 4.4	27 ± 9.7
Mean (7)	**1**	**19 ± 1.9**	**44 ± 5.4**	**36 ± 3.8**	**27 ± 5.0**
RI#5 (15)*	2	11 ± 1.2	29 ± 9.0	31 ± 5.9	26 ± 8.0
RI#6 (14)	2	31 ± 1.6	30 ± 4.7	15 ± 4.9	13 ± 5.5
RI#9 (15)*	2	5.6 ± 0.5	33 ± 12	32 ± 8.8	36 ± 11
RI#11 (13)	2	17 ± 1.8	36 ± 5.5	14 ± 8.7	13 ± 9.5
RI#12 (15)	2	14 ± 1.2	33 ± 7.8	21 ± 6.8	35 ± 5.2
RI#13 (15)	2	16 ± 2.0	46 ± 4.1	35 ± 3.0	30 ± 4.5
RI#14 (15)	2	18 ± 1.6	38 ± 5.1	34 ± 5.3	28 ± 6.4
RI#15 (9)	2	14 ± 1.5	26 ± 5.7	18 ± 3.9	14 ± 6.3
RI#18 (15)	2	6.7 ± 0.6	59 ± 9.1	58 ± 5.7	60 ± 6.6
RI#22 (15)*	2	7.9 ± 0.7	49 ± 8.6	51 ± 6.1	36 ± 7.1
RI#23 (15)*	2	2.1 ± 0.5	—	—	—
Mean (10)	**2**	**14 ± 2.2**	**38 ± 3.1**	**31 ± 4.4**	**29 ± 4.2**
RI#8 (15)	3	10 ± 0.9	75 ± 3.8	65 ± 6.0	60 ± 6.6
RI#16 (15)	3	26 ± 2.4	22 ± 5.1	13 ± 4.4	9.8 ± 7.5
RI#19 (15)*	3	19 ± 1.0	34 ± 5.9	28 ± 7.0	8.4 ± 7.6
RI#21 (15)*	3	7.9 ± 1.0	39 ± 9.0	41 ± 9.9	45 ± 9.4
RI#24 (15)	3	26 ± 3.2	36 ± 4.4	24 ± 6.8	15 ± 5.4
RI#27 (15)	3	57 ± 4.7	22 ± 3.9	13 ± 2.4	4.9 ± 2.8
RI#32 (15)	3	18 ± 2.0	48 ± 4.9	26 ± 6.7	18 ± 6.9
DBA/2J (10)	3	14 ± 2.0	23 ± 5.1	16 ± 5.8	2.1 ± 8.0
Mean (8)	**3**	**24 ± 5.8**	**40 ± 6.4**	**30 ± 6.4**	**23 ± 7.4**
RI#20 (15)	N.A.	24 ± 2.1	51 ± 6.1	27 ± 5.7	23 ± 8.0
Split Halves	*r* = 0.97	*r* = 0.84	*r* = 0.79	*r* = 0.78	

Note: The RI strains were classified into three groups on the basis of the data provided in Willott and Erway (1998): Group 1 = adult-onset HFHL; Group 2 = intermediate-onset HFHL; Group 3 = juvenile-onset HFHL. Those strains indicated by an (*) were placed in the various groups on the basis of cochlear pathology only and not acoustic brain response. Because of the low startle response, strain 23 was not included in the analysis. The startle session consisted of 12 blocks of 5 trial types: startle stimulus only, startle stimulus preceded 100 ms by 56, 68, or 80 dB, 20 ms white noise-burst and a null trial. The ASR data are presented in mean ±SE grams of force. PPI data is presented as the mean ±SE percent inhibition of the ASR.

series to map complex behavioral traits is a relatively recent development that was formalized by McClearn, Plomin, and colleagues in the early 1990s (Gora-Maslek et al., 1991; Plomin and McClearn, 1993). The first step is to determine the phenotypic strain means (e.g., Figures 29.1 to 29.4) for each member of the RI series. These data are then subjected to a QTL analysis, which attempts to find associations between these strain means and the strain distribution patterns (SDPs) of marker loci with a known genomic location. These QTL associations are generally expressed as point-biserial correlation coefficients. The significance of such correlations is the same as the regression of phenotype on gene dosage for a particular locus (Crabbe and Belknap, 1992). The BXD RI series is particularly useful for this type of analysis because it has the most marker information, the series is composed of a large number of strains, the progenitor B6 and D2 strains are highly polymorphic (Taylor, 1978; 1989; Plomin and McClearn, 1993; Dietrich et al., 1992), and these strains differ markedly for a wide variety of behavioral phenotypes. Because the BXD series has been widely used in behavioral research, one can capitalize on the accumulative and integrative nature of the RI approach. The RI strain means are comparable across time and studies.

The major problem in using only the BXD RI series to detect behavioral QTLs is the lack of statistical power. Neumann (1992) termed "simultaneous search" the approach ... "to map several QTLs influencing a trait in a single analytical procedure. This entails independent, 'simultaneous' attempts to detect linkage between loci influencing the trait of interest and multiple marker loci distributed over as much of the genome as possible, without a preliminary modeling of the effects of individual loci or the mode of inheritance." When this approach is applied to the analysis of RI strain data, Neumann (1992) argued that very stringent criteria will be required to demonstrate linkage of a particular loci to a trait of interest. Bayesian analysis (see also Neumann, 1990; Neumann and Collins, 1991) estimates that a p value in the range of 0.0025 to 0.0003 will be the minimum criterion for 95% probability of linkage. For an RI series with 26 strains, a correlation coefficient of 0.65 would be required to meet the test criterion. In other words, greater than 40% of the between-strains variance would need to be explained by a single locus.

Belknap (1992) took a somewhat different position on the analysis of RI data, but in the end argued that if the RI data are used alone, the threshold will need to be set very high. Belknap et al. (1996) also noted that when the threshold is set lower (e.g., $p < 0.01$) so as not to miss any significant correlations, the false negative rate will be quite high ($\geq 50\%$). With these arguments in mind, a new strategy was developed for using RI series in behavioral QTL analysis, one that suggested that the RI approach should be integrated into a two-step strategy (Belknap, 1992; Plomin and McClearn, 1993; Kanes et al., 1996; Buck et al., 1997). These authors argued that the BXD data could serve as a screen to identify candidate map locations, which are then confirmed in other RI series, standard inbred (non-RI) strains (Goldman et al., 1987), congenic lines (Bailey, 1981), or by linkage analysis in F_2 or backcross populations (Lander and Botstein, 1989; Rise et al., 1991; Neumann and Collins, 1991). In such a two-step analysis, the α value for the RI step could be set at 0.01 or even 0.05, because it yields lower Type II error rates (failing to detect important map sites). The protection against such Type I errors resides in the confirmation test (Belknap, 1992). Assuming that a B6D2 F_2 analysis is used for confirmation, the advantage of the two-step procedure is that the genotyping in the F_2 cross is confined to only those chromosomal regions containing candidate QTLs. At $p < 0.01$, this typically involves 5 to 15% of the genome. A number of behavioral phenotypes, especially ones related to alcohol or other drugs of abuse, have been successfully analyzed using this two-step procedure (see e.g., Crabbe et al., 1999).

For most investigators, the two-step procedure had a relatively short half-life. As laboratories became more efficient in genotyping animals, phenotyping 3 to 400 expensive RI animals was no longer a cost-effective first step. Furthermore, it became clear as more and more QTLs were detected that, on average, the effect size was relatively small (a 5% effect size would be considered large by most investigators). Consequently, the number of Type II errors in the RI analysis increased; that is, important QTLs were not detected. Thus, today, most investigators begin directly with an F_2 analysis or backcross analysis. Depending on the assumptions made, an F_2 sample of 5 to 600

TABLE 29.2
Candidate QTLs for the ASR and PPI Detected in the BXD RI Series

Marker(s)	Chr (cM)	ASR	PPI-80	PPI-68	PPI-56
Mpmv6, Ren2, Upg2	1 (70)	0.28	−0.36	−0.50*	−0.52*
D2Mit6, Ntp	2 (9)	−0.40	0.44	0.59*	0.67**
D3Nds2, D3Mit15	3 (66)	−0.40	0.63**	0.41	0.47
D4Mit71, Slc9a1	4 (62)	−0.52*	0.47	0.51*	0.66**
Dvl, D4Bir1	4 (82)	−0.07	0.33	0.44	0.52*
D5Mit1, Pmv40i	5 (5)	0.52*	−0.60*	−0.64**	−0.53*
D9Mit20, Bgl_s	9 (61)	0.30	0.68**	0.73**	0.71**
Hmg1_rs2, D10Mit51	10 (9)	−0.28	0.54*	0.52*	0.57*
D11Mit38, Brp8	11 (45)	0.53*	−0.51*	−0.51*	−0.53*
D12h14s17, D12Nyu14	12 (55)	0.35	−0.29	−0.58*	−0.40
D18Byu2, Slc12a2	18 (28)	−0.52*	0.05	0.04	0.27

Note: Data are the correlation coefficients obtained for the intervals where a significant interaction was detected for the either the ASR and/or PPI. Representative markers for each of the intervals are listed. cM distance refers to the approximate location of the peak correlation. *, $p < 0.01$; **, $p < 0.001$.

is sufficient to detect a QTL with an effect size of 5%. Because the animals whose phenotypic scores lie 1 SD above and below the mean contain more than 80% of the genetic information (Lander and Botstein, 1989), it is necessary to only genotype the extreme phenotypes. For a sample size of 600, only the top and bottom 100 would be genotyped. For QTL detection, marker spacings of 20 cM are adequate (Darvasi, 1998); thus a total of 16,000 genotypings would be required.

Despite the paradigm shift over the past 10 years, the BXD RI series remains an important mechanism for testing genetic hypotheses (e.g., Table 29.1). Furthermore, even given the limitations noted above, important information regarding QTLs can be extracted, especially if the effect size is moderate to large. A summary of the RI QTL analysis is found in Table 29.2; in this analysis, α was set at 0.01 because of the multiple comparisons being made. Furthermore, it has been our experience that QTLs detected at $p < 0.05$ but $p > 0.01$ have a false positive rate of greater than 90%. Eleven different QTLs were detected on ten different chromosomes. Several general observations of these data can be made.

1. Only one QTL (Chr 18) was specific for the ASR.
2. The sign of the QTLs for the ASR and PPI were generally opposite. The meaning of the sign builds from the convention of coding the D2 alleles as 1 and the B6 alleles as 0 in the point by serial correlation. Thus, for both the ASR and PPI, a positive sign indicates that the D2 allele is increasing the response, while a negative sign indicates that the B6 allele is increasing the response.
3. On chromosomes 2, 3, 4, 5, and 9, QTLs for PPI were detected that were significant at $p < 0.01$ or better.

To confirm the candidate QTLs from the RI analysis and to detect additional QTLs, a standard F_2 intercross QTL analysis was conducted (see Koyner et al., 2000, for details). A total of 600 male mice were used. Females were not used because of the variable effect the estrous cycle has on PPI (Swerdlow et al., 1997). The results obtained are illustrated in Figures 29.5 and 29.6. The threshold for suggestive QTLs was set at LOD $\geq$ 3, and the threshold for significant QTLs was set at LOD $\geq$ 4.3 (see Lander and Krugylak, 1995). For the ASR, significant or very significant (LOD > 6) QTLs were detected on chromosomes 5, 11, and 18. Thus, three of the four candidate QTLs detected in

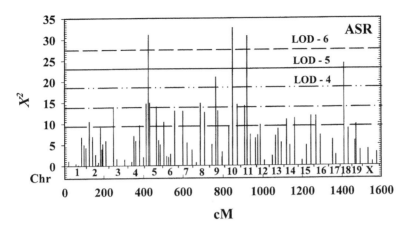

FIGURE 29.5   Summary of the genome-wide scan for the acoustic startle response in a B6xD2 F_2 intercross (N = 600). Details for the genome wide-scan are similar to those found in Koyner et al. (2000). Note that only male animals were used. A significant association was set at LOD ≥ 4.3.

the RI analysis for the ASR were confirmed (the QTL on chromosome 4 was not confirmed). In addition, QTLs were detected on chromosomes 9 and 10 that were not detected in the RI analysis. For PPI, the situation was more complex. The QTL on proximal chromosome 5 was confirmed for all prepulse conditions. In addition, the QTL for PPI 80 on chromosome 11 was confirmed. However, a comparison of Tables 29.2 and 29.3, illustrates that numerous QTLs were not confirmed, including what appeared to be a major QTL for PPI on the distal region of chromosome 9. For PPI 80, two new QTL were detected at the suggestive level on chromosomes 2 and 6. Finally, significant QTLs were detected on chromosomes 13 and 14 for PPI 68, but not for PPI 56 or 80.

For the QTLs detected in both the RI and F_2 analysis, some potential candidate genes in the regions of interest are listed in Table 29.3. Of these candidates, one of particular interest is reelin (*Reln*) found in the proximal region of chromosome 5. The *Reln* locus encodes a secreted extra-celluar glycoprotein involved in the migration of neurons in the developing brain. Briefly, in the cortex, neurons destined to occupy the wall of the embryonic cerebrum are generated in the cerebral ventricles and migrate radially along the neuroepithelial glial cells (Goffinet, 1995). As the neurons reach the marginal zone, the neurons secrete reelin to act as a matrix adhesion molecule that organizes the post-migratory neurons into appropriate cell patterns (Rakic and Caviness, 1995). The reelin protein was identified using the reeler mutant, first described by Falconer (1951). In the mutant, functional reelin is absent, resulting in altered patterns of cortical, hippocampal and cerebellar organization (Goffinet, 1984; 1995). Of particular interest to the current study is the observation that there are marked behavioral traits associated with reelin haplo-insufficiency in the heterozygous mouse (rl+/−). Importantly, these mice show a decrease in PPI and neophobic behavior on the elevated plus maze (Tueting et al., 1999). These data led the authors to conclude that there may be possible analogues between the rl+/− phenotypes and vulnerability to develop psychosis. This laboratory has also observed that reelin protein levels and mRNA levels are reduced in the brains of schizophrenic subjects (Impagnatiello et al., 1998); associated with the reelin decrease was a marked decrease in glutamic acid decarboxylase 67 protein content. The role(s) reelin may have in the organization of the adult brain has also been examined (Fatemi et al., 1999; Rodriguez et al., 2000). Overall, we conclude that reelin is a logical candidate gene in the chromosome 5 QTL. However, it is not the only candidate. For example, near *Reln* is *Tac1*, which encodes the hormones substance P, neurokinin A, and neuropeptide K. The role(s) of these hormones in the ASR and PPI is not difficult to imagine; further, there are numerous transcript variants of *Tac1*, although it is not known if there is a polymorphism between the B6 and D2 strains. Given the

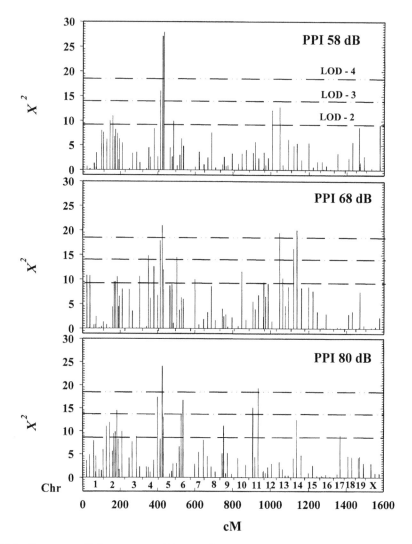

FIGURE 29.6 Summary of the genome-wide scan for prepulse inhibition (PPI) of the acoustic startle response in a B6xD2 F_2 intercross (N = 600). Data is presented for all prepulse intensities. Details for the genome-wide scan are similar to those found in Koyner et al. (2000). Note that only male animals were used. A significant association was set at LOD ≥ 4.3.

potential candidates on chromosome 5 and elsewhere, the question arises as to what will be the best strategy for actually identifying the gene or genes within a confirmed QTL interval.

IDENTIFYING GENES IN THE QTL INTERVAL

The basic elements of QTL analysis are independent of the phenotype, except for the assumption that one is dealing with a complex trait (i.e., the involvement of multiple genes). Thus, regardless of whether one is mapping QTLs for the ASR, PPI, or any phenotype associated with hearing performance, the basic process remains the same. As noted in this chapter and elsewhere (e.g., Crabbe et al., 1999), the approach has been very successful in detecting QTLs. However, the next stage, actually finding the relevant genes has been more difficult. Most investigators have begun this process by forming congenic lines for the interval(s) of interest. Consider the QTL for the ASR on chromosome 9 (Figure 29.6). The QTL was detected only in the F_2 analysis and the strength

TABLE 29.3
Summary of Combined QTL Analyses in the BXD RI Series and
B6D2 F$_2$ Intercross: QTLs Significant in the RI Analysis ($p < 0.01$)
and in the F$_2$ Analysis at LOD ≥3 or Better

Phenotype	(Chr[cM])[a]	Human Synteny	Candidate Genes[b]
ASR	5 (5)	7q21-q22	*Cacna2d1, Reln, Tac1, Nos3*
PPI 58			
PPI 68			
PPI 80			
ASR	11 (45)	17p13; 5q21,q35	*Acrb, Acre, Htt, ti, Sex6*
PPI 80		17q11-q13; q22-q23	
ASR	18 (30)	5q21-q34	*Slc2a2, Camka2, Adrb2*

[a] The cM position is intended to describe the approximate center of the QTL; with the sample sizes used, the 95% confidence intervals will be 15 to 25 cM.

[b] Candidate Genes: acetylcholine receptor epsilon *(Acre)*; acetylcholine receptor beta *(Acrb)*; adrenergic receptor beta 2 *(Adrb2)*; calcium/calmodulin-dependent protein kinase II alpha *(Camka2)*; calcium channel, voltage dependent, alpha2/delta subunit 1 *(Cacna2d1)*; nitric oxide synthase 3 *(Nos3)*; reelin *(Reln)*; seizure related gene 6 *(Sex6)*; serotonin transporter *(Htt)*; solute carrier family 12, member 2 *(Slc12a2)*; tachykinin precursor *(Tac1)*; tipsy *(ti)*.

of the association just met the LOD threshold; thus, there was some concern as to whether or not a QTL is actually present on chromosome 9.

To use congenic lines to test that the QTL is real, one introgresses the interval of interest from one of the parent strains onto the background of the other parent. The process begins with either a male F$_1$ hybrid (or a male from a RI strain that is homozygous for the donor strain across the interval). The male is then backcrossed to a recipient female. The progeny from this first cross are then tested to find animals heterozygous for the interval of interest; genotyping for three or four microsatellite markers across the interval is sufficient to find the appropriate animals (this first genotyping step is not necessary if a RI male is used, because all the progeny will be heterozygous for the interval). A heterozygous male is then backcrossed to a recipient female and the process continues for ten generations, at which point the homozygous animals are selfed (i.e., brothers and sisters with identical genotypes in the chromosomal region of interest are mated) to produce the congenic line. The amount of donor DNA, including the region of interest, will be about 2%.

For the chromosome 9 QTL, the region of interest stretched from about 10 to 40 cM. A summary of the data obtained for the reciprocal congenics (B6.D2 and D2.B6) formed for this interval is found in Figure 29.7; for both lines, the extent of the introgressed interval was such that the interval did not include the *dilute* or *Myo5* locus (which is easily checked by monitoring coat color). Focusing on the males, the B6.D2 congenic showed the expected decrease in the ASR, while the D2.B6 congenic showed the expected decrease. For the female mice, the situation was more complex; the B6.D2 females showed the expected decrease in the ASR but no effect was found in the D2.B6 animals, pointing to a gender x congenic interaction. However, overall, we conclude that the congenic data confirmed the presence of an ASR QTL on chromosome 9.

Congenic lines can serve as an important resource for reducing the QTL interval. To begin the process, the congenic animal is backcrossed to the recipient strain to produce mice with recombinations within the introgressed interval. By producing a sufficient number of animals, one can obtain a series of overlapping recombinant animals, which in turn are inbred to form new congenics. Darvasi (1998) formalized the design and termed the new strains, interval specific congenic strains

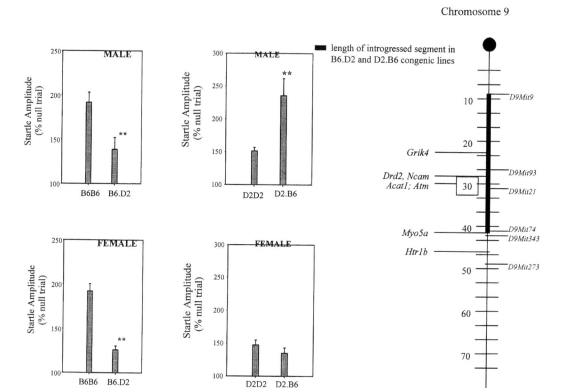

FIGURE 29.7 Acoustic startle response in the B6.D2 and D2.B6 congenic mouse lines and their respective controls. Controls were formed in the same way as the congenic lines (see text) except that the recipient alleles were maintained. Data are presented as the mean + S.E. increase in the startle amplitude above the null trial. **, significantly different from control; $p < 0.01$.

(ISCSs). Given the density of the mouse microsatellite map (see e.g., Dietrich et al., 1994; 1996), it is possible to construct a series of ISCSs which can give 1-cM resolution for QTL mapping.

The first step in this process is to determine which ISCSs contain the QTL. This process, as described by Darvasi (1998), occurs in two steps: the first step is to screen the ISCSs with sufficient power to avoid a Type II error; the second step retests at $p < 10^{-4}$ the strains that define the QTL location. The number of animals required at each of these steps can be easily calculated. Consider a QTL interval for which ten interval-specific congenic strains have been constructed at approximately 1-cM intervals and for which $h^2_{QTL} = 0.05$ (the QTL is associated with 5% of the phenotypic variance). Because the genetic variance in each ISCS is essentially 0, the standardized difference d^* between the two homozygous QTL genotypes is given by $2d^* = 2d/(1 - h^2_B)$. $h^2_B =$ broad sense heritability, which for the ASR is approximately 0.7. For $h^2_{QTL} = 0.05$, $d_{QTL} = 0.324$; thus, $d^* = 0.59$. The number of animals required per ISCS at a confidence level α, is given by $N = (Z_{1-\alpha}/d^*)^2$, where $Z_{1-\alpha}$ has the usual meaning. It should be noted that because the two alternative hypotheses (donor QTL retained vs. not retained) are symmetrical, α represents both the Type I and II errors. Since in this example there are 10 ISCSs, we set α for the first step at 0.005, and the number of animals required per strain is $(2.576/0.59)^2 = 19$ (or a total of 190 animals). In the second step, we set α at 10^{-4} and compare the two strains that most unambiguously define the QTL location; the number of animals required per strain is 46 (or a total of 92 animals). Overall, this strategy provides an efficient and cost-effective "phenotypic" mechanism for reducing the QTL interval to a size suitable for gene searching.

The mouse genome has an estimated length of between 1360 and 1500 cM and probably contains between 50,000 and 100,000 genes (Dietrich et al., 1996). Thus, a 1-cM interval is likely to contain between 30 and 75 genes. Assuming that the genes within a given interval are already known or will soon be known, one is faced with the task of locating functional polymorphisms (between the parental strains) within the interval of interest. The most efficient strategy for polymorphism screening remains to be determined. However, differences in gene expression can be monitored using the new micro-array technology.

CONCLUSION

The data presented here and elsewhere leave little doubt of the marked genetic effects on both the ASR and PPI. The question arises as to what are the genetic substrates? One possibility is the auditory threshold. Among inbred strains, there are significant differences in the acoustic brainstem response (e.g., Henry, 1983; Willott et al., 1994b; 1997), which to a significant extent are associated with cochlear pathology. However, there does not appear to be a clear relationship between auditory thresholds and the ASR. For example, the SJL/J, C3H/HeJ, CBA/J, and AKR/J inbred mouse strains have excellent (low) auditory thresholds (Henry, 1983; Trune et al., 1996) but yet relatively poor ASRs (Logue et al., 1997; Paylor and Crawley, 1997; unpublished observations). The data in Table 29.1 extend this observation for the BXD RI series. The ASR in those RI strains with juvenile onset HFHL (group 3) was not significantly different from those RI strains with adult-onset HFHL (group 1). These data should not be interpreted to indicate that HFHL cannot affect the ASR and, in fact, significant effects have been reported (e.g., Parham and Willott, 1988; Carlson and Willott, 1996). Rather, the data suggest that under the experimental conditions employed here of (i) using young adolescent animals (6 to 8 weeks) and (ii) using a startle threshold (100 dB SPL) that is above the minimum threshold for eliciting an acoustic brainstem response even in the juvenile-onset HFHL group, the genetic variance in the ASR is largely independent of differences in auditory threshold. Finally, it should be noted that there are moderate (Logue et al., 1997) to excellent (Paylor and Crawley, 1997) correlations between the tactile startle response and the ASR for inbred strains, suggesting that the locus of the genetic variation is independent of the type of startle stimulus.

The evidence presented here and elsewhere also suggests that the genetic variation in auditory PPI is generally not related to HFHL. An examination of PPI among adolescent to young adult AKR/J, C3H/HeJ, B6, A/J, SJL/J, and LP/J strains illustrates this point. Despite a similar auditory profile, PPI in the AKR/J strain is considerably better than in either the B6 or C3H/He J strains (Paylor and Crawley, 1997). The A/J and LP/J strains that have relatively poor auditory thresholds (Henry, 1983) exhibit similar if not better PPI than the B6 strain (Logue et al., 1997; Paylor and Crawley, 1997). The albino SJL/J and A/J strains differ markedly in their auditory thresholds (Henry, 1983) but are similar in PPI (Logue et al., 1997). The data in Table 29.1 extend these observations to the BXD RI series. The data illustrate that when the prepulse tone was presented as a white noise-burst, PPI was not significantly different between the adult- and juvenile-onset HFHL groups. Further, the juvenile-onset group responds normally even to the barely audible 56-dB tone. (In contrast, we have noted that the LP/J strain, which suffers from an early-onset otosclerosis-like condition (Henry and Chole, 1987), does not respond to the 56-dB prepulse tone, but does respond well to the 80-dB tone [unpublished observations]).

Willott and colleagues (e.g., Carlson and Willott, 1996) have observed that the effect of HFHL on PPI is to increase the salience of the still audible middle-frequency (12 to 16 kHz) tones to produce PPI. It was this phenomenon that has been observed in the B6, D2, and BALB/c strains (Willott et al., 1998) that prompted us to test the frequency response of PPI in the BXD RI series (McCaughran et al., 1999). Unexpectedly, it was observed that the RI strains with juvenile-onset HFHL showed deficits in PPI across all frequencies when compared with the adult-onset group. The expected increase in salience at the still-audible tones was not observed. The reason(s) for the differences between our data and those of Willott and colleagues are not entirely clear. However, it should be noted that the increased salience of the middle-frequency tones reported for the B6 strain is not evident until after 4 months of age (Carlson and Willott, 1996). Further, over the period of 1 to 5 months, the D2 strain does not appear to show increased salience to a 80-dB prepulse stimulus (Figure 4 in Willott et al., 1994b) and, in general, increased salience at lower prepulse intensities is relatively modest when compared to the B6 strain. These data suggest that the potential confound of increasing salience can be overcome by using relatively young animals and by focusing on higher prepulse intensities.

Both the B6 and D2 strains appear to have at least one identical age-related hearing loss gene (*Ahl*) (Erway et al., 1993a), which has been recently mapped to mouse chromosome 10 (K.R. Johnson et al., 1997). It has been proposed that the D2 strains contains at least two additional *Ahl*-like genes, one of which (*Ahl2*) is also located on chromosome 10 (Erway et al., 1993a; 1996; but see Chapter 28). The data in Figure 29.6 suggest that a QTL for the ASR was detected in the general region of *Ahl*. The question of whether or not *Ahl* lies within the QTL cannot be determined from the present data, given the the ambiguity of the QTL approach; one can really only conclude for certain that there is a QTL on chromosome 10. Definitive information on whether or not the gene or genes associated with the chromosome 10 QTL affect hearing acuity awaits identification of the genes. However, in the interim, preliminary data for this and other QTLs could be obtained by examining the acoustic brainstem response in the relevant congenic and interval specific congenic strains.

ACKNOWLEDGMENTS

The authors wish to thank Dr. James Willott for invaluable advice and assistance during the course of this study. This study was supported in part by a grant from the U.S. Public Health Service (MH 51372), a grant from the Department of Veterans Affairs, and a grant from the National Alliance for Research on Schizophrenia and Affective Disorders.

30 Transgenic Mice: Genome Manipulation and Induced Mutations

Lina M. Mullen and Allen F. Ryan

INTRODUCTION

The use of mice in auditory research has been accelerated by the advent of techniques that allow controlled changes in the genetics of this species. Increasing information about the genome of the mouse paired with the insertion of artificial genes, or transgenes, into genomic DNA has permitted experiments that could only be dreamed of in the past. These methods allow the study of genes in the context of the entire organism, connecting the reductionist world of molecular biology with systems biology. Unlike the experiments of nature presented by natural mutations, changes in the genome can be designed to address specific questions. Because the use of these powerful techniques has not been easy in other species, transgenic mice have become a staple of modern biology.

Now in use for 20 years, transgenic mice have contributed a wealth of information regarding gene function and regulation. The accelerating rate of gene discovery has resulted in increasing numbers of transgenic mice, many of which display changes in the auditory system as part of their phenotype. Moreover, transgenic strategies and techniques continue to evolve, leading to expanded possibilities for their use in the field of auditory research. The purposes of this chapter are to describe transgenic techniques and applications, to broadly review auditory phenotypes of transgenic mice, and to discuss future directions in which this powerful methodology may take us.

In general, two methods are used to generate controlled mutations in mice. The first involves random insertion of a foreign gene (or "transgene") into the mouse genome, by micro-injection of the construct into a fertilized egg. The second involves the targeted insertion of a gene construct into a specific genetic locus, by homologous recombination in embryonic stem (ES) cells. In both cases, the ability to stably introduce constructs into the genome of an organism allows gene modification to be studied in the context of the organism, including both the interaction of complex physiological systems and the entire lifespan.

Insertional transgenics are frequently used to explore the ectopic expression of a gene, in which a sequence is misexpressed at an unnatural location and/or time, or is overexpressed at its normal site. Another common use of this method is the expression of a mutated protein. This includes models of mutations found in human disease, as well as dominant negative or constituitively active mutations to probe protein function.

Transgenes are also used to explore the structure and function of gene regulatory elements. Promoter constructs driving the expression of reporter genes are used in transgenic models to characterize the control of gene expression by defined DNA segments. While promoter analysis is frequently carried out in cell lines, it has been found that the behavior of promoters in the intact organism can vary markedly from what is seen in isolated, transformed cells.

The targeted insertion of transgenes to a particular genomic location by homologous recombination is most frequently used for gene deletion studies, which can be a powerful method of exploring gene function. In addition to gene "knockout" studies, targeted insertion can also be used to "knock in" a desired sequence, so that its expression will be controlled by the promoter of the substituted gene. Of course, there are many variations of these basic uses for transgenic technology, and new applications are constantly being developed.

METHODS FOR THE GENERATION OF TRANSGENIC MICE

TRANSGENE DESIGN AND CONSTRUCTION

The typical insertional transgenic construct includes a regulatory sequence that determines the site, duration, and extent of transcription. This sequence is chosen to produce a desired pattern of transgene expression. The promoter sequence may be constitutive; that is, expression is constant and occurs in virtually all cell types. Many constitutive promoters are derived from viral genes; others are derived from mammalian *housekeeping* genes that are expressed in all or most cells. Alternatively, the promoter can be derived from the regulatory elements of a mammalian gene with more restricted expression. Such promoters can direct expression to a particular cell type and/or time. The transgenic construct also includes an expressed sequence, encoding a normal or mutated protein of choice. Finally, a termination sequence, often virally derived, is included to end transcription and, often, to enhance expression levels.

Constructs for site-directed mutagenesis contain two fragments of genomic DNA flanking the portion of a gene that is to be deleted. For a short gene, this can consist of one fragment 5' to the expressed sequence, and a second fragment 3' to the expressed sequence. For large genes (some can be hundreds of kilobases in size), DNA flanking critical exons is chosen. These are the recombination sites. In between these two genomic DNA fragments, a positive selection element is ligated. This element confers resistance to a selection factor, such as an antibiotic, and its expression is driven by a constitutive promoter. On one or both ends of the entire construct are inducible negative selection elements such as thymidine kinase, used to eliminate constructs that integrate by random insertion rather than by recombination.

METHODS OF TRANSGENE INTEGRATION

By far, the most common means of creating insertional transgenics is oocyte injection. In this method, oocytes are harvested from superovulating females and fertilized *in vitro*. Before pronuclear fusion, each egg is held with a suction pipette, and many copies of the purified insertional transgenic construct are injected into the male pronucleus. The eggs are then transferred to the uterus of a pseudopregnant female. In a fraction of these eggs, one or more copies of the transgene will integrate at random into the genome, and the result will be a transgenic mouse in which all cells carry the transgene.

An alternative method for the generation of transgenics, less commonly employed, is based on retroviral vectors. A transgene inserted into a modified retrovirus is injected into a mouse blastocyst *in vitro*. The virus infects cells of the blastocyst and is integrated into the genome of these cells. Viral integration is not random, but tends to occur preferentially at certain chromosomal locations. Because not all cells in the blastocyst are affected, the result is a chimeric animal. Only if the germ cells are affected will the transgenic line be propagated.

Site-directed mutagenesis is carried out in cultured embryonic stem (ES) cells. These are pleuripotent cell lines derived from the inner cell mass of blastomeres. Constructs are introduced into the cells in culture, usually by electroporation. Over the course of subsequent cell divisions, a very small proportion of the cells undergo recombination in both genomic DNA fragments flanking the positive selection element at the appropriate genomic locus, thereby deleting the targeted genomic segment. To select for this very rare event, the ES cells are treated with lethal levels of antibiotic. Only the tiny fraction of cells that have integrated the construct, and thus express the resistance gene, survive. The promoter driving thymidine kinase is then activated, which destroys any cells in which the negative selector has not been eliminated by recombination. The surviving ES cells are expanded and injected into blastocysts, where they integrate into the developing embryo to produce a chimera. If the germ cells of the chimera are derived from the genetically altered cells, the modification will be transmitted to future generations. The mutation can then be bred to homozygosity.

ADVANTAGES AND LIMITATIONS OF TRANSGENIC RESEARCH

The greatest strength of transgenic models is the ability to manipulate gene expression in context. Experiments carried out in cell lines or even in organotypic culture systems provide a limited and/or altered subset of the conditions that are present *in vivo*, and can be influenced by the effects of tissue culture itself. In a transgenic, the effects of a specific genetic change are observed with all of the normal cell types and processes present, and across the entire lifespan.

There are many disadvantages of transgenic techniques. One of the most important limitations is the requirement to work in a mouse model. While transgenic techniques can be applied to other species, for most investigators the mouse is the only practical model. This can be a disadvantage in studying phenomena that either do not occur in the mouse (e.g., hair cell regeneration) or are more difficult to study in this species than in other models (e.g., behavior). However, as the many chapters of this volume attest, an increasing number of standard auditory methods have been adapted for use in the mouse.

A second limitation is the expense and time required to generate transgenics, which is especially true of recombinant models. This limits the number of experiments that can be performed, and the speed with which research can progress. Not only are transgenics expensive to produce, but maintenance of transgenic lines becomes expensive if very many lines are generated and preserved.

Insertional transgenics require the use of an appropriate promoter to provide the specific cellular or temporal specificity needed. In the case of the auditory system, relatively few specific promoter constructs are available at the present time. However, such promoters are being and will be developed at an increasing rate. If a promoter fragment is relatively short, another possible problem is influence by DNA adjacent to the random integration site. This may cause expression to vary, sometimes dramatically, between different lines bearing the same construct.

Another potential problem with insertional transgenics is mutagenesis. It is estimated that between 2 to 20% of random transgene insertions disrupt an endogenous gene. In many cases, this leads to embryonic lethality and is undetected. However, in other cases in which the animals survive to adulthood, insertional mutations must be separated from the phenotype induced by the transgene itself. Of course, insertional mutations that affect the auditory system can be informative, and have even led to identification of the affected gene.

Transgenics that affect development of the early embryo can be lethal. This makes the study of certain genes impossible by standard transgenic techniques. Alternatively, many gene knockouts have little or no phenotype, or a completely unexpected phenotype. This reflects the functional redundancy that is a characteristic of the genome. However, it is has also been argued that this is a powerful statement regarding how little we understand regarding the function of genes. It is also true that phenotypes have been overlooked by focusing only on systems in which a phenotype is expected or desired by an investigator. In addition, phenotypes may be too subtle to detect with the methods employed. Finally, it must be remembered that the constrained environment of a research animal facility may not reveal phenotypes that could be critical to behavior or survival in the wild.

MOUSE STRAINS COMMONLY USED IN TRANSGENIC RESEARCH

Transgenic techniques have evolved in those mouse strains that are best adapted to the specific procedures required. The most favored strain for insertional transgenics is the C57BL/6 mouse, because this strain superovulates well, tolerates implantation of oocytes, and subsequently breeds well with large litter size. Recombinant transgenics are almost invariably produced in strain 129 mice, because ES cells derived from 129 strains reproduce well in culture and are much more tolerant of transfection and selection procedures than ES cells from other strains. These are unfortunate facts of life for the auditory researcher using transgenic mice, because both C57BL/6 and 129 mice display recessive, early-onset, inherited hearing loss that is severe (Chapter 28).

This problem can be overcome in an F1 generation by breeding founder mice to an inbred strain that does not display abnormal hearing (or to a strain that is not allelic to the deafness gene of either 129 or C57BL/6. However, if F2 mice are generated by crossing these offspring (as would be required in breeding knockouts to homozygosity), the deleterious gene would be expected to segregate to produce deafness in 1/4 of the offspring. Repeated crosses into a normal-hearing strain such as CBA are required to eliminate the contaminating gene.

TRANSGENICS AFFECTING THE DEVELOPMENT, ANATOMY, AND FUNCTION OF THE AUDITORY SYSTEM

The study of transgenic mice has advanced the auditory field and has revealed the identity of many genes involved in the development of the auditory system. This chapter section reviews the data obtained from transgenic mouse models in which auditory development, anatomy, and/or function are altered. The genes altered include those encoding transcription factors, transmembrane channels, transporters and receptors, and structural proteins. We have arranged this review based on gene family. However, within these families, we have also ordered studies by site of defect because this segregation is also informative (Fekete et al., 1998). Most of the investigations reviewed have utilized homologous recombination to generate null mutations. However, some insertional transgenics have auditory phenotypes, and in a few cases random insertional mutations affecting hearing have arisen as a by-product of the creation of transgenic mice. The information in this section is summarized in Table 30.1.

TRANSCRIPTION FACTORS

The process of development involves at its heart the precise regulation of the expression of thousands of genes. Gene expression is ultimately controlled by the interaction of many DNA-binding proteins with the regulatory elements present in each gene. These transcription factors modulate the levels of transcription of other (downstream) genes by binding to the DNA and enhancing or repressing their expression. Protein transcription factors can interact with the promoters of many genes, and it is the combination of factors present in a cell that determine which genes will be expressed at a given time. Development and function of the auditory system similarly relies on precise control of gene activity and the activity of regulatory transcription factors. A number of transcription factor encoding genes have been shown to be involved in auditory development by targeted mutagenesis. In particular, transcription factors have been found to play critical roles in tissue patterning, cell fate determination, and differentiation.

Transcription Factor Transgenics Affecting Primarily the Outer Ear

The structures of the outer ear arise largely from the first and second branchial arches, and their development involves epithelial/mesenchymal interactions. Mutations of genes encoding transcription factors that are expressed in these embryonic structures preferentially affect the outer ear.

The basic helix-loop-helix (bHLH) transcription factor *dHAND* is expressed in the distal portion of the first and second branchial arch mesenchyme beginning on embryonic day 9 (E9). Deletion of these genes is embryonic lethal at embryonic day (E)11. However, at this stage, the branchial

TABLE 30.1
Transgenic Mutations Affecting Inner Ear Development

Protein	Expression Site[a]	Site of Defect[a]	Ref.
	Transcription Factors		
dHAND	Branchial arches	OE, ME	Srivastava et al. (1997)
Goosecoid	Auditory meatus	OE, ME	Yamada et al. (1995)
AP-2	Neural crest	OE, ME	Schorle et al. (1996)
Msx1	Mesenchyme near otocyst	ME ossicles	Satokata and Maas (1994)
Dlx2	Branchial arches, otocyst	ME	Qui et al. (1997)
Dlx5	Branchial arches	ME, vestibular IE	Acampora et al. (1999)
Fkh10	Otocyst	IE	Hulander et al. (1998)
Otx1	Otocyst	Lateral SSC	Acampora et al. (1996)
Otx2	Otocyst	Enhances Otx1 defect	Morsli et al. (1999)
Eya 1	Otocyst	Otocyst	Xu et al. (1999)
Hoxa1	Rhombencephalon	IE, ME	Chisaka (1992)
Hoxb1	Rhombencephalon	Enhances Hoxa1 defects	Gavalas et al. (1998)
Hoxa2	Branchial arch mesenchyme	OE, ME	Barrow and Capecchi (1999)
Pax2	Otocyst	IE	Torres et al. (1996)
Hmx2	Otic placode, otocyst	Vestibular IE	Hadrys e al. (1998)
Hmx3	Otic placode, otocyst	Vestibular IE	Wang (1998)
Gbx2	Branchial arch, otocyst	Vestibular IE	Wassarman et al. (1997)
Prx1	Branchial arch	IE capsule	Martin et al. (1995)
Prx2	Branchial arch	w. Prx2, vestibular IE	ten Berge (1998)
RARα	All IE cells	w. RARg, IE	Lohnes et al. (1994)
RARγ	Developing cartilate	w. RARa, IE	Lohnes et al. (1994)
TRb1	Widely expressed	w. TRb2, cochlea	Rüsch et al. (1998)
TRb2	Cochea	Less age-related HL	Wang et al. (2000)
Math1	IE sensory epithelia	Hair cells	Bermingham et al. (1999)
Brn-3.1	Hair cell	Hair cell	Erkman et al. (1996)
Brn-3.0	Spiral/vestibular ganglion	Spiral/vestibular ganglia	McEvilly et al. (1996)
Brn-4	Mesenchyme	IE capsule	Phippard et al. (1998; 1999)
Neurogenin1	Otic placode	Spiral, vest. ganglion	Ma et al. (1998)
Twist	Ant. head mesenchyme	Middle ear bones	Bourgeois et al. (1998)
MITF	Neural crest	IE secretory epithelia	Tachibana et al. (1994)
	Ligands/Receptors		
Endothelin1	Branchial arch neural crest	EE, ME	Clouthier et al. (1998)
Endothelin RA	Branchial arch neural crest	EE, ME	Clouthier et al. (1998)
Endothelin CE-1	Branchial arch neural crest	EE, ME	Clouthier et al. (1998)
Int2/FGF3	Rhombencephalon	IE fluid spaces	Mansour et al. (1993)
FGFR3	IE capsule, organ of Corti	Organ of Corti	Colvin et al. (1996)
TGFβ2	Sensory epithelia	IE epithelia	Sanford (1997)
BMP-4	Sensory epithelia	IE	Winnier (1995)
Jagged 2	Hair cells	Organ of Corti	Lanford et al. (1999)
NT-3	Organ of Corti	Spiral ganglion	Farinas et al. (1994)
BDNF	Sensory epithelia	Vestibular ganglion	Pirvola et al. (1992)
TrkC	IE ganglia	Spiral ganglion	Ernfors et al. (1994)
TrkB	IE ganglia	Vestibular spiral ganglia	Klein et al. (1991; 1993)
α9 AChR	IE sensory epithelia	No HC efferent response	Vetter et al. (1999)
GABA(A) R	IE ganglia	Spiral ganglion	Porter et al. (1998)
Nociceptin R	Superior olivary complex	More NIHL	Nishi et al. (1997)
Integrin α8b1	Hair cells	HC stereocilia	Littlewood (2000)

TABLE 30.1 (continued)
Transgenic Mutations Affecting Inner Ear Development

Protein	Expression Site[a]	Site of Defect[a]	Ref.
	Channels/Transporters		
Na$^+$-K$^+$-2Cl$^-$ co-trans.	Stria vascularis	Stria, endolymph	Delpire et al. (1999)
IsK	Stria vascularis	Stria, endolymph	Vetter et al. (1996)
KVLQT	Stria vascularis	Stria, endolymph	Drici et al. (1998)
PMCA2	HCs, spiral ganglion	HCs, spiral ganglion	Kozel et al. (1998)
D-L Ca^{2+} channel	Cochlea	?	Platzer et al. (2000)
	Structural Proteins		
COL4A3	Basement membranes	Basement membranes	Cosgrove et al. (1998)
Mysosin 15	HCs	HCs	Probst et al. (1998)
Alpha-tectorin	Tectorial, vestibular membranes	Tectorial, vestibular membranes	Logan et al. (2000)
Otogelin	Tectorial, vestibular membranes	Tectorial, vestibular membranes	Simmler et al. (2000)
Netrin	Otocyst	SSCs	Salminen et al. (2000)
	Miscellaneous		
Hdh	Widely expressed	EE	White et al. (1997)
p27^{kip1}	Widely expressed	HCs	Chen and Segil (1999)
SOD	Widely expressed	More NIHL	McFadden et al. (2000)
Glutathione peroxidase	Widely expressed	More NIHL	Ohlemiller et al. (2000)
MPV17	Spiral ligament	Spiral ligament, endolymph	Meuller et al. (1997)
p-Glycoprotein	Capillary endothelium	IE	Zhang et al. (2000)
Rab 3A	IE sensory epithelium	IE	Durand et al. (1998)

[a] OE, outer ear; ME, middle ear; IE, inner ear; SSC, semicircular canal; HL, hearing loss; EE, external ear; HC, hair cell; NIHL, noise-induced hearing loss.

arches are hypoplastic (Srivastava et al., 1997), suggesting that this factor may play a role in early outer and middle ear development.

Goosecoid, a homeobox-containing gene resembling the anteriorizing *bicoid* of *Drosophila*, is thought to be a gastrula organizing gene as well as a gene involved in mesoderm induction in vertebrates. In the mouse, it is expressed in the gastrula and then again during craniofacial development in the base of the auditory meatus (Gaunt et al., 1993; Rivera-Perez et al., 1995; Yamada et al., 1995). *Goosecoid* null mutants are born with numerous external ear defects, including an absent tympanic ring and membane, and reduced external pinna and gonial bone (Yamada et al., 1995). In addition, middle ear development is abnormal. Of the middle ear bones, the manubrium of the malleus is severely shortened and the processus brevis is completely absent (Yamada et al., 1995; Rivera-Perez et al., 1995).

The helix-span-helix transcription regulator, activator protein 2 (AP-2), is expressed in both ectoderm and neural crest cells. Mice deficient in AP-1 have absent pinnae and underdeveloped middle and inner ear structures. This implicates AP-2 in craniofacial patterning (Schorle et al., 1996).

Transcription Factor Transgenics Affecting Primarily the Middle Ear

The structures of the middle ear are also derived from the first and second branchial arches, with contributions from the first pharyngeal pouch.

Msx genes, homeobox-containing genes related to a *Drosophila* muscle segment homeobox gene, have been proposed to be involved in epithelial/mesenchymal interactions (Davidson, 1995). *Msx1* is expressed in mesenchyme surrounding the otocyst and is strong during bone formation of the middle ear (MacKenzie et al., 1991). Mice deficient in *Msx1* display abnormalities in the middle ear consisting of a small malleus with an absent short process (Satokata and Maas, 1994). This effect is restricted to the first arch derivative and suggests that the expression of *Msx2* may substitute for an absent *Msx1* in these mutants.

The *Dlx* gene family members are related to the *Drosophila Distal-less* gene. *Dlx1* and *Dlx2* are expressed in the entire mesenchyme of branchial arches 1 and 2, while *Dlx3*, *Dlx5*, and *Dlx6* are restricted to the distal mesenchyme of these arches (Simeone et al., 1994; Qiu et al., 1997). *Dlx2* and *3* are expressed at low levels in the otic vesicle (Robinson and Mahon, 1994), and become restricted to the vestibular portion in overlapping but distinct domains. Mice lacking *Dlx1* display abnormalities in maxillary derivatives. Mice lacking the *Dlx2* gene die shortly after birth and have gross craniofacial abnormalities such as deletion of the alisphenoid, malformed incus and stapes, and styloid-derivatives of the first and second branchial arches (Qiu et al., 1995). Disruption of the *Dlx5* gene with *LacZ* ORF (cre-lox system) results in mice that have a reduced tympanic ring, a misshapen alisphenoid, and a reduced vestibular portion of the labyrinth including severe malformations of the semicircular canals (Acampora et al., 1999).

Transcription Factor Transgenics Affecting Primarily the Formation and Morphogenesis of the Inner Ear

The structures of the inner ear arise almost exclusively from a neuroectodermal placode that arises adjacent to the developing rhombencephalon. The placode invaginates to form the otocyst on around E10. The otocyst, responding to internal genetic programs as well as the inductive influences of the brainstem and other adjacent structures, develops a complex series of outpouchings that mature into the endolymphatic, cochlear, and the several vestibular compartments of the labyrinth. Mutations of genes expressed in and around the inner ear during the early stages of inner ear development can have dramatic influences on the patterning of the labyrinth.

Fkh10, a member of the forkhead family of the winged helix transcription factors, is expressed exclusively in the otocyst at E9.5. Mice in which this gene has been deleted show gross abnormalities in the development of both the vestibular and auditory labyrinth. In these animals, the labyrinth is represented by a simple cavity without identifiable sensory epithelia. This is associated with complete deafness and absence of vestibular responses (Hulander et al., 1998).

Otx1 and *Otx2* are homeobox-containing mouse cognates of *Drosophila* orthodenticle, involved in anterior central nervous system and head development. *Otx1* and *Otx2* are expressed in the developing ear in non-sensory areas. *Otx1* is found in the lateral canal, lateral ampulla, utricle, and pars inferior, while *Otx2* is expressed mainly in the developing pars inferior. Mice lacking *Otx1* show circling and head-bobbing behavior, and are missing their lateral semicircular canals (Acampora et al., 1996). Mice with a targeted disruption of *Otx2* demonstrate a loss of anterior neural structures and die at E10.5 (Ang et al., 1996). *Otx1*(–/–) and *Otx2*(+/–) double mutants have abnormalities that are more severe than the single *Otx1* mutants, including absent pars superior, utriculosaccular duct, and cochleosaccular duct (Morsli et al., 1999). This implies that these genes act cooperatively during auditory development.

The leucine zipper encoding *Eya* factors are homologs of the eyes absent gene in *Drosophila*. Mutations in *Eya1* cause branchio-oto-renal (BOR) syndrome in humans (Abdelhak et al., 1997). In mice, Eya1 protein is expressed in the otic placode and otocyst, and later in the ganglia, neuroepithelia, and adjacent mesenchyme of the developing labyrinth. Mice heterozygous for *Eya1* deletion show middle ear abnormalities, including disruption of the ossicular chain and a conductive hearing loss, despite the fact that no branchial arch expression of *Eya1* is observed. Homozygous null animals show an absent external and middle ear, as well as failure of inner ear development past the otocyst stage (Xu et al., 1999).

Members of the *Hox* gene family define the identity of rhombomeres by overlapping expression patterns along the developing neuraxis. Deletion of a member of this family leads to alterations in the development of rhombomeres and their associated structures. The ear develops adjacent to and under the influence of rhombomeres 5 and 6. Deletion of *Hoxa1* causes abnormal development of rhombomeres 4 to 6 affecting the middle and inner ear. The mutant mice have severe dysmorphology of the labyrinth with an absent cochlea, abnormal semicircular canals, lack of the VIIIth nerve, and reductions in the middle ear structures with a stapes either fused to the otic capsule or absent altogether (Chisaka et al., 1992; Gavalas et al., 1998; Mark et al., 1993; Barrow and Capecchi, 1999).

Deletion of *Hoxa2* possess severe defects in the external and middle ear, including nearly absent pinnae and mirror-image duplications of first-arch derived structures including the malleus, incus, tympanic ring, and gonial bone. *Hoxa1/Hoxa2* double mutants demonstrate all the duplication of *Hoxa2* single mutants as well as the defects found in *Hoxa1* mutants, including reduced or absent second arch elements (Barrow and Capecchi, 1999).

Although no ear defects have been reported in Hoxb1 null homozygotes (Goddard et al., 1996; Studer et al., 1996), null mutations of both Hoxa1 and *Hoxb1* result in early disruption of second arch development and full disruption of ear development. *Hoxa1*(–/–)/*Hoxb1*(+/–) double mutants showed more patterning defects in the ear than the *Hoxa1* null homozygous animals, suggesting a functional synergy between these two genes (Gavalas et al., 1998).

Members of the paired box containing transcription factor family *Pax2* and *Pax3* are involved in inner ear development. *Pax2* is expressed in the ventral otocyst, from which the saccular and cochlear regions derive. In *Pax2* loss-of-function mutants, the cochlea fails to develop and the cochlear ganglion is absent. (Torres et al., 1996). *Pax3* is expressed in neural crest cells, including those involved in endolymph generation in the labyrinth. Mutations in the *Pax3* gene that disrupt the binding of *Pax3* protein to target DNA cause deafness in the *Splotch* mouse (Epstein et al., 1993) and in Waardenburg Syndrome Type I (Tassabehji et al., 1993).

Two members of the *Hmx* homeobox gene family, *Hmx2* and *Hmx3* (formerly *Nkx5.2* and *Nkx5.1*, respectively and related to the *Drosophila NK* gene family), are expressed in the otic placode and then in restricted regions of the otocyst associated with vestibular structures (Rinkwitz-Brandt et al., 1995; 1996). Inactivation of *Hmx3* in mice leads to severe vestibular dysfunction due to deletion of large parts of the vestibular apparatus, including ablation of the semicircular canals (Wang, 1998). *Hmx3* appears to play no role in cochlear development.

The homeodomain homeobox protein gene *Gbx2* (gastrulation brain homeobox) is related to *Drosophila unplugged*, a gene involved in axial specification in the fly. *Gbx2* is involved in establishing the midbrain/hindbrain border and patterning of the anterior hindbrain, and it is expressed in the branchial arches and the developing otocyst. Null mutants of the *Gbx2* gene display abnormal development of the pars superior, a structure that gives rise to the vestibular portion of the inner ear (Wassarman et al., 1997).

Members of the vertebrate family of paired-class homeobox genes, *Prx1* and *Prx2* (formerly *Mhox* and *S8*, respectively), are expressed in the mesenchyme in largely overlapping patterns during early craniofacial and inner ear development. While they are both expressed in the second pharyngeal arch and in mesenchyme surrounding the otocyst, *Prx2* is present within the otocyst in the location of the future vestibule (Opstelten et al., 1991), and *Prx1* is not found in the otocyst. *Prx1* homozygous null mutant mice have numerous skeletal defects, including displacement of the stapes and oval window (Martin et al., 1995). *Prx2* mutants have no defects in the inner ear; however, *Prx1* (–/–) *Prx2* (–/–) double mutants fail to develop the lateral semicircular canal (ten Berge et al. 1998).

Transcription Factor Transgenics Affecting Primarily Cell Phenotypes of the Inner Ear

Many transcription factors function as determinants of cell fate and/or differentiation, and mutations in their genes can lead to quite specific abnormalities in one or a few cell types. Given the large number of cell types that comprise the inner ear, it is not surprising that transgenics involving a number of transcription factors have discrete effects on restricted cell populations.

The RAR family of nuclear receptors for retinoic acid are one of two groups of DNA binding proteins that are activated by interaction with this ligand. They serve as ligand-inducible regulators of transcription by activating RA responsive promoters. There are three *RAR* gene isotypes (*RARα*, *RARβ*, and *RARγ*), each with their own isoforms, and they have widespread expression patterns in the developing inner ear. *RARα* expression is ubiquitous in cochlear sensory and non-sensory structures. *RARβ* is expressed mainly in structures of mesenchyme origin and in vestibular sensory epithelia. *RARγ* is located in the cochlear and vestibular compartments in the epithelium of the inner ear (Romand et al., 1998). Because of functional redundancy, deletion of individual receptor isoforms has relatively little effect on the development of the auditory system. However, deletion of both *a* and *g* isotypes results in absence of the stapes, abnormal incus, a small and incomplete cartilaginous otic capsule, and absent organ of Corti and spiral ganglion of the cochlea (Lohnes et al., 1994).

The thyroid hormone receptors (TRs) represent another family of ligand-activated DNA binding factors necessary for hearing. Thyroid hormone deficiency and excess have both been associated with hearing loss (Meyerhoff, 1974; Ritter, 1967). The *TRβ1* isoform is expressed in many cell types, including those in the cochlea during embryonic and postnatal development. The *TRβ2* isoform is expressed in a much more restricted pattern, being found only in the cochlea and a few other sites. The *TRα1* isoform is widely expressed. Mice null for *TRβ2* have a permanent deficit in auditory function (Forrest et al., 1996), but do not exhibit a loss of hearing (Abel et al., 1999). Moreover, a recent study has shown less age-related hearing loss in these mutants on a C57BL/6 background than wild-type littermates (Wang et al., 2000b). Whereas *TRα1* absence does not affect function of the auditory system, mice deficient in both *TRβ1* and *TRβ2* show elevated thresholds and delayed expression of K^+ conductance in hair cells (Rüsch et al., 1998a,b).

The bHLH protein Math1 is a mouse homolog of the *Drosophila* neurogenic gene *atonal*. *Math1* is expressed in the developing sensory epithelia of the inner ear, prior to hair cell development, and becomes restricted to hair cells as development proceeds. Deletion of this gene results in lack of hair cells, although supporting cells are present. This is likely due to the inability of progenitor cells to differentiate into hair cells, and identifies *Math1* as a possible pro-hair-cell gene (Bermingham et al., 1999).

POU-domain genes encode proteins with a highly conserved N-terminal region (the POU-specific domain) and conserved C-terminal domain (the POU homeodomain), and are divided into six classes, I–VI (Wegner et al., 1993). They are highly conserved across evolution. Of particular interest for sensory-neuronal development is the *Brn-3* family. *Brn-3.1* (also called *Brn 3c*) is expressed in hair cell precursors just after commitment to the hair cell lineage, and continue to the be expressed by hair cell throughout life. *Brn3.1* null mice (Erkman et al., 1996) show complete failure of hair cell differentiation in both the organ of Corti and vestibular labyrinth. In addition, all vestibular and most spiral ganglion neurons degenerate. A mutation in the human gene for this factor that results in a truncated protein causes a dominant form of progressive hearing loss, DFNA 15 (Vahava et al., 1998), suggesting that haploinsufficiency of *Brn-3.1* might cause progressive hearing loss. However, mice heterozygous for a null mutation of *Brn3.1* show hearing comparable to wild-type littermates even at 24 months. This suggests that the truncated *Brn-3.1* in DFNA15 may have dominant negative function.

Brn-3.0 (also called *Brn-3a*) null mice have reduced spiral and vestibular ganglion populations, and spiral ganglion neurons fail to migrate into Rosenthals canal (McEvilly et al., 1996). The related factor *Brn-4* is expressed throughout the mesenchyme of the developing ear (Phippard et al., 1998), and mice lacking this gene have a gross malformation in the footplate of the stapes resulting in reduced movement. In addition, mutants suffer from cochlear hypoplasia and malformation of the superior semicircular canals (Phippard et al., 1999).

Neurogenins are neural-specific bHLH transcription factors more distantly related to the *Drosophila* neurogenic gene *atonal*. *Neurogenin1* (*ngn1*) is expressed in the otic placode, presumably in precursor cells of the cochleo/vestibular ganglion. Mice null for the *ngn1* gene fail to develop acoustic or vestibular ganglia (Ma et al., 1998).

Transcription factors of the bHLH family regulate the determination and differentiation of many cell types. The bHLH factor *twist* was identified in *Drosophila* as a gene required for mesoderm cell patterning in the developing fly. In humans, mutations in this gene are associated with diseases marked by severe skeletal abnormalities. In mice, it is expressed in the branchial arches in the area where the faciacoustic crest will form, in mesenchymal cells of the otic capsule, and in primordia of otic ossicles. A null mutation of *twist* is embryonic lethal by E11.5. Animals heterozygous for this mutation show delayed growth of the tympanic ring and other otic bones, and an absent malleus (Bourgeois et al., 1998; Chen and Behringer, 1995).

An insertional mutation in a series of transgenic mice resulted in a phenotype similar to that of the human hereditary disorder, Waardenburg syndrome type II. Isolation and characterization of the transgene integration site in this line resulted in identification of the *microphthalmia* (*mi*) gene, a transcription factor containing a helix-loop-helix-leucine-zipper (bHLH-ZIP) domain (Tachibana et al., 1994). This gene is the homolog of human *MITF*. The neural crest makes a small but critical contribution to the developing inner ear. The melanocytes involved in fluid transport epithelia, including the stria vascularis, are derived from neural crest cells. *mi* is expressed in the neural crest, including cells destined to become the intermediate cells of the stria vascularis. Mice with mutations at this site show abnormal development of strial intermediate and dark cells, resulting in abnormal endolymph and endocochlear potential. These mice lack cochlear pigment cells and are deaf (Hodgkinson et al., 1993).

Gene Hierarchies

Relatively little is known about the molecular mechanisms governing the interpretation and integration of multiple gene signals during development of the auditory and vestibular systems. Within this complex developmental process, transcription factors, which regulate the expression of particular downstream genes, are themselves regulated by other transcription factors in an intricate cascade. The identification of genes within this hierarchy requires data from transgenic studies, in addition to the understanding of spatio-temporal expression patterns of each of these genes. In *Eya* mutant animals, for example, *Pax2* expression is normal and is therefore upstream or acts independently from the *Eya1* gene. However, expression of *Six1* in the otic vesicle and facioacoustic ganglion in *Eya1* mutants is reduced, in agreement with the pattern seen in *Drosophila* (Xu et al., 1999). In *Hmx3* mutant otocysts, *Pax2* usually expresses in a complementary fashion with *Hmx3*, remains unchanged, as does *Msx1* expression. This indicates independent pathways for these genes (Hadrys et al., 1998). *Neurogenin1* is found to positively regulate a number of downstream genes. *NeuroD*, for example, is an *atonal* related gene necessary for neuronal differentiation, and is expressed in columnar epithelial cells in the otic placode as well as in cells migrating toward the vestibulo-cochlear ganglion. *ngn1* mutant mice have lost *NeuroD* expression despite the presence of placodal precursor cells that would normally express *ngn1*. *delta1* expression in the otic placode is also eliminated in *ngn1* mutant mice (Ma et al., 1998). Data such as these will help us to define a sequential expression pattern for these and other genes during otogenesis.

LIGANDS/RECEPTORS

Ligand/receptor binding subserves many cell-cell and cell-environment interactions. During development, these interactions are important determinants of cellular patterning, survival, and apoptosis. Post-developmentally, these interactions are critical for neurotransmission, cell signaling, and tissue homeostasis. Many mutations that affect signaling between cells by specific ligand/receptor interaction influence the development and/or adult function of the auditory system.

A member of the G-protein coupled receptor family, the endothelin receptor is involved in the development of neural crest derived tissues (Baynash et al., 1994; Hosoda et al., 1994). It is expressed in the facio-acoustic neural crest complex and in mesenchyme of arches 1, 2, and 3

(Clouthier et al., 1998). Inactivation of the *endothelin receptor A* (ET_A) gene by targeted mutation results in multiple defects in the pharyngeal arches as well as their associated arteries (Clouthier et al., 1998). In the middle ear, the malleus, incus, and tympanic ring are completely absent in the mutant, while the inner ear remains normal. Endothelin-1 (ET-1) and one of its activating enzymes, ECE-1 (endothelin converting enzyme), are expressed in the pharyngeal arches, and deletion of either *ET-1* or *ECE-1* also results in a loss of most of the middle ear structures. It is thus highly probable that the loss of these arch derived structures is a result of the loss of ET-1 signaling via endothelin receptor A (Clouthier et al., 1998).

The *int-2* gene (also known as *Fgf-3*) is expressed in the otic placode and in the rhombencephalon adjacent to the developing inner ear (Wilkinson et al., 1989), and has been proposed as a candidate for the otocyst-inducing signal (Wilkinson et al., 1988). Inner ear defects in *int-2* null mutants include abnormal endolymphatic duct, abnormal osseous and membranous labyrinth structure, hydrops resulting in enlarged cochlear duct and semicircular canals, and reduced ganglia (Mansour et al., 1993). However, the structure of the otic vesicle at E9.5 in these null mutants appears normal in comparison to wild-type controls, suggesting that *int-2* is not required for otocyst induction (Mansour et al., 1993) and instead may be necessary for induction of the endolymphatic duct.

FGF signaling may also play a role in targeting or maintaining neurons projecting to the outer hair cells (OHCs). Fibroblast growth factor receptor 3 (Fgfr3), a tyrosine kinase receptor family member, is expressed in developing cochlea, including the cartilaginous capsule and organ of Corti, and targeted disruption of *Fgfr3* results in many inner ear defects and deafness (Colvin et al., 1996). *Fgfr3* mutant mice have no identifiable inner and outer pillar cells, and the tunnel of Corti is missing. There is also a reduced innervation of the OHCs, and these mutant mice show no auditory brainstem response (ABR). In these mice, the cochlea of adults closely resembles that of newborn mice (Colvin et al., 1996). Although null mutations of another FGF receptor, *Fgfr2*, are peri-implantation lethal, mice deficient for the IIIb isoform of Fgfr2 created using the cre-lox recombination system, are viable until birth. These animals have grossly abnormal semicircular canals and a cystic inner ear, possibly due to a failure in endolymphatic duct formation (DeMoerlooze et al., 2000).

The activation by growth factors is known to regulate many aspects of cell behavior during development. Members of the TGFβ (transforming growth factor beta) ligand protein family can promote or inhibit cell growth (Sporn et al., 1987; Massagué, 1990) and modulate cell migration and location during development. TGFβ2 RNA is expressed in the sensory epithelia of the developing ear (Frenz et al., 1992), while TGFβ2 peptide is present in the underlying mesenchyme (Pelton et al., 1990). TGFβ2 null mutants fail to form a spiral limbus in the basal cochlear turn and, as a result, the spiral ganglion lies close to the sensory epithelium. In addition, the greater epithelial ridge with its basal lamina is separated from the underlying basilar membrane in the mutant (Sanford et al., 1997). These results and previous studies suggest that TGFβ2 plays a role in epithelial-mesenchymal interactions that are important for development of the cochlea.

Bone morphogenetic proteins (BMPs) are members of the decapentaplegic (dpp) subgroup within the TGFβ superfamily. In *Drosophila*, these genes regulate the patterning of anterior structures during development. In vertebrates, the BMPs regulate mesenchymal condensations, proliferation, differentiation, and apoptosis, and their activity has been implicated in development of almost all vertebrate tissues and organs (Hogan, 1996). *BMP4* is expressed in the presumptive vestibular sensory organs as well as in the Claudius' cells of the cochlea, and later it is found in mesenchyme surrounding the cochlea (Takemura et al., 1996; Morsli et al., 1998). *BMP2* is expressed in the developing spiral limbus as well as interdentate cells of the cochlea (Thomadakis et al., 1999). Inactivation of *BMP4* results in embryonic lethality (Winnier et al., 1995); however, mice heterozygous for *BMP4* deletion exhibit abnormal vestibular behavior and malformations of the lateral semicircular canal (Teng et al., 2000), suggesting a role in labyrinthine patterning.

The differentiation of hair cells in the inner ear can be accomplished by the process of lateral inhibition, in which a hair cell signals its neighbors and inhibits them from differentiating into hair cells. The neighboring cells would instead become supporting cells (Corwin et al., 1991; Lewis, 1991). This signal may be mediated by the transmembrane protein Notch, acting as the receptor in cells of the developing cochlear duct. The transmembrane protein Jagged 2, acting as the ligand, is restricted to cells that will develop as hair cells (Lanford et al., 1999). Mice that contain a null mutation of *Jagged 2* have cochleae with multiple inner hair cell duplications in both the inner and outer hair cell rows. This increase in the number of hair cells leads to a defect in patterning, including a misorientation of hair cell stereociliary bundles, pairs of contacting inner hair cells, and loss of individual supporting cells (Lanford et al., 1999). Deletion of another Notch ligand, Delta 1, had no effect on the cochlear epithelium (Morrison et al., 1999).

Brain-derived neurotrophic factor (BDNF) is a member of the neurotrophin family of growth factors. It enhances the differentiation and survival of sensory neurons and their target innervations. It is expressed by cells of the sensory epithelia of the vestibular labyrinth (Pirvola et al., 1992). Targeted disruption of the *BDNF* gene results in loss of neurons in the vestibular ganglion and excessive cell death in primary sensory neurons (Ernfors et al., 1994), leading to abnormal vestibular behavior. Neurotrophin 3 (NT-3), another neurotrophin, is expressed in the sensory epithelia of both the vestibular and auditory labyrinth. In mice with a targeted disruption of the *NT-3* gene, a dramatic loss of spiral ganglion neurons is seen, with a complete loss of neurons in the basal turn (Fritzsch et al., 1997a). Mice with a double mutation in *NT-3* and *BDNF* show nearly complete loss of cochlear and vestibular neurons (Ernfors et al., 1995).

Signaling from the neurotrophins, including BDNF and NT-3, is mediated primarily by the Trk family of high-affinity protein-tyrosine kinase receptors (Barbacid, 1993). Of the three, trk loci, trkB, and trkC are expressed in the cochlear and vestibular ganglia before and during sensory epithelial innervation (Represa et al., 1991). The *trkB* gene product, expressed in both vestibular and auditory ganglia, is a receptor primarily for BDNF (Klein et al., 1991) and neurotrophin 4 (NT-4; Meakin and Shooter, 1992). Mice with targeted mutations of *trkB* demonstrate numerous neurological defects (Klein et al., 1993). In the inner ear, these mice have a reduced number of vestibular neurons, as well as a preferential loss of innervation to the OHCs in the apex and middle turn of the cochlea (Schimmang et al., 1995; Fritzsch, 1998). TrkC, expressed in the spiral ganglion, is a high-affinity receptor primarily for NT-3. *TrkC* null mutants show a complete absence of basal turn spiral neurons (Fritzsch, 1998). Another study was performed in which targeted mutations of both *trkB* and *trkC* were present in a double knockout, the results of which suggest the existence of a regional effect of neurotrophins or their receptors in the cochlea. That is, TrkB activity preferentially supports middle and apical turn spiral ganglion neurons, while TrkC activity supports basal turn neurons (Fritzsch, 1998).

TrkA is a high-affinity receptor for nerve growth factor (NGF) and is expressed in the cochlear and vestibular ganglion before and during innervation at very low levels (Vazquez et al., 1994), and well before these neurons become dependent on neurotrophins for their survival (Schecterson and Bothwell, 1994). In *trkA* mutant mice, the inner ear is normal (Crowley et al., 1994).

The α9 nicotinic acetylcholine (nACh) receptor is involved in the cholinergic efferent synapses on hair cells and is expressed in OHCs of the cochlea. In α9 knockout mice, most OHCs are innervated by one large terminal instead of multiple smaller terminals as in wild-types. This suggests a role for the α9 nACh in development of mature synaptic connections. *Alpha9* deletion also leads to absence of efferent responses in the cochlea (Vetter et al., 1999).

Activity of the inhibitory neurotransmitter gamma-aminobutyric acid (GABA) is mediated by two receptor types: the $GABA_A$ and $GABA_B$ receptors. $GABA_A$ receptors are expressed in afferent nerves and in cell bodies of the vestibular ganglion. Deletion of the beta-3 subunit of the $GABA_A$ receptor results in hearing loss and vestibular disfunction associated with spiral ganglion cell atrophy in the basal turn and aberrant morphology of vestibular organs (Porter et al., 1998).

The opioid receptors, members of the G-protein coupled receptor superfamily, are comprised of d, m, and k opioid receptors subtypes and the receptor for nociceptin, designated orphanin FQ. The opioid receptors mediate a number of cellular inhibitory effects, including inhibition of adenylate cyclase, activation of potassium channels, and inhibition of calcium channels (Loh and Smith, 1990). The nociceptin system has not been well characterized, but it has been implicated in locomotor activity, immunologic responses, and neuronal development. The nociceptin receptor precursor message is detected in the periolivary region which marks the origin of the olivocochlear bundle (Vetter et al., 1991; M.C. Brown, 1993; Simmons et al., 1996a), the sites involved in brainstem auditory relay and centrifugal control of the cochlear OHCs. In mice lacking the nociceptin receptor (–/–), the thresholds of ABRs show a rise following exposure to intense sound (Nishi et al., 1997). This suggests an insufficient recovery of hearing ability from the adaptation to sound exposure in the mutant mice, indicating that this system is involved in hearing regulation following sound exposure.

Extracellular matrix components are known to affect the behavior of many cell types, and their effects can be mediated via integrin receptors. Integrin α8β1, a receptor for fibronectin, is located on the apical hair cell surface, where stereocilia are forming. Mice with a disruption of the α8 subunit gene, *Itga8*, show perturbations of hair cells in the utricle, lack stereocilia, or possess abnormal steriocilia. Activity of this integrin may be necessary for the differentiation and maturation of stereocilia (Evens and Muller, 2000).

CHANNELS/TRANSPORTERS

All cells depend on the maintenance of ionic gradients across their plasma membranes and between intracellular compartments, and utilize the movement of ions in signaling. A large number of transmembrane proteins mediate the movement of ions, from transporters to gated channels. The movement of other substances across the cell membrane is also mediated by transmembrane proteins. The inner ear is particularly dependent for its function on controlling the distribution of ions. Potassium is the dominant ion in the transduction process of the hair cell, while control of intracellular calcium appears to be especially tightly regulated in these cells. Thus, it is perhaps not surprising that mutations in genes encoding transporters and channels can influence auditory function.

The secretion of K^+ from the stria vascularis is required for normal cochlear function. Several mutations that affect this function have been created in transgenic mice. The Na^+-K^+-$2Cl^-$ co-transporter, encoded by the *Slc12a1* gene, is expressed in the stria vascularis and is critical for transport of K^+ into the epithelium. Deletion of *Slc12a1* results in collapse of the endolymph compartment, and deafness (Delpire et al., 1999). The *isk* gene is expressed in the stria vascularis, where it encodes one subunit of the channel responsible for the slow component of a delayed rectifier potassium current I_Ks. This channel is necessary for release of K^+ ions from the marginal cells of the stria into endolymph. As with the Na^+-K^+-$2Cl^-$ co-transporter, deletion of the *isk* gene results in failure to develop high K^+ concentration in endolymph, collapse of the endoplymph space soon after birth, and deafness (Vetter et al., 1996). A similar phenotype results from deletion of KVLQT-1, another subunit of this channel (Francis et al., 2000). In humans, mutations in either the *isk* or *KVLQT-1* genes can result in Jervell and Lange-Neilsen syndrome, which includes deafness (Drici et al., 1998).

The OHC contains a number of proteins that control intracellular calcium, including plasma membrane Ca^{2+}-ATPase (PMCA) located at the tips of the stereocilia. This appears to be the PMCA2 isoform, which is preferentially expressed in OHCs (Furuta et al., 1998). Deletion of the *Pmca2* gene results in loss of hair cells, spiral ganglion neurons, and deafness (Kozel et al., 1998). The D-L-type Ca^{2+} channel consists of several subunits. This class of channels (formed by alpha1D) is expressed in a variety of cell types, including the cochlea. Deletion of the gene encoding the alpha1D subunit results in deafness (Platzer et al., 2000).

STRUCTURAL PROTEINS/MATRIX MOLECULES

A number of structural genes that influence the ear have been deleted in mice. Mutations in genes encoding subunits of the basement membrane component collagen 4A cause Alport syndrome, a genetic disease in humans characterized by glomerulonephritis and progressive, high-frequency hearing loss. A mouse model of this condition was created by targeted deletion of the *col4A3* gene (Cosgrove et al., 1998). Ultrastructural changes in the basement membranes of cochlear epithelia were also noted, as was a modest hearing loss. The cochlear phenotype was therefore less severe in humans than in mice.

Mutations in genes encoding unconventional myosins cause several forms of inherited deafness. Naturally occurring *myosin VIIa* mutations cause Usher syndrome type 1B (Weil et al., 1995) and nonsyndromic deafness (Liu et al., 1997a) in humans, and the *shaker-1* phenotype in mice (Gibson et al., 1995), while a natural mutation in *myosin VI* causes the Snell's waltzer phenotype (Avraham et al., 1995). These mutations were identified by standard gene localization and candidate gene approaches. However, Probst et al. (1998) used a transgenic approach to identify changes in the gene encoding myosin 15 as causing the *shaker-2* mutation. After initial localization of the defect, transenic mice were created using BAC (bacterial artificial chromosome) inserts (which typically range from 100 to 300 kb) from the approximate genomic location. One of these inserts corrected the defect, and was found to include the gene encoding mysoin 15.

The tectorins are proteins involved in the structure of the acellular membranes overlying sensory epithelia in the inner ear, including the tectorial and vestibular membranes. Impaired tectorin protein is associated with autosomal dominant nonsyndromic hearing impairment in humans (Verhoeven et al., 1998). Mice with a targeted deletion in the *tecta* gene are deaf. Their tectorial membranes are detached from the reticular lamina, and the otolithic membranes are severely reduced in extent (Legan et al., 2000).

The gene *otog* encodes otogelin, an N-glycosylated protein in the acellular membranes covering the cochlea, the tectorial membrane, the vestibule, the otoconial membranes, and the cupulae of the semicircular canals. Mice with a deletion of *otog* demonstrate vestibular dysfunction as early as P4 (Simmler et al., 2000). However, the acellular membranes of the vestibule and the tectorial membrane appeared normal. A severe hearing loss in both ears was detected in *Otog–/–* mice. Results indicate that the organization of the fibrillar network and mechanical stability of the tectorial membrane is compromised in the absence of otogelin, and as a result in these mutant animals, the otoconial membranes and cupulae detach from the neuroepithelia. (Simmler et al., 2000)

The netrins are a family of secreted proteins related to laminins. Members of this family are involved in axon guidance and cell migration (Hedgecock and Norris, 1997). In mice, *netrin1* expression is found in the inner ear, and in outpocketings of the otic vessicle that form the semicircular ducts. Expression persists in semicircular ducts in the epithelium until birth. The transcript is also detected in non-sensory areas of the utricle during development. *Netrin-1* mutant mice are marked by complete absence of posterior and lateral semicircular canals. It is possible that netrin 1 is necessary for disruption of the basement membrane and rearrangement of the epithielia of the otocyst, and that loss of this component inhibits the fusion of epithelia that is necessary for the formation of the semicircular ducts (Salminen et al., 2000).

Tenascin is expressed in the developing inner ear, especially in the osseus spiral lamina and organ of Corti. However, *tenascin* knockout mice, (Saga et al., 1992), in which the *lacZ* gene replaces most of the *tenascin* gene, exhibits no abnormalities of the inner ear, and hearing is not altered.

MISCELLANEOUS GENES

Mutations in many other genes have been shown to influence the auditory system. There may be no obvious reason for the auditory phenotype. For example, complete or partial inactivation of

Hdh, which is the mouse cognate of the Huntington's disease gene encoding a presumed *housekeeping* gene, results in CNS abnormalities, but also displacement of the external ear (White et al., 1997).

The cyclin-dependent kinase inhibitor, p27^{kip1}, functions as a cell cycle inhibitor. It is strongly expressed in the primordial organ of Corti. Mice null for this gene possess supernumerary hair cells in the inner and outer rows and suffer from severe hearing impairment (Chen and Segil, 1999).

The *Mos* protooncogene was identified as an oocyte maturation factor in *Xenopus*. In mice, it is expressed in the brain in low levels. Overexpression of the *Mos* protooncogene under the control of a constitutive promoter results in widespread neuropathies, including degeneration of hair cells and spiral ganglion neurons, with resultant deafness (Propst et al., 1990).

The production of free radicals is thought to be an important component of cell damage mechanisms in many systems, including the auditory system. Both glutathione peroxidase and superoxide dismutase (SOD) function as intracellular free radical scavengers. Deletion of either gene increases the sensitivity of the cochlea to noise damage (Salvi et al., 1998; McFadden et al., 2000; Ohlemiller et al., 2000).

The *Mpv17* gene, encoding a peroxisomal membrane protein involved in reactive oxygen metabolism, is expressed in type II fibroblasts of the spiral ligament, which play a critical role in the recirculation of K$^+$ ions from the organ of Corti to the stria vascularis. A null mutation of this gene leads to loss of ion transporter gene expression in these cells, followed by their degeneration. Abnormalities in endolymph composition produce deafness. (Meuller et al., 1997; Schubert et al., 1999).

P-glycoprotein (p-gp) is a drug transporter membrane protein that is restricted to capillary endothelial cells of the brain and inner ear. It acts as an efflux pump to prevent drug-induced ototoxicity. Deletions of the gene encoding this protein lead to higher accumulation of p-gp transported drugs, adriamycin and vinblastin, in the inner ear tissues. (Zhang et al., 2000).

Rab3A is a protein of the presynaptic complex involved in recruitment of synaptic vessicles prior to exocytosis. Mice with a null mutation of the *Rab3A* gene exhibit decreased amplitude of auditory brainstem response to clicks at high repetition rates, suggesting that vessicle recruitment has been hampered in auditory neurons (Durand et al., 1998).

Transgenic Mutations that Do Not Affect the Auditory System

Many transgenic animals are reported that exhibit no detectable abnormalities in auditory structure or function, although the genes involved are expressed in the auditory system. In fact, many gene knockouts have been found to show no phenotype of any kind. However, it should be noted that absence of a detectable phenotype in null mutants does not mean that the gene plays no role in the auditory or any other system. An important consideration is the depth of analysis employed. Few of the transgenic mice created to date have been generated specifically to study the auditory system. In fact, most groups that generate transgenic animals detect an inner ear deficit only when mice exhibit an obvious phenotype such as vestibular dysfunction, or a noticeable defect in auditory morphology prior to birth (the period during which the inner ear is likely to be analyzed, since the size of the head and the need for decalcification exclude the inner ear in most postnatal analysis by non-auditory groups). It is thus quite likely that many induced mutations that affect the auditory system in isolation and in subtle ways have gone unrecognized.

Another issue discussed above is gene redundancy. For example, the POU-domain genes *Brn3.0* and *Brn3.2* are both expressed in the developing ganglia of the inner ear. However, only deletion of *Brn3.0* results in ganglion abnormalities. Detailed analysis of the mutants revealed that *Brn3.0* deletion results in failure of *Brn-3.2* expression in inner ear ganglion cells, creating a functional double-knockout. In contrast, *Brn3.2* deletion does not affect *Brn-3.0* expression by inner ear ganglion cells. Presumably, *Brn-3.0* is able to subserve ganglion development alone. Thus, the inner ear ganglia appear to be rescued by redundancy in one case, but not in the other. It is likely that role of other genes that influence the inner ear are masked by redundancy when they are deleted. This may be revealed when the mutations of related genes are combined.

Another issue of importance is embryonic lethality. Deletion of some genes results in early embryonic or postnatal death, before certain aspects of auditory structural or functional development occur. The role of such genes in the auditory system must be studied by conditional transgenic approaches, as discussed below.

TRANSGENIC ANALYSIS OF GENE EXPRESSION, MUTATIONS, AND DISEASE

Transgenic technology is also employed to study the biological activity of gene regulatory regions using reporter gene strategies. By linking a putative regulatory region (usually the DNA 5′ to the CAP site) to a reporter gene that produces a detectable product such as beta-galactosidase (*lac-Z*) or green fluorescent protein (GFP), the activity of specific regulatory regions can be assessed by comparing transgene expression with endogenouse gene expression. A member of the opioid receptor subfamily of G protein-coupled receptors, the k opioid receptor is an example of such a study. Expression of a transgene that includes the kOR 5′ upstream regulatory region, splicing control and translational signal, driving *lacZ* (Hu et al., 1999). The whole-mount staining of transgenic embryos revealed that *kOR-lacZ* is expressed in the developing ear.

Another example of promoter analysis by transgenic mouse techniques is the study of calcitonin receptor (CTR) promoter (Jagger et al., 1999). CTR is a member of the G protein coupled receptor superfamily that is know to inhibit osteoclast-mediated bone resorption and calcium excretion by the kidney (Friedman and Raisz, 1965). Analysis was done with the CTR promoter fragment driving *lacZ* expression, and results revealed CTR promoter activity in the developing external ear.

A Notch promoter-GFP construct was used to determine the expression patterns of *Notch* in transgenic mice (Lewis et al., 1998). This construct shows low-level expression in mesenchymal tissues of the inner ear, while the other *Notch* forms do not, suggesting that Notch 1 may be involved in the specification of sensory cells of the inner ear. GFP expression is detected in the otic vessicle, facio-acoustic ganglion, and cells migrating into this ganglion. GFP-Notch expression is detected at low levels, later in the sensory epithelia during HC differentiation, and in terminally differentiated hair cells, an unconventional pattern of expression for this receptor (Lewis et al., 1998). These results suggest a very complex mechanism for sensory hair cell differentiation as a result of the complicated expression of multiple Notch ligands within the developing cochlea.

Creation of a *Delta 1:lac Z* knock-in mouse, in the process of creating the *Delta1* knockout discussed above, was used to study the Notch signaling pathway controlling production of sensory hair cells in the mouse inner ear (Morrison, 1999). *lacZ* is expressed in the anteroventral region of the otic vessicle, corresponding to the site where neuroblasts form the VIIIth cranial ganglion, and later in vestibular sensory patches. In the cochlea, expression is restricted to the future inner and OHCs of the organ of Corti. Hair cell-specific expression suggests that Delta 1 might participate in lateral inhibition. However, because (as noted above) the knockout did not affect sensory epithelium morphogenesis, Delta 1 is not required for hair cell/supporting cell differentiation.

The enzyme alcohol dehydrogenase 4 (ADH4), while a poor metabolizer of alcohol, is an efficient retinol dehydrogenase, which is probably its endogenous function. Regulatory sequences from the *ADH4* gene were fused to *lacZ*. The resultant transgenic mice show high levels of expression in the otic vesicle at E9.5 (Haselbeck and Deuster, 1998).

In addition to the use of relatively large promoter constructs to mimic endogenous gene regulation, promoter deletion analysis can be performed in transgenics to identify critical regulatory elements. This is especially useful in tissues for which cell lines are not well developed, such as the inner ear. In addition, promoter function in cell lines can be quite different from that *in vivo*, due to loss of expression of critical transcripion factors during the process of immortalization and passaging. Thus, it is important to verify promoter analysis obtained in cell lines *in vivo* systems such as transgenics. Deletion analysis of several promoters that operate in the auditory system is currently in progress.

Demyelinating diseases lead to widespread neuropathies that can also involve the auditory system. Transgenic mice with intentionally disrupted peripheral myelination show hearing loss and vestibular dysfunction. Expression of diphtheria toxin (Assouline et al., 1994), SV40 large-T antigen (Assouline et al., 1995), or interleukin 3 (Woolf et al., 1997) under the control of a promoter active in Schwann cells produces a similar phenotype consisting of spiral ganglion dendrite and neuron degeneration, with hearing loss. A naturally occurring shiverer mutation, caused by mutation of a myelin subunit, has been corrected by expression of the subunit under the control of a Schwann cell promoter in transgenic mice (Fujiyoshi et al., 1994).

Inactivation of BMP2 and BMP4 is early embryonic lethal. However, inactivation of BMP2/4 signaling was targeted to neural crest cells of the second and more caudal branchial arches by creating animals in which *Xenopus noggin* (*XNoggin*), an inhibitor of signaling by physical interaction (Zimmerman et al., 1996), is driven by an enhancer of the *Hoxa2* gene. These transgenic embryos are missing second arch elements, the stapes, and styloid process, and the oval window is smaller than in normal embryos (Kanzler et al., 2000).

Overexpression of genes can reduce the severity of otologic disorders. Expression of the bacterial *Neo* gene, under the control of a constitutive promoter in transgenic mice, renders the hair cells of these animals resistant to ototoxicity (Dulon et al., 1998). One implication of this finding is that caution must be used in evaluating ototoxicity in transgenic mice. Because the *Neo* and other antibiotic resistance genes are frequently used as positive selection elements in the generation of knockout animals, these animals may be quite different in their sensitivity to certain ototoxins. Overexpression of *superoxide dismutase*, driven by a constitutive promoter, also protects hair cells against ototoxicity (Sha et al., 1997).

FUTURE DIRECTIONS IN TRANSGENIC AUDITORY RESEARCH

As noted above, most transgenic mice have not been generated specifically to study the auditory system. This will change rapidly as more auditory scientists adopt transgenic techniques to develop models that are meant to influence the auditory system in a targeted manner.

The study of auditory structures with transgenic technology can be approached in a variety of ways. For example, a promoter construct derived from a gene that is expressed in specific tissue or cell type, or over a specific period, an auditory structure can be used to limit transgene expression in time and space. Promoters that target gene expression to particular inner ear cell types are under active development in several laboratories. A construct derived from the *Brn3.1* gene drives GFP expression limited to hair cell precursors and in hair cells (Ryan et al., 1998). A drawback of this method is that in some cases the regulatory region may be too large to isolate.

Another means of targeting expression is a gene knock-in, in which the desired coding sequence is substituted for the natural coding sequence of a gene that is expressed in the tissue of interest, as used by Lewis et al. (1998) to study *Delta1* expression in the inner ear. Of course, this method has the drawback that it is sensitive to any haplo-insufficiency effects resulting from deletion of one copy of the target gene. A variant of this method uses homologous recombination to substitute gene coding regions in a BAC construct, which is then used to generate a transgenic mouse. The size of BAC inserts (100 to 300 kb) greatly increases the probability that the relevant regulatory regions are included in the transgene. This method was used by Zuo et al. (1999) to drive GFP expression in hair cells using the $\alpha 9$ promoter.

Targeted deletion of genes can also be accomplished in a tissue-specific manner using Cre-lox recombination. A tissue-specific promoter is used to drive the expression of Cre recombinase in a target tissue or cell population in transgenic mice. Using homologous recombination, the target gene is then flanked by lox sites that are recognized by Cre recombinase. In offspring of crosses between the two strains, the floxed gene is deleted only in cells expressing Cre recombinase. Mice expressing Cre recombinase in auditory tissues are currently under development.

Transgenic techniques also permit the study of a variety of mutations that are more restricted than gene deletions or ectopic expression. A small number of studies utilizing dominant negative function to explore the role of proteins in the auditory system were reviewed above. Studies that exploit our ability to induce very specific mutations in genes will undoubtedly see more common application to the auditory system. For one thing, many additional genes important to the auditory system will be identified, providing targets for intervention. Moreover, the study of such genes will evolve beyond the identification stage, to the study of protein structure/function relationships. Dominant negative and gain-of-function mutations are examples of this approach. However, other mutations within sequences encoding specific domains of proteins will allow quite detailed analysis. For example, transgenics based on mutations of individual phosphorylation sites in signaling molecules will allow quite specific studies of the role of phosphorylation in determining protein function at the cell and systems levels. Similarly, mutations affecting interaction domains can help to dissect the roles of protein/protein and protein/DNA binding.

Finally, the use of inducible promoters in transgenics will further refine our ability to dissect gene function, by allowing transgene sequences to be expressed only during a period of interest. For example, inducible promoters will allow the study of critical periods in development. The cochlea in particular is particularly amenable to this technique, because soluble inducers can be introduced to most cochlear tissues via perilymphatic perfusion.

CONCLUSION

The power of transgenic techniques is increasingly being applied to study the function of genes in the auditory system.

Section V

Murine Models of Diseases or Conditions Affecting the Auditory System

We end the book with chapters focusing on mouse models for a variety of conditions that affect hearing in humans. The application of murine subjects to research on the ubiquitous problem of noise-induced hearing loss is discussed in Chapter 31 (Davis). This is followed by a range of topics including oxygen free radical damage to the ear studied with SOD1 knockout mice (Chapter 32; McFadden, Ding, Ohlemiller, and Salvi), mouse models of immunologic diseases (Chapter 33; Trune), muscular distrophy (Chapte 34; Pillers and Trune), and hypothyroidism (Chapter 35; Walsh and McGee).

Mouse models of Allport's and Usher's syndromes are the topics of Chapter 36 (McGee and Walsh). Chapter 37 (Ohlemiller, Vogler, Daly, and Sands) reviews work on a mouse model of lysosomal storage disease and the potential for treament, while Chapter 38 (Burkard, Durand, Secor, and McFadden) describes research on a mouse with deletion of the RAB-3A gene.

Finally, Chapter 39 (Crenshaw) focuses on mutations of the BRN4/POU3F4 locus.

Many syndromes and conditions affect hearing and the auditory system, but only a portion have been discussed in this final section because it is not feasible to have chapters representing all areas of research in detail. Nonetheless, the array of research topics and approaches presented here provide a nice overview of how various conditions can be explored using mouse models.

31 Noise-Induced Hearing Loss

Rickie R. Davis

INTRODUCTION AND BACKGROUND

Noise has been a universal problem from the time man first put hammer to stone. Our lives have not gotten any quieter. On-the-job hearing loss due to noise is the most common form of occupational injury in the United States. Estimates by the National Institute for Occupational Safety and Health (NIOSH) in the early 1980s estimated that about four million workers were exposed to noise in excess of 85 dBA (NIOSH, 1998). NIOSH calculates that a lifetime exposure to noise in excess of 85 dBA will cause an excess risk of 15% of those workers suffering a disabling hearing loss. With exposure to 90 dBA over a working lifetime, the estimated risk almost doubles to 29%. Current thinking is that every ear is vulnerable to noise — given enough acoustic energy at the right frequency for enough time.

NIOSH (1988) identified noise-induced hearing loss as one of its top ten priorities. In the 1990s, it was again identified as a major public health priority by ASHA (Cherow, 1991). Based on testimony from industry, private organizations, and governmental agencies, the National Occupational Research Agenda (NIOSH, 1996) identified noise-induced hearing loss as a priority area for research.

Hearing loss is common in the general population and appears to be becoming more so (Ries, 1985). With the introduction of high-power audio systems, boom boxes, and car stereos, noise-induced hearing loss is here to stay. Civilian and military firearms use is an important contributor to loss of hearing (Ylikoski, 1994; Prosser et al., 1988).

It is well known among practicing audiologists that all humans are not equally susceptible to the damaging effects of noise. Noise researchers know that noise susceptibility in experimental animals is quite variable (e.g., Cody and Robertson, 1983). The inbred mouse, while still variable from one mouse to another, appears to be less variable within strains. Between strains, the mouse shows great differences in susceptibility to noise as well as differences in prebycusis.

The goal of this chapter is to review mouse noise-induced hearing loss research and speculate about organizing principles. Most noise-induced hearing loss research has not been done in the mouse, but rather in the chinchilla, guinea pig, cat, and even rabbit. In the past 10 years, there has been a renaissance in noise studies in mice. It is believed that mechanisms of noise-induced hearing loss cross species, but exceptions will be noted. For additional background information, the reader is referred a review of the literature on physiological effects of noise-induced hearing loss by Borg, Canlon, and Engstrom (1995).

EQUAL ENERGY HYPOTHESIS

The equal energy hypothesis (EEH) was first proposed by Eldred et al. (1955) and elaborated later by Ward et al. (1958). This hypothesis implies that the ear acts as an integrator of acoustical energy. Hearing loss is equal to the product of accumulated time and acoustic intensity. In addition, time and intensity may be traded. By doubling the exposure time, the noise dose is increased by 3 dB (because decibels are log units, 3 dB represents a doubling of energy; e.g., see Vernon, Katz, and Meikle, 1976). In recent years, the EEH has been shown to be a reasonable first approximation within certain limits of times and energies. However, Henderson's group (Henderson et al., 1991,

Danielson et al., 1991) has shown that once a specific sound level is exceeded, equal energy no longer holds. This appears to be the point at which acoustic energy stops damaging the neural elements of the cochlea, and mechanical damage is being done to the cochlear partition. The equal energy limits for time remain unknown. However, when you begin to think about doubling time, you soon realize that it does not take many doublings to exceed the lifespan of the subject. Thus, time is bounded by the lifespan of the organism. Extremely short, high-level sounds (i.e., impacts and impulses) do not appear to obey the EEH (Henderson et al., 1991).

The EEH has been incorporated into U.S. occupational hearing conservation regulations. However, rather than utilizing 3 dB as the doubling and halving factor for time, 5 dB is used, under the premise that most workers are not exposed to continuous noise over an entire work shift. Rest breaks from sound appear to be more beneficial than one would predict based on the EEH (Price, 1974). For example, Clark et al. (1987) exposed two groups of chinchillas to a 95-dB octave band of noise centered on 500 Hz. A periodic rest group was exposed round-the-clock to 15 minutes of noise and 45 minutes quiet; a continuous group was exposed to 6 hours of continuous noise and 18 hours of quiet. When compared, the periodic rest group had less permanent threshold shift and less cochlear damage than the continuous group, although both groups had equal energy exposures. The effect of rest seems to begin almost immediately after the cessation of the sound (Price, 1976).

CONDITIONING

In some species, daily exposure to loud sound seems to protect the ear from a later, intense sound (Henderson et al., 1996a; Canlon et al., 1988; Canlon and Dagli, 1996). This is the so-called conditioning or toughening (or more recently, priming) effect which can provide 10 to 20 dB of protection against noise. Although demonstrated in the chinchilla, rabbit, gerbil, and guinea pig, some accounts have not been able to demonstrate the conditioning effect in mice (Fowler et al., 1995). In a very complex report, Fowler et al. (1995) exposed groups of CBA/Ca mice to a number of different conditioning paradigms (Table 31.1). They then exposed the mice to a traumatic noise of either 107, 110, or 117 dB for either 6 or 24 hours. They were not able to demonstrate any protective effect due to any of the pre-exposures.

From our experience, the spectral frequency of these exposures may have been too low to damage the mouse ear (R.R. Davis et al., 1994; Fay, 1988; see also Figure 31.2). On the other hand, in the chinchilla, low-frequency conditioning exposures are much more protective for the ear than high-frequency conditioning exposures (Henderson et al., 1996a). A recent article by Yoshida et al. (2000) has demonstrated conditioning in the CBA/CaJ mouse to an 81 dB (for one week) or 89 dB (for 15 minutes) conditioning stimulus consisting of 8-16 kHz octave-band noise. The traumatic noise exposure was 2 hours at 100 dB. The long-term conditioning exposure narrowed the range of frequencies affected by the trauma, while the short-term conditioning reduced peak PTS by 22 dB. This conditioning result is qualitatively different from that seen in other species. Conditioning

TABLE 31.1
Exposure Paradigm and Exposure Levels Used to Attempt Auditory Conditioning in CBA/Ca Mice

Exposure Paradigm	Exposure Level
4.5 kHz centered narrow-band noise 6 h/day for 10 days	86, 91, or 96 dB
Continuous noise 24 h/day for 24 days	80 or 86 dB
1-kHz tone for 10 days	75 dB

From Fowler et al., 1995. With permission.

may be a fruitful area to look at comparative species differences, and the mouse may be a valuable animal model to examine the mechanisms underlying conditioning.

Ohlemiller et al. (1999a; b) have produced a series of papers in C57BL/6J (B6) mice demonstrating hydroxyl free radicals are generated after a 110-dB broadband noise exposure for 1 hour. There is some evidence in chinchillas that points to the basis of conditioning as increases in levels of a protective enzyme (catalase) and scavenger (glutathione) to protect against oxygen free radicals (Jacono et al., 1998). Mice have the same enzyme and scavenger present in the ear and should condition equally well.

Along the same lines, Willott and Turner (1999) have demonstrated a reduction in age-related hearing loss in B6 and DBA/2J strains of mice to a low-level noise exposure (broadband noise bursts, 70 dB 12 h/day; see Chapter 14). These inbred mice strains possess the *Ahl* gene, which accelerates presbycusis (see Chapter 28). Assuming conditioning is acting upon oxygen free radical metabolism in the cochlea, the procedure described by Willott and Turner may be modifying oxygen free radical metabolism affecting aging in the ear.

TTS vs. PTS

The relationship between temporary threshold shift (TTS) and permanent threshold shift (PTS) to noise exposure is still being actively debated. (In some reports, TTS is referred to as *combined threshold shift* or CTS — having both temporary and permanent components.) TTS is an immediate post-exposure increase in auditory threshold which resolves over time, to either pre-exposure threshold levels or to a PTS. PTS is defined as a post-exposure increase in auditory threshold that remains relatively stable over time. The debate centers around whether TTS is an early, reversible form of PTS; or whether TTS and PTS are two separate processes. Most recent evidence points to two separate processes, although the U.S. occupational noise regulations are based on TTS being a predictor of PTS. There is evidence to support the view that TTS may be related to swelling of the VIIIth nerve fibers in the cochlea, perhaps due to neurotransmitter excitotoxicity (Puel et al., 1996), or it may be due to changes in hair cell or stereocilia stiffness (Husbands et al., 1999; Saunders et al., 1986). PTS appears to be due to cell death due to oxygen free-radical production, calcium influx, or mechanical disruption of the hair cell. Much effort and many resources have been expended on the TTS vs. PTS question over the past 40 years. It is a problem awaiting a clever new tool or technique. Recently, Bohne and colleagues (Bohne et al., 1999; Nordmann et al., 2000) have developed a technique in chinchillas allowing for temporal snapshots of cochlear changes in the same subject. This technique uses fixation of one ear immediately after exposure, and recovery and fixation of the second ear a number of days later. This procedure may be of use in teasing out differences between TTS and PTS and may be adaptable to the mouse.

DISADVANTAGES OF THE MOUSE IN STUDYING NIHL

Each species has its advantages and disadvantages as a model of noise-induced hearing loss (NIHL). The major disadvantage of using the mouse for NIHL is the frequency range of its audiogram. First, as the acoustic stimulus climbs above the frequency range of human audition, it becomes difficult to troubleshoot exposure and measurement systems. The experimenter becomes more dependent on test equipment and microphones to solve problems.

Second, the physics of the high-frequency acoustic wave become more complex above 10 to 15 kHz. As the acoustic wavelength becomes shorter, it becomes possible for reflecting sound waves to interfere both constructively and destructively with the main wavefront, producing standing waves (Appendix A).

Third, most equipment readily available off-the-shelf for measuring the auditory brainstem response (ABR) and distortion product otoacoustic emissions (DPOE) is designed to be used on humans. This limits the upper test frequency to 8 kHz (but see Chapter 4).

Finally, calibration at these frequencies becomes a challenge, often with two consecutive measures differing by many dB. Noise bands are easier to calibrate than pure tones, so noise exposures are usually more consistent, while calibrating ABR sources can be frustrating. A statistical approach should be taken. Measurements should be made often enough to get a good sample so that it can be assumed that the mean (or median or mode) is the normal situation. Moreover, the measuring method should be standardized. Five-dB steps are about the smallest ABR increment possible at the higher frequencies. In noise experiments, threshold shifts rather than absolute thresholds are usually the data of interest.

MEASURING NIHL

Generally, noise-induced hearing loss is measured by the ABR, although the cochlear microphonic or N_1 can also be used. The advantage of the ABR is that an animal may be measured a number of times, and this technique is discussed in detail in Chapters 4 and 38. Mice are typically anesthetized in order to obtain clear recordings. Restraint without anesthesia works well in chinchillas and rabbits with indwelling electrodes (Snyder and Salvi, 1994) and reduces complications due to multiple sessions of anesthesia; however this method has proven difficult with mice. Anesthetized mice should have their body temperatures externally supported by a heating pad.

We test using tone pips at 8, 16, and 32 kHz and a click. The 0.1-ms click results seem to be highly correlated with the results from the 8-kHz tone. Tones are tested with an envelope of 1-ms rise time, 1-ms decay time, and 1-ms steady state. The ABR is obtained by averaging 128 to 1024 presentations of the stimulus at 31 presentations per second. We have found that the most noise damage occurs at 16 kHz and have debated omitting other test frequencies to reduce test time but so far continue testing all frequencies. It is possible that maximum damage may occur at different frequencies in other mouse strains.

THRESHOLD CHANGES

In our experience, 1 week after a noise exposure, the mouse still shows a small amount of TTS. By 9 days any PTS predominates. We have seen a 40-dB TTS at 16 kHz measured at day 1 resolve to no measurable PTS at day 30 post-exposure (R.R. Davis et al., 1994). Because the ABR tends to be a rather crude measure of hearing loss, one cannot say that there was *no* PTS, only that none was detectible.

THE EXPOSURE ACOUSTIC STIMULUS

The damaging stimuli most commonly used for mice are tones, octave bands of noise, or broadband noise. Our experience is that exposures in which the stimulus energy is low in the 16-kHz region do not produce significant PTS (Figure 31.2) (R.R. Davis et al., 1994). Calibration of the exposure stimulus is paramount. The accompanying appendix (How We Do It) provides a tutorial for making and measuring sound.

When publishing exposure conditions, broadband exposures should include the spectrum of the exposure stimulus as well as the intensity. It is very difficult to replicate an exposure condition without a graphic description. It is helpful in the case of tonal exposures to indicate the amplitude of any harmonics. Anything unusual about the acoustic environment should be included in the methods section. For example, for long exposures, access to water is required. Sources of water can be water bottles, pieces of potato or apple, pans of water, etc. Each of these objects may interact with the sound field and could be important for replicating an exposure condition.

GENETICS OF NIHL SUSCEPTIBILITY

Although speculated in the human literature for a long time, the genetic basis of susceptibility to NIHL has only recently come under study, probably because an experimental animal model has become available only in the past 5 years. The discovery by Erway et al. (1993a) of a single recessive gene (*Ahl*) in the B6 mouse strain which increased the rate of presbycusis led to our current research. As discussed below and in Chapter 28, *Ahl* in the homozygous condition contributes to increased susceptibility to noise-induced hearing loss (Erway et al., 1996; Davis et al., 1999; Newlander et al., 1995).

Shone et al. (1991a) first showed differences in susceptibility to noise in B6 and CBA/Ca mice but hypothesized those differences were due to the underlying presbycusis. They exposed their mice to 101-dB broadband noise for 45 minutes. Their B6 mice were old enough so that they were already showing high-frequency hearing loss at pre-exposure testing.

Erway et al. (1996) noise exposed four groups of mice with four different genotypes prior to the detection of any presbycusis. C57BL/6J mice (B6) are homozygous for the *Ahl* gene (*Ahl/Ahl*). The CBA/CaJ inbred mouse strain (CB) have wild-type alleles in the corresponding position (+/+). A hybrid was generated from crossbreeding the CBA/CaJ and C57BL6J inbred strain (CB × B6), which are heterozygous at the *Ahl* allele (*Ahl/+*). Finally, a hybrid was generated from crossbreeding the inbred strain B6 with the inbred strain DBA/2J (B6 × DB). DBA/2J mice are known for their loss of hearing very early in life — earlier than even the B6. We hypothesized based on Erway et al. (1993a) that these hybrid offspring are homozygous for *Ahl* (*Ahl/Ahl*). Mice were exposed to 110 dB of broadband noise for 1 hour and tested at various times after exposure. There was a statistically significant difference between the two genotypes: the CB and CB×B6 strains showed no NIHL, and B6 and B6 × DB strains did show NIHL. This indicated that mice homozygous at the *Ahl* locus were more susceptible to noise than wild-type or heterozygotes.

Newlander et al. (1995) and Davis et al. (2001) were able to show in backcross mice that the *Ahl* gene followed Mendelian laws of genetics. In the parent generation, C57 mice were bred with CBA/CaJ mice. The resulting F1 generation mice (CB × B6) all have the *Ahl/+* genotype. These F1 hybrids are then back-bred to the inbred C57 stock. This backcross generation now had 50% of offspring with the *Ahl/+* genotype and 50% with the *Ahl/Ahl* genotype. Noise exposures were made in the backcross generation mice to define their phenotype. DNA markers for specific alleles defined their genotype. Newlander et al. (1995) were able to demonstrate a high level of predictability of noise susceptibility for certain DNA markers (presumably the *Ahl/Ahl* genotype). This is a strong logical argument that the changes seen in noise susceptibility are modulated by this gene. Due to hybrid vigor, these backcross mice required significantly greater noise exposures than the inbred strains (Table 31.2).

Davis et al. (1999) exposed groups of CB and B6 mice to increasing levels of noise (Table 31.2 and Figure 31.1) to produce a dose-response curve for the two strains. B6 mice were about 6 dB more sensitive to noise, and the slope of their dose-response curve was shallower than the dose-response curve for CB. It was speculated that the B6 mouse ears were being damaged through metabolic mechanisms, while the CB mouse ears were being damaged through direct acoustic trauma.

It now appears that the *Ahl* gene is present in a number of strains exhibiting early presbycusis (Q.Y. Zheng et al., 1999a; b). These strains include but are not limited to DBA/2J, BUB/BnJ, NOD/LtJ, A/J, and SKH2/J. Johnson and colleagues (see Chapter 28) mapped the *Ahl* gene to the inbred strains 129/ReJ, A/J, BALB/cByJ, BUB/BnJ, C57BRLtJ, DBA/2J, NOD/LtJ, SKH/2J, and STOCK760. They were able to demonstrate age-related hearing loss in 50% of offspring in a backcross generation, indicating a recessive gene.

Q.Y. Zheng et al. (1999b) cataloged 80 inbred mouse strains (see Chapter 28), and this should provide fertile ground for discovering other mouse strains that are highly susceptible to NIHL. For

TABLE 31.2
Exposure Parameters for Some Noise Studies in Mice

Authors	Strains	Stimuli[a]	Results	Notes
Davis et al., 1999	C57BL/6J and CBA/CaJ	BBN 1–30kHz 0, 98, 101, 104, 107, 110, 113, 116, and 119 dB, 1 h	Two noise dose-response curves	Exposed awake
Davis, Shiau, and Erway, 1994	CBA/CaJ × C57BL/6J and C57BL/6J	BBN 1–30kHz 110 dB, 1 h vs. BBN 7–24kHz, 110 dB, 1h	Low-freq. exposure produced TTS but not PTS; high-freq. produced equal TTS and significant PTS	Exposed awake
Henry, 1982b	CBA/J, AUS/sJ and SJL/J	Octave band 12–24 kHz, 124 dB, 5 min.	15–50 dB PTS depending on age and strain	Exposed awake, 3 inbred strains
Li and Borg, 1992a	CBA/Ca and C57BL/6J	BBN 2–7 kHz, 120 dB, 5 min	C57BL/6J more susceptible	Exposed anesthetized
Newlander et al., 1995; Davis et al., 2001	C57BL/6J × (C57BL/6J × CBA/J)	BBN 1–30 kHz 110 dB 8 h	Separated phenotypes into two groups	Exposed away, hybrid vigor
Ohlemiller, Wright, and Dugan, 1999	C57BL/6J	BBN 4–45 kHz, 110 dB 1h	Oxygen free radicals measured in perilymph	Exposed awake(?)
Shone et al., 1991a	CBA/Ca and C57BL/6	BBN 500–40 KHz, 101 dB, 45 min	30–35 dB TTS, 17 dB PTS in B6, 0 dB PTS in CB	Exposed awake, no hair cell differences between groups
Yanz et al., 1985	C56BL6J wild-type and albino	BBN 3.8–16 kHz, 125 dB, 10 min	20–52 dB PTS	Exposed awake, only measured to 8 kHz; no difference between albino and wild-type
Yoshida et al., 2000	CBA/CaJ and 129/SvEv	Octave band 8–16 kHz, 97 dB, 2 h; 100 dB, 2h; 103 dB, 2h; 103 dB, 8h; 106 dB, 8h	129/SvEv shows less damage than CBA/CaJ	Exposed awake measured via compound action pot and DPOE

[a] BBN = broadband noise.

example, it would be worthwhile to determine if NIHL susceptibility and age-related hearing loss are truly coupled. Of 19 strains that have late-onset hearing loss, only B6 has been studied for NIHL.

Yoshida et al. (2000) reported that the inbred strain 129/SvEv is much less sensitive to noise damage than the inbred strain CBA/CaJ. They exposed young mice to 97 to 106 dB for 2 to 8 hours (Table 31.2) and incorporated a slow onset of noise to prevent sensitive 129/SvEv mice from developing autogenic seizures. They were able to demonstrate that the differences between the strains were due to the inner ear and not middle ear transmission of vibration. This is a puzzling result because Johnson et al. (2000) listed a closely related substrain, 129/ReJ, as mapping the *Ahl* gene. Q.Y. Zheng et al. (1999b) also showed that 129/ReJ demonstrates early presbycusis. Yoshida et al. speculated that perhaps age-related hearing loss and susceptibility to noise-induced hearing loss may not be linked. Based on Newlander's data, this would require two closely linked genes on chromosome 10: one encoding susceptibility to AHL, the other encoding susceptibility to NIHL.

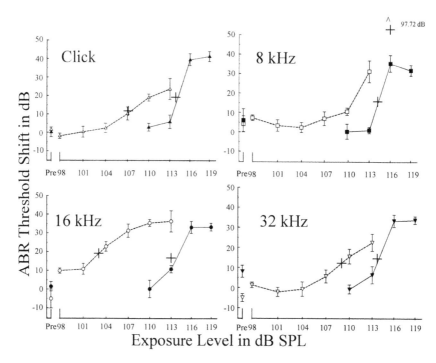

FIGURE 31.1 Dose-response curves for noise effects on ABR threshold. Open symbols are B6 data, filled symbols are CB data. Left-most points on all graphs are unexposed control levels. Each point represents the mean ABR threshold shift of one group of mice exposed to one noise level once, recorded 2 weeks after exposure. Each individual graph represents a different ABR test frequency. The cross represents the inflection point for each curve — the half effect point. Error bars indicate standard error. From Davis et al., 1999, with permission.

OTHER FACTORS AFFECTING NOISE SUSCEPTIBILITY

There are other agents that interact with noise to produce increased susceptibility to hearing loss. The following are some of the more commonly studied variables, a number of which have been studied in mice.

SEX

Although we routinely include sex as part of our analysis model, a statistically significant effect of gender has not yet been found in mice. However, others using chinchillas have seen a difference in susceptibility to noise between males and females, depending on the test frequency. McFadden et al. (1999d) showed a significant difference in auditory threshold between males and females prior to impulse noise exposure and a significant difference in hearing loss between sexes after exposure. The female chinchillas had about 10 dB more loss in the high frequencies and 5 dB less loss in the low frequencies than males.

Q.Y. Zheng et al. (1999b) statistically tested the thresholds measured in their mice and found no differences between males and females for any of the strains showing congenital or age-related hearing loss.

Although there are many confounding factors, human males tend to show hearing loss in excess of their female counterparts. They also tend to engage in noisier activities.

ANESTHETIZED VS. UNANESTHETIZED

There are advantages to using an anesthetized animal for noise-exposure studies. First, the stimulus can be introduced into the animal's ear canal with a minimum of variation. Sleeping animals do not change orientation, cover ears, or locate acoustic nulls in their environment. Second, monaural exposures can be done with the unexposed ear serving as a within-subject control. Third, a major physiological or surgical manipulation may require the subject to be anesthetized. However, whenever the animal is anesthetized, a non-physiological subject is being used. Anesthetic agents can alter breathing, blood pressure, and the ability to maintain body temperature (J.N. Brown et al., 1988). There may be changes in middle ear muscle activity and ventilation. Also, neurological activity changes with reduction in protective mechanisms, including middle ear muscles. In guinea pigs, noise exposure during anesthesia leads to *less* TTS than in awake subjects (Hildesheimer et al., 1991). However, if body temperature is maintained, TTS is about 11 dB *greater* in the anesthetized guinea pigs. This may be an interesting area of inquiry for mouse researchers.

BODY TEMPERATURE

Physiological systems operate best at normal body temperature for the species. Some animal data have indicated that lowering the subject's body temperature makes them less vulnerable to noise (e.g., Hildesheimer et al., 1991). There are also some human data indicating that working in hot environments increases vulnerability to noise (Pekkarinen, 1995).

OTOTOXIC AGENTS

It has been known for at least 20 years that the aminoglycoside antibiotics (i.e., kanamycin, neomycin, streptomycin, gentamicin, and amikacin) interact with noise in guinea pigs to increase noise-induced hearing loss (Brown et al., 1980; Brummett et al., 1992). It appears that asphyxiates such as carbon monoxide also act to increase the damaging effect of noise in rats (Young et al., 1987; Fechter et al., 1988b; Chen and Fechter, 1999; G.D. Chen et al., 1999). In rats and mice, industrial solvents such as toluene have been shown to interact with noise (Johnson and Canlon, 1994; Li, 1992b). Ototoxins that do not appear to interact with noise include loop-inhibiting diuretics (ethacrynic acid and furosemide; Vernon et al., 1977) and aspirin (sodium salicylate; Spongr et al., 1992).

PIGMENTATION

Conlee et al. (1986) and Creel (1980) have proposed that true albino rats and mice are more vulnerable to noise damage because they lack melanin in the stria vascularis of the cochlea. Some researchers have demonstrated a difference in hearing level between human races based on skin pigment. Members of dark-skinned races have greater hearing sensitivity than members of light-skinned races. Others discount this finding as a difference in recreational activity — suggesting that whites are more often involved in hunting and other noisy activities (Clark and Bohl, 1996). In probably the best test of this question to date, Yanz et al. (1985) exposed wild-type B6 and c-locus albino C57BL/6J(c^{2j}/c^{2j}) mice to 10 minutes of a 125-dB broadband noise. These inbred strains differed only in the absence or presence of tyrosinase. They found no difference between groups but only tested their mice to 8 kHz, which is not the most sensitive frequency for mice. Also, B6 mice tend to be sensitive to the traumatic effects of noise (Davis et al., 1999). A lower intensity exposure might have been able to separate the phenotypes. There are other, better models of albinism (e.g., CBA/J-Tyr[c-11J] strain) for hearing that might help to clarify the issue.

Until this controversy has been settled, it is probably better to use strains with the same amount of pigmentation for comparisons — either all albino or all pigmented. Care must be exercised in testing the effects of pigmentation in mice; although some strains are pigmented and others not, there are significant genetic and physiologic differences between inbred strains other than coat color.

AGE

Numerous papers have been written on aging in the mouse auditory system (Chapters 24 and 28). The average laboratory mouse lives to about 2 years. Henry (1982b) exposed three mouse strains

(Table 31.2) to noise at 20, 180, and 360 days. He found strain differences in susceptibility to the damaging effects of the noise. In addition, the younger mice were more sensitive to the noise than the older animals. Results of coat color were opposite to that predicted for melanin: the albino strain was least sensitive to noise, the agouti was intermediate, and the black strain was the most sensitive to noise.

FUTURE DIRECTIONS

The mouse is the premier subject for mammalian genetic studies and will be the basis for numerous future projects investigating the role of genes and noise susceptibility. The National Institute on Deafness and Other Communication Disorders has encouraged the use of inbred mice to study diseases of the ear and hearing. Some interesting topics include the following.

FREE-RADICAL SCAVENGERS AND SUSCEPTIBILITY

Free radicals have been implicated in hearing damage. Ototoxic and noise damage seem to be modulated, if not directly caused, by oxygen free radicals. It would be very useful to understand the mechanisms of free-radical generation, damage and repair, if any, in the ear. Very little is known about repair mechanisms in the organ of Corti.

One problem with hearing research in the mouse — and all animals for that matter — concerns the tools for detecting damage. The ABR, DPOE, behavioral audiogram, and even microscopy are all very gross techniques. Often, these tools do not agree well with one another. It would be very useful to have a much finer-grained tool for detecting cochlear changes. This would permit the study of noise exposures in the 80 to 95 dB range — the range normally encountered on the job. There is some evidence that the transient otoacoustic emission may be more useful for detecting organ of Corti changes. Histochemical and immunological techniques should be developed to probe subtle changes in hair cell physiology.

AGE-RELATED HEARING LOSS AND NOISE SUSCEPTIBILITY

At this time, it appears that mice with an increased susceptibility to age-related hearing loss are also more susceptible to noise-induced hearing loss. This question needs to be explored in greater detail. Is an ear susceptible to presbycusis also more susceptible to noise, or just more vulnerable to *any* trauma? Is presbycusis a form of cumulative noise damage? Are some ears predestined to die early in life? How can susceptible ears be rescued? For this effort, it would be very useful to discover an inbred mouse strain that *exhibits presbycusis* but does not map for the *Ahl* gene. Yoshida et al. (2000) report that inbred strain 129/SvEv is not as susceptible to noise as CBA/CaJ.

Also, how do changes in the mitochondrial genome affect noise susceptibility?

GENE THERAPY FOR SUSCEPTIBLE INDIVIDUALS

If single genes can be associated with noise-induced hearing loss, it may be reasonable to contemplate the modification of these genes. Although the current costs of such procedures are prohibitive, one cannot predict what the future prices may be. These gene modifications should first be tried on mice susceptible to noise and presbycusis.

We are probably living in the golden age of ear research. We are beginning to understand how it is built and how it works. The mouse provides numerous models for abnormal development and functioning. The mouse also provides a unique model for learning about the pathology of the ear due to noise, genetics, and chemical agents.

ACKNOWLEDGMENTS

Thanks to my collaborators at the University of Cincinnati: Lawrence C. Erway, J. Kelly Newlander, Michael L. Cheever, and Yea-Wen (Wendy) Shiau. And to my NIOSH collaborators: Ed Krieg, Bill Murphy, and John Franks.

APPENDIX A: HOW WE DO IT

Making Noise

Procurement

The researcher in noise-induced hearing loss often finds the most suitable acoustic generating equipment at the professional audio store (i.e., the same place local rock-and-roll bands purchase or lease their equipment). That is because to obtain the levels of noise necessary, without distortion, requires many watts of electrical energy. Generally, a minimum audio amplifier will be 300 watts.

Speakers

The weakest link in the chain is speakers. Tweeters and super-tweeters are used to produce the frequencies necessary for mouse or rat exposures. The ideal speaker should respond linearly up to an output of about 130 dB, require less than 100 watts of drive, should be inexpensive, and should be available at the local electronics store. Unfortunately, this speaker has not yet been invented (or if it has, no one has told this author). Because of the physics of their high-frequency response, tweeters must have minimum mass. This implies thin diaphragms and thin wire voice coils. As the driving force increases, the thin wire starts to heat up like an incandescent lamp and eventually opens.

We have used a number of speakers. Our chinchilla work utilized Altec-Lansing 504 high-frequency drivers with horns. However, unless high-pass filtered, most of the noise energy is located in the frequencies below those effective for mouse hearing (Figure 31.2) (R.R. Davis et al., 1994). In fact, Altec-Lansing has discontinued this line of driver but does provide replacement voice coils. Radio Shack has the Realistic 1310B Supertweeter (Ft. Worth, TX), which currently costs about U.S. $20.00 each. They can be purchased at the local Radio Shack store or ordered in bulk from their toll-free number or Web page. We remove them from their plastic case and install them in a sheet of plywood that fits over the exposure chamber, four speakers per chamber. They are wired two in a series, then two series in parallel, so that the effective impedance is still 8 ohms. We utilize the factory-provided high-pass filter to keep DC and low frequencies off of the voice coils. Using an acoustic foam-lined exposure chamber (Davis and Franks, 1989), we can comfortably produce 116 dB for over 8 hours. With the foam out and a more reflective situation, we can easily produce over 120 dB. Going above that level requires some experimentation. We have found that placing heat sinks on the voice coil housing during exposure allows us a few more dB before speakers are damaged.

For one experiment, we were called upon to produce an octave band of noise centered on 20 kHz. We found that the Radio Shack supertweeters were not able to produce much effective output at these high frequencies. We resorted to using piezoelectric Motorola Bullet Supertweeters. We have not found them very useful for everyday use, but they are great at higher frequencies. Our impression is that the piezoelectrics do not appear to be as capable of surviving a short bout of being overdriven as voice-coil speakers. Motorola makes a piezoelectric driver/horn assembly that is rated at 400 watts (Powerline®). However, we have found that this driver still tops out at 110 dB, and more power does not result in more acoustic output. The piezoelectrics are very high impedance (2000 to 4000 ohms). This is often problematic for power amplifiers that are designed to drive 1 to

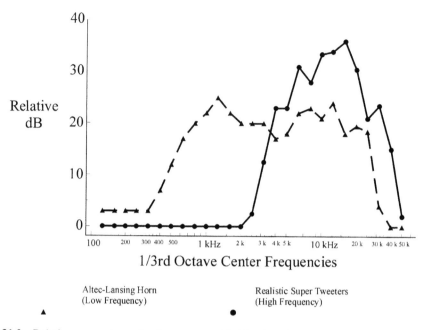

FIGURE 31.2 Relative comparison of noise spectra with Altec-Lansing 504 High Frequency Drivers (producing a broader, lower frequency) and Realistic 1310B Supertweeters (producing a narrower, higher frequency). Initial attempts at noise exposing CBA/CaJ and C57BL/6J strains with the Altec-Lansing speakers resulted in 40-dB TTS, which resolved into no measurable PTS. Mouse ears are sensitive to the acoustic energy present at 16 kHz. Our laboratory currently uses the Realistic Supertweeters in a four-speaker array wired in a series-parallel configuration to develop 8 ohms of load. The standard 5-kHz high-pass filter is maintained. (Adapted from Davis et al., 1994.)

16 ohms. Many power amplifiers are able to produce greater wattage the lower the load impedance, so they are unable to acceptably drive piezoelectrics.

Noise

Our signal source is an old General Radio 1382 Random Noise Generator. These can be purchased on the secondary equipment market (Tucker Electronics, Tucker, TX). We have had some experience with the Tucker Davis Technologies (Gainesville, FL) Noise Generators, along with programmable filters and headphone amplifiers as a noise source and they are viable.

We then control the signal with Wavetek turret attenuators in 1-dB steps. The signal is then passed into a Mackie 1202 pre-amplifier, usually utilized in the unity gain mode, although sometimes used to add a few dB of gain. We moved to the Mackie 1202 after we had a number of failures of our power amplifier. We decided that impedance mismatches in the signal path were causing problems. The Mackie, in effect, acts as an impedance match between the signal level equipment and the power amplifier.

The Physical Surround

At higher frequencies, the short-wavelength acoustic signal reflecting off of a flat, hard surface can result in standing waves. Standing waves result in nulls and peak intensity levels that can allow the subject to be exposed in unpredictable ways. Generally, an absorptive chamber should be used for exposure. This reduces standing waves. A broadband noise source is not as likely to generate noticeable standing waves as tonal sources.

Care should be taken to ensure that subjects are at least 1/4 wavelength from any reflective surface. Cages should be on short legs to boost them up from flooring material. Also, cages should be made of wires or tubing that is less than 1/4 wavelength in diameter. Trays to catch feces and urine should be avoided. We use plastic-backed absorbent paper to catch droppings. Monitoring microphones should be about the same height off the chamber floor as the mouse ears.

To reduce stress, apple or potato slices, or water bottles can be placed in the cage as sources of water. Although this reduces the homogeneity of the sound field, it may be required to maintain animal health.

Depending on the quality and quantity of the power available, an uninterruptable power source may be recommended. This will allow the exposure to continue even if the power should fail.

Pilot Studies

Although hours can be devoted to planning an exposure, the best way to discover errors in logic and hardware is to pilot test. We often pilot test exposure setups overnight without subjects. If a system will survive a 12- or 18-hour run, it will survive a shorter 2-, 4-, or 8-hour run the next day. The most likely element to fail is a speaker; thus, backups should be available.

A short pilot run with subjects, if possible, will indicate whether the exposures are producing the amount of TTS and PTS desired. Every effort should be taken to ensure that these pilot subjects are similar to one's study animals. It appears that every new strain requires some effort to generate acceptable levels of PTS. We usually start out with around a 110-dB 1-hour exposure and adjust from there. Usually, it is better to double the exposure (i.e., increase levels by +3 dB or double time) or quadruple the exposure (i.e., +6 dB or quadruple the time) as necessary.

Also, care should be taken not saturate the mouse's ear. For example, one is exposing two strains of mice to 125 dB for an hour; and upon completion, the TTS and PTS are similar in both groups. An additional group or two at some lower exposure intensities may reveal some interesting differences between the two strains. There is a level below which neither strain will show a PTS, and there is an upper level at which both strains will show maximum PTS. To demonstrate no differences between the strains, one must look at exposure levels between those extremes.

32 The Role of Superoxide Dismutase in Age-Related and Noise-Induced Hearing Loss: Clues from SOD1 Knockout Mice

Sandra L. McFadden, Dalian Ding, Kevin Ohlemiller, and Richard J. Salvi

INTRODUCTION

The two most common causes of hearing loss in adults are (1) acoustic overexposure, resulting in noise-induced hearing loss (NIHL), and (2) age-related cochlear degeneration, resulting in age-related hearing loss (AHL), or presbycusis. The mechanisms underlying NIHL and AHL are not well understood. However, recent investigations implicate a common etiological factor in NIHL and AHL: an imbalance between levels of reactive oxygen species (ROS) produced during cellular metabolism, and the body's defenses against them. Produced in excess of the body's ability to remove them, ROS can cause extensive cellular damage. One important ROS is the superoxide radical ($\cdot O_2^-$). Superoxide has many important functions in the body, but it can also be cytotoxic under certain conditions (Halliwell and Gutteridge, 1999). In addition, $\cdot O_2^-$ can be easily converted to other ROS that have greater potential for causing cellular damage, such as peroxynitrite (ONOO–) and the extremely reactive hydroxyl ($\cdot OH$) free radical molecule. Superoxide dismutase (SOD), an antioxidant enzyme present in virtually every cell of the body, plays a crucial role in regulating $\cdot O_2^-$ levels. An imbalance between $\cdot O_2^-$ generation and SOD availability would be expected to have serious consequences for cellular function and survival. We have been exploring the effects of such an imbalance on AHL and NIHL, using mutant mice with a targeted deletion of *Sod1*, the gene that codes for one copper/zinc isoform of SOD, Cu/Zn SOD, or SOD1. Our experiments with *Sod1* knockout mice (129/CD1-*Sod1*^{tm1Cep}) have provided us with insights into possible chemical pathways underlying NIHL and AHL.

Before describing our experiments with *Sod1* knockout mice, it may be useful to provide a broad overview of ROS and cellular defenses against them. What are ROS and how are they generated? What do they do, and when are they harmful? How are ROS levels normally regulated in the body?

ROS AND CELLULAR DEFENSES AGAINST THEM

WHAT ARE ROS?

The term "reactive oxygen species" refers to a large class of oxygen-containing chemicals that are either free radicals (i.e., atoms, ions, or molecules with one or more unpaired electrons) or non-radical molecules with oxidizing properties. (Note: The chemical term "oxidation" refers to the

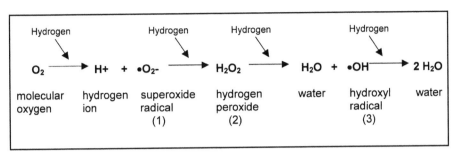

FIGURE 32.1   Formation of three oxygen intermediates during the univalent reduction of oxygen to water.

loss of electrons. Its counterpart is "reduction," i.e., the gain of electrons. A "reducing agent" donates electrons to an "oxidizing agent." Conversely, an oxidizing agent accepts electrons from a reducing agent. Reduced molecules are energy-rich, and they release their energy when they are oxidized.) Examples of common ROS produced in the human body include the free radicals $\cdot O_2^-$ and $\cdot OH$, and the non-radicals hydrogen peroxide (H_2O_2) and ONOO–. Free radicals are denoted by a dot in their chemical formula, preferably located next to the element with the unpaired electron.

How Are ROS Formed?

ROS are formed in a variety of ways *in vivo*. A major source of $\cdot O_2^-$ is the activity of electron transport chains during the coupled processes of cellular respiration and oxidative phosphorylation. (Note: Cellular respiration is a step-wise catabolic process whereby organic food molecules, such as glucose, are oxidized to carbon dioxide and water. The energy released during respiration is used by mitochondria to form energy-rich molecules of ATP in the anabolic process, oxidative phosphorylation.) Some electrons passing through the respiratory chains "leak" from intermediate electron carriers onto molecular oxygen (O_2) to form $\cdot O_2^-$. Figure 32.1 illustrates the process of ROS generation during the step-wise reduction of O_2 to water (H_2O) (a simplified version of cellular respiration). Each successive univalent reduction creates a different reactive oxygen intermediate: first superoxide, then hydrogen peroxide, then hydroxyl. The greater the metabolic activity of the cell, the more ROS it will produce.

Superoxide is also generated through basic chemical reactions in the body, including the oxidation of thiols (sulfur-containing compounds such as cysteine, methionine, and glutathione), the activity of various enzymes (e.g., xanthine oxidase and cytochrome P450, myeloperoxidase), and the auto-oxidation of biomolecules such as catecholamines and hemoglobin. The body typically produces more than 2 kg of $\cdot O_2^-$ per year; $\cdot O_2^-$ production can be increased as a result of heavy exercise, certain drugs and toxins, infections, and various disease states (Evans and Halliwell, 1999). $\cdot O_2^-$ production is also increased during the reperfusion phase of ischemia/reperfusion. The burst of ROS during reperfusion is now thought to be a major source of damage in ischemic episodes (Halliwell, 1992) and noise trauma (Yamane et al., 1995a; b).

Table 32.1 shows several ways in which $\cdot O_2^-$ participates in the formation of other ROS. The formation of the hydroxyl radical is particularly important to consider, because $\cdot OH$ is one of the most aggressive and dangerous radicals known. $\cdot O_2^-$ can be a substrate in the formation of $\cdot OH$ from H_2O_2 in Haber-Weiss reactions (Table 32.1). More importantly, it can facilitate Fenton reactions, in which transition metal ions (i.e., metal ions with one or more unpaired electrons) catalyze the formation of $\cdot OH$ from H_2O_2. $\cdot O_2^-$ facilitates Fenton reactions by liberating iron from iron-sulfur clusters (Keyer et al., 1995; Keyer and Imlay, 1996), and by acting as an electron donor to reduce ferric iron back to ferrous iron, in effect "recycling" it to participate in more $\cdot OH$ generation. The recycling of iron by $\cdot O_2^-$ enables trace levels of iron to catalyze the formation of large quantities of $\cdot OH$. Other heavy metals ions, such as copper and platinum ions, can also take part in Fenton

TABLE 32.1
Formation of Other ROS from Superoxide ($\cdot O_2^-$)
(ROS are listed in order of increasing chemical reactivity)

ROS (Chemical Formula)	Reaction Involving $\cdot O_2^-$
Hydrogen peroxide (H_2O_2)	$2 \cdot O_2^- + 2H^+ \rightarrow H_2O_2 + O_2$ (spontaneous dismutation)
	SOD $\curvearrowright$
	$2 \cdot O_2^- + 2H^+ \rightarrow H_2O_2 + O_2$ (catalyzed dismutation)
Peroxynitrite (ONOO–)	$\cdot O_2^- + NO \rightarrow ONOO-$
Hydroxyl radical ($\cdot OH$)	$\cdot O_2^- + H_2O_2 \rightarrow O_2 + \cdot OH + OH^-$ (Haber-Weiss reaction)
	$\cdot O_2^- + Fe^{3+} \rightarrow O_2 + Fe^{2+}$ $Fe^{2+} + H_2O_2 \rightarrow Fe^{3+} + OH- + \cdot OH$ (Fenton reaction)
	$\cdot O_2^- + HOCl \rightarrow \cdot OH + Cl^- + O_2$

reactions. Thus, intracellular levels of free heavy metal "radicals" are extremely important in determining how much $\cdot OH$ is produced from $\cdot O_2^-$ and H_2O_2.

WHAT DO ROS DO?

Many ROS perform useful functions in the body, such as regulating vascular tone, acting as intra- and intercellular signaling molecules, promoting cell proliferation, and acting as antimicrobial and antiparasitic agents (Babior, 1999; Crawford, 1999; Gutteridge and Halliwell, 1999). For example, activated phagocytes (e.g., monocytes, neutrophils, eosinophils, and macrophages) produce $\cdot O_2^-$ which plays a role in killing engulfed bacteria. Neutrophils also use the enzyme myeloperoxidase to catalyze the formation of hypochlorous acid (HOCl) from chloride (Cl$^-$) and H_2O_2 (formed from $\cdot O_2^-$; see Table 32.1). HOCl, commonly known as bleach, is a powerful bacteriocidal agent that neutrophils use against foreign invaders.

The useful functions of ROS derive from their ability to react rapidly with appropriate chemical substrates. Unfortunately, this same chemical reactivity, when directed indiscriminately at inappropriate targets, can result in harmful effects as well. $\cdot O_2^-$ is capable of decreasing the activity of many enzymes (Gutteridge and Halliwell, 1999; Halliwell and Gutteridge, 1999; McCord and Russell, 1988; Zhang et al., 1990), including enzymes of the electron transport chain in mitochondria (e.g., NADH dehydrogenase, NADH oxidase, and succinate dehydrogenase), antioxidant enzymes (e.g., catalase and glutathione peroxidase), and enzymes that contain or depend on sulfhydryls (e.g., glutamic acid decarboxylase, acetylcholinesterase, and Na,K-ATPase). As shown in Table 32.1, $\cdot O_2^-$ can also be converted to more reactive ROS. For example, $\cdot O_2^-$ reacts at an extremely fast rate at physiological pH with nitric oxide ($\cdot NO$) to generate ONOO–, which can produce cell damage directly by oxidizing lipids, proteins, and DNA. Presumably, ONOO– can also act indirectly, by decomposing to form other toxic ROS such as $\cdot OH$. However, the extent to which decomposition of ONOO– is a physiologically relevant pathway for $\cdot OH$ production is currently a matter of debate.

There is a wide range of reactivity among ROS. Superoxide is one of the least reactive species. Its negative charge inhibits movement across membranes, and it reacts rapidly with only a few molecules, such as $\cdot$NO. The protonated form of $\cdot O_2^-$, the hydroperoxyl radical ($HO_2\cdot$), exists in equilibrium with $\cdot O_2^-$ at physiological pH and is favored at more acidic pH. $HO_2\cdot$ is slightly more reactive than $\cdot O_2^-$; it can cross membranes and initiate lipid peroxidation directly (Halliwell and Gutteridge, 1999). ROS such as ONOO– have intermediate chemical reactivity. $\cdot$OH is at the extreme end of the reactivity spectrum. It will react almost instantaneously with any substance (DNA, proteins, lipids, and carbohydrates) near its site of generation. $\cdot$OH reacts by addition to unsaturated bonds, hydrogen abstraction, and electron transfer. When $\cdot$OH reacts with other biological molecules, most of which are non-radicals, it can initiate and propagate chain reactions that lead to extensive cell and membrane damage.

One of the best characterized chain reactions initiated and propagated by ROS is lipid peroxidation. This occurs when an initiator, often $\cdot$OH, interacts with the polyunsaturated fatty acid side chains of membrane phospholipids. The $\cdot$OH abstracts a hydrogen atom from one of the carbon atoms in the fatty acid side chain to form water, leaving a carbon-centered radical behind in the membrane. The carbon-centered radical can have various fates, the most common one being the formation of yet another ROS, the peroxyl radical ($RO_2\cdot$; e.g., $LipidO_2\cdot$, $HO_2\cdot$), that continues the lipid peroxidation chain reaction. Peroxyl radicals also attack membrane proteins (including receptors and membrane-bound enzymes), oxidize cholesterol, and modify DNA (Evans and Halliwell, 1999). Through this type of chemical cascade, one molecule of $\cdot$OH can result in the conversion of many hundred fatty acid side chains into membrane-disrupting lipid hydroperoxides ($LipidO_2H$). The lipid hydroperoxides accumulate in the membrane, destabilizing it and causing ion leakage. They can also decompose into cytotoxic by-products such as aldehydes (e.g., malondialdehyde) which, like $RO_2\cdot$, can damage membrane proteins directly. To make matters worse, lipid peroxidation is enhanced in the presence of transition metal ions such as iron or copper, primarily because the metal ions can catalyze the decomposition of $LipidO_2H$ into $LipidO_2\cdot$.

Lipid peroxidation is only one example of the damage that can be caused by ROS. ROS can also induce protein oxidation, attack DNA and disrupt protein synthesis, alter cytoskeletal components, disrupt ionic balance, interfere with cellular signaling and calcium homeostasis, and damage DNA repair and transcription processes (Adams et al., 1996; Halliwell, 1992; Orrenius and Nicotera, 1994). Oxidative stress can also trigger the generation of excitatory amino acids such as glutamate, leading to excitotoxic damage to neurons.

What Defenses Do Cells Have Against ROS?

Given the potential harm caused by ROS, it is not surprising that the body maintains a complex set of defenses against them. These defenses include agents that (1) sequester or bind free metal ions that stimulate ROS formation or convert less reactive species to more reactive ones (see Fenton reaction in Table 32.1); (2) help repair DNA, proteins, and membranes after they are damaged; and (3) either prevent the formation of ROS or scavenge them once they are formed. Antioxidants of the defense system include "chain-breaking" molecules such as vitamin C, vitamin E, and reduced glutathione (GSH) that inhibit lipid and protein peroxidation chain reactions by donating either an electron or a hydrogen atom to cellular components after they have been oxidized by ROS. Antioxidants also include enzymes that remove ROS after they are formed, such as SOD and glutathione peroxidase (GPx). SOD and GPx are located in the cytosol and mitochondria of virtually all cells. They work together to regulate levels of $\cdot O_2^-$, H_2O_2, and $\cdot$OH. SOD removes $\cdot O_2^-$ through a dismutation reaction in which one $\cdot O_2^-$ is oxidized to molecular oxygen, and another is reduced to H_2O_2. (Note: dismutation is defined as a chemical reaction in which the same species is both oxidized and reduced.) Although $\cdot O_2^-$ dismutation also occurs in the absence of SOD (see Table 32.1), the rate of non-enzymatic dismutation is approximately four orders of magnitude less than the SOD-catalyzed reaction at pH 7.4. GPx removes H_2O_2 created by $\cdot O_2^-$ dismutation by using it to convert GSH to oxidized GSH (GSSG).

Ideally, the body would be able to maintain a balance between ROS generation and the availability of antioxidant defenses. Unfortunately, endogenous defenses are not completely effective, and some oxidative damage occurs constantly in the human body (Gutteridge and Halliwell, 1999). Oxidative damage is exacerbated when cells are metabolically challenged or defense mechanisms are impaired. These events disrupt the normal balance between ROS and antioxidants; that is, they produce "oxidative stress." If mild oxidative stress occurs as a result of slightly increased ROS generation, cells and tissues may be able to compensate by making more antioxidants. However, severe or prolonged oxidative stress can easily cause cell injury and death through either apoptosis (programmed cell death) or necrosis.

THE ROS/ANTIOXIDANT PICTURE IS COMPLICATED

Many factors complicate our understanding of ROS damage and the actions of antioxidants in the body. Several important factors that should be kept in mind when conducting or evaluating ROS research are mentioned here.

1. An antioxidant that exerts protection in one biologic system may cause damage in another, and levels of antioxidants that exceed immediate physiological needs may themselves be harmful (Bar-Peled et al., 1996; Michiels et al., 1994; Nelson et al., 1994; Yim et al., 1993). For example, when SOD is used therapeutically in high doses, it either loses its ability to protect against myocardial ischemia, or actually exacerbates the injury (McCord, 1993).
2. The balance between different types of antioxidants in a cell, tissue, or organ can be very important. An excess of one in relation to another may have deleterious effects. For example, an age-related increase in SOD activity that is not matched by an increase in GPx activity has been implicated as a source of cell damage in some organs during aging (Cristiano et al., 1995; de Haan et al., 1995; Park et al., 1996).
3. Some antioxidants scavenge one ROS, only to generate others. SOD, which removes $\cdot O_2^-$, but creates H_2O_2 in the process, is one example. A second example is glutathione, which reacts extremely rapidly with oxygen to produce $\cdot O_2^-$ when it is in its oxidized form. The bottom line is that cells must often choose between the lesser of two evils — because the process of removing one radical may produce a different type of oxidative stress through the generation of another radical.
4. It is important to bear in mind that ROS do not have fixed values of toxicity. Rather, the toxicity of an ROS is influenced by its biological milieu, including the presence of transition metals, other biomolecules and ROS, and the pH of the chemical environment. For example, OONO- and $\cdot O_2^-$ are stable in strongly alkaline solutions. At physiological pH, the lifetime of OONO- is on the order of a second. The lifetime of $\cdot O_2^-$ increases by a factor of 10 per pH unit with increasing pH above pH 6.

Different reactions leading to the same end point can proceed at vastly different rates. For example, both HOCl and H_2O_2 can oxidize ferrous iron (Fe^{2+}) to ferric iron (Fe^{3+}) and liberate hydroxyl radicals through analogous reactions:

$$HOCl + Fe^{2+} \qquad Fe^{3+} + Cl^- + \cdot OH$$

$$H_2O_2 + Fe^{2+} \qquad Fe^{3+} + OH^- + \cdot OH$$

However, the former reaction is about a thousand times faster than the latter reaction, and consequently may be much more deleterious in a living system.

An extremely important example of how balances between different ROS can affect their toxicity is provided by Brüne et al. (1999). During their studies with rat mesangial cells, they were surprised to find that $\cdot$NO-mediated apoptotic cell death was antagonized by the simultaneous formation of $\cdot O_2^-$. In subsequent experiments, they found that balanced and simultaneous generation $\cdot$NO and $\cdot O_2^-$ was actually protective for mesangial cells, presumably because the diffusion-controlled interaction redirected the apoptotic initiating activity of $\cdot$NO toward protection. If the generation of either $\cdot$NO or $\cdot O_2^-$ was offset relative to the other, protection was less efficient. This type of interaction may be relevant for understanding the effects of SOD1 deficiency on NIHL.

The examples given above emphasize that the study of ROS and ROS-mediated damage is not simple or straightforward. We have a long way to go before we truly understand the complex contributions of ROS to health and disease. Focusing on a single ROS or antioxidant, as we have done in our studies with *Sod1* knockout mice, is a simplistic approach to a complex system. However, we view it as a necessary beginning.

WHAT CAN WE LEARN BY MANIPULATING SOD GENES IN MICE?

Mammals have two other isoforms of SOD in addition to the soluble Cu/Zn SOD or SOD1 isoform that is found in the cytosol of every cell: a manganese isoform (Mn-SOD or SOD2) that is bound to the matrix of the mitochondrial inner membrane in all cells except erythrocytes; and an extracellular secreted glycoprotein Cu/Zn isoform (EC-SOD or SOD3) found on the surface of some cells. The three SOD isoforms are coded by separate genes on different chromosomes. Cu/Zn SOD is encoded by SOD1 on human chromosome 21 (*Sod1* on mouse chromosome 16); Mn-SOD by SOD2 on chromosome 6 (*Sod2* on mouse chromosome 17); and EC-SOD by SOD3 on chromosome 4 (*Sod3* on mouse chromosome 5). All SODs appear to have evolved for the purpose of catalyzing the dismutation of $\cdot O_2^-$ to H_2O_2 (McCord and Fridovich, 1969). However, they can participate gratuitously in other reactions as well. For example, reduced copper from Cu/Zn SOD can be used to oxidize H_2O_2 to $\cdot$OH in a Fenton reaction. This reaction occurs spontaneously at high pH (pH > 9), and at physiological pH in the presence of bicarbonate ($HCO3^-$) or structurally similar anions (Sankarapandi and Zweier, 1999). With advances in genetic technology, it is now possible to manipulate SOD genes and observe the consequences of SOD protein overexpression, alteration, or elimination on development and susceptibility to oxidative stress. Transgenic mice carrying the normal human SOD1 gene express increased levels of SOD1 in blood, brain, and fibroblasts. SOD1 overexpressors show less age-related oxidative damage to protein and DNA in the brainstem (Cardozo-Pelaez et al., 1998), and we might speculate that they would show decreased susceptibility to AHL and NIHL as well. However, because overexpression of Cu/Zn SOD also enhances formation of $\cdot$OH (Peled-Kamar et al., 1997), increased susceptibility to AHL and NIHL is equally likely. Transgenic mice that express mutant human SOD1 (e.g., SOD1 containing a glycine to alanine substitution at position 93) develop paralysis as a result of loss of spinal cord motor neurons; these mice are used as models for human amylotrophic lateral sclerosis (e.g., Dal Canto and Gurney, 1994; Gurney et al., 1994; Gurney, 1997a; b).

Mice with targeted mutations that reduce or eliminate SOD activity provide a perspective on the relative physiological importance of the three isoforms of SOD during development. Homozygous knockout mice lacking Mn-SOD (Lebovitz et al., 1996; Li et al., 1995) show early cardiomyopathy, lipid accumulation in skeletal muscles and the liver, and acidosis. Succinate dehydrogenase and aconitase activities are severely reduced, especially in the heart, and lifespan is very short (approximately 10 to 21 days). In contrast, mice lacking Cu/Zn isoforms of SOD develop relatively normally, showing no overt signs of pathology unless subjected to conditions of increased oxidative stress (Carlsson et al., 1995; Kondo et al., 1997; Ohlemiller et al., 1999a; Reaume et al., 1996).

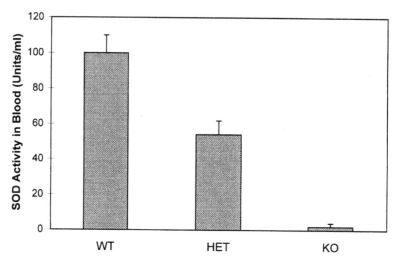

FIGURE 32.2 Mean SOD activity (units/mL) + sd from whole blood samples as a function of genotype. Genotype was determined by PCR analysis of tail DNA, using separate sets of primers for the *Sod1* gene and the neomycin resistance gene. (Data from Ohlemiller et al., 1999a.)

Our research has focused on the effects of Cu/Zn SOD deficiency and, by implication, the effects of increased $\cdot O_2^-$ (and decreased H_2O_2) in the cytosol of cochlear cells. Our subjects, 129/CD1-*Sod1*[tm1Cep] mice, were produced at Cephalon, Inc. (West Chester, PA) by replacing the *Sod1* gene with the neomycin resistance gene in embryonic stem cells derived from an F1 cross of 129/Sv and 129/Re mice (Reaume et al., 1996). The modified stem cells were inserted into donor embryos of CD-1 females (Charles River Laboratories). Germline-positive chimeric males were mated with CD-1 females, and their heterozygous *Sod1* offspring were used to produce WT, heterozygous knockout (HET), and homozygous knockout (KO) mice. As shown in Figure 32.2, SOD activity is virtually eliminated in KO mice, and reduced by 50% in HET mice. There are no significant differences among genotypes (KO, HET, WT) in levels of Mn-SOD activity or in GSH/GSSG ratio that would suggest a compensatory increase in related antioxidants (Reaume et al., 1996).

There are two primary reasons to suspect that *Sod1* deletion would have a major impact on the cochlea. First, the cochlea is one of the most metabolically active organs of the body. As a result, $\cdot O_2^-$ production is likely to be substantial, even when the cochlea is not stressed by noise or ototoxic drugs. Some of the pathways by which superoxide might cause damage in the cochlea are shown in Figure 32.3. Proposed pathways include direct damage to cell and vesicle membranes, direct inactivation of enzymes that are essential to cochlear function, and indirect damage through the generation of other ROS such as $\cdot OH$ and ONOO–. Given this model, it is reasonable to predict decreased damage via the $H_2O_2/\cdot OH$ pathway, and increased damage via all other $\cdot O_2^-$ pathways in SOD1-deficient mice. Second, Cu/Zn SOD is the most prevalent form of SOD in the cochlea (Pierson and Gray, 1982; Rarey and Yao, 1996; Yao and Rarey, 1996). As shown in Figure 32.4, SOD1 levels are highest in the metabolically active stria vascularis, followed by the spiral ligament and the organ of Corti. In the rat organ of Corti, Rarey and Yao (1996) observed intense Cu/Zn SOD immunostaining in Reissner's membrane, inner hair cells (IHCs), outer hair cells (OHCs), and supporting cells, and lighter staining in the spiral ganglion cells. *Sod1* deletion should have important consequences for tissues with high endogenous levels of Cu/Zn SOD.

The *Sod1* knockout mouse was developed from parent strains that show progressive cochlear pathology and hearing loss. Interestingly, the CD-1 parent strain (originally derived from a group of non-inbred albino Swiss mice) is maintained as an outbred strain by Charles River Laboratories, yet every CD-1 mouse exhibits progressive high-frequency hearing loss (LeCalvez et al., 1998a;

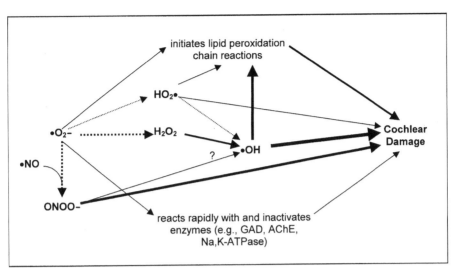

FIGURE 32.3 Some pathways whereby superoxide ($\cdot O_2^-$) could initiate damage in the cochlea. $\cdot O_2^-$ can initiate damage indirectly (represented by dashed lines) or directly (represented by solid lines). Indirect routes involve the formation of more toxic ROS, e.g., the protonated form of superoxide ($HO_2\cdot$), hydrogen peroxide (H_2O_2), peroxynitrite (ONOO–), and hydroxyl radicals ($\cdot OH$). $\cdot O_2^-$ can also cause damage directly, e.g., by initiating lipid peroxidation and deactivating enzymes essential for normal cochlear function. Line thickness is proportion to the amount of damage hypothesized to occur through each pathway.

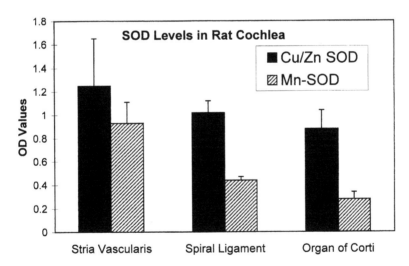

FIGURE 32.4 Levels of Cu/Zn SOD and Mn-SOD in three regions of the rat cochlea. SOD protein levels were determined by ELISA using polyclonal antibodies against Cu/Zn-SOD and Mn-SOD. Optical density (OD) of the color reaction of each sample was detected at 490 nm in an ELISA plate reader. Values shown are means + sd. (Data from Yao and Rarey, 1996.)

Shone et al., 1991b). Given the CD-1 background of the *Sod1* knockout mice (see above), we expected that both KO mice and their WT controls might show AHL. We hypothesized that Cu/Zn SOD would act as a modulating factor, leading to earlier and/or more severe AHL in the KO mice. We also predicted that KO mice would exhibit much greater damage after acoustic overexposure due to increased levels of $\cdot O_2^-$. An additional prediction was that KO mice would show greater cochlear hair cell loss after treatment with carboplatin, a commonly used platinum-based anti-cancer drug that can have ototoxic and nephrotoxic side effects. Unfortunately, our attempt to test this last prediction was only partially successful. We injected 18 2-month-old mice with carboplatin (100 mg/kg i.p.), and observed no adverse effects until 7 days later, when 11 of the mice developed severe diarrhea and died. The remaining seven mice were immediately sacrificed for cochlear histology. No additional hair cell loss attributable to carboplatin was observed in any of the cochleae. This could be due to the short survival time after carboplatin treatment, a masking of carboplatin ototoxicity by pre-existing hair cell loss in the base of the cochlea, or a general lack of sensitivity to carboplatin in the mouse cochlea. We favor the last explanation, because we obtained similar results using CBA and C57BL/6 mice (i.e., no cochlear hair cell losses from carboplatin treatment in young mice).

EXPERIMENTS WITH *SOD1* KNOCKOUT MICE

GENERAL METHODS

All procedures were conducted in accordance with the *NIH Guide for the Care and Use of Laboratory Animals* and approved by the appropriate Institutional Animal Care and Use Committees. Auditory brainstem responses (ABRs) were recorded from mice anesthetized with Avertin (2,2,2-tribromoethanol from Aldrich Chemical, dissolved in saline; approximately 0.35 mg/g body weight, i.p.) or ketamine+xylazine (80 mg/kg + 15 mg/kg, i.p.). The mice were placed on a homeothermic blanket inside a sound chamber, and core temperature was maintained at 37.5 ± 1°C. Subdermal recording electrodes were placed at the midline of the animal's head, posterior to the left ear, and at the back. Responses to pure-tone stimuli were amplified, filtered, digitized, and averaged for 250 to 1000 stimulus presentations. The lowest SPL at which a replicable response could be discerned was considered threshold. Immediately after ABR testing, the cochleae were removed and prepared for counting vestibular or cochlear hair cells (see Chapter 13) or spiral ganglion cells and auditory nerve fibers.

DOES CU/ZN SOD DEFICIENCY EXACERBATE AHL?

As shown in Figure 32.5, both WT and KO mice exhibited an age-related base-to-apex gradient of cochlear hair cell loss. This pattern of cochlear degeneration is attributable to the genetic background of the strain. To determine if *Sod1* deletion exacerbates inner ear pathology, we compared counts of IHCs and OHCs in the cochlea, ganglion cell bodies in Rosenthal's canal, nerve fibers passing through the habenula perforata in the osseous spiral lamina, and hair cells in the vestibular portion of the inner ear (see Chapter 13 for examples of surface preparations and details of the various staining techniques). We also measured ABR thresholds to determine the effects of SOD1 deficiency on auditory sensitivity. In all cases, SOD1 deficiency exacerbated cochlear pathology.

Inner Ear Pathology

One consistent finding in our histological material has been greater IHC and OHC losses in cochleae of KO mice compared to WT controls — irrespective of age (McFadden et al., 1999b; c). OHC losses of 2-month-old, 7-month-old, and 17–19-month-old mice are shown in Figure 32.5. KO mice also had greater loss of ganglion cells and auditory nerve fibers than WT controls, as shown in Figures 32.6 and 32.7, respectively. The average number of fibers passing through each habenula perforata decreased significantly between 2 and 13 months of age, with significantly greater losses in aged KO mice compared to aged WT mice. Interestingly, the effects of SOD1 deficiency on hair cell loss were confined to the cochlea, at least in mice as old as 7 months. We examined the vestibular end organs of 7-month-old WT and KO mice, and found no significant differences in vestibular hair cell density (Figure 32.8). By contrast, cochlear hair cell losses were dramatically different in these same mice (see Figure 32.5).

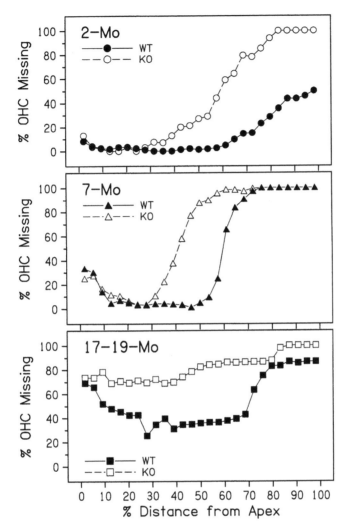

FIGURE 32.5 Mean cochleograms showing outer hair cell (OHC) loss for young mice (top panel), middle-aged mice (middle panel), and aged mice (bottom panel). Note the progression of cochlear pathology with increasing age in both wild-type (WT) and homozygous *Sod1* knockout (KO) mice, and the more severe cochlear pathology in KO mice at all ages. Inner hair cell losses (not shown) were smaller, but followed a similar pattern of loss with age and genotype. (Data from McFadden et al., 1999c.)

Cochleograms from WT mice were indistinguishable from those of C57BL/6 mice of similar age, whereas KO mice appeared to have accelerated cochlear pathology compared to C57BL/6 mice (see Chapter 13; and Spongr et al., 1997a). A simple question that arises is whether 129 and CD-1 mice share the *Ahl* gene that is responsible for age-related cochlear degeneration in C57BL/6J mice (K.R. Johnson et al., 1997).

Auditory Sensitivity

ABR thresholds were consistent with cochlear histopathology in showing the effects of age and *Sod1* deletion. All mice tended to have hearing loss at the highest frequencies tested (32 to 40 kHz), irrespective of genotype. Young (1- to 3-month-old) mice had thresholds of approximately 70 dB SPL at 40 kHz, and middle-aged (6-month-old) mice had thresholds that were 80 dB SPL at 32 kHz. The high-frequency hearing loss is consistent with the basal cochlear pathology shown in

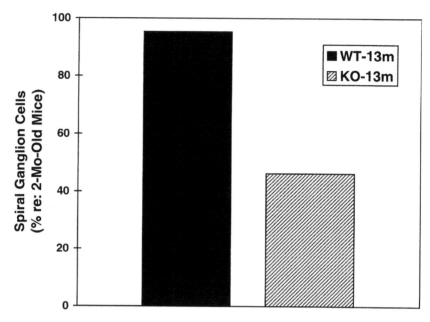

FIGURE 32.6   Percentage of spiral ganglion cells remaining in cochleae of wild-type (WT) and homozygous knockout (KO) mice at 13 months of age, relative to 2-month-old WT mice. KO mice had significantly greater loss of spiral ganglion cells than WT mice. (Data from McFadden et al., 1999b.)

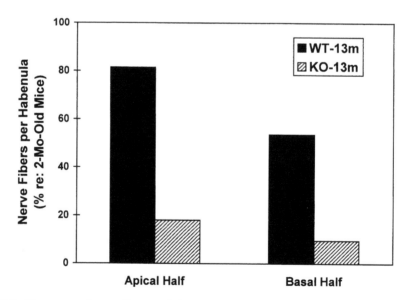

FIGURE 32.7   Percentage of nerve fibers per habenular opening in cochleae of wild-type (WT) and homozygous knockout (KO) mice at 13 months of age, relative to 2-month-old WT mice. The mean number of fibers per habenula decreased significantly for both groups, and KO mice had a significantly fewer fibers than WT mice. (Data from McFadden et al., 1999b.)

Figure 32.5. Consequently, our comparisons among genotypes in this section will focus on thresholds at frequencies below 32 kHz.

The influence of age and SOD1 deficiency on auditory sensitivity can be seen by comparing threshold curves of young, middle-aged, and "old" (13-month-old) mice (Figure 32.9). KO mice

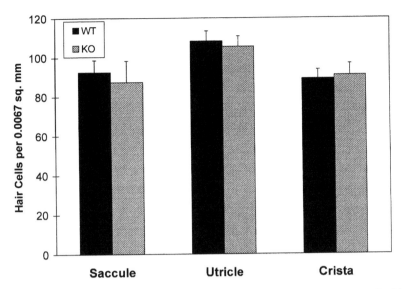

FIGURE 32.8   Hair cell density (cells/0.0067 sq. mm) in vestibular end organs of 7-month-old WT and KO mice. Saccule and utricle counts are for striola and marginal regions combined. Cochlear OHC loss for this group was shown previously in Figure 32.5. Bars show standard deviations.

had higher thresholds than WT and HET mice at all ages. In addition, age-related threshold shifts of KO mice were disproportionately large, e.g., increasing by 20 to 35 dB between 1–3 and 6 months of age, compared to 15 to 20 dB for WT and HET mice. At 13 months of age, KO mice had mean thresholds exceeding 80 dB SPL at all frequencies, whereas WT mice had thresholds that were 20 to 45 dB lower. It is interesting that a dose effect of the *Sod1* gene was observed only in the oldest mice tested. Thresholds of WT and HET mice were indistinguishable in the young and middle-aged groups. At 13 months of age, however, HET mice had thresholds that were higher than those of WT mice, but lower than those of KO mice at all frequencies. Thus, a 50% reduction of SOD1 was deleterious to cochlear function in the oldest age group, but less so than total elimination of SOD1.

One explanation for the delayed appearance of a dose effect of *Sod1* deletion revolves around the concept of a threshold for oxidative damage. It has been proposed that every cell has a threshold of oxidative damage beyond which repair and recovery are not possible (Michiels et al., 1994). The ability of a cell to survive oxidative stress depends on many factors, including the antioxidant enzyme activities of the cell and the duration and intensity of the oxidative stress. It may be that the effects of SOD1 deficiency accumulate over time in HET mice, resulting in late and variable onset of cochlear dysfunction.

One interpretation of the data from aging mice is that Cu/Zn SOD deficiency exacerbates AHL in genetically susceptible individuals. However, we must stress that we do not yet know if SOD deficiency produces damage independently of genetic background, or whether it specifically modulates the expression of AHL genes. Would SOD deficiency lead to AHL in CBA mice? Would SOD deficiency accelerate AHL in C57BL/6 mice? These are interesting questions with implications regarding the mechanisms of AHL.

DOES CU/ZN SOD DEFICIENCY EXACERBATE NIHL?

Several recent studies have focused on the role of ROS in NIHL. Yamane et al. (1995a; b) observed increased levels of $\cdot O_2^-$ along the luminal surface of the marginal cell membrane of the stria vascularis after a 3-h exposure to high-level noise. Cochlear antioxidant activities change following

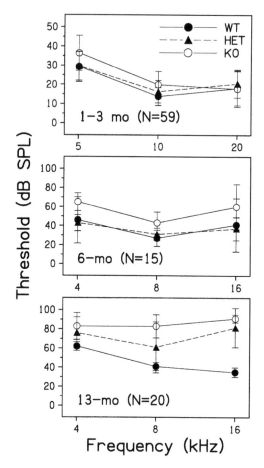

FIGURE 32.9 Thresholds of young mice (top panel), middle-aged mice (middle panel), and aged mice (bottom panel) as a function of genotype. Note the progression of hearing loss with age, and the consistent differences between KO mice and WT/HET mice. Differences between HET mice and WT mice were significant at 13 months only. Differences between HET and KO mice were not significant at 13 months of age. (Data from McFadden et al., 1999a; c).

exposure to noise (Bobbin et al., 1995; Jacono et al., 1998). Rats treated with polyethylene glycol-conjugated SOD developed less noise-induced temporary threshold shifts than non-treated noise-exposed controls (Seidman et al., 1993). Chinchillas treated with a round window application of R-N6-phenyl-isopropyladenosine, a selective adenosine receptor agonist that can up-regulate SOD and other antioxidant enzymes (Maggirwar et al., 1994), showed faster recovery of sensitivity and less OHC loss after exposure to high-level noise (Hu et al., 1997). Ohlemiller et al. (1999b) observed a significant increase in the production of hydroxyl radicals in cochleae of C57BL/6J mice following an acute noise exposure that produced permanent threshold shifts (PTS). Collectively, these studies strongly support a role of ROS in cochlear damage caused by noise exposure. Nevertheless, the pathways underlying ROS generation and damage during noise exposure are poorly understood.

There are at least three routes for the formation of ROS in the noise-exposed cochlea. One is through the increased activity of mitochondria to meet the increased energy demands of cells in the organ of Corti and stria vascularis. The second is through recruitment of ROS-generating phagocytes to areas of cellular injury. The third is through mechanical or chemical injury to tissues that leads to cell rupture and the release of transition metal ions into the surrounding fluid (Halliwell et al., 1992). The increased availability of metal ions could facilitate ROS formation through Fenton reactions.

We investigated the influence of SOD1 deficiency on NIHL in a series of experiments in which subject age and acoustic bandwidth and duration were relevant variables. Experiments used broad-band noise at 110 dB SPL for 1 h (Ohlemiller et al., 1999a), 4-kHz octave band noise at 110 dB SPL for 2 h (McFadden et al., 1999a), and a 4-kHz sine wave at 105 dB SPL for 7 days (McFadden et al., 2000). All noise-exposure conditions produced significant noise-induced PTS, with maximum PTS in the 10 to 24 kHz region. PTS values of young mice were similar to those of C57BL/6J mice, and less than those of CBA/CaJ mice, under similar exposure conditions (Davis et al., 1999). However, SOD1 deficiency had surprisingly little influence on the magnitude of PTS.

The largest deleterious effect of *Sod1* deletion was seen in young mice following the 1-h broadband exposure (Ohlemiller et al., 1999a). PTS measured 28 days after the exposure was graded according to genotype, but the only statistically significant difference was between KO and WT/HET mice at 20 kHz. There were no notable differences among genotypes in the pattern or magnitude of hair cell loss after exposure. Thus, the ABR data, but not the histological data, showed a reliable — but surprisingly small (approximately 10 dB overall) — effect of homozygous *Sod1* deletion on NIHL in young mice.

We explored two possible reasons for the small effect of *Sod1* deletion on NIHL. The first factor we considered was the age of the subjects, reasoning that older mice might be more vulnerable to noise damage and the influence of SOD1 deficiency than young mice. Six-month-old mice were exposed to 4-kHz, octave-band noise at 110 dB SPL for 2 h, and PTS was measured 14 days later. There were no significant differences in PTS (although HET mice developed approximately 15 dB more PTS than WT or KO mice), or hair cell loss as a function of genotype. Thus, it appears that young mice may be more deleteriously affected by SOD1 deficiency than older mice.

The second factor we considered was the duration of the exposure, reasoning that differences among genotypes would be enhanced under conditions of chronic acoustic overstimulation and prolonged oxidative stress. Young (3-month-old) and middle-aged (7-month-old) mice were exposed to a 4-kHz tone at 105 dB SPL for 168 h, and PTS was measured 14 days later (McFadden et al., 2000). The results were similar to those obtained with acute noise exposure. Middle-aged mice showed no differences in thresholds after exposure; consequently, PTS values were actually lowest for KO mice. Thresholds of young mice differed at a single frequency after exposure: at 12 kHz, thresholds of young KO mice were approximately 20 dB higher than those of WT and HET mice. In terms of PTS, young KO mice developed 5 to 15 dB more PTS at 12 and 24 kHz, but 15 to 20 dB less PTS at 3 and 6 kHz. The results support that notion that young KO mice are slightly more susceptible to NIHL at high frequencies, whereas middle-aged KO mice are not. Because cochleograms of noise-exposed mice showed relatively greater hair cell losses in WT and HET cochleae (all cochleograms were similar after exposure), it could be argued that KO mice were actually less susceptible to NIHL than WT and HET mice. Clearly, our predictions regarding the effects of *Sod1* deletion on NIHL were not supported. We turn now to some possible implications of these results for understanding the role of superoxide dismutase and ROS in AHL and NIHL.

IMPLICATIONS FOR UNDERSTANDING THE MECHANISMS OF AHL AND NIHL

Our data provide strong evidence that SOD1 deficiency exacerbates hearing loss and cochlear hair cell, ganglion cell, and nerve fiber loss in 129/CD1-*Sod1*[tm1Cep] mice during aging. Deletion of one *Sod1* gene in HET mice produced variable and delayed effects, suggesting that damage accumulates over time until a critical threshold for phenotypic expression is reached. Deletion of both *Sod1* genes in KO mice resulted in early cochlear pathology that became more pronounced with age, particularly in the base. In contrast to these results, our noise-exposure experiments yielded surprisingly small effects of SOD1 deficiency. Homozygous *Sod1* deletion produced a modest 10-dB enhancement of noise-induced hearing loss but no additional cochlear hair cell loss in 1- to 3-month-old mice, and no enhancement in 6- to 7-month-old mice, irrespective of exposure duration. In fact, there was some evidence that KO mice were actually less affected by acoustic overexposure than WT and HET mice.

One interpretation of our experimental results is that SOD1 deficiency exacerbates AHL but not NIHL. Before accepting this conclusion, however, several factors should be considered. First, it is possible that the results we obtained are strain-specific; that is, they may depend on the specific genetic background of the 129/CD-1 mice. SOD1 deficiency in a different strain (e.g., C57BL/6 or CBA) might have effects that are more or less deleterious with respect to AHL and NIHL. Second, the pre-existing (age-related) cochlear pathology may have masked the effects of SOD1 deficiency on NIHL. If the cochlea is already damaged, then additional damage from acoustic overexposure is not possible. This could explain why increased susceptibility to NIHL was seen in 1- to 3-month-old mice, but not older mice, and why acoustic overexposure made middle-aged WT and HET mice more like KO mice in terms of hair cell loss and PTS. The above considerations underscore the importance of testing the influence of SOD1 deficiency in other models, including murine models developed from strains without AHL.

A third factor to consider is the effect of SOD1 deficiency on other antioxidant molecules in the cochlea: there may be compensatory mechanisms in the KO mice to deal with increased levels of $\cdot O_2^-$ generated during noise exposure. Indeed, Ghoshal et al. (1999) recently reported that levels of metallothionein-I and -II are elevated in livers of homozygous *Sod1* knockout mice. If metallothioneins or other antioxidants are overexpressed in the cochleae of *Sod1* knockout mice as well, this might contribute to protection from ROS damage during noise exposure. However, if compensatory mechanisms protect KO mice from acoustic trauma but not from aging, then this implies that different mechanisms mediate ROS damage in AHL vs. NIHL.

Does SOD1 deficiency increase susceptibility to both AHL and NIHL? We cannot answer this question from the current data, primarily because the pre-existing (age-related) pathology in all of the mice complicates the interpretation of the noise-exposure data. There is no question that SOD1 deficiency was deleterious with regard to cochlear pathology and hearing loss during aging. With respect to NIHL, however, the effect of SOD1 deficiency could be interpreted as being either deleterious, protective, or inconsequential. We use these observations as the basis for some bold speculations regarding the role of SOD1 and ROS in the etiology of AHL and NIHL.

SOD1 deficiency altered the rate and severity of age-related cochlear pathology, but not its basic pattern or base-to-apex gradient. This is consistent with a role of $\cdot O_2^-$ in the etiology of AHL. We can speculate that $\cdot O_2^-$ contributes to AHL by directly inactivating important cochlear enzymes, directly initiating lipid peroxidation and membrane damage, and enhancing the generation of cytotoxic peroxynitrite (see Figure 32.2). Promoting these events by increasing $\cdot O_2^-$ generation or decreasing the availability of SOD1 might place individuals at risk for developing earlier or more severe AHL.

With respect to NIHL, we can propose three alternative hypotheses:

1. Assuming SOD1 deficiency increased susceptibility to NIHL, we can speculate that the NIHL pathway involves direct $\cdot O_2^-$ damage and/or generation of peroxynitrite. An important implication is that the NIHL pathway is not necessarily mediated by the hydroxyl radical, because $\cdot OH$ is presumably reduced in SOD1-deficient cochleae.

2. Assuming SOD1 deficiency was protective, we can speculate that $\cdot OH$ is a major source of noise-induced damage. Ohlemiller et al. (1999b) reported that increased $\cdot OH$ production is an early consequence of noise exposure in C57BL/6 mice. If $\cdot OH$ is a primary contributor to NIHL, then an ear with decreased ability to generate $\cdot OH$ due to SOD1 deficiency would be relatively protected from damage.

3. Assuming SOD1 deficiency had no effect on susceptibility, we can speculate that noise damage can be mediated equally by $\cdot OH$ and ONOO–. In the SOD1 deficient mice, a decrease in $\cdot OH$ production might be offset by an increase in ONOO– generation.

ACKNOWLEDGMENTS

The authors acknowledge Cephalon, Inc., for providing the *Sod1* knockout mice to R.J.S. We would like to thank Robert Burkard, Marlene Shero, and Haiyan Jiang from University at Buffalo, and James Wright and Girish Putcha at Central Institute for the Deaf for their contributions in collecting the data described in this chapter.

33 Mouse Models for Immunologic Diseases of the Auditory System

Dennis R. Trune

BACKGROUND

SIGNIFICANCE OF MOUSE IMMUNE MUTANT STRAINS AND MODELS

Although the impact of the immune system on the middle and inner ear has been studied for half a century, the use of mice as experimental models is a relatively recent development. The virtual explosion in our understanding of the immune system in general over the past 25 years has made it possible to identify several immunologic mouse models that have application to the auditory system. As a result, most mouse research in auditory immunology has been conducted in the past two decades and their study is rapidly increasing. Most mouse models currently under investigation for auditory immunology have been standard models for decades in other fields of immunologic research, such as the systemic lupus erythematosus mouse models in autoimmune hearing loss (New Zealand Black, MRL/MpJ-*Fas^{lpr}*, C3H.MRL-*Fas^{lpr}*, and Palmerston North).

As with other models of hearing research described elsewhere in this book, the consistent genotype of mouse inbred strains offers significant advantages to immunologic research as well. This not only permits reliable comparison of research results with one strain over time within a single laboratory, but also between laboratories. No other animal model offers this degree of immunologic consistency and comparability of study outcomes. An additional advantage of mouse immunologic models is that their genome is better understood than any other laboratory animal, thus facilitating correlation with human genes and diseases. Also, the ability to knock out (or in) specific mouse genes offers advantages for immunologic research that are unparalleled in other animal models.

Immunologic mouse models currently being investigated generally have application to one specific anatomic portion of the auditory pathway, with little or no overlap between them. Therefore, this review is organized with regard to the respective regions of the auditory periphery (internal, middle, and external ear). The origins and backgrounds of the relevant mice are discussed in their respective areas throughout the chapter.

SYSTEMIC IMMUNOLOGIC MECHANISMS AND HYPERSENSITIVITY

Throughout this chapter, reference are made to different types of immune reactions and processes that impact different portions of the auditory system. A thorough understanding of the basic immunologic mechanisms underlying disease would be helpful, but unfortunately beyond the scope and space of this chapter. For more details of basic immunology and hypersensitivity, some excellent and inexpensive introductory texts available are those by Abbas et al. (2000), Male et al. (1996), Roitt (1997), and Roitt et al. (1998).

0-8493-2328-2/01/$0.00+$.50
© 2001 by CRC Press LLC

Immunity is a very specific and normal systemic process for eliminating antigens, such as microbes and foreign substances. If a person is said to be immune to something, it means that he/she has *sensitivity* to it and will react with an immunologic response to rid the body of it. Normally this happens with little or no pathology. The problems occur when the normal immunologic responses are uncontrolled and an excessive or exaggerated immune reaction results, leading to local tissue damage and destruction. Thus, the person is said to have a *hypersensitivity* response, which is the underlying principle in many immunologic diseases. Not only are immune responses to foreign antigens exaggerated to cause pathology, but the person's own tissues may be perceived as foreign antigens and attacked by the hypersensitive immune system (i.e., autoimmune reactions). Unfortunately, it is often difficult to identify the boundary between a normal and hypersensitive immune response.

The ear is no exception to hypersensitive immune reactions. The hypersensitivity mechanisms that lead to exaggerated and destructive immune responses affect the ear as much as any other organ. For example, otitis media is a complex, multifactorial immunologic response and hypersensitivity reactions may play a role in exacerbating some aspects of this disease (Ogra et al., 1998). Also, losing one's hearing because of elevated levels of circulating immune complexes would have to be considered an immune reaction that is a bit exaggerated. In fact, the anatomical isolation of the middle ear and inner ear that is required to make them function properly also makes them more susceptible to pathology in these hypersensitivity immune mechanisms. That is why a thorough understanding of immunologic disease mechanisms is necessary — first to counteract or minimize the extent of pathology, and secondly to prevent the damaging immune reaction from occurring again. Otitis media is a classic example. Once we understand the processes of the immune system that cause middle ear disease, we take steps to counteract them with antibiotics or ear tubes, then move to the development of a vaccine to prevent the disease processes from occurring in the first place.

A brief summary below provides the basics of the types of hypersensitivity immune reactions, their mechanisms of action, and how they might impact the auditory system. Then a discussion follows of the mouse models employed to research the immunologic disorders and pathology of the ear.

TYPES OF HYPERSENSITIVITY IMMUNE REACTIONS AND DISEASES

TYPE I: ANAPHYLACTIC HYPERSENSITIVITY

Anaphylaxis and allergy are examples of a Type I hypersensitivity reaction. The natural immune response is an acute inflammatory reaction to an offending antigen that has entered the body. This response is rapid (minutes) and is caused by B cell production of IgE antibody. The IgE attaches to the antigen and then the mast cell, leading to its degranulation. The mast cells (effector cells) secrete various mediators (vasoactive amines and cytokines) to cause recruitment of neutrophils and eosinophils, macrophage activation, vascular dilatation, and edema. The danger arises when the reaction is excessive and released mediators compromise lung and vasomotor control. This type of hypersensitivity generally occurs on the external ear or within the external auditory meatus, and is an immediate response to an allergen to which the person is already sensitized. There is evidence that otitis media may involve some allergic responses (Hurst et al., 1999), but it probably is only one of many immunologic mechanisms contributing to the disease. Allergy is suspected in some cases of Meniere's disease as well (Derebery, 1996).

TYPE II: ANTIBODY MEDIATED HYPERSENSITIVITY

This mechanism occurs within hours and is caused by circulating (humoral) IgM and IgG antibodies secreted by B lymphocytes against tissue or cell surface antigens. The antibodies attach to the offending antigen and recruit other immune system cells to destroy it. Because this reaction often involves the complement-fixing classes of IgG, it results in local tissue injury due to complement activation, recruitment and activation of neutrophils and macrophages, and inflammation. Activated neutrophils and macrophages elicit local tissue injury through production of hydrolytic enzymes, reactive oxygen species, arachidonic acid metabolism, and cytokine release. Because the antigen attacked is often the tissue of the host, autoimmune diseases are the predominant immunologic disease in this category. Often, the antibody originally may have been created against a foreign antigen, but cross-reactivity with similar epitopes on host tissues or cells results. This immunologic process is generally tissue or organ specific and not systemically widespread. The inner ear may be the target of antibody-specific reactions (autoimmune reactions) if the antigen occurs within the labyrinth. Antibodies also can attach to a particular cell surface receptor and interfere with a cellular function (downregulation) without causing destruction of the cell. The anti-DNA antibodies of systemic lupus erythematosus have been proposed to down-regulate DNA receptor function within the ear and cause the significant hearing loss seen in lupus patients and mice (Trune et al., 1997). This mechanism may be involved in some otitis media if systemic antibodies to microbes are recruited when colonization occurs within the middle ear space (Lim et al., 1988; Ryan et al., 1986). The reported coincidence of hearing loss with serum antibodies to type II collagen (Joliat et al., 1992; Helfgott et al., 1991), endothelial cells (Ottaviani et al., 1999), or myelin (Cao et al., 1996a; b) may also be an example of this type of hypersensitivity.

Type III: Immune Complex Mediated Hypersensitivity

This type of immunologic injury also is caused by IgG and IgM antibodies, but in this case they are bound to the antigen and freely circulating systemically. This hypersensitivity reaction is different from Type II because the antigen is extracellular and the excessive immune complexes formed are not cleared normally. The actual pathological process is initiated when these immune complexes (antigen-antibody complexes) deposit on vascular walls or mucous membranes and initiate the same complement cascade through recruitment and activation of neutrophils and macrophages. From this point on, the disease process is similar to Type II hypersensitivity. This type of immunologic reaction is not organ specific because the antibody is already coupled with its antigen, so the detrimental effect can be seen anywhere the antigen is in excess and immune complexes deposit. This generally affects blood vessels and not tissues, and thus, the delicate blood-labyrinth barrier of the inner ear is a susceptible target. Because autoimmune diseases (systemic lupus erythematosus, polyarteritis nodosa) also have high levels of circulating immune complexes, this type of vascular immune injury is suspected in autoimmune sensorineural hearing loss (Sperling et al., 1998; Andonopoulos et al., 1995), as well as some cases of Meniere's disease (Hsu et al., 1990; Derebery et al., 1991; Brookes, 1986). There also is some evidence this type of hypersensitivity reaction contributes to chronic otitis media because immune complexes of host antibodies and invading pathogens within the middle ear space lead to excessive inflammatory reactions, often prolonged due to slow clearing (Lim et al., 1988; Krekorian et al., 1990; 1991).

Type IV: T Cell-Mediated Hypersensitivity

The type of immune injury is mediated directly by T lymphocytes and their products. The T cell may be reacting against a foreign antigen (virus) or a self-antigen (autoimmunity). Furthermore, the antigen has to be processed and presented to the T cell by an antigen presenting cell, which can be a macrophage, activated B cell, vascular endothelial cell, skin Langerhans cell, or lymph node dendritic cell. There are two major T cell populations that underlie cell mediated immunologic disease, the CD4+ T cell and the CD8+ T cell.

CD4+ T Cells

This cell type is involved in delayed-type hypersensitivity reactions that often lead to tissue destruction. Exposure of cutaneous tissues to foreign antigens (microbes, chemicals, drugs, cosmetics, environmental antigens) will cause recruitment of CD4+ T cells leading to inflammation within hours or days. Langerhans cells within the dermis serve as the antigen presenting cell by attaching the antigen to its surface or endocytosing the antigen to break it down and traffic the antigenic peptides to its surface in combination with the class II major histocompatibility complex (MHC) molecules. The T cell responds by attaching and secreting numerous cytokines, such as tumor necrosis factor, lymphotoxin, interleukin-4, interleukin-5, gamma-interferon (IFN-γ), and interleukin-2. These act on vascular endothelial cells and macrophages, leading to vascular leakage, edema, lymphocyte and macrophage infiltration, inflammation, antigen destruction, and possibly even fibrin deposition due to leakage of plasma proteins. Fibrosis also occurs due to local CD4+ T cell cytokine production that up-regulates fibroblasts to produce collagen. Often, the vascular endothelial cells will aid in the recruitment of CD4+ T cells by also expressing the antigenic peptides on their surface with class II MHC molecules. This T cell activation essentially creates an immune reaction center through secretion of cytokines for up-regulation of macrophages and CD8+ T cells. External ear delayed type hypersensitivity would be an example of CD4+ T cell-mediated immunity. Because of CD4+ T cell infiltration into organs, this mechanism is also implicated in some autoimmune reactions. For example, the high incidence of sclerosing labyrinthitis and fibrin deposition that occurs within the cochlea of autoimmune patients (systemic lupus erythematosus, polyarteritis nodosa) may reflect the fibrosis in this response (Schuknecht, 1993; Keithley et al., 1998; Sone et al., 1999; Khan et al., 2000). The chronic granuloma due to the fibrosis and necrosis within the middle ear leads to the hearing loss in Wegener's granulomatosis, occasionally progressing to the point it invades the inner ear (Schuknecht, 1993). Also, experimental autoimmune encephalitis is a CD4+ T cell-mediated reaction against myelin and considered similar to multiple sclerosis, a confirmed central auditory pathway disease (Jerger et al., 1986; Furst et al., 2000). There is a significant recruitment of T lymphocytes to the middle ear space immediately upon endotoxin inoculation of the ear to cause otitis media (Krekorian et al., 1990; 1991), but their source appears to be non-specific (Ryan et al., 1990). Therefore, this type of cell-mediated hypersensitivity probably contributes to acute otitis media and may be employable in the development of vaccines for otitis media (Ogra et al., 1994). Also, some cases of Meniere's disease have been shown to have elevated cellular antibodies to viral antigens, suggesting that the inner ear deficit is related to an underlying cell mediated response to infection (Williams et al., 1987).

CD8+ T Cells

The CD8+ T cells are mainly involved in lysing cells by differentiating into cytotoxic T lymphocytes. Their main antigenic targets are cells infected with intracellular viruses, but cytotoxic T lymphocytes are also involved with graft and tumor rejection. Virus peptides synthesized within the antigen presenting cells are trafficked to the cell surface associated with class I MHC molecules. These are recognized by CD8+ T cells, leading to lysis of the cell, even if the virus is not harming the cell. Often, cytokines secreted by local CD4+ T cells aid in this process. Compared to the CD4+ T cell-mediated processes of delayed type hypersensitivity above, the cytotoxic CD8+ T cells exhibit much more precision by destroying only the target cell (virus infected cell). Viral-induced tumor cells will be destroyed by the cytotoxic T cells because of the class I MHC-virus antigen complexes. However, some tumor cell destruction is MHC-unrestricted and involves natural killer cells, a more primitive cytotoxic T lymphocyte that does not have a T cell receptor for antigen recognition. Eighth nerve tumors presumably develop due to failure of the CD8+ T cell and natural killer cell-mediated responses to eliminate the tumor cells. Also, tumors on the external ear develop due to failure of an adequate immune response to tumor cell surface antigens.

Type V: Stimulatory Hypersensitivity

Occasionally, the receptor for a hormone or enzyme can be stimulated directly by a circulating antibody. This up-regulates the cell to perform its normal function, but now excessively, because it is no longer under normal systemic control. An example is the thyroid stimulating antibody that up-regulates the thyroid cell function like thyroid stimulating hormone would. A B cell is normally up-regulated by an antigen attaching to its surface receptor, which is an antibody (immunoglobulin). The anti-immunoglobulin antibodies that occur in rheumatoid arthritis could also attach to this immunoglobulin receptor to cause B cells to produce even more antibody. This may be a factor in the rheumatoid arthritis of middle ear ossicle joints (Schuknecht, 1993).

INNATE HYPERSENSITIVITY

Many infections elicit responses of the innate immune system, which is independent of the various acquired immune processes described above. The innate immune response provoked is a toxic shock syndrome mechanism that leads to recruitment of cellular immune elements and release of various cytokines, such as tumor necrosis factor. The immune reaction is further intensified by activation of the alternative complement pathway. The eliciting agents are generally the structural components of bacteria, such as the endotoxins (lipopolysaccharides) of Gram-negative bacteria and the peptidoglycans of both Gram-positive and Gram-negative organisms. The inability to clear these pathogens, and the release of more toxins when bacteria are killed, lead to excessive and prolonged hypersensitivity reactions to these microbes. The best example of innate hypersensitivity in the auditory system is the massive effusions of otitis media. Numerous studies have shown that endotoxin alone can elicit severe middle ear disease (Ichimiya et al., 1990; Krekorian et al., 1990) and endotoxins can reside within the middle ear space for prolonged periods, contributing to the chronic inflammatory status of the disease (DeMaria and Murwin, 1997; DeMaria, 1988).

These various forms of immune hypersensitivity encompass most immunologic disease in the auditory system. Often, more than one type of immune reaction can be operating to exacerbate the detrimental effects, such as otitis media. This makes it more difficult to ascertain exactly what immunologic process is interfering with auditory structure or function, and therefore, how to either counter the immediate immune effects or prevent them from occurring. The survey below describes, as best we know, the immunologic mechanisms underlying various diseases of the human auditory system. Nearly all experimental immunologic studies of the ear have been conducted in the past 20 years and, therefore, most research is only at a very early stage. This makes this field of immunologic auditory research a fertile one indeed, and one that has the potential to elucidate, and eradicate, numerous auditory immune diseases over the next 20 years. The mouse has contributed significantly to this research objective.

MOUSE EXPERIMENTAL IMMUNOLOGIC RESEARCH

RELATIONSHIP OF MOUSE STUDIES TO HUMAN DISEASE

The review that follows is an attempt to distill years of mouse research that is of relevance to immunologic diseases of the human ear. Some studies are purely basic and endeavor only to better understand the natural immune processes operating within the auditory system. Others are an attempt to describe, through experimental animal investigation, the actual immunologic processes involved in clinical disorders of the ear. It is this latter category where one needs to be careful in interpretation. Important questions to *always* keep in mind are: How do the experimental results apply to human disease? Does the model being investigated have anything to do with the actual human disease process to which it is being applied? Do the experimental techniques of immune induction mimic induction of the actual human disease? Is the animal's immune response the same as the human response, including anatomical changes? Thus, provoking an immune response in a mouse may not place the investigator any closer to determining the immune process underlying human disease. For example, getting middle ear inflammation and effusion is not evidence for mechanisms of human otitis media unless the offending pathogen, natural immune response, hypersensitivity reaction, local tissue response, and recovery process are similar. Doyle (1989) best summed up the applicability of animal models for insights into human otitis media by encouraging researchers to agree on protocols for evaluating pathogenicity of organisms. He also encouraged establishment of criteria that:

1. The organism must induce pathologies similar to that seen in patients with the disease.
2. The pathologies can be objectively documented by otomicroscopy, tympanometry, and histopathology.
3. The organism is shown to reproduce in the middle ear space.
4. The challenge organism should be dictated by a reasonable possibility that it has a role in the pathogenesis of the disease in humans.

Similar criteria must also be upheld for immunologic inner ear disease. Does the demonstration of a hearing loss in an experimentally inoculated animal actually tell you anything about the actual disease process in patients? Just because one can induce a hearing loss in animals does not mean one has reliably explained spontaneous human hearing loss. If the causative agent in experimental hearing loss is one that never invades or affects a person, applicability to human hearing disease is severely limited. Also, as we have available more and more sensitive detection techniques (e.g., Western blot, ELISA), the likelihood of false positives, and therefore misinterpretation, increases. For example, the presence of an autoreactive antibody on a Western blot does not necessarily offer evidence of a true autoimmune disease process. In other words, *an autoantibody does not an autoimmune disease make.*

This is not to say that animal research has no application. Quite the contrary. We will see that investigators have made great strides in our understanding of how the immune system affects the various components of the ear. Often, we understand more about the animal immunologic basis for disease than we do the human condition, simply because the latter is so difficult to investigate. In fact, animal studies can often show us where to look next in clinical studies for better understanding disease processes of the ear. Some findings from animal studies have changed our thinking of clinical disease processes and therapies, such as steroid responsive hearing loss. Nevertheless, critical thought must be given to making the leap from interpretation of experimental results to clinical application of findings.

Immunologic Variability among Mouse Strains and Substrains

Another complicating factor when reviewing mouse research is that there is considerable strain variability in disease susceptibility (resistance). In the early 1940s, it was recognized that the mouse strains available for research differed in their susceptibility to murine typhoid, with survival ranging from 2 to 84% (Gowan, 1963). This makes direct application of animal study results to human disorders very difficult, not to mention comparisons between mouse strains. The majority of immunological studies of the mouse ear use the normal strains (and substrains) of CBA/J, BALB/c, C57Bl/6J, and C3H. However, it is imperative that one realizes there are significant immunologic differences not only among strains, but even among the substrains within a strain. The Mouse Genome Informatics review in the Jackson Labs Database (www.informatics.jax.org/external/festing/mouse/docs) summarizes extensive immunologic and infectious disease information for these "normal" mice, and it is imperative that one be familiar with strain differences before selecting a mouse for study.

For example, the four strains above vary significantly with regard to susceptibility or resistence to infection of Salmonella, Pneumococcus, Streptococcus, and Mycobacteria. Streptococcus-induced meningitis occurs more readily in BALB/c mice than in the C57 strain (Kataoka et al., 1991). On the other hand, experimental autoimmune encephalomyelitis (EAE) is moderately successful in C57 mice, but BALB/c and DBA/J are resistant. Their susceptibility to measles virus-induced encephalomyelitis is consistent with EAE, with C3H now being added to the resistant group. If you are studying the effects of UV light-induced immunosuppression, you will have better luck with C57 than with BALB/c, which is resistant. Do not use C57 mice for keyhole limpet hemocyanin antibody responses, use BALB/c instead. The C57 is also a poor choice for Lyme disease studies because it is resistant to the spirochete-induced carditis, whereas C3H and BALB/c are more susceptible. If you are studying hemodynamics, keep in mind that C3H mice generally have lower than normal leukocyte and erythrocyte counts, in contrast to DBA mice that have higher than normal counts. C57 mice naturally have lower numbers of hematopoetic stem cells. To complicate immune response studies even further, C3H and C57 mice often have accessory spleens. Induction of anaphylaxis with passive subcutaneous inoculation will work much better in C3H mice than it will in C57 and DBA mice because the latter two have naturally low IgE responses. CBA mice are resistant to antigen-induced arthritis, while BALB/c mice respond so well that they are considered a good model for human rheumatoid arthritis and ankylosing spondylitis. Finally, C3H mice are insensitive to histamine; thus, they probably would not be a good choice for the study of vascular inflammatory changes.

What mouse best suits a particular study may depend on the objective of the study. For example, C3H/HeJ mice have a gene defect (Lps^d) that prevents or reduces activation of the CD14 receptors on lymphocytes, particularly B cells (Mitchell et al., 1997). This is the receptor for bacterial lipopolysaccharide, the endotoxin component of the cell wall, making these mice hyporesponsive to Gram-negative bacterial infections such as *Hemophilus influenzae*. This is one of the predominant bacteria responsible for otitis media (DeMaria, 1988); thus, the C3H/HeJ mouse probably would not be a good animal to use for studies of the middle ear immune responses to this microbe. On the other hand, if one wanted to investigate the middle ear immune responses that are due specifically to the bacterial endotoxin and not other bacterial antigens, this mouse would provide a valuable control. The substrain C57Bl/10CR also carries this gene defect, although other C3H and C57 substrains do not.

This short review of strain differences should not discourage us from using mice for immunologic research, but rather caution us to use extreme care in strain selection. The value of the inbred strain (substrain) lies in the fact that its genetic consistency offers considerable value and confidence in comparing results between laboratories *with the same substrain*. However, making comparisons of results between strains, or even between substrains, can be difficult and possibly misleading. Therefore, as we progress through the review of mouse ear immunologic studies below, conflicting results should not automatically be interpreted as improper science. Nevertheless, care should be exercised in making automatic application to human otologic disease by assuming parallel processes are operating in patients.

The various immunologic diseases and disorders that affect the ear are unique to either the inner ear (cochlea, vestibule), middle ear, or external ear (pinna, external auditory meatus). Therefore, the mouse models that have application to diseases in these respective regions are also unique. Categorization of immunologic problems of the inner ear is difficult at best, but current research in this quickly developing field has focused mostly on autoimmune reactivity as a significant underlying cause of hearing loss. Otitis media is generally a reaction to colonization by bacteria or viruses, while the external ear has problems related more to inflammatory and allergic hypersensitivity reactions.

INNER EAR

The inner ear is often perceived as an immunologically isolated or privileged site because of the tight junctions of the blood-labyrinth barrier. For the most part this is true and serum-borne cells seldom penetrate the endolymphatic space (scala media) through the blood vessels of the stria vascularis. However, there are other inner ear sites where the blood vessels readily permit the movement of immunocompetent cells, such as in the endolymphatic sac and the spiral modiolar vein adjacent to the perilymphatic spaces. These vessels do not possess tight junctions, and antigenic challenges of the ear elicit antibody production and inflammatory cell movement from these vessels (possibly Type II and Type IV hypersensitivity, respectively). The inner ear is also quite susceptible to systemic autoimmune diseases (Type III hypersensitivity) and mouse models probably offer the most to this specific area of inner ear immunologic research.

IMMUNE COMPETENCE OF THE INNER EAR

The normal inner ear does not have a significant number of resident immune cells, much like the middle ear. It is only when the ear is challenged by pathogens or foreign antigens that intrinsic immune response mechanisms are activated to elicit antibody production and/or an inflammatory cell infiltration reaction. The two major anatomical structures that bring this into play are the endolymphatic sac and the spiral modiolar vein, neither of which possesses vascular tight junctions. Studies of the normal mouse inner ear have shown there are no lymphocytes, macrophages, immunoglobulin, or secretory component, although occasionally very small numbers of T cells or macrophages are seen in the endolymphatic sac (Takahashi and Harris, 1988a; b; 1993; Kawauchi et al., 1992). Kawauchi et al. (1992) provided the most insight into these normal populations of resident cells by examining mice held in germ-free, pathogen-free, and conventional housing conditions. The endolymphatic sac was devoid of any immunocompetent cells under germ-free conditions, with populations of such cells increasing as mice were raised in conventional animal housing quarters. They concluded that the endolymphatic sac is only populated by immune cells if the mouse (and systemic circulation) has been exposed to pathogens. This is borne out by studies of secondary antigen challenge of the inner ear with keyhole limpet hemocyanin (KLH) after systemic sensitization (Takahashi and Harris, 1988a; 1993; Kawauchi et al., 1992). This leads to extensive inflammatory reactions within the mouse inner ear and endolymphatic sac, comprised mostly of macrophages, T helper cells, immunoglobulin bearing cells, and secretion of free immunoglobulin.

The inflammatory cells that traffic to the ear presumably infiltrate these regions via the vasculature because donor mouse T cells are found within the endolymphatic sac of the host (Iwai et al., 1995). More advanced studies in the guinea pig have shown that removing the endolymphatic sac prior to challenge leads to less antibody and fewer immune cells in the same ear (Tomiyama and Harris, 1987) and the sac may actually play a role in presenting inner ear antigen to the immune system (Yeo et al., 1995). The endolymphatic sac appears to sequester antigen, whether it is presented to the perilymphatic spaces (Yeo et al., 1995) or middle ear (Ikeda and Morgenstern, 1989), without violating the endolymphatic space of the scala media. The route of immunocompetent cells appears to be the vascular channels connecting marrow spaces with the endolymphatic sac (Yamanobe et al., 1993) or the spiral modiolar vein (Stearns et al., 1993; Fukuda et al., 1992; Ichimiya et al., 1998), possibly through the expression of intercellular adhesion molecule-1 (ICAM-1) on the endothelial cells (Suzuki and Harris, 1995).

AUTOIMMUNE INNER EAR DISEASE

Human Autoimmune Ear Disease

Numerous reports over the past 20 years have shown significant hearing loss in patients with systemic autoimmune diseases. Although McCabe (1979) is often cited for identifying "autoimmune sensorineural hearing loss," he simply was the first to use the term in discussing a series of patients. Autoimmune-related hearing loss has actually been known since the 1940s with Cogan's first reports of interstitial keratitis, eventually designated as Cogan's syndrome (Cogan, 1945; Lindsay and Zuidema, 1950). However, McCabe did help raise the awareness of this form of hearing loss and dozens of clinical papers have been published in the past two decades describing its diagnosis, treatment, and correlated serum markers (Harris and Ryan, 1995). Autoimmune diseases with correlated hearing loss include polyarteritis nodosa, Cogan's syndrome, Wegener's granulomatosis, Behçet's syndrome, relapsing polychondritis, systemic lupus erythematosus, rheumatoid arthritis, and Alport's syndrome (Trune, 1997; Harris and Ryan, 1995). Furthermore, autoreactive antibodies and elevated immune complexes have been associated with a high proportion of patients with Meniere's disease, rapidly progressing sensorineural hearing loss, and sudden hearing loss (Harris and Ryan, 1995; Hsu et al., 1990; Derebery et al., 1991; Brookes, 1986). Perhaps the best relationship between systemic autoimmune disease and hearing loss is seen in systemic lupus erythematosus. As many as 50 to 60% of lupus patients have some degree of hearing loss (Andonopoulos et al., 1995; Sperling et al., 1998) and nearly all lupus mouse models have elevated cochlear thresholds (see Table 33.1).

Spontaneous Autoimmune Disease Mouse Models

There are numerous mouse models for systemic lupus erythematosus that have been studied for several decades. Excellent reviews comparing the molecular genetics, immunology, pathology, and history of these various autoimmune mice have been written by Theofilopoulos and Dixon (1985) and Theofilopoulos et al. (1989), as well as the summaries within the Jackson Laboratory Database. The more commonly studied autoimmune mice are the New Zealand Black variants (Yoshida et al., 1990), Palmerston North (Walker, 1988; Walker et al., 1978), BXSB (Theofilopoulos and Dixon, 1985; Theofilopoulos et al., 1989), and mice carrying a defective gene for the Fas receptor (Fas^{lpr} and Fas^{lpr-cg}) or Fas ligand ($Fasl^{gld}$) (Kimura et al., 1992; Cohen and Eisenberg, 1991; 1992; Nagata and Suda, 1995; Watanabe-Fukunaga et al., 1992). All these mice have been evaluated for the hearing loss that often accompanies systemic autoimmune disorders (see Table 33.1).

The major advantage of these mouse models is that the systemic disease and hearing loss are spontaneous, as in autoimmune disease patients. This spontaneous onset is quite significant if one is attempting to understand the systemic immune mechanisms that impact the ear, the actual ear pathology underlying the hearing loss in autoimmune disease patients, the mechanisms of steroid and immunosuppressive therapy employed to counter the hearing loss in autoimmune inner ear disease, and the relative efficacies of different steroids. We will see below that numerous attempts have been made to elicit hearing loss in normal mice with various immunization protocols (see Table 33.2) to explain putative autoimmune hearing loss mechanisms. However, these protocols often fall short because they do not replicate the consistency of hearing loss, serum correlates, and inner ear pathology of actual autoimmune hearing loss patients. Thus, the autoimmune mouse models eliminate considerable confusion regarding the actual systemic autoimmune mechanisms that underlie the inner ear dysfunction.

A summary of all autoimmune mouse inner ear studies to date is provided in Table 33.1. Studies of hearing loss in autoimmune disease mice were begun by this author in 1984 with the screening of NZB, BXSB, MRL.MpJ, MRL.MpJ-Fas^{lpr}, C3.MRL-Fas^{lpr}, and Palmerston North. Nearly all models demonstrated some degree of hearing loss, but research efforts focused mainly on the MRL.MpJ-Fas^{lpr} and C3.MRL-Fas^{lpr} mice because of consistency of hearing loss, identified gene defect, and availability of critical controls for hearing level comparisons. Since that time, nearly all of these strains have been extensively studied by other laboratories and a remarkably consistent picture of auditory pathology among these strains has emerged. Although these are discussed in detail below, the basic findings of all autoimmune strains has been elevated auditory thresholds that begin with systemic autoimmune disease onset, stria vascularis edema and breakdown, little or no hair cell loss, and virtually no cellular inflammation of the ear.

Fas receptor and fas ligand defects

These mutant autoimmune mice have defects in the Fas receptor or Fas ligand, which normally interact to eliminate self reactive lymphocytes through apoptosis. Defects in these genes lead to increased populations of both T and B cells (lymphoproliferation) that produce autoreactive antibodies (hypergammaglobulinemia, anti-DNA) and elevated systemic immune complexes (Cohen and Eisenberg, 1991; Nagata and Suda, 1995; Watanabe-Fukunaga et al., 1992). The Fas gene

TABLE 33.1

Investigations of the Auditory System in Spontaneous Autoimmune Disease Mice

Autoimmune Strain [Former designations]	Major Findings	Ref.
C3.MRL-*Fas*^{lpr}	Stria edema, elevated thresholds	Trune et al., 1989; 1996; McMenomey et al., 1992
[C3H/*lpr*,	Elevated immune complexes, ANA	Trune et al., 1989; 1996
C3H/He-*lpr/lpr*,	Breakdown of blood-labyrinth barrier	Lin and Trune, 1997
C3H.MRL-*Fas*^{lpr}]	Stria pericapillary immunoglobulin	Wong et al., 1992; Trune, 1997
MRL.MpJ-*Fas*^{lpr}	Stria edema, elevated thresholds	Ruckenstein et al., 1993; 1999a,b; Ferber et al., 1992; Kusakari et al., 1992; Trune et al., 1997
[MRL/*lpr*,	Lower endocochlear potential	Ruckenstein et al., 1999a
MRL-*lpr/lpr*]	Elevated immune complexes, ANA	Tago and Yanagita, 1992; Nariuchi et al., 1994; Trune et al., 1997; 1999a; b
	Stria capillary immunoglobulin	Tago and Yanagita, 1992; Ruckenstein and Hu, 1999
	Steroid responsive hearing loss	Wobig et al., 1999; Ruckenstein et al., 1999d; Trune et al., 1999a; b; 2000; 2001
	Cochlear DNA receptor involvement	Trune et al., 1997; Kaylie et al., 2001
	No otic capsule lesions	Sørensen et al., 1988
	Female greater hearing loss than male	Trune (unpublished)
	Spleen cell transfer of hearing loss	Iwai et al., 1998
MRL/MpJ	Lessened or no stria pathology	Ruckenstein et al., 1993; 1999b; Ferber et al., 1992; Ruckenstein and Hu, 1999
[MRL/++; MRL-J+]		
C3.MRL-*Fas*^{lpr} x	Stria edema	Delaney-Soldevilla et al., 1992
MRL.MpJ-*Fas*^{lpr} F1	Elevated immune complexes and serum immunoglobulins	Delaney-Soldevilla et al., 1992
	Elevated thresholds	Trune (unpublished)
C3H/HeJ-*Fasl*^{gld}	Elevated thresholds	Trune (unpublished)
[C3H/HeJ–gld/gld]		
CBA/KlJms-*Fas*^{lpr-cg}	No elevated thresholds	Trune (unpublished)
[CBA/*lpr*,		
CBA/KlJms-*lpr*^{cg}]		
Palmerston North	Stria edema, elevated thresholds	Trune et al., 1991
	Cochlear tissue mineralization	Hertler and Trune, 1990; Trune et al., 1990; 1994; Traynor et al., 1992; Khan et al., 2000
	Fibroblast growth factor	Pedersen et al., 1993
BXSB/MpJ Yaa	Stria edema	Ferber et al., 1992
[BXSB]	No elevated thresholds	Nariuchi et al., 1994
	Possible elevated thresholds	Trune (unpublished)
NZB/BlNJ	Stria edema	Ferber et al., 1992
[NZB,	Elevated thresholds	Trune (unpublished)
New Zealand Black]		
(NZB x NZW) F1	Stria edema	Ruckenstein et al., 1999c
NZB/kl	Stria edema, elevated thresholds	Tago and Yanagita, 1992; Nariuchi et al., 1994; Sone et al., 1995
	Elevated immune complexes, ANA	Sone et al., 1995
	Stria capillary immunoglobulin	Tago and Yanagita, 1992; Nariuchi et al., 1994; Sone et al., 1995
	Spiral ganglion immunoglobulin	Tago and Yanagita, 1992
NZB/san	No stria edema	Nariuchi et al., 1994; Sone et al., 1995
	No elevated thresholds	Sone et al., 1995
	Elevated immune complexes, ANA	Nariuchi et al., 1994
NZW/n	Normal thresholds	Tago and Yanagita, 1992

TABLE 33.2
Putative Cochlear Antigens Underlying Autoimmune Hearing Loss

Mouse Immunization with:	Major Finding	Ref.
DNA receptor	Induces hearing loss, immune complexes	Trune et al., 1998b
Heat shock protein 70	No hearing loss, but immune complexes	Trune et al., 1998a
Collagen II	Elevated thresholds, ear degeneration	Yoo et al., 1987; Takeda et al., 1996; Yoo et al., 1997
	Tympanic membrane thickening	Yoo et al., 1997; Fujiyoshi et al., 1997
Human otosclerotic tissue	No otic capsule bone effects	Bretlau et al., 1987
Myelin protein P0 (PNS)	Elevated thresholds, cochlear nerve inflammation	Matsuoka et al., 1999
Myelin basic protein (CNS)	Elevated thresholds, central inflammation	Watanabe et al., 1996; Suzuki et al., 1998
Inner ear homogenates:		
Bovine inner ear	Inner ear inflammation	Tomiyama et al., 1999
Guinea pig inner ear	Antibodies transferred to normal mice cause: elevated thresholds, cochlea degeneration	Orozco et al., 1990; Nair et al., 1995
	Antibodies transferred to guinea pigs cause: elevated thresholds, cochlea degeneration	Nair et al., 1997; 1999
Chicken inner ear	Elevated thresholds, cochlea degeneration	Orozco et al., 1990

defect originated in the MRL strain, although it is now available on several strains, such as C3H, CBA, MRL, B6, and CPt (Jackson Laboratory). Most auditory work has been done on the C3H and MRL.

The first demonstration of hearing loss in autoimmune mice was by this author in studies of the Fas gene defect on the C3H strain (Trune et al., 1989). Beginning in the early 1990s, several laboratories reported similar findings in MRL.MpJ mice with the same defect (Table 33.1). The consistent findings among all these studies was the elevation of auditory thresholds that coincided with the development of systemic disease, as demonstrated by elevated serum immune complexes, immunoglobulin, and anti-nuclear antibodies (ANA). The only pathology within the inner ear was edema and breakdown of the stria vascularis with virtually no inflammation or significant hair cell loss. These changes in the stria lead to disruption of the blood-labyrinth barrier (Lin and Trune, 1997). The impact of this stria pathology on hearing was recently demonstrated by Ruckenstein et al. (1999a) when they showed lowered endocochlear potentials in the autoimmune disease mice.

In a effort to isolate the Fas gene defect and determine if the genetic backgrounds of C3H or MpJ mice were responsible for the cochlear damage, F1's of a cross between the MRL.MpJ-Fas^{lpr} and C3.MRL-Fas^{lpr} mice were evaluated. These mice also showed similar auditory and systemic pathology to their parents (Delaney-Soldevilla et al., 1992), demonstrating that the autoimmunity due to the Fas gene defect was responsible for the inner ear problems. Hearing loss was created in other mice by transfer of spleen cells from MRL.MpJ-Fas^{lpr} mice, providing further evidence of the autoimmune basis of the hearing loss (Iwai et al., 1998).

Autoimmune CBA/KlJms-Fas^{lpr-cg} mice were spontaneously derived on the CBA/klJms sub-strain in Tokyo (Kimura et al., 1992; Matsuzawa et al., 1990) and only recently have been available in this country at Jackson Labs. The technical description of this gene defect is "lymphoproliferation complementing gld." Although these mice have significant autoimmune disease with regard to serum autoantibodies, the impact on organs is less severe than that of the Fas^{lpr} receptor mice above. Recent preliminary studies in the author's laboratory have failed to detect any elevation in cochlear thresholds (Table 33.1) in this milder form of autoimmunity. Disease impact is greater if the gene defect is transferred to the MRL/MpJ strain, probably because its autoimmune background contributes to development of disease (Kimura et al., 1992).

C3H/HeJ-*Fasl^{gld}* mice have a defective Fas ligand instead of Fas receptor, and T cells are the predominant cell type affected (Cohen and Eisenberg, 1991; 1992; Nagata and Suda, 1995). Binding of this ligand with the Fas receptor normally leads to apoptosis of these self-reactive T cells, so their survival essentially leads to the same lupus phenotype as defects on the Fas receptor. Not surprisingly, these mice appear to have elevated auditory thresholds, based on very preliminary studies (Trune, unpubublished, Table 33.1).

New Zealand Black

The NZB mouse has been an autoimmune model since the 1950s, although its background was not established when it originated in New Zealand (Theofilopoulos and Dixon, 1985). Its autoimmunity is largely due to hemolytic anemia; but when the mice are crossed with normal New Zealand White mice, the resultant F1 develops spontaneous autoimmune disease similar to human systemic lupus erythematosus (Theofilopoulos et al., 1989; Yoshida et al., 1990). Several variants of the NZB line have been examined in Japan, such as the NZB/san and NZB/kl, the latter apparently derived from the Karolinska Institute in Sweden (Sone et al., 1995).

Table 33.1 reviews what is known about the auditory system within the various substrains of the NZB mice. Our early observations of the NZB demonstrated auditory threshold elevations and stria edema (Ferber et al., 1992) and Ruckenstein et al. (1999c) found similar pathology in the NZB x NZW F1. The various Japanese laboratories have reported elevated auditory thresholds, stria edema and immunoglobulin, and elevated circulating immune complexes and anti-DNA antibodies in the NZB/kl, but little change in NZB/san (Table 33.1).

Palmerston North

Ancestors of the Palmerston North mice were albino mice purchased from a pet shop in New Zealand in 1948 and raised in the Pathology Department at Palmerston North Hospital (Walker et al., 1978). Their eventual breeding by selection for anti-nuclear antibodies began in 1964 for their development as an inbred line with lupus-like symptoms. These mice have the typical lupus symptoms of systemic vasculitis, immune complex-mediated glomerulonephritis, abnormal T and B cell function, antinuclear autoantibodies (ANA), and anti-DNA antibodies (Handwerger et al., 1999). These mice are not commercially available and most used in studies have been derived from a private stock at the University of Missouri (Dr. Sara E. Walker).

The Palmerston North mice have coincident autoimmune disease and hearing loss (Trune et al., 1991). Like other autoimmune mice, they typically have stria edema and elevated auditory thresholds that coincide with systemic disease development. This group also has some degree of hair cell loss, but the lack of a normal control makes it difficult to judge whether the hair cell loss is due to the autoimmune disease or to an underlying genotype. A unique feature of the Palmerston North mouse is the development of cochlear connective tissue mineralization or sclerification with advancing age (Table 33.1). More will be addressed about this below in the section on otosclerosis.

BXSB

The BXSB/Mp mouse was derived from a C57BL/6J female and SB/Le male in 1976 at the Jackson Laboratory (Theofilopoulos and Dixon, 1985). The defect on, or linked to, the Y chromosome (*Yaa*) causes more pronounced lupus symptoms in males than females. A few studies have shown they do have stria edema but results on elevated auditory thresholds are not consistent (Table 33.1).

MECHANISMS OF AUTOIMMUNE INNER EAR DISEASE

The exact cause of cochlear (stria) pathology due to systemic autoimmune disease has not been established. However, consistent findings among various Fas defect mouse studies is the deposition of immunoglobulin along the vessels of the stria vascularis (Table 33.1). In fact, Ruckenstein and Hu (1999) have shown that the MRL.MpJ-*Fas^{lpr}* stria blood vessels have increases of all major immunoglobulin isotypes and subclasses, as well as both complement fixing and non-complement fixing antibodies. Furthermore, nearly every investigation of autoimmune mice has specifically stated that no inflammatory cell infiltration is seen anywhere within the cochlea. These combined observations suggest that systemic immune complexes or autoantibodies are directly affecting the vasculature (and function) of the stria without T cell recruitment. This suggests that a Type II or III hypersensitivity reaction is operating in autoimmune hearing loss.

Observations of antibodies in the stria vasculature and the breakdown in stria structure (Lin and Trune, 1997) and function (Ruckenstein et al., 1999a) suggest that this is the site of pathology that underlies the hearing loss seen in autoimmune inner ear disease. This is further supported by the significant parallel with human autoimmune disease studies that have shown elevated anti-endothelial cell antibodies in most patients (Meroni et al., 1996). In particular, lupus patients (Faaber et al., 1986; Direskeneli et al., 1994; del Papa et al., 1994; Vismara et al., 1988) and lupus MRL.MpJ-Fas^{lpr} mice (Rauch et al., 1984; Faaber et al., 1986; Chan et al., 1992) have significant levels of antibodies that attack the endothelial cells. It is assumed that these anti-endothelial cell antibodies are probably the anti-DNA antibodies that are so prevalent in autoimmune disease (Eilat, 1985; Frampton et al., 1991; Faaber et al., 1986; Rauch et al., 1984). These antibodies appear to attach to negatively charged proteoglycans and phospholipids on and around the endothelial cells, including the extracellular matrix (Eilat, 1985; Vismara et al., 1988). These antibodies will attach to numerous cell surface antigens (heparin sulfate, cardiolipin), collagen type IV and laminin in the basement membrane, and antigens within the extracellular matrix (del Papa et al., 1994; Direskeneli et al., 1994; Ihrcke et al., 1993; Vismara et al., 1988). The stria vascularis has significant negatively charged molecules (Yamasoba et al., 1996) that appear to be the targets for circulating autoantibodies (Tomoda et al., 1992). Furthermore, clinical hearing loss has been correlated with anti-endothelial cell antibodies (Ottaviani et al., 1999), anti-cardiolipin antibodies (Tumiati and Casoli, 1995; Hisashi et al., 1993), anti-laminin antibodies (Klein et al., 1989b), and anti-collagen antibodies (Joliat et al., 1992; Helfgott et al., 1991; Tomoda et al., 1992). This is strong evidence that anti-endothelial cell autoantibodies cross-react with numerous antigens on the stria vessel wall, basement membrane, and/or extracellular matrix.

Loss of heparin sulfate from the endothelial cell occurs with anti-endothelial cell antibody attachment and this leads to breakdown of endothelial cell integrity and loss of function, as well as initiation of certain immune responses (Ihrcke et al., 1993). This is probably why autoimmune mouse ears demonstrate breakdown of stria endothelial cell tight junctions and the blood-labyrinth barrier (Lin and Trune, 1997) and loss of stria controlled endocochlear potentials (Ruckenstein et al., 1999a). There is also evidence the anti-DNA autoantibodies (or their anti-idiotypes) that occur in this disease interfere with the DNA receptor and DNA binding within the autoimmune mouse inner ear (Trune et al., 1997; Kaylie et al., 2000). In fact, preliminary studies have shown that systemically inoculating normal mice with this receptor protein will raise circulating antibodies against it and cause elevated thresholds (Trune et al., 1998b) (see Table 33.2). Furthermore, just the attachment of anti-endothelial cell antibodies to the endothelial cells can interfere with receptors that are in close proximity to the antibodies and down-regulate their respective cell processes (Meroni et al., 1996; Ihrcke et al., 1993). These various observations suggest that the anti-endothelial cell antibodies seen along the stria vessels in autoimmune mice, which also occur in autoimmune hearing loss patients, can sufficiently compromise stria endothelial cell function. Thus, the anti-endothelial cell antibody impact may eventually prove to be the connection between systemic autoimmune diseases and impairment of cochlear function through stria disruption. We will see below that steroid treatment reverses autoimmune hearing loss in these mice and it probably is accomplishing this by restoring stria structure and function.

Complement is not needed for anti-endothelial cell antibody induced cytotoxicity of endothelial cells (Meroni et al., 1996; Savage et al., 1991; del Papa et al., 1992; Chan et al., 1993). This would explain the lack of T cells in the severely compromised autoimmune mouse stria vascularis. This suggests the autoimmune inner ear disease is a Type II and/or III hypersensitivity reaction. Autoimmune hearing loss and stria vascular (anti-endothelial cell?) immunoglobulin were also created in

SCID (immunodeficient) mice by transferring MRL.MpJ-*Fas^lpr* spleen cells (Iwai et al., 1998). The observation of stria damage and immunoglobulin without inflammatory cells also led them to conclude that the hearing loss is due to circulating autoantibody, again implying a Type II or III hypersensitivity process. Although these numerous observations of the lack of inflammatory cells within the stria may cause some question about actual autoimmune mechanisms, this does parallel observations of human temporal bones. Arnold (1987) found serum antibodies against the stria in all patients with Meniere's disease and yet saw no inflammation within the stria of temporal bones from Meniere's patients. This lack of temporal bone inflammation in Meniere's disease was also reported by Nadol and McKenna (1987). These human observations reinforce the observations in mice that inflammation does not have to occur in sites of autoantibody impact. This is similar to findings in other organs of autoimmune mice that vascular immune complex deposition and cytotoxic degeneration can occur without lymphocytic infiltration and inflammation (Accini and Dixon, 1979; Berden et al., 1983).

STEROIDS AND AUTOIMMUNE INNER EAR DISEASE

Steroids play multiple roles in the development and treatment of autoimmune diseases. Estrogen increases the normal immune responses by up-regulating B cell activity. This essentially causes hyperactive immune responses in women and underlies the higher incidence of autoimmune diseases in women (Ansar Ahmed et al., 1999). Compounding this problem is that postmenopausal estrogen therapy is associated with increased risk of autoimmune disease (Mayes, 1999). Female autoimmune mice usually show lupus symptoms earlier and stronger than male mice (except BXSB). This is why one must be careful about gender selection for autoimmune mouse ear studies and drawing conclusions about levels of hearing impairments. Although male and female mice are often used in inner ear investigations, no published study has specifically set out to determine if hearing loss is more prevalent in female mice than male mice. The author has compared auditory thresholds in male and female MRL.MpJ-*Fas^lpr* mice, and preliminary results suggest that females lose hearing earlier than males (unpublished results). This should be kept in mind when evaluating investigations that use male mice or do not even mention what gender was used. Mouse studies have shown considerable estrogen receptors within the inner ear (Stenberg et al., 1999).

Corticosteroid treatment is the standard therapy for autoimmune hearing loss and the glucocorticoids (prednisone, dexamethasone) are generally prescribed because of their immunosuppressive and anti-inflammatory effects. Recent studies of the MRL.MpJ-*Fas^lpr* mice (Table 33.1) have shown that treatment with prednisolone prevents hearing loss if it is started before disease onset and reverses hearing loss once it occurs (Wobig et al., 1999; Trune et al., 1999a; b). Although glucocorticoids are prescribed clinically because of their immune suppression and anti-inflammatory functions, there is little evidence for inflammatory changes in the ear. If the stria is the main site of autoimmune pathology, then hearing loss is due to decreased stria function (i.e., abnormal ion transport). This was demonstrated by Ruckenstein et al. (1999a) with lower endocochlear potentials in the MRL.MpJ-*Fas^lpr* mice. This implies that restoring ion balances (sodium, potassium) in the endolymph is the key to hearing restoration. The glucocorticoids (prednisolone, not dexamethasone) not only have an anti-inflammatory/immune suppressor effect, but also up-regulate sodium transport functions (Rupprecht et al., 1993; Munck et al., 1990). On the other hand, the mineralocorticoids (aldosterone) have as their sole function the control of sodium transport. Ironically, the glucocorticoids have a higher affinity for the mineralocorticoid receptor than for the glucocorticoid receptor. If clinical hearing restoration with prednisone treatment is due to its ion transport role, then treating autoimmune mice with a mineralocorticoid should be just as effective. This is the case. Treatment of MRL.MpJ-*Fas^lpr* mice with the mineralocorticoid aldosterone, which increases sodium transport and has no anti-inflammatory function, also restored or prevented the hearing loss as effectively as prednisolone (Trune et al., 2000; 2001). In fact, those autoimmune mice treated with aldosterone had a better appearing stria than those treated with prednisolone, providing further evidence that stria dysfunction and sodium transport defects underlie autoimmune hearing loss. This is supported by the findings of Ruckenstein et al. (1999d) who investigated the effects of the glucocorticoid dexamethasone on these mice and found immune suppression, but little change in stria appearance. Dexamethasone is an anti-inflammatory/immune suppressor glucocorticoid, but has no sodium transport function. This finding of aldosterone treatment for autoimmune hearing loss may have application to other types of clinical hearing loss that have a suspected stria pathology that is not immune related. Glucocorticoid receptors have been demonstrated in the mouse inner ear (Erichsen et al., 1996), as have mineralocorticoid receptors (D.R. Trune, unpublished).

One further note on experimental steroid treatment of mice is the recent demonstration that putting steroids in the drinking water is just as effective as injections (Zhou et al., 1994; Hunneyball et al., 1986; Van der Kraan et al., 1993). This technique has been employed successfully by this author in several studies of treatment of autoimmune mice (Wobig et al., 1999; Trune et al., 1999a; b; 2000). The mice tolerate the steroid in drinking water very well and show no adverse effects. If the steroid is not water soluble and one must use alcohol, such as for aldosterone, the steroid can be prepared in small quantities of alcohol first and then diluted with water (Hausler et al., 1992; Trune et al., 2000). In this way an effective steroid treatment can be achieved and the final alcohol concentration can be kept below significant levels. The delivery of steroids in the drinking water not only replicates the oral administration of steroids to patients, but eliminates all animal discomfort due to daily injections and excessive handling. To administer the required dose, one simply prepares the steroid concentration based on the animal drinking 3 to 5 mL water per day. This technique should provide a valuable experimental tool for future mouse auditory studies in which steroid treatment is necessary.

INDUCED IMMUNE HEARING LOSS MOUSE MODELS

Autoimmune inner ear disease is well established, both clinically and experimentally. However, from time to time, autoantibodies to specific proteins are observed in hearing loss patients and attempts are made to determine if these represent a disease etiology. For example, hearing loss has been reported in patients with elevated antibodies to heat shock proteins (Shin et al., 1997; Bloch et al., 1999), collagen (Helfgott et al., 1991; Joliat et al., 1992), myelin protein P0 (Matsuoka et al., 1999), and organ of Corti supporting cells (Disher et al., 1997). These conditions are labeled as types of "autoimmune hearing loss" strictly on the basis of antibody presence and the fact that many of these patients respond to steroids. This significantly broadens the original definition of autoimmune inner ear disease, but may not be warranted if evidence for an autoimmune process cannot be demonstrated. Nevertheless, numerous studies in mice have been conducted to establish if hearing loss does occur with inoculation of these antigens, demonstrating in some cases that an immune relationship exists (see Table 33.2).

Before any discussion of induced autoimmune hearing loss, it is critical that we clarify what constitutes a true autoimmune reaction. The classic concept of an autoimmune process is based on meeting certain immunologic conditions, as originally outlined by Witebsky et al. (1957) and recently redefined by Rose and Bona (1993). Table 33.3 lists these criteria, which remain generally accepted as requisite for demonstration of an autoimmune reaction, whether it be organ specific or

---

TABLE 33.3
Criteria for Classification of Autoimmune Disease

1. Identify self-recognizing antibody, either freely circulating or on self-reactive T cells
2. Identify the self-antigen to which antibodies are directed
3. Produce disease in normal animal by passive transfer of autoantibody or self-reactive T cells
4. Produce disease in normal animal by immunization with self-antigen
5. Generate autoantibody or self-reactive T cells in normal animal by immunization with self-antigen

systemic. Basically, to demonstrate an autoimmune etiology, one must identify the autoantibody and autoantigen in the patient, then immunize a normal animal with both independently and recreate the disease. As we shall see with many of the purported autoimmune hearing loss mechanisms, some fare better than others in meeting these criteria. Table 33.2 summarizes the mouse models used to identify the potential autoantigens that have been proposed to underlie some forms of clinical hearing loss. The criteria of Table 33.3 should be carefully applied to the interpretation of whether these are experimentally valid demonstrations of an autoimmune basis for hearing loss.

DNA Receptor

Lupus patients and mice have antibodies against the DNA receptor and transfer of the mouse antibodies to normal mice creates similar systemic autoimmune disease symptoms (Hefeneider et al., 1993). The DNA receptor has been shown to predominantly occur in the stria and spiral ligament and autoimmune mice demonstrate different staining patterns than normal controls (Kaylie et al., 2001). Antibodies against the inner ear DNA receptor and decreased DNA binding have been shown to correlate with hearing loss in MRL.MpJ-Fas^{lpr} autoimmune mice (see Table 33.1). The presence of these antibodies has not been confirmed in hearing loss patients. Transfer of spleen cells from MRL.MpJ-Fas^{lpr} autoimmune mice to SCID mice also causes hearing loss, demonstrating the transfer of disease with transfer of antibody producing cells. Preliminary studies also showed that inoculation of normal mice with the DNA receptor antigen creates elevated autoantibodies and hearing loss in the recipient (Trune et al., 1998b). Thus, all five criteria (Table 33.3) for confirmation of an autoimmune mechanism have been met. The presence of the DNA receptor and anti-endothelial cell (anti-DNA) antibodies in the stria suggests that the DNA receptor may be the link between systemic autoimmune disease and cochlear dysfunction.

Heat Shock Proteins

The heat shock proteins (stress proteins or chaperone proteins) are responsible for intracellular trafficking of synthesizing proteins during stress responses and are found in virtually all cells, including bacteria. Several studies have shown antibodies to heat shock protein 70 in hearing loss patients, particularly those whose hearing loss was responsive to steroids (Shin et al., 1997; Bloch et al., 1999). However, inoculation of normal mice with heat shock protein 70 did raise antibodies against it, but did not cause hearing loss (Trune et al., 1998a). Inoculations of guinea pigs with heat shock protein 70 did not cause hearing loss either (Billings et al., 1998). Furthermore, recent studies of hearing loss patients have shown that 25% of normal-hearing people have measurable antibodies to this protein (Rauch et al., 2000) and others have shown that autoantibodies to heat shock protein 70 are no higher in lupus patients than in the normal population (Kindås-Mügge et al., 1993). There is increasing evidence that the presence of such antibodies may be an epiphenomenon of bacterial or viral infection because the antigen presenting cells use heat shock proteins to traffic foreign antigen to the cell surface within the MHC complex for interaction with other immune cells (Winfield and Jarjour, 1991). Therefore, cell surface heat shock proteins are not only available to T cells, but are also released into the circulation upon destruction of antigen bearing cells. Also, because bacterial heat shock proteins have significant homology to human sequences and comprise the vast majority of bacterial intracellular proteins, antibodies to bacterial proteins generated during infections lead to significant self-reactive autoantibodies (Winfield and Jarjour, 1991; Jones et al., 1993; Van Eden, 1991; Yi et al., 1997). When all factors are considered, there is limited compelling evidence that autoantibodies heat shock proteins are the cause of hearing loss.

Supporting Cells (KHRI-3 Antibody)

Inoculation of normal mice with guinea pig hair cells and supporting cells created monoclonal antibodies that reacted with specific cochlear proteins (Zajic et al., 1991). One in particular, KHRI-3, specifically reacted with supporting cells under the hair cells and immunization of mice with this antibody created hearing loss and elevated serum immunoglobulin (Nair et al., 1995). Subsequent examination of hearing loss patient sera also demonstrated antibodies to this same cochlear antigen (Disher et al., 1997). Thus, although this autoantibody in humans was originally identified in a mouse model, there does appear to be some correlation with hearing loss in humans. The antigenic protein in the supporting cells is unidentified.

Collagen

Autoimmunity to collagens as a cause of hearing loss has been debated more than any other inner ear antigen. Clinical evaluations have shown the incidence of anti-collagen antibodies in hearing loss patients to range from 50 to 60% to no measurable levels (Helfgott et al., 1991; Joliat et al., 1992; Sutjita et al., 1992; Fattori et al., 1994; Lopez-Gonzalez et al., 1999). The observation of low incidence of patients with antibodies prompted the speculation that anti-collagen antibodies within the serum were the result of the hearing loss, not the cause (Fattori et al., 1994). Also, Sutjita et al. (1992) cautioned that the level of collagen autoantibodies in patients with hearing loss may be artifactually high because of improper use of the ELISA technique. Furthermore, it has been reported that normal patients also have significant levels of autoantibodies and T cells that are specific for type II collagen (Lacour et al., 1990; Sutjita et al., 1992). Animal immunization studies have not settled the matter much, as results have varied from no observable effect to significant threshold elevations, cochlear degeneration, and elevated serum antibodies to collagen (Yoo et al., 1983b; Cruz et al., 1990; Harris et al., 1986; Soliman, 1990). Immunization of mice with either the whole type II collagen molecule or just the autoreactive epitope has been reported to cause hearing loss and degeneration of the organ of Corti and spiral ganglion (Takeda et al., 1996), as well as increase the thickness of healing tympanic membranes (Fujiyoshi et al., 1997). Interestingly, Tomoda et al. (1992) showed that inoculating normal guinea pigs with collagen caused alteration of the negative charge barrier of the stria capillary basement membrane, leading to stria dysfunction and endolymphatic hydrops. This establishes significant parallels with the anti-endothelial cell antibodies in autoimmune disease above that cross-react with negatively charged stria endothelial cell membrane proteins to cause hearing loss.

Protein P0 (Peripheral Nervous System)

Myelin protein P0 is a major Schwann cell membrane protein and has been shown to be the antigenic target of antibodies in patients with idiopathic progressive hearing loss and Meniere's disease (Cao et al., 1996a; b; Joliat et al., 1992). These antibodies were also seen in a small percentage of controls. Its potential relationship to the ear is demonstrated by the hearing loss associated with its genetic defect in Charcot-Marie-Tooth disease and hearing loss correlated with antibodies to it in Guillain-Barre syndrome (Cao et al., 1996b). P0's sequence homology with several viruses suggests that antibodies that form against invading microbes may elicit cross-reactive antibody reactions against self-myelin (Cao et al., 1996b). The inoculation of normal mice with P0 elicited inflammation of spiral ganglion and cochlear nerve, elevated cochlear thresholds, and extended brainstem evoked peak latencies in 25% of the animals (Matsuoka et al., 1999). Antibodies to a peripheral nerve myelin glycosphingolipid antigen have been shown to be elevated in patients with Meniere's disease and progressive hearing loss (Lake et al., 1997), although it is presumed to be different from P0.

Myelin Basic Protein (Central Nervous System)

Multiple sclerosis is an autoimmune disease that has been associated with significant deficits in hearing and central auditory processing (Jerger et al., 1986; Furst et al., 2000). To study the central manifestations of multiple sclerosis, the experimental allergic encephalomyelitis (EAE) mouse model was developed. Mice are immunized with myelin basic protein to elicit central nervous system demyelination and motor deficits. EAE is also shown to cause elevated auditory thresholds and inflammation of the mouse central auditory pathways (Watanabe et al., 1996; M. Suzuki et al., 1998). This process is T cell mediated and antibodies against T cells will prevent the severe demyelination and hearing loss (M. Suzuki et al., 1998). MRL.MpJ-*Fas^lpr* autoimmune mice also show central nervous system inflammation and leakage of IgG into brain tissue (Vogelweid et al., 1991). This presumably occurs because autoimmune anti-endothelial cell antibodies interfere with blood-brain barrier integrity (McIntyre et al., 1990), which up-regulates vascular cell adhesion molecules for lymphocyte attraction and extravasation into the brain tissue (Barten and Ruddle, 1994; Raine et al., 1990). These anti-endothelial cell antibodies also are commonly seen in patients with multiple sclerosis and neuro-Behçet's disease (Tsukada et al., 1989) and inoculating normal guinea pigs with endothelial cells essentially reproduced EAE (Tsukada et al., 1987). Thus, the breakdown of the blood-brain barrier is the first stage in autoimmune CNS disease and EAE, which establishes significant parallels with breaking the blood-labyrinth barrier in autoimmune diseases that cause hearing loss.

OTOSCLEROSIS AND AUTOIMMUNE COCHLEAR OSTEOGENESIS

Active otosclerosis is often correlated with elevated antibodies, either total IgG (Shrader et al., 1990) or specifically against collagen Type II (Joliat et al., 1992; Bujía et al., 1994). Others have shown no significant elevation of collagen antibodies in otosclerosis patients (Lopez-Gonzalez et al., 1999; Sørensen et al., 1988). If autoimmunity does underlie some otosclerotic development, it is probably humoral (Type II or II) and not cell mediated (Type IV) because inflammatory cells are not seen around otosclerotic centers within human temporal bones (Nadol and McKenna, 1987). Animal studies have not clarified the issue as both positive (Yoo et al., 1983a) and negative (Harris et al., 1986; Bretlau et al., 1987; Sørensen et al., 1988) otospongiotic responses to collagen immunization have been seen. Injection of autoimmune NZB mice with human otosclerotic tissue did not result in capsule lesions (Bretlau et al., 1987) and such lesions were not reported in normal mice inoculated with collagen (Takeda et al., 1996). Bony lesions within the middle ear of LP/J mice have some features in common with otosclerosis and evidence for its immune-mediated basis has been provided (Brodie and Chole, 1987; Chole and Henry, 1985; Chole and Tinling, 1987).

Autoimmune disease (Schuknecht and Nadol, 1994; Keithley et al., 1998) and bacterial infections (Axon et al., 1998) have been shown to result in cochlear ossification and ossifying labyrinthitis. This is different from otosclerosis in that the scala tympani and vestibuli fill with fibrous connective tissue that ossifies. Autoimmune Palmerston North mice also have been shown to develop small sclerotic foci within the modiolus (Table 33.1), although the degree of ossification is much less than that seen in human temporal bones. It may simply be a factor of time, because the mice live only 18 to 24 months and patients presumably develop these ossifying lesions over many years. A recent investigation of the Palmerston North mouse suggests that the ossification results from laying down of new fibrous material by activated fibroblasts, mineralization of these fibers in small foci, and merging of these foci as they enlarge by continued mineralization (Khan et al., 2000). The Palmerston North is the only autoimmune mouse reported to have such lesions, as examination of NZB and MRL.MpJ-*Fas^lpr* have not revealed them, despite having autoantibodies to type II collagen (Sørensen et al., 1988; Bretlau et al., 1987). Ultrastructurally, the lesions seen in the Palmerston North mouse (Khan et al., 2000; Trune et al., 1994) are quite similar to the LP/J (Chole and Tinling, 1987).

FUTURE AREAS OF STUDY

The study of autoimmune disease mice will undoubtedly continue to provide insight into the mechanisms of autoimmune inner ear disease. The parallels between human and mouse immunology and spontaneous cochlear pathology are quite striking and suggest that similar cellular processes are involved in their respective disorders. The recent demonstration of steroid efficacy in mice also emphasizes the overlap of disease processes between the mice and clinic patients. Efforts to identify other putative inner ear autoantigens have met with varied success. Some antigens have been studied more completely and their roles (or lack thereof) are more clearly defined. Future research should concentrate on identifying the antigenic target(s) within the ear of the various hearing loss mice models to clarify potential ear antigens attacked in human autoimmune disease. It is quite possible that several antigens within the ear are affected, possibly related to multiple immunologic origins of disease. The relationship of these antigenic targets to steroid treatment reversal will also add to our understanding of the mechanisms potentially involved in this universal, but poorly understood, steroid treatment in patients.

MIDDLE EAR

MIDDLE EAR IMMUNE MECHANISMS

The middle ear has an extensive immune response capability, some of which is brought into play during otitis media. Because of the significant medical and economic impact of this disease, it is the research focus of numerous laboratories (Ogra et al., 1998). The mouse is simply one of many experimental animal models used to better understand the potential mechanisms of this disease. However, to understand otitis media, one must first identify the immune mechanisms of the middle ear. Research in the mouse has probably contributed more to our understanding of middle ear immunology than any other animal, simply because the basic immunology of the mouse is better understood than any other research animal. This is particularly true when drawing genomic comparisons with humans.

Although most studies cite otitis media as their underlying rationale, the experimental approaches are quite varied. Thus, some findings actually make a more direct contribution to our understanding of the immunology of the middle ear than actual disease mechanisms of otitis media. This is not to downplay the value of these studies. Quite the contrary. Any insight gained into the basic immune biology of the middle ear contributes significant information about antigen presentation, inflammation development and control, trafficking of immunocompetent cells, microenvironment requirements, cytokine up-regulation and release, pathology, healing, and vaccine efficacy. Therefore, the review of mouse research studies below, while presented under the topic of otitis media, includes numerous studies that contribute significantly more to our understanding of basic middle ear immunology than otitis media. Special care has been taken to make this distinction where it is relevant, with the caveat that all studies are building a critical knowledge base of immunology of the middle ear. They are discussed together because they all have a common goal, but represent a continuum of direct otitis media applicability.

OTITIS MEDIA

Most middle ear immunologic research conducted in the mouse has been related to otitis media. Although there have been a number of significant studies conducted in the mouse, the vast majority of otitis media research uses either the chinchilla or guinea pig. It is not because the mouse is not a suitable immunologic model, it is simply a factor of size. Because microbes enter the middle ear through the eustachian tube, the experimental animal must be large enough to inoculate either the oropharynx or nasopharynx, sample these same areas, as well as the effusions from the middle ear space, and not be susceptible to naturally occurring middle ear disease to confound findings. The chinchilla offers these significant advantages as well as an incredibly large middle ear or bulla that has sufficiently thin bone to permit easy middle ear inoculations and sampling (DeMaria, 1989). The guinea pig is also a well-accepted animal model for middle ear research (Ryan et al., 1986; Ryan and Catanzaro, 1983), but its susceptibility to otitis media, thicker bullar bone, and smaller middle ear space makes the guinea pig more challenging experimentally. An excellent review of the current status of otitis media research in general is by Ogra et al. (1998).

The development of otitis media follows a progression of microbe attachment and colonization within the nasopharynx, their movement through the eustachian tube into the middle ear space, colonization and resultant immunologic reactions by the host, possible prolonged residence within the middle ear space for chronic otitis media, and host systemic reactions to provide long-term protection from that particular microbe strain (Lim et al., 1988; Lim and DeMaria, 1987; Ogra et al., 1994). The predominant bacterial species underlying middle ear disease are *Hemophilus influenzae* and *Streptococcus pneumoniae*, and less frequently *Moraxella (Branhamella) catarrhalis*, *Streptococcus pyogenes*, and *Staphylococcus aureus* (Giebink, 1989). Antigens within the bacterial cell membranes, or their surface proteins, are generally regarded as the antigenic stimulants that elicit the immune response of the host. These include the endotoxin (lipopolysaccharides) of Gram-negative bacteria (*Hemophilus influenzae*) or other cell wall proteins (DeMaria, 1988; Ogra et al., 1994).

The reaction of the host system to this bacterial invasion probably centers more on the innate hypersensitivity reaction described above, with possibly some Type III hypersensitivity reactions due to immune complex and antibody concentration within the middle ear space. However, during the acute phase of otitis media infection, both local secretory immunoglobulin and serum-derived immunoglobulin are found within 12 hours of infection onset, implying that Type II hypersensitivity is also a mechanism (Karjalainen et al., 1990). This study also demonstrated that during a middle ear infection with a particular bacterium, it is common to find antibodies to the other bacteria within the middle ear effusions. This presumably reflects previous infections with the other bacteria that resulted in systemic immune memory. Because lymphocytes enter the middle ear from all systemic lymphoid organs (Ryan et al., 1990), it is not surprising that T and B cells specific for a previous microbial infection transudate into the middle ear and provide their relevant antibodies when that antigen is present within the middle ear (Type IV hypersensitivity).

Efforts to better understand the pathogenesis of otitis media focus on why nasopharynx colonization occurs in the first place, what controls the extreme inflammatory reactions within the middle ear once infection occurs, and what can be done to immunize or vaccinate individuals to prevent the detrimental inflammatory reactions from occurring in the first place. A number of studies have used the mouse to better understand the immunologic parameters of these phases of disease and its prevention.

Colonization of Nasopharynx

The nasopharynx has certain mechanisms in place to prevent the colonization of bacteria. These include production of IgA to prevent bacterial attachment, innate immune responses of enzymes and immune cells that are bactericidal, ciliary mechanisms to expel bacteria, and an open eustachian tube to drain bacteria from the middle ear space (Lim and DeMaria, 1987). The normal mouse nasopharynx has a full array of immunocompetent cells that serves as the first line of defense against bacterial invasion (Ichimiya et al., 1991). For example, attachment of *Hemophilus influenzae* bacteria to the mouse respiratory epithelium induces epithelial cell production of interleukin-8 (IL-8) and intercellular adhesion molecule-1 (ICAM-1), both of which promote neutrophil adherence for defense against the bacteria (Frick et al., 2000). However, this up-regulation of ICAM-1 production appears to vary with different bacteria as these authors noted that *Staphylococcus aureus* and *Streptococcus pneumoniae* did not have the same effect.

For bacteria to colonize the nasopharynx, innate defensive mechanisms must be compromised. The most common cause of compromise of nasopharynx defenses is viral infection (Giebink, 1989). Viral infection often predisposes mice to otitis media because bacterial colonization occurs in the absence of normal defenses (Ward et al., 1976). Influenza A virus inoculation intranasally in the mouse leads to changes in the glycoconjugate linings of nasopharynx epithelium and bacterial clearance is reduced (Hirano et al., 1999). The virus itself can invade the middle ear space and be found in the otitis media effusions (Meek et al., 1999), although the presence of viral antigen cannot automatically be assumed to have directly caused the inflammatory response. It has been shown, however, that otitis media effusion cultures often demonstrate virus without bacteria (Giebink, 1989). Whether virus alone can elicit the dramatic middle ear inflammatory response remains to be determined, although mouse studies certainly should make that possible.

Cigarette smoke exposure contributes to otitis media development in children (Klein et al., 1998; McCormick and Uchida, 1999), and research in C57XC3H F1 mice has shown it probably occurs due to destruction of ciliated epithelium and loss of ability to clear bacteria (Henry and Kouri, 1986). Eustachian tube blockage, even in the absence of microbial infection, has been shown to increase the cytokine interleukin-1 in the middle ear space and cause pathology similar to otitis media effusion (Johnson et al., 1994). The principle of eustachian tube blockage to enhance otitis media has always been assumed to be due to failure of bacteria to drain from the middle ear.

One of the most remarkable things about nasopharyngeal bacterial colonization, or its prevention, is that bacteria are not passive victims of whatever defenses the host employs. The substrains of *Hemophilus influenzae* bacteria show considerable genetic and phenotypic variability and can even adapt to the host pharyngeal environment to enhance their colonization and chances of successful invasion of the middle ear. *In vivo* and *in vitro* mouse models have shown that bacterial surface lipooligosaccharide (LOS), membrane proteins, and secreted proteins can change the host epithelium to maximize attachment and increase bacterial survival by preventing expulsion by normal pharyngeal mechanisms (Foxwell et al., 1998).

Middle Ear Immune Response

The normal middle ear of the mouse is considered a potential organ immunologically because it contains cells that could be recruited for a local immune response (Ichimiya et al., 1990; Takahashi et al., 1989). Immune potential cells include predominantly mast cells, macrophages, and granulocytes, followed in number by helper T cells, suppressor T cells, and cells bearing IgG, IgM, and IgA. Within the lymphocyte group, B cells were found in higher concentration, followed by CD4$^+$ T cells and CD8$^+$ T cells (Suenaga et al., 1999). To simulate otitis media development as closely as possible with human infections, mice are generally given injections of bacteria, or the endotoxin from bacteria, directly into the middle ear space. Such otitis media has been induced in BALB/c or C3H mice with *Hemophilus influenzae* or endotoxin (Krekorian et al., 1990; 1991; Ichimiya et al., 1990). Immediately, the immunoglobulin bearing cells, differentiated T cells (CD4$^+$ T and CD8$^+$ T), macrophages, and granulocytes increase significantly. These cell populations remain elevated for 7 to 10 days, at which time all cellular populations subside. The combined observations in these mouse studies indicate relatively consistent immune responses of otitis media, whether inoculation was with live bacteria or the just endotoxin of the bacteria. The middle ear effusions were presumed to be due to the increased vascular permeability, which also would increase the number of immunocompetent cells beyond those up-regulated locally. The round window membrane shows severe thickening and infiltration with leukocytes within 24 hours, progressing back to normal within a few days after that (Krekorian et al., 1990; 1991). This offers some explanation for the infiltration of immunocompetent cells into the inner ear spaces and endolymphatic sac. New bone formation is also seen in the middle ear within 3 weeks (Krekorian et al., 1991).

Some insight into the long-term (chronic) effects of a single middle ear inoculation was also provided by these mouse studies. Following clearance of the acute phase, immunoglobulin (IgA, IgG, IgM) bearing cells (plasma cells and lymphocytes) remained as the dominant immune feature 2 to 3 weeks after the initial inoculation, suggesting residual immunostimulation and effusion production (Krekorian et al., 1990; 1991; Ichimiya et al., 1990). The populations of immunocompetent cells within the middle ear appear higher long term with endotoxin inoculation than with viable bacteria inoculation (Ichimiya et al., 1990), but whether this was due to differences in the absolute amount of endotoxin in the two inoculates is not clear. This effect of endotoxin inoculation shows significant parallels with human studies, in which high levels of endotoxin have been measured in the middle ear in chronic otitis media (DeMaria, 1988; DeMaria et al., 1984a), and chinchilla studies showing inoculation with dead bacteria or endotoxin alone is sufficient to elicit otitis media (DeMaria et al., 1984b; 1988; 1992).

Chronic otitis media is a significant problem and it is not clear why such prolonged inflammation occurs, particularly in light of such a pronounced immune response to get rid of it. Studies of effusions in children have shown endotoxin within the middle ear space long after the bacteria have been killed; and in fact, destruction of the bacteria may actually increase the release of endotoxin from the bacterial wall (DeMaria et al., 1984a). It has been shown that *Hemophilus influenzae* bacteria reside and multiply intracellularly in human adenoids (Forsgren et al., 1994), and there is a correlation between *Hemophilus influenzae* DNA presence in adenoids and nasopharyngeal secretions (Sakamoto et al., 1996). The mouse may be a suitable model in which to study this relationship of intracellular resident bacteria in the nasopharynx and otitis media development, the relative effectiveness of antibiotic treatments to reach intracellular populations, and potential vaccines that will increase nasopharyngeal IgA to prevent bacterial up-regulation and colonization.

Although the role of endotoxin (lipopolysaccharide) in middle ear inflammation has been well demonstrated, it is not clear what role other bacterial membrane proteins play in the middle ear response. C3H/HeJ mice have a gene defect that makes them hyporesponsive to the lipopolysaccharide (Lps) component of the bacterial wall. Mitchell et al. (1997) showed a high incidence of otitis media in C3H/HeJ mice, but not in the C3H/HeSnJ substrain. The fact that these mice showed extensive middle ear disease, despite this hyporesponsiveness, at first glance appears incongruous. However, if the innate hypersensitivity reaction to Lps does not occur upon initial infection, then the bacteria would not be cleared quickly and therefore allowed to colonize the middle ear. The other antigens within the bacterial wall could elicit an inflammatory response, but the systemic reaction may not be adequate to clear the infection without the endotoxin-induced immune response. These mice may be valuable in research efforts to differentiate those immunologic reactions generated against the endotoxin vs. reactions against the other antigenic proteins. McGinn et al. (1992) reported a higher incidence of otitis media in CBA/J mice than in CBA/CaJ similarly housed; however, it has not been determined if there is a genotypic difference between the two substrains to cause a difference in susceptibility.

Secondary middle ear challenge of BALB/c mice with keyhole limpet hemocyanin (KLH) after systemic immunization (Takahashi et al., 1992), or challenge of C3H/HeN middle ear with ovalbumin after systemic immunization (Ichimiya et al., 1989), also manifested similar immune cell recruitment in the middle ear response. Ichimiya et al. (1997) also showed that KLH secondary challenge increased the number of lymphocytes and antigen presenting cells within the tympanic membrane, suggesting a basis for its inflammatory changes during otitis media. This is a common experimental method for generating otitis media, that is, systemic sensitization with antigen (KLH or ovalbumin), followed several days later with direct inoculation of the middle ear with the same antigen. Because this experimental approach elicits middle ear disease, it is often concluded that delayed-type hypersensitivity may be a potential immunologic mechanism for the disease. However, it must be borne in mind that KLH and ovalbumin are not microbial pathogens; they are not factors in human otitis media; and once a person is infected with a particular strain (isotype) of bacteria, recurrent otitis media does not generally result from that same strain or isotype because of protective immunity (Ogra et al., 1994). Therefore, using systemic immunization with non-bacterial antigen, followed by subsequent middle ear challenge, may not necessarily be replicating the actual middle ear disease conditions or systemic immunologic processes in human otitis media. However, Ueyama et al. (1988) showed that transferred T suppressor cells from mice immunized with ovalbumin could prevent otitis media in immunologically naive mice that were challenged in the middle ear with ovalbumin. This could be interpreted as a potential mechanism by which systemic immunity is actually achieved once a person has been infected with a particular strain of bacteria. Thus, although this particular mouse sensitization/challenge immunologic model does not exactly replicate human infections, it does offer insight into the systemic control over inflammatory reactions within the ear and vaccine protective mechanisms.

Because one of the inflammatory cytokines, interleukin-1 beta, is produced by macrophages and monocytes, BALB/c otitis media due to endotoxin inoculation was examined for its presence (Kurono et al., 1998). Not only was interleukin-1 beta present within the middle ear effusions, but inoculation with this cytokine alone without endotoxin replicated the otitis media inflammatory changes (Watanabe et al., 1999). Another prominent inflammatory cytokine, interleukin-8, is responsible for leukocyte recruitment to sites of bacterial infection. Inoculation of the ICR mouse middle ear with this cytokine alone also induces inflammatory changes comparable to bacterial inoculation, suggesting it may play a role in the hypersensitivity reactions of the middle ear infections (M. Johnson et al., 1997). Bikhazi and Ryan (1995) have attempted to distinguish potential cytokine involvement in acute vs. chronic otitis media in the mouse. They found that interleukin-2 and interleukin-4 predominated in acute otitis media and possibly related to the higher IgG production, whereas interleukin-5 was correlated with chronic otitis media and its associated IgA production. The effusions of chronic otitis media were also shown to be derived predominantly from vascular transudation because middle ear goblet cells in BALB/c mice did not occur in sufficiently high numbers long term to provide the fluid levels usually seen in chronic disease (Maeda et al., 1999). Also, hydrogen peroxides released by inflammatory cells within the middle ear are presumed to contribute to the chronic disease state. Treatment of mouse neutrophils with s-carboxymethylcysteine appears to reduce peroxide release and may underlie the improvement in clinical otitis media seen with carbocysteine treatment (Ohga et al., 1999).

Middle ear inflammatory changes require a dynamic interaction of cytokines and vascular integrity. It has been shown in the mouse (and other mammals) that calcitonin gene related peptide (CGRP) positive nerve fibers are prevalent within the middle ear mucosa (Uddman et al., 1985). This suggests local neural control of glandular secretions and vasculature, possibly through afferent nerve fiber stimulation and release of vasoactive peptides. Thus, the stimulation of pain receptors within the inflamed middle ear could exacerbate the already uncontrolled edema by causing neurogenic inflammatory responses.

Inner Ear Manifestations

Inner ear inflammation secondary to otitis media has been described clinically (Schuknecht, 1993), making labyrinthitis and permanent hearing loss a potential sequella to middle ear disease. The route of entry to the mouse inner ear in otitis media is generally assumed to be either the oval or round window. The round window membrane is one of the first structures to become infiltrated with inflammatory cells (Krekorian et al., 1990; 1991; Takahashi and Kanai, 1992), but whether this protects the inner ear or increases its chances for infection is not yet clear. Another interesting observation was the bulging of the stapes footplate into the inner ear with middle ear inflammation (Krekorian et al., 1991), which also may jeopardize the protection of the inner ear from infiltration of inflammatory cells. Inflammatory cells were reported in the BALB/c inner ear following *Streptococcus pneumoniae* (Ichimiya et al., 1999) or *Hemophilus influenzae* (Krekorian et al., 1991) inoculation of the middle ear. These cells were predominantly T helper cells and macrophages in the perilymphatic spaces and elevated immunolgobulin was seen in the endolymphatic sac. Ohya et al. (1999) also reported inflammatory cells within the inner ear and elevated fibrinogen staining in the spiral ligament, leading them to conclude that the blood labyrinth barrier may have been disrupted.

Otitis Media Vaccine Development

A goal of many otitis media researchers is to develop a vaccine to protect children from this virtual epidemic of middle ear disease. Efforts to develop a universal immunization protocol have thus far proven unfruitful, mainly because of the numerous bacteria species, and substrains within a species, that can elicit the disease. Vaccination studies have focused largely on prevention of disease through two main mechanisms: prevention of colonization in the first place, or creation of systemic immunity to the bacteria to prevent the exaggerated middle ear inflammatory response upon its invasion.

Streptococcal Pneumoniae

Bacterial adherence within the nasopharynx is the first stage of disease development. Preventing this adherence and colonization through immunization is one potential mechanism for interference with disease development. Secretory IgA from the salivary glands and oral mucosa is a major inhibitor of bacterial adherence. Immunizing mice orally with *Streptococcal pneumoniae* increased the secretion of IgA and IgG in their saliva, which decreased the number of adherent bacteria on subsequent ELISA binding (Kurono et al., 1993). The 90 different capsular subtypes of this bacteria make it difficult to identify one protein antigen that will create cross-protection across all heterologous strains. One of the mouse models being explored for vaccines against this bacteria is concentrating on the common surface proteins (surface protein A) to create host antibodies that will be suitably reactive across all subtypes (Briles et al., 1998).

Hemophilus Influenzae

Similar surface proteins are being explored for vaccines against *Hemophilus influenzae*. Oral immunizations of BALB/c mice with whole killed *Hemophilus influenzae* bacteria will elicit sufficient salivary and serum IgA (and IgG) to significantly reduce nasopharyngeal colonization on subsequent challenge with live bacteria (Kurono et al., 1992; Mogi and Kurono, 1996). Furthermore, nasopharyngeal colonizations by homologous and heterologous strains of bacteria were also reduced, indicating that immunity to one strain can provide protection against other strains. These results have encouraged efforts to identify specific bacterial antigens to be used in vaccines that will provide patient protection from a maximum number of other strains. Again, surface proteins are the most likely antigenic determinants in raising systemic antibodies in the host. Oral immunization of BALB/c mice with just the outer membrane proteins of *Hemophilus influenzae* increases IgA and IgG in saliva and sera and decreases nasopharyngeal bacterial growth on subsequent challenge with live bacteria (Kodama et al., 1996).

P6 is one of these outer membrane proteins that is ubiquitous to nearly all *Hemophilus influenzae* strains; thus, efforts to use this specific protein have been based on the hope that if one can generate antibodies to P6, it will provide immunity against all strains. Intranasal immunization of mice with the P6 outer membrane protein of *Hemophilus influenzae* elicited P6-specific secretory IgA and IgG, which led to less colonization of the bacteria to the nasopharynx epithelium (Yamanaka et al., 1997; Hotomi et al., 1996; Mogi et al., 1999). Furthermore, oral immunization even leads to lymphocytes in the middle ear that secrete P6-specific IgA and IgG (Mogi et al., 1999). Recombinant P6 instead of natural bacterial P6 would be required for human clinical immunization and this has been shown in mice to be equally effective (Ikeda et al., 1999). If the P6 protein was coupled with cholera toxin during the intranasal immunization of the mouse, nasopharyngeal antibody responses were significantly better (Hotomi et al., 1998). Other mouse studies have shown that coupling different toxins to bacterial antigen vaccines enhances different CD4+ T cells and their respective cytokines, which would contribute regulatory effects on mucosal IgA production (VanCott et al., 1996). Kurono et al. (1999a) showed this IgA response to *Hemophilus influenzae* membrane proteins and impaired bacterial adherence was due to increased numbers of CD4+ cells and their production of interferon-gamma and interleukins IL-6 and IL-10. Also, interferon-gamma knockout mice show less antibody production compared to controls, demonstrating its role in antibody production (Kurono et al., 1999b). Another *Hemophilus influenzae* surface membrane protein is lipooligosaccharide, which also has been shown in mice to elicit sufficient secretory IgA to suppress bacterial attachment (Gu et al., 1996; Wu and Gu, 1999).

Moraxella (Branhamella) catarrhalis

The third most common pathogen in otitis media is *Moraxella (Branhamella) catarrhalis.* Similar surface proteins, such as CD, UspA, and lipooligosaccharide (LOS), have all been shown to elicit sufficient antibody responses in the immunized mouse to serve as potential immunogens (Yang et al., 1997; Gu et al., 1998; D. Chen et al., 1996). LOS is the Moraxella membrane antigen most extensively studied as a vaccine candidate. Gu et al. (1998; 1999) have shown that immunization of NIH Swiss mice with detoxified LOS coupled with tetanus toxin (or high molecular weight proteins) elicited an immune response that was bactericidal in some mice. These results are encouraging because Moraxella is a human pathogen, not a mouse pathogen. Getting sustained or effective immunoprotection in mice similar to the natural human antibody response indicates that an effective vaccine is potentially achievable.

FUTURE AREAS OF STUDY

These various mouse middle ear studies have provided a great deal of information about the immunologic properties of the ear and how these relate to certain disease processes. There are numerous mouse models that may be of value in furthering our understanding of specific auditory immune processes, such as otitis media inflammation, vaccine development, systemic immune memory, required immunocompetent cells, transfer of immune factors (cells, cytokines) to the inner ear, therapeutic treatments, etc. By using mice deficient in specific immune responses, the respective roles of those immune mechanisms can be identified. Many immune defect mice are outlined within the Jackson Laboratory Database (www.informatics.jax.org/external/festing/mouse/docs). The C3H/HeJ mouse is hyporesponsive to bacterial endotoxin (Mitchell et al., 1997), and its use may permit differentiation of middle ear immune responses that are endotoxin dependent vs. those due to other bacterial components. The specific role of endotoxin-induced inflammatory changes in the middle ear can also be evaluated in the recently developed mouse model using endotoxin-binding peptides to prevent its deleterious effects (Dankesreiter et al., 2000). CBA/CaHn-Btk^{xid}/J mice have an X-linked B cell defect that prevents antibody responses to bacterial polysaccharides, again possibly having some application to clarifying B cell functions in otitis media. T cell receptor defects in the RIIIS/J mouse could distinguish T cell mediated immune mechanisms in middle ear disease. Both B and T cell defects lead to severely reduced immunoglobulin production in C57BL/6J-$Prkdc^{scid}$/SzJ mice. More general immune system defects are found in the athymic nude mouse (Hfh11^{nu}/Hfh11^{nu}), which is available on several standard inbred strains. FVB/NJ mice are resistant to histamine and could have application to the study of vasoactive peptides in the transudation of immune cells from the vasculature in middle ear disease. Inbred DBA/1LacJ mice have a susceptibility to arthritis if immunized with collagen type II and a congenic inbred line has been generated that is deficient in C5 complement, although all other immune responsive cells are fully functional (Wang et al., 2000a). These mice may be applicable to studies of how complement is involved in middle ear disease inflammatory reactions.

EXTERNAL EAR

Although there have been literally thousands of investigations into mouse external ear immunology, virtually none have dealt with hearing. Instead, the mouse pinna has provided an excellent model system to study the immunology of allergy, delayed hypersensitivity, inflammation, and tumor biology. The pinna is easily evaluated and monitored because it is mostly hairless, has typical dermis, numerous blood vessels, and is anatomically sequestered.

HYPERSENSITIVITY REACTIONS, ALLERGY, AND TUMOR DEVELOPMENT

The Mouse Ear Swelling Assay (MESA) is a recommended procedure to evaluate inflammatory responses to skin irritants, chemical allergens, allergic contact dermatitis, contact hypersensitivity, and delayed hypersensitivity reactions (Kimber and Dearman, 1993; Thorne et al., 1991). The antigen presenting cells for antigens on the skin are the epidermal Langerhans cells (Cavanagh et al., 1997). They endocytose the antigen, modify it, combine it with the MHC complex, and traffic both together to the cell surface for presentation to the relevant T cell within the draining lymph node. It is generally accepted that the Langerhans cell becomes the nodal dendritic cell that serves as an attachment site for immune complexes and activation of memory T cells in the immune response (Abbas et al., 2000; Male et al., 1996). This mouse pinna model is used to evaluate the immunologic responses in contact hypersensitivity, the animal model equivalent to human allergic contact dermatitis (L.F. Wang et al., 1999; DiIulio, 2000; Garssen et al., 1994). This is a delayed hypersensitivity reaction (Type IV) in which CD4$^+$ T cells are involved in antigen-antibody complexing, inflammation, and recruitment and up-regulation of relevant accessory immune cells (macrophage, neutrophil, mast cell, lymphocyte) for release of cytokines, vasoactive mediators, and leakage of serum proteins (Kondo et al., 1994; McHale et al., 1999). Irritant stimulation of afferent nerve endings also contributes to inflammation through release of vasoactive neuropeptides (substance P, somatostatin, and calcitonin gene-related peptide) that cause vessel leakage (Gutwald et al., 1991). This pinna model system also has contributed to our understanding of the immunology of Lyme disease (Lyme borreliosis), such as cytokine control of inflammation (Anguita et al., 1996; Zeidner et al., 1996), antibiotic treatment (Barthold, 1999), genetic susceptibility (Barthold et al., 1992), and vaccine development (Gern et al., 1994; Zhong et al., 1997; Simon et al., 1996).

The mouse external ear also serves an excellent model system for evaluating the immunologic factors underlying tumor development. Ultraviolet radiation exposure of the skin depletes the Langerhans cells responsible for antigen presentation, which suppresses contact hypersensitivity reactions upon subsequent challenge (Burnham and Bey, 1991). Their depletion from the epidermis also suppresses anti-tumor immunity, suggesting a relationship between sun exposure and skin tumor development (Cavanagh et al., 1996; 1997; Donawho and Kripke, 1992; Hammerberg et al., 1994). Thus, this mouse external ear tumor model directly applies to the high incidence of ear and nose skin tumors in sunny regions of the country.

FUTURE AREAS OF STUDY

Future research on immunology of the middle and inner ear may be able to capitalize on some of these very sophisticated mouse pinna research models. For example, neuropeptide control of cochlear blood flow would presumably involve similar vasomotor control to the afferent nerve endings and neuropetides within the pinna. Thus, vasoactivity within the pinna could serve as a valuable control for studies of inner or middle ear blood flow and neurogenic inflammation or serve as a test site for preliminary studies before engaging in the more technically difficult inner ear studies. The hypersensitivity reactions of the pinna also may offer preliminary insights into the immunology of middle ear inflammation, otitis media vaccine development, or the putative inner ear antigens in autoimmune hearing loss. For example, recent studies of Meniere's disease have suggested that allergy plays a role (Derebery, 1996) and the pinna offers a simple model to first evaluate systemic reactivity of putative allergens. Finally, the vascularized pinna is an excellent topical delivery site for drugs, allergens, microbes, vaccines, or antigens that may have implications for middle or inner ear immunology.

SUMMARY

There are numerous immunologic diseases that affect the auditory system, including otitis media, autoimmune inner ear disease, labyrinthitis, and possibly immune complex disease in some cases of sudden hearing loss, idiopathic rapidly progressing hearing loss, and Meniere's disease. The mouse has served as a valuable experimental model to better understand the immune-mediated pathology underlying these clinical disorders. This is due to the wealth of basic information about the mouse immune and auditory systems, the immunologic consistency offered by inbred strains, and the availability of immunologic mutant strains that have applicability to particular immune disorders of the auditory system. Mouse studies conducted to date have provided us with a better understanding of the normal immune responses of the ear, the exaggerated or hypersensitive immune reactions that compromise auditory system structure and function, the therapeutic methods employed to counteract immune-mediated damage to the ear, and the efficacy of vaccines and other preventive measures employed to protect the ear. Although most research of mouse auditory immunology has been conducted in the past 20 years, research findings are already significantly impacting clinical otolaryngology.

ACKNOWLEDGMENT

The author would like to thank Dr. David Lim for providing published material from recent otitis media conferences.

34 Focus: Muscular Dystrophy Mouse Models and Hearing Deficits

De-Ann M. Pillers and Dennis R. Trune

Hearing loss has been demonstrated in association with various forms of muscular dystrophy. A unifying hypothesis regarding the relative roles of structural proteins in the etiology of the various muscular dystrophies has been emerging which may have an impact on the understanding of mechanisms involved in sensorineural deafness. Dystrophin, the product of the DMD gene, is thought to play a structural role in cells by linking the actin cytoskeleton to a transmembrane cluster of proteins known as the "dystrophin glycoprotein complex" or DGC. The DGC, in turn, is linked to the basement membrane via laminin (Ervasti and Campbell, 1991). Proteins at each level of the association have been linked to muscular dystrophy phenotypes (Bonneman et al., 1996) and may also be necessary for cochlear function.

Evidence suggesting that the most common form of muscular dystrophy, Duchenne muscular dystrophy (DMD), has associated hearing loss is tenuous, as there have been few investigations into hearing in DMD patients. Allen (1973) reported delayed responses to tones but no alterations in thresholds. The delay was attributed to motor problems resulting in slow movement rather than an actual delay in the electrophysiology. Raynor and Mulroy (1997) found abnormal brainstem auditory evoked responses in the *mdx* mouse model for DMD, but investigations by our group using a more sensitive pure-tone auditory brainstem response (ABR) method demonstrated normal hearing thresholds in this same animal model (Pillers et al., 1999a). Indirect evidence for hearing abnormalities in DMD is based on linkage to Xp21.2 and the DMD gene in two families (Lalwani et al., 1994; Pfister et al., 1998; 1999). Although no muscular dystrophy phenotype and no specific DMD gene defect have been identified in either family, abnormal electroretinography typical of that associated with dystrophin defects has been shown in one Xp21.2-linked family (Pillers et al., 1993; Cibis et al., 1993; Pfister et al., 1999).

Fascioscapulohumeral muscular dystrophy (FSHD) maps to 4q35 in man and is associated with impaired hearing (Taylor et al., 1982; Meyerson et al., 1984; Voit et al., 1986; Brouwer et al., 1991; 1994; Verhagen et al., 1995). A mouse model for FSHD, the *myd* mouse, has sensorineural hearing loss which maps to the syntenic region on the mouse chromosome 8q (Mathews et al., 1995). Neurosensory hearing loss has also been reported in patients with limb-girdle muscular dystrophy (LGMD) due to adhalin deficiency (Oexle et al., 1996), and with a variant of congenital muscular dystrophy (CMD) (Seidahmed et al., 1996).

We investigated the *dy* mouse, which is a model for one form of congenital muscular dystrophy (CMD). The *dy* mouse has a defect in the gene encoding laminin-α2, a subunit of the protein heterotrimer laminin-2, as its underlying basis for muscular dystrophy (Xu et al., 1994). The goal was to determine whether defects in laminin might also be implicated in sensorineural hearing loss. Expression of the laminin defect in the *dy/dy* mice caused considerable muscle weakness and reduced motor activity. Although motor activity was significantly impaired, there was no indication of vestibular dysfunction in the mice. ABR thresholds were tested according to the method of

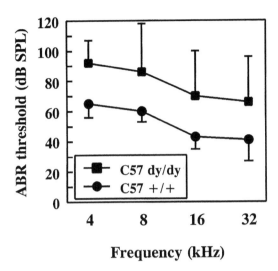

FIGURE 34.1   Average ABR threshold responses for the *dy/dy* mouse and C57 age-matched controls. Thresholds were significantly elevated in the *dy/dy* mice at all frequencies (F = 20.27, $p < 0.0001$), suggesting compromised cochlear function. Vertical lines represent 1 standard deviation.

Mitchell and colleagues (1996) and were significantly elevated in the *dy/dy* mice compared to C57 controls (F = 20.27, $p < 0.0001$). Comparison of the average thresholds showed consistent 25- to 27-dB increases in *dy/dy* mice across all frequencies tested (Figure 34.1) (Pillers et al., 1999b).

The physiologic basis of hearing loss in the *dy* mouse most likely relates directly to the site of localization of laminin-α2 within the inner ear. Laminin proteins have been studied extensively and have been detected at various sites within the inner ear, including the basement membrane of endothelial, epithelial, and spiral ganglion cells, the strial capillaries, cochlea, endolymphatic sac, and vestibular end organs (Hemond and Morest, 1991a; Yamashita et al., 1991; Takahashi et al., 1992; Hokunan et al., 1994; Sagara et al., 1995; Cosgrove et al., 1996a; Sakaguchi et al., 1997). However, the panoply of different laminin proteins and subunits leaves some confusion as to the actual contribution of the laminin-α2 chain that is defective in the *dy* mouse. It is well established that laminin-α2 is one of three monomeric subunits (in addition to laminin-β1 and laminin-γ1) that form the large trimeric basement membrane protein laminin-2 (formerly known as merosin) (Jucker et al., 1996). Additional studies are indicated to clarify the specific localization of laminin proteins containing the laminin α2 chain, as opposed to the more generic protein grouping of "laminin," within the inner ear.

The mechanism by which defects in laminin-2 might lead to hearing loss is not well understood. Laminin-2 is localized to the cell membrane/extracellular matrix interface, where it acts as a receptor for α-dystroglycan (an extracellular component of the dystrophin-associated protein complex) (Ervasti and Campbell, 1991; Bonneman et al., 1996). α-Dystroglycan, in turn, binds to β-dystroglycan and dystrophin. Thus, laminin-2 acts as a bridge to the extracellular matrix, which may stabilize the cellular integrity of the hair cells of the cochlea or other components of the inner ear.

In summary, mouse models for inherited muscular dystrophies have proven to be useful models for the study of inherited hearing deficits. As is the case for these proteins when expressed in muscle, their role in normal hearing remains to be elucidated. It is likely, however, that the lessons learned from muscle research regarding the interactions of proteins within and between cells will be equally applicable in hearing research, and will provide fruitful candidate genes for studies in congenital deafness and hearing loss.

ACKNOWLEDGMENTS

This work was supported in part by the Foundation Fighting Blindness, the Medical Research Foundation of Oregon, and by research grants EY10084 from the National Eye Institute and DC03573 from the National Institute on Deafness and Other Communication Disorders. This work was presented in part at the annual meetings of the American Society for Human Genetics, Denver, CO, October 1998; and the Association for Research in Otolaryngology, St. Petersburg Beach, FL, February, 1999.

35 Hypothyroidism in the Tshr Mutant Mouse

Edward J. Walsh and JoAnn McGee

INTRODUCTION

Having described a feline model of congenital deafness that implicates the olivocochlear (OC) system as an etiological factor (Walsh et al., 1998a; b), we recently turned our attention to the search for a murine model that will support experiments designed to further test the basic hypothesis that abnormalities of the OC system contribute to the auditory pathophysiology observed in congenital deafness, and support investigations designed to determine the molecular and genetic basis of congenital deafness in general. To that end, we have screened several strains of mice in an effort to identify appropriate murine equivalents of the condition that we refer to as Deefferentation Deafness Syndrome (DDS). The signs of DDS include general loss of acoustic sensitivity, response recruitment, and diminished frequency-resolving power. However, the two most important provisions are that sensory cells retain their morphological integrity, and passive aspects of transduction operate normally in affected individuals. All physiological indices point to a defect in the cochlear amplifier, and outer hair cells (OHCs) by association, as the source of an enduring pathophysiological state following neonatal deefferentation.

Because OHCs, the presumptive source of amplification, are paradoxically normal at both the light and electron microscopic levels in adult cats deefferented early in postnatal life, one is naturally drawn to consider the possibility that the cellular defect may be molecular. It is difficult, for example, to avoid speculating over the possibility that the protein comprising the molecular motor of OHCs (prestin perhaps), or an essential channel subunit necessary for an OHC conductance that determines the dynamic operating range (and thereby sets the gain of the cochlear amplifier) is not expressed in animals "deefferented" just as they enter the final stage of development during which function is acquired. Such speculation is, at the moment, pure conjecture but underlines the importance of an animal model that can be exploited to answer these and other even more vexing questions. Although a number of plausible OC abnormalities could theoretically produce the effect created by surgically transecting the bundle, failure of the OC system to develop would seem to be the most parsimonious parallel that might occur in nature.

Approximately 20 years ago, Uziel and his colleagues (Uziel et al., 1980; 1983a; b; 1985a; b) described such a condition in an experimental animal model of hypothyroidism. This suggested to us that genetically hypothyroid animals may be naturally "deefferented" and we were subsequently motivated to seek the murine equivalent of Uziel's hypothyroid rats.

Prominent among candidates thus far studied is the Tshr[hyt] mutant, commonly referred to as the "hyt" mouse. Hyt mice exhibit a naturally occurring genetic defect in the gene that encodes the thyrotropin receptor (Tshr), and the phenotype of individuals that are homozygous for the *hyt* allele is profound hypothyroidism. The hyt defect is a point mutation located on chromosome 12 that is transmitted as an autosomal recessive trait (Beamer et al., 1981; Stein et al., 1994). The physiological characteristics of hyt mice, as well as the consequences of thyroxin replacement, have been studied in some detail (O'Malley et al., 1995; Li et al., 1999; Sprenkle et al., 1997; 2001a; b; c; Walsh et al., 2000; Farrell et al., 2000).

The physiological studies described later in this chapter support one clear conclusion: namely, that cochlear amplification and/or its expression are abnormal in hypothyroid Tshr mutants. While this finding is encouraging in the context of our search for a murine representative of DDS, preliminary anatomical findings are confusing. Although preliminary data from our laboratory suggest that development of the OC system in Tshr mutants is delayed relative to normal animals, abnormalities, if they exist at all, are far less evident than those described by Uziel et al. (1985a) in the rat. The difference raises an interesting question: are mice, and the Tshr mouse in particular, different from rats in their response to congenital hypothyroidism? While preliminary findings suggest that the inconsistency reflects species difference, it is nonetheless surprising to find significant differences between two groups so closely related in phylogeny.

This chapter is divided into three sections. The first section reviews the relationship between hypothyroidism and deafness; the second section reviews relevant aspects of olivocochlear (OC) system-development that provide a background against which our thinking can be more clearly seen; and the final section considers the physiological characteristics of the Tshr mouse and explains the rationale underlying our view that homozygous Tshr mice might suffer from DDS.

HYPOTHYROIDISM AND DEAFNESS

Although estimates of hypothyroidism-induced deafness among humans vary greatly (20 to 80%), the fact that there is a relationship between thyroxin deficiency and deafness is unambiguous (Meyerhoff, 1979; Hébert et al., 1985a; b; Legrand et al., 1988; Gil-Loyzaga et al., 1990). The diversity of abnormalities resulting from hypothyroidism reported in the literature is extensive, and depends at least in part on the etiology of the disease. In humans suffering from thyroid deficiency, abnormalities ranging from osteoblastosis of the bony cochlear wall to ossicular abnormalities have been described, along with tectorial membrane (TM) and lateral wall defects (Meyerhoff, 1979). The highly variable nature of pathology associated with hypothyroidism clarifies the need for controlled animal studies. In that context, Uziel et al. (1985a) reported a veritable constellation of cochlear abnormalities associated with rat pups rendered congenitally hypothyroid by treatment with the goitrogenic compound propylthiouracil (PTU). PTU is a thiocarbamide that interferes with the iodination of monoiodotyrosine and blocks the coupling of iodide to tyrosine, producing hypothyroidism in a dose-dependent manner. Abnormalities in these animals were associated with Kolliker's organ, cytoskeletal features associated with the tunnel of Corti pillar cells (Gabrion et al., 1984), the opening of fluid compartments, and innervation patterns, especially in the case of OC projections. Of the many abnormalities presumably associated with hypothyroidism, perhaps the two most obvious and frequently reported are TM malformation and failure of the OC pathway to develop normally.

INNERVATION AND HYPOTHYROIDISM

The observation that efferent innervation is disrupted in at least some forms of experimentally induced hypothyroidism is unambiguous. Perhaps the strongest testimonial of that position was made by Uziel et al. (1985a), who stated that, "The main feature of the 30-day-old [PTU treated] animal is the incomplete development of efferents which never reach the base of OHCs and never establish synapses with them."* The same authors found remarkable differences between hypothyroid animals and normal controls when thyroxin was administered for brief, 2-day periods during development. For example, axodendritic contacts between OC efferents and primary afferent fibers connected to OHCs were observed in 14- and 20-day-old animals that had received thyroxin on

---

* Reprinted from *Developmental Brain Research,* 1985, Uziel, A., Legrand, C., and Rabie, A., Corrective effects of thyroxine on cochlear abnormalities induced by congenital hypothyroidism in the rat. I. Morphological study, 111-122, Copyright 1985. With permission from Elsevier Science.

the 3rd and 4th postnatal days. While some efferents occasionally approached the base of an OHC under these conditions, clear axosomatic synapses were never observed. Equally remarkable was their observation that normal efferent innervation was restored when thyroxin was administered to hypothyroid animals between the 12th and 17th postnatal days.

On the basis of these findings, we set out to determine whether or not the same was true in the Tshr mutant (a process that is ongoing in our laboratory), presuming that profound hypothyroidism should produce the same pathological consequences regardless of etiology. Because virtually nothing is known about developmental anatomy in the Tshr mouse, and because of the obvious importance of morphological data in the argument raised earlier, we break with traditional protocol and include a discussion of anatomical findings from a limited set of preliminary studies that suggest that there may be significant differences between the two groups. Anomalies associated with the OC system of homozygous Tshr mutants are far less evident than those observed in PTU-treated rat pups. It is clear, for example, that efferent fibers have made their way into the organ of Corti by 16 postnatal days in at least some *hyt/hyt* individuals, as revealed by the presence of dense acetylcholinesterase (AChE) reaction product throughout the apical-basal length of the organ of Corti from a 16-day-old shown in Figure 35.1. Although efferent OC fibers are clearly present in the OHC region, and their presence would seemingly undermine the basic premise being tested, our interest shifted toward the possibility that the projection, although present, may be immature. Specifically, we entertained the notion that the arrival and intracochlear organization of efferents might be delayed in Tshr mutant animals. In addition, the delay might lead to a missed window of opportunity to trigger a key developmental event(s) necessary for the full cytodifferentiation of the end organ; that the delay might effectively "deefferent" the end organ during a critical period of development. On preliminary grounds, it appears that efferents do indeed arrive at their intracochlear targets relatively late in hypothyroid Tshr mutants.

For example, the sample shown in Figure 35.1 was taken from a region approximately 4.5 mm from the cochlear apex in a *hyt/hyt* animal and shows dense staining in the periphery of the osseous spiral lamina where the efferent fibers emerge to enter the organ of Corti. Dense AChE reaction product is also visible beneath the inner hair cells (IHCs), in tunnel crossing fibers, and beneath the first row of OHCs. However, the pattern of reaction product observed surrounding OHCs populating the second and third rows is irregular, both in terms of the size and distribution of labeled fibers and terminals. This suggests that not every hair cell has received its expected full and uniform complement of efferent innervation by P16. In contrast, clear punctate deposits of AChE reaction product have been observed in association with all three rows of OHCs in normal, age-matched control animals. This finding is consistent with the commonly held view that the OCB is essentially adult-like by this age. According to the findings of Sobkowicz and Emmerling (1989), in the normal HA/ICR mouse the basal turn exhibits a virtually mature pattern of AChE reaction product that mirrors the natural array of the three rows of OHCs by P12 (see Figure 11, in Sobkowicz and Emmerling, 1989).

Therefore, these preliminary findings support the notion that the efferent system develops abnormally, although it is clear that OC fibers project into the OHC domain relatively early in life. The heavy deposit of AChE reaction product that completely occupies the habenula perforata in animals thus far studied suggests that the majority of the OC projection has just arrived and accumulated at that level of the system at or around postnatal day 16. This pilot finding is consistent with the hypothesis that OC fibers project into and organize within the organ of Corti later in Tshr mutants than in normal animals.

Based on anatomical data alone, it might appear that the Tshr mutant mouse is not a particularly good candidate in our search for a murine model of DDS; efferent innervation appears normal in hypothyroid animals treated with thyroxin between 12 and 17 postnatal days (Uziel et al., 1985a), and preliminary data from our lab indicate that the OCB projects into the OHC domain relatively early in the development of Tshr mutant animals. Aside from the observation that OC fibers appear to arrive in the domain of OHCs late, there is little reason to be encouraged about the prospect of the Tshr mouse as a DDS equivalent on anatomical grounds, at least on the surface.

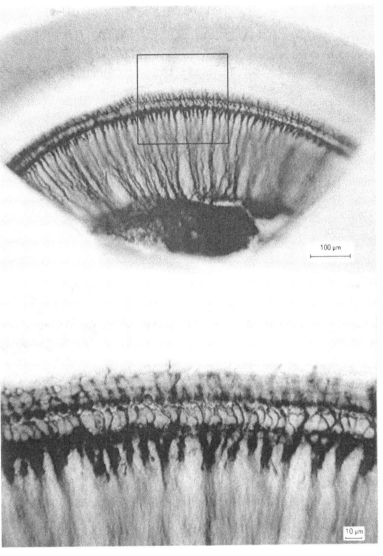

FIGURE 35.1 Surface view of acetylcholinesterase (AChE) reaction product in the basal turn (approx. 4.5 mm from the apex) in a 15-day-old homozygous hyt mouse at low and high magnifications (upper and lower frames, respectively). The rectangle indicated in the upper frame indicates the approximate region from where the lower panel was taken. Imaged with Zeiss 16× objective (top) and 63× oil objective, DIC (bottom).

However, the picture changes critically when function is considered. In the same hypothyroid rats showing complete anatomical recovery following thyroxin treatment, physiological recovery is limited (Uziel et al., 1985b). Compound action potential (CAP) thresholds are elevated relative to controls in T4-treated hypothyroid animals. Cochlear microphonic (CM) potentials, on the other hand, are essentially normal, according to Uziel et al. (1985b). While not explaining how CM thresholds could be normal under these circumstances, the authors suggest that tectorial membrane abnormality in general, and the coupling of OHC stereocilia to the TM in particular, is the evident explanation of this finding. They based this conclusion on their view that TM distortion was the only *apparent* abnormality observed under these conditions. However, both physiological and anatomical findings in our laboratory suggest otherwise. We present preliminary data in the following section, suggesting that TM abnormalities are not evident in homozygous Tshr mutants.

As in the work of Uziel et al. (1985b), evoked potential thresholds elicited from *hyt/hyt* animals are elevated relative to heterozygous euthyroid littermates (O'Malley et al., 1995; Sprenkle et al., 2001a). However, distortion product otoacoustic emission (DPOAE) thresholds are elevated as well (see below for a detailed summary) (Li et al., 1999; Walsh et al., 2000; Farrell et al., 2000), and this finding may add a critical piece to the puzzle. The observation that both evoked potential and DPAOE thresholds are elevated suggests that the transduction defect lies at the level of the cochlear amplifier; DPOAEs reflect the activity level of OHCs directly and, consequently, serve as an ideal index of the OHC's functional status.

Although OHC innervation patterns are clearly abnormal in hypothyroidism, Uziel et al. (1983b) claim that IHC innervation patterns are normal and mature in rat pups less than 1 week old. However, clear axosomatic contact between efferents and an IHC are evident in the photomicrograph used by Uziel to illustrate this finding, suggesting that the efferent projection to the region of IHCs is also immature at this stage of development. While this issue is not the focus of this chapter, the question is significant, thereby raising the possibility that naturally occurring OC abnormalities might affect development of the inner hair cell domain as well as the outer.

The Tectorial Membrane and Kolliker's Organ in Hypothyroid Tshr Mutants

While we question the significance of TM malformation as a source of otopathology in homozygous Tshr mutants, it remains one of the most commonly reported cochlear defects reported uniformly from laboratory to laboratory (Deol, 1973a; 1976; Uziel et al., 1981; 1985a; b; Anniko and Rosenkvist, 1982; Rabie et al., 1988; Remezal and Gil-Loyzaga, 1993). Whether or not the TM is abnormal in living hypothyroid animals to the extent that it is in fixed tissue remains an open question. The rationale underlying our skepticism regarding the commonly held view that the TM plays a major role in Tshr otopathology is addressed in the following paragraphs. We focus here on the TM and its relationship with Kolliker's organ (KO).

KO is a bed of primordial pseudostratified columnar epithelium that occupies the inner spiral sulcus in developing mammals, and it is commonly held that the tissue contributes to the secretion of the TM (Lim, 1986; 1987; 1992; Hinojosa, 1977). A primitive version of the TM is itself intimately associated with the surface of KO early in its development (Hinojosa, 1977). During the first postnatal week, KO in mice, presumably finished with its secretory responsibilities, is transformed to its adult cuboidal form, as the developing TM organizes over progressively more lateral aspects of the primitive organ of Corti. The distribution of organelles in Kolliker's epithelial cells, along with the observation that their apical surfaces are covered in a dense field of microvilli, strongly suggest that they are secretory in character. These cytological features are lost during the transformation of KO, and it appears that the conversion process is influenced by thyroxin, in that the immature epithelium persists in hypothyroidism. Uziel et al. (1985a) conclude that the tissue never transforms to its adult state in hypothyroid animals. However, subjects were sacrificed on the 30th postnatal day as a part of the protocol in those experiments, making it impossible to comment on KO's long-term fate. Preliminary data from our laboratory suggest that the KO does eventually acquire normal, adult-like morphology in the hypothyroid Tshr mutant. Nonetheless, when thyroxin is administered to a hypothyroid animal in whom KO persists, even for a brief 2-day period during inner ear development, the tissue regresses and assumes an adult configuration rapidly (Uziel et al., 1985a).

Given the role that the KO apparently plays in the formation of the TM, and the abnormal status of KO in hypothyroidism, it is not surprising that there are many reports claiming that the TM is abnormal in hypothyroid individuals (Prieto et al., 1990a; b; Anniko, 1980; Anniko and Rosenkvist, 1982; Anniko and Wroblewski, 1981). However, the issue is complicated by the fact that the nature of TM defects are variable, as reported from lab to lab, and animal model to animal model. For example, Uziel et al. (1985a) comment on the fact that the defect is severe in PTU-treated

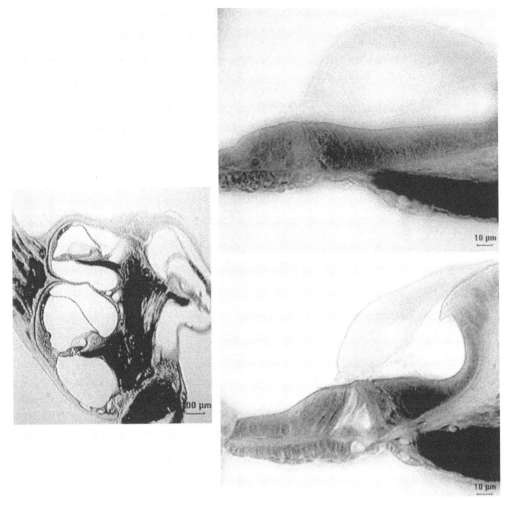

FIGURE 35.2   Cross-section of the cochlea in a 16-postnatal day-old homozygous Tshr mutant mouse. Left: mid-modiolar section showing radial profiles through the organ of Corti in the basal (lower left) and apical (upper left) turns. Top right: high magnification view of the apical turn. Bottom right: high magnification view of the basal turn.

rat pups, such that the leading edge of the TM remains attached to the lateral aspect of the KO, while the main body separates, producing a humped up and grossly distorted appearance (see Figure 1 in Uziel et al., 1985a). Contrary to this finding, Li et al. (1999) studied the morphology of the TM in the *hyt/hyt* mouse and, although they report that the TM is smaller than normal, a finding that is itself contrary to most other reports (Uziel et al., 1985a; Meyerhoff, 1979), it is notable that its overall form was not distorted.

Preliminary data from our laboratory support the view that the TM of the Tshr homozygous mutant is not obviously abnormal in either adult or developing *hyt/hyt* animals, although its development is notably delayed. To demonstrate this, developmental differences within apical and basal turns of the cochlea from a P16 homozygous Tshr mutant are shown in a mid-modiolar section through the organ of Corti in Figure 35.2. A high-magnification view of the apical turn reveals that the organ of Corti is grossly immature. Neither the tunnel of Corti nor space of Nuel has developed, and the TM still has a primitive form in that the minor TM is not yet organized in the area overlying the lesser epithelial ridge. A high-magnification view of the basal turn reveals that, although still somewhat immature, hair cells are present in the organ of Corti, as are presumptive stereocilia, and the TM is far more mature than it is in the apical turn. The tunnel of Corti and space of Nuel are clearly present and the limbus (Kolliker's organ) has converted from an immature pseudostratified columnar epithelium to its mature, cuboidal form. This 16-day-old cochlea closely resembles tissue taken from normal 10- to 12-day-old animals (Kraus and Aulbach-Kraus, 1981), and there is no clear evidence of distinctive pathology, aside from the developmental delay. On the contrary, it clear that the chemical composition of the TM in hypothyroid animals is abnormal (Prieto et al., 1990b). That finding, along with physiological observations presented later that discount the contribution of the TM to hypothyroidism-induced pathophysiology, suggest the possibility that the morphological anomalies observed in hypothyroidism may reflect an unusual reaction to fixation, and that the TM in living tissue may not appear distorted. The observation that the TMs of normal and hypothyroid individuals differ chemically offers an especially attractive explanation of an interesting observation made by Li et al. (1999). These authors observed that the tips of a subpopulation of stereocilia from adjacent OHCs in *hyt/hyt* mice are bound together by an apparently glue-like material of unknown composition. It is possible that a residue of the TM is left behind when processing tissue from hypothyroid animals, but not under normal circumstances. This potentially important issue clearly requires additional work.

Interestingly, cochlear malformations, including innervation patterns, are not observed in mice with null mutations in the gene encoding TRβ, the beta form of the T_3 receptor, although affected animals are hearing impaired (Forrest et al., 1996; and Chapter 10 in this volume). These data also support the notion that the gross morphology of the TM is unaffected in hypothyroidism.

In the last section we show that the physiological data support the argument that the TM is not an etiological factor in the expression of the disease; that is, electrophysiological data suggest that passive aspects of transduction in hypothyroid Tshr mutants are normal.

THE OCB AND DEVELOPMENT

The purpose of this section is to provide a background against which our claim that the OC system plays a role in cochlear development can be more easily seen. Very few efforts have been made to determine the role of the efferent OC system in inner ear development, although it innervates intracochlear targets during the period that the cochlea achieves maturity. Nonetheless, a composite, common view of efferent OCB development, derived from several laboratories and integrating findings from several mammals, has recently emerged. In it, fibers that most experts agree constitute the medial division of the OC system, arrive in the domain of the IHC at roughly the time that airborne sounds first elicit peripheral auditory responses in altricial mammals (Perkins and Morest, 1975; Pujol and Abonnenc, 1977; Pujol et al., 1978; 1979; Lenoir et al., 1980; Shnerson and Pujol, 1982; Jones and Eslami, 1983; Ginzberg and Morest, 1984; Walsh and McGee, 1986; 1987; Roth et al., 1991; Walsh and Romand, 1992; Roth and Bruns, 1993; Simmons et al., 1990; 1996a,b; 1998). These fibers form both axosomatic and axodendritic synapses with IHCs and primary afferent dendrites, respectively, during this period, much like those observed in 30-day-old, PTU-treated rat pups (Uziel et al., 1985a). It is notable that this is the only time in the life of a normal mammal that efferent fibers routinely make synaptic contact with IHCs in large numbers.

At an age corresponding to this early stage of functional development, Walsh and McGee (1997) studied auditory nerve fiber (ANF) responses from acutely deefferented 6-day-old kittens in an effort to determine the role of the OC system in this unique configuration. After cutting the tract, we noted — among other things — the conversion of spike train temporal firing patterns from immature, rhythmic sequences that are characteristic of neonatal cats (Walsh and McGee, 1988; 1997) to adult-like patterns that are characterized by their sustained steady-state peristimulus behavior (Figure 35.3).

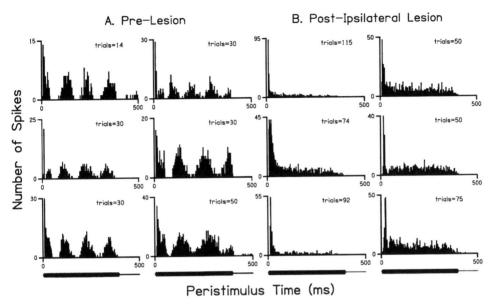

FIGURE 35.3 Peristimulus time histograms (PSTHs) from cochlear nucleus (CN) neurons recorded prior to an olivocochlear bundle lesion (A), and following a laterally placed lesion at the floor of the IVth ventricle, ipsilateral to the recording site (B). Data shown are from a 6-day-old kitten. Each panel represents responses from different CN neurons to stimuli in the range of 1.1 to 2.2 kHz. The repetition interval was 800 ms, and stimulus duration is indicated by the bars located below the bottom row of histograms. Number of trials for each PSTH is indicated in each panel.

On the basis of these findings, we suggested that the bursting character observed in immature ANF responses might reflect the direct modulation of IHC currents by OC efferents. The action may lead to the refinement of IHC innervation patterns by influencing the pruning back of supernumerary connections between IHCs and primary afferents, much like neuronal and sensory cell bursting in the visual system refines retinal and central innervation patterns (Shatz, 1990). Recording from individual efferent fibers in perinatal animals strengthened the view that the OCB is the source of rhythmic ANF activity in immature animals. Immature efferents have very high thresholds in neonates, and their temporal response properties are classically immature. Peristimulus time histograms (PSTHs) exhibited unambiguous regularity that corresponded temporally to the bursting pattern observed in immature neurons along the ascending pathway (Walsh and McGee, 1988; 1997).

After this relatively brief transitional period of IHC innervation, fibers of the MOC detach from IHCs in response to an as-yet-unknown signal, migrate across the tunnel of Corti, and eventually establish contact with OHCs (Pujol et al., 1978; Simmons et al., 1996a; Merchán-Pérez et al., 1990a; b; c; 1993; 1994; Pirvola et al., 1991; Echteler, 1992). It is at this stage that Walsh et al. (1998a; b) made off-midline cuts to the floor of the IVth ventricle of neonatal cats and determined the chronic consequences of deefferentation in the study that led to the formulation of the DDS model of congenital deafness. The chief findings in that study were that (1) the acoustic thresholds of ANFs at their characteristic frequencies (CFs) were elevated, sometimes rising into the profound loss category; (2) tuning curve tail thresholds, on the other hand, were the same as in controls, and in some cases tip thresholds actually exceeded tail thresholds, making tip-to-tail ratios less than 1; (3) the frequency-resolving power of ANFs in the relatively high CF range was diminished; and (4) DPOAE thresholds were also elevated. These findings suggest that processing abnormalities associated with neonatally deefferented animals occur in the context of active mechanics and not in relation to passive transduction; that is, only the gain of the cochlear amplifier is affected in neonatally deefferented animals.

All in all, ANFs from sectioned animals look a great deal like those recorded from acoustically traumatized animals, suggesting that cutting the OCB may leave individuals vulnerable to their environment. However, the one finding that contradicts this otherwise straightforward explanation is the status of hair cells in deefferented animals. Both OHCs and IHCs appear normal in both light and electron microscopic analyses. This finding is clearly inconsistent with expected anatomical correlates of acoustic trauma and led us to conclude that, under normal circumstances, the OCB triggers an important developmental event leading to the acquisition of normal auditory function. More specifically, we conclude that the cochlear amplification system develops abnormally as a consequence of neonatal deefferentation.

Aside from the Walsh and McGee (1997) and Walsh et al. (1998a; b) studies, the only other effort to experimentally determine the role of the OCB during development came from the laboratory of Pujol (Carlier and Pujol, 1976; Pujol and Carlier, 1982). The chief finding from Pujol and Carlier was that, after cutting the OCB in immature kittens and examining inner ear tissues under the electron microscope 2 months later, the number of afferent terminals was not reduced in deefferented cases. According to earlier work from Pujol's laboratory, the number of afferent contacts with OHCs is reduced during development as the result of competition for cell membrane space between in-growing efferents and existing afferents, leading to the pruning back of afferent contacts. Carlier and Pujol also studied CM and CAP responses from acutely deefferented neonates, showing that stimulation of what was assumed to be the lateral olivocochlear (LOC) system affected cochlear output even in perinatal animals (see Walsh and Romand, 1992, for a more thorough review of this work). The conclusions of Pujol and Carlier appear to be inaccurate in the vision of hindsight. Based on what is now known about OCB innervation patterns during development, the effects produced by stimulating the immature OC system were most likely mediated through the MOC, and not the LOC. Additionally, the results of a recent quantitative analysis of tissue from adult cats that were deefferented as neonates indicates that the number of primary afferent terminals on OHCs is not significantly different from control animals, raising a serious question about the efferent competition model of synapse refinement during development (Liberman et al., 2000). However, their pioneering efforts provided clear evidence that the descending OC system was in a position to affect cochlear mechanics in immature mammals.

THE OCB AS A MATURATIONAL FACTOR

Efferent OCB fibers, along with afferents, find their way into the otocyst at a surprisingly early stage of development, long before the cell masses comprising sensory and non-sensory primordia are distinguishable as differentiated tissues (Tello, 1931; Fritzsch and Nichols, 1993; Bruce et al., 1997). The importance of early innervation remains unclear, although current thinking suggests that otocyst differentiation is independent of afferent or efferent influences (Van De Water and Repressa, 1991). Growing neurites may play a role quite aside from their role in mature nervous systems. It may be that perinatal OCB fibers release substances that affect support/secretory cells that consequently produce substances leading to differentiation and morphogenesis of the end organ. In that context, work from the laboratory of Knipper et al. (1999) suggest that thyroid hormones regulate a variety of neurotrophic factors important to the differentiation of inner ear tissues.

At about the time that Walsh and McGee (1997) were studying the consequences of neonatal deefferentation, He and colleagues (He et al., 1994; He, 1997) published two reports indicating that OHCs taken from neonatal gerbils develop normal function *in vitro* (i.e., motility developed normally, as did certain receptor currents) when isolated from OCB influences prior to the time of their harvesting. While the details of that report are interesting and important, we suggest that two recent findings compromise their conclusions. First, and most important, Rontal and Echteler (1999) revised an earlier finding reported by Echteler (Echteler, 1992) that OCB efferents in gerbils arrive relatively late in development. In the more recent study, Rontal and Echteler show that the tract tracer DiI was transported from the OHC region into OCB fibers in neonates. This finding complicates the assumption that OHCs harvested from perinatal gerbils were free of OC system influences, suggesting instead that projections of the OC system are in a position to affect inner ear development at the time hair cells were harvested by He et al.

Sobkowicz and colleagues also address this question by harvesting the otocyst and growing it under *in vitro*, organotypic conditions (Emmerling and Sobkowicz, 1988; Sobkowicz and Emmerling, 1989; Whitlon and Sobkowicz, 1989; Emmerling et al., 1990; Sobkowicz, 1992). It is presumed that this tissue develops in the unambiguous absence of a brain influence. However, as mentioned above, it has been clear since as far back as Tello (1931) that efferent fibers probe the cell masses of the embryonic ear, and their influence cannot be ignored in the interpretation of *in vitro* work related to this question.

PHYSIOLOGICAL CHARACTERISTICS OF Tshr MUTANTS AND THE CONSEQUENCES OF T4 REPLACEMENT THERAPY

We have attempted in the preceding sections to make the case supporting our contention that the Tshr mutant mouse may be a murine equivalent of DDS. In this section, we summarize what is known about the auditory physiology of this strain by reviewing the findings of three relevant studies recently concluded in our laboratory, as well as those of O'Malley and co-workers (O'Malley et al., 1995; Li et al., 1999), and directly compare the physiological characteristics of neonatally deefferented cats and Tshr mutants.

AUDITORY CAPACITY IN TSHR MUTANT MICE

In addition to confirming the prior observation that audition in *hyt* animals is severely impaired (O'Malley et al., 1995; Sprenkle et al., 1997; Li et al., 1999), we recently extended that work by studying *hyt/hyt* individuals that were treated with thyroxin from birth through P10. The purpose of the study, at least in part, was to determine whether or not the thyroxin-dependent critical development period described by Deol (1973a) could be identified in hypothyroid Tshr animals. Progeny of sires that were homozygous for the trait and heterozygous dams (a condition that assures us that subjects were exposed to maternal thyroxin, a necessary condition to compare with Deol's findings) were treated with T4 or placebo between birth and P10, and ABRs to acoustic clicks and tone-bursts were recorded from young adults. *Hyt/hyt* animals exhibited a distinctive pattern of sensory pathology similar to that observed in neonatally deefferented cats: they were insensitive to sound (Figure 35.4), response latencies were prolonged, peak amplitudes were reduced (Figure 35.5), and latency-intensity curves were steep relative to euthyroid, *hyt/+* littermates.

One of the most interesting, if not important, findings from Sprenkle et al. (2001a) is illustrated in Figure 35.5. Amplitude-level curves representing ABR wave I were shifted to the right relative to those derived from heterozygotes in the majority of saline-treated homozygotes. While average wave I amplitudes associated with thyroxin-treated homozygotes were indistinguishable from those of normal euthyroid animals at relatively high stimulus levels, function was not restored to the threshold levels observed in heterozygotes. This finding is consistent with the view that the pathology underlying hypothyroidism affects the gain of the cochlear amplifier and, most important, that thyroxin-dependent intracochlear developmental events blocked by hypothyroidism cannot be prevented by thyroxin therapy during the first 10 postnatal days. This indicates that thyroxin is an important developmental factor beyond the period identified by Deol (1973a).

Nonetheless, as in other animal models (Deol, 1973a; Uziel et al., 1985a; b), thyroxin also promotes the recovery of function in *hyt/hyt* mice. In general, affected animals responded to acoustic stimuli more frequently, and were more sensitive to tone-bursts throughout their audiometric range following treatment with thyroxin. Although acoustic thresholds were improved relative to the untreated group, thyroxin-treated homozygotes were always less sensitive than their normal euthyroid counterparts (Figure 35.4).

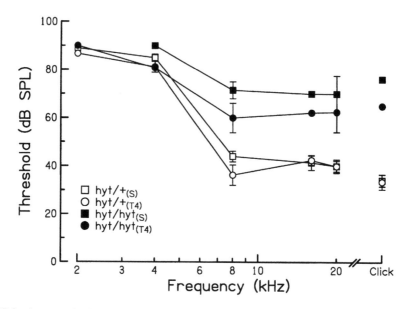

FIGURE 35.4 Average ABR thresholds in response to click and tone-burst stimuli obtained from each experimental group of hyt mice indicated in the symbol key. Mice were generated from paternal *hyt/hyt* and maternal *hyt/+* pairings, and recordings were made when animals were 75 to 90 postnatal days old. The (S) and (T4) subscripts denote that animals were treated with saline (placebo) or thyroxin (T4) during the first 10 postnatal days. Error bars represent the SEM of 8 to 12 mice tested per group. (Adapted from Sprenkle et al., 2001a.)

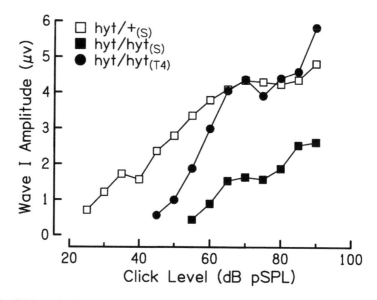

FIGURE 35.5 Click-evoked ABR wave I amplitudes as a function of level for three experimental groups of hyt mice. Genetic types and treatments, indicated in the key, are the same as those shown in Figure 35.4. Values represent averages obtained from 8 to 12 mice per group. (Adapted from Sprenkle et al., 2001a.)

In summary, the combined physiological and pharmacological findings, which include recruitment-like behavior and the restoration of response magnitude at high but not low levels, support our view that the cochlear amplifier is the primary locus of an enduring otological defect associated with hypothyroidism in Tshr mutant mouse development.

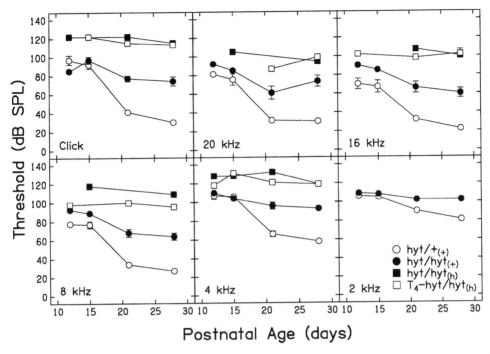

FIGURE 35.6 Development of ABR thresholds in response to clicks and tone-bursts are shown for four experimental groups of hyt mice. The symbol key is located in the lower right frame. The (+) and (h) subscripts denote progeny born to euthyroid and hypothyroid dams, respectively; those designated with (+) were generated from paternal *hyt/hyt* and maternal *hyt/+* pairings, whereas those designated with (h) were generated from paternal *hyt/hyt* and maternal *hyt/hyt* pairings. The unfilled squares represent hypothyroid animals that were treated with thyroxin (T4) between birth and 10 postnatal days. Values represent averages ± SEM of 6 to 13 mice. (Adapted from Sprenkle et al., 2001b.)

DEVELOPMENT OF FUNCTION IN TSHR MUTANTS

Although hypothyroidism is congenital in *hyt* mice, the development of auditory function had not been studied at the time that we became interested in its potential as a neonatal deefferentation substitute. Consequently, we recorded ABRs to clicks and tone-bursts on P12, P15, P21, and P28, tracking the development of auditory function and hoping to more thoroughly understand the extent to which pre- and postnatal thyroid hormones influence the development of auditory function in this strain of mice. To that end, experimental subjects were offspring of euthyroid and hypothyroid dams. Basic developmental trends are shown in Figure 35.6.

Nothing remarkable was observed in the development of heterozygotes, in that they followed a perfectly normal sequence of maturation based on similar studies of other mammals (Jewett and Romano, 1972; Walsh et al., 1986a; b; c; Pettigrew and Morey, 1987; Schweitzer, 1987; McFadden et al., 1996) and other mice (Henry and Haythorn, 1978; Hunter and Willott, 1987). Clear responses to high-level stimuli were observed for most stimulus conditions on P12; and thresholds, response amplitudes, interpeak intervals, and latencies developed normally, achieving adult-like properties by P21. Predictably, development was fundamentally abnormal in *hyt/hyt* mice born to hypothyroid dams. In effect, development simply did not occur in these severely diseased animals, all of whom remained insensitive to acoustic stimulation throughout the period of the investigation.

On the other hand, grossly immature responses were occasionally observed in *hyt/hyt* animals born to euthyroid dams (i.e., pups were exposed to thyroxin *in utero*) on day 15, although clear, low-amplitude responses were not routinely observed until day 21. As with heterozygotes, thresholds generally improved with age, and intensity-latency curves that were relatively steep in young animals developed normally among representatives of this group. The most significant developmental changes occurred unambiguously between P15 and P21, at which time latency-intensity slopes were essentially the same in heterozygotes and homozygotes. Some, but not all, *hyt/hyt* animals born to euthyroid dams exhibited prolonged latencies and central conduction times (the I–IV interpeak interval) throughout the observed intensity range. Response amplitudes were generally larger in heterozygotes than in *hyt/hyt* mice, regardless of level, but were highly variable, as observed in other mammals. Based on these findings, we conclude that the need for thyroxin during development is extensive. Animals exposed to prenatal thyroxin develop partial function, but never achieve normal, or even near-normal, acoustic sensitivity. Combined with the finding that *hyt/hyt* individuals fail to develop normal auditory capacity, even when thyroxin is replaced for the first 10 postnatal days, leads to the conclusion that the thyroxin-dependent critical period extends further into postnatal life than Deol (1973a) described, setting the stage for the follow-up study that is summarized in the following chapter section.

THYROXIN IS EFFICACIOUS THROUGHOUT DEVELOPMENT

Motivated by our interest to better understand the limits of thyroxin-dependent critical periods, we attempted to determine the relative importance of prenatal and postnatal thyroxin in the treatment of hypothyroidism-induced deafness by examining experimental subjects born to *hyt/hyt* breeders that were implanted either with thyroxin or placebo controlled-release pellets prior to mating. All subjects were homozygous for the *hyt* allele, and all were born to *hyt/hyt* dams, and subjects received exogenous thyroxin or saline placebo injections from birth through P14 or the time of testing on P28.

The overall findings are summarized in Figure 35.7. In the absence of exogenous thyroxin, very high stimulus intensities were required to elicit ABRs, revealing a severe to profound (>80 dB) hearing loss in this hypothyroid group that had never been exposed to thyroxin. Auditory performance was not significantly improved when thyroxin treatment was confined to the postnatal period. In contrast, ABR thresholds, latencies, and amplitudes of mice born to dams that had received thyroxin during pregnancy were significantly improved relative to both of the other groups. ABR thresholds were improved even more (relative to mice in whom treatment was stopped at birth) when prenatal thyroxin replacement was followed by treatment during the first 14 days after birth, and animals treated throughout prenatal and postnatal life were comparable to those of age-matched euthyroid *hyt/+* mice.

These data illustrate the fact that treatment of *hyt/hyt* mice with exogenous thyroxin significantly attenuates hypothyroid-induced otopathology in a developmental, sequential stage dependent manner. In addition, we show that the critical thyroxin-dependent period of development includes a key prenatal influence plus an extended postnatal influence, in contrast to the findings of Deol, firmly establishing the Tshr mutant mouse as a model system for the study of thyroid hormone influences on the developing auditory system.

A COMPARISON OF DDS AND HYPOTHYROIDISM

Having summarized what is known about the basic anatomy and physiology of the Tshr mouse, we now turn attention to a direct comparison of data acquired from neonatally deefferented cats that served as the basis of the DDS concept and data from hypothyroid Tshr mice acquired under similar experimental conditions.

The primary purpose for studying DPOAEs in adult animals lesioned as neonates was to directly test the primary conclusion in Walsh et al. (1998a) that OCB transection early in life blocked the development and/or expression of active transduction. The approach used in that study was to compare DPOAEs, an indicator of the state of active transduction mechanics, in affected and normal animals. The outcome of that study is shown in the upper panels of Figure 35.8, in which CAP

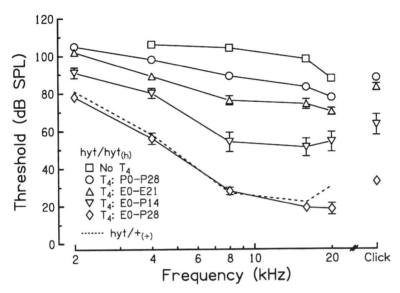

FIGURE 35.7   ABR thresholds as a function of stimulus frequency of *hyt/hyt* mice generated from *hyt/hyt* breeding pairs and tested at P28. Mice received T4 supplementation during the periods indicated in the key, with E0 designating embryonic day 0, P0 designating birth, etc. T_4 treatment during the gestational period was accomplished by implanting dams with a 60-day controlled-release pellet 2 weeks prior to mating. Control dams received placebo. Postnatally, animals were injected with L-thyroxin subcutaneously using the following dosing strategy to achieve normal age-matched serum values: 4 ng/g, P0–5; 5.8 ng/g, P6–8; 9.1 ng/g, P9–10; and 14 ng/g thereafter. The dashed line represents thresholds obtained from heterozygotes born to euthyroid dams. The means ± SEM are depicted for the 9 to 12 mice tested per group. (Adapted from Sprenkle et al., 2001c.)

and DPOAE thresholds representing control and lesion cases are compared directly. Average CAP threshold differences were on the order of 20 dB, except for the highest frequencies studied. DPOAE threshold differences, on the other hand, while always elevated in lesioned animals, were smaller for stimulus frequencies in the vicinity of 10 kHz than they were for either lower or higher frequencies, suggesting that the OCB has a differential effect on the development of active mechanics.

As in cats deefferented as neonates, insensitivity to sound was a uniform property of hypothyroid Tshr mutants. Average ABR thresholds are plotted as a function of stimulus frequency for a group of 2-month-olds in the lower panel of Figure 35.8 and it is clear that Tshr mutant mice are between 30 and 40 dB less sensitive than their euthyroid counterparts. This degree of insensitivity is similar to that observed in adult cats deefferented as neonates and we conclude that Tshr mice and deefferented cats are the same in this dimension.

Physiological differences separating homozygotes and heterozygotes were not limited to acoustic sensitivity. The insensitivity of *hyt/hyt* animals is illustrated in a plot of ABR wave I amplitude vs. level in Figure 35.9. In addition to high thresholds, amplitude growth near threshold among hypothyroid animals was steeper than in euthyroid animals than in hypothyroid individuals, thereby exhibiting the characteristics of response recruitment, a well-recognized indicator of sensorineural hearing loss.

Although ABRs are useful indicators of the overall status of auditory system function, the possibility that abnormal ABRs reflect abnormal neural, rather than, or in addition to abnormal sensory elements in hypothyroidism, must be considered to acquire a thorough understanding of the pathophysiology of this disease. Clear evidence that the pathophysiology observed in hypothyroidism in Tshr animals is primarily otological can be found by considering DPOAE production, because DPOAEs reflect the OHC contribution to active transduction mechanics. In Figure 35.10, DPOAE input-output curves from a homozygous individual and a heterozygous individual are

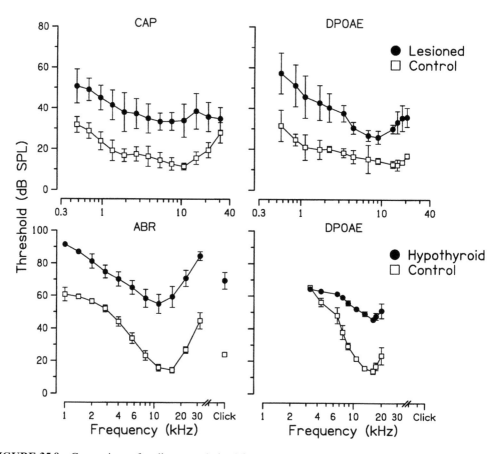

FIGURE 35.8 Comparison of audiograms derived from evoked potentials (left panels) and DPOAEs (right panels) in adult cats that had surgical lesions of the olivocochlear bundle as neonates vs. controls (top panels), and *hyt/hyt* (hypothyroid) and *hyt/+* (control) mice (bottom panels). Evoked potentials were either compound action potentials (CAP) of the auditory nerve (used for cats) or auditory-evoked brainstem responses (used for mice). (Data from cats are adapted from Walsh et al., 1998b, and those from mice are adapted from Walsh et al., 2000.)

shown. The relative insensitivity of DPOAEs representing hypothyroid individuals relative to the euthyroid individuals is clear, and threshold differences are in the same general range as those observed in ABRs. Interestingly, DPOAE input-output curves representing homozygous individuals do not exhibit the clear recruitment-like behavior noted in ABR input-output curves (i.e., slopes were not significantly different). This suggests that DPOAEs are either poor indicators of recruitment-like behavior or that the locus of recruitment-associated pathology occurs at a retrocochlear site or involves transduction at the level of the inner hair cell. Whether or not this observation reflects a characteristic difference between the two response types is not clear at this time.

As with audiograms based on ABR recordings, threshold vs. frequency plots representing homozygotes and heterozygotes show the same basic differences when DPOAEs are used to estimate thresholds. Average differences between the euthyroid and hypothyroid cases are approximately 40 dB in the region of the hyt mouse's greatest sensitivity, but trail off above and below 18 kHz. This is a most interesting finding because it essentially matches the characteristic separation between CAP and DPOAE estimated thresholds observed in deefferented cats.

In summary, the relevant frequency-threshold relationships between deefferented cats and hypothyroid mice are illustrated in Figure 35.8. Threshold estimates derived from CAP measurements in the case of chronically lesioned cats and from ABR wave I in hypothyroid mice are shown

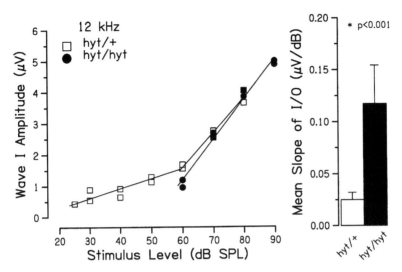

FIGURE 35.9 Amplitude of ABR wave I as a function of stimulus level for *hyt/+* and *hyt/hyt* mice. Stimulus frequency was 12 kHz. Slopes of the amplitude-level curves were fitted by least squares linear regression of the values near threshold and mean slopes at 12 kHz are shown in the right panel. (Adapted from Walsh et al., 2000.)

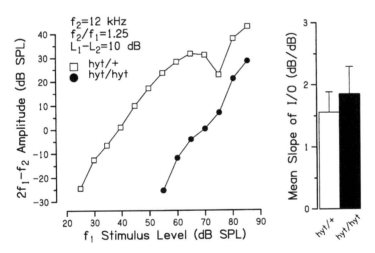

FIGURE 35.10 Amplitude of the distortion product, $2f_1-f_2$, as a function of f_2 level for *hyt/+* and *hyt/hyt* mice. F_2 frequency = 12 kHz, f_2/f_1 ratio = 1.25, and L_1 was held 10 dB greater than L_2. Slopes of the near-threshold amplitude-level curves were fitted by least-squares linear regression and mean slopes at 12 kHz are shown in the right panel. (Adapted from Walsh et al., 2000.)

in the left panels, and DPOAE estimates are shown in the right panels. Although species differences are evident, it is clear that the same basic relationships are found in both models.

TUNING CURVES REVEAL THE SOURCE OF PATHOPHYSIOLOGY IN *HYT/HYT* MICE

Having shown that the response properties of *hyt/hyt* mice and neonatally deefferented cats are similar, one comparison of interest yet to be considered is tuning curves tip and tail thresholds. If tip thresholds associated with hypothyroidism are significantly higher than those of euthyroid animals, and tail thresholds are not significantly different, we can conclude that hypothyroidism causes a form of congenital deafness affecting active mechanics alone, as in DDS. If both tip and tail

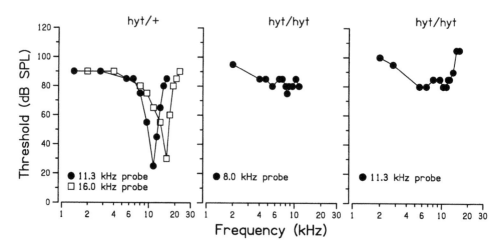

FIGURE 35.11 Tuning curves (TC) generated using a forward masking paradigm of ABRs for *hyt/+* and *hyt/hyt* mice, plotted as a function of masker frequency and the masker level that produced approximately 50% reduction in the amplitude evoked by a probe stimulus. Probe stimuli were approximately 15 dB above threshold. (Adapted from Walsh et al., 2000.)

thresholds are significantly elevated when compared to control animals, we can conclude that both active and passive aspects of transduction are affected by hypothyroidism. If tail thresholds are significantly lower (i.e., hypersensitive) in hypothyroid animals when compared to euthyroid animals, we can conclude that either OHCs or their stereocilia, or the association between the tectorial membrane and sensory cells, are abnormal, based on the findings of Liberman and Dodds (1984).

Tuning curves from a heterozygous, euthyroid individual are shown in the left panel of Figure 35.11. Quality factor estimates of sharpness are clearly adult, and tip-to-tail ratios are also normal, a property that generalizes among heterozygotes. Tuning curves with identical probe or center frequencies collected from animals that were homozygous for the *hyt* allele are shown in the right-hand panels. These tuning curves are unmistakably abnormal. Tips are completely missing in both examples (although in some cases poorly tuned, insensitive tips are observed) and broad, insensitive, but normal low-frequency tails are evident. Tuning curves of ANFs from animals lesioned as neonates exhibited similar characteristics. In contrast, tail thresholds are the same in euthyroid and hypothyroid individuals; the average tail threshold was approximately 85 to 90 dB in heterozygotes and approximately 85 dB in homozygotes, providing evidence that passive mechanics are unaffected by the disease.

CONCLUSION

Although it is too early to conclude that the Tshr mutant mouse suffers from DDS and can now be put into service as a model system in the search for the molecular basis of at least certain forms of congenital deafness, a compelling argument can be made. The reasoning behind this claim is based on the observation that the OC system plays a critical role in the final differentiation of intracochlear elements that produce cochlear amplification (Walsh et al., 1998a; b), that the physiological characteristics of deefferented cats and hypothyroid Tshr animals are very similar, and that outer hair cells are morphologically normal in both neonatally deefferented cats and Tshr homozygotes (see Figure 35.12).

One remaining question is whether or not the delayed outgrowth of the OC projection in homozygous Tshr animals leads to a missed opportunity to interact with intracochlear tissues necessary for the final stage of cytodifferentiation leading to active mechanics and cochlear amplification. Preliminary data suggest that such is the case, but the final answer is pending, awaiting

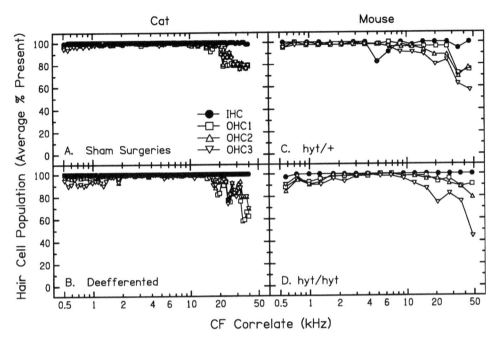

FIGURE 35.12 Comparison of cytocochleograms in adult cats that had surgical lesions of the olivocochlear bundle as neonates vs. controls (left panels), and *hyt/hyt* (hypothyroid) and *hyt/+* (control) mice (right panels). The percentage of hair cells present is plotted for each row of hair cells as a function of cochlear location expressed as characteristic frequency (CF) correlate. Three mice were tested within each group at 6 months of age. The loss of hair cells at the basal end of the cochlea was also observed in age-matched wild-type animals, and is indicative of age-related hair cell loss. (Data from cats are adapted from Walsh et al., 1998a, and data from mice are adapted from Walsh et al., 2000.)

the completion of that study. Anticipating the outcome, we offer the following conceptual model of thyroxin's influence on cochlear development.

The final stage of development, during which function is acquired, can be divided into two stages, one regulated directly by thyroxin and a second through OCB-dependent mechanisms. In stage I, we suggest that thyroxin mediates critical aspects of inner ear morphogenesis that culminate in the acquisition of a primitive form of peripheral auditory function characterized by passive mechanoelectrical transduction. It is during this period that immature responses are first elicited from the peripheral auditory system by a limited set of high-level, low-frequency airborne sounds. Anatomical correlates of this developmental dynamic include the secretion of the tectorial membrane, the sculpting of the inner spiral sulcus, the thinning of the tympanic epithelial cover layer, and the overall maturation of the organ of Corti's electroanatomy. IHCs acquire normal characteristics during this period.

In the second stage of development, characterized by the appearance of adult sensitivity and frequency selectivity, we suggest that thyroxin regulates neurite extension in the OCB, that in turn plays a significant role in the final differentiation of the inner ear. The central tenent of the conceptual model is that active transduction is acquired through OC interactions with an as yet unknown inner ear element(s). At least two crucial events in OC system development appear to be vulnerable to thyroxin deficiency: neurite outgrowth and synaptogenesis at the level of OHCs. We suggest that blockage of either, or both, of these events interferes with the cytodifferentiation of OHCs that subsequently and irreversibly leads to ineffective cochlear amplification.

ACKNOWLEDGMENTS

This project was supported by grants from the Deafness Research Foundation and the NIH (DC00215 and DC00982). The authors wish to gratefully acknowledge collaborations with Dr. M.C. Liberman and Dr. Bruce Warr in preliminary efforts to assess the anatomical characteristics of the TSHR mouse.

36 Mouse Models for Usher and Alport Syndromes

JoAnn McGee and Edward J. Walsh

INTRODUCTION

Syndromic deafness may account for as much as 30% of all inherited forms of deafness, and the identification of genetic defects associated with specific conditions has been a major goal of biomedical scientists for some time. Although mouse models are commonly exploited to understand human disease, few animal models of syndromic deafness have been developed or identified. However, for two major diseases, Usher and Alport syndromes, there are well-defined mouse models available at this time that harbor mutations in the orthologous genes that cause human deafness, and they are the focus of this chapter.

USHER SYNDROME

DISEASE CHARACTERISTICS

Usher syndrome is inherited as an autosomal recessive disorder that is characterized by sensorineural hearing loss and the progressive degradation of vision due to retinitis pigmentosa (RP). RP is one of the most common forms of hereditary retinal disease. It produces night blindness in its early stages, progressing to visual field constriction and loss of visual acuity as the ultimate consequence of degenerating photoreceptors and pigmented retinal epithelium (Villa, 1997). Usher syndrome is the leading cause of deafness/blindness in the United States and accounts for 3 to 6% of the congenitally deaf population. Although the condition is rare, having a prevalence of approximately 4.4 to 5.0 individuals per 100,000, approximately 1/70 to 1/100 are thought to carry affected alleles in the general population (Vernon, 1969; Boughman et al., 1983; Rosenberg et al., 1997).

From a clinical perspective, there are three primary categories of Usher syndrome, and group affiliation has historically been determined on the basis of phenotype. The chief symptoms used to assign individuals to appropriate diagnostic groups include (1) the severity of associated auditory and visual impairments, (2) the age that symptoms first appear, and (3) whether or not individuals manifest vestibular system comorbidity (McLeod et al., 1971; Moller et al., 1989; Keats et al., 1992; Smith et al., 1994; Wagenaar et al., 1999). Usher syndrome type I (USH1) is the most extreme form of the disease. Patients with USH1 suffer from bilateral, severe to profound congenital hearing loss, rapidly progressing retinitis pigmentosa that begins in childhood or adolescence, as well as congenital vestibular dysfunction. Usher type II (USH2) patients exhibit mild to moderate congenital hearing loss at low frequencies and severe to profound loss at high frequencies; RP begins relatively late in life, usually sometime in the second and third decades, and patients show no signs of vestibular system abnormality. Some USH2 patients also show progressive hearing loss. Finally, hearing loss in USH3 patients is progressive, the onset of RP is variable, and vestibular dysfunction is observed in approximately 50% of the diseased population (Karjalainen et al., 1989; Pakarinen et al., 1995; Joensuu et al., 1996).

0-8493-2328-2/01/$0.00+$.50
© 2001 by CRC Press LLC

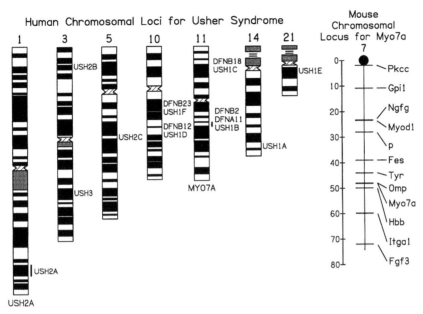

FIGURE 36.1   Human chromosomal loci associated with Usher syndrome are shown on ideograms, along with non-syndromic genes associated with deafness that map to overlapping regions: USH1A (Kaplan et al., 1992; Larget-Piet et al., 1994); USH1B (Kimberling et al., 1992; Bonne-Tamir et al., 1994); USH1C (Smith et al., 1992; Keats et al., 1994); USH1D (Wayne et al., 1996); USH1E (Chaib et al., 1997); USH1F (Wayne et al., 1997); USH2A (Kimberling et al., 1990; 1995; Lewis et al., 1990); USH2B (Hmani et al., 1999); USH2C (Pieke-Dahl et al., 2000); USH3 (Sankila et al., 1995; Joensuu et al., 1996); DFNB23 (Van Camp and Smith, 2000); DFNB12 (Chaib et al., 1996); DFNB18 (Jain et al., 1998); DFNB2 (Guilford et al., 1994; Weil et al., 1997; Liu et al., 1997c); and DFNA11 (Tamagawa et al., 1996; Liu et al., 1997d). Below chromosomes 1 and 11 are the genes associated with Usher syndrome that have been identified to date. The relative chromosomal locus for Myo7a in the mouse is shown schematically on the right (Gibson et al., 1995). Distances are in cM from the centromere. Locations of other genes located on mouse chromosome 7 were obtained from the Mouse Genome Database (http://www.informatics.jax.org).

The variability of phenotype in Usher syndrome patients clearly indicates that the genetic basis of the disease is heterologous. Defective genes located on at least seven chromosomes have been implicated as etiological factors and genetic linkage studies have mapped USH1 to six different chromosomal loci (USH1A to USH1F; 14q32, 11q13.5, 11p15.1, 10q, 21q, 10, respectively), USH2 to three loci (USH2A to USH2C; 1q41, 3p23-24.2, 5q14.3-21.3); and USH3 to a single location on chromosome 3 at the 3q21-25 locus (Figure 36.1)* (Kimberling et al., 1990; 1992; 1995; Lewis et al., 1990; Kaplan et al., 1992; Smith et al., 1992; Bonne-Tamir et al., 1994; Keats et al., 1994; Larget-Piet et al., 1994; Sankila et al., 1995; Joensuu et al., 1996; Wayne et al., 1996, 1997; Chaib et al., 1997; Hmani et al., 1999; Pieke-Dahl et al., 2000). Recently, a mutation in the mitochondrial MTTS2 gene was identified in an Irish family in which affected members present with retinitis pigmentosa and progressive hearing loss (Mansergh et al., 1999). It is likely that more loci will emerge since families with known victims that are not linked to any of the established loci have been identified (Larget-Piet et al., 1994; Pieke-Dahl et al., 1996; 2000; Chaib et al., 1997; Saouda et al., 1998).

USH1B accounts for the majority of patients falling into the type I category, and the condition affects families from a variety of ethnic backgrounds (Weil et al., 1995; Kimberling et al., 1992;

---

* The Usher syndromes mapped to chromosomal locations 3p23-24.2 and 5q14.3-21.3 have both been designated USH2B (Hmani et al., 1999; Pieke-Dahl et al., 2000); however, the locus on 5q14.3-21.3 has been officially designated USH2C by the Human Genome Organization nomenclature committee.

Bonne-Tamir et al., 1994). Conversely, USH1A is less widely distributed, having been observed exclusively in families located in a restricted region of France (Kaplan et al., 1992). Thus far, only French Acadians and a Lebanese family are known to harbor the gene underlying USH1C (Smith et al., 1992; Saouda et al., 1998). USH1D and USH1F have been observed in solitary families from Pakistan (Wayne et al., 1996; 1997) and USH1E in a single family from Morocco (Chaib et al., 1997).

The vast majority of Usher syndrome type II cases reflect mutations at the USH2A locus (Bessant et al., 1998) and, like USH1B, this disorder has been identified in a variety of ethnic groups (Kimberling et al., 1990; Lewis et al., 1990). USH2B has been described in a Tunisian family (Hmani et al., 1999) and USH2C in nine unrelated families of diverse origin (Pieke-Dahl et al., 2000). Among the three Usher phenotypes, Usher type II is most prevalent, accounting for more than half of the cases thus far discovered (Hope et al., 1997; Rosenberg et al., 1997). While only 2 to 3% of all Usher syndrome patients are identified as type III on the basis of phenotype, 42% of Finnish families have Usher syndrome classified as type III (Sankila et al., 1995; Joensuu et al., 1996; Gasparini et al., 1998).

Several of the chromosomal loci associated with Usher syndrome map to similar chromosomal regions as other forms of non-syndromic deafness. For example, USH1C is known to overlap the locus identified for the recessive form of non-syndromic deafness commonly known as DFNB18 (Smith et al., 1992; Jain et al., 1998). In addition, USH1D overlaps the DFNB12 locus (Chaib et al., 1996) and USH1F with DFNB23 (Van Camp and Smith, 2000). The gene responsible for USH1B is the same gene that causes a dominant form of non-syndromic deafness, DFNA11, *as well as* a recessive, non-syndromic form of deafness, DFNB2 (Guilford et al., 1994; Tamagawa et al., 1996; Liu et al., 1997c; d; Weil et al., 1997). These allelic relationships suggest that genetic variants associated with at least some of these loci are responsible for both syndromic and isolated forms of deafness, as well as different modes of inheritance.

Although numerous chromosomal loci have been mapped for Usher syndrome, only two genes have been identified:* MYO7A, which is responsible for Usher syndrome type 1B (Weil et al., 1995), and USH2A, which is responsible for Usher syndrome type 2A (Eudy et al., 1998). Mutations in the MYO7A gene are responsible for DFNA11 and DFNB2 (Weil et al., 1997; Liu et al., 1997c; d), as well as "atypical" Usher syndrome in which hearing loss is progressive rather than stable over time, thereby resembling Usher type III (Liu et al., 1998a).

The USH2A gene encodes a protein called usherin, a novel extracellular matrix protein (Eudy et al., 1998), and the mouse ortholog maps to chromosome 1 (Sumegi et al., 2000). USH2A transcripts are located in bipolar cells of the mouse retina as well as spiral ganglion cells. The protein itself is expressed in the interphotoreceptor cell matrix of the retina, in addition to the matrix surrounding spiral ganglion cells and their processes (Bhattacharya et al., 2000; Sumegi et al., 2000). A mouse model of Usher syndrome type 2A is not yet available. It is interesting that a mutation in the human USH2A gene has been reported that causes RP without affecting hearing, suggesting that this gene may be responsible for a number of cases of non-syndromic retinitis pigmentosa (Rivolta et al., 2000).

In pursuit of appropriate animal models of Usher syndrome, several candidate mice have been considered. For example, *rd3* mice that harbor a mutation on the retinal dystrophy gene located on chromosome 1, exhibit severe retinal degeneration when the allele is expressed in the homozygous state. However, auditory brainstem response (ABR) thresholds appear normal in affected animals, suggesting that the *rd3* mutation does not influence auditory function (Pieke-Dahl et al., 1997). In addition, recessive mutations of the *rd5* (*tub*) gene on mouse chromosome 7, lead to late-onset obesity and insulin resistance, early progressive retinal degeneration, and early hearing loss with progressive cochlear degeneration (Heckenlively et al., 1995; Ohlemiller et al., 1995; 1997). However, hearing loss only occurs when *tub* mutant mice are also homozygous for a mutation in the

---

* See **Notes Added in Proof**.

moth1 gene (modifier of tubby hearing 1), located on chromosome 2 (Ikeda et al., 1999). Recessive mutations in related genes, such as the *tulp-1* gene (tubby-like protein 1), lead to early-onset retinal degeneration but do not affect auditory function (Ikeda et al., 2000). Clearly, animal models for the study of Usher syndrome will require the development of new models or the identification of impaired genes responsible for deafness in existing models. Currently, the only mouse model of Usher syndrome that has been identified with mutations in the orthologous gene causing human deafness is the shaker-1 mouse, and that model is the focus of the remainder of this section.*

SHAKER-1 MOUSE: HOMOLOG OF USHER SYNDROME TYPE 1B, DFNB2, DFNA11, AND ATYPICAL USHER SYNDROME

A naturally occurring mutation that is inherited as an autosomal recessive trait, called shaker-1 (*sh-1*), causes choreic head movements, hyperactivity, circling behavior, and progressive deafness in affected animals. It was originally identified in the BALB/c mouse strain by Lord and Gates in 1929. Other spontaneous mutations at the shaker-1 locus have been identified, including *sh1^{6J}*, which arose on the C57BL/KsJ-*dbm* strain (Letts et al., 1994). Several forms of *shaker* mutations have been chemically induced in the BALB/cR1 strain using the mutagenic agent N-ethyl-N-nitrosourea (ENU), including *sh1^{26SB}*, *sh1^{816SB}*, *sh1^{3336SB}*, *sh1^{4494SB}*, and *sh1^{4626SB}* (Rinchik et al., 1990). After the gene responsible for the shaker-1 phenotype, Myo7a, was discovered, the nomenclature changed to reflect the gene's identity and that system is used in the remainder of the chapter to differentiate among the shaker-1 mice (e.g., *Myo7a^{sh1}* to represent the original shaker-1 mouse, and *Myo7a^{6J}*, *Myo7a^{26SB}*, *Myo7a^{816SB}*, *Myo7a^{3336SB}*, *Myo7a^{4494SB}*, and *Myo7a^{4626SB}* to represent the other mutations).

The genetic defect in the original shaker-1 mouse has been located on chromosome 7 and is closely linked to the tyrosinase (*Tyr*) gene (Gates, 1929) that is located between the *Tyr* marker and the β-globin (*Hbb*) gene. Further refinement of the *sh-1* gene location placed it just distal to the gene that encodes the olfactory marker protein (*Omp*) (K.A. Brown et al., 1992), which is itself closely linked to the Usher syndrome 1B gene (Evans et al., 1993), although the nucleotide sequence of the *Omp* gene is normal in *sh-1* mice (K.A. Brown et al., 1994). In a major breakthrough, Gibson et al. (1995) identified the *sh-1* gene (Figure 36.1) and discovered that it encoded the myosin VIIa protein. That work led to the subsequent identification of the human MYO7A gene responsible for Usher type 1B (Weil et al., 1995), which was the first of the Usher syndrome genes to be cloned.

MYOSIN VIIA

Unlike conventional myosins that form bipolar filaments and are partially responsible for contractile events in muscle cells, unconventional myosins, including myosin VIIa, appear to be involved in numerous other intracellular activities, including service as molecular motors that drive the movement of subcellular elements along actin filaments, a phenomenon that occurs primarily within non-muscle cells (Mooseker and Cheney, 1995; Cope et al., 1996; Hasson and Mooseker, 1997; Weil et al., 1997; Baker and Titus, 1998; Mermall et al., 1998; Hasson, 1999). Myosin VIIa (Figure 36.2) is a polypeptide composed of 2215 amino acids, has a molecular weight of about 250 kDa, and consists of an N-terminal motor, or head domain, where the binding sites for ATP and actin are located. Contiguous with the head domain is the regulatory, or neck, region consisting of a light chain-binding domain (the IQ motif) that includes five repeats and binds with calcium binding proteins, possibly calmodulin. At the carboxy-terminal end is a long tail domain (1359 amino acids) consisting of a short coiled-coil region that is contiguous with the IQ domain that allows formation of a two-headed dimer, that is followed by a direct repeat of two elements: a proximal MyTH4 (myosin tail homology 4) domain and a distal talin-like domain, which are thought to target the myosin molecule to the plasma membrane or some other cellular constituent. An SH3

---

* See **Notes Added in Proof**.

Myosin VIIa and Shaker−1 Mutations

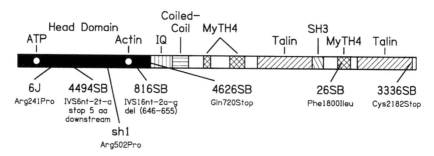

FIGURE 36.2 Schematic representation of myosin VIIa domain structure (adapted from Mooseker and Cheney, 1995; Z.Y. Chen et al., 1996; Cope et al., 1996; Baker and Titus, 1998; Hasson and Mooseker, 1997; Hasson, 1999), along with the relative locations of the shaker-1 mutations (Gibson et al., 1995; Mburu et al., 1997). The myosin VIIa protein consists of a head (motor) domain, where the ATP and actin binding sites are located, a neck region consisting of the IQ motif that binds with calcium-binding proteins, and a tail region consisting of a coiled-coil region that allows the formation of a molecule with two motor domains. This region is followed by two sections, each containing a MyTH4 (myosin tail homology 4) domain and a talin-like domain, which likely target the myosin molecule to the plasma membrane or cellular organelles. Between these two sections lies an SH3 (Src homology 3) domain, which may serve as a ligand binding site.

(Src homology 3) domain is interleaved between the two repeated tail elements and may serve as a ligand binding site.

The gene that encodes myosin VIIa spans approximately 114 kb of genomic DNA, is composed of 7465 base pairs, and includes 49 exons (Weil et al., 1995; 1996; Hasson et al., 1995; Z.Y. Chen et al., 1996; Levy et al., 1997; Kelley et al., 1997). Two products have been transcribed from the MYO7A gene. The largest is 7.4 kb, which encodes the 250-kDa protein described above; and the other is 4.2 kb segment, which encodes a smaller polypeptide (138 kDa) that has the same motor and regulatory domains but includes a truncated and, consequently, distinct tail region. The smaller transcript has not been detected in the cochlea or retina and therefore appears to be unrelated to the pathology associated with Usher syndrome type IB.

Numerous mutations of the MYO7A gene in Usher type Ib patients have been identified that affect the head, neck, or tail region of the protein (Weil et al., 1995; Weston et al., 1996; Adato et al., 1997; Liu et al., 1997a; Levy et al., 1997; Espinos et al., 1998; Cuevas et al., 1998; 1999; Janecke et al., 1999). Although most mutations have been localized in the motor domain (Figure 36.2), it is important to point out that analyses have been largely restricted to this region in many of the published reports. Of the mutations thus far identified for USH1B patients, most reflect nucleotide substitutions, including missense (~45%), nonsense (~28%), and splice-site (~11%) mutations. The remaining mutations are due to small deletions (<21 bp) that constitute about 13% of the population studied, with one example each of a small insertion and a gross deletion. In one affected individual from a family mapped to the USH3 locus, a single allele containing a mutated MYO7A gene resulting from a complex rearrangement appeared to exacerbate the phenotype associated with USH3, resulting in congenital deafness and vestibular dysfunction (Adato et al., 1999). Moreover, examination of a family exhibiting an USH3 phenotype, but not linked to the USH3 locus, led to the identification of two siblings that were compound heterozygotes for two missense mutations in the MYO7A gene (atypical Usher syndrome) (Liu et al., 1998a).

In addition, it has been determined that two DFNB2-affected families harbor missense mutations in the MYO7A gene that are unique from those described thus far in USH1B individuals, and in one DFNB2 family affected individuals were compound heterozygotes for a splice acceptor site mutation in the motor domain and a small insertion in a MyTH4 region (Weil et al., 1997; Liu et al., 1997c). DFNB2-affected individuals are characterized by their severe to profound hearing loss, the onset of which is variable, and variable vestibular system dysfunction (Guilford et al., 1994; Liu et al., 1997c). In the DFNA11-affected family, 9 bp are deleted from the location encoding the coiled-coil region of the MYO7A gene, producing a moderate, but slowly progressing hearing loss (Liu et al., 1997d; Tamagawa et al., 1996); interestingly, this is the only mutation in the coiled-coil region thus far identified.

The amino acid sequence for myosin VIIa is highly conserved among mammals, in that 96% of the sequence is identical in humans and mice, and 98% is similar (Mburu et al., 1997; Chen et al., 1996; Weil et al., 1996). In addition, a splice variant is alternatively transcribed, producing a smaller molecule that has a shorter myosin tail region as described in humans.

In the seven sh-1 mutants, five Myo7a mutations are located in the portion of the gene that encodes the head region of the myosin VIIa protein and include two missense mutations ($Myo7a^{sh1}$ and $Myo7a^{6J}$), a nonsense mutation ($Myo7a^{4626SB}$) and two splice-site mutations ($Myo7a^{4494SB}$ and $Myo7a^{816SB}$) (Figure 36.2). Mutations in the gene domain that encodes the protein tail are caused by one missense mutation ($Myo7a^{26SB}$) and one nonsense mutation ($Myo7a^{3336SB}$) leading to a premature stop codon that causes truncation of the molecule (Gibson et al., 1995; Mburu et al., 1997). While the mutation found in the original sh-1 mouse is located in a nonconserved region of the head domain near the actin binding site, the mutation in the $Myo7a^{6J}$ mouse is in a highly conserved region located closer to the ATP binding site, suggesting that both mutations interfere with myosin's capacity to carry out its cytological roles(s), but through different mechanisms. The splice site mutation in the $Myo7a^{4494SB}$ mouse leads to a stop codon 5 amino acids downstream from the mutation, whereas the splice site mutation of $Myo7a^{816SB}$ leads to a 10 amino acid deletion that includes a highly conserved amino acid residue located in the head domain of the gene.

Myosin VIIa mRNA is expressed in a variety of tissues. Using Northern blot analyses, myosin VIIa transcript is detected primarily in mouse testis, kidney, and lung (Gibson et al., 1995). Using RT-PCR analyses, the transcript is detected in adult human liver, kidney, and retina (Weil et al., 1995). The RT-PCR expression profile is similar in the mouse, in that myosin VIIa transcript is detected in the liver, kidney, cochlea, and retina (Weil et al., 1995). Both cochlear and vestibular neuroepithelial tissues express myosin VIIa, as do olfactory sensory cells, RPE and photoreceptor cells, although photoreceptor cells appear to express myosin VIIa later than RPE cells in human embryos, as determined using in $situ$ hybridization procedures (Weil et al., 1996). It is especially interesting that in the mouse embryo, expression of the myosin VIIa gene is primarily restricted to epithelial cells decorated with microvillus extensions, including cochlear and vestibular hair cells, RPE cells, olfactory epithelium, epithelial cells of the small intestine, hepatocytes, renal cells, adrenal cells, testicular cells, and cells of the choroid plexus (Weil et al., 1996; Sahly et al., 1997). Antibodies to the myosin VIIa protein stain the same tissues (Sahly et al., 1997) and are concentrated primarily in the microvilli (Wolfrum et al., 1998).

Not surprisingly, based on estimates of mRNA expression, the myosin VIIa protein is also detected in adult rat cochlea, retina, kidney, and testis, with the highest levels measured in the testis, followed by the kidney (Hasson et al., 1995). The results of immunostaining studies indicate that the protein is localized exclusively in inner and outer hair cells (OHCs), and specifically in stereocilia, the cuticular plate and cell bodies in the guinea pig cochlea, and inner hair cells (IHCs) are more heavily stained than OHCs in adult animals. Similar localization profiles are observed in mouse and rat cochlear and vestibular hair cells (el-Amraoui et al., 1996). The protein is found uniformly throughout stereocilia, the cuticular plate, and in hair cell bodies of both IHCs and OHCs, as well as type I and II hair cells of the utricle and semicircular canals (Hasson et al., 1997a). Moreover, myosin VIIa has been localized in the cell body and stereocilia of frog saccular hair cells. However, unlike mammalian hair cells, more intense labeling is observed near the base of the stereociliary bundle at the level of the horizontal links that connect adjacent stereocilia, and in the pericuticular necklace. Staining is also more intense in undifferentiated saccular hair cells than in maturity (Hasson et al., 1997a), and kinocilia of immature mouse cochlear hair cells also label with antibodies to the protein (Wolfrum et al., 1998).

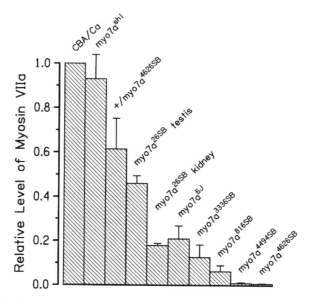

FIGURE 36.3   Relative levels of myosin VIIa protein in shaker-1 mutant mice compared to wildtype controls (CBA/Ca). Samples were obtained from testis and kidneys, which showed similar levels, except in the *Myo7a^{26SB}* mutant, which showed different levels, as indicated. All samples were obtained from animals homozygous for the mutant allele, except for *Myo7a^{4626SB}*, in which heterozygotes are also shown. Values represent means ± S.D. (Adapted from Hasson et al., 1997b.)

Although species differences in the retinal distribution of myosin VIIa were originally thought to exist (el-Amraoui et al., 1996), that does not appear to be the case. Instead, in the retina, antibodies to myosin VIIa stain the RPE in the region of apically located microvilli (Hasson et al., 1995; el-Amraoui et al., 1996), as well as rods and cones where staining is concentrated near the plasma membrane of the connecting cilium linking the inner and outer segments across species thus far studied (Liu et al., 1997b).

Myosin VIIa mRNA levels are normal in the testes of all *sh-1* mutants based on Northern blot analysis; however, protein expression levels vary greatly in mutated animals in a mutation-dependent manner (Hasson et al., 1997b). While near-normal levels of protein are expressed in the original *sh-1*, expression levels are reduced, in some cases dramatically, in all other homozygous mutants, as well as in the *Myo7a^{4626SB}* heterozygote (Figure 36.3). The extremely low levels of protein detected in *Myo7a^{4494SB}* and *Myo7a^{4626SB}* homozygous mutants suggest that these mutations are, in effect, null mutations. As observed previously for rats and other mice, myosin VIIa is located in the microvilli of RPE cells of the retina for both wild-type and *sh-1* mice, with the level of staining, when observed, consistent with protein expression levels (Hasson et al., 1997b; Liu et al., 1998b) and in the connecting cilium of photoreceptors of *sh-1* mice, as in normal mice (Liu et al., 1999).

ANATOMY

Based on the Preyer reflex, the shaker-1 mouse is completely deaf by 3 postnatal weeks and, although the cochlea appears morphologically normal through the 6th week at the light level of microscopy, evidence of OHC and spiral ganglion cell degeneration can be observed at the ultra-structural level as early as postnatal day 3 and at the level of IHCs as early as postnatal day 6 (Kikuchi and Hilding, 1965b; Shnerson et al., 1983). As with many forms of otopathology involving sensory cells, hair cell loss is first observed in the base and progressively advances in an apical direction. The stria vascularis is the next structure to undergo atrophy, at about 1 month of age, after which spiral ganglion cells are progressively lost in affected individuals (Gruneberg et al.,

1940; Deol, 1956; Mikaelian and Ruben, 1964). By the end of week 3, the majority of afferent endings on IHCs have atrophied (Kikuchi and Hilding, 1965b; Shnerson et al., 1983). Kikuchi and Hilding (1965b) reported that intraganglionic spiral bundle fibers and olivocochlear efferent endings were virtually absent, except for a few endings that appear late in development and subsequently degenerate, in mutant animals. Shnerson et al. (1983), on the other hand, suggested that efferent fibers originally contact their sensory targets during development, and that the abnormal efferent OHC innervation pattern observed later reflects secondary changes associated with the degeneration of their targets. Consistent with the view of Shnerson et al., Emmerling and Sobkowicz (1990a) observed normal levels of acetylcholinesterase (AChE) activity and the presence of AChE-stained efferent endings on OHCs in cochleae of shaker-1 mice, which show signs of degeneration around 1 postnatal month. In addition to these changes, the spiral vessel below the tunnel of Corti atrophies early in development, and although the stria vascularis starts to degenerate after about 1 postnatal month, the distribution of ATPase staining is normal in mutant animals (Kikuchi and Hilding, 1967).

In addition to degenerative changes, development is delayed in diseased individuals. Hair cell differentiation and spiral ganglion cell myelination lag behind in mutant animals, the tunnel of Corti and spaces of Nuel are slow to develop, and the tectorial membrane retains its attachments to the reticular lamina as late as postnatal day 18.

Interestingly, hair cell stereocilia from the original shaker-1 mouse look normal under the scanning electron microscope, even at 15 postnatal days, although the number of stereociliary rows decorating OHCs is frequently reduced to two relative to the three rows observed in normal animals (Self et al., 1998). In contrast to this relationship, stereociliary bundles of $Myo7a^{6J}$ and $Myo7a^{816SB}$ mutants develop abnormally. Although stereociliary patterns appear to be normal relatively late in prenatal life, by approximately 18 gestational days, bundles are found in a state of disarray and kinocilia, when identifiable, are misplaced. Stereociliary disarray, which is more extreme in $Myo7a^{816SB}$ mutants, is observed first in the base of the cochlea and involves both IHCs and OHCs. The pathology is progressive, such that the first abnormality, stereociliary clumping, is followed by almost complete stereociliary loss by postnatal day 20, as well as the eventual loss of hair cells.

OHC stereocilia are also disorganized in 1-day-old organotypic cochlear cultures obtained from $Myo7a^{6J}$ mice between postnatal days 1 and 3, whereas cells taken from the original shaker-1 mouse appear normal (Richardson et al., 1997). Horizontal cross-links that bind adjacent stereocilia to one another, and the distance between adjacent stereocilia are normal in both $Myo7a^{sh1}$ and $Myo7a^{6J}$ mutant mice (Self et al., 2000). The localization of myosin VIIa in hair cells is also normal in $Myo7a^{6J}$ mutants, but immunocytochemical staining is less dense than in CBA controls (Self et al., 2000), consistent with the reduction of levels found in other organs of mutant animals (Hasson et al., 1997b). Interestingly, OHCs obtained from $Myo7a^{6J}$ mice lack the ability to accumulate aminoglycosides, unlike normal heterozygotes and $Myo7a^{sh1}$ mice. This suggests that myosin VIIa may play a role in the transport of aminoglycosides and related compounds into sensory cells (Richardson et al., 1997).

Unlike Usher type IB patients, retinal anatomy is normal for all seven sh-1 mutants at 18 months of age. Retinal thickness is normal and there is no evidence of pathology among pigmented cells (Hasson et al., 1997b). In addition, photoreceptor density and ultrastructure appear normal in the original sh-1, $Myo7a^{4494SB}$, $Myo7a^{4626SB}$, and littermate controls through 6 months of age (Liu et al., 1999). At the ultrastructural level, the RPE is also normal in the original sh-1 mutant, as are phagosomes; however, unlike heterozygotes, melanosomes are excluded from the apical processes in mutant animals, suggesting that normal myosin VIIa may participate in the intracellular transportation of melanosomes in the RPE (Liu et al., 1998b). In addition, opsin, a protein that is synthesized in the inner segment and transported to the outer segment, is abnormally distributed within the photoreceptors of mutant animals according to immunogold labeling studies recently reported (Liu et al., 1999). Specifically, in control animals, staining for opsin is concentrated in the outer segment and little label is found in the connecting cilium. Contrary to this finding, dense opsin stains are found in the connecting cilium, or at the base of the connecting cilium, in mutant

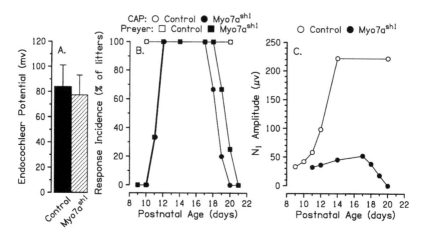

FIGURE 36.4 (A) Comparison of endocochlear potentials in the original shaker-1 (*Myo7a^sh1*) mouse compared to CBA-J controls. Values represent mean values for 10 to 11 mice per group ± S.D. Recordings were made from the basal turn of the cochlea in animals 6 months of age or older. (Adapted from Brown and Ruben, 1969.) (B) Comparison of response incidence between controls and *Myo7a^sh1* mutant mice, expressed as the percentages of litters producing a Preyer reflex or a compound action potential (CAP) as a function of age. (Adapted from Mikaelian and Ruben, 1964b.) (C) Growth of N1 of the CAP evoked by click stimuli as a function of postnatal age for controls and *Myo7a^sh1* mutants. Controls were normal CBA-J mice. (Adapted from Mikalian and Ruben, 1964.)

animals who express relatively low amounts of the myosin VIIa protein, although the same amount of opsin is present in the outer segment domain in these individuals. In addition, three *sh-1* mutants renew disc membranes at reduced rates relative to normal animals. Because, the distribution of the protein, peripherin/*rds*, which is also transported from the inner to outer segments, is normal in the *sh-1* mutants, Liu et al. (1999) propose that myosin VIIa plays a role in the transport of opsin through the connecting cilium to the outer segment, and that the absence of retinal degeneration in mice compared to humans may be due to differences in genetic background or the rates of photoreceptor degeneration.

PHYSIOLOGY

As expected on the basis of anatomical delays observed in developing mutant animals, the development of cochlear function is delayed as well. Compound auditory nerve action potentials (CAPs), as well as Preyer's reflex, are first elicited with airborne sounds 2 days later than normal (Figure 36.4B) and CAP amplitudes are greatly reduced compared to age-matched controls (Figure 36.4C) (Mikaelian and Ruben, 1964). After 17 days, CAP amplitudes decline and cannot be elicited after postnatal day 20. Despite the degenerative changes observed in stria vascularis, endocochlear potentials are normal in shaker-1 mice (Figure 36.4A) (Brown and Ruben, 1969).

The first cochlear microphonic (CM) potentials that can be elicited acoustically are also delayed by a day, and although the responsive frequency range expands during the first 14 postnatal days, the bandwidth over which responses are observed in age-matched groups is relatively small, with insensitivity to high frequencies limiting the audiometric range (Figure 36.5) (Mikaelian and Ruben, 1964). During the first 17 postnatal days, thresholds decrease, although they never achieve the degree of sensitivity observed in normal age-matched controls and certainly never reach adult values. Thresholds begin to deteriorate after postnatal day 17, and shaker-1 animals rapidly become unresponsive to acoustic stimulation by postnatal day 22 (Figure 36.5).

When shaker-1 animals are compared to heterozygous littermates, CM thresholds develop normally through postnatal day 14, and subsequently deteriorate (Figure 36.6A) (Steel and Harvey,

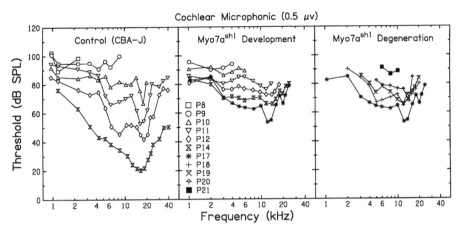

FIGURE 36.5 Changes in threshold of the cochlear microphonic (CM) potentials as a function of stimulus frequency in control animals (left panel) and *Myo7a*[sh1] mutant mice (middle and right panels). Threshold of the CM was determined using an amplitude criterion of 0.5 μV. Symbol key for all panels is located in the middle panel. (Adapted from Mikalian and Ruben, 1964.)

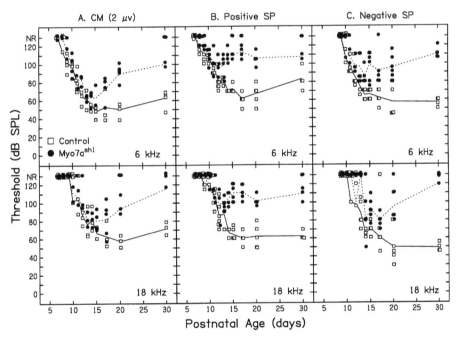

FIGURE 36.6 Changes in thresholds of the cochlear microphonic (CM) (left panels), positive summating potential (SP) (middle panels), and negative SP (right panels) for control and *Myo7a*[sh1] mutant mice as a function of age. Data were obtained in response to 6 kHz (upper row) and 18 kHz (lower row). Threshold of the CM was determined using an amplitude criterion of 2 μV. Symbol key for all panels is located in the upper left panel. (Adapted from Steel and Harvey, 1992.)

1992). In contrast, thresholds of positive summating potentials (SPs) develop normally through the 11th day only, and become relatively insensitive when compared with heterozygotes, who continue to develop normally. Negative SPs, on the other hand, develop at a slower rate than in heterozygotes (Figure 36.6C), according to Steel and Harvey (1992). Note, however, that threshold estimates are highly variable in shaker-1 animals, and in the case of positive SPs produced by 6 kHz

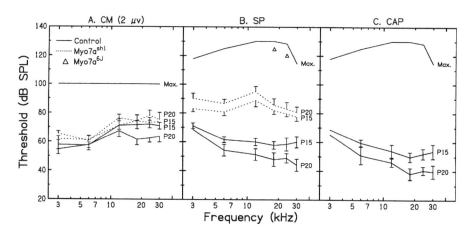

FIGURE 36.7 Thresholds of cochlear microphonic (CM), summating potential (SP), and compound action potential (CAP) for control, $Myo7a^{sh1}$, and $Myo7a^{6J}$ mutant mice as a function of stimulus frequency, shown in (A) to (C), respectively. For control and $Myo7a^{sh1}$ animals, thresholds are shown for 15 and 20 postnatal days (P15 and P20) and the maximum stimulus levels used for each measure are indicated by the solid lines (labeled "Max.") in each frame. Key for all frames is shown in (A). Values represent means ± S.E.M. (Adapted from Self et al., 1998.)

(Figure 36.6B), at least one heterozygote was almost as insensitive as the most sensitive mutant and the mean SP threshold at 30 days was considerably higher than that observed on day 20, most likely reflecting the low number of observations per condition.

Examination of CM, SP, and CAP thresholds across frequency revealed substantial differences among different shaker-1 mutants, as well as among response measures (Figure 36.7) (Self et al., 1998). In the original shaker-1 mutant, CM differed only slightly, if at all, from controls at 15 and 20 postnatal days (Figure 36.7A), whereas SP was significantly elevated (Figure 36.7B), and CAPs were never observed in mutant animals (Figure 36.7C). Responses from $Myo7a^{816SB}$ mutants were not observed under any circumstances, and although most $Myo7a^{6J}$ mutants were also unresponsive, SP was elicited in two cases, but only in response to very intense stimuli. These findings are interesting in the context of the finding that the myosin VIIa protein is more heavily expressed in IHCs than OHCs (Hasson et al., 1995). Because the SP presumably represents the voltage generated by activated OHCs and CAP preferentially reflects the output of IHCs, one might conclude that the protein plays a more vital role in IHCs than in OHCs on the basis of the findings illustrated in Figure 36.7.

Surprisingly, despite the stereociliary disarray associated with the $Myo7a^{6J}$ mutant, mechano-electrical transduction currents recorded from OHCs of $Myo7a^{6J}$ and original shaker-1 mutants that were maintained in culture are, in general, comparable to those of heterozygous littermates (Richardson et al., 1997). Moreover, resting membrane potentials, linear leak conductances, and basolateral membrane currents (e.g., outward K^+ currents and sustained inward Ca^{++} currents) are the same in heterozygous and homozygous $Myo7a^{6J}$ mice, although, unlike heterozygotes, little or no transducer current is detected at rest and greater stereociliary displacement is required to produce transducer currents in homozygotes (Kros et al., 1999). Consistent with vestibular hair cell abnormalities, in shaker-1 mice there is no evidence that affected animals have a vestibulo-ocular reflex, but they do exhibit an optokinetic reflex, although the gain of the system is significantly reduced (Sun et al., 1999).

While it is relatively clear that the structural integrity of hair cell stereocilia is dependent on myosin VIIa, the mechanism of its action has not been determined. However, that picture is beginning to change as a better understanding of the kinds of intracellular cargo that the myosins target and sometimes transport, and as the nature of effective ligands becomes clear, to mention just two currently productive avenues of research. It is especially interesting that stereociliary abnormalities are not observed at the ultrastructural level in the original shaker-1 mouse, although animals that are homozygous for the trait are essentially deaf. Those findings suggest that myosin VIIa may influence molecular aspects of cellular function that are themselves not understood. For example, myosin VIIa may affect the stiffness of the stereocilia, each of which is tightly packed with actin filaments, and consequently may alter transduction dynamics. It is also important to remember that myosin VIIa is but one of many proteins implicated in the pathogenesis of Usher syndromes. Nonetheless, based on recent progress, it is clear that our understanding of the biological mechanisms underlying Usher syndrome will be advanced and refined in the upcoming years, a situation that will greatly serve the victims of this heterogeneous disease.

ALPORT SYNDROME

DISEASE CHARACTERISTICS

Alport syndrome is an inherited disorder caused by the mutation of one of several genes that encode the α form of Type IV collagen that is an integral component of the glomerular basement membrane. While the disease is generally characterized by progressive nephropathy, sensorineural hearing loss, and ocular abnormalities, kidney dysfunction is the primary pathological feature and patients frequently achieve end-stage renal disease (ESRD) in early adulthood, requiring either kidney transplantation or dialysis, particularly in the case of males with the X-linked form of the disease. The clinical course of the most common form of Alport syndrome is characterized by persistent, life-long hematuria and progressive proteinuria. Otopathology associated with Alport syndrome is generally bilateral and sensorineural in character. Although hearing loss progresses from mild to moderately severe in the mid- and high-frequency range, affecting 55% of males and 45% of females, the extent and frequency range of hearing loss are highly variable and tend to expand as the disease progresses (Wester et al., 1995). Ocular defects include retinal anomalies (e.g., typically dot-and-fleck retinopathy) in the majority of patients (85% of males) and anterior lenticonus, characterized by the protrusion of the lens into the anterior chamber of the eye, and numerous other corneal pathologies (Govan, 1983; Colville and Savige, 1997) that become more common and severe with age (Jacobs et al., 1992; Pajari et al., 1999).

Alport syndrome is genetically heterogeneous and may be inherited as X-linked, autosomal recessive, or autosomal dominant (Figure 36.8) (Feingold et al., 1985; Feingold and Bois, 1987). Approximately 80% of all cases are X-linked, 15% are autosomal recessive, and the remainder are autosomal dominant (Kashtan, 1999). The X-linked form of Alport syndrome is dominant in males and frequently leads to ESRD, whereas the phenotype in females is widely variable, ranging from microscopic hematuria to ESRD. In the population at large, the prevalence of Alport syndrome is 1:5000 (Flinter, 1997), and the syndrome accounts for approximately 1% of all forms of genetic hearing loss (Wester et al., 1995).

The X-linked form of the disease has been mapped to the long arm of the X-chromosome (Xq22.3) (Atkin et al., 1988; Szpiro-Tapia et al., 1988; Flinter et al., 1988; 1989; Hertz et al., 1991), and mutations in the COL4A5 gene, which encodes the α5 chain of type IV collagen (see below) are responsible for the X-linked version of Alport syndrome (Barker et al., 1990). Numerous mutations have been identified in the COL4A5 gene, affecting all regions (Barker et al., 1990; Boye et al., 1991; 1993; 1995; Zhou et al., 1991; 1992a; b; 1993; Antignac et al., 1994; Knebelmann et al., 1992; 1995; 1996; Netzer et al., 1992; 1993; Renieri et al., 1992a; b; 1994b;c; 1995; 1996; Smeets et al., 1992; Vetrie et al., 1992; Guo et al., 1993; 1995; Lemmink et al., 1993; 1994; 1997; Nakazato et al., 1993; 1994; Nomura et al., 1993; Ding et al., 1994; Hertz et al., 1995; Turco et al., 1995; 1997; Heiskari et al., 1996; Kawai et al., 1996a; b; Martin et al., 1998; Mazzucco et al., 1998; Neri et al., 1998; Cruz-Robles et al., 1999; Inoue et al., 1999; Plant et al., 1999). Mutations include

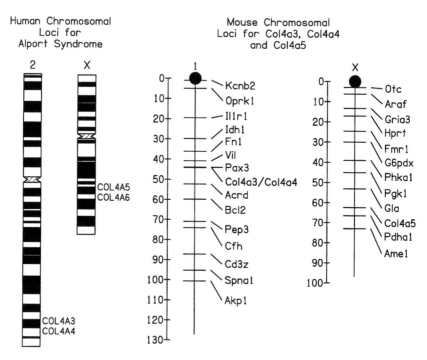

FIGURE 36.8 Ideograms of human chromosomes 2 and chromosome X, indicating the relative locus of the COL4A3/COL4A4 and COL4A5 genes, responsible for autosomal recessive and X-linked Alport syndrome, respectively (Barker et al., 1990; Hostikka et al., 1990; Mariyama et al., 1992; Mochizuki et al., 1994; Sugimoto et al., 1994). The relative location of the COL4A6 gene, which is responsible in part for Alport syndrome with diffuse leiomyomatosis, is shown as well (Zhou et al., 1993). The relative locations of *Col4a3* and *Col4a4* are shown on mouse chromosome 1 (Lu et al., 1999), and *Col4a5* is shown on mouse chromosome X. Distances are in cM from the centromere. Locations of genes other than *Col4a3* and *Col4a4* were obtained from the Mouse Genome Database (http://www.informatics.jax.org).

missense mutations, nonsense mutations, small and large deletions, splice-site mutations, and complete deletions of the gene.

Some Alport syndrome patients have also been diagnosed with diffuse leiomyomatosis (DL), which is characterized by the benign proliferation of smooth muscle cells primarily affecting the wall of the esophagus and trachea (Grunfeld et al., 1987; Antignac et al., 1992; Lonsdale et al., 1992; Hudson et al., 1993; Van Loo et al., 1997; Federici et al., 1998). The genetic basis of Alport syndrome with DL is a large deletion mutation that disrupts the 5′ end of both the COL4A5 and the COL4A6 genes, which are located contiguously on the X-chromosome (Zhou et al., 1993). While always associated with the 5′ end of the gene, the size of the deletion affecting COL4A5 is variable, although the deletion consistently affects the COL4A6 gene within intron 2 (Garcia-Torres and Orozco, 1993; Renieri et al., 1994a-c; 1995; Heidet et al., 1995; 1997; Dahan et al., 1995; Antignac and Heidet, 1996; Ueki et al., 1998; Segal et al., 1999). Another variant of Alport syndrome, called AMME syndrome, characterized by Alport syndrome (A), mental retardation (M), midface hypoplasia (M), and elliptocytosis (E), is caused by a contiguous gene deletion on chromosome X, including COL4A5, FACL4 (which encodes a long-chain acyl-CoA synthetase) and AMMECR1 (Piccini et al., 1998; Vitelli et al., 1999), and the orthologous genes in the mouse have recently been identified (Vitelli et al., 2000).

Mutations within the COL4A3 and/or COL4A4 genes are responsible for the autosomal recessive forms of the syndrome, and have been mapped to chromosome 2q35-37 (Mochizuki et al., 1994). These genes encode the α3 and α4 chains of type IV collagen and, like COL4A5 and

COL4A6, they reside contiguously on the chromosome (Mariyama et al., 1992). Genetic defects include missense and nonsense mutations, small deletions, and splice-site mutations (Mochizuki et al., 1994; Lemmink et al., 1994; 1997; Ding et al., 1995; Knebelmann et al., 1995; Boye et al., 1998; Torra et al., 1999). The autosomal dominant form of Alport syndrome is also linked to defects in COL4A3 and COL4A4 genes (Jefferson et al., 1997), and COL4A4 mutations have been identified in autosomal dominant familial benign hematuria (Lemmink et al., 1996). In the mouse, the *Col4a3* and *Col4a4* genes have been mapped to chromosome 1 (Figure 36.8), at a location that is distal to villin and proximal to *Acrd*, and close to the *Pax3* gene (Lu et al., 1999).

Fechtner syndrome is a rare autosomal dominant condition that is commonly thought of as a variant of Alport syndrome. Fechtner syndrome is characterized by nephropathy, deafness, and eye abnormalities, just like Alport syndrome. However, in addition to these common symptoms, Fechtner syndrome patients exhibit macrothrombocytopenia and cytoplasmic inclusion bodies have been identified in the leukocytes of affected individuals. Fechtner syndrome is especially interesting because the mutation has been mapped to chromosome 22q11-13, a region that does not contain genes that encode collagen or basement membrane proteins (Toren et al., 1999). Epstein syndrome, another closely related variant of Alport syndrome, resembles Fechtner syndrome in many ways; however, inclusion bodies have not been observed in Epstein syndrome patients and the distribution of the α1(IV) through α6(IV) collagen chains is normal in kidney biopsies (Naito et al., 1997). Identification of the genes responsible for these disorders, as well as the proteins that they encode, will undoubtedly lead to a better understanding of the pathological variants of Alport syndrome.

Abnormalities in the basement membrane of the renal glomerulus have been observed under the electron microscope in biopsies from patients associated with both X-linked and autosomal forms of Alport syndrome (Hinglais et al., 1972; Spear and Slusser, 1972; Spear, 1974; Churg et al., 1974; Gubler et al., 1980; Habib et al., 1982; Bernstein, 1987; Rumpelt, 1987; Kashtan et al., 1998). When compared to normal glomerular capillary basement membranes, differences are clear. Diffuse thickened and lamellated areas are evident in basement membranes from Alport syndrome patients, giving the membrane the appearance of a "weaved-basket" and producing glomerulosclerotic lesions.

TYPE IV COLLAGENS

Type IV collagen is a primary constituent of basement membranes (Timpl et al., 1981; Timpl, 1989; 1996; Hudson et al., 1993; Sado et al., 1998; Gunwar et al., 1998), and six genes have been identified (COL4A1 through COL4A6) that encode the polypeptide chains comprising the molecule. These are identified as α1(IV) through α6(IV), respectively. The genes are arranged in pairs, in a head-to-head configuration, as described above for the genes that are defective in Alport syndrome. COL4A3 and COL4A4 are found on chromosome 2, COL4A5 and COL4A6 on the X-chromosome, and COL4A1 and COL4A2 are located on chromosome 13q34.

Each chain consists of a large collagenous domain (~1400 amino acids) composed of Gly-x-y repeats situated between a noncollagenous domain (NC1) located at the carboxy-terminal end (~230 amino acids), and a 7S domain (~15 amino acids) at the amino-terminal end (Figure 36.9). The chains aggregate into groups of three and form a triple-helix, with two α1 chains and one α2 chain forming one trimer; α3, α4, and α5 another; and a mix of α5 and α6 chains forming a third. Trimers aggregate through novel disulfide bonds at the NC1 domain and by ionic and hydrophobic interactions via the 7S domain, forming the complex network of type IV collagens that provide structural support for basement membranes. Laminin, the other major component of basement membranes, binds to the glycoprotein entactin (nidogen), which also binds to type IV collagen.

The amino acid homology between human and mouse type IV collagen chains is high, in that at least 90%, or more, of the amino acids in the sequence are identical in the NC1 domains, depending on the chain (Figure 36.10A) (Miner and Sanes, 1994). In addition, the identity of the amino acid sequence among the NC1 domains is high among α-chains (Figure 36.10B), indicating

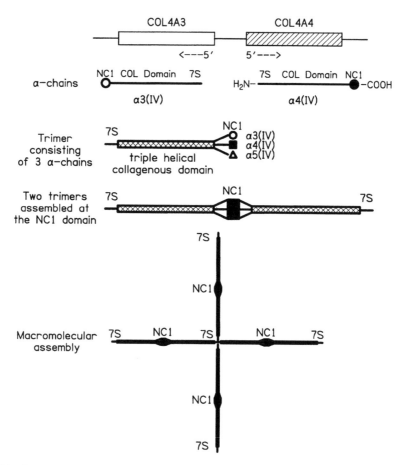

FIGURE 36.9 Schematic of the head-to-head arrangement of the COL4A3 and COL4A4 genes (note adjacent 5′ ends) (Mariyama et al., 1992), and schematic structure of the α-chains, with the 7S domain located at the amino-terminal end, the NC1 domain at the carboxyl-terminal end, and the interposed long collagen domain consisting of Gly-x-y repeats. Three α-chains aggregate in specific combinations to form a triple helix (trimer) [α3α4α5; (α1)2α2; or (α5)2α6]. Trimers self-assemble by bonding at the NC1 domain where two trimers can bond, and at the 7S domain where four trimers can bond, creating complex macromolecular assemblies. (Adapted from Timpl et al., 1981; Timpl, 1989; 1996; Gunwar et al., 1998; Sado et al., 1998; and Kashtan, 1999.)

that they are closely related, with one group comprised of α1(IV), α3(IV), and α5(IV) chains, and a second group including α2(IV) and α4(IV) chains.

The distribution of the type IV collagen chains is tissue specific, such that α1(IV) and α2(IV) are present in all basement membranes, while α3(IV) to α6(IV) are components in a more limited set of tissues (Butkowski et al., 1989; Kleppel et al., 1989; 1992; Kleppel and Michael, 1990; Hostikka et al., 1990; Gunwar et al., 1991; Takahashi and Hokunan, 1992; Miner and Sanes, 1994; Zhu et al., 1994; Cosgrove et al., 1996c; Ding et al., 1997; Kahsai et al., 1997; Sakaguchi et al., 1997; Kalluri et al., 1998). Based on immunostaining studies in the kidney, α3(IV) to α5(IV) are found in the glomerular basement membrane, Bowman's capsule, and the distal and collecting tubule basement membranes, whereas α6(IV) is present only in Bowman's capsule and the distal and collecting tubule basement membranes. In the eye, α3(IV) to α5(IV) are localized in the lens capsule, and Descemet's, Bruch's, and internal limiting membranes, whereas in the cochlea, α1(IV) and α2(IV) are concentrated in the osseous spiral lamina, and vasculature of the spiral ligament and stria vascularis, and Reissner's membrane, and α3(IV) to α5(IV) are concentrated in the spiral

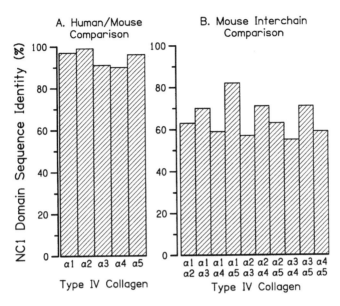

FIGURE 36.10 A. Comparison of amino acid sequence identity for five of the type IV collagen NC1 (non-collagenous) domains of the α1 through α5 chains between human and mouse (A) and among the five cloned domains in the mouse (B). (Adapted from Miner and Sanes, 1994.)

limbus, inner sulcus, basilar membrane, spiral prominence, and the spiral ligament, particularly in the region of type II fibrocytes. Basement membranes associated with the vessels of the stria vascularis also stain for α3(IV) to α5(IV) chains. While other investigators have not observed staining for type IV collagen in the tectorial membrane (Takahashi and Hokunan, 1992; Cosgrove et al., 1996a; c; Satoh et al., 1998), Kalluri et al. (1998) reported that the tectorial membrane stained for all α1(IV) to α6(IV) chains. Type IV collagen has also been observed in basement membranes of the mammalian endolymphatic sac (Harada et al., 2000) and during early development of the avian otic placode and its association with the neural ectoderm (Hilfer and Randolph, 1993).

In the guinea pig cochlea, a semi-quantitative study of type IV collagens using ELISA revealed greater immunoreactivity to α1(IV) and α2(IV) chains (Figure 36.11), compared to α3(IV) to α6(IV) chains (Kalluri et al., 1998). In addition, Kalluri et al. (1998) found that solubilized cochleae also bind to serum from Alport syndrome patients who develop antibodies to transplanted kidneys, primarily against the α3(IV) chain, as well as to serum from patients with Goodpasture syndrome (anti-glomerular basement membrane disease), an autoimmune disease in which the α3(IV) chain has been identified as the offending autoantigen (Turner et al., 1992).

The α1(IV) and α2(IV) forms of collagen type IV found in glomerular basement membrane of neonatal mice are transiently expressed during development. During the first postnatal week or so, a transitional stage occurs in which α1(IV) through α5(IV) chains are generally expressed, and this phase is eventually followed by a stage in which α1(IV) and α2(IV) are replaced by α3(IV) through α5(IV) (Kashtan and Kim, 1992; Miner and Sanes, 1994). A similar developmental pattern has been observed in the mouse cochlea (Cosgrove et al., 1996a). At birth, α1(IV) and α2(IV) chains are widely distributed in the cochlea. This is followed by a transitional state between postnatal days 4 and 10, in which α3(IV) through α5(IV) chains are broadly distributed, after which the expression profiles of α3(IV) through α5(IV) are refined to produce the adult pattern.

Furthermore, X-linked and autosomal recessive forms of Alport syndrome can be distinguished on the basis of the forms of type IV collagen present in various tissues (Kashtan et al., 1986; 1989; Kashtan and Kim, 1992; Cheung et al., 1994; Nakanishi et al., 1994; 1996; 1998; Yoshioka et al., 1994; Gubler et al., 1995; Peissel et al., 1995; Hino et al., 1996; Naito et al., 1996; Kagawa et al., 1997; Nomura et al., 1998; Seki et al., 1998). In most males with X-linked Alport syndrome, staining

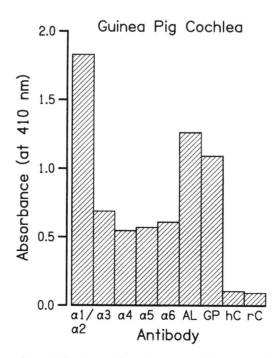

FIGURE 36.11 Presence of type IV collagens in guinea pig cochleae determined semi-quantitatively by direct ELISA (enzyme-linked immunosorbent assay) on collagenase digested tissue extracts. Antibodies were directed to the NC1 domains of α1(IV)/α2(IV) collagen and toward those for the α3(IV) through α6(IV) chains. In addition, cochlear extracts bind to antibodies obtained from the serum of a subset of Alport syndrome patients following kidney transplants (AL), as well as to antibodies from patients with Goodpasture syndrome (GP); whereas a small extent of non-specific binding is observed to control sera from humans (hC) and from rabbits (rC). (Adapted from Kalluri et al., 1998.)

for the α3(IV) through α5(IV) chains is absent in the glomerular basement membrane, Bowman's capsule, and distal tubular basement membranes, although these proteins are detected in some patients and in other cases may even appear normal. This otherwise paradoxical finding suggests that a variety of mutated forms of the COL4A3 through COL4A5 genes are represented in the population at large. Typically, when α5(IV) immunoreactivity is absent, staining for the α6(IV) chain is also negative. A mosaic pattern of staining for α3(IV) through α5(IV) in the glomerular basement membrane, and for α6(IV) in Bowman's capsule and tubular basement membranes, is often observed in females with X-linked Alport syndrome. Basement membranes of the epidermis normally stain for α5(IV) and α6(IV), but not for α3(IV) or α4(IV) chains. However, in X-linked males, α5(IV) and α6(IV) do not appear to be expressed, whereas a mosaic pattern of staining is observed in females. In patients with autosomal recessive Alport syndrome, staining for the α3(IV) and α4(IV) chains is also absent throughout the kidney, and the α5(IV) chain is absent in the glomerular basement membrane; but in contrast to X-linked forms, the α5(IV) chain is present in Bowman's capsule and distal tubular basement membranes. In addition, epidermal basement membranes stain normally for α5(IV) and α6(IV) in autosomal recessive Alport syndrome patients.

MOUSE MODEL FOR AUTOSOMAL RECESSIVE ALPORT DISEASE

Two mouse models of autosomal recessive Alport syndrome have been developed using the targeted mutagenesis approach. In both cases, the 3′ end that encodes the NC1 domain of the *Col4a3* gene, an area of the gene that is essential for macromolecular assembly, was the target (Cosgrove et al., 1996b; Miner and Sanes, 1996). The success of the "knockout" was determined using Southern blot analysis of genomic DNA. The result of that analysis clearly indicated that a relatively small

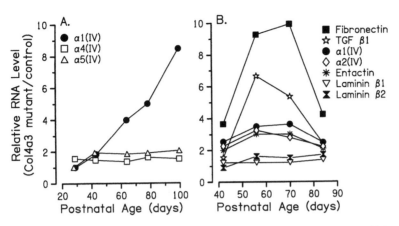

FIGURE 36.12 (A) Relative RNA levels for α1(IV), α4(IV), and α5(IV) collagen in kidneys of *Col4a3* homozygous mutant mice compared to littermate controls as a function of postnatal age. Expression of RNA was assessed by ribonuclease protection analyses. (Adapted from Miner and Sanes, 1996.) (B) Relative RNA levels of fibronectin, transforming growth factor β1 (TGF-β1), α1(IV), and α2(IV) collagen, entactin, laminin β1 and laminin β2 in kidneys of *Col4a3* homozygous mutants compared to littermate controls as a function of postnatal age. Levels were determined from Northern blot analyses. (Adapted from Sayers et al., 1999.)

molecular weight fragment was observed in place of what is normally observed when the *Col4a3* gene is intact (Cosgrove et al., 1996b; Miner and Sanes, 1996).

Having a prospective Alport syndrome mouse in hand, one of the first questions of interest was, naturally, the determination of expression differences between normal and mutated animals. Not surprisingly, clear differences were observed. Based on Northern blot analyses, mRNA for *Col4a3* is not expressed in the kidney of mice that are homozygous for the *Col4a3* mutation, whereas mRNAs of *Col4a1*, *Col4a2*, *Col4a4*, and *Col4a5* are detectable (Cosgrove et al., 1996b). Another key difference is observed during development. Instead of the typical developmental sequence in which α1(IV) and α2(IV) chains are replaced by the α3(IV) through α5(IV) chains in glomerular basement membranes (Miner and Sanes, 1994; Kashtan and Kim, 1992), the conversion never occurs in mutant animals and the relative amount of α1(IV) RNA progressively increases with age when compared to control animals (Figure 36.12A) (Miner and Sanes, 1996). In the alternative *Col4a3* mutant model, levels of α1(IV) RNA initially increased, then plateaued at about 10 weeks of age, and subsequently declined slightly at 11 weeks, much like the developmental profile reported for α2(IV) RNA (Figure 36.12B) (Sayers et al., 1999). The reason for this difference is not clear; however, the answer may be technical. The Northern blot analyses used by Sayers et al. (1999) may be more susceptible to RNA degradation than the RNase protection method used by Miner and Sanes (1996).

Clinically, the progression of renal disease observed in the knockout mouse mimics that observed in Alport syndrome patients, although the disease progresses more rapidly in the mouse than in humans (Cosgrove et al., 1996b; Miner and Sanes, 1996). Microscopic hematuria is detected as early as postnatal week 2 in affected mice and continues throughout the remainder of the animal's life. Proteinuria is first detected around postnatal week 5 and rapidly increases in severity until about week 6. Albumin is the major constituent protein and can be used as a marker of glomerular degeneration. These stages are followed by the uremia stage. Serum titers of creatinine and blood-urea-nitrogen (BUN) concentrations are used to determine whether or not an individual is uremic. That condition becomes evident at about 8 postnatal weeks and becomes more and more pronounced over the following 4 weeks. Animals start losing weight between 8 and 12 weeks, and ESRD is reached by approximately 14 postnatal weeks.

Ultrastructurally, the histopathology observed in glomerular basement membranes of *Col4a3* knockout mice is similar to that observed in humans (Cosgrove et al., 1996b; Miner and Sanes,

1996). Immunohistochemical analyses indicate that staining patterns for antibodies to $\alpha1,\alpha2(IV)$ collagen are relatively normal in the knockout mouse, although $\alpha1,\alpha2(IV)$ collagen continues to be expressed in the glomerular basement membrane in adult mutant mice. In contrast, the $\alpha3(IV)$ through $\alpha5(IV)$ chains are not expressed in the glomerular basement membrane. Staining for other basement membrane associated proteins typically found in the glomerulus, such as perlecan and heparan sulfate proteoglycan, increase, while extracellular matrix proteins such as fibronectin and collagen VI that are not found in basement membranes under normal conditions accumulate in mutant animals (Miner and Sanes, 1996). Levels of entactin, laminin-1, and the major integrin cell membrane receptors that bind to type IV collagen and laminin are the same in mutant and control animals, according to Miner and Sanes (1996). Like Miner and Sanes, Cosgrove et al. (1996b) observed an increase in the staining of the glomerular basement membrane to fibronectin and heparan sulfate proteoglycan, but the latter authors also observed an increase in staining to entactin, as well as transforming growth factor $\beta1$ (TGF-$\beta1$), and it was later determined that increases in fibronectin, entactin, and TGF-$\beta1$ (Figure 36.12B) are due to increased transcription activity (Sayers et al., 1999). Changes in protein levels most likely contribute to fibrotic lesions observed in glomerular basement membranes in mutant animals.

As observed in the glomerular basement membrane, immunostaining for $\alpha1(IV)$ and $\alpha2(IV)$ collagen is normal and staining is absent for the $\alpha3(IV)$ through $\alpha5(IV)$ chains in the seminiferous tubule basement membrane in *Col4a3* mutant mice (Kalluri and Cosgrove, 2000). In contrast, in the anterior capsule of the lens, while staining is present for $\alpha1(IV)$ and $\alpha2(IV)$ collagen and absent for $\alpha3(IV)$ and $\alpha4(IV)$ chains, there is immunological evidence that the $\alpha5(IV)$ chain is expressed. Using a semi-quantitative approach based on ELISA analysis, relatively high levels of binding are found for the $\alpha1(IV)$ and $\alpha2(IV)$ chains, and low levels are observed for $\alpha3(IV)$ through $\alpha6(IV)$ chains in the kidney of *Col4a3* mutants compared to wild-type controls (Figure 36.13A); whereas in the lens, normal levels of $\alpha1(IV)$, $\alpha2(IV)$, $\alpha5(IV)$, and $\alpha6(IV)$ chains are detected and low levels of the $\alpha3(IV)$ and $\alpha4(IV)$ chains are observed (Figure 36.13B).

Another autosomal recessive Alport syndrome model was recently produced transgenically by inserting a tyrosinase minigene that disrupts the 5' ends of *Col4a3* and *Col4a4* and the shared

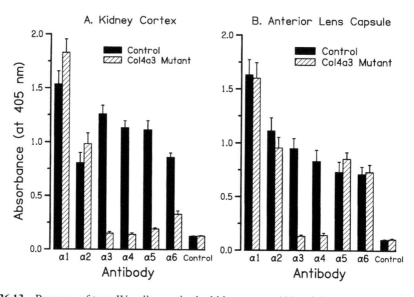

FIGURE 36.13 Presence of type IV collagens in the kidney cortex (A) and the anterior lens capsule (B) of *Col4a3* mutant mice and littermate controls. Levels were determined semi-quantitatively by direct ELISA (enzyme-linked immunosorbent assay) on collagenase digested tissue extracts. Antibodies were directed to the NC1 domains of the $\alpha1(IV)$ through $\alpha6(IV)$ collagens. Values represent means ± S.E.M. (Adapted from Kalluri and Cosgrove, 2000.)

promotor region (Lu et al., 1999). Hematuria and proteinurea were detected at 2 postnatal weeks, and by 4 weeks protein levels in the urine increased tenfold. By 12 weeks, blood-urea-nitrogen (BUN) was elevated tenfold, and ESRD was observed between 10 and 14 postnatal weeks. Ultrastructurally, the glomerular basement membrane resembled that found in the *Col4a3* mutants. Glomeruli were larger than normal, due in part to the proliferation of parietal epithelial cells and other unidentified cells that could be either endothelial cells, mesangial cells, or inflammatory cells. Transcripts for *Col4a3* and *Col4a4* were not detected in the kidneys of mutant mice, whereas the *Col4a5* transcript was evident. Normal expression of $\alpha1$ and $\alpha2(IV)$ collagen was observed and immunostaining to the $\alpha3$ through $\alpha5(IV)$ chains was not detected in glomerular basement membranes.

Using light microscopy, obvious differences were not observed in the cochleae of *Col4a3* knockout mice when compared with normal mice (Cosgrove et al., 1998). However, ultrastructurally, basement membrane thinning is observed in tissues of the limbus, inner sulcus, basilar membrane, external sulcus, and spiral prominence. In contrast, basement membranes associated with vessels of the stria vascularis are thicker than normal, endothelial cells are edematous, and glomerulosclerosis is evident as early as 5 postnatal weeks. These degenerative changes are consistent with pathology reports in Alport syndrome patients (Weidauer and Arnold, 1976; Johnsson and Arenberg, 1981). In addition, the distribution of $\alpha1(IV)$ and $\alpha2(IV)$ collagen appears normal in mutant mice, based on immunohistochemical staining studies, but may be more heavily expressed in vessels of the stria vascularis when compared with normal individuals. In contrast, $\alpha3(IV)$ and $\alpha4(IV)$ chains are not detected in the cochleae of mutant animals. Similarly, the $\alpha5(IV)$ chain is not expressed in basement membranes of the cochlea, with the notable exception of blood vessels in the stria vascularis. The persistence of the $\alpha5(IV)$ chain in capillaries of the stria, as well as in the basement membrane of the anterior lens capsule, suggest that this chain may constitute novel macromolecular assemblies in the absence of the $\alpha3(IV)$ and $\alpha4(IV)$ chains in at least some tissues (Kalluri and Cosgrove, 2000).

From a physiological point of view, ABRs suggest that, on average, there is little, if any, difference in the auditory capacity of mutant and normal animals for at least the first 8 postnatal weeks (Cosgrove et al., 1998). While it is true that the sensitivity of mutant animals to acoustic stimulation degrades slightly between 6 and 8 postnatal weeks, significant threshold differences are never observed (Figure 36.14). This point notwithstanding, auditory performance is clearly degraded in some mutant animals, as shown in a series of ABR waveforms recorded from the same animal between the 6th and 8th postnatal weeks (Figure 36.15). However, in an effort to relate the mouse model to the patient, the truly relevant question is: how often is a significant threshold difference observed? Then the similarity of the groups comes into focus. Alport syndrome patients exhibit relatively clear otopathology in the high-frequency domain in approximately 50% of patients (Wester et al., 1995). Although too few Alport mice have been studied to reliably estimate the frequency of otopathology among affected animals, audiograms derived from responses of five Alport animals studied by Cosgrove et al. (1998) are shown in Figure 36.16, and it appears relatively clear that roughly half the sample exhibit hearing loss that would be detectable in the clinic. It is also interesting that thresholds tend to be elevated in a frequency-independent manner in Alport mice, unlike humans suffering from the disease, although at least some individuals appear to lose sensitivity in response to "low" frequencies preferentially. This somewhat tentative finding may reflect the fact that the audiometric range of mice tends to be much higher than that of humans.

Because uremia is observed between $6\frac{1}{2}$ and $7\frac{1}{2}$ postnatal weeks in mutant mice, it is reasonable to consider the possibility that the loss of acoustic sensitivity constitutes an ototoxic response secondary to advanced glomerulonephritis. Ohashi et al. (1999) tested this possibility directly by considering changes in CAP and CM thresholds following a large-scale kidney resection in guinea pigs. Although endocochlear potential was not affected, both CAP and CM thresholds were progressively elevated in operated animals over the course of the 3 postsurgical months. It is interesting that otopathological changes observed by these authors were relatively minor at the end of the first postsurgical month, suggesting that the toxic otological reaction takes a fairly long time

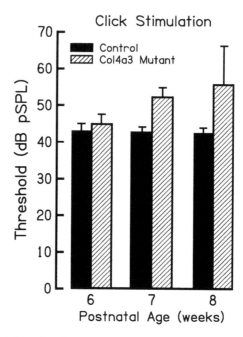

FIGURE 36.14 Mean thresholds of auditory-evoked brainstem responses (ABRs) obtained to click stimulation from *Col4a3* homozygous mutant mice and littermate controls (wild-type) at 6, 7, and 8 postnatal weeks of age. Values represent means ± S.E.M. (Adapted from Cosgrove et al., 1998.)

to develop and raising a question about whether or not nephrotoxicity was a factor in the Cosgrove et al. (1998) study. However, additional support for this view can also be found in the clinical literature. In at least one example, Alport-related hearing loss was reversed in a patient that received a kidney transplant, and hearing loss observed in four other Alport syndrome patients stabilized following the procedure (McDonald et al., 1976).

CONCLUSION

Although great progress is being made in the search for an understanding of the genetic and molecular basis of auditory development and function, as well as the molecular genetics of deafness, we remain on the proverbial tip of the iceberg in our depth of knowledge on almost every relevant front in this area. In the case of Usher syndrome, not only are there eight known genes yet to identify, but it is highly likely that there are more, and we have only begun to understand the subcellular function of the gene products. We may, for example, suspect that myosin VIIa works to traffic intracellular cargo around the organelles of cells in the retina and the cochlea, or establish and maintain the structural and functional integrity of stereocilia, but we have a long way to go before it will be possible to precisely identify their roles in hearing. Likewise, although we are beginning to appreciate the role of collagen IV in the basement membranes of the inner ear, there is much to learn about many aspects of the basement membrane and its function; for example, the nature of interaction(s) between cellular receptors and the matrix. The next 10 years should prove to be especially interesting as this field develops.

ACKNOWLEDGMENT

Supported in part by the NIDCD.

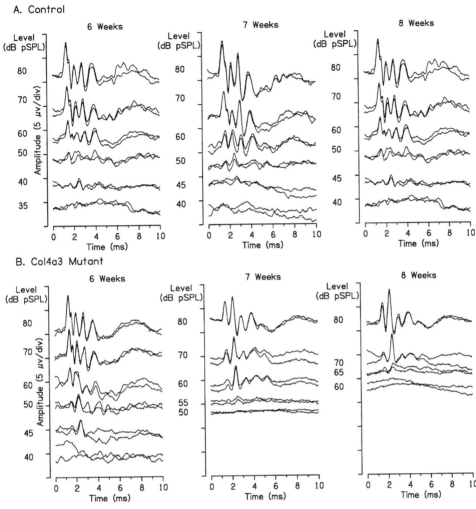

FIGURE 36.15 Examples of auditory-evoked brainstem responses (ABRs) obtained from a wild-type control (A) and from a *Col4a3* homozygous mutant (B) at 6, 7, and 8 postnatal weeks of age (left, middle, and right columns, respectively). Stimuli were alternating polarity clicks presented at a repetition interval of 115 ms, and 200 trials were averaged for each waveform. Two waveforms are shown overlapping at each stimulus level (in dB peak SPL) presented, which is indicated to the left of each pair of waveforms. (Adapted from Cosgrove et al., 1998.)

NOTES ADDED IN PROOF

Since this chapter was written, the gene underlying Usher's type 1C was identified as USH1C, which encodes harmonin, a protein expressed in the cytoplasm and sterocilia of auditory and vestibular hair cells and which harbors a PDZ domain (Verpy et al., *Nat. Gen.* 26:51-55, 2000). In addition, the gene underlying Usher's type 1D, as well as DFNB12, was identified as CDH23, which encodes a novel cadherin protein (cadherin 23) (Bolz et al., *Nat. Gen.* 27:108-112, 2001; Bork et al., *Am. J. Hum. Gen.* 68:26-37, 2001). The orthologous gene, Cdh23, encoding, otocadherin, is also defective in three different mutant forms of the waltzer (*v*) mouse (v^{6J}, v^{A1b}, and v^{2J}), and in the mutant v^{2J} variant, the hair cell stereocilia are disorganized (Di Palma et al., *Nat. Gen.* 27:103-107, 2001).

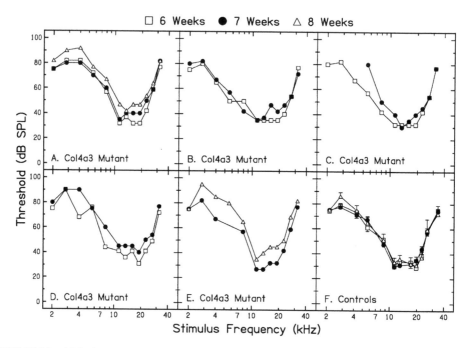

FIGURE 36.16 ABR thresholds across stimulus frequency for five individual *Col4a3* homozygous mutant mice recorded at more than one age (A through E) and mean thresholds (± s.e.m.) of littermate controls recorded at each of those ages (F). (Adapted from Cosgrove et al., 1998.)

37 Preventing Sensory Loss in a Mouse Model of Lysosomal Storage Disease

Kevin K. Ohlemiller, Carole A. Vogler, Thomas M. Daly, and Mark S. Sands

INTRODUCTION

THE LYSOSOMAL STORAGE DISEASES

The lysosomal storage diseases (LSDs) include more than 40 genetic disorders in the function of specific hydrolytic enzymes that catabolize glycosaminoglycans (GAGs), glycoproteins, and lipids (Gieselman, 1995; Sands et al., 1997b; Daly and Sands, 1998; Meikle et al., 1999). Typically, the degradation of these cellular components involves the sequential action of many hydrolases, each of which remove specific terminal residues. Thus, when a specific lysosomal enzyme is defective, macromolecules containing its substrate residue will accumulate, and any cells normally degrading these will show abnormal lysosomal storage. If the affected macromolecules are normally located extracellularly, then the cells showing lysosomal storage may be of a different type than those involved in synthesis, and have a phagocytic function. Individually, LSDs are rare. As a group, however, they occur with an incidence estimated at 1 in 6700 live births (Meikle et al., 1999). Because any single enzyme defect can impair the breakdown of several types of macromolecules that are likely to be widely distributed across organs and tissues, LSDs are syndromes. At least 12 LSDs are associated with hearing loss (the mucopolysaccharidoses, Tay-Sachs, GM_1 gangliosidosis, Neimann-Pick, Fabry, galactosialidosis, and aspartylglucosamineuria) (Schuknecht, 1993; Gorlin, 1995).

The mucopolysaccharidoses are characterized by the inability to degrade glycosaminoglycans, which are carbohydrate chains of the extracellular matrix. Including subtypes, there are at least 11 different mucopolysaccharidoses, with the major forms designated MPS I through MPS VII (Schuknecht, 1993; Gorlin, 1995). All MPSs have been linked to hearing loss. This chapter focuses on MPS VII (Sly syndrome) (Sly et al., 1973). MPS VII is associated with a defect in β-D-glucuronidase, an enzyme that normally removes glucuronic acid residues from dermatan sulfate, heparan sulfate, and chondroitan 4- and 6-sulfate. MPS VII is autosomal recessively transmitted. Although there is considerable variability of presentation (depending on the specific mutation), this disease typically features skeletal dysplasias, enlargement of liver and spleen, moderate mental retardation, corneal clouding, and retinal degeneration, in addition to mixed hearing loss and recurrent otitis media (Vogler et al., 1994; Gieselman, 1995; Gorlin, 1995). Often, life span is markedly shortened.

Otologic evaluations of patients with any of the MPSs are relatively few (Keleman, 1966; Hayes et al., 1980; Peck, 1984; Wallace et al., 1990; Bredenkamp et al., 1992; Papsin et al., 1998). Hearing loss in MPS is present at the earliest ages tested and progressive in nature. A substantial conductive component is often found, consistent with more general effects of the disease on bone and cartilage, although the hearing loss is usually mixed. Temporal bone evaluations reveal sclerosis of the cochlear capsule and ossicles, with hypertrophy of the middle ear mucosal lining. Most histopathological assessment of the sensorineural component is confounded by poor tissue preservation, and by variability of life history and genetic background. Evidence for hair cell loss is contradictory, as is evidence for involvement of the stria vascularis and spiral ganglion.

Published descriptions of ocular component of MPS include no cases of MPS VII. Retinal degeneration in MPS is generally characterized as rod-cone (Caruso et al., 1986), referring to the order in which the two types of photoreceptors become affected. Age of onset and extent and rate of photoreceptor loss are highly variable, being dependent on the type of MPS and the specific mutation.

Research on potential treatments for LSDs has been facilitated by two factors. The first factor is the ability of cells to take up lysosomal enzymes from the extracellular space (Neufeld and Fratantoni, 1970). Most lysosomal enzymes are post-translationally modified in the endoplasmic reticulum by the addition of carbohydrate groups. The enzymes are then further modified in the Golgi apparatus by the addition of a phosphate moiety to the terminal mannose residues. This modification allows them to bind to specific receptors for targeting to lysosomes. Fortuitously, the same receptors may also reside in the cell membrane (Kornfeld, 1992). Thus, a cell unable to make a given enzyme can obtain it from a potentially remote source, a phenomenon known as cross-correction (Neufeld and Fratantoni, 1970). Cross-correction means that any one of a number of means of introducing a missing enzyme into affected tissues has the potential to correct a genetic defect (Sands et al., 1997b; Daly and Sands, 1998). The second factor is the development or discovery of suitable animal models for converting the principal of cross-correction into effective therapies. Feline, canine, and murine models exist for many LSDs. Mouse models have the advantage of economy, short life spans and genetic homogeneity. The MPS VII mouse was among the first to be discovered and characterized (Birkenmeier et al., 1989; Vogler et al., 1990; Sands and Birkenmeier, 1993), and has led to rapid growth of research on MPS VII as an experimental vehicle for establishing broad principles in the treatment of genetic metabolic disorders.

THE MPS VII MOUSE MODEL

The MPS VII mouse model originated with an irradiated female C57BL/6By mouse at The Jackson Laboratory. Mice homozygous for the null mutation (mps) the of the β-D-glucuronidase gene (gus, hence gus^{mps}/gus^{mps}) have no β-D-glucuronidase activity, and show essentially all the features of human MPS VII (Birkenmeier et al., 1989). Affected animals appear normal at birth, but by 21 days begin to show characteristic features of shortened stature, facial dysmorphisms, and respiratory problems. Later, they develop an enlarged spleen, liver, and heart. Microscopic examination reveals lysosomal storage in many organs and tissues, including glial cells. Few mice live longer than 8 months. Hearing is never normal; eyes appear normal to about 4 weeks of age. The progression of sensory deficits is described in the following chapter sections.

DESIGNING TREATMENT STRATEGIES

The phenomenon of cross-correction has provided the foundation for several treatment strategies for MPS VII, with potentially wider applicability. These are presented in the following pages, and include direct injection of β-D-glucuronidase (enzyme replacement therapy, or ERT), bone marrow transplantation (BMT), viral mediated gene therapy using adeno-associated virus (AAV), and combined therapies. Each of these has been shown to have both advantages and limitations.

Subjects in the experiments to be described were B6.C-H-2^{bml}/ByBir mice that were wild-type, heterozygous, or homozygous for the gus^{mps} allele. Because wild-type and heterozygous mice are identical by most measures, they are not distinguished here, and "normal control" and "wild-type" are not intended to signify different genotypes. Mice were derived from stocks originally obtained from The Jackson Laboratory, and sustained by heterozygous matings at Washington University. To assess hearing, ABR thresholds were obtained using two different arrangements. Recording methods applied in ERT and BMT studies are described in Sands et al. (1995) and O'Connor et al. (1998). Methods used for characterization of the MPS mouse model and in AAV-therapy studies are described in Ohlemiller et al. (1999a) and Daly et al. (2001). The noninvasive flash electroretinogram was used as functional measure of the health of the photoreceptors and inner retina, excluding retinal ganglion cells (see Figure 37.6). It is easy to record and may find increasing use as workers in many disciplines attempt to characterize knockout and transgenic models. Histological evaluations were made on the cochlea and eye. Details about the electroretinogram and histological method are presented in the Appendix of this chapter.

PATHOPHYSIOLOGY OF THE MPS VII MOUSE

Middle and Inner Ears

By 4 weeks of age, considerable differences can be found in the auditory sensitivities of MPS VII and normal control mice (Figure 37.1). Disparities in ABR thresholds range from 30 to 40 dB at 5 to 20 kHz, to over 50 dB at 40 kHz. With the exception of 40 kHz, controls show little change in sensitivity to 30 weeks of age, while hearing in MPS VII mice continues to deteriorate. Elevation of thresholds at the highest frequency, observed in the controls, is probably related to the age-related hearing loss gene *Ahl*, known to be carried by C57BL/6 mice (K.R. Johnson et al., 1997). For purposes of quantitation, frequencies for which no response was found have been assigned a value of 110 dB, so that Figure 37.1 indicates better hearing at high frequencies in mutant mice than is often the case. In fact, seven of ten MPS VII mice tested at ages 16 weeks or older showed no response at 40 kHz.

The anatomical bases of conductive hearing loss in MPS VII mice have been well described (Berry et al., 1994). Affected animals as young as 1 month show thickening of the tympanic

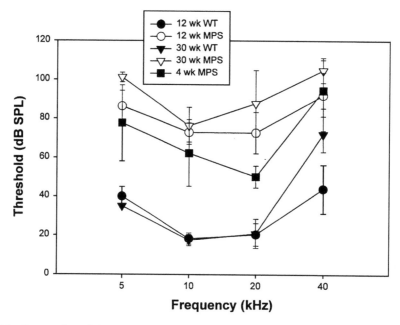

FIGURE 37.1 Progression of ABR threshold elevation in untreated MPS VII mice. Sensitivity in mutants is never normal and undergoes further declines, while that in wild-type controls (WT) remains unchanged to 30 weeks of age, except at high frequencies.

membrane, hypertrophy of the middle ear musosa, and sclerosis of middle ear walls and cochlear capsule. Osteocytes and chondrocytes show cytoplasmic vacuoles. Ossicles are thickened and often encased in connective tissue. The ossicular joint capsules are similarly thickened and show lysosomal storage in fibrocytes. The constriction of the bulla, sometimes accompanied by blocking of the eustachian tube, is conducive to otitis media, which is frequently present.

Comparison of cochleae from five normal mice (Figure 37.2) and five MPS VII mice (Figure 37.3) at 30 weeks of age by light microscopy also revealed striking differences. Abnormalities found in both base and apex of mutant cochleae only (see labels and legends, Figures 37.2 and 37.3) include cytoplasmic vacuolation of both endothelial and mesothelial cells of Reissner's membrane (a); diffuse vacuolated cells of the spiral limbus (especially along the medial endothelial surface) (b); vacuolated osteocytes in the cochlear capsule (c); distention of mesothelial cells lining scala vestibuli and tympani (d and f); distention of fibrocytes throughout the spiral ligament (e); and distention of the epithelial cells of the spiral prominence (g, not apparent at this magnification). Higher magnification of the MPS VII cochlea (Figure 37.4) reveals distended glial cell bodies and processes throughout the osseous spiral lamina and Rosenthal's canal (B, stars show examples). The obvious thickening of the basilar membrane (Figure 37.4A) appears to be a continuation of the distended mesothelial cells lining scala tympani. Cytoplasmic vacuolation of affected cells, including mesothelial cells lining the lower surface of the basilar membrane and ganglion cells (arrows in Figure 37.4A; stars in Figure 37.4B.) imparts a "foamy" character to these. Surprisingly, the organ of Corti appears normal. Outer hair cells (OHCs) did not show cytoplasmic vacuoles. No vacuoles were found in any supporting cells of the organ of Corti, spiral ganglion cell bodies or processes, nor were any clear anomalies of the tectorial membrane noted. Although radial views of the organ of Corti are not optimal for assessing stereocilia, stereociliary bundle profiles were similar in mutant and wild-type mice. It is likely that the stereocilia of MPS VII mice are normal.

Hair cell counts were performed in four MPS VII and four normal mice at 30 weeks, in the opposite cochleae to those described above. No difference was found in the extent of OHC loss (Figure 37.5B). Both mutants and controls exhibited severe loss in the hook region, in keeping with their high-frequency hearing loss and the probable influence of the *Ahl* gene (Spongr et al., 1997a). Both groups showed a relatively abrupt transition about 0.8 to 1.2 mm from the cochlear base, wherein near-normal numbers of hair cells gave rise to patches of loss, moving basally. Somewhat paradoxically, the only significant difference found was that MPS VII mice showed essentially no loss of inner hair cells (IHCs) in the hook, where controls had lost about half of theirs (Figure 37.5A). This finding was mirrored in the gross appearance of the hook region. Cochlear surface preparations from all 4 mutants stained darkly with osmium for nerve fibers. By contrast, preparations from three of four control mice showed staining that was patchy or absent. MPS VII mice may therefore lose fewer IHCs than would otherwise occur in the presence of *Ahl*, and avoid secondary nerve fiber loss. This result merits further examination with a larger sample.

The pattern of cochlear pathology in MPS VII mice shows good agreement with the distribution of heparan sulfate and chondroitan sulfate reported in mice, guinea pigs, and gerbils. At least one of these glycosaminoglycans (GAGs) has been localized to the tectorial membrane, Reissner's membrane, spiral limbus, spiral ligament, basilar membrane, spiral prominence epithelium, and osseous spiral lamina (Munyer and Schulte, 1994; Torihara et al., 1995; Cosgrove et al., 1996; Hultcrantz and Bagger-Sjoback, 1996; Satoh et al., 1998). Thus, there is close spatial overlap between the synthesis and degradation of these GAGs, although these processes may not occur in the same cells. Notably, previous studies do not indicate that heparan sulfate and chondroitan sulfate are present in the hair cell stereociliary bundle, in keeping with their generally normal appearance structures in our preparations. We view cytoplasmic vacuolation of the mesothelial cells of the basilar membrane and Reissner's membrane within the context of the distention of mesothelial cells throughout the perilymphatic spaces, where GAGs have not been reported. These mesothelial cells normally have a very narrow profile, however, so that such labeling may have been missed.

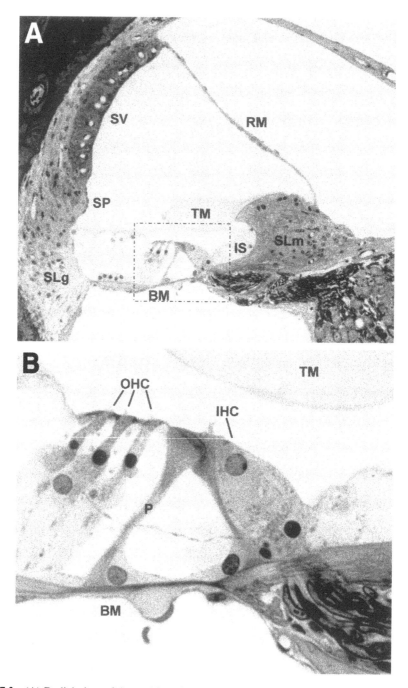

FIGURE 37.2   (A) Radial view of the cochlear duct in a 30-week-old normal control mouse. (B) Expanded view of the boxed region in (A). BM: basilar membrane; TM: tectorial membrane; IS: inner sulcus; RM: Reissner's membrane; SV: stria vascularis; SP: spiral prominence; SLg: spiral ligament; SLm: spiral limbus; IHC: inner hair cell; OHC: outer hair cell.

In summary, MPS VII mice show abnormalities of both middle and inner ears, supporting a mixed hearing loss that is consistent with human MPS. The pattern of elevation in ABR threshlolds in affected animals does not clearly point to conductive vs. sensorineural contributions, except for how one interprets the loss of sensitivity at high frequencies. The expectation that this might be

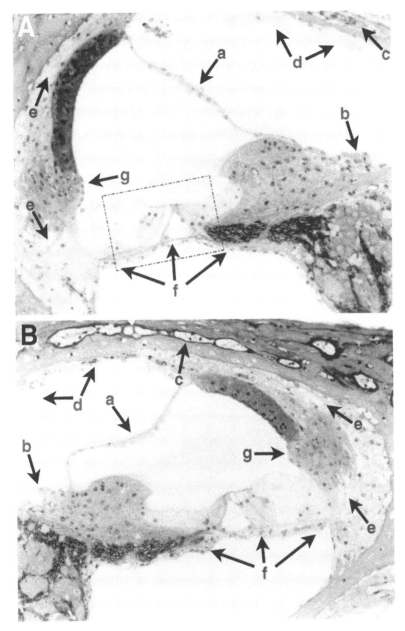

FIGURE 37.3 (A) Radial view of the cochlear duct in the upper basal turn in an untreated 30 week old MPS VII mouse. (B) Upper apex. Highlighted features: (a) thickened Reissner's membrane with distention of endothelial and mesothial layers; (b) hypertrophy and vacuolation of cells of the spiral limbus; (c) vacuolated osteocytes of the cochlear capsule; (d) vacuolated mesothelial cells lining perilymphatic spaces; (e) vacuolated fibrocytes of the spiral ligament; (f) vacuolated mesothelial cells of the basilar membrane; and (g) vacuoles in epithelial cells of the spiral prominence.

explained in terms of greater basal hair cell loss in the mutants is not supported. This feature may instead have its cause in the middle ear. MPS-associated changes in the middle ear may be expected to lead not only to increased damping of ossicular motion, but also to mass and stiffness increases in the ossicles, giving rise to steeper cutoffs at both low and high frequencies. Although the cochlea

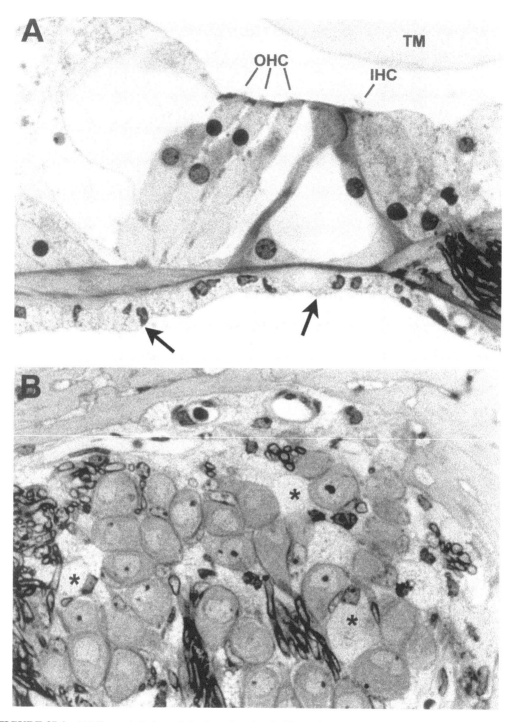

FIGURE 37.4 (A) Expanded view of the boxed region in Figure 37.3A taken from an untreated 30-week-old MPS VII mouse. The organ of Corti appears normal, except for vacuolated mesothelial cells lining the lower surface of the basilar membrane (arrows). (B) Vacuolated glia (stars indicate examples) of the spiral ganglion from a 30-week-old MPS VII mouse. Spiral ganglion cells appear normal.

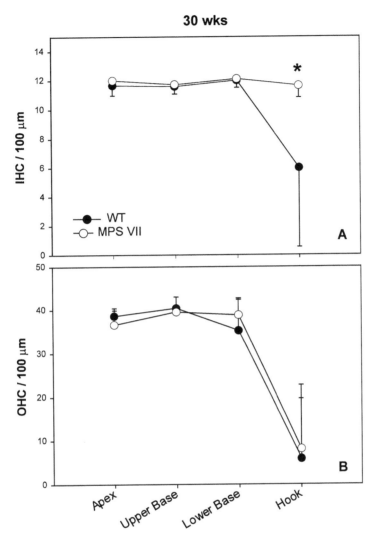

FIGURE 37.5 Cochlear hair cell density at 30 weeks in four untreated MPS VII mice and four normals (WT) (A). Inner hair cells; (B) outer hair cells. Mutants differed from controls only with respect to inner hairs cells in the extreme base, where controls lost significantly more (*t-test, $p < 0.009$). Both genotypes lose most outer hair cells in the extreme base.

shows many abnormal features, the only features that should clearly impact hearing sensitivity are the abnormal thickness (and possibly mass) of both basilar and Reissner's membranes, which would be expected to alter macromechanics. Histopathologic changes we noted also raise the possibility of altered fluid homeostasis, altered permeabilty of scala media, and an abnormal endocochlear potential. Finally, despite the normal appearance of hair cells and afferent neurons, it remains to be shown that these function normally. Mouse models of MPS VII and other MPSs can provide consistent functional and anatomical hallmarks that should be useful in guiding clinical assessments.

RETINA

The flash electroretinogram (ERG) consists of a negative-going "a-wave," followed by a positive-going "b-wave" (Figure 37.6). On the b-wave is also superimposed a series of rapid fluctuations known as oscillatory potentials (OPs). Although these components reflect different cells and processes,

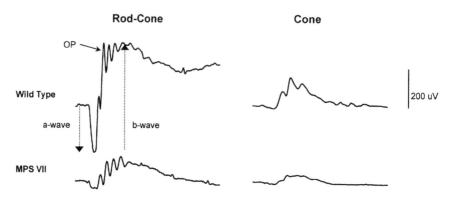

FIGURE 37.6 Example electroretinograms obtained in response to a bright white flash in 20-week-old MPS VII wild-type and mutant mice. Rod-cone responses are obtained by presenting flashes in the dark, following typically 2 or more hours of dark adaptation. Cone responses are obtained by presenting the same flash against a brightly lit rod-suppressing background. By convention, a-wave and b-wave components (see text) are measured as indicated. OP: oscillatory potentials.

the fact that they partially cancel has led to their use (particularly in rodents) as a general measure of inner and outer retinal functional integrity (Dowling, 1987). By convention, the b-wave is measured as the total peak-to-peak extent of the waveform, and thus includes the a-wave and sometimes the OPs (the approach adopted here). After an hour or more of dark adaptation, a bright flash presented in darkness elicits a b-wave that is considered to reflect contributions of both rods and cones. After 10 minutes or more of exposure of the eye to a brightly lit background, which suppresses rod responses, the same flash elicits a b-wave considered to be dominated by cones. For gross potentials, rod-cone ERG responses to a bright flash are quite large in mice, and can exceed 1.0 mV, depending on electrode type and location. Flash ERGs have been found to be an effective functional diagnostic, yielding functional information that complements anatomical measures. Notably, in contrast with ABR waveforms, flash ERGs provide no information about the function of ganglion cells or central pathways.

The flash ERG waveform of MPS VII mice has a normal shape, but is reduced in amplitude compared to similar-aged normal controls (Figure 37.6). This is true of both rod-cone and cone responses. Rod-cone responses in MPS VII mice and controls begin to diverge at about 4 weeks of age, while cone responses in the mutants may never be normal (Figure 37.7). The disparity between mutant and control mice progresses with age, but the ERG is typically still recordable at 30 weeks, above which age there are few survivors to test.

Anatomical signs of retinal degeneration in MPS VII mice are apparent by about 4 weeks (Lazarus et al., 1993). The first indications include shortening of photoreceptor outer segments and lysomal storage in the retinal pigment epithelium (RPE). By 4 months, some loss of photoreceptors is apparent, which accelerates after about 6 months. Initial losses reportedly are limited to cones. The inner retina, including retinal ganglion cells, retains a normal appearance in the oldest MPS VII mice examined. Figure 37.8 compares typical retinas of a 20-week-old MPS VII mouse (A, C) with a normal control of the same age (B, D). Mutants show reduction in the number of photoreceptors (a), shortened outer segments (b), and thickening of the retinal pigment epithelium, corresponding to increased lysosomal storage (c). The inter-photoreceptor matrix (not shown at this magnification) contains undigested cellular debris.

The RPE is involved in support functions for the photoreceptors, including turnover of materials at the distal outer segments (Nguyen-Legros and Hicks, 2000). Accordingly, the RPE normally contains β-D-glucuronidase, while GAGs chondroitan sulfate and heparan sulfate are found in the

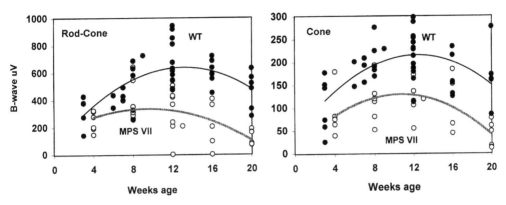

FIGURE 37.7   Scatter plot of flash electroretinogram b-wave amplitudes in MPS VII wild-type and mutant mice at different ages. Lines are best-fit polynomials. Each data point in each plot represents one animal. Rod-cone responses begin to diverge at about 8 weeks. Cone responses in mutants are never normal. Both responses are still recordable in some mutants at 30 weeks of age. (Adapted from Ohlemiller et al., 2000.)

inter-photoreceptor matrix (Lazarus et al., 1993). The histopathology of the MPS VII retina therefore fits well with the distribution of these components and functions. Reduced photoreceptor function and number presumably result from a lack of maintenance of outer segments by the RPE, although it is not clear why this should lead to photoreceptor loss. The cone-rod pattern of degeneration in the MPS VII mouse differs from the rod-cone pattern associated with other MPSs as desribed in humans (Caruso et al., 1986), and with other retinal degenerations known to originate with the RPE (Dowling and Sidman, 1962).

TREATMENT STRATEGIES

ENZYME REPLACEMENT THERAPY

The simplest treatment suggested for MPS VII by the phenomenon of cross-correction is direct enzyme replacement by intravenous injection. β-D-glucuronidase that is tagged with the mannose-6-phosphate (Man 6-P) receptor recognition moiety and injected via the superficial temporal vein (Sands and Barker, 1999) is taken up to a degree that is correlated with the distribution of Man 6-P receptors in the body (Vogler et al., 1993). Several factors argue for beginning such injections soon after birth. First, because MPS VII becomes evident in the first few weeks of life, early treatment will lead to fewer irreversible effects of the disease. Second, the distribution of Man 6-P receptors appears less restricted during development, potentially facilitating access of the free enzyme to affected tissues (Matzner and Van Figura, 1992). Third, the blood-brain barrier may be more permeable in developing animals, permitting access to the CNS (Vogler et al., 1999). Mice given weekly injections of enzyme beginning at birth and examined at 6 weeks of age (Sands et al., 1994) showed enzyme activities roughly 3% of normal levels in kidney and spleen, up to 12% of normal in brain, and 28% of normal in liver. Treated mice had an overall normal appearance, with near-normal bone length. Lysosomal storage was markedly reduced in liver, bone, spleen, heart, kidney, RPE of the eye, and some CNS neurons and glia. Apparently, even small amounts of β-D-glucuronidase are adequate to correct the MPS VII phenotype in many tissues. After injections are terminated, enzyme activity can be demonstrated in MPS VII mice for at least 14 days. Increased signs of lysosomal storage begin to appear in some tissues by roughly 1 month (Vogler et al., 1996).

    ABR thresholds obtained at 6 weeks of age in normal controls and treated and untreated MPS VII mice revealed that normal hearing sensitivity was maintained in the mutants in the mid-frequency range (8 to 16 kHz), although there was hearing loss at high frequencies (Figure 37.9)

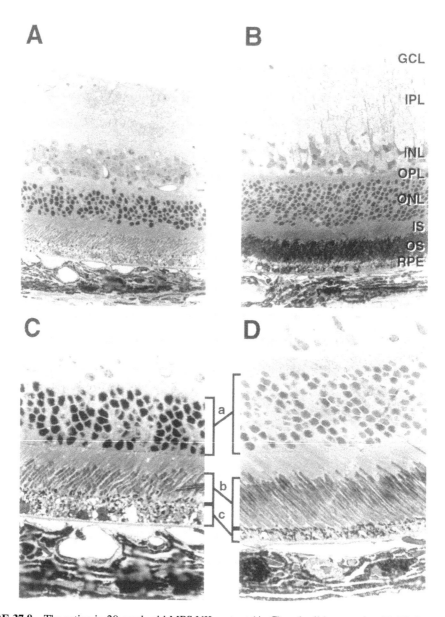

FIGURE 37.8 The retina in 20-week-old MPS VII mutant (A, C) and wild-type mice (B, D). Lower panels show an expanded view. Anatomical features differ in three key respects: (a) the thickness of the outer nuclear layer (number of photoreceptors); (b) the length of photoreceptor outer segments; and (c) the thickness of the retinal pigment epithelium (reflecting cytoplasmic vacuolation). GCL: ganglion cell layer; IPL: inner plexiform layer; INL: inner nuclear layer; OPL: outer plexiform layer; ONL: outer nuclear layer; IS: inner segments; OS: outer segments; RPE: retinal pigment epithelium. (Adapted from Ohlemiller et al., 2000.)

(O'Connor et al., 1998). Anatomical evaluation of the middle ear showed considerable improvement of MPS VII mice over sham-treated mutants, but the former still had some thickening of the tympanic membrane, lysosomal storage within ossicles, and distention of the ossicular joints. Although cochleae were not examined, the remaining abnormalities of the ossicular chain and tympanic membrane appear adequate to explain the difference in hearing sensitivity between treated mutant and normal mice, and it is likely that the cochlea itself was largely corrected.

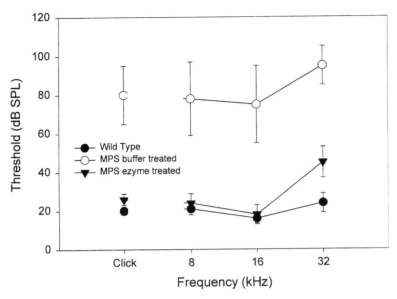

FIGURE 37.9 ABR thresholds in 6-week-old MPS VII wild-type mice, and in mutant mice that received intravenous injections of β-D-glucuronidase or buffer at birth. Mice were injected through the superficial temporal vein with 28,000 U of enzyme in 100 μL buffer, beginning on the day of birth, then at weekly intervals to 5 weeks. Treated mutants differed from normals only at high frequencies. (Adapted from O'Connor et al., 1998.)

BONE MARROW TRANSPLANTATION

Because β-D-glucuronidase circulating in the bloodstream can be taken up by tissues throughout the body, one possible strategy is to create stable resident populations of hematopoietic stem cells that can generate the enzyme. Bone marrow cells obtained from a compatible donor and injected intravenously can become established and serve in this capacity. Moreover, bone marrow-derived macrophages should be able to cross the blood-brain barrier, although perhaps after some delay (Gieselman, 1995; Kennedy and Abkowitz, 1997), potentially providing an advantage over ERT in preventing the disease within the CNS. Before bone marrow transplantation (BMT) can be performed, native bone marrow cells must be ablated, typically with high doses of radiation. Just as for enzyme replacement therapy, the early onset of MPS VII and increased permeability of the blood-brain barrier early in life favor early treatment. Yet, radiation is particularly toxic to cells undergoing division, and can permanently damage developing epithelia whose cells have not yet undergone terminal mitoses. The early "safe" age varies with organ, and of course with species. MPS VII mice are ideal for determining optimal BMT strategies because syngeneic donor stem cells are easy to obtain.

BMT in MPS VII mice at a few months of age corrects many of the features of the disease and leads to a near-normal life span, but fails to reverse skeletal abnormalities or lysosomal storage in CNS neurons (Birkenmeier et al., 1991). By contrast, BMT performed at birth prevents skeletal defects and reduces lysosomal storage in the meninges of the CNS at least to 10 months (Sands et al., 1993). The amount of enzyme expressed in brain, spleen, and kidney increases with the level of pre-treatment irradiation (^{137}Cs source) over the range of 200 to 800 rads, achieving up to 80% of normal levels in spleen. However, irradiation in newborn mice that is sufficient to promote therapeutic levels of reconsition of hematopoietic cells was found to lead to disruption of the cerebellum, producing ataxia in some cases. There was also extensive loss of retinal photoreceptors, probably reflecting the fact that terminial mitoses within the retina are not complete until about 1 week of age (Young, 1985).

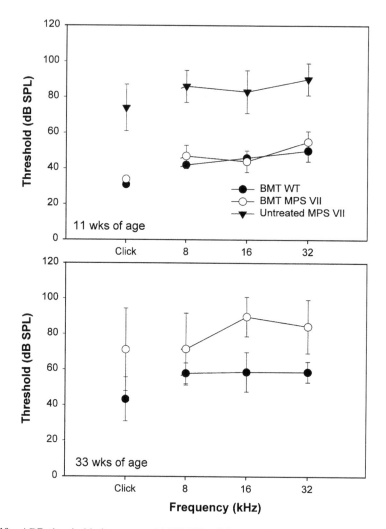

FIGURE 37.10   ABR thresholds in untreated MPS VII wild-type mice, and in mutant and wild-type mice that underwent bone marrow transplantation (BMT) at birth. On the day of birth, mice were exposed to 200 rads by a ^{137}Cs irradiator, then received an intravenous injection of 100 µL buffer containing 10^6 bone marrow cells from syngeneic wild-type mice. Testing at 11 weeks of age (upper) showed no difference between treated normals and mutants. Repeat testing at 33 weeks (lower) showed some loss of sensitivity in BMT-treated mutants. (Adapted from Sands et al., 1995.)

By contrast with retina, terminal mitoses in the cochlea of mice are complete at birth (Kikuchi and Hilding, 1965a). BMT performed at birth in MPS VII mice yields ABR thresholds that are indistinguishable from those in treated normal mice at 11 weeks of age (Figure 37.10) (Sands et al., 1995). By 33 weeks, however, the same treated MPS VII mice were 10 dB or more less sensitive than treated normals at all frequencies. Evaluation of middle ears of these animals revealed pathology similar to MPS VII mice undergoing ERT. Because cochleae were not examined, it is not clear whether the hearing loss in treated mutants at 33 weeks was solely attributable to the middle ear, or whether return of lysosomal storage in cells of the inner ear was involved.

To provide benefit for the eye in MPS VII, BMT must be delayed at least beyond the first week of life. In a separate study, MPS VII mice underwent BMT at 4 weeks, followed by flash ERG testing at 8, 12, and 20 weeks. Rod-cone responses in treated mutants showed gradual improvement and were essentially identical to those in normal mice by 20 weeks (Figure 37.11). Cone responses

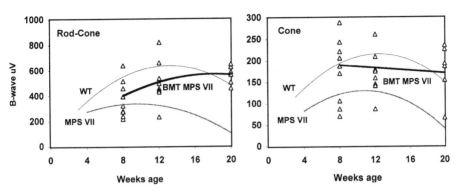

FIGURE 37.11 Scatter plot of flash electroretinogram b-wave amplitudes in BMT treated MPS VII mice, compared with averaged data from wild types and untreated mutants at different ages. At 4 weeks of age, mice were exposed to 650 rads by a ^{137}Cs irradiator, then received an intravenous injection of 100 μL buffer containing 5×10^6 bone marrow cells from syngeneic wild-type mice. Rod-cone responses improved to normal after 12 weeks of age. Cone responses reached normal amplitudes more quickly. Both responses were statistically indistinguishable from normals to at least 20 weeks of age. Thin lines are taken from Figure 37.7; heavy lines are best-fit polynomials to treated mutant data. Each data point in each plot represents one animal. (Adapted from Ohlemiller et al., 2000.)

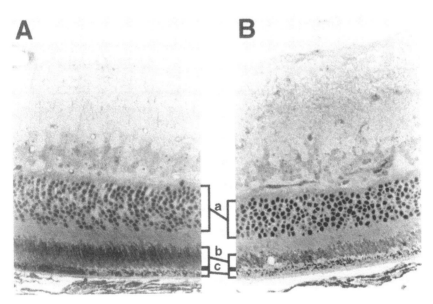

FIGURE 37.12 Example retinas from 20-week-old BMT treated MPS VII wild-type (A) and mutant mice (B). Animals received BMT at 4 weeks, as described in Figure 37.11 Differences include shortened photoreceptor outer segments (b) and possibly fewer photoreceptors (a) in the mutants. Retinal pigment epithelium (c) appears normal in each case. (Adapted from Ohlemiller et al., 2000.)

in treated mutants appeared to improve more rapidly and were similar to normals by 8 to 12 weeks. Histological examination at 20 weeks (Figure 37.12) showed normal appearance of the retinal pigment epithelium (c), and improved (possibly complete) preservation of photoreceptors (a). The only consistent difference found was moderate shortening of photoreceptor outer segments (b). BMT performed at 8 weeks of age yielded functional and histopathologic results similar to those for BMT at 4 weeks. Functional preservation of retina in the MPS VII mouse by BMT, as determined by ERG, appears to be somewhat more complete than that of hearing. It remains to be determined whether this preservation is stable for longer periods. Although the retina appears largely normal in MPS VII mice at 4 weeks of age (Lazarus et al., 1993), and produces near-normal ERG responses, there occurred a lag in the functional correction of the retina in mutants (Figure 37.11). Rod-cone responses did not achieve normal amplitudes until 12 to 16 weeks post treatment, probably reflecting the time required for hematopoietic stem cells to become sufficiently reconstituted. During this time, however, the disease may progress. The disparity between functional correction of the retina and histopathologic correction (Figure 37.12) may arise because shortening of photoreceptor outer segments occurs during the delay period and is not reversible.

BMT has been applied clinically in MPS and other lysosomal storage diseases for over a decade (Gieselman, 1995; Sands et al., 1997b; Daly and Sands, 1998). The majority of cases show reduction in the multisystemic effects of the disease, including the ear. In an otologic follow-up study of patients with MPS I, II, and VI, 11 patients undergoing BMT by age 10, then evaluated 4 to 14 years later, showed consistent improvement relative to an untreated control sample (Papsin et al., 1998), although mixed hearing loss was usually still present. Limited benefits of BMT for vision in MPS have been demonstrated. A clinical follow-up study of 23 patients undergoing treatment by age 15 (Summers et al., 1989) showed functional improvement (as determined by ERG) in 81% of the patients within the first year. However, longer term follow-up data obtained up to 11 years later indicated that these benefits often did not persist (Gillingsgrud et al., 1998). Complicating this analysis were potential adverse effects of BMT itself, which appear more pronounced for the eye than for the ear. Variability of host engraftment of transplanted tissue, stem cell incompatibility, and adverse effects of treatment protocols still pose hurdles for successful application of BMT in humans. As a potentially useful variant on this approach, bone marrow-derived macrophages express relatively high levels of β-D-glucuronidase. Transplantation of fully differentiated macrophages into non-irradiated MPS VII mice resulted in relatively persistent ($\geq$30 days) enzyme activity in several tissues and a corresponding reduction in lysosomal storage (Freeman et al., 1999). With further development, this strategy may provide therapeutic levels of enzyme to tissues that are sensitive to radiation during development.

COMBINED ENZYME REPLACEMENT THERAPY (ERT) AND BONE MARROW TRANSPLANTION (BMT)

In the MPS VII mouse, ERT and BMT both reduce lysosomal storage in many tissues. Both approaches improve the function of the ear, and the function and/or appearance of the eye. ERT at birth poses fewer complications than BMT, and provides nearly complete preservation of hearing sensitivity to 6 weeks of age (O'Connor et al., 1998). However, the benefits of ERT are temporary, requiring re-injection at intervals of one to a few months. The sheer expense of such treatments is likely to limit the application of ERT in MPS. Combining ERT and BMT has therefore been proposed as an alternative strategy (Sands et al., 1997a). MPS VII mice receiving Man 6-P-tagged β-D-glucuronidase injections during the first 5 weeks of life, followed by BMT, showed additional benefits compared with animals receiving enzyme alone, when examined at 6 months to 1 year of age. Increased protection from lysosomal storage was noted for the meninges, bone, and cornea and retinal pigment epithelium of the eye. Middle and inner ears were not examined.

VIRAL-MEDIATED GENE TRANSFER

The transient character of the benefits of ERT and potential complications of BMT (especially for clinical applications) have encouraged the development of more efficient yet safe means of getting stable sources of β-D-glucuronidase into the body. Additional motivations include the incomplete correction of MPS VII within CNS neurons and glia, incomplete correction of the appearance of the eye, and the recurrence or persistence of middle ear abnormalities. Viral-mediated gene therapy has been intensively explored for the treatment of many diseases (Sands et al., 1997b; Daly and Sands, 1998). Again, because of the potential for cross-correction, lysosomal storage diseases may be particularly suitable for this approach. AAV has many features desired of an optimal vector for treatment of LSDs, including persistent expression, the ability to transduce many tissues and organs, and non-pathogenicity.

Two different approaches for treating MPS VII mice using AAV have been examined to date, both in neonates. In the first approach, mice received injections of AAV containing human β-D-glucuronidase cDNA into both quadriceps muscles on a single occasion (Daly et al., 1999a). Histochemical and quantitative analysis showed increased enzyme activity near the injection site to over 50 times normal levels during the following 6 weeks, and stable to at least 16 weeks of age. Enzyme activity was also found at a few distant sites; β-D-glucuronidase activity in both liver and spleen rose to approximately 1% of normal levels over the 16-week period. Liver expression of enzyme appeared to result from viral transduction of hepatocytes. Therapeutic response to the treatment in terms of reduced lysosomal storage was limited, however, even within liver and spleen.

More impressive results have been obtained by a much simpler approach, namely intravenous injection of the same AAV vector (Daly et al., 1999b). Newborn MPS VII mice receiving AAV containing human β-D-glucuronidase cDNA via the superficial temporal vein showed activity of the enzyme up to 10% of normal in brain, kidney, and lung, and more than tenfold elevated over normal levels in heart. These elevations were stable to at least 16 weeks of age. Accordingly, lysosomal storage was largely or completely eliminated in these organs, as well as in liver, spleen, and retina. Particularly striking was the virtual elimination of lysosomal storage within neurons and glia of the CNS, where relatively little evidence for improvement has been seen using alternative therapy methods. Elevated enzyme activity within brain, heart, kidney, and lung correlated with the amount of human β-D-glucuronidase cDNA, suggesting that local viral infection rather than cross-correction from distant sites was responsible for the enzyme activity.

The benefits of neonatal AAV treatment for hearing and vision have subsequently been examined functionally (Daly et al., 2001). At 16 weeks of age, by which time untreated MPS VII mice may retain little hearing, treated mutants showed hearing sensitivity approaching that of wild-type mice (Figure 37.13). Threshold sensitivity observed at 16 weeks in treated mutants does not differ from that seen at 4 weeks of age, suggesting that correction of hearing might persist for much longer periods. Although differences between treated mutants and normal mice were significant overall, they exceeded 15 dB only at the highest frequencies. Three of six cochleae of treated mutants used for ABR testing appeared normal when examined by light microscopy at 20 weeks. (Mice were euthanized after an additional ERG recording at 20 weeks.) The others showed some abnormalities characteristic of MPS VII, including an increase in thickness of Reissner's membrane and slight distention of mesothelial cells lining the basilar membrane (Figure 37.14). Notably, the extent of these features was not predictive of hearing loss. The animal represented in Figure 37.14, which illustrates the maximum extent of MPS-like features in the AAV-treated mice, had hearing thresholds that were within 10 dB of mean wild type thresholds (Figure 37.13) at all test frequencies. Although middle ears in these animals have not yet been examined, we therefore speculate that persisting middle ear problems can account for sensitivity differences between controls and treated MPS VII mice.

Flash ERG responses were obtained at 20 weeks of age. Treated MPS VII mice showed both rod-cone and cone responses that were indistinguishable from those in normal controls (Figure 37.15). This finding is consistent with the elimination of lysosomal storage in the retinal pigment epithelium of treated animals, as observed by light microscopy (Daly et al., 1999b). It has not yet been determined whether or not photoreceptor outer segments were normal in length.

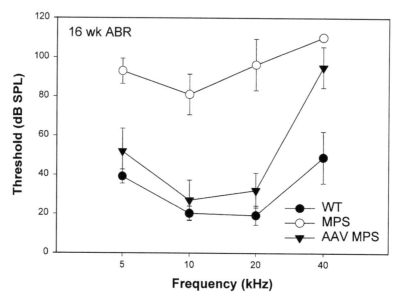

FIGURE 37.13 ABR thresholds compared in 16 week old MPS VII wild type, untreated mutant, and mutant mice receiving intravenous AAV containing human β-D-glucuronidase cDNA. One day after birth, mice received a single injection through the superficial temporal vein of 100 μL of buffer containing 5×10^9 IU/kg of recombinant virus. Minor differences appear between wild-type and AAV-treated mutant mice, except at high frequencies, where treated mutants more closely resemble untreated mice. (Adapted from Daly et al., 2001.)

CONCLUSIONS

TREATMENT OF MPS IN MICE AND HUMANS

The MPS VII mouse closely models its human counterpart and provides an excellent model for developing treatments of the MPSs and other lysosomal storage diseases. Not all murine genetic diseases produce features that closely resemble their human homologs; nevertheless, those that disrupt basic metabolism often may. Thus, detailed functional and anatomical studies of the ear in murine LSD models (Daly and Sands, 1998) may point to specific features to look for in clinical assessments and temporal bone studies. Although other animal models have been found for some LSDs, developing therapies in mouse models offers advantages of economy and genetic standardization.

Some of the earliest features of MPS VII, including shortening of photoreceptor outer segments and skeletal anomalies (including mass and stiffness changes in the ossicles), may be largely irreversible, once established. These changes, which are somewhat resistant to treatment even in mice, may reflect slow turnover of GAGs within the retina, and limitations of the capacity for bone remodeling. Prevention, rather than remediation, of the characteristic features of MPS by early treatment appears critical. Because mice are altricial, treatments that are effective when applied postnatally may have limited clinical potential unless they can be applied before birth (Sands et al., 1997b).

Three major treatment strategies were compared, with an emphasis on efficacy in the inner ear and retina. Enzyme replacement therapy is noninvasive, and can be applied soon after birth. ERT can restore hearing sensitivity to near normal, although it remains to be determined whether this efficacy is sustained with repeated dosing into adulthood. Early doses of enzyme in ERT may have more lasting benefits than later doses, particularly within the brain (Vogler et al., 1998). Among

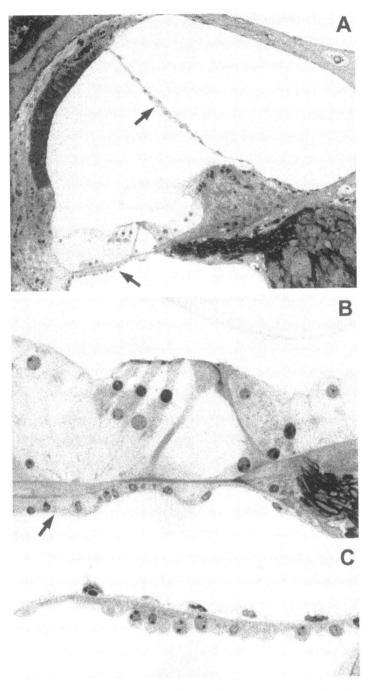

FIGURE 37.14 (A) Radial view of the cochlear duct in the upper basal turn of a 20-week-old MPS VII mutant mouse that underwent AAV therapy at birth (see Figure 37.13). The cochlea appears completely corrected except for modest thickening of Reissner's membrane and distention of epithelial cells lining the basilar membrane (arrows, compare with Figure 37.3). These features were seen only in some treated animals. (B) and (C) show expanded views of indicated regions in (A) taken from an adjacent section. At 16 weeks, this animal's ABR thresholds were within 10 dB of wild-type thresholds at all test frequencies.

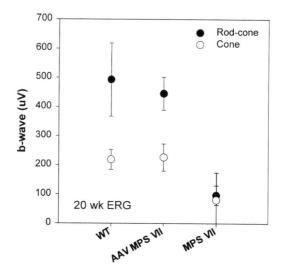

FIGURE 37.15 Comparison of flash electroretinogram amplitudes in MPS VII wild-type and AAV-treated mutant mice (see Figure 37.13). Both rod-cone and cone responses of treated mutants are in the normal range. (Adapted from Daly et al., 2000.)

the disadvantages, ERT is potentially expensive, and may provide relatively poor correction within the CNS when applied in adults. Bone marrow transplantation with irradiation preconditioning provides long-term protection against MPS for many tissues and organs. Hearing sensitivity can approach normal for at least a few months after treatment, but eventually degrades somewhat. If BMT is delayed to the fourth week of life, the electrical responses of the the retina can recover to normal amplitudes. Presumably, certain MPS-related changes in photoreceptor function not apparent by light microscopy can be reversed. It is not yet presently clear what the implications are for visual perception. Because application of BMT is precluded during development, when it might otherwise be most beneficial, the promise of ERT may lie in its role as a "bridge" technique. ERT at birth, followed by BMT at a few weeks of age, was shown to be more effective than either treatment alone. In any configuration that has been examined, however, ERT and BMT typically provide only partial correction within the CNS. Intravenous AAV-mediated gene therapy appears particularly promising for reducing the ensemble of features of MPS, notably including lysosomal storage within the CNS. Because it is quickly effective, is noninvasive, and provides stable correction, this approach may find wide application. However, it appears to work less well in resolving the conductive component of MPS VII compared to either ERT or BMT. For all three forms of treatment, most evidence is consistent with greater responsiveness of the inner ear than the middle ear. The middle ear is either less responsive initially, or may more readily revert to a diseased state, than the inner ear. Middle ear problems, however, may be amenable to other relatively simple strategies, such as trans-tympanic application of enzyme or viral vectors.

RELEVANCE TO OTHER GENETIC DISORDERS OF HEARING

In the cochlea as elsewhere, lysosomal storage diseases involve disruption of metabolism. The functions of lysosomal enzymes include cellular repair and protective responses to xenobiotics (e.g., Ishii et al., 1968). Thus, in addition to known LSDs, related deficits may impact the ability of cochlear sensory cells to withstand insults and survive injury. Changes in the appearance of lysosomes and peroxisomes have long been associated with aging and possible exhaustion of maintenance and repair capabilities (Schuknecht, 1993). Secretion of lysosomal enzymes and recapture by distant cells is an adaptive product of evolution with the secondary benefit of promoting several promising treatment strategies for LSDs. Yet the phenomenon of cross-correction and its molecular bases would not have been predicted based on simple assumptions about the system. One implication is that other factors found to be deficient in congenital or age-related/progressive deafness may have unexpected access to affected cells of the cochlea. Intravenous viral-mediated gene therapy could be effective in treating such diseases, either by non-selectively establishing local cells as producers of missing factors, or by specifically targeting certain cell types. Nearly all attempts at getting genes into the cochlea have focused on direct introduction of vectors into cochlear fluids (e.g., Lalwani et al., 1996; Derby et al., 1999; Stover et al., 1999; Waering et al., 1999; Yagi et al., 1999), which requires invasive procedures in animal models, and probably more so in humans. Successes in treating MPS VII mice indicate that non-surgical approaches may be possible in some cases.

ACKNOWLEDGMENTS

We thank Marie Roberts and Jaclynn Lett for assistance and Dr. Ann Hennig for helpful discussions. This work is supported by grants from the Edward Mallinckrodt Jr. Foundation to KKO, NIH HD35671, DK53920, and DK50158 to MSS, and DK41082 to CAV.

APPENDIX: METHODS

All procedures in the studies reported by our group were approved by the Animals Studies Committees of Washington University Medical School (WUMS) or CID.

FLASH ELECTRORETINOGRAM

Mice were anesthetized, mounted, and maintained identically to ABR recordings. Animals were dark adapted for at least 2 hours, then prepared for recording under dim red light. All recordings were obtained from the left eye. A 2.0-mm-diameter stainless steel loop positioned gently on the eye by a micromanipulator served as the recording electrode. Pupillary dilation was maintained by perfusing the cornea with a solution of pH-adjusted 2.0% xylazine, delivered via a length of PE10 tubing terminating directly above the recording loop, and connected at its other end to a 20-cc syringe. Dilation measured at the end of each experiment was usually 1.5 mm or greater. The reference electrode (inactive) was a stainless steel needle inserted into the skin behind the right ear. A stainless steel needle in the skin of the back served as ground. Electrodes were led to a Grass P55 battery-powered differential amplifier (0.3 to 300 Hz, 1000X). Responses were acquired at 3 kHz and stored using a CED micro1401 and Cambridge software, as for ABR recording. Responses were averaged online and stored for later analysis.

Flashes were generated by a Grass PS33-Plus photic stimulator set at I16, triggered by the computer. The 13-cm-diameter xenon flash source was positioned in front of a white background, 25 cm from the eye, and 30° anterior to the medial-lateral axis of the eyes. Flashes were 10 μs in duration and had an intensity of 2.3 cd-s/m^2, measured at the position of the eye. Rod-cone responses were obtained by presenting flashes in darkness and averaging the response over 5 to 10 presentations at 0.1 Hz. Cone responses were obtained by presenting flashes against a light background (34 cd/m^2) at 1 Hz and averaging the response over 50 presentations.

ANATOMICAL ASSESSMENT

For euthanasia, animals were injected with sodium pentobarbital (60 mg/kg i.p.) and perfused transcardially with 2.0% paraformaldehyde/2.0% glutaraldehyde in 0.1 M phosphate buffer. Both cochleae were isolated, immersed in fixative, and the stapes removed. Cochleae were decalcified in sodium EDTA, post-fixed in buffered 1.0% osmium tetroxide, dehydrated in an ascending acetone series, and embedded in Epon. They were then cut in 4-μm midmodiolar sections for light microscopy evaluation, or cut into segments for hair cell counts. For cell counts, one cochlea from each animal was dissected into roughly half-turn segments, and these segments were viewed as surface preparations under mineral oil using Nomarski optics and a calibrated ocular. For each cochlea, three separate IHC and OHC counts were obtained from non-overlapping 100-μm segments at four locations: apical (0.0–1.0 mm from the apex), upper base (2.0–3.0 mm from the apex), lower base (3.5–4.5 mm from the apex), and hook (most basal 1.0 mm).

Eyes were removed and immersed in 2.0% glutaraldehyde/4.0% paraformaldehyde in phosphate buffer. They were embedded in Spurr's resin and sectioned at 0.5 μm, then stained with toluidine blue.

38 Auditory Brainstem Responses in CBA Mice and in Mice with Deletion of the RAB3A Gene

Robert Burkard, Blanca Durand, Carrie Secor, and Sandra L. McFadden

INTRODUCTION

Neurotransmitter secretion is the primary means of intercellular communication within the nervous system. The process of neurotransmitter release involves a complex series of biochemical events that includes regulation of the synaptic vesicle cycle (see Figure 38.1). As defined by Schiavo and Stenbeck (1998), the essential steps of the synaptic vesicle cycle include transport of vesicles to the plasma membrane, followed by their docking, priming, and finally their fusion with the plasma membrane. These events are triggered by calcium entry through specific calcium channels. All of the steps in the synaptic vesicle cycle are regulated by proteins and protein-lipid interactions.

Recent studies have concentrated on identifying the proteins involved in vesicle trafficking at the presynaptic nerve terminal. These studies have shown that three proteins comprising the SNARE complex — synaptobrevin, SNAP-25, and syntaxin — are essential for membrane fusion, and that synaptotagmin is the major calcium sensor for calcium-regulated exocytosis at the synapse. Other important proteins include a family of approximately 30 low molecular weight GTP-binding proteins, called Rab proteins. The Rab3 isoforms are vesicle-associated GTPases that are highly expressed in neural tissue. Rab3a, one of four known Rab3 isoforms, controls a late step in the vesicle docking and fusion process. The precise point at which Rab3a acts in the process is not known. It has been suggested that Rab3a plays a role in sequestering vesicles near their release sites (Nonet et al., 1997) or recruiting synaptic vesicles for exocytosis during repetitive stimulation in neurons (Geppert et al., 1994). However, recent experiments suggest that the function of Rab3a is to regulate neurotransmitter release from the synaptic vesicle by restricting exocytosis to a single vesicle per releasing site (Schiavo and Stenbeck, 1998). Using electrophysiological analysis of neurotransmitter release, Geppert et al. (1997) found that the size of the readily releasable pool of vesicles was normal in mutant mice lacking Rab3a, but calcium-triggered fusion was altered. Specifically, more exocytic events occurred within a brief time after arrival of the nerve impulse than normal.

Rab3a distribution has not been investigated in the cochlea. However, the protein has been detected in the vestibular end-organs of fetal and adult CBA/C57 mice, using immunocytochemical techniques (Dechesne et al., 1997). Dechesne et al. (1997) detected Rab3a immunoreactivity in the sensory cells, the efferent nerve endings at the base of the sensory cells, and the calyces of afferent nerve fibers innervating type I hair cells. During fetal development, Rab3a was first detected on embryonic day 16 (E16). At E16 and E17, intense Rab3a staining was observed in the afferent neurites and at the base of the vestibular hair cells all along the utricles and in the central zones of the cristae. At E19, Rab3a labeling was denser in the afferent endings in the utricle and cristae, and the labeled fibers formed a dense plexus at the base of the sensory cells. A few hair cells in

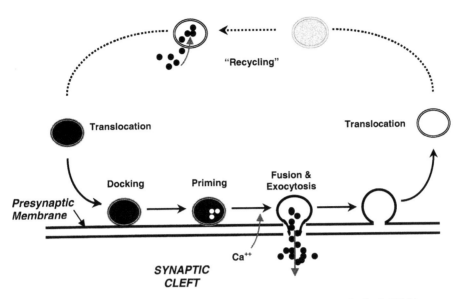

FIGURE 38.1   Schematization of the synaptic vesicle cycle. (Adapted from Sudhof, 1995.)

the utricle were very faintly stained at E17. At birth, strong labeling was observed in numerous afferent neurites and in some, but not all sensory cells. Beginning at postnatal day 2 (P2), Rab3a was detected in the afferent nerve calyces around the type I sensory cells (see Chapter 13). Between P5 and P17, intense staining was observed in the upper part of the afferent calyces, and moderate-to-intense staining was present in the hair cell cytoplasm. In the adult mouse, the apical part of the nerve calyces surrounding the type I hair cells, and the efferent nerve endings at the base of the sensory cells of the cristae and maculae, were strongly labeled. Most type I and type II hair cells had light labeling in their cytoplasm, but not their nuclei. No Rab3a immunolabel was observed in supporting cells.

A major gap in our knowledge of synaptic proteins involves their functional significance. It is necessary to have techniques available for evaluating the functional consequences of gene and protein alteration. One way to evaluate the results is to stimulate and record from isolated synapses. A second technique is to use gross stimulation and recording techniques in live animals. The auditory brainstem response (ABR) is one such technique.

THE AUDITORY BRAINSTEM RESPONSE

The ABR method is discussed in detail in Chapter 4. Several aspects of the ABR technique favor its use for the investigation of the Rab3a gene. Onset responses such as ABR are critically dependent on the synchrony of the underlying biomechanical and subsequent neural events in response to an acoustic transient, and its exquisite sensitivity to various stimulus manipulations make it a useful measure of neural synchrony. For the study of neural synchrony, it is useful to evaluate peak latencies and amplitudes in response to stimuli presented at suprathreshold levels.

The ABR is a series of peaks emanating from the auditory nerve and auditory structures of the brainstem. The first ABR peak arises from the auditory nerve (humans: Møller, 1994; cats: Buchwald and Huang, 1975; gerbils: Burkard et al., 1993) and hence represents the contribution of the auditory system up to and including the synapse between the cochlear hair cells and auditory nerve fibers. The later ABR peaks are generated by more rostral auditory structures, with the generators contributing to these later peaks differing across animal species. For example, the fifth positive peak of the human ABR, typically labeled wave V, is thought to reflect primarily activity from the lateral lemniscus (Møller, 1994), while the fifth positive peak from the cat ABR is thought to reflect mostly activity from the inferior colliculus (Buchwald and Huang, 1975). These later waves thus reflect activity of both the auditory periphery and auditory brainstem. One can calculate the time interval between waves to determine brainstem conduction time.

Changes in click level produce similar changes in the early and later ABR peaks for animal species such as humans (Starr and Achor, 1975; Cox, 1985; Stockard et al., 1978) and gerbils (Burkard and Voigt, 1989a; 1990). In contrast, increases in click rate produce a greater ABR peak latency shift for the later than the earlier peaks (Burkard and Hecox, 1987; Burkard and Voigt, 1989a; 1990). Similarly, in response to a constant-level click stimulus in the presence of a continuous broadband noise, there is a greater increase in the latency of the later ABR peaks than the earlier peaks with increasing noise level (Burkard and Hecox, 1987; Burkard and Voigt, 1989b, 1990). Decreasing click level, increasing click rate, and increasing level of masking noise all produce a decrease in ABR peak amplitudes.

The greater increase in latency of the later ABR peaks, as compared to the earlier peaks, to manipulations of click rate and noise level presumably results from an increase in brainstem conduction time. Such increases in brainstem conduction time cannot be the result of changes in the peripheral hair-cell/eighth-nerve synapse, as this time would be reflected in the first ABR peak. This greater latency shift in the later ABR waves (relative to the first peak) must reflect mechanisms central to the site of action potential discharge in the VIIIth nerve. It is unlikely that the nerve conduction velocity in the auditory nerve or the central auditory nervous system is influenced by click rate or level of masking noise, making synaptic events a likely place to seek the underlying mechanisms for these rate- and masking-induced latency shifts. ABR changes resulting from repeated stimulation to click trains (rate effects) or to stimulation with a continuous masking noise could be the result of either pre- or post-synaptic changes with repeated stimulation. Presynaptic limitations in neurotransmitter synthesis, storage, or release could lead to changes in the magnitude or the time course of post-synaptic spike discharge. It is also feasible that the latency changes with rate and masking noise are the result of limitation in discharge rate due to post-synaptic membrane characteristics that are related to refractory period. Regardless of the specific cause, rate and masking paradigms might be useful to probe disorders of the central auditory nervous system. For example, Jacobson et al. (1987) found that human ABR peak latency was increased beyond the normal range in a larger number of multiple sclerosis patients when using high click stimulation rates, as compared to low click rates. In addition, increasing click rate produces a greater increase in ABR peak latencies in human infants than adults (Lasky, 1984), and kittens show greater ABR peak latency increases with increasing rate than young-adult cats (Burkard et al., 1996a). These developmental data suggest that the "synaptic machinery" of the immature auditory system is more susceptible to rate manipulations than the adult system.

ABRS IN MICE LACKING THE GENE CODING FOR THE RAB3A PROTEIN

Work described here evaluated the effects of click stimulation rate, level of background noise, and click level on mice lacking the gene coding for the Rab3a protein. We hypothesized that compared to normal-hearing CBA/CaJ mice, these mice would show greater ABR peak latency shifts and amplitude reductions at higher rates and noise levels, as these conditions would stress synaptic function. Assessing the effects of click rate, click level, and noise level on ABRs of CBA mice provided normative data on the CBA strain, as well as providing a backdrop for evaluating the responses from Rab3a knockout (KO) mice.

B6,129S-*Rab3a*^{tm1Sud} mice, referred to henceforth as Rab3a KO (or simply Rab3a) mice, were created in the laboratory of Dr. Thomas C. Sudhof at the University of Texas Medical Center at Dallas through homologous recombination. Homozygous Rab3a KO mice do not express Rab3a protein, but are viable, fertile, and comparable in health and weight to normal (wild-type) littermates.

Because Rab3a mice are maintained by homozygote x homozygote mating, wild-type siblings are not available as controls. The most appropriate control strain, B6129F2/J, was not commercially available at the time our studies were conducted; consequently, we compared responses from Rab3a KO mice to those of normal-hearing CBA/CaJ mice.

Young adult Rab3a and CBA female mice (approximately 2 months old, 8 mice per strain) were purchased from Jackson Laboratories for use in this investigation. Animals weighed between 13 and 24 grams. Animals were anesthetized with Avertin and core temperature was maintained at 38°C. Three stimulus protocols were performed: a click-rate series, a noise-level series, and a click-level series. For the click-rate series, both conventional and maximum length sequence (MLS) ABRs were obtained. For MLS ABRs, responses to a train of clicks are averaged, with a specified minimum time between pulses in a train. This minimum time between pulses is called the minimum pulse interval (MPI). When the MPI is sufficiently short, the ABR to sequential clicks overlap. Following signal averaging, the overlapped responses are disentangled by use of a cross-correlation procedure. The average time between pulses is approximately twice the MPI; and thus for an MPI of 1 ms, the average interval is approximately 2 ms, resulting in an average stimulation rate of roughly 500 Hz. For conventional ABRs, all responses are the averaged response to 200 click presentations. For MLS ABRs, responses were averaged to 15 pulse trains. As each train was composed of 64 pulses, MLS ABRs are the averaged response to 960 clicks. Two ABRs were collected for each condition for all studies reported herein. For a detailed review of the procedures used to obtain MLS ABRs, the reader is referred to Burkard et al. (1990a).

For the click-rate series, click level was 80 dB pSPL. For conventional ABRs, click rates included 10, 25, 50, 75, and 100 Hz. For MLS ABRs, MPIs of 5, 3, 2, 1, and 0.5 ms were used, providing average click rates of approximately 100, 167, 250, 500, and 1000 Hz, respectively. For the noise-level series, click level was 80 dB pSPL, click rate was 25 Hz, and noise level varied from 20 to 80 dB SPL in 10-dB steps. For the click-level series, clicks were presented at a rate of 25 Hz, and click level decreased from 80 dB pSPL to 20–30 dB pSPL, in 10-dB steps.

Dependent variables investigated include the peak latencies and amplitude of the various ABR peaks. In the summary plots that follow, mean latencies and amplitudes are only shown when at least four of eight mice showed that particular peak for that specific stimulus condition.

Effects of Click Rate

Figure 38.2 shows ABRs to a click-rate series in each mouse strain. The upper left and right panels show conventional ABRs for CBA and Rab3a mice, respectively. MLS ABRs are shown in the lower left and right panels of Figure 38.2 for CBA and Rab3a mice, respectively. ABRs were present in all CBA and Rab3a mice at all rates. For each strain, click-evoked ABRs consisted of a series of five or more peaks occurring within 5 to 6 ms of click onset. The relative prominence of the peaks varied across individual mice. We labeled the five most consistently observed positive peaks as waves i, ii, iii, iv, and v. These are labeled for each strain for the 10-Hz condition for conventional ABRs (Figure 38.2, upper panels). MLS ABRs are grossly similar in morphology to conventional ABRs in both CBA and Rab3a mice. Waves i and ii were present in all CBA and Rab3a mice at all rates. In CBA mice, wave iii was present at all rates; while in Rab3a mice, wave iii was missing in several mice at the 1000-Hz rate. In CBA mice, wave iv was missing in several animals for rates of 250, 500, and 1000 Hz. Wave iv was missing in one animal at a 75-Hz rate, and in 2, 1, and 4 mice for MLS rates of 167, 500, and 1000 Hz, respectively. Finally, for both CBA and Rab3a mice, wave v was missing for some animals at all rates, and for most animals at the higher rates.

Mean ABR peak latencies across click rate are shown in Figure 38.3. In this and all subsequent figures, panel A shows data from CBA mice, while panel B shows data from Rab3a mice. For each mouse strain, the majority of animals showed waves i through iv at click rates up to 1000 Hz. Wave v was only present in half of the animals for clicks rates up to 75 Hz for CBA mice and 100 Hz for the Rab3a mice. For both CBA and Rab3a mice, ABR peak latencies increase with increasing

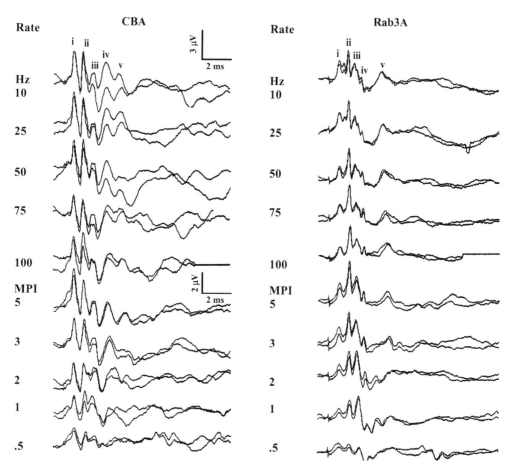

FIGURE 38.2 ABRs are shown across click rate from one CBA and one Rab3a mouse. The upper left and right panels show conventional ABRs for a CBA and Rab3a mouse, respectively. ABR waves i through v are labeled for CBA and Rab3a mice for the 10-Hz rate. MLS ABRs from one CBA and one Rab3a mouse are shown in the lower left and right panels, respectively.

click rate, with this increase being more prominent for the later ABR peaks. Mean rate-induced peak latency shift increases with increasing peak number for CBA mice. In Rab3a mice, rate-induced latency shift increases with increasing peak number for waves i through iii, but mean wave iv latency shift is less than wave iii. Finally, mean rate-induced latency shift is greater for CBA mice for waves i, ii, and iv, with rate-induced latency shift greater for Rab3a mice only for wave iii.

Mean ABR peak amplitudes across click rate are shown in Figure 38.4. For each mouse strain, there is a decrease in ABR peak amplitudes with increasing click rate, although wave v in Rab3a mice is small in amplitude at all rates, and appears to increase with increasing rate from 10 to 75 Hz, and decrease for higher rates. Rab3a mouse ABR peak amplitudes are generally smaller than those seen in the CBA mouse. At the lowest rate shown (10 Hz), the mean amplitudes of waves i through v were 7.415, 3.573, 6.506, 3.239, and 1.568 μV, respectively, for CBA mice, and 2.171, 3.011, 3.284, 1.443 and 0.763 μV, respectively, for Rab3a mice. In all cases, the mean peak amplitudes were smaller for the Rab3a than the CBA at higher click levels, but these differences were greatest for waves i, iii, and iv. Mean amplitudes of waves i and iv were larger for CBA mice at all rates, while mean wave iii amplitude was larger for CBA mice at all rates up to 500 Hz. In contrast, mean wave ii amplitude was larger for CBA mice at low rates (up to 100 Hz conventional

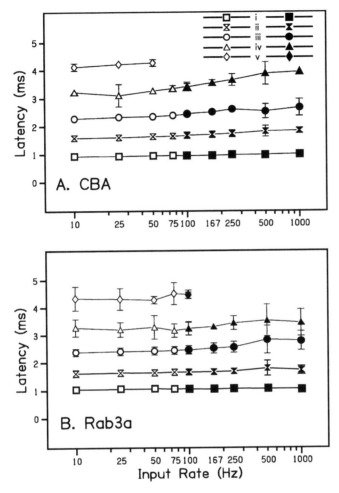

FIGURE 38.3 Mean ABR peak latency is plotted across click rate. Open symbols show conventional ABR data, while filled symbols show MLS-ABR data. (a) Mean latency data for CBA mice; and (B) mean latency data for Rab3a mice.

rate), but was larger for Rab3a mice for the higher rates. Thus, ABR peak amplitudes across rate behaved similarly in both strains, although peak amplitudes were generally smaller in Rab3a mice.

The observations that latency shift with rate is minimal for wave i, but is larger for the later ABR peaks parallel those reported in humans (Debruyne, 1986; Chiappa et al., 1979; Burkard and Hecox, 1987; Burkard et al., 1990a), cats and kittens (Burkard et al., 1996a; b), gerbils (Burkard and Voigt, 1989a; 1990; Burkard, 1994) and ferrets (Kelly et al., 1989). ABRs were seen in the majority of mice of each strain for click rates as high as 1000 Hz. ABRs have been reported to click rates as high as 1000 Hz in gerbils (Burkard, 1994) and cats (Burkard et al., 1996a; b).

EFFECTS OF NOISE LEVEL

Figure 38.5 shows ABRs across level of masking noise for one CBA and one Rab3a mouse. Clearly, with increasing noise level, there is a decrease in ABR peak amplitudes, with responses difficult to observe for masker levels above 50 to 60 dB SPL. Figure 38.6 plots mean ABR peak latencies across level of masking noise. For CBA mice, wave iii was the only peak seen in half or more of the animals for 60 dB SPL of masking noise. Waves i, ii, and iv were seen in half or more animals for masker levels up to 50 dB SPL, while wave v was seen in half or more animals only up to

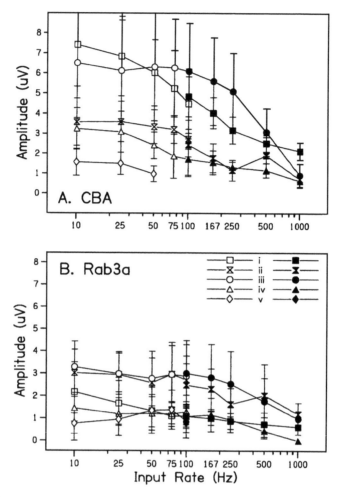

FIGURE 38.4   Mean ABR peak amplitude is plotted across click rate. Open symbols show conventional ABR data, while filled symbols show MLS-ABR data. (A) Mean amplitude data for CBA mice; and (B) mean amplitude data for Rab3a mice.

20 dB SPL of masking noise. For Rab3a mice, waves i through iv were seen in half or more of the animals for masker levels up to 60 dB SPL, while wave v was only seen in half or more mice up to 40 dB SPL of noise. In both CBA and Rab3a mice, ABR peak latencies generally increased with increasing level of masking noise, with little latency shift for wave i, and generally larger shifts for the later ABR peaks. For CBA mice, wave i shows a very small increase with noise level, while in Rab3a mice, there is a small mean decrease in wave i latency for the 50 dB SPL noise condition, when compared to the no-noise condition. In Rab3a mice, however, there was a small mean wave i latency increase (0.045 ms) for the 60 dB SPL noise condition relative to the latency seen for the no-noise condition. ABR peak latency shifts with noise were greater for waves ii, iii, and iv than wave i for both CBA and Rab3a mice. In both CBA and Rab3a mice, latency shift was largest for wave iii. In addition, for any given peak, mean ABR peak latency increase due to masking noise was greater for CBA than for Rab3a mice.

Figure 38.7 plots ABR peak amplitudes across masker level. ABR peak amplitudes decrease with increasing level of masking noise for both strains. As seen in the click rate data, peak amplitudes were generally larger for CBA mice, with this effect most obvious for waves i and iii. For the CBA mouse, wave i amplitude is substantially reduced for noise levels of 30 dB SPL and above, while wave ii is little affected by masking noise until masking noise equals or exceeds 40 dB SPL. Similar

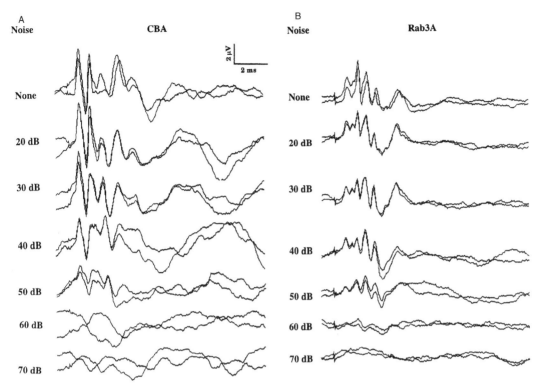

FIGURE 38.5   ABRs are shown across noise level from one CBA and one Rab3a mouse. (A, B) Conventional ABRs for a CBA and Rab3a mouse, respectively.

trends are seen for Rab3a mice, with mean wave i amplitude decreasing monotonically with increasing level of masking noise, and wave ii changing little in amplitude until masker levels of 40 dB SPL or greater are used. Again, ABR peak amplitudes behave similarly with noise level for CBA and Rab3a mice, but with Rab3a mice generally showing smaller ABR peak amplitudes.

These effects of masking noise seen in CBA and Rab3a mice are similar to those reported in humans (Burkard and Hecox, 1983; 1987; Burkard et al., 1990b) and gerbils (Burkard and Voigt, 1989b; 1990). Masking noise appears to have little effect on peak latencies or amplitudes of the mouse ABR until the level of masking noise was 30 dB SPL and above (see Figures 38.6 and 38.7). In humans, ABR peak latencies and amplitudes are relatively unaffected by masking noise until it equals or exceeds 30 to 40 dB SPL (Burkard and Hecox, 1983; 1987), with similar results observed in the gerbil (Burkard and Voigt, 1989b; 1990).

EFFECTS OF CLICK LEVEL

Figure 38.8 plots a click intensity series from one CBA and one Rab3a mouse. Response amplitudes decrease with decreasing click levels, with small or absent responses for click levels below 40 dB pSPL, in these examples. Figure 38.9 shows mean peak latencies across click level. For CBA mice, waves i through iv were seen in half or more of the animals for click levels as low as 40 dB pSPL, while wave v was seen for half or more CBA mice only for click levels as low as 50 dB pSPL. For Rab3a mice, waves i, iii, and iv are present in half or more animals down to 40 dB pSPL, and waves ii and v are seen in half or more mice down to 50 dB pSPL. For both CBA and Rab3a mice, ABR peak latencies decrease with increasing click level. For CBA mice, latency/intensity function slopes for waves i-iv range from –5.33 to –10.6 μs/dB, with waves i and iv showing the steepest slopes. For Rab3a mice, latency/intensity function slopes for waves i-iv range from –6.82 to –17.12 μs/dB, with the slope systematically increasing with increasing ABR peak.

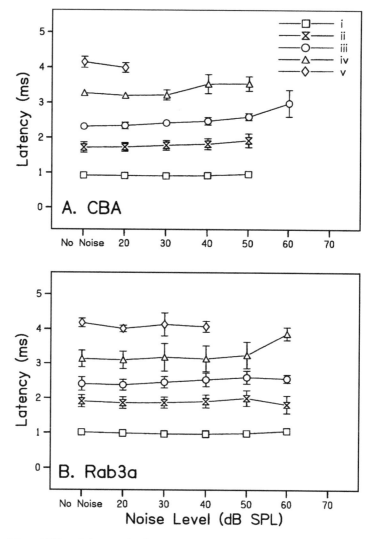

FIGURE 38.6 Mean ABR peak latency is plotted across noise level: (A) mean latency data for CBA mice; and (B) mean latency data for Rab3a mice.

Figure 38.10 shows that ABR peak amplitudes increase with increasing click level, although there is little change in mean amplitude with click level for wave v in CBA mice and wave iv in Rab3a mice. Again, peak amplitudes are generally larger for CBA than Rab3a mice.

Let us consider ABR threshold as the lowest click level at which any ABR peak could be identified. Using this criterion, ABR threshold in CBAs was 30 dB pSPL in three mice and 40 dB pSPL in five mice, with a mean threshold of 36.25 dB pSPL. For Rab3a mice, two had thresholds of 30 dB pSPL, five had thresholds of 40 dB pSPL, and one had a threshold of 50 dB pSPL, with a mean threshold of 38.75 dB pSPL. Thus, click thresholds were very similar for the two strains of mice.

Unlike the effects of clicks rate and noise level, where the latency shifts are minimal for wave i and greater for the later ABR peaks, with decreasing click level, the latency shift of all ABR peaks is quite substantial with increasing click level. For CBA mice, the slopes of the latency/intensity functions are steepest for waves i and iv (−8.5 and −10.6 μs/dB, respectively), with the latency/intensity function slopes somewhat smaller for waves ii and iii (−6.02 and −5.33 μs/dB, respectively). In Rab3a mice, there is an increase in latency/intensity function slope with increasing peak number,

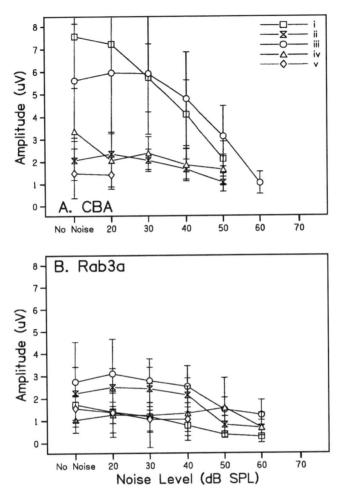

FIGURE 38.7 Mean ABR peak amplitude is plotted across noise level: (A) mean amplitude data for CBA mice; and (B) mean amplitude data for Rab3a mice.

increasing from −6.82 µs/dB for wave i to −17.12 µs/dB for wave iv. Parallel changes in the various ABR peaks across click level (i.e., similar latency/intensity function slopes) have been reported in humans (Cox, 1985; Starr and Achor, 1975), cat (Huang and Buchwald, 1978), gerbil (Burkard and Voigt., 1989a; 1990), and ferret (Kelly et al., 1989). The slopes of the latency/intensity functions seen for CBA and Rab3a mice are similar to those seen in gerbils (−8.1 to −8.6 µs/dB: Burkard and Voigt, 1989a; −4.9 to −5.3 µs/dB: Burkard and Voigt, 1990) and ferrets (−7.7 to −10.4 µs/dB: Kelly et al., 1989), somewhat less than those reported in cats (roughly −14 to −16 µs/dB: Huang and Buchwald, 1978; Fullerton et al., 1987), and substantially less than those reported for humans (e.g., −40 µs/dB: Burkard and Hecox, 1983).

RAB3A VS. CBA

Responses from the two strains of mice were remarkably similar, except that Rab3a mice showed smaller ABR peak amplitudes than the CBA mice. In addition, the effects of various stimulus manipulations on the ABR of CBA and Rab3a were very similar. We had proposed that ABR peak latency shifts with increasing rate and/or masking noise would be greater in the Rab3a than in the CBA mice. This hypothesis was not supported (see Figures 38.3 and 38.6). Indeed, CBA mice

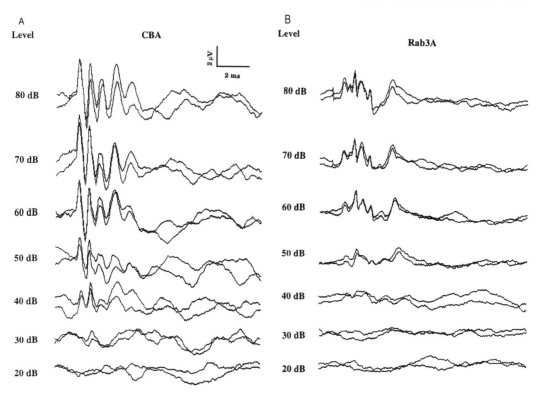

FIGURE 38.8   ABRs are shown across click level from one CBA and one Rab3a mouse: (A, B) conventional ABRs for a CBA and Rab3a mouse, respectively.

typically show greater ABR peak latency shifts with increasing rate and noise level. As reviewed above, with increasing click rate and level of masking noise, there is a greater effect on the latency of the later ABR peaks. This greater latency shift with rate and masking noise for the later ABR peaks suggests that these paradigms place demands on either the presynaptic events involving the synaptic vesicle cycle (see Figure 38.1), or post-synaptically result in a decreased probability of discharge and/or delay in neural discharge. Herein, we refer to these changes as "stressing synaptic transmission." Several lines of evidence seem to support this interpretation of rate and noise paradigms as stressing synaptic transmission. For example, Jacobson et al. (1987) reported that high click rates sensitized the ABR (i.e., resulted in more abnormalities) in patients suspected of having multiple sclerosis. Similarly, Antonelli et al. (1986) found that using ipsilateral masking noise sensitized the ABR in the identification of subclinical brainstem involvement in patients suspected of having multiple sclerosis. In a separate line of evidence, high click presentation rates produce greater ABR peak latency shifts in human infants as compared to human adults (Lasky, 1984), and in kittens as compared to adult cats (Burkard et al., 1996a).

ABRs were present in both CBA and Rab3a mice at click rates as high as 1000 Hz, and responses were seen in over half of the CBA and Rab3a mice for masker levels as high as 60 dB SPL. Geppert et al. (1994) reported that the Rab3a knockout mouse did not express Rab3a, and they found no compensatory increases in 20 associated synaptic proteins. When studying pyramidal cells of hippocampus, Rab3a mouse neurons showed apparently normal discharge patterns, except that there was a greater decrease in discharge rate with repeated stimulation (15 to 30 stimuli at a rate of 14 Hz), as compared to responses from wild-type mice. The authors concluded that Rab3a is not necessary for exocytosis.

It seems clear that the deletion of Rab3a has little effect on ABR peak latencies across a range of click levels, rate, and background masking noise levels. Perhaps Rab3a deletion truly has no effect on the ABR. There is no direct evidence that Rab3a is expressed in the auditory nervous

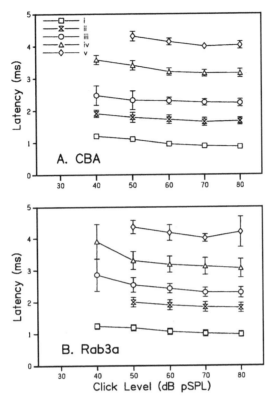

FIGURE 38.9   Mean ABR peak latency is plotted across click level: (A) mean latency data for CBA mice. and (B) mean latency data for Rab3a mice.

system, although there is evidence of Rab3a expression in the peripheral vestibular system (Dechesne et al., 1997). If Rab3a is not expressed in the auditory nervous system, then there would be no reason to expect to observe differences in rate- and masking-induced latency shift for CBA and Rab3a mice. It should also be noted that the CBA mouse is not the ideal control group for Rab3a KO mice. If wild-type and Rab3a KO mice were compared, it is possible that the hypothesized effects with rate and noise level would be seen. A second possibility is that our lowest click rate (10 Hz) was already a "high" rate as far as the Rab3a mouse auditory system was concerned. Geppert et al. (1994) found synaptic rundown after 15 to 30 stimuli at a rate of 14 Hz. As we used continuously presented stimuli at a minimum rate of 10 Hz, perhaps whatever effects this rundown would have on latency was already present in the 10-Hz rate, and thus could not be seen as a rate effect in the present study.

Perhaps the effect of Rab3a deficiency is a substantial reduction in ABR amplitude. ABR peak amplitudes (especially waves i and iii) were much smaller for Rab3a than CBA mice, even for higher click levels, lower click rates, and low levels of background noise. As already stated, our 10-Hz rate may have already been a high stimulus rate for the Rab3a mice, and hence may have resulted in a substantial decrement in response amplitude. It is interesting that kittens not only show increased rate-induced latency shifts (as compared to the adult cat), but also show decreasing ABR peak amplitudes with decreasing age (below 30 days post-partum) for either a constant click level (80 dB pSPL) or at 20 dB above threshold (Burkard et al., 1996b). Geppert et al. (1997) reported that the pool of available synaptic vesicles was normal in Rab3a knockout mice. They also reported that more exocytic events occurred within a short time period following the arrival of a nerve impulse. Following repeated stimulation, this would in all probability lead to a substantial depletion in the availability of synaptic vesicles pre-synaptically. This would likely result in a

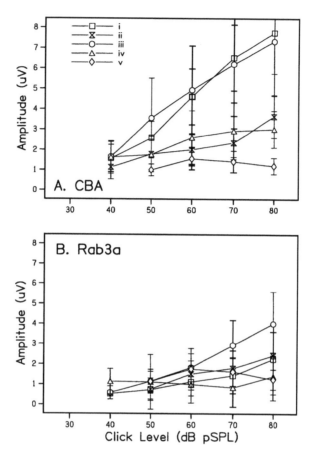

FIGURE 38.10   Mean ABR peak amplitude is plotted across click level: (A) mean amplitude data for CBA mice; and (B) mean amplitude data for Rab3a mice.

decrease in the number of synaptic vesicles undergoing exocytosis per stimulus, and thus could conceivably reduce the probability of discharge post-synaptically. This, in turn, would lead to a decrease in the amplitude of the ensemble auditory nerve response, resulting in a decrease in ABR wave i amplitude. Further, this would likely cause a decrease in amplitude of the later ABR peaks. Were we to run another group of Rab3a mice, we would further reduce click presentation rate (down to 1 Hz or less) to see if this would cause a substantial increase in their ABR peak amplitudes.

It is also possible that the Rab3a mice have a high-frequency hearing loss, causing a reduction of the amplitude of the click-evoked ABR. We did not obtain ABR thresholds to a range of tone-burst frequencies in these mice, and hence cannot rule out the possibility of a hearing loss. Furthermore, we know of no other studies that have evaluated ABR threshold across tone-burst frequency in Rab3a mice. It should be noted, however, that the similarity in ABR thresholds to click stimuli for CBA and Rab3a mice would suggest that the thresholds of these strains are similar for at least some frequencies.

ACKNOWLEDGMENTS

This work was supported, in part, by NIH-NIA AG09524. Renee Kee is thanked for her assistance with figure preparation.

39 Focus: Mutations of the *Brn4/Pou3f4* Locus

E. Bryan Crenshaw, III

INTRODUCTION

Mutations in the *Brn4/Pou3f4* gene cause congenital hearing loss in man and mouse. This chapter introduces the phenotype of each species, then compares and contrasts the developmental phenotypes in the two species. Analyses of the *Brn4* mouse mutant pedigrees demonstrate that this is a useful animal model for understanding the pathology of the mutation in man, as well as characterizing the regulation and function of the *Brn4* gene during inner ear development.

MUTATIONS OF THE *POU3F4* GENE RESULT IN X-LINKED MIXED DEAFNESS WITH PERILYMPHATIC GUSHER (DFN3)

X-linked deafness type III (DFN3) is most often characterized by mixed conductive and sensorineural deafness associated with a perilymphatic gusher upon stapedectomy (McKusick, 1998). However, there is variability of the phenotype among pedigrees with some patients demonstrating sensorineural deafness alone (Bitner-Glindzicz et al., 1994; Bitner-Glindzicz et al., 1995). DFN3 is the most common form of X-linked deafness, and constitutes between 1 and 2% of congenital deafness in humans (Nance et al., 1971). In DFN3 patients in which an exploratory tympanotomy has been performed, perilymphatic gusher is associated with removal or even disturbance of the stapes (Cremers et al., 1985; Glasscock, 1973; Nance et al., 1971). The stapes footplate in these patients lacks the annular rim of the stapes footplate (Glasscock, 1973; Nance et al., 1971), which is formed from the otic capsule during development (Anson et al., 1960). Although some patients demonstrate stapes fixation, others demonstrate brisk acoustic reflexes, suggesting that the conductive component of hearing loss may be due to mechanisms other than stapes fixation (Cremers, 1985; Cremers et al., 1985). Radiological examination typically demonstrates a bulbous enlargement of the internal auditory meatus (IAM) at its lateral extent (Glasscock, 1973; Phelps et al., 1991). Additional radiological features include small cochleae, enlarged vestibule, and reduced diameter of the semicircular canals (Cremers et al., 1985; Phelps et al., 1991). A reduction of vestibular function in affected individuals has been demonstrated (Cremers et al., 1985; Phelps et al., 1991). *In toto*, these observations suggest that the phenotype of these patients results from developmental anomalies affecting the otic capsule during the ontogeny of the inner ear.

In 1995, Cremers and colleagues demonstrated that the DFN3 locus resulted from mutations in the POU-domain gene, POU3F4, which maps to position Xq21.1 (de Kok et al., 1995). This gene is a member of the POU-domain gene family, which are transcriptional factors that regulate developmental and/or differentiation events (for review, Herr and Cleary, 1995; Ryan and Rosenfeld, 1997). The term "POU-domain" is an acronym derived from the first four members of the family that were characterized: Pit-1, a pituitary transcription/developmental regulatory factor; Oct-1, a widely expressed transcription factor; Oct-2, an immune system transcription/developmental regulatory factor; and *unc-86*, a factor that regulates the development of the peripheral nervous system in the nematode, *C. elegans* (Herr et al., 1988). The POU-domain is a bipartite DNA-binding domain that is composed of a POU-specific domain, which shares structural homology to helix-turn-helix DNA-binding proteins, and the POU-homeodomain, which shares structural homology to the "classical" 60 amino acid homeodomain. Several mutant alleles of the POU3F4 result from point mutations that are invariably found within the POU-domain (Bitner-Glindzicz et al., 1995; de Kok et al., 1995; Friedman et al., 1997; Hagiwara et al., 1998). Approximately 60% of the mutations in affected individuals result from large deletions, and many of these deletions encompass the protein coding sequences. However, a number of these deletions lie upstream of the POU3F4 coding sequences (de Kok et al., 1996). Cremers and colleagues have demonstrated that the smallest of these nested deletions (8 kb [kilobases]) lies 900 kb upstream and centromeric to the coding sequence of the POU3F4 gene (de Kok et al., 1996). These data suggest that either there are two closely linked genes that result in the DFN3 phenotype, or that the upstream deletions encompass upstream transcriptional regulatory elements of the POU3F4 gene.

EXPRESSION PROFILE OF THE *BRN4/POU3F4* GENE DURING MOUSE OTIC DEVELOPMENT

To further characterize the function of the POU3F4 gene, analysis of its mouse ortholog, *Brn4/Pou3f4*, has been undertaken. The *Brn4* gene is expressed early in the development of the mouse inner ear, and is associated with the initial mesenchymal condensation events that give rise to the otic capsule (Phippard et al., 1998). Mesenchymal condensation, as well as *Brn4* gene expression are initially restricted to the ventral aspect of the otic vesicle at stages 10.5 to 11.5 dpc. Later during embryogenesis, *Brn4* gene expression is detected in all parts of the otic capsule, which completely surround the otic vesicle by 14.5 dpc. Expression in the late fetal and early neonatal stages continues to be widespread in the otic capsule until about P12, at which time the expression of *Brn4* is largely restricted to the strial fibrocytes and spiral limbus (Friedman et al., 1997; Minowa et al., 1999; our unpublished observations). Additionally, the *Brn4* gene is expressed throughout most of the neural tube, as well as the pituitary gland, pancreas, and whisker follicles (Alvarez-Bolado et al., 1995; Phippard et al., 1998; Schonemann et al., 1995; our unpublished observations). Although less well characterized, the available evidence suggests that similar patterns of expression are found in rat and man (de Kok et al., 1996; Le Moine and Young, 1992).

TARGETED MUTAGENESIS OF THE ORTHOLOGOUS *BRN4/POU3F4* GENE IN MICE

To generate an animal model for DFN3 mutations, the mouse ortholog, *Brn4/Pou3f4*, has been mutagenized using mouse embryonic stem (ES) cell technology by two different laboratories (Minowa et al., 1999; Phippard et al., 1999). The phenotype of these "knockout" mutations demonstrate many similarities with the human POU3F4 mutations. Although there appear to be differences in the mouse models, they share several characteristics (Minowa et al., 1999; Phippard et al., 1999). Most importantly, both animal models demonstrate hearing loss, although the magnitude of hearing loss is apparently different. This apparent disparity may be due to the different methods used to assess hearing loss (Preyer's reflex vs. auditory brain response [ABR]). Alternatively, the hearing loss may vary depending on the genetic background of the ES cells used to generate the mutant animals (Minowa et al., 1999; Phippard et al., 1999; Steel, 1999). If the differences are due to genetic background, then it will be possible to characterize modifying loci that enhance or suppress the mutant phenotype and provide greater insight into the role of *Brn4/Pou3f4* during otic development. In either case, light and electron microscopy demonstrate that both mouse models have dysplastic strial fibrocytes, characterized by unusual intercellular spaces and cytoplasmic extensions. These fibrocytes underlie the stria vascularis, a structure that is responsible for maintaining the ionic composition of endolymph in the scala media. The ionic composition of the endolymph consists of high K^+ and low Na^+, which is maintained by the high rate of K^+ pumped into the endolymph by the stria vascularis (for review, see Steel, 1999). Alteration in the ionic composition of the endolymph in the *Brn4* mutants is suggested by two observations. First, the mice have hydrops (Phippard et al., 1999). Second, the endocochlear potential in the mutant mice is lowered (Minowa et al., 1999). Steel (1999) has proposed that the dysplastic nature of the fibrocytes compromises a K^+ recycling pathway that removes K^+ ions from the hair cells through the supporting cells of the organ of Corti, then through the strial fibrocytes, and finally through the stria vascularis into the endolymph. This hypothesis is supported by a number of deafness mutations which should act along the proposed cellular highway (Steel, 1999). The dysplastic strial fibrocytes and the hypothesized defect in the K^+ recycling pathway provide a good explanation for the sensorineural component of hearing loss in the human patients.

The conductive component of deafness in the DFN3 patients is recapitulated in one of the two mouse knockout pedigrees (Phippard et al., 1999). Defects in the stapes were reported by Phippard et al. (Phippard et al., 1999), particularly in the stapedial footplate, which is derived from the otic capsule (Anson et al., 1960). Interestingly, expression of *Brn4* was detected in the mouse otic capsule, but not in the mesenchymal condensations from Reichert's cartilage, which gives rise to most of the stapes (Anson et al., 1960; Langman, 1982). A definitive demonstration that embryonic cells that express *Brn4* contribute to the formation of the stapes await cell lineage analyses.

Other malformations of the temporal bone have been detected in the mouse models generated by Phippard et al. (1999). Enlargement of the foramina of the IAM are seen in this mouse model, which roughly correspond to the bulbous IAM observed in DFN3 patients. Additional malformations occurring in the mice that have been observed in DFN3 patients include hypoplasia of the cochlea resulting from a reduction in the size of the perilymphatic scalae, as well as a reduction in the number of turns of the cochlea. In the vestibule, the mutant mice demonstrate a narrowing of the superior semicircular canal, which likely explains the vertical head-bobbing phenotype observed in the mutants (Phippard et al., 1999). Interestingly, this vestibular defect does not interfere with the animals' swimming ability, a standard test of vestibular function in mice (Minowa et al., 1999; our unpublished observations).

SEX-LINKED FIDGET MUTATION ELIMINATES EXPRESSION OF *BRN4* IN THE OTIC CAPSULE, BUT NOT THE NEURAL TUBE

There is an additional mouse pedigree that is apparently an allele of the *Brn4* gene called sex-linked fidget (*slf*), which arose in a screen for X-linked lethal mutations (Phillips and Fisher, 1978). The phenotype of these animals consists of vertical head-bobbing, similar to that observed in the *Brn4* knockout animals. *slf*, which was induced by X-irradiation, results from an inversion of the middle region of the X chromosome (Phippard et al., 2000). The distal breakpoint of this inversion does not fall within the *Brn4* coding sequences or within ~10 kb flanking the coding sequence. However, it does appear to lie within several hundred kilobases upstream (centromeric) of the *Brn4* coding sequences. Intercross breeding experiments between *slf* and the *Brn4* knockout demonstrate that the *slf* mutation does not genetically complement the *Brn4* gene, which is consistent with the interpretation that *slf* is an allele of the *Brn4* gene. Non-complementation is found in the phenotypes of fibrocyte dysplasia and constriction of the semicircular canals, thereby demonstrating that these two phenotypes are present in *Brn4* null mutants on disparate genetic backgrounds (B6/129 vs. 3H1). Other phenotypes that differ between the Minowa et al. *Brn4* knockout (Minowa et al., 1999) and the Phippard et al. (1999) mutant have not been explored in the *slf* mutants. Comparison of *Brn4* mutations on different genetic backgrounds should provide insight into the genetic contribution of phenotype variability found in man and mouse. Interestingly, the expression of the *Brn4* protein is eliminated in the otic capsule of presumptive *slf* embryos, but this expression is unaffected in the neural tube of these embryos. We have demonstrated that the transcriptional regulatory elements that direct expression to the neural tube lie within 6 kb of the *Brn4* coding sequence in a region of the gene that is not grossly rearranged in the *slf* mutant (our unpublished data). Therefore, these data indicate that the *slf* chromosomal inversion eliminates the function of the transcriptional regulatory elements that direct expression to the otic capsule. The nature and position of the *slf* mutation parallel the deletion mutations in the human POU3F4 locus that lie 900 kb upstream of the coding sequence. Therefore, these data suggest that the architecture of the cis-active transcriptional regulatory elements is conserved in mouse and human. Although 900 kb is a considerable distance over which cis-active transcriptional regulatory elements must function, there are examples in other genes in which regulatory elements are found hundreds of kilobases from the coding sequences of a gene (for review, see Bedell et al., 1996). Definitive demonstration of this presumptive transcriptional enhancer awaits the cloning of this element and testing of its ability to direct otic capsule specific expression in transgenic mice.

In summary, mutant alleles of the *Brn4/Pou3f4* gene in mice have provided a powerful means to investigate the molecular mechanisms that result in deafness from mutations in the orthologous human locus, POU3F4. Because of the many parallels in the phenotype of man and mouse, both the underlying developmental defects, as well as the variability in phenotypes observed in these mutants, can be examined. Ongoing characterization of the genes that are regulated by the *Brn4* gene should provide insight into the molecular mechanisms that regulate inner ear development and function.

References

Abbas, A. K., Lichtman, A. H., Pober, J. S. 2000. *Cellular and Molecular Immunology*. Saunders, Philadelphia.

Abdelhak, S., Kalatzis, V., Heilig, R., Compain, S., Samson, D., Vincent, C., Weil, D., Cruaud, C., Sahly, I., Leibovici, M., Bitner-Glindzicz, M., Francis, M., Lacombe, D., Vigneron, J., Charachon, R., Boven, K., Bedbeder, P., Van Regemorter, N., Weissenbach, J., Petit, C. 1997. A human homologue of the Drosophila eyes absent gene underlies branchio-oto renal (BOR) syndrome and identifies a novel gene family. *Nature Genet.*, 15, 157-164.

Abel, E. D., Boers, M. E., Pazos-Moura, C., Moura, E., Kaulbach, H., Zakaria, M., Lowell, B., Radovick, S., Liberman, M. C., Wondisford, F. 1999. Divergent roles for thyroid hormone receptor beta isoforms in the endocrine axis and auditory system. *J. Clin. Invest.*, 104, 291-300.

Abel, E. L. 1991. Alarm substance emitted by rats in the forced-swim test is a low volatile pheromone. *Physiol. Behav.*, 50, 723-727.

Abel, E. L. 1992. Response to alarm substance in different rat strains. *Physiol. Behav.*, 51, 345-347.

Abel, E. L. 1994. The pituitary mediates production or release of an alarm chemosignal in rats. *Horm. Behav.*, 28, 139-145.

Acampora, D., Mazan, S., Avantaggiato, V., Barone, P., Tuorto, F., Lallemand, Y., Brulet, P., Simeone, A. 1996. Related articles: epilepsy and brain abnormalities in mice lacking the Otx1 gene. *Nature Genet.*, 14, 218-222.

Acampora, D., Merlo, G. R., Paleari, L., Zerega, B., Postiglione, M. P., Mantero, S., Bober, E., Barbieri, O., Simeone, A., Levi, G. 1999. Craniofacial, vestibular and bone defects in mice lacking the Distal-less-related gene Dlx5. *Devel.*, 126, 3795-809.

Accinni, L., Dixon, F. J. 1979. Degenerative vascular disease and myocardial infarction in mice with lupus-like syndrome. *Am. J. Pathol.*, 96, 477-492.

Achor, L. J., Starr, A. 1980. Auditory brain stem responses in the cat. II. Effects of lesions. *Electroenceph. Clin. Neurophysiol.*, 48, 174-190.

Adams, J. C. 1979. Ascending projections to the inferior colliculus. *J. Comp. Neurol.* 183, 519-538.

Adams, J. C. 1983. Multipolar cells in the ventral cochlear nucleus project to the dorsal cochlear nucleus and the inferior colliculus. *Neurosci. Lett.* 37, 205-208.

Adams, J. C. 1997. Projections from octopus cells of the posteroventral cochlear nucleus to the ventral nucleus of the lateral lemniscus in cat and human. *Aud. Neurosci.* 3, 335-350.

Adams, J. D., Mukherjee, S. K., Klaidman, L. K., Chang, M. L., Yasharel, R. 1996. Apoptosis and oxidative stress in the aging brain. *Ann. N.Y. Acad. Sci.*, 786, 135-151.

Adato, A., Kalinski, H., Weil, D., Chaib, H., Korostishevsky, M., Bonne-Tamir, B. 1999. Possible interaction between USH1B and USH3 gene products as implied by apparent digenic deafness inheritance. *Am. J. Hum. Genet.*, 65, 261-265.

Adato, A., Weil, D., Kalinski, H., Pel-Or, Y., Ayadi, H., Petit, C., Korostishevsky, M., Bonne-Tamir, B. 1997. Mutation profile of all 49 exons of the human myosin VIIA gene, and haplotype analysis, in Usher 1B families from diverse origins. *Am. J. Hum. Genet.*, 61, 813- 821.

Adler, R., Landa, K. B., Manthorpe, M., Varon, S. 1979. Cholinergic neuronotrophic factors: Intraocular distribution of trophic activity for ciliary neurons. *Science*, 204, 1434-1436.

Aebischer, P., Salessiotis, A. N., Winn, S. R. 1989. Basic fibroblast growth factor released from synthetic guidance channels facilitates peripheral nerve regeneration across long nerve gaps. *J. Neurosci. Res.*, 23, 282-289.

Aizenman, Y., de Vellis, J. 1988. Brain neurons develop in a serum and glial free environment: effects of transferrin, insulin, CW. Basic fibroblast growth factor prevents death of lesioned cholinergic neurons *in-vivo*. *Nature*, 332, 360-361.

Airaksinen, L., Virkkala, J., Aarnisalo, A., Meyer, M., Ylikoski, J., Airaksinen, M. S. 2000. Lack of calbindin-D28k does not affect hearing level or survival of hair cells in acoustic trauma. *J. Oto-Rhino-Laryngol.,* 62, 9-12.

Albone, E. S. 1984. *Mammalian Semiochemistry: The Investigation of Chemical Signals Between Mammals.* John Wiley & Sons, New York.

Alford, B. R., Ruben, R. J. 1963. Physiological, behavioral and anatomical correlates of the development of hearing in the mouse. *Ann. Otol. Rhinol. Laryngol.,* 72, 237-247.

Allen, J. B., Fahey, P. F. 1993. A second cochlear-frequency map that correlates distortion product and neural tuning measurements. *J. Acoust. Soc. Am.,* 94, 809-816.

Allen, N. R. 1973. Hearing acuity in patients with muscular dystrophy. *Devel. Med. Child. Neurol.,* 15, 500-506.

Altman, F. P. 1974. Studies on the reduction of tetrazolium salts. 3. The products of chemical and enzymic reduction. *Histochemistry,* 38, 155-171.

Altman, F. P. 1976. Tetrazolium salts: a consumer's guide. *Histochem. J.,* 8, 471-485.

Altschuler, R. A., Parakkal, M. H., Rubio, J. A., Hoffman, D. W., Fex, J. 1984. Enkephalin-like immunoreactivity in the guinea pig organ of Corti: ultrastructural and lesion studies. *Hear. Res.,* 16, 17-31.

Alvarez-Otero, R., Anadón, R. 1992. Golgi cells of the cerebellum of the dogfish, Scyliorhinus canicula (elasmobranchs): a GOLGI and ultrastructural study. *J. Hirnforsch.,* 33, 321-327.

Alvarez-Bolado, G., Rosenfeld, M. G., Swanson, L. W. 1995. Model of forebrain regionalization based on spatiotemporal patterns of POU-III homeobox gene expression, birthdates, and morphological features. *J. Comp. Neurol.,* 355, 237-295.

Anday, E. K., Cohen, M. E., Hoffman, H. S. 1991. Comparison of reflex modification procedures and auditory brainstem response in high-risk neonates. *Devel. Med. Child Neurol.,* 33, 130-137.

Anderson, J. W. 1954. The production of ultrasonic sounds by laboraory rats and other mammals. *Science,* 119, 808-809.

Anderson, S. D. 1980. Some ECMR properties in relation to other signals from the auditory periphery. *Hear. Res.,* 2, 273-296.

Anderson, S. D., Kemp, D. T. 1979. The evoked cochlear mechanical response in laboratory primates. *Arch. Otorhinolaryngol.,* 224, 47-54.

Andonopoulos, A. P., Naxakis, S., Goumas, P., Lygatsikas, C. 1995. Sensorineural hearing disorders in systemic lupus erythematosus. A controlled study. *Clin. Exp. Rheum.,* 13, 137-141.

Andressen, C., Blümcke, I., Celio, M. R. 1993. Calcium-binding proteins: selective markers of nerve cells. *Cell Tissue Res.,* 271, 181-208.

Ang, S. L., Jin, O., Rhinn, M., Daigle, N., Stevenson, L., Rossant, J. 1996. A targeted mouse Otx2 mutation leads to severe defects in gastrulation and formation of axial mesoderm and to deletion of rostral brain. *Devel.,* 122, 243-252.

Angelborg, C., Hultcrantz, E., Agerup, B. 1977. The cochlear blood flow. *Acta Otolaryngol.,* 83, 92-97.

Anguita, J., Persing, D. H., Rincon, M., Barthold, S. W., Fikrig, E. 1996. Effect of anti-interleukin 12 treatment on murine lyme borreliosis. *J. Clin. Invest.,* 97, 1028-1034.

Angulo, J. A., McEwen, B. S. 1994. Molecular aspects of neuropeptide regulation and function in the corpus striatum and nucleus accumbens. *Brain Res. Rev.,* 19, 1-28.

Anniko, M. 1980. Embryogenesis of the inner ear. III. Formation of the tectorial membrane of the CBA/CBA mouse *in vivo* and *in vitro. Anat. Embryol.,* 160, 301-313.

Anniko, M. 1983. Cytodifferentiation of cochlear hair cells. *Am. J. Otolaryngol.,* 4, 375-388.

Anniko, M., Bagger-Sjöbäck, D. 1987. Freeze fracture and numerical analyses of the spiral ganglion cells. *Arch. Otorhinolaryngol.,* 243, 407-410.

Anniko, M., Rosenkvist, U. 1982. Tectorial and basal membranes in experimental hypothyroidism. *Arch. Otolaryngol.,* 108, 218-220.

Anniko, M., Thornell, L.-E., Virtanen, I., Ramaekers, F. C. S. 1990. Freeze fracture and immunomorphological analysis of the spiral ganglion cells. *J. Electron Microsc. Tech.,* 15, 155-164.

Anniko, M., Wroblewski, R. 1981. Elemental composition of the developing inner ear. *Ann. Otol.,* 90, 25-32.

Ansar Ahmed, S., Hissong, B. D., Verthelyi, D., Donner, K., Becker, K., Karpuzoglu-Sahin, E. 1999. Gender and risk of autoimmune diseases: possible role of estrogenic compounds. *Environment. Health Perspect.,* 107, 681-686.

Anson, B. J., Hanson, J. R., Richany, S. F. 1960. Early embryology of the auditry ossicles and associated structures in relation to certain anomalies observed clinically. *Ann. Otol., Rhinol. Laryngol.,* 69, 427-447.

Antignac, C., Heidet, L. 1996. Mutations in Alport syndrome associated with diffuse esophageal leiomyomatosis. *Contrib. Nephrol.,* 117, 172-182.

Antignac, C., Knebelmann, B., Drouot, L., Gros, F., Deschenes, G., Hors-Cayla, M. C., Zhou, J., Tryggvason, K., Grunfeld, J. P., Broyer, M. 1994. Deletions in the COL4A5 collagen gene in X-linked Alport syndrome. Characterization of the pathological transcripts in nonrenal cells and correlation with disease expression. *J. Clin. Invest.,* 93, 1195-1207.

Antignac, C., Zhou, J., Sanak, M., Cochat, P., Roussel, B., Deschenes, G., Gros, F., Knebelmann, B., Hors-Cayla, M. C., Tryggvason, K. 1992. Alport syndrome and diffuse leiomyomatosis: deletions in the 5' end of the COL4A5 collagen gene. *Kidney Int.,* 42, 1178-1183.

Antonelli, A., Bellotto, R., Bertazzoli, M., Busnelli, G., Castro, M., Felisati, G., Romagnoli, M. 1986. Auditory brain stem response test battery for multiple sclerosis patients: Evaluation of test findings and assessment of diagnostic criteria. *Audiology,* 25, 227-238.

Antonopoulos, J., Pappas, I. S., Parnavelas, J. G. 1997. Activation of the $GABA_A$ receptor inhibits the proliferative effects of bFGF in cortical progenitor cells. *Eur. J. Neurosci.,* 9, 291-298.

Arakawa, Y., Sendtner, M., Thoenen, H. 1990. Survival effect of ciliary neurotrophic factor (CNTF) on chick embryonic motoneurons in culture: comparison with other neurotrophic factors and cytokines. *J. Neurosci.,* 10, 3507-3515.

Ard, M. D., Morest, D. K. 1984. Cell death during development of the cochlear and vestibular ganglia of the chick. *Int. J. Neurosci.,* 2, 535-547.

Ard, M., Morest, D., Haugher, S. 1985. Trophic interactions between the cochleovestibular ganglion of the chick embryo and its synaptic targets in culture. *Neuroscience,* 16, 151-170.

Arnold, A. P., Breedlove, S. M. 1985. Organizational and activational effects of sex steroids on brain and behavior: a reanalysis. *Horm. Behav.,* 19, 469-498.

Arnold, W. J. 1987. Oto-immunology. Facts or fantasy? In Veldman, J. E. (Ed.), *Immunobiology, Histophysiology, Tumor Immunology in Otolaryngology.* Kugler Publications, Amsterdam, 39-45.

Artavanis-Tsakonas, S., Matsuno, K., Fortini, M. E. 1995. Notch signaling. *Science,* 268, 225-268.

Artavanis-Tsakonas, S., Rand, M. D., Lake, R. J. 1999. Notch signaling: cell fate control and signal integration in development. *Science,* 284, 770-776.

Assouline, J., Zhang, M., Abbas, P., Messing, A., Gantz, B. 1995. Hypomyelinated acoustic nerve in transgenic mice expressing SV40 T-antigen causes hearing deficits. *Assoc. Res. Otolaryngol. Abstr.*

Assouline, J., Zhou, R., Abbas, P., Messing, A., Gantz, B. 1994. A transgenic myelin deficient model to evaluate the role of peripheral myelin in the auditory system. *Assoc. Res. Otolaryngol. Abstr.*

Atkin, C. L., Hasstedt, S. J., Menlove, L., Cannon, L., Kirschner, N., Schwartz, C., Nguyen, K., Skolnick, M. 1988. Mapping of Alport syndrome to the long arm of the X chromosome. *Am. J. Hum. Genet.,* 42, 249-255.

Attanasio, G., Spongr, V. P., Henderson, D. 1994. Localization of F-actin and fodrin along the organ of Corti in the chinchilla. *Hear. Res.,* 81, 199-207.

Avila M. A., Varela-Nieto I., Romero G., Mato J. M., Giraldez F., Van De Water T. R., Represa J. 1993. Brain-derived neurotrophic factor and neurotrophin-3 support the survival and neuritogenesis response of developing cochleovestibular ganglion neurons. *Devel. Biol.,* 159, 266-275.

Avraham, K. B., Hasson, T., Steel, K. P., Kingsley, D. M., Russell, L. B., Mooseker, M. S., Copeland, N. G., Jenkins, N. A. 1995. The mouse Snell's waltzer deafness gene encodes an unconventional myosin required for structural integrity of inner ear hair cells. *Nature Genet.,* 11, 369-375.

Axon, P. R., Temple, R. H., Saeed, S. R., Ramsden, R. T. 1998. Cochlear ossification after meningitis. *Am. J. Otol.,* 19, 724-729.

Babior, B. M. 1999. The Production and Use of Reactive Oxidants by Phagocytes. In Gilbert, D. L., Colton, C. A. (Eds.), *Reactive Oxygen Species in Biological Systems: An Interdisciplinary Approach.* Kluwer Academic/Plenum Publishers, New York, 503-526.

Bahn, S., Jones, A., Wisden, W. 1997. Directing gene expression to cerebellar granule cells using gamma-aminobutyric acid type A receptor alpha6 subunit transgenes. *Proc. Natl. Acad. Sci. USA,* 94, 9417-9421.

Bailey, D. W. 1981. Recombinant inbred strains and bilineal congenic strains. In Foster, H. L., Small, J. D., Fox, J. G. (Eds.), *The Mouse in Biomedical Research,* Vol 1. Academic Press, New York, 223-239.

Baimbridge, K. G., Celio, M. R., Rogers, J. H. 1992. Calcium-binding proteins in the nervous system. *Trends Neurosci.,* 15, 303-308.

Baker, J. P., Titus, M. A. 1998. Myosins: matching functions with motors. *Curr. Opin. Cell Biol.,* 10, 80-86.

Bal, R., Oertel, D. 2000. Hyperpolarization-activated, mixed-cation current (Ih) in octopus cells of the mammalian cochlear nucleus. *J. Neurophysiol.*, in press.

Bancroft, J. D., Cook, H. C. 1984. *Manual of Histological Techniques.* Churchill Livingstone, Edinburgh, Scotland.

Bar-Peled, O., Korkotian, E., Segal, M., Groner, Y. 1996. Constitutive overexpression of Cu/Zn superoxide dismutase exacerbates kainic acid-induced apoptosis of transgenic-Cu/Zn superoxide dismutase neurons. *Proc. Natl. Acad. Sci. USA*, 93, 8530-8535.

Barbacid, M. 1993. Nerve growth factor: a tale of two receptors. *Oncogene*, 8, 2033-2042.

Barbin, G., Manthorpe, M., Varon, S. 1984. Purification of the chick eye ciliary neurotrophic factor. *J. Neurochem.*, 43, 1468-1478.

Barde, Y. A., Edgar, D., Thoenen, H. 1982. Purification of a new neurotrophic factor from mammalian brain. *EMBO J.*, 1, 549-553.

Barfield, R. J., Geyer, L. A. 1975. The ultrasonic postejaculatory vocalization and the postejaculatory refractory period of the male rat. *J. Comp. Physiol. Psychol.*, 88, 723-724.

Barfield, R. J., Geyer, L. A. 1972. Sexual behavior: ultrasonic postejaculatory song of the male rat. *Science*, 176, 1349-1350.

Barker, D. F., Hostikka, S. L., Zhou, J., Chow, L. T., Oliphant, A. R., Gerken, S. C., Gregory, M. C., Skolnick, M. H., Atkin, C. L., Tryggvason, K. 1990. Identification of mutations in the COL4A5 collagen gene in Alport syndrome. *Science*, 248, 1224-1227.

Barker, J. L., Nicoll, R. A. 1972. Gamma-aminobutyric acid: role in primary afferent depolarization. *Science*, 176, 1043-1045.

Barros, A. C., Erway, L. C., Krezel, W., Curran, T., Kastner, P., Chambon, P., Forrest, D. 1998. Absence of thyroid hormone receptor beta-retinoid X receptor interactions in auditory function and in the pituitary-thyroid axis. *NeuroRep.*, 14, 2933-2937.

Barrow, J. R., Capecchi, M. R. 1999. Compensatory defects associated with mutations in Hoxa1 restore normal palatogenesis to Hoxa2 mutants. *Devel.*, 126, 5011-5026.

Barsz, K., Walton, J. P., Ison, J. R., Snell, K. B. 2000. Changes in gap detection in the aging mouse: behavioral measures and their correlates in the inferior colliculus. *Assoc. Res. Otolaryng. Abstr.*, 23.

Barten, D. M., Ruddle, N. H. 1994. Vascular cell adhesion molecule-1 modulation by tumor necrosis factor in experimental allergic encephalomyelitis. *J. Neuroimmunol.*, 51, 123-33.

Barthold, S. W. 1999. Specificity of infection-induced immunity among Borrelia burgdorferi sensu lato species. *Infect. Immun.*, 67, 36-42.

Barthold, S. W., Sidman, C. L., Smith, A. L. 1992. Lyme borreliosis in genetically resistant and susceptible mice with severe combined immunodeficiency. *Am. J. Trop. Med. Hygiene*, 47, 605-613.

Baskin, D. G. 1987. Insulin in the brain. *Annu. Rev. Physiol.*, 49, 335-347.

Batini, C., Palestini, M., Thomasset, M., Vigot, R. 1993. Cytoplasmic calcium buffer, calbindin-D28k, is regulated by excitatory amino acids, *NeuroRep.*, 4, 927-930.

Battey, J., Jordan, E., Cox, D., Dove, W. 1999. An action plan for mouse genomics. *Nature Genet.*, 21, 73-75.

Baynash, A. G., Hosoda, K., Giaid, A., Richardson, J. A., Emoto, N., Hammer, R. E., Yanagisawa, M. 1994. Interaction of endothelin-3 with endothelin-B receptor is essential for development of epidermal melanocytes and enteric neurons. *Cell*, 79, 1277-1285.

Beamer, W. G., Eicher, E. M., Maltais, L. J., Southard, J. L. 1981. Inherited primary hypothyroidism in mice. *Science*, 212, 61-63.

Bean, N. J. 1982. Olfactory and vomeronasal mediation of ultrasonic vocalizations in male mice. *Physiol. Behav.*, 28, 31-37.

Bean, N. J., Nunez, A. A., Wysocki, C. J. 1986a. 70-kHz vocalizations by male mice do not inhibit aggression in lactating mice. *Behav. Neural Biol.*, 46, 46-53.

Bean, N. J., Nunez, A. A., Conner, R. 1981. Effects of medial preoptic lesions on male mouse ultrasonic vocalizations and copulatory behavior. *Brain Res. Bull.*, 6, 109-112.

Bean, N. J., Nyby, J., Kerchner, M., Dahinden, Z. 1986b. Hormonal regulation of chemosignal-stimulated precopulatory behaviors in male housemice (*Mus musculus*). *Horm. Behav.*, 20, 390-404.

Beauchamp, G. K., Doty, R. L., Moulton, D. G., Mugford, R. A. 1976. The pheromonal concept in mammalian communication: a critique. In R. L. Doty (Ed.), *Mammalian Olfaction, Reproductive Processes, and Behavior.* Academic Press, New York, 144-157.

Beaulieu, C., Kisvarday, Z., Somogyi, P., Cynader, M., Cowey, A. 1992. Quantitative distribution of GABA-immunopositive and -immunonegative neurons and synapses in the monkey striate cortex (Area 17). *Cereb. Cort.,* 2, 295-309.

Bedell, M. A., Jenkins, N. A., Copeland, N. G. 1996. Good genes in bad neighbourhoods [news; comment]. *Nature Genet.,* 12, 229-232.

Behar, T. N., Schaffner, A. E., Scott, C. A., O'Connell, C., Barker, J. L. 1998. Differential response of cortical plate and ventricular zone cells to GABA as a migration stimulus. *J. Neurosci.,* 18, 6378-6387.

Behar, T., Schaffner, A., Laing, P., Hudson, L., Komoly, S., Barker, J. 1993. Many spinal cord cells transiently express low molecular weight forms of glutamic acid decarboxylase during embryonic development. *Devel. Brain Res.,* 72, 203-218.

Beilharz, R. G., Beilharz, V. C. 1975. Observations on fighting behaviour of male mice (*Mus musculus* L.). *Z. Tierpsychol.,* 39, 126-140.

Belendiuk, K., Butler, R. A. 1975. Monaural localization of low-pass noise bands in the horizontal plane. *J. Acoust. Soc. Am.,* 58, 701-705.

Belknap, J. D. 1992. Empirical estimates of Bonferroni corrections for use in chromosome mapping studies with the BXD recombinant inbred strains. *Behav. Genet.,* 22, 677-684.

Belknap, J. K., Mitchell, S. R., O'Toole, L., A, Helms, M. L., Crabbe, J. C. 1996. Type I and type II error rates for quantitative trait loci (QTL) mapping studies using recombination inbred mouse strains. *Behav. Genet.,* 26, 149-160.

Benson, T. E, Brown, M. C. 1990. Synapses formed by olivocochlear axon branches in the mouse cochlear nucleus. *J. Comp. Neurol.,* 295, 52-70.

Benson, T. E., Berglund, A. M., Brown, M. C. 1996. Synaptic input to cochlear nucleus dendrites that receive medial olivocochlear synapses. *J. Comp. Neurol.,* 365, 27-41.

Berden, J. H., Hang, L., McConahey, P. J., Dixon, F. J. 1983. Analysis of vascular lesions in murine SLE. I. Association with serologic abnormalities. *J. Immunol.,* 130, 1699-1705.

Berglund, A. M., Brown, M. C. 1994. Central trajectories of type II spiral ganglion cells from various cochlear regions in mice. *Hear. Res.,* 75, 121-130.

Berglund, A. M., Benson, T. E., Brown, M. C. 1996. Synapses from labeled type II axons in the mouse cochlear nucleus. *Hear. Res.,* 94, 31-46.

Berglund, A. M., Ryugo, D. K. 1987. Hair cell innervation by spiral ganglion neurons in the mouse. *J. Comp. Neurol.,* 255, 560-570.

Berkemeier, L. R., Winslow, J. W., Kaplan, D. R. 1991. Neurotrophin-5: a novel neurotrophic factor that activates trk and trk B. *Neuron,* 991, 857-866.

Berlin, C. I. 1963. Hearing in mice via GSR audiometry. *J. Speech Hear. Res.,* 6, 359-368.

Berlin, C. I., Gill, A., Leffler, M. 1968. Hearing in mice by GSR audiometry. I. Magnitude of unconditioned GSR as an index of frequency sensitivity. *J. Speech and Hear. Res.,* 11, 159-168.

Bermingham, N. A., Hassan, B. A., Price, S. D., Vollrath, M. A., Ben-Arie, N., Eatock, R. A., Bellen, H. J., Lysakowski, A., Zoghbi, H. Y. 1999. Math1: an essential gene for the generation of inner ear hair cells. *Science,* 284, 1837-1841.

Bernd, P., Zhang, D., Yao, L., Rozenberg, I. 1994. The potential role of nerve growth factor, brain-derived neurotrophic factor and neurotrophin-3 in avian cochlear and vestibular ganglia development. *Int. J. Devel. Neurosci.,* 12, 709-723.

Bernstein, J. 1987. The glomerular basement membrane abnormality in Alport's syndrome. *Am. J. Kidney Dis.,* 10, 222-229.

Bernstein, J. M. 1988. Middle ear mucosa: histologic, histochemical, immunochemical, and immunological aspects. In A. F. Jahn and J.Santos-Sacchi (Eds.), *Physiology of the Ear.* New York, Raven Press, 59-80.

Berrebi, A. S., Morgan, J. I., Mugnaini, E. 1990. The Purkinje cell class may extend beyond the cerebellum. *J. Neurocytol.,* 19, 643-654.

Berrebi, A. S., Mugnaini, E. 1991. Distribution and targets of the cartwheel cell axon in the dorsal cochlear nucleus of the guinea pig. *Anat. Embryol.,* 183, 427-454.

Berry, C. J., Vogler C., Galvin N., J., Birkenmeier E. H. Sly W. S. 1994. Pathology of the ear in murine mucopolysaccharidosis type VII. Morphological correlates of hearing loss. *Lab. Invest.,* 71, 438-445.

Bertilson, H. S., Mead, J. D., Morgret, M. K., Dengerink, H. A. 1977. Measurement of mouse squeals for 23 hours as evidence of long-term effects of alcohol on aggression in pairs of mice. *Psychol. Rep.,* 41, 247-250.

Bessant, D. A., Payne, A. M., Plant, C., Bird, A. C., Bhattacharya, S. S. 1998. Further refinement of the Usher 2A locus at 1q41. *J. Med. Genet.,* 35, 773-774.

Bhattacharya, G., Sumegi, J., Usami, S.-I., Kimberling, W., Cosgrove, D. 2000. Structural characterization and expression of Usherin, the protein encoded by the gene defective in Usher syndrome type IIa. *Assoc. Res. Otolaryngol. Abstr.* 23, 119-120.

Bianchi, L. M. 1999. Eph molecules in the embryonic inner ear. *Soc. Neurosci. Abstr.,* 25.

Bianchi, L. M. 2000. Role of ephrin-B and EphB molecules in statoacoustic nerve fiber development. *Assoc. Res. Otolaryngol. Abstr.* 23.

Bianchi, L. M., Cohan, C. S. 1991. Developmental regulation of a neurite-promoting factor influencing statoacoustic neurons. *Devel. Brain Res.,* 64, 167-174.

Bianchi L. M., Cohan C. S. 1993. The effects of neurotrophins and CNTF on developing statoacoustic neurons: comparison with an otocyst-derived factor. *Devel. Biol.,* 159, 353-365.

Bianchi L. M., Conover, J. C., Fritzsch, B., DeChiara, T., Lindsay, R. M. Yancopoulos, G. D. 1996. Degeneration of vestibular neurons in late embryogenesis of both heterozygous and homozygous BDNF null mutant mice. *Devel.,* 122, 1965-1973.

Bianchi, L. M., Dolnick, R., Medd, A. M., Cohan, C. S. 1998. Developmental changes in growth factors released by the embryonic inner ear. *Exp. Neurol.,* 150, 98-106.

Bianchi, L. M., Gale, N. W. 1998. Distribution of Eph-related molecules in the developing and mature cochlea. *Hear. Res.,* 117, 161-172.

Bianchi, L. M., Liu, H. 1999. Comparison of Ephrin-A ligand and EphA receptor distribution in the developing inner ear. *Anat. Rec.,* 254, 127-134.

Bichler., E., Spoendlin, H., Rauchegge, H. 1983. Degeneration of cochlear neurons after amikacin intoxication in the rat. *Arch. Otolaryng.,* 237, 201-207.

Bikhazi, P., Ryan, A. F. 1995. Expression of immunoregulatory cytokines during acute and chronic middle ear immune response. *Laryngoscope,* 105, 629-34.

Billings, P. B., Shin, S. O., Harris, J. P. 1998. Assessing the role of anti-hsp70 in cochlear impairment. *Hear. Res.,* 126, 210-213.

Birch, L. M., Warfield, D., Ruben, R. J., Mikaelian, D. O. 1968. Behavioral measurements of pure tone thresholds in normal CBA-J mice. J. Aud. Res. 8, 459-468.

Birkenmeier, E. H., Barker, J. E., Vogler, C. A., Kyle, J. W., Sly, W. S., Gwynn, B., Levy, B., Pegors, C. 1991. Increased life span and correction of metabolic defects in murine mucopolysaccharidosis Type VII after syngeneic bone marrow transplantation. *Blood,* 11, 3081-3092.

Birkenmeier, E. H., Davisson, M. T., Beamer, W. G., Ganschow, R. E., Vogler, C. A., Gwynn, B., Lyford, K. A., Maltais, L. M., Wawrzyniak, C. J. 1989. Murine Mucopolysaccharidosis Type VII: characterization of a mouse with beta-glucuronidase deficiency. *J. Clin. Invest.,* 83, 1258-1266.

Bitner-Glindzicz, M., de Kok, Y., Summers, D., Huber, I., Cremers, F. P., Ropers, H. H., Reardon, W. et al. 1994. Close linkage of a gene for X linked deafness to three microsatellite repeats at Xq21 in radiologically normal and abnormal families. *J. Med. Genet.,* 31, 916-921.

Bitner-Glindzicz, M., Turnpenny, P., Hoglund, P., Kaariainen, H., Sankila, E. M., van der Maarel, S. M., de Kok, Y. J. et al. 1995. Further mutations in Brain 4 (POU3F4) clarify the phenotype in the X-linked deafness, DFN3. *Hum. Molec. Genet.,* 4, 1467-1469.

Blackburn, C. C., Sachs, M. B. 1990. The representations of the steady-state vowel/e/in the discharge patterns of cat anteroventral cochlear nucleus neurons. *J. Neurophysiol.,* 63, 1191-1212.

Blackburn, C. C., Sachs, M. B. 1989. Classification of unit types in the anteroventral cochlear nucleus: PST histograms and regularity analysis. *J. Neurophysiol.,* 62, 1303-1329.

Blanchard, R. J., Hebert, M. A., Ferrari, P., Palanza, P., Figueira, R., Blanchard, D. C., Parmigiani, S. 1998. Defensive behaviors in wild and laboratory (Swiss) mice: the mouse defense test battery. *Physiol. Behav,* 65, 201-209.

Blizard, D. A. 1992. Recombinant-inbred strains: general methodological considerations relevant to the study of complex characters. *Behav. Genet.,* 22, 621-633.

Bloch, D. B., Gutierrez, J. A., Guerriero, V., Jr., Rauch, S. D., Bloch, K. J. 1999. Recognition of a dominant epitope in bovine heat-shock protein 70 in inner ear disease. *Laryngoscope,* 109, 621-625.

Blumberg, B., Evans, R. M. 1998. Orphan nuclear receptors--new ligands and new possibilities. Genes Devel. 12, 3149-3155.

Blumberg, M. S. 1992. Rodent ultrasonic short calls: locomotion, biomechanics, and communication. *J. Comp. Psychol.,* 106, 360-365.

Bobbin, R. P., Fallon, M., LeBlanc, C. Baber, A. 1995. Evidence that glutathione is the unidentified amine (Unk 2.5) released by high potassium into cochlear fluids. *Hear. Res.,* 87, 49-54.

Bohne, B. A. 1976. Safe level for noise exposure. *Ann. Otol. Rhinol. Laryngol.,* 85, 711-724.

Bohne, B. A., Bozzay, D. G., Harding, G. W. 1986. Interaural correlations in normal and traumatized cochleas: length and sensory cell loss. *J. Acoust. Soc. Am.,* 80, 1729-1736.

Bohne, B. A., Carr, C. D. 1985. Morphometric analysis of hair cells in the chinchilla cochlea. *J. Acoust. Soc. Am.,* 77, 153-158.

Bohne, B. A., Clark, W. W. 1982. Growth of hearing loss and cochlear lesion with increasing duration of noise exposure. In Hamernik, R. P., Henderson, D., Salvi, R. (Eds.), New *Perspectives on Noise-Induced Hearing Loss.* Raven Press, New York, 283-302.

Bohne, B. A., Harding, G. W. 1997. Processing and analyzing the mouse temporal bone to identify gross, cellular and subcellular pathology. *Hear. Res.,* 109, 34-45.

Bohne, B. A., Harding, G. W., Nordmann, A. S., Tseng, C. J., Liang, G. E., Bahadori, R. S. 1999. Survival-fixation of the cochlea: A technique for following time-dependent degeneration and repair in noise-exposed chinchillas. *Hear. Res.,* 134, 163-178.

Bonne-Tamir, B., Korostishevsky, M., Kalinsky, H., Seroussi, E., Beker, R., Weiss, S., Godel, V. 1994. Genetic mapping of the gene for Usher syndrome: linkage analysis in a large Samaritan kindred. *Genomics,* 20, 36-42.

Bonneman, C. G., McNally, E. M., Kunkel, L. M. 1996. Beyond dystrophin: current progress in muscular dystrophies. *Curr. Opin. Pediatr.,* 8, 569-582.

Bonner, R., Nossal, R. 1981. Model for laser Doppler measurements of blood flow in tissue. *Appl. Optics,* 20, 2097-2107.

Borg, E., Canlon, B., Engstrom, B. 1995. Noise induced hearing loss: literature review and experiments in rabbits. *Scand. Audiol.,* 24, Suppl. 40, 9-59.

Boughman, J. A., Vernon, M., Shaver, K. A. 1983. Usher syndrome: definition and estimate of prevalence from two high-risk populations. *J. Chronic. Dis.,* 36, 595-603.

Bourgeois, P., Bolcato-Bellemin, A. L., Danse, J. M., Bloch-Zupan, A., Yoshiba, K., Stoetzel, C., Perrin-Schmitt, F. 1998. The variable expressivity and incomplete penetrance of the twist-null heterozygous mouse phenotype resemble those of human Saethre-Chotzen syndrome. *Hum. Molec. Genet.,* 7, 945-957.

Bowditch, H. P., Warren, J. W. 1890. The knee-jerk and its physiological modifications. *J. Physiol.,* 11, 25-64.

Boye, E., Flinter, F. A., Bobrow, M., Harris, A. 1993. An 8 bp deletion in exon 51 of the COL4A5 gene of an Alport syndrome patient. *Hum. Molec. Genet.,* 2, 595-596.

Boye, E., Flinter, F., Zhou, J., Tryggvason, K., Bobrow, M., Harris, A. 1995. Detection of 12 novel mutations in the collagenous domain of the COL4A5 gene in Alport syndrome patients. *Hum. Mutat.,* 5, 197-204.

Boye, E., Mollet, G., Forestier, L., Cohen-Solal, L., Heidet, L., Cochat, P., Grunfeld, J. P., Palcoux, J. B., Gubler, M. C., Antignac, C. 1998. Determination of the genomic structure of the COL4A4 gene and of novel mutations causing autosomal recessive Alport syndrome. *Am. J. Hum. Genet.,* 63, 1329-1340.

Boye, E., Vetrie, D., Flinter, F., Buckle, B., Pihlajaniemi, T., Hamalainen, E. R., Myers, J. C., Bobrow, M., Harris, A. 1991. Major rearrangements in the alpha 5(IV) collagen gene in three patients with Alport syndrome. *Genomics,* 11, 1125-1132.

Bradley, D. J., Towle, H. C., Young, W. S. 1994. Alpha and beta thyroid hormone receptor (TR) gene expression during auditory neurogenesis: evidence for TR isoform-specific transcriptional regulation *in vivo. Proc. Natl. Acad. Sci. USA,* 91, 439-443.

Brady, K. P., Rowe, L. B., Her, H., Stevens, T. J., Eppig, J., Sussman, D. J., Sikela, J., Beier, D. R. 1997. Genetic mapping of 262 loci derived from expressed sequences in a murine interspecific cross using single-strand conformational polymorphism analysis. *Genome Res.,* 7, 1085-1093.

Braff, D. L., Grillon, C., Geyer, M. A. 1992. Gating and habituation of the startle reflex in schizophrenic patients. *Arch. Genet. Psychol.,* 49, 206-215.

Braff, D. L., Stone, C., Callaway, E., Geyer, M., Glick I., Bali, L. 1978. Prestimulus effects on human startle reflex in normals and schizophrenics. *Psychophysiology,* 15, 339-343.

Brain, P. F., Benton, D., Cole, C., Prowse, B. 1980. A device for recording submissive vocalizations of laboratory mice. *Physiol. Behav.,* 24, 1003-1006.

Brambilla, R., Klein, R. 1995. Telling axons where to grow: a role for Eph receptor tyrosine kinases in guidance. *Molec. Cell. Neurosci.,* 6, 487-495.

Braun, K., Scheich, H., Schachner, M., Heizmann, C. W. 1985. Distribution of parvalbumin, cytochrome oxidase activity and ^{14}C-2 deoxyglucose uptake in the brain of zebra finch. *Cell Tissue Res.,* 240, 117-127.

Brawer, J. R., Morest, D. K. 1975. Relations between auditory nerve endings and cell types in the cat's anteroventral cochlear nucleus seen with the Golgi method and Nomarski optics. *J. Comp. Neurol.,* 160, 491-506.

Brawer, J. R., Morest, D. K., Kane, E. C. 1974. The neuronal architecture of the cochlear nucleus of the cat. *J. Comp. Neurol.,* 155, 251-300.

Bray, S. 1998. Notch signalling in Drosophila: three ways to use a pathway. *Semin. Cell. Devel. Biol.,* 9, 591-597.

Brechtelsbauer, P. B., Nuttall, A. L., Miller, J. M. 1994. Basal nitric oxide production in regulation of cochlear blood flow. *Hear. Res.,* 77, 38-42.

Bredberg, G. 1968. Cellular pattern and nerve supply of the human organ of Corti. *Acta Otolarygol. Suppl.,* 236, 1-135.

Bredberg, G., Hunter-Duvar, I. M. 1975. Behavioral tests of hearing and inner ear damage. In Keidel, W. D., Neff, W. D. (Eds.), *Handbook of Sensory Physiology,* Springer Verlag, Berlin, 261-306.

Bredenkamp, J. K., Williams J. C., Smith M. E., Crumley R. L., Dudley J. P. Crockett D. M. 1992. Otolaryngologic manifestations of the mucopolysaccharidoses. *Ann. Otol. Rhinol. Laryngol.,* 101, 472-478.

Breedlove, S. M. 1992. Sexual differentiation of the brain and behavior. In Becker, J. B., Breedlove, S. M., Crews, D. (Eds.), *Behavioral Endocrinology.* The MIT Press, Cambridge, MA, 39-68.

Bretlau, P., Balle, V., Causse, J. B., Hørslev-Petersen, K., Sørensen, C. H., Sølvsteen, M. 1987. Is otosclerosis an autoimmune disease? In Veldman, J. E. (Ed.), *Immunobiology, Histophysiology, Tumor Immunology in Otolaryngology.* Kugler Publications, Amsterdam, 201-206.

Briles, D. E., Tart, R. C., Swiatlo, E., Dillard, J. P., Smith, P., Benton, K. A., Ralph, B. A., Brooks-Walter, A., Crain, M. J., Hollingshead, S. K., McDaniel, L. S. 1998. Pneumococcal diversity: considerations for new vaccine strategies with emphasis on pneumococcal surface protein A (PspA). *Clin. Microbiol. Rev.,* 11, 645-657.

Briner, W., Willott, J. F. 1989. Ultrastructural features of neurons in the C57BL/6J mouse anteroventral cochlear nucleus: young mice versus old mice with chronic presbycusis. *Neurobiol. Aging,* 10, 295-303.

Britt, R., Starr, A. 1976. Synaptic events and discharge patterns of cochlear nucleus cells. II. Frequency-modulated tones. *J. Neurophysiol.,* 39, 179-194.

Brodie, H. A., Chole, R. A. 1987. The possible role of immunologic injury in the dysplastic bony lesion in LP/J mice. *Am. J. Otolaryngol.,* 8, 342-350.

Bronson, F. H. 1979. The reproductive ecology of the house mouse. *Quart. Rev. Biol.,* 54, 265-299.

Brookes, G. B. 1986. Circulating immune complexes in Meniere's disease. *Arch. Otolaryngol. Head Neck Surg.,* 112, 536-540.

Brouwer, O. F., Padberg, G. W., Ruys, C. J. M., Brand, R., deLaat, J. A. P. M. 1991. Hearing loss in fascioscapulohumeral muscular dystrophy. *Neurology,* 41, 1878-1881.

Brouwer, O. F., Padberg, G. W., Wijmenga, C., Frants, R. R. 1994. Facioscapulohumeral muscular dystrophy in early childhood. *Arch. Neurol.,* 51, 387-394.

Brown, A. M. 1976. Ultrasound and communication in rodents. *Comp. Biochem. Biophys.,* 53, 313-317.

Brown, A. M. 1987. Acoustic distortion from rodent ears: comparison of response from rats, guinea pigs and gerbils. *Hear. Res.,* 31, 25-38.

Brown, A. M., Gaskill, S. A. 1990. Can basilar membrane tuning be inferred from distortion measurement? In Dallos, P., Geisler, C. D., Mathews, J. W., Ruggero, M. A., Steele, C. R. (Eds.), *Mechanics and Biophysics of Hearing,* Springer Verlag, New York, 164-169.

Brown, A. M., Gaskill, S. A., Williams, D. M. 1992. Mechanical filtering of sound in the inner ear. *Proc. R. Soc. Lond.,* B250, 29-34.

Brown, A. M., Kemp, D. T. 1984. Suppressibility of the $2f_1-f_2$ stimulated acoustic emissions in gerbil and man. *Hear. Res.,* 13, 39-46.

Brown, A. M., McDowell, B., Forge, A. 1989. Acoustic distortion products can be used to monitor the effects of chronic gentamicin treatment. *Hear. Res.,* 19, 191-198.

Brown, J. J., Brummett, R. E., Fox, K. E., Bendrick, T. W. 1980. Combined effects of noise and kanamycin: cochlear pathology and pharmacology. *Arch. Otolaryngol.,* 106, 744-750.

Brown, J. N., Miller, J. M., Nuttall, A. L. 1995. Age-related changes in cochlear vascular conductance in mice. *Hear. Res.,* 86, 189-194.

Brown, J. N., Thorne, P. R., Nuttall, A. L. 1988. Effects of anesthesia on guinea pig blood pressure. *Abstracts of the Eleventh Midwinter Research Meeting of the Association for Research in Otolaryngology,* Abstract 154.

Brown, J. S., Kalish, H. I., Farber, I. E. 1951. Conditioned fear as revealed by magnitude of startle response to an auditory stimulus. *J. Exp. Psychol.,* 41, 317-328.

Brown, K. A., Sutcliffe, M. J., Steel, K. P., Brown, S. D. 1994. Sequencing of the olfactory marker protein gene in normal and shaker-1 mutant mice. *Mamm. Genome,* 5, 11-14.

Brown, K. A., Sutcliffe, M. J., Steel, K. P., Brown, S. D. 1992. Close linkage of the olfactory marker protein gene to the mouse deafness mutation shaker-1. *Genomics,* 13, 189-193.

Brown, M. C. 1993. Fiber pathways and branching patterns of biocytin-labeled olivocochlear neurons in the mouse brainstem. *J. Comp. Neurol.,* 337, 600-613.

Brown, M. C., Berglund, A. M., Kiang, N. Y. S., Ryugo, D. K. 1988a. Central trajectories of type II spiral ganglion neurons. *J. Comp. Neurol.,* 278, 581-590.

Brown, M. C., Ledwith J. V. 1990. Projections of thin (type-II) and thick (type-I) auditory-nerve fibers in the cochlear nucleus of the mouse. *Hear. Res.,* 49, 105-118.

Brown, M. C., Liberman, M. C., Benson, T. E., Ryugo, D. K. 1988b. Brainstem branches from olivocochlear axons in cats and rodents. *J. Comp. Neurol.,* 278, 591-603.

Brown, P. G., Ruben, R. J. 1969. The endocochlear potential in the Shaker-1 (sh-1/sh-1) mouse. *Acta Otolaryngol.,* 68, 14-20.

Brown, R. Z. 1953. Social behavior, reproduction, and population changes in the house mouse (*Mus musculus* L.). *Ecol. Mon.,* 23, 217-340.

Brown, S. D., Nolan, P. M. 1998. Mouse mutagenesis-systematic studies of mammalian gene function. *Hum. Molec. Genet.,* 7, 1627-1633.

Brown, S. D., Steel, K. P. 1994. Genetic deafness — progress with mouse models. *Hum. Molec. Genet.,* 3, 1453-1456.

Brownell, W. E. 1983. Observations on a motile response in isolated outer hair cells. In Webster, W. R., Aitkin, L. M. (Eds.), *Mechanisms of Hearing,* Monash University Press, 5-10.

Brownell, W. E., Bader, C. R., Bertrand, D., de Ribaupierre, Y. 1985. Evoked mechanical responses of isolated cochlear outer hair cells. *Science,* 227, 194-196.

Browner, R. H., Baruch, A. 1982. The cytoarchitecture of the dorsal cochlear nucleus of the 3-month- and 26-month-old C57BL/6 mouse: a Golgi impregnation study. *J. Comp. Neurol.,* 211, 115-138.

Bruce, L. L., Kingsley, J., Nichols, D. H., Fritzsch, B. 1997. The development of vestibulocochlear efferents and cochlear afferents in mice. *Int. J. Devel. Neurosci.,* 15, 671-692.

Bruckner, K., Pasquale, E. B., Klein, R. 1997. Tyrosine phosphorylation of transmembrane ligands for Eph receptors. *Science,* 275, 1640-1643.

Brummett, R. E., Fox, K. E., Kempton, J. B. 1992. Quantitative relationships of the interaction between sound and kanamycin. *Arch. Otolaryngol. Head Neck Surg.,* 118, 498-500.

Brundin, L., Flock, A., Khanna, S. M., Ulfendahl, M. 1991. Frequency-specific position shift in the guinea pig organ of Corti. *Neurosci. Lett.,* 128, 77-80.

Brüne, B., von Knethen, A., Sandau, K. B. 1999. Nitric oxide (NO): an effector of apoptosis. *Cell Death Diff.,* 6, 969-975.

Brunjes, P. C., Alberts, J. R. 1981. Early auditory and visual function in normal and hyperthyroid rats. *Behav. Neural Biol.,* 31, 393-412.

Buchman, V. L., Davies, A. M. 1993. Different neurotrophins are expressed and act in a developmental sequence to promote the survival of embryonic sensory neurons. *Devel.,* 118, 989-1001.

Buchwald, J. S., Huang, C.-M. 1975. Far-field acoustic response: origins in the cat. *Science,* 189, 382-384.

Buck, K. J., Metten, P., Belknap, J. K., Crabbe, J. C. 1997. Quantitative trait loci involved in genetic predisposition to acute alcohol withdrawal in mice. *J. Neurosci.,* 17, 3946-3955.

Buckland, G., Buckland, J., Jamieson, C., Ison, J. R. 1969. Inhibition of the startle response to acoustic stimulation produced by visual prestimulation. *J. Comp. Physiol. Psychol.,* 67, 493-496.

Bueker, E. D. 1948. Implantation of tumors in the hind limb field of the embryonic chick and the developmental response of the lumbosacral nervous system. *Anat. Rec.,* 102, 369-390.

Bujía, J., Alsalameh, S., Jerez, R., Sittinger, M., Wilmes, E., Burmester, G. 1994. Antibodies to the minor cartilage collagen type IX in otosclerosis. *Am. J. Otol.,* 15, 222-224.

Burian, M., Gestoettner, W. 1988. Projection of primary vestibular afferent fibres to the cochlear nucleus in the guinea pig. *Neurosci. Lett.,* 84, 13-17.

Burkard, R. 1984. Sound pressure level measurement and spectral analysis of brief acoustic transients. *Electroenceph. Clin. Neurophysiol.,* 57, 83-91.

Burkard, R. 1994. Gerbil brainstem auditory evoked responses (BAERs) to maximum length sequences. *J. Acoust. Soc. Am.,* 95, 2126-2135.

Burkard, R., Hecox, K. 1983. The effect of broadband noise on the human brainstem auditory evoked response. I. Rate and intensity effects. *J. Acoust. Soc. Am.,* 74, 1204-1213.

Burkard, R., Hecox, K. 1987. The effect of broadband noise on the human brainstem auditory evoked response. III. Anatomic locus. *J. Acoust. Soc. Am.,* 81, 1050-1063.

Burkard, R., McGee, J., Walsh, E. 1996a. The effects of stimulus rate on the feline BAER during development. I. Peak latencies. *J. Acoust. Soc. Am.,* 100, 978-990.

Burkard, R., McGee, J., Walsh, E. 1996b. The effects of stimulus rate on the feline BAER during development. II. Peak amplitudes. *J. Acoust. Soc. Am.,* 100, 991-1002.

Burkard, R., Shi, Y., Hecox, K. 1990a. A comparison of maximum length and Legendre sequences to derive BAERs at rapid rates of stimulation. *J. Acoust. Soc. Am.,* 87, 1656-1664.

Burkard, R., Shi, Y., Hecox, K. 1990b. The effects of masking noise on BAERs obtained by deconvolution. *J. Acoust. Soc. Am.,* 87, 1665-1672.

Burkard, R., Voigt, H. 1989a. Stimulus dependencies of the gerbil brainstem auditory evoked response (BAER). I. Effects of click level, rate and polarity. *J. Acoust. Soc. Am.,* 85, 2514-2525.

Burkard, R., Voigt, H. 1989b. Stimulus dependencies of the gerbil brainstem auditory evoked response (BAER). II. Effects of broadband noise level and high-pass masker cutoff frequency across polarity. *J. Acoust. Soc. Am.,* 85, 2526-2536.

Burkard, R. Voigt, H. 1990. Stimulus dependencies of the gerbil brainstem auditory evoked response. III. Additivity of click level and rate with noise level. *J. Acoust. Soc. Am.,* 88, 2222-2234.

Burkard, R., Voigt, H., Smith, R. 1993. A comparison of N1 of the whole nerve action potential and wave i of the brainstem auditory evoked response in Mongolian gerbil. *J. Acoust. Soc. Am.,* 93, 2069-2076.

Burnham, K., Bey, M. 1991. Effects of crude oil and ultraviolet radiation on immunity within mouse skin. *J. Toxicol. Envir. Health,* 34, 83-93.

Buss, E., Hall, 3rd, J. W., Grose, J. H., Hatch, D. R. 1998. Perceptual consequences of peripheral hearing loss: do edge effects exist for abrupt cochlear lesions? *Hear. Res.,* 125, 98-108.

Bussoli, T. J., Kelly, A., Tucher, J. B., Steel, K. P. 1998. New, atypical hair cells in the Bronx waltzer mouse mutant. *Molec. Biol. Hear. Deafness Abstr.,* 3, 135.

Butkowski, R. J., Wieslander, J., Kleppel, M., Michael, A. F., Fish, A. J. 1989. Basement membrane collagen in the kidney: regional localization of novel chains related to collagen IV. *Kidney Int.,* 35, 1195-1202.

Byatt, S., Nyby, J. 1986. Hormonal regulation of chemosignals of female mice that elicit ultrasonic vocalizations from males. *Horm. Behav.,* 20, 60-72.

Cable, J., Barkway, K., Steel, K. P. 1992. Characteristics of stria vascularis melanocytes of viable dominant spotting (W^v/W^v) mouse mutants. *Hear. Res.,* 64, 6-20.

Cai, Y., McGee, J., Walsh, E. J. 2000. Contributions of ion conductances to the onset responses of octopus cells in the ventral cochlear nucleus: simulation results. *J. Neurophysiol.,* 83, 301-314.

Caicedo, A., d'Aldin, C., Eybalin, M., Puel, J.-L. 1997. Temporary sensory deprivation changes calcium-binding proteins levels in the auditory brainstem. *J. Comp. Neurol.,* 378, 1-15.

Caicedo, A., d'Aldin, C., Puel, J.-L., Eybalin, M. 1996. Distribution of calcium-binding protein immunore-activities in the guinea pig auditory brainstem. *Anat. Embryol.,* 194, 465-487.

Caicedo, A., Herbert H. 1993. Topography of descending projections from the inferior colliculus to auditory brainstem nuclei in the rat. *J. Comp. Neurol.,* 328, 377-392.

Cajal, S. R. 1928. *Degeneration and Regeneration of the Nervous Sysytem,* translated by Raoul May. Oxford Press, London, 1928.

Cajal, S. R, 1909. Histologie du Système Nerveux de I'Homme et des Vertébrés. Consejo Superior de Investigaciones Cientificas, Instituto Ramón y Cajal, Madrid.

Cajal S. R. 1892. La rétine des vertébrés. *La Cellule,* 9, 121-246.

Calford, M. B., Rajan, R., Irvine, D. R. F. 1993. Rapid changes in the frequency tuning of neurons in cat auditory cortex resulting from pure-tone-induced temporary threshold shift. *Neuroscience, 55, 953-964.*

Campbell, J. P., Henson, M. M. 1988. Olivocochlear neurons in the brainstem of the mouse. *Hear. Res., 35,* 271-274.

Campeau, S., Davis, M. 1992. Fear-potentiation of the acoustic startle reflex in rats using noises of various spectral frequencies. *Anim. Learn. Behav., 20, 177-186.*

Campeau, S., Davis, M. 1995. Involvement of subcortical and cortical afferents to the lateral nucleus of the amygdala in fear conditioning measured with fear-potentiated startle in rats trained concurrently with auditory and visual conditioned stimuli. *J. Neurosci., 15, 2312-2327.*

Campos-Barros, A., Amma, L. L., Faris, J. S., Shailam, R., Kelley, M. W., Forrest, D. 2000. Type 2 iodothyronine deiodinase expression in the cochlea before the onset of hearing. *Proc. Natl. Acad. Sci. USA, 97,* 1287-1292.

Canlon, B. 1996. The effects of sound conditioning on the cochlea. In Salvi, R. J., Henderson, D. H., Colletti, V., Fiorino, F. (Eds.), *Auditory Plasticity and Regeneration.* Thieme Medical Publishers, New York, 118-127.

Canlon, B., Borg, E., Flock, Å. 1988. Protection against noise trauma by pre-exposure to a low level acoustic stimulus. *Hear. Res., 34, 197-200.*

Canlon, B., Dagli, S. 1996. Protection against temporary and permanent noise-induced hearing loss by sound conditioning. In Axelsson, A., Borchgrevink, H. M., Hamernik, R. P., Hellström, P.-A, Henderson, D. Salvi, R. J. (Eds.), *Scientific Basis of Noise-Induced Hearing Loss.* Thieme Medical Publishers, New York, 172-180.

Canlon, B., Schacht, J. 1981. The effect of noise on deoxyglucose uptake into inner ear tissues of the mouse. *Arch. Otorhinolaryngol., 230, 171-176.*

Canlon, B., Schacht, J. 1983. Acoustic stimulation alters deoxyglucose uptake in the mouse cochlea and inferior colliculus. *Hear. Res., 10, 217-226.*

Cant, N. B. 1981. The fine structure of two types of stellate cells in the anterior division of the anteroventral cochlear nucleus of the cat. *Neuroscience, 6, 2643-2655.*

Cant, N. B. 1982. Identification of cell types in the anteroventral cochlear nucleus that project to the inferior colliculus. *Neurosci. Lett., 32, 241-246.*

Cant, N. B., Casseday, J. H. 1986. Projections from the anteroventral cochlear nucleus to the lateral and medial superior olivary nuclei. *J. Comp. Neurol., 247, 457-476.*

Cant, N. B., Gaston, K. C. 1982. Pathways connecting the right and left cochlear nuclei. *J. Comp. Neurol.,* 212, 313-326.

Cant, N. B., Morest, D. K. 1979a. Organization of the neurons in the anterior division of the anteroventral cochlear nucleus of the cat. Light-microscopic observations. *Neuroscience, 4, 1909-1923.*

Cant, N. B., Morest, D. K. 1979b. The bushy cells in the anteroventral cochlear nucleus of the cat. A study with the electron microscope. *Neuroscience, 4, 1925-1945.*

Cao, M. Y., Deggouj, N., Gersdorff, M., Tomasi, J. P. 1996a. Guinea pig inner ear antigens: extraction and application to the study of human autoimmune inner ear disease. *Laryngoscope, 106, 207-212.*

Cao, M. Y., Dupriez, V. J., Rider, M. H., Deggouj, N., Gersdorff, M. C., Rousseau, G. G., Tomasi, J. P. 1996b. Myelin protein Po as a potential autoantigen in autoimmune inner ear disease. *FASEB J., 10, 1635-1640.*

Cardozo-Pelaez, F., Song, S., Parthasarathy, A., Epstein, C. J. 1998. oxidative damage to DNA and protein in brainstem of Tg Cu/Zn SOD mice. *Neurobiol. Aging, 19, 311-316.*

Carlier, E., Pujol, R. 1976. Early effects of efferent stimulation on the kitten cochlea. *Neurosci. Lett., 3, 21-27.*

Carlisle, L., Aberdeen, J., Forge, A., Burnstock, G. 1990a. Neural basis for regulation of cochlear blood flow, peptidergic and adrenergic innervation of the spiral modiolar artery of the guinea pig. *Hear. Res., 43,* 107-113.

Carlisle, L., Steel, K., Forge, A. 1990b. Endocochlear potential generation is associated with intercellular communication in the stria vascularis, structural analysis in the viable dominant spotting mouse mutant. *Cell Tissue Res., 262, 329-337.*

Carlson, S., Willott, J. F. 1998. Caudal pontine reticular formation of C57BL/6J mice: responses to startle stimuli, inhibition by tones, plasticity. *J. Neurophysiol., 79, 2603-2614.*

Carlson, S., Willott, J. F. 1996. The behavioral salience of sounds as indicated by prepulse inhibition of the startle response: relationship to hearing loss and central neural plasticity in C57BL/6J mice. *Hear. Res.,* 99, 168-175.

Carlsson, L. M., Jonsson, J., Edlund, T. Marklund, S. L. 1995. Mice lacking extracellular superoxide dismutase are more sensitive to hyperoxia. *Proc. Natl. Acad. Sci. USA,* 92, 6264-6268.

Caruso, R. C., Kaiser-Kupfer M. I., Meunzer J., Ludwig I. H., Zasloff M. A. Mercer P. A. 1986. Electrotretinographic findings in the mucopolysaccharidoses. *Ophthalmology,* 93, 1612-1616.

Caspary, D. M., Backoff, P. M., Finlayson, P. G., Palombi, P. S. 1994. Inhibitory inputs modulate discharge rate within frequency receptive fields of anteroventral cochlear nucleus neurons. *J. Neurophysiol.,* 72, 2124-2133.

Caspary, D. M., Holder, T. M., Hughes, L. F., Milbrandt, J. C. McKernan, R. M, Naritoku, D. K. 1999. Age-related changes in GABAa receptor subunit composition and function in rat auditory system. *Neuroscience,* 93, 307-312.

Caspary, D. M., Milbrandt, J. C, Helfert, R. H. 1995. Central auditory aging: GABA changes in the inferior colliculus. *Exp. Gerontol.,* 30, 349-360.

Caspary, D. M., Raza, A., Armour, B. A. L., Pippin, J., Arneric, S. P. 1990. Immunocytochemical and neurochemical evidence for age-related loss of GABA in the inferior colliculus: implications for neural presbycusis. *J. Neurosci.,* 10, 2363-2372.

Cavanagh, L. L., Barnetson, R. S., Basten, A., Halliday, G. M. 1997. Dendritic epidermal T-cell involvement in induction of CD8+ T cell-mediated immunity against an ultraviolet radiation-induced skin tumor. *Int. J. Cancer,* 70, 98-105.

Cavanagh, L. L., Sluyter, R., Henderson, K. G., Barnetson, R. S., Halliday, G. M. 1996. Epidermal Langerhans' cell induction of immunity against an ultraviolet-induced skin tumour. *Immunology,* 87, 475-480.

Caviness, V. S., Jr., Frost, D. O. 1980. Tangential organization of thalamic projections to the neocortex in the mouse. *J. Comp. Neurol.,* 194, 335-367.

Caviness, V. S., Jr., 1975. Architectonic map of neocortex of the normal mouse. *J. Comp. Neurol.,* 164, 247-264.

Celio, M. R. (Ed.), Pauls, T., Schwaller, B. (Co-Eds.). 1996. *Guidebook to the Calcium-Binding Proteins.* A Sambrook & Tooze Publication at Oxford University Press.

Celio, M. R. 1990. Calbindin D-28k and parvalbumin in the rat nervous system. *Neuroscience,* 35, 375-475.

Celio, M. R., Schärer, L., Morisson, J. H., Norman, A. W., Bloom, F. E. 1986. Calbindin immunoraectivity alternates with cytochrome c-oxidase-rich zones in some layers of the primate visual cortex. *Nature,* 323, 715-717.

Chaib, H., Kaplan, J., Gerber, S., Vincent, C., Ayadi, H., Slim, R., Munnich, A., Weissenbach, J., Petit, C. 1997. A newly identified locus for Usher syndrome type I, USH1E, maps to chromosome 21q21. *Hum. Molec. Genet.,* 6, 27-31.

Chaib, H., Place, C., Salem, N., Dode, C., Chardenoux, S., Weissenbach, J., El Zir, E., Loiselet, J., Petit, C. 1996. Mapping of DFNB12, a gene for a non-syndromal autosomal recessive deafness, to chromosome 10q21-22. *Hum. Molec. Genet.,* 5, 1061-1064.

Chan, T. M., Frampton, G., and Cameron, J. S. 1993. Identification of DNA-binding proteins on human umbilical vein endothelial cell plasma membrane. *Clin. Exp. Immunol.,* 91, 110-114.

Chan, T. M., Frampton, G., Staines, N. A., Hobby, P., Perry, G. J., Cameron, J. S. 1992. Different mechanisms by which anti-DNA MoAbs bind to human endothelial cells and glomerular mesangial cells. *Clin. Exp. Immunol.,* 88, 68-74.

Chard, P. S., Bleakman, D., Christakos, S., Fullmer, C. S., Miller, R. J. 1993. Calcium buffering properties of calbindinD28k and parvalbumin in rat sensory neurones. *J. Physiol.,* 472, 341-357.

Charron, F., Nemer, M. 1999. GATA transcription factors and cardiac development. Semin. Cell *Devel. Biol.,* 10, 85-91.

Chen G. D. Fechter, L. D. 1999. Potentiation of octave-band noise induced auditory impairment by carbon monoxide. *Hear. Res.,* 132, 149-59.

Chen, G. D., McWilliams, M. L. Fechter, L. D. 1999. Intermittent noise-induced hearing loss and influence of carbon monoxide. *Hear. Res.,* 138, 181-191.

Chen, L., Kelly, J. B., Wu, S. H. 1999. The commissure of probst as a source of GABAergic inhibition. *Hear. Res.,* 138, 106-114.

Chen, P., Segil, N. 1999. p27(Kip1) links cell proliferation to morphogenesis in the developing organ of Corti. *Devel.,* 126, 1581-1590.

Chen, Q.-C., Cain, D., Jen, P. H.-S. 1995. Sound pressure transformation at the pinna of *Mus domesticus. J. Exp. Biol.,* 198, 2007-2023.

Chen, Z. F., Behringer, R. R. 1995. Twist is required in head mesenchyme for cranial neural tube morphogenesis. *Genes Devel.,* 9, 686-699.

Chen, Z. Y., Hasson, T., Kelley, P. M., Schwender, B. J., Schwartz, M. F., Ramakrishnan, M., Kimberling, W. J., Mooseker, M. S., Corey, D. P. 1996. Molecular cloning and domain structure of human myosin-VIIa, the gene product defective in Usher syndrome 1B. *Genomics*, 36, 440-448.

Chen, D., McMichael, J. C., VanDerMeid, K. R., Hahn, D., Mininni, T., Cowell, J., Eldridge, J. 1996. Evaluation of purified UspA from *Moraxella catarrhalis* as a vaccine in a murine model after active immunization. *Infect. Immunol.*, 64, 1900-1905.

Cheng, A. G., Huang, T., Stracher, A., Kim, A., Liu, W., Malgrange, B., Lefebvre, P. P., Schulman, A., Van de Water, T. R. 1999. Calpain inhibitors protect auditory sensory cells from hypoxia and neurotrophin-withdrawal induced apoptosis. *Brain Res.*, 850, 234-243.

Cheng, A. K., Niparko, J. K. 1999. Cost-utility of the cochlear implant in adults: a meta-analysis. *Arch. Otolaryngol. Head Neck Surg.*, 125, 1214-1218.

Cheong, H. I., Kashtan, C. E., Kim, Y., Kleppel, M. M., Michael, A. F. 1994. Immunohistologic studies of type IV collagen in anterior lens capsules of patients with Alport syndrome. *Lab. Invest.*, 70, 553-557.

Cherow, E. (Ed.) 1991. Combatting noise in the '90s: a national strategy for the United States. American Speech-Language-Hearing Association, Washington, D.C.

Cherubini, E., Gaiarsa, J. L., Ben-Ari, Y. 1991. GABA: an excitatory transmitter in early postnatal life. *Trends Neurosci.*, 14, 515-519.

Chiappa, K., Gladstone, K., Young, R. 1979. Brain stem auditory evoked responses. Studies of waveform variations in 50 normal human subjects. *Arch. Neurol.*, 36, 81-87.

Chin, K., Kurian, R., Saunders, J. C. 1997. Maturation of tympanic membrane layers and collagen in the embryonic and post-hatch chick (*Gallus domesticus*). *J. Morphol.*, 233, 257-266.

Chisaka, O., Musci, T. S., Capecchi, M. R. 1992. Developmental defects of the ear, cranial nerves and hindbrain resulting from targeted disruption of the mouse homeobox gene HOX-1.6. *Nature*, 355, 516-520.

Chitnis, A. B. 1999. Control of neurogenesis — lessons from frogs, fish and flies. *Curr. Opin. Neurobiol.*, 9, 18-25.

Chole R. A., Henry, K. R. 1985. Ossicular and otic capsule lesions in LP/J mice. *Ann. Otol. Rhinol. Laryngol.*, 94, 366-372.

Chole, R. A., Tinling, S. P. 1987. Fine morphology of bony dysplasia of the murine ear: comparisons with otosclerosis. *Am. J. Otolaryngol.*, 8, 325-331.

Christakos, S., Gabrielides, C., Rhoten W. B. 1989. Vitamin D-dependent calcium-binding proteins. Chemistry, distribution, functional considerations and molecular biology. *Endocr. Rev.*, 10, 3-26.

Churg, J., Strauss, L., Sherman, R. L. 1974. Electron microscopic studies in hereditary nephritis. *Birth Defects Orig. Article Series*, 10, 89-92.

Cibis, G. W., Fitzgerald, K. M., Harris, D. J., Rothberg, P. G., Rupani, M. 1993. The effects of dystrophin gene mutations on the ERG in mice and humans. *Invest. Ophthalmol. Vis. Sci.*, 34, 3646-3652.

Ciossek, T., B. Millauer, Ullrich, A. 1995. Identification of alternatively spliced mRNAs encoding variants of MDK1, a novel receptor tyrosine kinase expressed in the murine nervous system. *Oncogene*, 9, 97-108.

Clark, L. H., Schein, M. W. 1966. Activities associated with conflict behavior in mice. *Anim. Behav.*, 14, 44-49.

Clark, W. W., Bohl, C. D. 1996. Hearing levels of US industrial workers employed in low-noise environments. In Axelsson, A., Borchgrevink, H. M., Hamernik, R. P., Hellström, P.-A., Henderson, D. Salvi, R. J. (Eds.), *Scientific Basis of Noise-Induced Hearing Loss*. Thieme Medical Publishers, New York, 397-414.

Clark, W. W., Bohne, B. A., Boettcher, F. A. 1987. Effect of periodic rest on hearing loss and cochlear damage following exposure to noise. *J. Acoust. Soc. Am.*, 82, 1253-1264.

Clarke, D. D., Lajtha, A. L., Maker, H. S. 1989. Intermediary metabolism. In G. J. Siegel (Ed.), *Basic Neurochemistry: Molecular, Cellular, and Medical Aspects*, Raven Press, 565-590.

Clemens, L. G., Gladue, B. A., Coniglio, L. P. 1978. Prenatal endogenous androgenic incluences on masculine sexual behavior and genital morphology in male and female rats. *Horm. Behav.*, 10, 40-53.

Clouthier, D. E., Hosoda, K., Richardson, J. A., Williams, S. C., Yanagisawa, H., Kuwaki, T., Kumada, M., Hammer, R. E., Yanagisawa, M. 1998. Cranial and cardiac neural crest defects in endothelin-A receptor-deficient mice. *Devel.*, 125, 813-824.

Coble, J. 1972. The relative contributions of genotype and environment to the production of ultrasounds by adult *Mus musculus* in male-female pairings. Unpublished Doctoral dissertation, Florida State University, Tallahassee, FL.

Cockerell, T., Miller, I., Printz, M. 1914. The auditory ossicles of American rodents. *Bull. Am. Museum Nat. Hist.*, 33, 347-369.

Cody, A. R., Robertson, D. 1983. Variability of noise-induced damage in the guinea pig cochlea: electrophysiology and morphological correlates after strictly controlled exposures. *Hear. Res.,* 9, 55-70.

Cogan, D. G. 1945. Syndrome of nonsyphilitic interstitial keratitis and vestibuloauditory symptoms. *Arch. Ophthalmol.,* 33, 144-149.

Cohen, L. H., Hilgard, E. R., Wendt, G. R. 1933. Sensitivity to light in a case of hysterical blindness studied by reinforcement-inhibition and conditioning methods. *Yale J. Biol. Med.,* 34, 61-67.

Cohen, M. E., Cranney, J., Hoffman, H. S. 1983. Motor and cognitive factors in the modification of a reflex. *Perc. Psychophys.,* 34, 214-220.

Cohen, P. L., Eisenberg, R. A. 1991. *Lpr* and *gld*: single gene models of systemic autoimmunity and lymphoproliferative disease. *Annu. Rev. Immunol.,* 9, 243-269.

Cohen, P. L., Eisenberg, R. A. 1992. The *lpr* and *gld* genes in systemic autoimmunity: life and death in the Fas lane. *Immunol. Today,* 13, 427-428.

Cohen, S., Levi-Montalcini, R., Hamburger, V. 1954. A nerve growth stimulating factor isolated from sarcoma 37 and 180. *Proc. Soc. Nat. Acad. Sci. USA,* 40, 1014-1018.

Cohen, S. 1960. Purification of a nerve growth promoting protein from the mouse salivary gland and its neurocytotoxic antiserum. *Proc. Natl. Acad. Sci. USA,* 46, 302-311.

Cohen, Y. E, Knudsen, E. I. 1999. Maps versus clusters: different representations of auditory space in the midbrain and forebrain (review). *Trends Neurosci.,* 22, 128-135.

Cohn, E. S., Kelley, P. M., Fowler, T. W., Gorga, M. P., Lefkowitz, D. M., Kuehn, H. J., Schaefer, G. B., Gobar, L. S., Hahn, F. J., Harris, D. J., Kimberling, W. J. 1999. Clinical studies of families with hearing loss attributable to mutations in the connexin 26 gene (GJB2/DFNB1). *Pediatrics,* 103, 546-550.

Colburn, H. S., Zurek, P. M., Durlach, D. I. 1987. Binaural directional hearing impairments and aids. In W. A. Yost, G. Gourevitch (Eds.). *Directional Hearing.* Springer-Verlag, New York, 261-278.

Coleman, J. K., Lee, J. I., Miller, J. M., Nuttall, A. L. 1998. Changes in cochlear blood flow due to intraarterial infusions of angiotensin II (3-8) (angiotensin IV) in guinea pigs. *Hear. Res.,* 119, 61-68.

Colville, D. J., Savige, J. 1997. Alport syndrome. A review of the ocular manifestations. *Ophthal. Genet.,* 18, 161-173.

Colvin, J. S., Bohne, B. A., Harding, G. W., McEwen, D. G., Ornitz, D. M. 1996. Skeletal overgrowth and deafness in mice lacking fibroblast growth factor receptor 3. *Nature Genet.,* 12, 390-397.

Conlee, J. W., Abdul-Baqi, K. J., McCandless, G. A., Creel, D. J. 1986. Differential susceptibility to noise induced permanent threshold shift between albino and pigmented guinea pigs. *Hear. Res.,* 23, 81-91.

Contreras, N. E., Bachelard, H. S. 1979. Some neurochemical studies on auditory regions of mouse brain. *Exp. Brain Res.,* 36, 573-584.

Cope, M. J. T., Whisstock, J., Rayment, I., Kendrick-Jones, J. 1996. Conservation within the myosin motor domain: implications for structure and function. *Structure,* 4, 969-987.

Cordeiro, P. G., Seckel, B. R., Lipton, S. A. 1989. Acidic fibroblast growth factor enhances peripheral nerve regeneration *in-vivo. Plast. Reconstr. Surg.,* 83, 1013-119.

Corwin, J. T., Jones, J. E., Katayama, A., Kelley, M. W., Warchol, M. E. 1991. Hair cell regeneration: the identities of progenitor cells, potential triggers and instructive cues. *Ciba Found. Symp. 160,* 103-120; discussion 120-130.

Cosgrove, D., Kornak, J. M., Samuelson, G. 1996a. Expression of basement membrane type IV collagen chains during postnatal development in the murine cochlea. *Hear. Res.,* 100, 21-32.

Cosgrove, D., Meehan, D. T., Grunkemeyer, J. A., Kornak, J. M., Sayers, R., Hunter, W. J., Samuelson, G. C. 1996b. Collagen COL4A3 knockout: a mouse model for autosomal Alport syndrome. *Genes Devel.,* 10, 2981-2992.

Cosgrove, D., Rodgers, K. D. 1997. Expression of the major basement mebrane-associated proteins during development of the murine cochlea. *Hear. Res.,*105, 159-170.

Cosgrove, D., Samuelson, G., Meehan, D. T., Miller, C., McGee, J., Walsh, E. J., Siegel, M. 1998. Ultrastructural, physiological, and molecular defects in the inner ear of a gene-knockout mouse model for autosomal Alport syndrome. *Hear. Res.,* 121, 84-98.

Cosgrove, D., Samuelson, G., Pinnt, J. 1996c. Immunohistochemical localization of basement membrane collagens and associated proteins in the murine cochlea. *Hear. Res.,* 97, 54-65.

Cotman, C. W., Neeper, S. 1996. Activity-dependent plasticity and the aging brain. In: Schneider, E. L., Rowe, J. W. (Eds.), *Handbook of the Biology of Aging* (4th ed.). Academic Press, San Diego, 284-299.

Covey, E., Casseday, J. H. 1991. The monaural nuclei of the lateral lemniscus in an echolocating bat: parallel pathway for analyzing temporal features of sound. *J. Neurosci.,* 11, 3455-3470.

Covey, E., Casseday, J. H. 1999. Timing in the auditory system of the bat. *Annu. Rev. Physiol.,* 61, 457-476.

Cowan, C. A., Yokoyama, N., Bianchi, L. M., Henkemeyer, M., Fritzsch, B. 2000. EphB2 guides axons at the midline and is necessary for normal vestibular function. *Neuron,* 26, 417-430.

Cox, G. A., Lutz, C. M., Yang, C. L., Biemesderfer, D., Bronson, R. T., Fu, A., Aronson, P. S., Noebels, J. L., Frankel, W. N. 1997. Sodium/hydrogen exchanger gene defect in slow-wave epilepsy mutant mice [published erratum appears in *Cell,* 91(6), 861, 1997]. *Cell,* 91, 139-148.

Cox, L. 1985. Infant assessment: developmental and age-related considerations. In Jacobson, J. (Ed.), *The Auditory Brainstem Response.* College Hill Press, San Diego, 200-230.

Crabbe, J. C., Belknap, J. K., Buck, K. J. 1994. Genetic animal models of alcohol and drug abuse. *Science,* 264, 1715-1723.

Crabbe, J. C., Belknap, J. K. 1992. Genetic approaches to drug dependence. *Trends Pharmacol. Sci.,* 13, 212-219.

Crabbe, J. C., Phillips, T. J., Buck, K. J., Cunningham, C. L., Belknap, J. K. 1999. Identifying genes for alcohol and drug sensitivity: recent progress and future directions. *Trends Neurosci.,* 22, 173-179.

Crace, R. 1970. Morphologic Alterations with Age in the Human Cochlear Nuclear Complex. Ph.D. dissertation, Ohio University.

Crawford, D. R. 1999. Regulation of mammalian gene expression by reactive oxygen species. In Gilbert, D. L., Colton, C. A. (Eds.), *Reactive Oxygen Species in Biological Systems: An Interdisciplinary Approach.* Kluwer Academic/Plenum Publishers, New York, 155-172.

Crawley, J. N. 2000. *What's Wrong with My Mouse? Behavioral Phenotyping of Transgenic and Knockout Mice.* Wiley-Liss, New York.

Crawley, J. N., Belknap, J. K., Collins, A., Crabbe, J. C., Frankel, W., Henderson, N., Hitzemann, R. J., Maxson, S. C., Miner, L. L., Silva, A. J., Wehner, J. M., Wynshaw-Boris, A., Paylor, R. 1997. Behavioral phenotypes of inbred mouse strains: implications and recommendations for molecular studies. *Psychopharmacology,* 132, 107-124.

Creel, D. 1980. Inappropriate use of albino animals as models in research. *Pharmacol. Biochem. Behav.,* 12, 969-977.

Cremers, C. W. 1985. Audiologic features of the X-linked progressive mixed deafness syndrome with perilymphatic gusher during stapes gusher. *Am. J. Otol.,* 6, 243-246.

Cremers, C. W., Brown, S. D., Steel, K. P., Brunner, H. G., Read, A. P., Kimberling, W. J. 1995. Gene linkage and genetic deafness. *Int. J. Pediatr. Otorhinolaryngol.,* 32, S167-174.

Cremers, C. W., Hombergen, G. C., Scaf, J. J., Huygen, P. L., Volkers, W. S., Pinckers, A. J. 1985. X-linked progressive mixed deafness with perilymphatic gusher during stapes surgery. *Arch. Otolaryngol.,* 111, 249-254.

Crispens, Jr., C. G. 1975. *Handbook on the Laboratory Mouse.* Charles C. Thomas, Springfield, IL.

Cristiano, F., de Haan, J. B., Iannello, R. C., Kola, I. 1995. Changes in the levels of enzymes which modulate the antioxidant balance occur during aging and correlate with cellular damage. *Mech. Ageing Devel.,* 80, 93-105.

Crowley, C., Spencer, S. D., Nishimura, M. C., Chen, K. S., Pitts-Meek, S., Armanini, M. P., Ling, L. H., MacMahon, S. B., Shelton, D. L., Levinson, A. D., et al. 1994. Mice lacking nerve growth factor display perinatal loss of sensory and sympathetic neurons yet develop basal forebrain cholinergic neurons. *Cell,* 76, 1001-1011.

Cruz, O. L., Miniti, A., Cossermelli, W., Oliveira, R. M. 1990. Autoimmune sensorineural hearing loss: a preliminary experimental study. *Am. J. Otol.,* 11, 342-346.

Cruz-Robles, D., Garcia-Torres, R., Antignac, C., Forestier, L., de la Puente, S. G., Correa-Rotter, R., Garcia-Lopez, E., Orozco, L. 1999. Three novel mutations in the COL4A5 gene in Mexican Alport syndrome patients. *Clin. Genet.,* 56, 242-243.

Cuevas, J. M., Espinos, C., Millan, J. M., Sanchez, F., Trujillo, M. J., Ayuso, C., Beneyto, M., Najera, C. 1999. Identification of three novel mutations in the MYO7A gene. *Hum. Mutat.,* 14, 181.

Cuevas, J. M., Espinos, C., Millan, J. M., Sanchez, F., Trujillo, M. J., Garcia-Sandoval, B., Ayuso, C., Najera, C., Beneyto, M. 1998. Detection of a novel Cys628STOP mutation of the myosin VIIA gene in Usher syndrome type Ib. *Molec. Cell Probes,* 12, 417-420.

D'Hooge, R., Coenen, R., Gieselmann, V., Lullmann-Rauch, De Deyn, P. P. 1999. Decline in brainstem auditory-evoked potentials coincides with loss of spiral ganglion cells in arylsulfatase A-deficient mice. *Brain Res.,* 847, 353-356.

Dahan, K., Heidet, L., Zhou, J., Mettler, G., Leppig, K. A., Proesmans, W., David, A., Roussel, B., Mongeau, J. G., Gould, J. M. 1995. Smooth muscle tumors associated with X-linked Alport syndrome: carrier detection in females. *Kidney Int.,* 48, 1900-1906.

Dal Canto, M. C., Gurney, M. E. 1994. Development of central nervous system pathology in a murine transgenic model of human amyotrophic lateral sclerosis. *Am. J. Pathol.,* 145, 1271-1279.

Dallos, P. 1973. *The Auditory Periphery: Biophysics and Physiology.* Academic Press, New York.

Daly, T. M., Ohlemiller, K. K., Roberts, M. S., Vogler, C. A., Sands, M. S. 2001. Prevention of clinical disease in MPS VII mice following systemic AAV-mediated neonatal gene transfer. *Gene Ther.* (In press).

Daly, T. M., Okuyama, T., Vogler, C., Haskins, M. E., Muzyczka, N., Sands, M. S. 1999a. Neonatal intramuscular injection with recombinant adeno-associated virus results in prolonged beta-glucuronidase expression *in situ* and correction of liver pathology in mucopolysaccharidosis Type VII mice. *Hum. Gene Ther.,* 10, 85-94.

Daly, T. M., Sands, M. S. 1998. Gene therapy for lysosomal storage diseases. *Exp. Opin. Invest. Drugs,* 7, 1673-1682.

Daly, T. M., Vogler, C., Levy, B., Haskins, M. E., Sands, M. S. 1999b. Neonatal gene transfer leads to widespread correction of pathology in a murine model of lysosomal storage disease. *Proc. Natl. Acad. Sci.,* 96, 2296-2300.

Danielson, R., Henderson, D., Gratton, M. A., Bianchi, L., Salvi, R. 1991. The importance of "temporal pattern" in traumatic impulse noise exposures. *J. Acoust. Soc. Am.,* 90, 209-218.

Dankesreiter, S., Hoess, A., Schneider-Mergener, J., Wagner, H., Miethke, T. 2000. Synthetic endotoxin-binding peptides block endotoxin-triggered TNF-α production by macrophages *in vitro* and *in vivo* and prevent endotoxin-mediated toxic shock. *J. Immunol.,* 164, 4804-4811.

Dannhof, B. J., Roth, B., Bruns, V. 1991. Anatomical mapping of choline acetyltransferase (ChAT)-like and glutamate decarboxylase (GAD)-like immunoreactivity in outer hair cell efferents in adult rats. *Cell Tissue Res.,* 266,89-95.

Darvasi, A. 1998. Experimental strategies for the genetic dissection of complex traits in animal models. *Nature Genet.,* 18, 19-24.

Davidson, D. 1995. The function and evolution of Msx genes: pointers and paradoxes. *Trends Genet.,* 11, 405-411.

Davis, K. A., Miller, R. L., Young, E. D. 1996. Effects of somatosensory and parallel-fiber stimulation on neurons in dorsal cochlear nucleus. *J. Neurophysiol.,* 76, 3012-3024.

Davis, K. A., Young E. D. 1997. Granule cell activation of complex spiking neurons in the dorsal cochlear nucleus. *J. Neurosci.,* 17, 6798-6806.

Davis, M. (Ed.). (1992). The role of the amygdala in conditioned fear. Wiley-Liss, New York.

Davis, M. 1974. Signal-to-noise ratio as a predictor of startle amplitude and habituation in the rat. *J. Comp. Physiol. Psychol.,* 8, 812-826.

Davis, M. 1979. Diazepam and flurazepam: effects on conditioned fear as measured with the potentiated startle reflex. *Psychopharmacol.* (Berlin), 61, 1-7.

Davis, M., Astrachan, D. I. 1978. Conditioned fear and startle magnitude: effects of different footshock or backshock intensities used in training. *J. Exp. Psychol. Anim. Behav. Proc.,* 4, 95-103.

Davis, M. 1984. The mammalian startle response. In Eaton, R. C. (Ed.), *Neural Mechanisms of Startle Behavior.* Plenum Publishing, New York, 287-351.

Davis, M., Campeau., S., Kim, M., Falls, W. A. 1995. Neural systems of emotion: the amygdala's role in fear and anxiety. In McGaugh, J. L., Weinberger, N. M., Lynch, G. (Eds.), *Brain and Memory: Modulation and Mediation of Neuroplasticity.* Oxford University Press, New York, 3-40.

Davis, M., Falls, W. A., Campeau, S., Kim, M. 1993. Fear-potentiated startle: a neural and pharmacological analysis. *Behav. Brain Res.,* 58, 175-198.

Davis, M., Gendelman, D. S., Tischler, M. D., Gendelman, P. M. 1982. A primary acoustic startle circuit: lesion and stimulation studies. *J. Neurosci.,* 2, 791-805.

Davis, R. R., Cheever, M. L., Krieg, E. F., Erway, L. C. 1999. Quantitative measure of genetic differences in susceptibility to noise-induced hearing loss in two strains of mice. *Hear. Res.,* 134, 9-15.

Davis, R. R., Franks. J. R. 1989. Design and construction of a noise exposure chamber for small animals. *J. Acoust. Soc. Amer.,* 85, 963-966.

Davis, R. R., Newlander, J. K., Ling, X.-B., Cortopassi, G., Krieg, E. F., Erway, L. C. (In press.) A common genetic basis for susceptibility to age-related and noise-induced hearing loss. *Hear Res.*

Davis, R. R., Shiau, Y.-W., Erway, L. C. 1994. Temporary threshold shift does not predict permanent threshold shift in a "low frequency" exposure of mice. *Effects of Noise on Hearing: Vth International Symposium,* Gothenberg, Sweden, May 12-14, 1994.

Davis, S., Gale, N. W., Aldrich, T. H., Maisonpierre, P. C., Lhotak, V., Pawson, T., Goldfarb, M., Yancopoulos, G. D. 1994. Ligands for the Eph-related receptor tyrosine kinases that require membrane attachment or clustering for activity. *Science,* 266, 816-819.

Davisson, M. T. 1999. The future of animal models. *Lab. Anim.,* 28, 53-56.

de Haan, J. B., Cristiano, F., Iannello, R. C., Kola, I. 1995. Cu/Zn-superoxide dismutase and glutathione peroxidase during aging. *Biochem. Molec. Biol. Int.,* 35, 1281-1297.

de Kok, Y. J., van der Maarel, S. M., Bitner-Glindzicz, M., Huber, I., Monaco, A. P., Malcolm, S., Pembrey, M. E. et al. 1995. Association between X-linked mixed deafness and mutations in the POU domain gene POU3F4. *Science,* 267, 685-688.

de Kok, Y. J., Vossenaar, E. R., Cremers, C. W., Dahl, N., Laporte, J., Hu, L. J., Lacombe, D. et al. 1996. Identification of a hot spot for microdeletions in patients with X-linked deafness type 3 (DFN3) 900 kb proximal to the DFN3 gene POU3F4. *Human Molec. Genet.,* 5, 1229-1235.

Debruyne, F. 1986. Influence of age and hearing loss on the latency shift of the auditory brainstem response as a result of increased stimulus rate. *Audiol.,* 25, 101-106.

Dechesne, C., Kauff, C., Stettler, O., Tavitan, B. 1997. Rab3A immunolocalization in the mammalian vestibular end organs during development and comparison with synaptophysin expression. *Devel. Brain Res.,* 99, 103-111.

deJong, G., Telenius, A. H., Telenius, H., Perez, C. F., Drayer, J. I., Hadlaczky, G. 1999. Mammalian artificial chromosome pilot production facility: large-scale isolation of functional satellite DNA-based artificial chromosomes. *Cytometry,* 35, 129-133.

del Cerro, M., Ison, J. R., Bowen, G. P., Collier, R. J., Lazar, E., Grover, D. A., del Cerro, C. 1991. Intraretinal grafting restores visual function in light-blinded rats. *NeuroRep.,* 2, 529-532.

del Papa, N., Conforti, G., Gambini, D., La Rosa, L., Tincani, A., D'Cruz, D., Khamashta, M., Hughes, G. R., Balestrieri, G., Meroni, P. L. 1994. Characterization of the endothelial surface proteins recognized by anti-endothelial antibodies in primary and secondary autoimmune vasculitis. *Clin. Immunol. Immunopathol.,* 70, 211-216.

del Papa, N., Meroni, P. L., Barcellini, W., Sinico, A., Radice, A., Tincani, A., D'Cruz, D., Nicoletti, F., Borghi, M. O., Khamashta, M. A., Hughes, G. R. V., Balestrieri, G. 1992. Antibodies to endothelial cells in primary vasculitides mediate *in vitro* endothelial cytotoxicity in the presence of normal peripheral blood mononuclear cells. *Clin. Immunol. Immunopathol.,* 63, 267-274.

Delaney-Soldevilla, J., Morton, J. I., Trune, D. R. 1992. Cochlear pathology following autoimmune (*lpr*) gene isolation in F1 hybrids of C3H/*lpr* and MRL/*lpr* mice. *Otolaryngol. Head Neck Surg.,* 107, 231.

Dell Anna, E., Geloso, M. C., Magarelli, M., Molinari, M. 1996. Development of GABA and calcium binding proteins immunoreativity in the rat hipocampus following neonatal anoxia. *Neurosci. Lett.,* 211, 93-96.

DelPezzo, E. M., Hoffman, H. S. 1980. Attentional factors in the inhibition of a reflex by a visual stimulus. *Science,* 210, 673-674.

Delpire, E., Lu, J., England, R., Dull, C., Thorne, T. 1999. Deafness and imbalance associated with inactivation of the secretory Na-K-2Cl co-transporter. *Nature Genet.,* 22, 192-195.

Demarest, K., Koyner, J., McCaughran, J. Jr., Cipp, L., Hitzemann, R. 2000. Further characterization and high resolution mapping of quantitative trait loci for ethanol-induced locomotor activity. *Behav. Genet.,* in press.

DeMaria, T. F., Murwin, D. M. 1997. Tumor necrosis factor during experimental lipopolysaccharide- induced otitis media. *Laryngoscope,* 107, 369-372.

DeMaria, T. F. 1988. Endotoxin and otitis media. *Ann. Otol. Rhinol. Laryngol.,* Suppl. 132, 31-3.

DeMaria, T. F. 1989. Animal models for nontypable *Haemophilus influenzae* otitis media. *Ped. Infect. Dis. J.,* 8, S40-42.

DeMaria, T. F., Briggs, B. R., Lim, D. J., Okazaki, N. 1984b. Experimental otitis media with effusion following middle ear inoculation of nonviable *H. influenzae. Ann. Otol. Rhinol. Laryngol.,* 93, 52-56.

DeMaria, T. F., Prior, R. B., Briggs, B. R., Lim, D. J., Birck, H. G. 1984a. Endotoxin in middle ear effusions from patients with chronic otitis media with effusion. In Lim, D. J., Bluestone, C. D., Klein, J. O., Nelson, J. D. (Eds.), *Recent Advances in Otitis Media with Effusion.* B. C. Decker, Philadelphia, 123-125.

DeMaria, T. F., Yamaguchi, T., Bakaletz, L. O., Lim, D. J. 1992. Serum and middle ear antibody response in the chinchilla during otitis media with effusion induced by nonviable nontypeable *Haemophilus influenzae*. *J. Infect. Dis.*, 165, Suppl. 1, S196-197.

DeMaria, T. F., Yamaguchi, T., Lim, D. J. 1988. Quantitative cytologic and histologic changes in the middle ear after injections of nontypeable *Haemophilus influenzae* endotoxin. In Lim, D. J., Bluestone, C. D., Klein, J. O., Nelson, J. D. (Eds.), *Proc. Fourth Int. Symp. Recent Advances in Otitis Media*. B. C. Decker, Philadelphia, 320-323.

DeMoerlooze, L., Spencer-Dene, B., Revest, J. M., Hajihosseini, M., Rosewell, I., Dickson, C. 2000. An important role for the IIIb isoform of fibroblast growth factor receptor-2 (FGFR-2) in mesenchymal-epithelial signalling during mouse organogenesis. *Devel.*, 127, 483-492.

Denoyelle, F., Martin, S., Weil, D., Moatti, L., Chauvin, P., Garabedian, E.-N, Petit, C. 1999. Clinical features of the prevalent form of childhood deafness, DFNB1, due to a connexin-26 gene defect: implications for genetic counseling. *Lancet*, 353, 1298-1303.

Deol, M. S. 1954. The anomalies of the labyrinth of the mutants varitint-waddler, shaker-2 and jerker in the mouse. *J. Genet.*, 52, 562-588.

Deol, M. S. 1956. The anatomy and development of the mutants pirouette, shaker-1 and waltzer in the mouse. *Proc. R. Soc. Lond. B. Biol. Sci.*, 145, 206-213.

Deol, M. S. 1964. The abnormalities of the inner ear in *kreisler* mice. *J. Embryol. Exp. Morphol.*, 12, 475-490.

Deol, M. S. 1966. Influence of the neural tube on the differentiation of the inner ear in the mammalian embryo. *Nature*, 209, 219-220.

Deol, M. S. 1968. Inherited diseases of the inner ear in man in the light of studies on the mouse. *J. Med. Genet.*, 5, 137-158.

Deol, M. S. 1970. The relationship between abnormalities of pigmentation and of the inner ear. *Proc. R. Soc. Lond. B Biol. Sci.*, 175, 201-217.

Deol, M. S. 1973a. An experimental approach to the understanding and treatment of hereditary syndromes with congenital deafness and hypothyroidism. *J. Med. Genet.*, 10, 235-242.

Deol, M. S. 1973b. An experimental approach to the understanding and treatment of hereditary syndromes with congenital deafness and hypothyroidism. *J. Med. Genet.*, 10, 235-242.

Deol, M. S. 1973c. Congenital deafness and hypothyroidism. *Lancet*, 2, 105-106.

Deol, M. S. 1976. The role of thyroxin in the differentiation of the organ of Corti. *Acta Otolaryngol.*, 81, 429-435.

Derby, M. L., Sena-Esteves M., Breakfield X. O. Corey D. P. 1999. Gene transfer into the mammalian inner ear using HSV-1 and vaccinia virus vectors. *Hear. Res.*, 134, 1-8.

Derebery, M. J. 1996. Allergic and immunologic aspects of Meniere's disease. *Otolaryngol. Head Neck Surg.*, 114, 360-365.

Derebery, M. J., Rao, V. S., Siglick, T. J., Linthicum, F. H., Nelson, R. A. 1991. Meniere's Disease: an immune complex-mediated illness? *Laryngoscope*, 101, 225-229.

Devaskar, S. U. 1991. A review of insulin/insulin like peptide in the central nervous system. In: Raizada, M. K., LeRoith, D. (Eds.), *Molecular biology and physiology of insulin and insulin like growth factors*. Plenum Press, New York.

Dietrich, W. F., Miller, J., Steen, R., et al. 1996. A comprehensive genetic map of the mouse genome. *Nature*, 380, 149-152.

Dietrich, W. F., Miller, J. C., Steen, R. G., Merchant, M., Damron, D., Nahf, R., Gross, A., Joyce, D. C., Wessel, M., Dredge, R. D., et al. 1994. A genetic map of the mouse with 4,006 simple sequence length polymorphisms. *Nature Genet.*, 7, 220-245.

Dietrich, W., Katz, H., Lincoln, S. E., Shin, H.-S., Friedman, J., Dracopoli, N. C., Lander, E. S. 1992. A genetic map of the mouse suitable for typing intraspecific crosses. *Genetics*, 131, 423-447.

Dieudonné, S. 1998. Submillisecond kinetics and low efficacy of parallel fibre — Golgi cell synaptic currents in the rat cerebellum. *J. Physiol.*, 510, 845-866.

DiIulio, N. A., Xu, H., Fairchild, R. L. 1996. Diversion of CD4+ T cell development from regulatory T helper to effector T helper cells alters the contact hypersensitivity response. *Eur. J. Immunol.*, 26, 2606-2612.

DiMaio, F. H. P., Tonndorf, J. 1978. The terminal zone of the external auditory meatus in a variety of mammals. *Arch. Otolaryngol.*, 104, 570-577.

Ding, D. L., McFadden, S. L., Wang, J., Hu, B. H., Salvi, R. J. 1999. Age-and strain-related differences in dehydrogenase activity and glycogen levels in CBA and C57 mouse cochleas. *Audiol. Neuro-Otol.*, 4, 55-63.

Ding, J., Benson, T. E., Voigt, H. F. 1999. Acoustic and current-pulse responses of identified neurons in the dorsal cochlear nucleus of unanesthetized decerebrate gerbils. *J. Neurophysiol.*, 82, 3434-3457.

Ding, J., Stitzel, J., Berry, P., Hawkins, E., Kashtan, C. E. 1995. Autosomal recessive Alport syndrome: mutation in the COL4A3 gene in a woman with Alport syndrome and posttransplant antiglomerular basement membrane nephritis. *J. Am. Soc. Nephrol.,* 5, 1714-1717.

Ding, J., Voigt, H. F. 1997. Intracellular response properties of units in the dorsal cochlear nucleus of unanesthetized decerebrate gerbil. *J. Neurophysiol.,* 77, 2549-2572.

Ding, J., Yang, J., Liu, J., Yu, L. 1997. Immunofluorescence study of type IV collagen alpha chains in epidermal basement membrane: application in diagnosis of X-linked Alport syndrome. *Chin. Med. J.,* 110, 584-586.

Ding, J., Zhou, J., Tryggvason, K., Kashtan, C. E. 1994. COL4A5 deletions in three patients with Alport syndrome and posttransplant antiglomerular basement membrane nephritis. *J. Am. Soc. Nephrol.,* 5, 161-168.

Direskeneli, H., D'Cruz, D., Khamashta, M. A., Hughes, G. R. 1994. Autoantibodies against endothelial cells, extracellular matrix, and human collagen type IV in patients with systemic vasculitis. *Clin. Immunol. Immunopathol.,* 70, 206-210.

Disher, M. J., Ramakrishnan, A., Nair, T. S., Miller, J. M., Telian, S. A., Arts, H. A., Sataloff, R. T., Altschuler, R. A., Raphael, Y., Carey, T. E. 1997. Human autoantibodies and monoclonal antibody KHRI-3 bind to a phylogenetically conserved inner-ear-supporting cell antigen. *Ann. N.Y. Acad. Sci.,* 830, 253-265.

Disterhoft, J., Perkins, R., Evans, S. 1980. Neuronal morphology of the rabbit cochlear nucleus. *J. Comp. Neurol.,* 192, 687-702.

Dixon, A. K., Mackintosh, J. H. 1971. Effects of female urine upon the social behavior of adult male mice. *Anim. Behav.,* 19, 138.

Dizinno, G., Whitney, G. 1977. Androgen influence on male mouse ultrasounds during courtship. *Horm. Behav.,* 8, 188-192.

Dizinno, G., Whitney, G., Nyby, J. 1978. Ultrasonic vocalizations by male mice (Mus musculus) in response to a female sex pheromone: effects of experience. *Behav. Biol.,* 22, 104-113.

Doan, D. E., Cohen, Y. E. Saunders, J. C. 1994. Middle-ear development. IV. Umbo motion in mice. *J. Comp. Physiol., A.,* 174, 103-110.

Doan, D. E., Erulkar, J. S., Saunders, J. C. 1996. Functional changes in the aging mouse middle ear. *Hear. Res.,* 97, 174-177.

Dodge, R. 1931. *Conditions and Consequences of Human Variability.* Yale, New York.

Doering, C. H., Leyra, P. T. 1984. Methyltrienolone (R1881) is not aromatized by placental microsomes or rat hypothalamic homogenates. *J. Steroid Biochem.,* 20, 1157-1162.

Donawho, C. K., Kripke, M. L. 1992. Lack of correlation between UV-induced enhancement of melanoma development and local suppression of contact hypersensitivity. *Exp. Derm.,* 1, 20-26.

Doucet, J. R., Ryugo, D. K. 1997. Projections from the ventral cochlear nucleus to the dorsal cochlear nucleus in rats. *J. Comp. Neurol.,* 385, 245-264.

Dowling, J. E. Sidman R. L. 1962. Inherited retinal dystrophy in the rat. *J. Cell Biol.,* 14, 73-103.

Dowling, J. E., 1987. *The Retina: An Approachable Part of the Brain,* Belknap Press, Cambridge, MA.

Doyle, W. J. 1989. Animal models of otitis media: other pathogens. *Ped. Infect. Dis. J.,* 8, S45-47.

Dreyer, D., Lagrange, A., Grothe, C., Unsicker, K. 1989. Basic fibroblast growth factor prevents ontogenetic neuron death *in-vivo. Neurosci. Lett.,* 99, 35-38.

Drici, M. D., Arrighi, I., Chouabe, C., Mann, J. R., Lazdunski, M., Romey, G., Barhanin, J. 1998. Involvement of IsK-associated K+ channel in heart rate control of repolarization in a murine engineered model of Jervell and Lange-Nielsen syndrome. *Circul. Res.,* 83, 95-102.

Drury, R. A. B., Wallington, E. A. 1980. *Carleton's Histological Technique.* Oxford University Press, Oxford.

Duan, M. L., Canlon, B. 1996. Forward masking is dependent on inner hair cell activity. *Audiol. Neuro-Otol.,* 1, 320-327.

Dublin, W. B. 1976. *Fundamentals of Sensorineural Auditory Pathology.* Charles C. Thomas, Springfield, IL.

Duling, B. R., Desjardins, C. 1987. Capillary hematocrit: What does it mean? *News Int. Physiol. Soc.,* 2, 66-69.

Dulon, D., Luo, L., Zhang, C., Ryan, A. F. 1998. Expression of small-conductance calcium-activated potassium channels (SK) in outer hair cells of the rat cochlea. *Eur. J. Neurosci.,* 10, 907-915.

Dumesnil-Bousez, N., Sotelo, C. 1993. The dorsal cochlear nucleus of the adult Lurcher mouse is specifically invaded by embryonic grafted Purkinje cells. *Brain Res.,* 622, 343-347.

Dunn, M. E., Vetter, D. E., Berrebi, A. S., Krider, H. M., Mugnaini, E. 1996. The mossy fiber-granule cell-cartwheel cell system in the mammalian cochlear nuclear complex. In Ainsworth, W. A., Evans, E. F., Hackney, C. M. (Eds.), *Advances in Speech, Hearing and Language Processing.* JAI, London, 63-87.

Durand, B., Secor, C., Burkard, R. 1998. The effects of click rate, click level and noise level on CBA and Rab3A transgenic mice ABR. *Assoc. Res. Otolaryngol. Abstr.*

Eberhard, M., Erne, P. 1994. Calcium and magnesium binding to rat parvalbumin. *Eur. J. Biochem.*, 222, 21-26.

Echteler, S. M. 1992. Developmental segregation in the afferent projections to mammalian auditory hair cells. *Proc. Natl. Acad. Sci. USA*, 89, 6324-6327.

Eckenstein, F. P., Esch, F., Holbert, T., Blacher, R. W., Nishi, R. 1990. Purification and characterization of a trophic factor for embryonic peripheral neurons: comparison with fibroblast growth factors. *Neuron*, 4, 623-631.

Edwards, R. H., Rutter, W. J., Hanahan, D. 1989. Directed expression of NGF to pancreatic beta cells in transgenic mice leads to selective hyperinnervation of the islets. *Cell*, 14, 58, 161-170.

Ehret, G. 1974. Age-dependent hearing loss in normal hearing mice. *Naturwissenschaften*, 61, 506.

Ehret, G. 1975a. Masked auditory thresholds, critical ratios, and scales of the basilar membrane of the housemouse (*Mus musculus*). *J. Comp. Physiol.*, 103, 329-341.

Ehret, G. 1975b. Frequency and intensity difference limens and nonlinearities in the ear of the housemouse (*Mus musculus*). *J. Comp. Physiol.*, 102, 321-336.

Ehret, G. 1976a. Development of the absolute auditory thresholds in the house mouse (*Mus musculus*). *J. Am. Audiol. Soc.*, 1, 179-184.

Ehret, G. 1976b. Temporal auditory summation for pure tones and white noise in the house mouse (*Mus musculus*). *J. Acoust. Soc. Am.*, 59, 1421-1427.

Ehret, G. 1977. Postnatal development in the acoustic system of the house mouse in the light of developing masked thresholds. *J. Acoust. Soc. Am.*, 62, 143-148.

Ehret, G. 1979. Quantitative analysis of nerve fibre densities in the cochlea of the house mouse (*Mus musculus*). *J. Comp. Neurol.*, 183, 73-88.

Ehret, G. 1983a. Peripheral anatomy and physiology. II. In Willott, J. F. (Ed.), *The Auditory Psychobiology of the Mouse*. Charles C. Thomas, Springfield, IL, 169-200.

Ehret, G. 1983b. Psychoacoustics. In Willott, J. (Ed.), *The Auditory Psychobiology of the Mouse*. Charles C. Thomas, Springfield, IL, 305-339.

Ehret, G. 1987. Left hemisphere advantage in the mouse brain for recognizing ultrasonic communication calls. *Nature*, 325, 249-251.

Ehret, G., Dreyer, A. 1984. Localization of tones and noise in the horizontal plane by unrestrained house mice (*Mus musculus*) *J. Exp. Biol.*, 109, 163-174.

Ehret, G., Frankenreiter, M. 1977. Quantitative analysis of cochlear structures in the house mouse in relation to mechanisms of acoustical information processing. *J. Comp. Physiol.*, 122, 65-85.

Ehret, G., Moffat, A. J. M. 1985b. Inferior colliculus of the house mouse III. Response probabilities and thresholds of single units to synthesized mouse calls compared to tone and noise bursts. *J. Comp. Physiol. A*, 156, 637-644.

Ehret, G., Moffat, A. J. M. 1984. Noise masking of tone responses and critical ratios in single units of the mouse cochlear nerve and cochlear nucleus. *Hear. Res.*, 14, 45-57.

Ehret, G., Moffat, A. J. M. 1985a. Inferior colliculus of the house mouse II. Single unit responses to tones, noise and tone-noise combinations as a function of sound intensity. *J. Comp. Physiol. A*, 156, 619-635.

Ehret, G., Romand, R. 1992. Development of tone response thresholds, latencies and tuning in the mouse inferior colliculus. *Devel. Brain Res.*, 67, 317-326.

Eibl-Eibesfeldt, I. 1970. *Ethology, The Biology of Behavior*. Holt, Rinehart and Winston, New York.

Eilat, D. 1985. Cross-reactions of anti-DNA antibodies and the central dogma of lupus nephritis. *Immunol. Today*, 6, 123-127.

Einsiedel, L. J., Luff, A. R. 1992. Alterations in the contractile properties of motor units within the aging rat medial gastrocnemius. *J. Neurol. Sci.*, 112, 170-177.

el-Amraoui, A., Sahly, I., Picaud, S., Sahel, J., Abitbol, M., Petit, C. 1996. Human Usher 1B/mouse shaker-1: the retinal phenotype discrepancy explained by the presence/absence of myosin VIIA in the photoreceptor cells. *Hum. Molec. Genet.*, 5, 1171-1178.

Eldred, K. M., Gannon, W. J., von Gierke, H. 1955. Criteria for Short Time Exposure of Personnel to High Intensity Jet Aircraft Noise, Rep. WADC-TN-355. Aerosp. Med. Lab., Wright AFB, Ohio.

Elledge, S. J. 1996. Cell cycle checkpoints: preventing an identity crisis. *Science*, 274, 1664-1672.

Ellis, J., Liu, Q., Breitman, M., Jenkins, N. A., Gilbert, D. J., Copeland, N. G., Tempest, H. V., Warren, S., Muir, E., Schilling, H., Fletcher, F. A., Ziegler, S. F., Rogers, J. H. 1995. Embryo brain kinase: a novel gene of the eph/elk receptor tyrosine kinase family. *Mech. Dev.*, 52, 319-341.

Emmerling, M. R., Sobkowicz, H. M. 1990a. Acetylcholinesterase-positive innervation in cochleas from two strains of shaker-1 mice. *Hear. Res.*, 47, 25-37.

Emmerling, M. R., Sobkowicz, H. M., Levenick, C. V., Scott, G. L., Slapnick, S. M., Rose, J. E. 1990. Biochemical and morphological differentiation of acetylcholinesterase-positive efferent fibers in the mouse cochlea. *J. Electron Microsc. Tech.*, 15, 123-143.

Emmerling, M. R., Sobkowicz, H. M. 1988. Differentiation and distribution of acetylcholinesterase molecular forms in the mouse cochlea. *Hear. Res.*, 32, 137-146.

Emmerling, M. R., Sobkowicz, H. M. 1990b. Intermittent expression of GAP-43 during the innervation of the cochlea in the mouse. *Assoc. Res. Otolaryngol. Abstr.* 13, 61.

Engström, H., Ades, H. W., Andersson, A. 1966. *Structural Pattern of the Organ of Corti: A Systematic Mapping of Sensory Cells and Neural Elements*. The Williams & Wilkins Company, Baltimore.

Epstein, D. J., Vogan, K. J., Trasler, D. G., Gros, P. 1993. A mutation within intron 3 of the Pax-3 gene produces aberrantly spliced mRNA transcripts in the splotch (Sp) mouse mutant. *Proc. Natl. Acad. Sci. USA*, 90, 532-536.

Erichsen, S., Bagger-Sjöbäck, D., Curtis, L., Zuo, J., Rarey, K., Hultcrantz, M. 1996. Appearance of glucocorticoid receptors in the inner ear of the mouse during devlopment. *Acta Otolaryngol.*, 116, 721-725.

Erkman, L., McEvilly, R. J., Luo, L., Ryan, A. K., Hooshmand, F., O'Connell, S. M., Keithley, E. M., Rapaport, D. H., Ryan, A. F., Rosenfeld, M. G. 1996. Role of transcription factors Brn-3.1 and Brn-3.2 in auditory and visual system development. *Nature*, 381, 603-606.

Ernfors, P., Lee, K. F., Jaenisch, R. 1994. Mice lacking brain-derived neurotophic factor develop with sensory deficits. *Nature*, 368, 147-150.

Ernfors, P., Ibanez, C. F., Ebendal, T., Olson, L., Persson, H. 1990. Molecular cloning and neurotrophic activities of a protein with structural similarities to nerve growth factor: Developmental and topographical expression in the brain. *Proc. Natl. Acad. Sci. USA*, 87, 5454-5458.

Ernfors, P., Van De Water, T., Loring, J., and Jaenisch, R. 1995. Complementary roles of BDNF and NT-3 in vestibular and auditory development. *Neuron*, 14, 1-20.

Ernfors, P., Van De Water, T. R., Loring, J., Jaenisch, R. 1995. Complementary roles of BDNF and NT-3 in vestibular and auditory development. *Neuron*, 14, 1153-1164.

Erskine, L., Stewart, R., McCaig, C. D. 1995. Electric field-directed growth and branching of cultured frog nerves: effects of aminoglycosides and polycations. *J. Neurobiol.*, 26, 523-536.

Ervasti, J. M., Campbell, K. P. 1991. Membrane organization of the dystrophin-glycoprotein complex. *Cell*, 66, 1121-1131.

Erway, L. C., Shiau, Y.-W., Davis, R., R, Krieg, E. F. 1996. Genetics of age-related hearing loss in mice. III. Susceptibility of inbred and F1 hybrid strains to noise-induced hearing loss. *Hear. Res.*, 93, 181-187.

Erway, L. C., Willott, J. F., Archer, J. R., Harrison, D. E. 1993a. Genetics of age-related hearing loss in mice. I. Inbred and F1 hybrid strains. *Hear. Res.*, 65, 125-132.

Erway, L. C., Willott, J. F. 1996. Genetic susceptibility to noise-induced hearing loss in mice. In A. Axelsson, H. Borchgrevink, R. P. Hamernik, P. A. Hellstrom, D. Henderson, R. J. Salvi (Eds.), *Scientific Basis of Noise-Induced Hearing Loss*. Thieme Medical Publishers, New York, pp. 56-64.

Erway. L. C., Willott, J. F., Cook, S. A. Johnson, K. R., Davission, M. T. 1993b. Segregation of genes for age-related hearing loss from C57BL/6J and DBA/2J inbred mice. *Assoc. Res. Otolaryngol. Abstr.* 16, 137.

Esch, F., Baird, A., Ling, N. 1985. Primary structure of bovine pituitary basic fibroblast growth factor (FGF) and comparison with the amino terminal sequence of bovine brain acidic FGF. *Proc. Natl. Acad. Sci. USA*, 82, 6507-6511.

Espinos, C., Millan, J. M., Sanchez, F., Beneyto, M., Najera, C. 1998. Ala397Asp mutation of myosin VIIA gene segregating in a Spanish family with type-Ib Usher syndrome. *Hum. Genet.*, 102, 691-694.

Estivill, X., Fortina, P., Surrey, S., Rabionet, R., Melchionda, S., D'Agruma, L., Mansfield, E., Rappaport, E., Govea, N., Mila, M., Zelante, L., Gasparini, P. 1998. Connexin-26 mutations in sporadic and inherited sensorineural deafness. *Lancet*, 351, 394-398.

Eudy, J. D., Weston, M. D., Yao, S., Hoover, D. M., Rehm, H. L., Ma-Edmonds, M., Yan, D., Ahmad, I., Cheng, J. J., Ayuso, C., Cremers, C., Davenport, S., Moller, C., Talmadge, C. B., Beisel, K. W., Tamayo, M., Morton, C. C., Swaroop, A., Kimberling, W. J., Sumegi, J. 1998. Mutation of a gene encoding a protein with extracellular matrix motifs in Usher syndrome type IIa. *Science*, 280, 1753-1757.

Evans, E. F., Nelson, P. G. 1973. The responses of single neurones in the cochlear nucleus of the cat as a function of their location and anesthetic state. *Exp. Brain Res.*, 17, 402-427.

Evans, E. F., Zhao, W. 1993. Varieties of inhibition in the processing and control of processing in the mammalian cochlear nucleus. *Prog. Brain Res.*, 97, 117-126.

Evans, K. L., Fantes, J., Simpson, C., Arveiler, B., Muir, W., Fletcher, J., van Heyningen, V., Steel, K. P., Brown, K. A., Brown, S. D. 1993. Human olfactory marker protein maps close to tyrosinase and is a candidate gene for Usher syndrome type I. *Hum. Molec. Genet.,* 2, 115-118.

Evans, P., Halliwell, B. 1999. Free radicals: cause, consequence and criteria. In Henderson, D., Salvi, R. J., Quaranta, A. McFadden, S. L., Burkard, R. F. (Eds.), *Ototoxicity: Basic Science and Clinical Applications.* The New York Academy of Sciences, New York, 19-40.

Evens A. L., Muller, U. 2000. Stereocilia defects in the sensory hair cells of the inner ear in mice deficient in integrin alpha8 beta1. *Nature Genet.,* 24, 424-428.

Everett, L. A., Glaser, B., Beck, J. C., Idol, J. R., Buchs, A., Heyman, M., Adawi, F., Hazani, E., Nassir, E., Baxevanis, A. D., Sheffield, V. C., Green, E. D. 1997. Pendred syndrome is caused by mutations in a putative sulphate transporter gene (PDS). *Nature Genet.,* 17, 411-422.

Eybalin, M. 1993. Neurotransmitters and neuromodulators of the mammalian cochlea. *Physiol. Rev.,* 73, 309-373.

Eybalin, M., Abou-Madi, L., Rossier, J., Pujol, R. 1985. Electron microscopic localization of N-terminal proenkephalin (synenkephalin) immunostaining in the guinea pig organ of Corti. *Brain Res.,* 358, 354-359.

Eybalin, M., Pujol, R. 1987. Choline acetyltransferase (ChAT) immunoelectron microscopy distinguishes at least three types of efferent synapses in the organ of Corti. *Exp. Brain Res.,* 65, 261-270.

Faaber, P., Rijke, T. P., van de Putte, L. B., Capel, P. J., Berden, J. H. 1986. Cross-reactivity of human and murine anti-DNA antibodies with heparan sulfate. The major glycosaminoglycan in glomerular basement membranes. *J. Clin. Invest.,* 77, 1824-1830.

Fahey, P. F., Allen, J. B. 1986. Characterization of cubic intermodulation distortion products in the cat external auditory meatus. In Allen, J. B., Hall, J. L., Hubbard, A., Neely, S. T., Tubis, A. (Eds.), *Development of Auditory and Vestibular Systems.* Academic Press, New York, 211-237.

Fahey, P. F., Allen, J. B. 1997. Measurement of distortion product phase in ear canal of the cat. *J. Acoust. Soc. Am.,* 2880-2891.

Falconer, D. S. 1951. Two new mutants, "trembler" and "reeler", with neurological actions in the house mouse. *J. Genet.,* 50, 192-201.

Falconer, D. S. 1960. *Introduction to Quantitative Genetics.* Oliver and Boyd, Ltd., Edinburgh.

Falls, W. A., Carlson, S., Turner, J. G., Willott, J. F. 1997. Fear potentiated startle in two strains of inbred mice. *Behav. Neurosci.,* 111, 855-861.

Falls, W. A., Davis, M. 1994. Fear-potentiated startle using three conditioned stimulus modalities. *Anim. Learn. Behav.,* 22, 379-383.

Farinas, I., Jones, K. R., Backus, C., Wang, X.-Y., Reichardt, L. F. 1994. Severe sensory and sympathetic deficits in mice lacking neurotrophin-3. *Nature,* 369, 658-661.

Farrell, P., McGee, J., Walsh, E. 2000. Mechanical inner ear filtering in Tshr mutant mice. *Assoc. Res. Otolaryngol.,* 23, 192.

Fatemi, S. H., Emamian, E. S., Kist, D., Sidwell, R. W., Nakajima, K., Akhter, P., Shier, A., Sheikh, S., Bailey, K. 1999. Defective corticogenesis and reduction in reelin immunoreactivity in cortex and hippocampus of prenatally infected neonatal mice. *Molec. Psychol.,* 4, 145-154.

Fattori, B., Ghilardi, P. L., Casani, A., Migliorini, P., Riente, L. 1994. Meniere's disease: role of antibodies against basement membrane antigens. *Laryngoscope,* 104, 1290-1294.

Fay, R. R. 1988. *Hearing in Vertebrates: A Psychophysics Databook.* Hill-Fay Associates, Winnetka, IL.

Fechter, L. D., Sheppard, L., Young, J. S., Zeger, S. 1988a. Sensory threshold estimation from a continuously graded response produced by reflex modification audiometry. *J. Acoust. Soc. Am.,* 84, 179-185.

Fechter, L. D., Young, J. S. Carlisle, L. 1988b. Potentiation of noise induced threshold shifts and hair cell loss by carbon monoxide. *Hear. Res.,* 34, 39-47.

Federici, S., Ceccarelli, P. L., Bernardi, F., Tassinari, D., Zanetti, G., Tani, G., Domini, R. 1998. Esophageal leiomyomatosis in children: report of a case and review of the literature. *Eur. J. Pediatr. Surg.,* 8, 358-363.

Feingold, J., Bois, E. 1987. Genetics of Alport's syndrome. *Pediatr. Nephrol.,* 1, 436-438.

Feingold, J., Bois, E., Chompret, A., Broyer, M., Gubler, M. C., Grunfeld, J. P. 1985. Genetic heterogeneity of Alport syndrome. *Kidney Int.,* 27, 672-677.

Fekete, D. M. 1999. Development of the vertebrate ear: insights from knockouts and mutants. *Trends Neurosci.,* 22, 263-269.

Fekete, D. M., Muthukumar, S., Karagogeos, D. 1998. Hair cells and supporting cells share a common progenitor in the avian inner ear. *J. Neurosci.,* 18, 7811-7821.

Feliciano, M., Saldaña, E., Mugnaini, E. 1995. Direct projection from the rat primary auditory neocortex to the nucleus sagulum, paralemniscal regions, superior olivary complex and cochlear nuclei. *Aud. Neurosci.,* 1, 287-308.

Feng, J., Kuwada, S., Ostapoff, E.-M., Batra, R., Morest, D. K. 1994. A physiological and structural study of neuron types in the cochlear nucleus. I. Intracellular responses to acoustic stimulation and current injection. *J. Comp. Neurol.,* 346, 1-18.

Ferber, D. E., Morton, J. I., Trune, D. R. 1992. Stria vascularis pathology in several strains of autoimmune disease mice. *Otolaryngol. Head Neck Surg.,* 107, 232.

Ferragamo, M. J., Oertel, D. 1998a. Shaping of synaptic responses and action potentials in octopus cells. *Assoc. Res. Otolaryngol. Abstr.,* 21, 96.

Ferragamo, M. J., Golding, N. L., Oertel, D. 1998b. Synaptic inputs to stellate cells in the ventral cochlear nucleus. *J. Neurophysiol.,* 79, 51-63.

Ferragamo, M. J., Golding, N. L., Gardner, S. M., Oertel, D. 1998c. Golgi cells in the superficial granule cell domain overlying the ventral cochlear nucleus: morphology and electrophysiology in slices. 400, 519-528.

Ferraro, J. A., Durrant, J. D. 1994. Auditory evoked potentials: overview and basic principals. In Katz, J. (Ed.), *Handbook of Clinical Audiology* (4th ed.). Williams & Wilkins, Baltimore, 317-338.

Fessenden, J. D., Coling, D. E., Schacht, J. 1994. Detection characterization of nitric oxide synthase in the mammalian cochlea. [published erratum appears in *Brain Res.,* 675(1/2), 394, 1995] *Brain Res.,* 668(1/2), 9-15.

Fex, J., Altschuler, R. A. 1984. Glutamic acid decarboxylase immunoreactivity of olivocochlear neurons in the organ of Corti of guinea pig and rat. *Hear. Res.,* 15, 123-131.

Fina, M., Popper, A., Honrubia, V. 1994. Survival and cell biologic changes in the vestibular ganglion cells following vestibular neuronectomy in the chinchilla. *Assoc. Res. Otolaryngol. Abstr.*

Finlayson, P. G., Caspary. D. M. 1991. Low frequency neurons in the lateral superior olive exhibit phase-sensitive binaural inhibition. *J. Neurophysiol.,* 65, 598-605.

Finlayson, P. G., Caspary, D. M. 1993. Response properties in young and old Fischer-344 rat lateral superior olive neurons: a quantitative approach. *Neurobiol. Aging,*14, 127-139.

Fitzpatrick, D. C., Batra, R., Stanford, T. R., Kuwada, S. 1997. A neuronal population code for sound localization. *Nature,* 388, 871-874.

Fleischer, G. 1978. Evolutionary principles of the mammalian middle ear. *Adv. Anat. Embryol. Cell Biol.,* 55, 1-70.

Fleshler, M. 1965. Adequate acoustic stimulus for startle reaction in the rat. *J. Comp. Physiol. Psychol.,* 60, 200-207.

Flint, J., Corley, R., DeFries, J. C., Fulker, D. W., Gray, J. A., Miller, S., Collins, A. C. 1995. A simple genetic basis for a complex psychological trait in laboratory mice. *Science,* 269, 1432-1435.

Flinter, F. 1997. Alport's syndrome. *J. Med. Genet.,* 34, 326-330.

Flinter, F. A., Abbs, S., Bobrow, M. 1989. Localization of the gene for classic Alport syndrome. *Genomics,* 4, 335-338.

Flinter, F. A., Cameron, J. S., Chantler, C., Houston, I., Bobrow, M. 1988. Genetics of classic Alport's syndrome. *Lancet,* 2, 1005-1007.

Floody, O. R., Pfaff, D. W. 1977a. Communication among hamsters by high-frequency acoustic signals. I. Physical characteristics of hamster calls. *J. Comp. Physiol. Psychol.,* 91, 794-806.

Floody, O. R., Pfaff, D. W. 1977b. Communication among hamsters by high-frequency acoustic signals. II. Determinants of calling by females and males. *J. Comp. Physiol. Psychol.,* 91, 807-819.

Floody, O. R., Pfaff, D. W. 1977c. Communication among hamsters by high-frequency acoustic signals. III. Responses evoked by natural and synthetic ultrasounds. *J. Comp. Physiol. Psychol.,* 91, 820-829.

Ford, J. M., Roth, W. T., Isaacks, B. G., White, P. M., Hood, S. H., Pfefferbaum, A. 1995. Elderly men and women are less responsive to startling noises: N1, P3 and blink evidence. *Biol. Psychol.,* 39, 57-80.

Forrest, D., Erway, L. C., Ng, L., Altschuler, R., Curran, T. 1996. Thyroid hormone receptor beta is essential for development of auditory function. *Nat. Genet.,* 13, 354-357.

Forrest, D., Vennstrom, B. 2000. Functions of thyroid hormone receptors in mice. *Thyroid,* 10, 41-52.

Forrest, T. G., Green, D. M. 1987. Detection of partially filled gaps in noise and the temporal modulation transfer funciton. *J. Acoust. Soc. Am.,* 82, 1933-1943.

Forsgren, J., Samuelson, A., Ahlin, A., Jonasson, J., Rynnel-Dagoo, B., Lindberg, A. 1994. Haemophilus influenzae resides and multiplies intracellularly in human adenoid tissue as demonstrated by *in situ* hybridization and bacterial viability assay. *Infect. Immunology,* 62, 673-679.

Forsmann, J. 1898. Ueber die ursachen welche die wachsthumsrichtung der peripheren nervenfasern beider regeneration bestimmen. *Beitr. Path. Anat. Allg. Path.,* 24, 56-100.

Förster, C. R., Illing, R. B. 2000. Plasticity of the auditory brainstem: cochleotomy-induced changes of calbindin-D28k expression in the rat. *J. Comp. Neurol.,* 416, 173-187.

Fowler, T., Canlon, B., Dolan, D. Miller, J. M. 1995. The effect of noise trauma following training exposures in the mouse. *Hear. Res.,* 88, 1-13.

Fox, J. E. 1979. Habituation and pre-stimulus inhibition of the auditory startle reflex in decerebrate rats. *Physiol. Behav.,* 23, 291-297.

Foxwell, A. R., Kyd, J. M., Cripps, A. W. 1998. Nontypeable Haemophilus influenzae: pathogenesis and prevention. *Micro. Molec. Biol. Rev.,* 62, 294-308.

Frampton, G., Hobby, P., Morgan, A., Staines, N. A. Cameron, J. S. 1991. A role for DNA in anti-DNA antibodies binding to endothelial cells. *J. Autoimmunol.,* 4, 463-478.

Francis, F., Zehetner, G., Hoglund, M., Lehrach, H. 1994. Construction and preliminary analysis of the ICRF human P1 library. *Genet. Anal. Tech. Appl.,* 11, 148-157.

Francis, H., Lustig, L., Gorelikow, M., Limb, C., Lee, M., Feinberg, A. 2000. Otopathology of the KVLQT-1 knockout mouse: a new murine model of deafness. *Assoc. Res. Otolaryngol. Abstr.,*

Francis, R. L. 1979., The Preyer reflex audiogram of several rodents and its relation to the "absolute" audiogram in the rat. *J. Aud. Res.,* 19, 217-233.

Franz, P., Hauser-Kronberger, C., Bock, P., Quint, C., Baumgartner, W. D. 1996. Localization of nitric oxide synthase I and III in the cochlea. *Acta Otolaryngol. (Stockholm),* 116, 726-731.

Fredelius, L., Johansson, B., Bagger-Sjöbäck, D., Wersäll, J. 1987. Qualitative and quantitative changes in the guinea pig organ of Corti after pure tone acoustic overstimulation. *Hear. Res.,* 30, 157-168.

Freeman, B. J., Roberts M. S., Vogler C. A., Nicholes A., Hofling A. A. Sands M. S. 1999. Behavior and therapeutic efficacy of B-glucuronidase-positive mononuclear phagocytes in a murine model of muco-ploysasccharidosis type VII. *Transplant,* 6, 2142-2150.

Frenz, D. A., Galinovic-Schwartz, V., Liu, W., Flanders, K. C., Van de Water, T. R. 1992. Transforming growth factor beta 1 is an epithelial-derived signal peptide that influences otic capsule formation. *Devel. Biol.,* 153, 324-336.

Friauf, E. 1994. Distribution of calcium binding protein calbindin-D28k in the auditory system of adult and developing rats. *J. Comp. Neurol.,* 349, 193-211.

Frick, A. G., Joseph, T. D., Pang, L., Rabe, A. M., St. Geme, J. W., III., Look, D. C. 2000. *Haemophilus influenzae* stimulates ICAM-1 espression on respiratory epithelial cells. *J. Immunol.,* 161, 4185-4196.

Fridberger, A., Flock, A., Ulfendahl, M., Flock, B. 1998. Acoustic overstimulation increases outer hair cell Ca^{2+} concentrations and causes dynamic contractions of the hearing organ. *Proc. Natl. Acad. Sci. USA,* 95, 7127-7132.

Friedman, J., Raisz, L. G. 1965. Thyrocalcitonin: inhibitor of bone resorption in tissue culture. *Science,* 150, 1465-1467.

Friedman, R. A., Bykhovskaya, Y., Tu, G., Talbot, J. M., Wilson, D. F., Parnes, L. S., Fischel-Ghodsian, N. 1997. Molecular analysis of the POU3F4 gene in patients with clinical and radiographic evidence of X-linked mixed deafness with perilymphatic gusher. *Ann. Otol. Rhinol. Laryngol.,* 106, 320-325.

Friedmann, I., Ballantyne, J. 1984. *Ultrastructural Atlas of the Inner Ear.* Butterworth, London.

Frisina, D. R., Frisina, R. D. 1997. Speech recognition in noise and presbycusis: relations to possible neural mechanisms. *Hear. Res.,* 106, 95-104.

Frisina, D. R., Frisina, R. D., Snell, K. B., Burkard, R., Walton, J. P, Ison, J. R. 2001. Auditory temporal processing during aging. In *Functional Neurobiology of Aging,* Hof, P. R., Mobbs, C. V. (Eds.), Academic Press, San Diego, Ch. 39, 565-579.

Frisina, R. D. 2001. Anatomical and neurochemical bases of presbycusis. In *Functional Neurobiology of Aging.* Hof, P. R., Mobbs, C. V. (Eds.), Academic Press, San Diego, Ch. 37, 531-547.

Frisina, R. D., Chamberlain, S. C., Brachman, M. L, Smith, R. L. 1982. Anatomy and physiology of the gerbil cochlear nucleus: an improved surgical approach for microelectrode studies. *Hear. Res.,* 6, 259-275.

Frisina, R. D., Karcich, K. J., Tracy, T. C., Sullivan, D. M, Walton, J. P. 1996. Preservation of amplitude modulation coding in the presence of background noise by chinchilla auditory-nerve fibers. *J. Acoust. Soc. Am.,* 99, 475-490.

Frisina, R. D., O'Neill, W. E, Zettel, M. L. 1989. Functional organization of mustached bat inferior colliculus. II. Connections of the FM_2 region. *J. Comp. Neurol.,* 284, 85-107.

Frisina, R. D., Smith, R. L., Chamberlain, S. C. 1990a. Encoding of amplitude modulation in the gerbil cochlear nucleus. I. A hierarchy of enhancement. *Hear. Res.,* 44, 99-122.

Frisina, R. D., Smith, R. L, Chamberlain, S. C. 1985. Differential encoding of rapid changes in sound amplitude by second-order auditory neurons. *Exp. Brain Res.,* 60, 417-422.

Frisina, R. D., Smith, R. L, Chamberlain, S. C. 1990b. Encoding of amplitude modulation in the gerbil cochlear nucleus. II. Possible neural mechanisms. *Hear. Res.,* 44, 123-141.

Frisina, R. D., Walton, J. P., Lynch-Armour, M. A., Byrd, J. D. 1998. Inputs to a physiologically characterized region of the inferior colliculus of the young adult CBA mouse. *Hear. Res.,* 115, 61-81.

Frisina, R. D., Walton, J. P., Lynch-Armour, M. A, Klotz, D. A. 1997. Efferent projections of a physiologically characterized region of the inferior colliculus of the young adult CBA mouse. *J. Acoust. Soc. Am.,* 101, 2741-2753.

Frisina, R. D., Walton, J. P, Karcich, K. J. 1994. Dorsal cochlear nucleus single neurons can enhance temporal processing capabilities in background noise. *Exp. Brain Res.,* 102, 160-164.

Frisina, R. D., Zettel, M. L., Walton, J. P., Kelley, P. E. 1995. Distribution of calbindin D28k immunoreactivity in the cochlear nucleus of the young adult chinchilla. *Hear. Res.,* 85, 53-68.

Fritzsch, B., Barbacid, M., Silos-Santiago, I. 1998. The combined effects of trkB and trkC mutations on the innervation of the inner ear. *Int. J. Devel. Neurosci.,* 16, 493-505.

Fritzsch, B., Beisel, K. 1998. Development and maintenance of ear innervation and function: lessons from mutations in mouse and man. *Am. J. Hum. Genet.,* 63, 1263-1270.

Fritzsch B., Farinas, I. Reichardt, L. F. 1997a. Lack of neurotrophin-3 causes losses of both classes of spiral ganglion neurons in the cochlea in a region-specific fashion. *J. Neurosci.,* 17, 6213-6225.

Fritzsch, B., Nichols, D. H. 1993. DiI reveals a prenatal arrival of efferents at the differentiating otocyst of mice. *Hear. Res.,* 65, 51-60.

Fritzsch, B., Silos-Santiago, I. Bianchi, L. M. Farinas, I. 1997b. Role of neurotrophic factors in regulating inner ear innervation. *Trends Neurosci.,* 20, 159-164.

Fritzsch B., Silos-Santiago, I., Smeyne, R., Fagan, A. M., Barbacid, M. 1995. Reduction and loss of inner ear innervation in trkB and trkC receptor knockout mice: a whole mount DiI and scanning electron microscope analysis. *Aud. Neurosci.,* 1, 401-417.

Frost, D. O, Caviness, Jr., F. S. 1980. Radial organization of thalamic projections to the neocortex in the mouse. *J. Comp. Neurol.,* 194, 369-393.

Frostholm, A., Rotter, A. 1985. Glycine receptor distribution in mouse CNS: autoradiographic localization of [3H]strychnine binding sites. *Brain Res., Bull.,* 15, 473-486.

Frostholm, A., Rotter, A. 1986. Autoradiographic localization of receptors in the cochlear nucleus of the mouse. *Brain Res., Bull.,* 16, 189-203.

Frotscher, M., Léránth, C. 1986. The cholinergic innervation of the rat fascia dentata: identification of target structures on granule cells by combining choline acetyltransferase immunocytochemistry and Golgi impregnation. *J. Comp. Neurol.,* 243, 58-70.

Fujiyoshi, T., Cheng, K. C., Krug, M. S., Yoo, T. J. 1997. Molecular basis of type II collagen autoimmune disease: observations of arthritis, auricular chondritis and tympanitis in mice. *ORL,* 59, 215-29.

Fujiyoshi, T., Hood, L., Yoo, T. J. 1994. Restoration of brain stem auditory-evoked potentials by gene transfer in shiverer mice. *Ann. Otol. Rhinol. Laryngol.,* 103, 449-456.

Fukuda, S., Harris, J. P., Keithley, E. M., Ishikawa, K., Kucuk, B., Inuyama, Y. 1992. Spiral modiolar vein: its importance in viral load of the inner ear. *Ann. Otol. Rhinol. Laryngol. Suppl.,* 157, 67-71.

Fullerton, B., Levine, R., Hosford-Dunn, H., Kiang, N. 1987. Comparison of cat and human brain-stem auditory evoked potentials. *Electroenceph. Clin. Neurophysiol.,* 66, 547-570.

Furst, M., Aharonson, V., Levine, R. A., Fullerton, B. C., Tadmor, R., Pratt, H., Polyakov, A., Korczyn, A. D. 2000. Sound lateralization and interaural discrimination. Effects of brainstem infacts and multiple sclerosis lesions. *Hear. Res.,* 143, 29-42.

Furuta, H., Luo, L., Hepler, K., Ryan, A. F. 1998. Evidence for differential regulation of calcium by outer versus inner hair cells: plasma membrane Ca-ATPase gene expression [published erratum appears in *Hear. Res.,* 126, 214] *Hear. Res.,* 123, 10-26.

Gabaizadeh, R., Staecker, H., Liu, W., Van De Water, T. R. 1997. BDNF protection of auditory neurons from cisplatin involves changes in intracellular levels of both reactive oxygen species and glutathione. *Molec. Brain Res.,* 50, 71-78.

Gabrion, J., Legrand, C., Mercier, B., Harricane, M. C., Uziel, A. 1984. Microtubules in the cochlea of the hypothyroid developing rat. *Hear. Res.,* 13, 203-214.

Gailly, P., Hermans, E., Octave, J. N., Gillis, J. M. 1993. Specific increase of genetic expression of parvalbumin in fast skeletal muscles of mdx mice. *FEBS Lett.,* 326, 272-274.

Gale, N. W., Holland, S. J., Valenzuela, D. M., Flenniken, A. M., Pan, L., Ryan, T. E., Henkemeyer, M., Strenhardt, K., Hirai, H., Wilkinson, D. G., Pawson, T., Davis, S., Yancopoulos, G. D. 1996. Eph receptors and ligands comprise two major specificity subclasses and are reciprocally compartmentalized during embryogenesis. *Neuron,* 17, 9-19.

Galinovic-Schwartz, V., Peng, D., Chiu, F. C., Van De Water, T. R. 1991. Temporal pattern of innervation in the developing mouse embryo: an immunohistochemical study of a 66 kD subunit of mammalian neurofilament. *J. Neurosci. Res.,* 30, 124-130.

Gandelman, R., Vom Saal, F. S., Reinisch, J. M. 1977. Contiguity to male foetuses affects morphology and behaviour of female mice. *Nature,* 266, 722-724.

Gantz, B., Tyler, R., Woodworth, G., Tye-Murray, N., Fryauf-Bertschy, H. 1994. Results of multichannel cochlear implants in congenital and acquired prelingual deafness in children: five year follow up. *Am. J. Otol.,* 15, 1-8.

Gao, W.-J., Newman, D. E., Wormington, A. B., Pallas, S. L. 1999. Development of inhibitory circuitry in visual and auditory cortex of postnatal ferrets: Immunocytochemical localization of GABAergic neurons. *J. Comp. Neurol.,* 409, 261-273.

Gao, W.-Q., Zheng, J. L., Lewis, A. K., Frantz, G. 1999. Heregulin promotes regenerative proliferation in rat utricular sensory epithelium following ototoxic damage and influences hair cell differentiation during development. *Assoc. Res. Otolaryngol. Abstr.,* 22, 896.

Garcia-Torres, R., Orozco, L. 1993. Alport-leiomyomatosis syndrome: an update. *Am. J. Kidney Dis.,* 22, 641-648.

Gardi, J. N., Bledsoe, S. C. 1981. The use of kainic acid for studying the origins of scalp-recorded auditory brainstem responses in the guinea pig. *Neurosci. Lett.,* 26, 143-149.

Gardner, S. M., Trussell, L. O., Oertel, D. 1999 Time course and permeation of synaptic AMPA receptors in cochlear nuclear neurons correlate with input. *J. Neurosci.,* 19, 8721-8729.

Garssen, J., Van Loveren, H., Kato, K., Askenase, P. W. 1994. Antigen receptors on Thy-1+ CD3- CS-initiating cell. *In vitro* desensitization with hapten-amino acid or hapten-Ficoll conjugates, versus hapten-protein conjugates, suggests different antigen receptors on the immune cells that mediate the early and late components of murine contact sensitivity. *J. Immunol.,* 153, 32-44.

Gaskill, S. A., Brown, A. M. 1990. The behavior of the acoustic distortion product $2f_1 - f_2$, from the human ear and its relation to auditory sensitivity. *J. Acoust. Soc. Am.,* 88, 821-839.

Gasparini, P., De Fazio, A., Croce, A. I., Stanziale, P., Zelante, L. 1998. Usher syndrome type III (USH3) linked to chromosome 3q in an Italian family. *J. Med. Genet.,* 35, 666-667.

Gates, G. R., Saunders, J. C., Bock, G. R., Aitkin, L. M., Elliot, M. A. 1974. Peripheral auditory function in the platypus (*Ornithorhynchus anathinus*). *J. Acoust. Soc. Am.,* 56, 152-156.

Gates, W. H. 1929. Linkage of the characters albinism and shaker in the house mouse. *Anat. Rec.,* 41, 104.

Gaunt, S. J., Blum, M., De Robertis, E. M. 1993. Expression of the mouse goosecoid gene during mid-embryogenesis may mark mesenchymal cell lineages in the developing head, limbs and body wall. *Devel.,* 117, 769-778.

Gavalas, A., Studer, M., Lumsden, A., Rijli, F. M., Krumlauf, R., Chambon, P. 1998. Hoxa1 and Hoxb1 synergize in patterning the hindbrain, cranial nerves and second pharyngeal arch *Devel.,* 125, 1123-1136.

Geisler, D. C. 1998. *From Sound to Synapse.* Oxford Press, New York.

Geppert, M., Bolshakov, V., Siegelbaum, S., Takei, K., Camilli, P., Hammer, R., Sudhof, T. 1994. The role of Rab3A in neurotransmitter release. *Nature,* 369, 493-497.

Geppert, M., Goda, Y., Stevens, C., Sudhof, T. 1997. The small GTP-binding protein Rab3A regulates a late step in synaptic vesicle fusion. *Nature,* 387, 810-814.

German, D. C., Ng, M. C., Liang, C. L., McMahon, A., Iacopino, A.M. 1997. Calbindin-D28k in nerve cells. *Neuroscience,* 81, 735-743.

Gern, L., Rais, O., Capiau, C., Hauser, P., Lobet, Y., Simoen, E., Voet, P., Petre, J. 1994. Immunization of mice by recombinant OspA preparations and protection against *Borrelia burgdorferi* infection induced by *Ixodes ricinus* tick bites. *Immunol. Lett.,* 39, 249-258.

Gerrard, R. L., Ison, J. R. 1990. Relative tonal frequency and the modulation of the acoustic startle reflex by background noise. *J. Exp. Psychol.: Anim. Behav. Processes,* 16, 106-112.

Gershenfeld, H. K., Neumann, P. E., Mathis, C., Crawley, J. N., Li, X., Paul, S. M. 1997. Mapping quantitative trait loci for open-field behavior in mice. *Behav. Genet.,* 27, 201-210.

Geyer, M. A. 1999. Assessing prepulse inhibition of startle in wild-type and knockout mice. *Psychopharmacology,* 147, 11-13.

Ghosh, A., Greenberg, M. E. 1995. Calcium signaling in neurons: molecular mechanisms and cellular consequences. *Science,* 268: 239-247.

Ghoshal, S., Kim, D. O. 1997. Marginal shell of the anteroventral cochlear nucleus: single-unit response properties in the unanesthetized decerebrate cat. *J. Neurophysiol.,* 77, 2083-2097.

Ghoshal, K., Majumder, S., Li, Z., Bray, T. M., Jacob, S. T. 1999. Transcriptional induction of metallothionein-I and -II genes in the livers of Cu,Zn-superoxide dismutase knockout mice. *Biochem. Biophys. Res. Commun.,* 264, 735-742.

Gibson, F., Walsh, J., Mburu, P., Varela, A., Brown, K. A., Antonio, M., Beisel, K. W., Steel, K. P., Brown, S. D. 1995. A type VII myosin encoded by the mouse deafness gene shaker-1. *Nature,* 374, 62-64.

Giebink, G. S. 1989. The microbiology of otitis media. *Ped. Infect. Dis. J.,* 8, S18-20.

Gieselman, V. 1995. Lysosomal storage diseases. *Biochem. Biophys. Act.,* 1270, 103-136.

Gil-Loyzaga, P., Menoyo Bueno, A., Poch Broto, J., Merchan Perez, A. 1990. Effects of perinatal hypothyroidism in the carbohydrate composition of cochlear tectorial membrane. *Hear. Res.,* 45, 151-156.

Gillespie, P. G. 1996. Feeling force: mechanical transduction by vertebrates and invertebrates. *Chem. Biol.,* 3, 223-227.

Gillingsgrud, E. O., Krivit W., Summers C. G. 1998. Ocular abnormalities in the mucopolysaccharidoses after bone marrow transplantation: longer follow-up. *Ophthalmology,* 105, 1099-1104.

Gimenez-Gallego, G., Conn, G., Hatcher, V. B., Thomas, K. A. 1986. Human brain derived acidic and basic fibroblast growth factors: amino terminal sequences and specific mitogenic activities. *Biochem. Biophys. Res. Commun.,* 135, 541-548.

Ginzberg, R. D., Morest, D. K. 1983. A study of cochlear innervation in the young cat with the Golgi method. *Hear. Res.,* 10, 227-246.

Ginzberg, R. D., Morest, D. K. 1984. Fine structure of cochlear innervation in the cat. *Hear. Res.,* 14, 109-127.

Glass, D. J., Nye, S. H., Hantzopoulos, P. 1991. Trk B mediates BDNF/NT-3 dependent survival and proliferation in fibroblasts lacking the low affinity NGF receptor. *Cell,* 66, 405-413.

Glasscock, M. E. D. 1973. The stapes gusher. *Arch. Otolaryngol.,* 98, 82-91.

Glendenning, K. K., Masterton, R. B. 1998. Comparative morphometry of mammalian central auditory systems: variation in nuclei and form of the ascending system. *Brain Behav. Evol.,* 51, 59-89.

Glowa, J. R., Hansen, C. T. 1994. Differences in response to an acoustic startle stimulus among forty-six rat strains. *Behav. Genet.,* 241, 79-84.

Goddard, J. M., Rossel, M., Manley, N. R., Capecchi, M. R. 1996. Mice with targeted disruption of Hoxb-1 fail to form the motor nucleus of the VIIth nerve. *Devel.,* 122, 3217-3228.

Godfrey, D. A., Kiang, N. Y. S., Norris, B. E. 1975. Single unit activity in the posteroventral cochlear nucleus of the cat. *J. Comp. Neurol.,* 162, 247-268.

Goffinet, A. M. 1984. Events governing organization of postmigratory neurons: studies on brain development in normal and reeler mice. *Brain Res.,* 19, 261-296.

Goffinet, A. M. 1995. Developmental neurobiology. A real gene for reeler [news, comment] *Nature,* 374, 675-676.

Gold, J. I, Knudsen, E. I. 2000. Abnormal auditory experience induces frequency-specific adjustments in unit tuning for binaural localization cues in the optic tectum of juvenile owls. *J. Neurosci.,* 20, 862-867.

Golding, N. L., Ferragamo, M. J., Oertel, D. 1999. Role of intrinsic conductances underlying responses to transients in octopus cells of the cochlear nucleus. *J. Neurosci.,* 19, 2897-2905.

Golding, N. L., Oertel, D. 1996. Context-dependent synaptic action of glycinergic and GABAergic inputs in the dorsal cochlear nucleus. *J. Neurosci.,* 16, 2208-2219.

Golding, N. L., Oertel, D. 1997. Physiological identification of the targets of cartwheel cells in the dorsal cochlear nucleus. *J. Neurophysiol.,* 78, 248-260.

Golding, N. L., Robertson, D., Oertel, D. 1995. Recordings from slices indicate that octopus cells of the cochlear nucleus detect coincident firing of auditory nerve fibers with temporal precision. *J. Neurosci.,* 15, 3138-3153.

Goldman, D., Lister, R. G., Crabbe, J. C. 1987. Mapping of a putative genetic locus determining ethanol intake in the mouse. *Brain Res.,* 420, 220-226.

Gonzalez-Hernandez, T. H., Meter, G., Ferres-Torres, R., Castaneyra-Perdomo, A, del Mar Perez Delgado, M. 1987. Afferent connections of the inferior colliculus in the albino mouse. *J. Hirnforsch,* 28, 315-323.

Gora-Maslak, G., McLearn, G. E., Crabbe, J. C., Phillips, T. J., Belknap, J. K., Plomin, R. 1991. Use of recombinant inbred strains to identify quantitative trait loci in psychopharmacology. *Psychopharmacology,* 104, 413-424.

Gorlin, R. J. 1995. Genetic hearing loss associated with endocrine and metabolic disorders. In Gorlin, R. J., Toriello, H. V., Cohen, M. M. (Eds.), *Hereditary Hearing Loss and Its Syndromes.* Oxford University Press, New York, 318-354.

Gosepath, K., Gath, I., Maurer, J., Pollock, J. S., Amedee, R., Forstermann, U., Mann, W. 1997. Characterization of nitric oxide synthase isoforms expressed in different structures of the guinea pig cochlea. *Brain Res.,* 747, 26-33.

Gospodarowicz, D. 1974. Localization of a fibroblast growth factor and its effect alone and with hydrocortisone on 3T3 cell growth. *Nature,* 249, 123-127.

Gospodarowicz, D., Cheng, J., Lui, G. M., Baird, A., Bohlen, P. 1984. Isolation of brain fibroblast growth factor by heparin-Sepharose affinity chromatography: identity with pituitary fibroblast growth factor. *Proc. Natl. Acad. Sci. USA,* 81, 6963-6967.

Gospodarowicz, D., Neufeld, G., Schweigerer, L. 1987. Fibroblast growth factor: structural and biological properties. *J. Cell. Physiol. (Suppl.),* 5, 15-26.

Gotz, R., Koster, R., Winkler, C. 1994. Neurotrophin-6 is a new member of the nerve growth factor family. *Nature,* 372, 266-269.

Govan, J. A. 1983. Ocular manifestations of Alport's syndrome: a hereditary disorder of basement membranes? *Br. J. Ophthalmol.,* 67, 493-503.

Gowan, J. W. 1963. Genetics of infectious diseases. In Burdette, W. J. (Ed.), *Methodology in Mammalian Genetics.* Holden-Day, San Francisco, 383-404.

Graf, R. A., Cooke, I. M. 1994. Outgrowth morphology and intracellular calcium of crustacean neurons displaying distinct morphologies in primary culture. *J. Neurobiol.,* 25, 1558-1569.

Green, E. 1999. The human genome project and its impact on the study of human disease. 8th ed. In Scriver, C. R., Beaudet, A. L., Sly, W. S., Valle, D., Childs, B., Vogelstein, B. (Eds.), *Metabolic and Molecular Bases of Inherited Disease.*

Greenwood, D. D. 1990. A cochlear frequency-position function for several species — 29 years later. *J. Acoust. Soc. Am.,* 87, 2592-2604.

Greybeal, A., Rosowski, J. J., Keten, D. R., Crompton, A. W. 1989. Inner-ear structure of *Morganucodon,* an early Jurassic mammal. *Zool. J. Linnean Soc.,* 96, 107-117.

Griffith, A., Friedman, T. B. 1999. Making sense out of sound. *Nat. Genet.,* 21, 347-349.

Grillon, C., Ameli, R., Charney, D. S., Krystal, J., Braff, D. 1992. Startle gating deficits occur across prepulse intensities in schizophrenic patients. *Biol. Psych.,* 32, 939-943.

Gruneberg, H. 1952. *The Genetics of the Mouse,* 2nd ed. Martinus Nijhoff, The Hague, The Netherlands.

Gruneberg, H. 1956. Hereditary lesions of the labyrinth in the mouse. *Br. Med. Bull.,* 12, 153-157.

Gruneberg, H., Hallpike, C. S., Ledoux, A. 1940. Observations on the structure, development and electrical reactions of the internal ear of the shaker-1 mouse (*Mus musculus*). *Proc. R. Soc. Lond. B. Biol. Sci.,* 129, 154-173.

Grunfeld, J. P., Grateau, G., Noel, L. H., Charbonneau, R., Gubler, M. C., Savage, C. O., Lockwood, C. M. 1987. Variants of Alport's syndrome. *Pediatr. Nephrol.,* 1, 419-421.

Gu, X. X., Chen, J., Gang, W. 1999. Development of conjugate vaccines against *Moraxella catarrhalis. Seventh International Symposium on Recent Advances in Otitis Media,* June 1–5, Fort Lauderdale, FL, 109.

Gu, X. X., Chen, J., Barenkamp, S. J., Robbins, J. B., Tsai, C. M., Lim, D. J., Battey, J. 1998. Synthesis and characterization of lipooligosaccharide-based conjugates as vaccine candidates for *Moraxella (Branhamella) catarrhalis. Infect. Immunol.,* 66, 1891-1897.

Gu, X. X., Tsai, C. M., Ueyama, T., Barenkamp, S. J., Robbins, J. B., Lim, D. J. 1996. Synthesis, characterization, and immunologic properties of detoxified lipooligosaccharide from nontypeable *Haemophilus influenzae* conjugated to proteins. *Infect. Immunol.,* 64, 4047-4053.

Gubler, M. C., Knebelmann, B., Beziau, A., Broyer, M., Pirson, Y., Haddoum, F., Kleppel, M. M., Antignac, C. 1995. Autosomal recessive Alport syndrome: immunohistochemical study of type IV collagen chain distribution. *Kidney Int.,* 47, 1142-1147.

Gubler, M. C., Levy, M., Naizot, C., Habib, R. 1980. Glomerular basement membrane changes in hereditary glomerular diseases. *Ren. Physiol.,* 3, 405-413.

Guilford, P., Ayadi, H., Blanchard, S., Chaib, H., Le Paslier, D., Weissenbach, J., Drira, M., Petit, C. 1994. A human gene responsible for neurosensory, non-syndromic recessive deafness is a candidate homologue of the mouse sh-1 gene. *Hum. Molec. Genet.,* 3, 989-993.

Gunwar, S., Ballester, F., Kalluri, R., Timoneda, J., Chonko, A. M., Edwards, S. J., Noelken, M. E., Hudson, B. G. 1991. Glomerular basement membrane. Identification of dimeric subunits of the noncollagenous domain (hexamer) of collagen IV and the Goodpasture antigen. *J. Biol. Chem.*, 266, 15318-15324.

Gunwar, S., Ballester, F., Noelken, M. E., Sado, Y., Ninomiya, Y., Hudson, B. G. 1998. Glomerular basement membrane. Identification of a novel disulfide-cross-linked network of alpha3, alpha4, and alpha5 chains of type IV collagen and its implications for the pathogenesis of Alport syndrome. *J. Biol. Chem.*, 273, 8767-8775.

Guo, C., Van Damme, B., Vanrenterghem, Y., Devriendt, K., Cassiman, J. J., Marynen, P. 1995. Severe alport phenotype in a woman with two missense mutations in the same COL4A5 gene and preponderant inactivation of the X chromosome carrying the normal allele. *J. Clin. Invest.*, 95, 1832-1837.

Guo, C., Van Damme, B., Damme-Lombaerts, R., Van den, B. H., Cassiman, J. J., Marynen, P. 1993. Differential splicing of COL4A5 mRNA in kidney and white blood cells: a complex mutation in the COL4A5 gene of an Alport patient deletes the NC1 domain. *Kidney Int.*, 44, 1316-1321.

Gurney, M. E. 1997a. Transgenic animal models of familial amyotrophic lateral sclerosis. *J. Neurol.*, 244(Suppl. 2), S15-20.

Gurney, M. E. 1997b. The use of transgenic mouse models of amyotrophic lateral sclerosis in preclinical drug studies. *J. Neurol. Sci.*, 152(Suppl. 1), S67-73.

Gurney, M. E., Pu, H., Chiu, A. Y., Dal Canto, M. C., Polchow, C. Y., Alexander, D. D., Caliendo, J., Hentati, A., Kwon, Y. W., Deng, H. X., et al. 1994. Motor neuron degeneration in mice that express a human Cu,Zn superoxide dismutase mutation. *Science*, 264, 1772-1775.

Gutierrez, C., Cusick, C. G. 1994. Effects of chronic monocular enucleation on calcium binding proteins calbindin-D28k and parvalbumin in the lateral geniculate nucleus of adult rhesus monkeys. *Brain. Res.*, 651, 300-310.

Gutteridge, J. M. C., Halliwell, B. 1999. Antioxidant protection and oxygen radical signaling. In Gilbert, D. L., Colton, C. L. (Eds.), *Reactive Oxygen Species in Biological Systems: An Interdisciplinary Approach.* Kluwer Academic/Plenum Publishers, New York, 189-218.

Gutwald, J., Goebeler, M., Sorg, C. 1991. Neuropeptides enhance irritant and allergic contact dermatitis. *J. Invest. Derm.*, 96, 695-698.

Haack, B., Markl, H., Ehret, G. 1983. Sound communication between parents and offspring. In Willott, J. F. (Ed.), *The Auditory Psychobiology of the Mouse.* Charles C. Thomas, Springfield, IL, 57-97.

Habib, R., Gubler, M. C., Hinglais, N., Noel, L. H., Droz, D., Levy, M., Mahieu, P., Foidart, J. M., Perrin, D., Bois, E., Grunfeld, J. P. 1982. Alport's syndrome: experience at Hopital Necker. *Kidney Int. (Suppl.)* 11, S20-S28.

Hack, M. H. 1968. The development of the Preyer reflex in the shaker-1 mouse. *J. Aud. Res.*, 8, 391-418.

Hackney, C. M., Furness, D. N., Sayers, D. L. 1988. Stereociliary cross-links between adjacent inner hair cells. *Hear. Res.*, 34, 207-212.

Hackney, C. M., Furness, D. N. 1995. Mechanotransduction in vertebrate hair cells: structure and function of the stereociliary bundle. *Am. J. Physiol.*, 268, C1-13.

Hackney, C. M., Osen, K. K., Kolston, J. 1990. Anatomy of the cochlear nuclear complex of guinea pig. *Anat. Embryol.*, 182,123-149.

Hackney, C. M., Furness, D. N., Benos, D. J. 1991. Localisation of putative mechanoelectrical transducer channels in cochlear hair cells by immunoelectron microscopy. *Scan. Microsc.*, 5, 741-746.

Hadrys, T., Braun, T., Rinkwitz-Brandt, S., Arnold, H. H., Bober, E. 1998. Nkx5-1 controls semicircular canal formation in the mouse inner ear. *Devel.*, 125, 33-39.

Hafidi, A., Romand, R. 1989. First appearance of type II neurons during ontogenesis in the spiral ganglion of the rat. An immunocytochemical study. *Devel. Brain Res.*, 48, 143-149.

Hagiwara, H., Tamagawa, Y., Kitamura, K., Kodera, K. 1998. A new mutation in the POU3F4 gene in a Japanese family with X-linked mixed deafness (DFN3). *Laryngoscope*, 108, 1544-1547.

Halbook, F., Ibanez, C. F., Persson, H. 1991. Evolutionary studies of the nerve growth factor family reveal a novel member abundantly expressed in Xenopus ovary. *Neuron*, 6, 845-858.

Haldi, M. L., Strickland, C., Lim, P., VanBerkel, V., Chen, X., Noya, D., Korenberg, J. R., Husain, Z., Miller, J., Lander, E. S. 1996. A comprehensive large-insert yeast artificial chromosome library for physical mapping of the mouse genome. *Mam. Genome*, 7, 767-769.

Halliwell, B. 1992. Reactive oxygen species and the central nervous system. *J. Neurochem.*, 59, 1609-1623.

Halliwell, B., Gutteridge, J. M. C. 1999. *Free Radicals in Biology and Medicine.* Oxford University Press, Oxford.

Halliwell, B., Gutteridge, J. M., Cross, C. E. 1992. Free radicals, antioxidants, and human disease: where are we now? *J. Lab. Clin. Med.,* 119, 598-620.

Hamburger, V. 1934. The effects of wing bud extirpation on the development of the central nervous system in chick embryos. *J. Exp. Zool.,* 68, 449-494.

Hamilton, B. A., Frankel, W. N., Kerrebrock, A. W., Hawkins, T. L., FitzHugh, W., Kusumi, K., Russell, L. B., Mueller, K. L., van Berkel, V., Birren, B. W., Kruglyak, L., Lander, E. S. 1996. Disruption of the nuclear hormone receptor RORalpha in staggerer mice [published erratum appears in *Nature,* 381, 346, 1996]. *Nature,* 379, 736-739.

Hammerberg, C., Duraiswamy, N., Cooper, K. D. 1994. Active induction of unresponsiveness (tolerance) to DNFB by *in vivo* ultraviolet-exposed epidermal cells is dependent upon infiltrating class II MHC+ CD11bbright monocytic/macrophagic cells. *J. Immunol.,* 153, 4915-4924.

Han, V. K. M., Lauder, J. M., D'Ercole, J. 1987. Characterization of somatomedin/insulin like growth factor receptors and correlation with biologic action in cultured neonatal rat astroglial cells. *J. Neurosci.,* 7, 505-511.

Handwerger, B. S., Storrer, C. E., Wasson, C. S., Movafagh, F., Reichlin, M. 1999. Further characterization of the autoantibody response of Palmerston North mice. *J. Clin. Immunol.,* 19, 45-57.

Harada, T., Juhn, S. K., Kim, Y., Sakakura, Y. 2000. Immunohistochemical localization of collagen types I, III, and IV, laminin, fibronectin, and keratin in the endolymphatic sac. *Ann. Otol. Rhinol. Laryngol.,* 109, 180-186.

Harper, S., Davies, A. M. 1990. NGF mRNA expression in developing cutaneous epithelium related to innervation density. *Devel.,* 110, 515-519.

Harper, J. W., Elledge, S. J. 1996. Cdk inhibitors in development and cancer. *Curr. Opin. Genet. Devel.,* 6, 56-64.

Harris, J. P., Ryan, A. F. 1995. Fundamental immune mechanisms of the brain and inner ear. *Otolaryngol. Head Neck Surg.,* 112, 639-653.

Harris, J. P., Woolf, N. K., Ryan, A. F. 1986. A reexamination of experimental type II collagen autoimmunity: middle and inner ear morphology and function. *Ann. Otol. Rhinol. Laryngol.,* 95, 176-180.

Harrison, D. E., Archer, J. R. 1983. Physiological assays for biological age in mice: relationship of collagen, renal function, and longevity. *Exp. Aging Res.,* 9, 245-251.

Harrison, J. M, Irving, R. 1965 The anterior ventral cochlear nucleus. *J. Comp. Neurol.,* 124, 15-41.

Harrison, J. M., Irving, R. 1966. The organization of the posterior ventral cochlear nucleus in the rat. *J. Comp. Neurol.,* 126, 391-401.

Hart, B. L., Leedy, M. G. 1985. Neurological basis of male sexual behavior. In Adler, N., Pfaff, D., Goy, R. W. (Eds.), *Handbook of Behavioral Neurobiology,* Vol. 7, Reproduction. Plenum Press, New York, 373-422.

Haselbeck, R. J., Duester, G. 1998. ADH4-lacZ transgenic mouse reveals alcohol dehydrogenase localization in embryonic midbrain/hindbrain, otic vesicles, and mesencephalic, trigeminal, facial, and olfactory neural crest. *Alc. Clin Exp. Res.,* 22, 1607-1613.

Hashimoto, S., Kimura, R. S., Takasaka, T. 1990. Computer-aided three dimensional reconstruction of the inner hair cells and their nerve endings in the guinea pig cochlea. *Acta Otolaryngol.,* 109, 228-234.

Hashitani, H., Windle, A., Suzuki, H. 1998. Neuroeffector transmission in arterioles of the guinea-pig choroid. *J. Physiol. (London),* 510(Pt 1), 209-223.

Hasson, T. 1999. Sensing a function for myosin-VIIa. *Curr. Biol.,* 9, R838-R841.

Hasson, T., Gillespie, P. G., Garcia, J. A., MacDonald, R. B., Zhao, Y., Yee, A. G., Mooseker, M. S., Corey, D. P. 1997a. Unconventional myosins in inner-ear sensory epithelia. *J. Cell Biol.,* 137, 1287-1307.

Hasson, T., Heintzelman, M. B., Santos-Sacchi, J., Corey, D. P., Mooseker, M. S. 1995. Expression in cochlea and retina of myosin VIIa, the gene product defective in Usher syndrome type 1B. *Proc. Natl. Acad. Sci. USA,* 92, 9815-9819.

Hasson, T., Mooseker, M. S. 1997. The growing family of myosin motors and their role in neurons and sensory cells. *Curr. Opin. Neurobiol.,* 7, 615-623.

Hasson, T., Walsh, J., Cable, J., Mooseker, M. S., Brown, S. D., Steel, K. P. 1997b. Effects of shaker-1 mutations on myosin-VIIa protein and mRNA expression. *Cell Motil. Cytoskel.,* 37, 127-138.

Haupt, H., Scheibe, F., Ludwing, C., Petzold. D, 1991. Measurements of perilymphatic oxygen tension in guinea pigs exposed to loud sound. *Eur. Arch. Otorhinolaryngol.,* 248, 413-416.

Hausler, A., Persoz, C., Buser, R., Mondadori, C., Bhatnagar, A. 1992. Adrenalectomy, corticosteroid replacement and their importance for drug-induced memory-enhancement in mice. *J. Ster. Biochem. Molec. Biol.,* 41, 785-789.

Hawkins, J. E., Jr. 1971. The role of vasoconstriction in noise-induced hearing loss. *Ann. Otol. Rhinol. Laryngol.*, 80, 903-913.

Hayes, E., Babin R. Platz C. 1980. The otologic manifestations of mucopolysaccharidoses. *Am. J. Otol.*, 2, 65-69.

He, D. Z. Z. 1997. Relationship between the development of outer hair cell electromotility and efferent innervation: a study of cultured organ of Corti of neonatal gerbils. *J. Neurosci.*, 17, 3634-3643.

He, D. Z. Z., Evans, B. N, Dallos, P. 1994. First appearance and development of electromotility in neonatal gerbil outer hair cells. *Hear. Res.*, 78, 77-90.

He, H. J., Schmiedt, R. A. 1993. Fine structure of the $2f_1$-f_2 acoustic distortion product: changes with primary level. *J. Acoust. Soc. Am.*, 94, 2659-2669.

Hébert, R., Langlois, J.-M., Dussault, J. H. 1985a. Effect of graded periods of congenital hypothyroidism on the peripheral auditory evoked activity of rats. *Electroenceph. Clin. Neurophysiol.*, 62, 381-387.

Hébert, R., Langlois, J.-M., Dussault, J. H. 1985b. Permanent defects in rat peripheral auditory function following perinatal hypothyroidism: Determination of a critical period. *Devel. Brain Res.*, 23, 161-170.

Heckenlively, J. R., Chang, B., Erway, L. C., Peng, C., Hawes, N. L., Hageman, G. S., Roderick, T. H. 1995. Mouse model for Usher syndrome: linkage mapping suggests homology to Usher type I reported at human chromosome 11p15. *Proc. Natl. Acad. Sci. USA*, 92, 11100-11104.

Hedgecock, E. M., Norris, C. R. 1997. Netrins evoke mixed reactions in motile cells. *Trends Genet.*, 13, 251-253.

Hefeneider, S. H., Brown, L. E., McCoy, S. L., Bakke, A. C., Cornell, K. A., Bennett, R. M. 1993. Immunization of BALB/c mice with a monoclonal anti-DNA antibody induces an anti-idiotypic antibody reactive with a cell-surface DNA binding protein. *Autoimmunology*, 15, 187-194.

Heffner, H. E., Heffner, R. S. 1986. Effect of unilateral and bilateral auditory cortex lesions on the discrimination of vocalizations by Japanese macaques. *J. Neurophysiol.*, 56, 683-701.

Heffner, H. E., Heffner, R. S. 1995. Conditioned avoidance. In Klump, G. M., Dooling, R. J., Fay, R. R., Stebbins, W. C. (Eds.), *Methods in Comparative Psychoacoustics*. Birkhäuser, Basel, 73-87.

Heffner, H. E. Heffner, R. S. 1998. Hearing. In Greenberg, G. and Haraway, M. M. (Eds.), *Comparative Psychology, A Handbook*. Garland, New York, 290-303.

Heffner, H. E., Masterton, B. 1980. Hearing in glires: domestic rabbit, cotton rat, feral house mouse, and kangaroo rat. *J. Acoust. Soc. Am.*, 68, 1584-1599.

Heffner, R. S., Heffner, H. E. 1983. Hearing in large mammals: Horses (*Equus caballus*) and cattle (*Bos taurus*). *Behav. Neurosci.*, 97, 299-309.

Heffner, R. S., Heffner, H. E. 1988a. Sound localization acuity in the cat: Effect of azimuth, signal duration, and test procedure. *Hear. Res.*, 36, 221-232.

Heffner, R. S., Heffner, H. E. 1988b. Sound localization and the use of binaural cues by the gerbil (*Meriones unguiculatus*). *Behav. Neurosci.*, 102, 422-428.

Heffner, R. S., Heffner, H. E. 1992a. Evolution of sound localization in mammals. In Popper, A. N., Fay, R. R., Webster, D. B. (Eds.). *The Evolutionary Biology of Hearing*. Springer-Verlag, New York, 290-303.

Heffner, R. S., Heffner, H. E. 1992b. Hearing in large mammals: sound-localization acuity in cattle (*Bos taurus*) and goats (*Capra hircus*). *J. Comp. Psychol.*, 106, 107-113.

Heffner, R. S., Heffner, H. E. 1992c. Visual factors in sound localization in mammals. *J. Comp. Neurol.*, 317, 219-232.

Heffner, R. S., Heffner, H. E., Kearns, D., Vogel, J., Koay, G. 1994. Sound localization in chinchillas. I. Left/right discriminations. *Hear. Res.*, 80, 247-257.

Heffner, R. S., Heffner, H. E., Koay, G. 1995. Sound localization in chinchillas. II. Front/back and vertical localization. *Hear. Res.*, 88, 190-198.

Hegarty J. L., Kay, A. R., Green, S. H. 1997. Trophic support of cultured spiral ganglion neurons by depolarization exceeds and is additive with that by neurotrophins or cAMP and requires elevation of [Ca2+]i within a set range. *J. Neurosci.*, 17, 1959-1970.

Heidet, L., Cohen-Solal, L., Boye, E., Thorner, P., Kemper, M. J., David, A., Larget, P. L., Zhou, J., Flinter, F., Zhang, X., Gubler, M. C., Antignac, C. 1997. Novel COL4A5/COL4A6 deletions and further characterization of the diffuse leiomyomatosis-Alport syndrome (DL-AS) locus define the DL critical region. *Cytogenet. Cell Genet.*, 78, 240-246.

Heidet, L., Dahan, K., Zhou, J., Xu, Z., Cochat, P., Gould, J. D., Leppig, K. A., Proesmans, W., Guyot, C., Guillot, M. 1995. Deletions of both alpha 5(IV) and alpha 6(IV) collagen genes in Alport syndrome and in Alport syndrome associated with smooth muscle tumours. *Hum. Molec. Genet.*, 4, 99-108.

Heiskari, N., Zhang, X., Zhou, J., Leinonen, A., Barker, D., Gregory, M., Atkin, C. L., Netzer, K. O., Weber, M., Reeders, S., Gronhagen-Riska, C., Neumann, H. P., Trembath, R., Tryggvason, K. 1996. Identification of 17 mutations in ten exons in the COL4A5 collagen gene, but no mutations found in four exons in COL4A6: a study of 250 patients with hematuria and suspected of having Alport syndrome. *J. Am. Soc. Nephrol.,* 7, 702-709.

Heitmann, J., Waldman, B., Schnitzler, H. U., Plinkert, P. K., Zenner, H.-P. 1998. Suppression of distortion product otoacoustic emissions near $2f_1-f_2$ removes DP-gram fine structure-Evidence for a secondary generator. *J. Acoust. Soc. Am.,* 103, 1527-1531.

Heizmann, C. W. 1984. Parvalbumin, an intracellular calcium-binding protein: distribution, properties and possible role in mammalian cells. *Experimentia,* 40, 910-921.

Heizmann, C. W., Berchtold, M. W. 1987. Expression of parvalbumin and other Ca^{2+}-binding proteins in normal and tumor cells: a topical review. *Cell Calcium,* 8, 1-41.

Heizmann, C. W., Braun, K., (Eds). 1995. *Calcium Regulation by Calcium-Binding Proteins in Nurodegenerative Disorders.* Springer-Verlag, Heidelberg, Germany.

Heizmann, C. W., Braun, K. 1992. Changes in Ca^{2+}-binding proteins in human neurodegenerative disorders. *Trends Neurosci.,* 15, 259-264.

Held, H. 1893. Die centrale Gehörleitung. *Arch. Anat. Physiol. Anat. Abt.,* 201-248.

Heldt, S. A., Falls, W. A. 1998. Destruction of the auditory thalamus disrupts the produciton of fear but not the inhibition of fear conditioned to an auditory stimulus. *Brain Res.,* 813, 274-282.

Heldt, S. A., Sundin, V., Willott, J. F., Falls, W. A. 2000. Post-training lesions of the amygdala interfere with fear-potentiated startle to both visual and auditory conditioned stimuli in C57BL/6J mice. *Behav. Neurosci.,* 114, 749-759.

Helfert, R. H., Sommer, T. J., Meeks, J., Hofstetter, P, Hughes, L. F. 1999. Age-related synaptic changes in the central nucleus of the inferior colliculus of Fischer-344 rats. *J. Comp. Neurol.,* 406, 285-298.

Helfgott, S. M., Mosciscki, R. A., San Martin, J., Lorenzo, C., Kieval, R., McKenna, M., Nadol, J., Trentham, D. E. 1991. Correlation between antibodies to type II collagen and treatment outcome in bilateral progressive sensorineural hearing loss. *Lancet,* 337, 387-389.

Hemond, S. G., Morest, D. K. 1991a. Ganglion formation from the otic placode and the otic crest in the chick embryo: mitosis, migration and the basal lamina. *Anat. Embryol.,* 184, 1-13.

Hemond, S. G., Morest, D. K. 1991b. Formation of the cochlea in the chicken embryo: sequence innervation and localization of basal lamina-associated molecules. *Devel. Brain Res.,* 61, 87-96.

Henderson, D., Subramaniam, M. Gratton, M. A. 1991. Impact noise: the importance of level, duration, and repetition rate. *J. Acoust. Soc. Am.,* 89, 1350-1357.

Henderson, D., Subramaniam, M., Henselman, L. W., Portalatini, P., Spongr, V. P. Sallustio, V. 1996a. Protection from continuous, impact or impulse noise provided by prior exposure to low level noise. In Axelsson, A., Borchgrevink, H. M., Hamernik, R. P., Hellström, P.-A., Henderson, D., Salvi, R. J. (Eds.), *Scientific Basis of Noise-Induced Hearing Loss.* Theime Medical Publishers, New York, 150-158.

Henderson, D., Subramaniam, M., Spongr, V., Attanasio, G. 1996b. Biological mechanisms for the "toughening" phenomenon. In Salvi, R. J., Henderson, D. H., Colletti, V., Fiorino, F. (Eds.), *Auditory Plasticity and Regeneration.* Theime Medical Publishers, New York, 143-154.

Henkemeyer, M., Marengere, L. E. M., McGlade, J., Olivier, J. P., Conlon, R. A., Holmyard, D. P., Letwin, K., Pawson, T. 1994. Immunolocalization of the Nuk receptor tyrosine kinase suggests roles in segmental patterning of the brain and axonogenesis. *Oncogene,* 9, 1001-1014.

Henry, C. J., Kouri, R. E. 1986. Chronic inhalation studies in mice. II. Effects of long-term exposure to 2R1 cigarette smoke on (C57BL/Cum x C3H/AnfCum)F1 mice. *J. Natl. Cancer Inst.,* 77, 203-212.

Henry, K. R. 1979a. Auditory nerve and brain stem volume-conducted potentials evoked by pure-tone pips in the CBA/J laboratory mouse. *Audiol.,* 18, 93-108.

Henry, K. R. 1979b. Auditory brainstem volume-conducted responses: origins in the laboratory mouse. *J. Am. Audiol. Soc.,* 4, 173-178.

Henry, K. R. 1982a. Age-related auditory loss and genetics: an electrocochleographic comparison of six inbred strains of mice. *J. Gerontol.,* 37, 275-282.

Henry, K. R. 1982b. Influence of genotype and age on noise-induced hearing loss. *Behav. Genet.,* 12, 563-573.

Henry, K. R. 1983. Ageing and audition. In Willott, J. F. (Ed.), *The Auditory Psychobiology of the Mouse.* Charles C. Thomas, Springfield, IL, 470-493.

Henry, K. R. 1992. Noise-induced auditory loss: influence of genotype, naloxone and methyl-prednisolone. *Acta Otolaryngol.,* 112, 599-603.

Henry, K. R., Buzzone, R. 1986. Auditory physiology and behavior in RB/1bg and RB/3bg, and their F1 hybrid mice (*Mus musculus*): influence of genetics, age, and acoustic variables on audiogenic seizure thresholds and cochlear functions. *J. Comp. Psychol.,* 100, 46-51.

Henry, K. R., Chole, R. A. 1980. Genotypic differences in behavioral, physiological and anatomical expressions of age-related hearing loss on the laboratory mouse. *Audiol.,* 19, 369-383.

Henry, K. R., Chole, R. A. 1987. Genetic and functional analysis of the otosclerosis-like condition of the LP/J mouse. *Audiol.,* 26, 44-55.

Henry, K. R., Haythorn, M. M. 1978. Effects of age and stimulus intensity on the far-field auditory brain stem potentials in the laboratory mouse. *Devel. Psychobiol.,* 11, 161-168.

Henry, K. R., Lepkowski, C. M. 1978. Evoked potential correlates of genetic progressive hearing loss. Age-related changes from the ear to the inferior colliculus of C57BL/6 and CBA/J mice. *Acta Otolaryngol.,* 86, 366-374.

Henry, K. R., McGinn, M. D., Carter, L. A., Savoska, E. A. 1992. Auditory brainstem function of the F1 offspring of the cross of CBA/CaJ and AU/SsJ inbred mice. *Audiol.,* 31, 190-195.

Hensen, V. (1863. Zur morphologie der schnedke des menschen und der saugetiere. *Z. Wiss. Zool.,* 13, 481-512.

Herr, W., Cleary, M. A. 1995. The POU domain: versatility in transcriptional regulation by a flexible two-in-one DNA-binding domain. *Genes Devel.,* 9, 1679-1693.

Herr, W., Sturm, R. A., Clerc, R. G., Corcoran, L. M., Baltimore, D., Sharp, P. A., Ingraham, H. A. et al. 1988. The POU domain: a large conserved region in the mammalian pit-1, oct-1, oct-2, and Caenorhabditis elegans unc-86 gene products. *Genes Devel.,* 2, 1513-1516.

Hertler, C. K., Trune, D. R. 1990. Otic capsule bony lesions in the Palmerston North autoimmune mouse. *Otolaryngol. Head Neck Surg.,* 103, 713-718.

Hertz, J. M., Heiskari, N., Zhou, J., Jensen, U. B., Tryggvason, K. 1995. A nonsense mutation in the COL4A5 collagen gene in a family with X-linked juvenile Alport syndrome. *Kidney Int.,* 47, 327-332.

Hertz, J. M., Kruse, T. A., Thomsen, A., Spencer, E. S. 1991. Multipoint linkage analysis in X-linked Alport syndrome. *Hum. Genet.,* 88, 157-161.

Hildesheimer, M., Henkin, Y., Muchnik, C., Anafi, R., Sahartov, E., Rubinstein, M. 1991. Sedation effect on temporary threshold shift induced by acoustic overstimulation. *Hear. Res.,* 51, 161-166.

Hilfer, S. R., Randolph, G. J. 1993. Immunolocalization of basal lamina components during development of chick otic and optic primordia. *Anat. Rec.,* 235, 443-452.

Hillerdal, M. 1987. Cochlear blood flow in the rat. A methodological evaluation of the microsphere method. *Hear. Res.,* 27, 27-35.

Hinglais, N., Grunfeld, J. P., Bois, E. 1972. Characteristic ultrastructural lesion of the glomerular basement membrane in progressive hereditary nephritis (Alport's syndrome). *Lab. Invest.,* 27, 473-487.

Hino, S., Takemura, T., Sado, Y., Kagawa, M., Oohashi, T., Ninomiya, Y., Yoshioka, K. 1996. Absence of alpha 6(IV) collagen in kidney and skin of X-linked Alport syndrome patients. *Pediatr. Nephrol.,* 10, 742-744.

Hinojosa, R. 1977. A note on the development of Corti's organ. *Acta. Otolaryngol.,* 84, 238-251.

Hirano, T., Kurono, Y., Ichimiya, I., Suzuki, M., Mogi, G. 1999. Effects of influenza A virus on lectin-binding patterns in murine nasopharyngeal mucosa and on bacterial colonization. *Otolaryngol. Head Neck Surg.,* 121, 616-621.

Hirsch, J. A., Oertel, D. 1988. Synaptic connections in the dorsal cochlear nucleus of mice, *in vitro. J. Physiol.,* (London), 396, 549-562.

Hisashi, K., Komune, S., Taira, T., Uemura, T., Sadoshima, S., Tsuda, H. 1993. Anticardiolipin antibody-induced sudden profound sensorineural hearing loss. *Am. J. Otolaryngol.,* 14, 275-277.

Hmani, M., Ghorbel, A., Boulila-Elgaied, A., Ben Zina, Z., Kammoun, W., Drira, M., Chaabouni, M., Petit, C., Ayadi, H. 1999. A novel locus for Usher syndrome type II, USH2B, maps to chromosome 3 at p23-24.2. *Eur. J. Hum. Genet.,* 7, 363-367.

Hodgkinson, C. A., Moore, K. J., Nakayama, A., Steingrimsson, E., Copeland, N. G., Jenkins, N. A., Arnheiter, H. 1993. Mutations at the mouse microphthalmia locus are associated with defects in a gene encoding a novel basic-helix-loop-helix-zipper protein. *Cell,* 74, 395-404.

Hofer, M. M., Barde, Y. A. 1988. Brain-derived neurotrophic factor prevents neuronal death *in-vivo. Nature,* 331, 261-262.

Hoffman, H. S., Fleshler, M. 1963. Startle reaction: modification by background acoustic stimulation. *Science,* 141, 928-930.

Hoffman, H. S., Fleshler, M. 1965. An apparatus for the measurement of the startle response in the rat. *Am. J. Psychol.,* 77, 307-308.

Hoffman, H. S., Ison, J. R. 1980. Principles of reflex modification in the domain of startle: I. Some empirical findings and their implications for the interpretation of how the nervous system processes sensory input. *Psychol. Rev.,* 87, 175-189.

Hoffman, H. S., Searle, J. L. 1965. Acoustic variables in the modification of the startle reaction in the rat. *J. Comp. Physiol. Psychol.,* 60, 53-58.

Hoffman, H. S., Searle, J. 1968. Acoustic and temporal factors in the evocation of startle. *J. Acoust. Soc. Am.,* 43, 269-282.

Hoffman, H. S., Stitt, C. L., Leitner, D. S. 1980. The optimum interpulse interval for inhibition of acoustic startle in the rat. *J. Acoust. Soc. Am.,* 68, 1218-1220.

Hoffman, H. S., Wible, B. L. 1969. Temporal parameters in startle facilitation by steady background signals. *J. Acoust. Soc. Am.,* 45, 7-12.

Hofstetter, K. M, Ehret, G. 1992. The auditory cortex of the mouse: connections of the ultrasonic field. *J. Comp. Neurol.,* 323, 370-386.

Hogan, B. L. 1996. Bone morphogenetic proteins: multifunctional regulators of vertebrate development. *Genes Devel.,* 10, 1580-1594.

Hogan, E., Ison, J. R. 2000. Temporal integration in the acoustic startle reflex in mice of different ages. *Assoc. Res. Otolaryng. Abstr.,* 23, 289.

Hohn, A., Leibrock, J., Bailey, K., Barde, Y. A. 1990. Identification and characterization of a novel member of the nerve growth factor/brain derived growth factor family. *Nature,* 344, 339-341.

Hokoc, J. N., Ventura, A. L. M., Gardino, P. F., De Mello, F. G. 1990. Developmental immunoreactivity for GABA and GAD in the avian retina: possible alternative pathway for GABA synthesis. *Brain Res.,* 532, 197-202.

Hokunan, K., Takahashi, M., Tomiyama, S. 1994. Alterations in the distributions of the basement membrane components after secondary inner ear immune reaction in guinea pigs. *Nippon Jibiinkoka Gakkai Kaiho,* 97, 226-232.

Holland S. J., Gale, N. W., Mbamalu, G., Yancopoulos, G. D., Henkemeyer, M., Pawson, T. 1996. Bidirectional signalling through the Eph-family receptor Nuk and its transmembrane ligands. *Nature,* 383, 722-725.

Holme, R. H., Steel, K. P. 1999. Genes involved in deafness. *Curr. Opin. Genet. Devel.,* 9, 309-314.

Hood, L. J. 1998. *Clinical Applications of the Auditory Brainstem Response.* Singular Publishing Group, San Diego.

Hood L. J, Berlin C. I, Allen, P. 1994. Cortical deafness: a longitudinal study. *J. Am. Acad. Audiol.,* 5, 330-342.

Hope, C. I., Bundey, S., Proops, D., Fielder, A. R. 1997. Usher syndrome in the city of Birmingham — prevalence and clinical classification. *Br. J. Ophthalmol.,* 81, 46-53.

Horn, J. M. 1974. Aggression as a component of relative fitness in four inbred strains of mice. *Behav. Genet.,* 4, 373-381.

Horner, K. C., Lenoir, M., Bock, G. R. 1985. Distortion product otoacoustic emission in hearing-imparied mutant mice. *J. Acoust. Soc. Am.,* 78, 1603-1611.

Hosoda, K., Hammer, R. E., Richardson, J. A., Baynash, A. G., Cheung, J. C., Giaid, A., Yanagisawa, M. 1994. Targeted and natural (piebald-lethal) mutations of endothelin-B receptor gene produce megacolon associated with spotted coat color in mice. *Cell,* 79, 1267-1276.

Hosokawa, Y., Sciancalepore, M., Stratta, F., Martina, M., Cherubini, E. 1994. Developmental changes in spontaneous $GABA_A$-mediated synaptic events in rat hippocampal CA3 neurons. *Eur. J. Neurosci.,* 6, 805-813.

Hostikka, S. L., Eddy, R. L., Byers, M. G., Hoyhtya, M., Shows, T. B., Tryggvason, K. 1990. Identification of a distinct type IV collagen alpha chain with restricted kidney distribution and assignment of its gene to the locus of X chromosome-linked Alport syndrome. *Proc. Natl. Acad. Sci. USA,* 87, 1606-1610.

Hotomi, M., Saito, T., Yamanaka, N. 1998. Specific mucosal immunity and enhanced nasopharyngeal clearance of nontypeable *Haemophilus influenzae* after intranasal immunization with outer membrane protein P6 and cholera toxin. *Vaccine,* 16, 1950-1956.

Hotomi, M., Yokoyama, M., Kuki, K., Yamamoto, R., Yamanaka, N. 1996. Induction of specific mucosal immunity by intranasal immunization of outer membrane protein P6 of *Haemophilus infuenzae* with the cholera toxin B subunit. In Lim, D. J., Bluestone, C. D., Casselbrant, M., Klein, J. O., Ogra, P. L. (Eds.), *Recent Advances in Otitis Media.* B. C. Decker, Hamilton, pp. 503-505.

Hou, T.-T., Johnson, J. D., Rall, J. A. 1991. Parvalbumin content and calcium and magnesium dissociation rates correlated with changes in relaxation rate of frog muscle fibers. *J. Physiol.*, 441, 285-304.

Hou, T.-T, Johnson, J. D., Rall, J. A. 1993. Role of parvalbumin in relaxation of frog skeletal muscle. In Sugi, H., Pollack, G. H. (Eds.), *Mechanism of Myofilament Sliding in Muscle Contraction*. Plenum Press, New York, 141-153.

Houseknect, C. R. 1968. Sonagraphic analyses of vocalizations of three species of mice. *J. Mammol.*, 49, 555-560.

Hoyle, G. W., Mercer, E. H., Palmiter, R. D., Brinster, R. L. 1993. Expression of NGF in sympathetic neurons leads to excessive axon outgrowth from ganglia but decreased terminal innervation within tissues. *Neuron*, 10, 1019-1034.

Hrabe de Angelis, M., McIntyre, J., Gossler, A. 1997. Maintenance of somite borders in mice requires the Delta homologue DlI1. *Nature*, 386, 717-721.

Hsu, L., Zhu, X.-N., Zhao, Y.-S. 1990. Immunoglobulin E and circulating immune complexes in endolymphatic hydrops. *Ann. Otol. Rhinol. Laryngol.*, 99, 535-538.

Hu, B. H., Zheng, X. Y., McFadden, S. L., Kopke, R. D., Henderson, D. 1997. R-phenylisopropyladenosine attenuates noise-induced hearing loss in the chinchilla. *Hear. Res.*, 113, 198-206.

Hu, X., Cao, S., Loh, H. H., Wei, L. N. 1999. Promoter activity of mouse kappa opioid receptor gene in transgenic mouse. *Molec. Brain Res.*, 69, 35-43.

Huang, C., Buchwald, J. 1978. Factors that affect the amplitudes and latencies of the vertex short latency acoustic responses in the cat. *Electroenceph. Clin. Neurophysiol.*, 44, 179-186.

Huang, J. M., Berlin, C. I., Lin, S. T., Keats, B. J. 1998. Low intensities and 1.3 ratio produce distortion product otoacoustic emissions which are larger in heterozygous (+/dn) than homozygous (+/+) mice. *Hear. Res.*, 117, 24-30.

Huang, J. M., Money, M. K., Berlin, C. I., Keats, B. J. 1995. Auditory phenotyping of heterozygous sound-responsive (+/dn) and deafness (dn/dn) mice. *Hear. Res.*, 88, 61-64.

Huang, J. M., Money, M. K., Berlin, C. I., Keats, B. J. 1996. Phenotypic patterns of distortion product otoacoustic emission in inbred and F1 hybrid hearing mouse strains. *Hear. Res.*, 98, 18-21.

Huangfu, M., Saunders, J. C. 1983. Auditory development in the mouse: structural maturation of the middle ear. *J. Morphol.*, 176, 249-259.

Hubel, D. H., Wiesel, T. N. 1963. Receptive fields, binocular interaction and functional architecture in the cat's visual cortex. *J. Physiol. (London)*, 160, 106-154.

Huck, S. 1983. Serum free medium for cultures of the postnatal mouse cerebellum: only insulin is essential. *Brain Res., Bull.*, 10, 667-674.

Hudson, B. G., Reeders, S. T., Tryggvason, K. 1993. Type IV collagen: structure, gene organization, and role in human diseases. Molecular basis of Goodpasture and Alport syndromes and diffuse leiomyomatosis. *J. Biol. Chem.*, 268, 26033-26036.

Hulander, M., Wurst, W., Carlsson, P., Enerbeck, S. 1998. The winged helix transcription factor Fkh10 is required for normal development of the inner ear. *Nature Genet.*, 20, 374-376.

Hultcrantz, M. 1995. Influence of prenatal irradiation on second generation mice. *Acta Otolaryngol.*, 115, 638-642.

Hulcrantz, M., Bagger-Sjoback D. 1996. Inner ear content of glycosaminoglycans as shown by monoclonal antibodies. *Acta Otolaryngol.*, 116, 25-32.

Hultcrantz, M., Spangberg, M. L. 1997. Pathology of the cochlea following a spontaneous mutation in DBA/2 mice. *Acta Otolaryngol.*, 117, 689-695.

Humason, G. L. 1972. *Animal Tissue Techniques*. W. H. Freeman, San Francisco.

Hunneyball, I. M., Crossley, M. J., Spowage, M. 1986. Pharmacological studies of antigen-induced arthritis in BALB/c mice. I. Characterization of the arthritis and the effect of steroidal and non-steroidal anti-inflammatory agents. *Agents Actions*, 18, 384-393.

Hunter, A. J., Nolan, P. M., Brown, S. D. 2000. Toward new models of disease and physiology in the neurosciences: the role of induced and naturally occurring mutations. *Hum. Molec. Genet.*, 9, 893-900.

Hunter, K. P., Willott, J. F. 1987. Aging and the auditory brainstem response in mice with severe or minimal prebyacusis. *Hear. Res.*, 30, 207-218.

Hunter-Duvar, I. M. 1978. Electron microscopic assessment of the cochlea. *Acta Otolaryngol. (Suppl.)*, 351, 3-23.

Hurd, L. B., Hutson, K. A., Morest, D. K. 1999. Cochlear nerve projections to the small cell shell of the cochlear nucleus: the neuroanatomy of extremely thin sensory axons. *Synapse*, 33, 83-117.

Hurst, D. S., Amin, K., Seveus, L., Venge, P. 1999. Evidence of mast cell activity in the middle ears of children with otitis media with effusion. *Laryngoscope*, 109, 471-477.

Husbands, J. M., Steinberg, S. A., Kurian, R., Saunders, J. C. 1999. Tip-link integrity on chick tall hair cell stereocillia following intense sound exposure. *Hear. Res.,* 135, 135-145.

Ichimiya, Y., Emson, P. C., Mountjoy, C. Q., Lawson, D. E. M., Heizmann, C. W. 1988. Loss of calbindin-D28k immunoreactive neurons from the cortex in Alzheimer-type dementia. *Brain Res.,* 475, 156-159.

Ichimiya, I., Kawauchi, H., Fujiyoshi, T., Tanaka, T., Mogi, G. 1991. Distribution of immunocompetent cells in normal nasal mucosa: comparisons among germ-free, specific pathogen-free, and conventional mice. *Ann. Otol. Rhinol. Laryngol.,* 100, 638-642.

Ichimiya, I., Kawauchi, H., Mogi, G. 1990. Analysis of immunocompetent cells in the middle ear mucosa. *Arch. Otolaryngol. Head Neck Surg.,* 116, 324-330.

Ichimiya, I., Kurono, Y., Hirano, T., Mogi, G. 1998. Changes in immunostaining of inner ears after antigen challenge into the scala tympani. *Laryngoscope,* 108, 585-591.

Ichimiya, I., Kurono, Y., Mogi, G. 1997. Immunological potential of the tympanic membrane. Observation under normal and inflammatory conditions. *Am. J. Otolaryngol.,* 18, 165-172.

Ichimiya, I., Suzuki, M., Hirano, T., Mogi, G. 1999. The influence of pneumococcal otitis media on the cochlear lateral wall. *Hear. Res.,* 131, 128-134.

Ichimiya, I., Suzuki, M., Mogi, G. 2000. Age-related changes in the murine cochlear lateral wall. *Hear. Res.,* 139, 116-122.

Ichimiya, I., Ueyama, S., Mogi, G. 1989. Experimental otitis media in mice. Immunohistochemical observations. *Acta Otolaryngol. (Suppl.),* 457, 148-153.

Idrizbegovic, E., Bogdanovic, N., Canlon, B. 1998. Modulating calbindin and parvalbumin immunoreactivity in the cochlear nucleus by moderate noise exposure in mice. A quantitative study on the dorsal and posteroventral cochlear nucleus. *Brain. Res.,* 800, 86-96.

Idrizbegovic, E., Bogdanovic, N., Canlon, B. 1999. Sound stimulation increases calcium-binding protein immunoreactivity in the inferior colliculus in mice. *Neurosci. Lett.,* 259, 49-52.

Ihrcke, N. S., Wrenshall, L. E., Lindman, B. J., Platt, J. L. 1993. Role of heparan sulfate in immune system-blood vessel interactions. *Immunol. Today,* 14, 500-505.

Ikeda, A., Zheng, Q. Y., Rosenstiel, P., Maddatu, T., Zuberi, A. R., Roopenian, D. C., North, M. A., Naggert, J. K., Johnson, K. R., Nishina, P. M. 1999. Genetic modification of hearing in tubby mice: evidence for the existence of a major gene (moth1) which protects tubby mice from hearing loss. *Hum. Molec. Genet.,* 8, 1761-1767.

Ikeda, M., Morgenstern, C. 1989. Immune response of the endolymphatic sac to horseradish peroxidase: immunologic route from the middle ear to the inner ear. *Ann. Otol. Rhinol. Laryngol.,* 98, 975-979.

Ikeda, S., Shiva, N., Ikeda, A., Smith, R. S., Nusinowitz, S., Yan, G., Lin, T. R., Chu, S., Heckenlively, J. R., North, M. A., Naggert, J. K., Nishina, P. M., Duyao, M. P. 2000. Retinal degeneration but not obesity is observed in null mutants of the tubby-like protein 1 gene. *Hum. Molec. Genet.,* 9, 155-163.

Ikeda, Y., Hotomi, M., Shimada, J., Suzumoto, M., Yamanaka, N., Green, B. 1999. Induction of specific mucousal immuity by intranasal application of recombinant outer membrane protein P6 mixed with cholera toxin. Presented at *Seventh International Symposium on Recent Advances in Otitis Media,* June 1–5, Fort Lauderdale, FL, 106.

Impagnatiello, F., Guidottti, A. R., Pesold, C., Dwivedi, Y., Caruncho, H., Pisu, M. G., Uzunov, D. P., Smalheiser, N. R., Davis, J. M., Pandey, G. N., Pappas, G. D., Tueting, P., Sharma, R. P., Costa, E. 1998. A decrease of reelin expression as a putative vulnerability factor in schizophrenia. *Proc. Natl. Acad. Sci. USA,* 95, 15718-15723.

Inoue, Y., Nishio, H., Shirakawa, T., Nakanishi, K., Nakamura, H., Sumino, K., Nishiyama, K., Iijima, K., Yoshikawa, N. 1999. Detection of mutations in the COL4A5 gene in over 90% of male patients with X-linked Alport's syndrome by RT-PCR and direct sequencing. *Am. J. Kidney Dis.,* 34, 854-862.

Ip, N. Y., Stitt, T. N., Tapley, P. 1993. Similarities and differences in the way neurotrophins interact with the trk receptors in neuronal and non-neuronal cells. *Neuron,* 10, 137-149.

Irvine, K. D. 1999. Fringe, Notch, and making developmental boundaries. *Curr. Opin. Genet. Devel.,* 9, 434-441.

Isaacson, J. S., Walmsley, B. 1995. Receptors underlying excitatory synaptic transmission in slices of the rat anteroventral cochlear nucleus. *J. Neurophysiol.,* 73, 964-973.

Ishii, T., Ishii, D., Balogh, K. 1968. Lysosomal enzymes in the inner ears of kanamycin-treated guinea pigs. *Acta-Otolaryngol.,* 65, 449-458.

Ison, J. R., Agrawal, P. 1998. The effect of spatial separation of signal and noise on masking in the free field as a function of signal frequency and age in the mouse. *J. Acoust. Soc. Am.,* 104, 1689-1695.

Ison, J. R., Agrawal, P., Pak, J., Vaughn, W. J. 1998. Changes in temporal acuity with age and with hearing impairment in the mouse: a study of the acoustic startle reflex and its inhibition by brief decrements in noise level. *J. Acoust. Soc. Am.,* 104, 1696-1804.

Ison, J. R. Bhullar, I., Castro, J., Hogan, E., Virag, T. 2000. Frequency-specific exaggeration of the acoustic startle reflex (ASR) and its modification in aging C57BL/6J mice with high-frequency hearing loss. *Assoc. Res. Otolaryng. Abstr.,* 23, 536.

Ison, J. R., Bhullar, I., Castro, J., O'Neill, W. E. 1999. Decay rates of excitation at noise offset as a function of age and hearing impairment in mouse models of presbycusis. *Soc. Neurosci. Abstr.,* 25, 33.

Ison, J. R., Bowen, G. P. 2000. Scopolamine reduces sensitivity to auditory gaps in the rat, suggesting a cholinergic contribution to temporal acuity. *Hear. Res.,* 145, 169-176.

Ison, J., Bowen, G. P., del Cerro, M. 1992. Impoverished stimulus input does not simulate the slowed visual kinetics of retinal damage. *Invest. Ophthalmol. Visual Sci.,* 33, 104-110.

Ison, J., Bowen, G. P., del Cerro, M. 1998b. A behavioral study of temporal processing and visual persistence in young and aged rats. *Behav. Neurosci.,* 112, 1273-1279.

Ison, J. R., Foss, J. A., Falcone, P., Sakovits, L., Adelson, A. A., Burton, R. I. 1986. Reflex modification: a method for assessing cutaneous dysfunction. *Percept. Psychophys.,* 40, 164-170.

Ison, J. R., Hammond, G. R. 1971. Modification of the startle reflex in the rat by changes in the auditory and visual environments. *J. Comp. Physiol. Psychol.,* 75, 435-452.

Ison, J. R., Hoffman, H. S. 1983. Reflex modification in the domain of startle: II. The anomalous history of a robust and ubiquitous phenomenon. *Psychol. Bull.,* 94, 3-17.

Ison, J. R., Krauter, E. E. 1975. Acoustic startle reflexes in the rat during consummatory behavior. *J. Comp. Physiol. Psychol.,* 89, 39-49.

Ison. J. R., McAdam, D. W., Hammond, G. R. 1973. Latency and amplitude changes in the acoustic startle reflex of the rat produced by variation in auditory prestimulation. *Physiol. Behav.,* 10, 1035-1039.

Ison, J. R., O'Connor, K., Bowen, G. P., Bocirnea, A. 1991. Temporal resolution of gaps in noise by the rat is lost with functional decortication. *Behav. Neurosci.,* 103, 33-40.

Ison, J. R., Payman, G. H., Palmer, M. J., Walton, J. P. 1997a. Nimodipine at a dose that slows ABR latencies does not protect the ear against noise. *Hear Res.,* 106, 179-183.

Ison, J. R., Pinckney, L. A. 1982. Reflex inhibition in humans: sensitivity to brief silent periods in white noise. *Percept. Psychophys.,* 34, 84-88.

Ison, J. R., Russo, J. M. 1990. Enhancement and depression of tactile and acoustic startle reflexes with variation in background noise level. *Psychobiology,* 18, 1, 96-100.

Ison, J. R., Sanes, J. R., Foss, J. A., Pinckney, L. A. 1990. Facilitation and inhibition of the human startle blink reflex by stimulus anticipation. *Behav. Neurosci.,* 104, 418-429.

Ison, J. R., Silverstein, L. 1978. Acoustic startle reactions, activity, and background noise intensity, before and after lesions of medial cortex in the rat. *Physiol. Psychol.,* 2, 245-248.

Ison, J. R., Taylor, M. K., Bowen, G. P., Schwarzkopf, S. B. 1997b. Facilitation and inhibition of the acoustic startle reflex in the rat after a momentary increase in background noise level. *Behav. Neurosci.,* 116, 1335-1352.

Itoh, K., Kamiya, H., Mitani, A., Yasui, Y., Takada, M., Mizuno, N. 1987. Direct projections from the dorsal column nuclei and the spinal trigeminal nuclei to the cochlear nuclei in the cat. *Brain Res.,* 400, 145-150.

Ivanova, A., Yuasa, S. 1998. Neural migration and differentiation in the development of the mouse dorsal cochlear nucleus. *Devel. Neurosci.,* 20, 495-511.

Iwahori, N. A. 1986. Golgi study on the dorsal nucleus of the lateral lemniscus in the mouse. *Neurosci. Res.,* 3, 196-212.

Iwai, H., Tomoda, K., Hosaka, N., Miyashima, S., Suzuka, Y., Ikeda, H., Lee, S., Inaba, M., Ikehara, S., Uamashita, T. 1998. Induction of immune-mediated hearing loss in SCID mice by injection of MRL/lpr mouse spleen cells. *Hear. Res.,* 117, 173-177.

Iwai, H., Tomoda, K., Inaba, M., Kubo, N., Tsujikawa, S., Ikehara, S., Yamashita, T. 1995. Evidence of cellular supplies to the endolymphatic sac from the systemic circulation. *Acta Otolaryngol.,* 115, 509-511.

Jackson Laboratory Database (www.informatics.jax.org/external/festing/mouse/docs).

Jacobs, M., Jeffrey, B., Kriss, A., Taylor, D., Sa, G., Barratt, T. M. 1992. Ophthalmologic assessment of young patients with Alport syndrome. *Ophthalmology,* 99, 1039-1044.

Jacobson, J., Murray, T., Deppe, U. 1987. The effects of ABR stimulus repetition rate in multiple sclerosis. *Ear Hear,* 8, 115-120.

Jacobson, R. D., Virag, L., Skene, J. H. P. 1986. A protein associated with axon growth, GAP-43, is widely distributed and developmentally regulated in rat CNS. *J. Neurosci.,* 6, 1843-1855.

Jacono, A. A., Hu, B., Kopke, R. D., Henderson, D., Van De Water, T. R., Steinman, H. M. 1998. Changes in cochlear antioxidant enzyme activity after sound conditioning and noise exposure in the chinchilla. *Hear. Res.,* 117, 31-38.

Jagger, C., Gallagher, A., Chambers, T., Pondel, M. 1999. The porcine calcitonin receptor promoter directs expression of a linked reporter gene in a tissue and developmental specific manner in transgenic mice. *Endocrinology,* 140, 492-499.

Jain, P. K., Lalwani, A. K., Li, X. C., Singleton, T. L., Smith, T. N., Chen, A., Deshmukh, D., Verma, I. C., Smith, R. J., Wilcox, E. R. 1998. A gene for recessive nonsyndromic sensorineural deafness (DFNB18) maps to the chromosomal region 11p14-p15.1 containing the Usher syndrome type 1C gene. *Genomics,* 50, 290-292.

Janecke, A. R., Meins, M., Sadeghi, M., Grundmann, K., Apfelstedt-Sylla, E., Zrenner, E., Rosenberg, T., Gal, A. 1999. Twelve novel myosin VIIA mutations in 34 patients with Usher syndrome type I: confirmation of genetic heterogeneity. *Hum. Mutat.,* 13, 133-140.

Jefferson, J. A., Lemmink, H. H., Hughes, A. E., Hill, C. M., Smeets, H. J., Doherty, C. C., Maxwell, A. P. 1997. Autosomal dominant Alport syndrome linked to the type IV collage alpha 3 and alpha 4 genes (COL4A3 and COL4A4). *Nephrol. Dial. Transpl.,* 12, 1595-1599.

Jerger, J. F., Oliver, T. A., Chmiel, R. A., Rivera, V. M. 1986. Patterns of auditory abnormality in multiple sclerosis. *Audiology,* 25, 193-209.

Jeskey, J., Willott, J. F. 2000. Modulation of prepulse inhibition in the DBA/2J mice by an augmented acoustic environment. *Behav. Neurosci.,* (in press).

Jewett, D. L. 1970. Volume-conducted potentials in response to auditory stimuli as detected by averaging in the cat. *Electroencephalogr. Clin. Neurophysiol.,* 28, 609-618.

Jewett, D. L., Romano, M. N. 1972. Neonatal development of auditory system potentials averaged from the scalp of rat and cat. *Brain Res.,* 36, 101-115.

Jiang, D., Palmer, A. R., Winter, I. M. 1996. The frequency extent of two-tone facilitation in onset units in the ventral cochlear nucleus. *J. Neurophysiol.,* 75, 380-395.

Jiang, R., Lan, Y., Chapman, H. D., Shawber, C., Norton, C. R., Serreze, D. V., Weinmaster, G., Gridley, T. 1998. Defects in limb, craniofacial, and thymic development in Jagged2 mutant mice. *Genes Devel.,* 12, 1046-1057.

Jiang, Z. G., Qiu, J., Ren, T., Nuttall, A. L. 1999. Membrane properties and the excitatory junction potentials in smooth muscle cells of cochlea spiral modiolar artery in guinea pigs. *Hear. Res.,* 138, 171-180.

Jimenez, A. M., Stagner, B. B., Martin, G. K., Lonsbury-Martin, B. L. 1999. Age-related loss of distortion product otoacoustic emissions in four mouse strains. *Hear. Res.,* 138, 91-105.

Joensuu, T., Blanco, G., Pakarinen, L., Sistonen, P., Kaariainen, H., Brown, S., Chapelle, A., Sankila, E. M. 1996. Refined mapping of the Usher syndrome type III locus on chromosome 3, exclusion of candidate genes, and identification of the putative mouse homologous region. *Genomics,* 38, 255-263.

Johansson, K., Ahn, H., Lindhagen, J., Lundgren, O. 1987. Tissue penetration and measuring depth of laser Doppler flowmetry in the gastrointestinal application. *Scand. J. Gastroenterol.,* 22, 1081-1088.

Johansson, K., Jakobsson, A., Lindahl, K., Lindhagen, J., Lundgren, O., Nilsson, G. E. 1991. Influence of fibre diameter and probe geometry on the measuring depth of laser Doppler flowmetry in the gastrointestinal application. *Int. J. Microcirc. Clin. Exper.,* 10, 219-229.

Johnson, A. C. 1993. The ototoxic effect of toluene and the influence of noise, acetyl salicylic acid, or genotype. A study in rats and mice. *Scand. Audiol.,* S39, 1-40.

Johnson, A. C. Canlon, B. 1994. Progressive hair cell loss induced by toluene exposure. *Hear. Res.,* 75, 201-208.

Johnson, A., Hawke, M. 1988. The non-auditory physiology of the external ear canal. In Jahn, A. F., Santos-Sacchi, J. (Eds.), *Physiology of the Ear.* Raven Press, New York, 41-58.

Johnson, D., Lanahan, A., Buck, C. R. 1986. Expression and structure of the human NGF receptor. *Cell,* 47, 545-554.

Johnson, K. R., Erway, L. C., Cook, S. A., Willott, J. F., Zheng, Q. Y. 1997. A major gene affecting age-related hearing loss in C57BL/6J mice. *Hear. Res.,* 114, 83-92.

Johnson, K. R., Zheng, Q. Y., Erway, L. C. 2000. A major gene affecting age-related hearing loss is common to at least ten inbred strains of mice. *Genomics,* 70, 171-180.

Johnson, M. D., Contrino, A., Contrino, J., Maxwell, K., Leonard, G., Kreutzer, D. 1994. Murine model of otitis media with effusion: immunohistochemical demonstration of IL-1 alpha antigen expression. *Laryngoscope,* 104, 1143-1149.

Johnson, M., Leonard, G., Kreutzer, D. L. 1997. Murine model of interleukin-8-induced otitis media. *Laryngoscope,* 107, 1405-1408.

Johnsson, L. G., Arenberg, I. K. 1981. Cochlear abnormalities in Alport's syndrome. *Arch. Otolaryngol.,* 107, 340-349.

Joliat, T., Seyer, J., Bernstein, J., Krug, M., Ye, X. J., Cho, J. S., Fujiyoshi, T., Yoo, T. J. 1992. Antibodies against a 30 kilodalton cochlear protein and type II and IX collagens in the serum of patients with inner ear diseases. *Ann. Otol. Rhinol. Laryngol.,* 101, 1000-1006.

Jones, D. B., Coulson, A. F., Duff, G. W. 1993. Sequence homologies between hsp60 and autoantigens. *Immunol. Today,* 14, 115-118.

Jones, D. G., Eslami, H. 1983. An ultrastructural study of the development of afferent and efferent synapses on outer hair cells of the guinea pig organ of Corti. *Cell Tissue Res.,* 231, 533-549.

Jones, E. G. 1985. *The Thalamus.* Plenum Press, New York.

Jones, E. G., Powell, T. P. S. 1969. Morphological variations in the dendritic spines of the neocortex. *J. Cell Sci.,* 5, 509-529.

Jones, K. R., Reichardt, L. F. 1990. Molecular cloning of a human gene that is a member of the nerve growth factor family. *Proc. Natl. Acad. Sci. USA,* 87, 8060-8064.

Joris, P. X. 1996. Envelope encoding in the lateral superior olive. II. Characteristic delays and comparison with responses in the medial superior olive. *J. Neurophysiol.,* 74, 2137-2156.

Joris, P. X. 1998. Response classes in the dorsal cochlear nucleus and its output tract in the chloralose-anesthetized cat. *J. Neurosci.,* 18, 3955-3966.

Joris, P. X., Carney, L. H., Smith, P. H., Yin, T. C. T. 1994b. Enhancement of neural synchronization in the anteroventral cochlear nucleus. I. Responses to tones at the characteristic frequency. *J. Neurophysiol.,* 71, 1022-1036.

Joris, P. X., Smith, P. H., Yin, T. C. T. 1992. Responses and projections of dorsal and intermediate stria axons labelled with HRP and Neurobiotin. *Assoc. Res. Otolaryngol. Abstr.,* 15, 58.

Joris, P. X., Smith, P. H., Yin, T. C. T. 1998. Coincidence detection in the auditory system: 50 years after Jeffress. *Neuron,* 21, 1235-1238.

Joris, P. X., Smith, P. H., Yin, T. C. T. 1994a. Enhancement of neural synchronization in the anteroventral cochlear nucleus. II. Responses in the tuning curve tail. *J. Neurophysiol.,* 71, 1037-1051.

Joris, P. X., Yin, T. C. T. 1995. Envelope encoding in the lateral superior olive. I. Sensitivity to interaural time differences. *J. Neurophysiol.,* 73, 1043-1062.

Josephson, E. M., Morest, D. K. 1999. A quantitative profile of the synapses on the stellate cell body and axon in the cochlear nucleus of chinchilla. *J. Neurocytol.,* 27, 841-864.

Jubilan, B. M., Nyby, J. G. 1992. The intrauterine position phenomenon and precopulatory behaviors of house mice. *Physiol. Behav.,* 51, 857-872.

Jucker, M., Tian, M., Norton, D. D., Sherman, C., Kusiak, J. W. 1996. Laminin α2 is a component of brain capillary basement membrane: reduced expression in dystrophic dy mice. *Neuroscience,* 71, 1153-1161.

Kaas, J. H. 1991. Plasticity of sensory and motor maps in adult mammals. *Annu. Rev. Neurosci.,* 14, 137-167.

Kagawa, M., Kishiro, Y., Naito, I., Nemoto, T., Nakanishi, H., Ninomiya, Y., Sado, Y. 1997. Epitope-defined monoclonal antibodies against type-IV collagen for diagnosis of Alport's syndrome. *Nephrol. Dial. Transpl.,* 12, 1238-1241.

Kageyama, R., Ohtsuka, T. 1999. The Notch-Hes pathway in mammalian neural development. *Cell Res.,* 9, 179-188.

Kahsai, T. Z., Enders, G. C., Gunwar, S., Brunmark, C., Wieslander, J., Kalluri, R., Zhou, J., Noelken, M. E., Hudson, B. G. 1997. Seminiferous tubule basement membrane. Composition and organization of type IV collagen chains, and the linkage of alpha3(IV) and alpha5(IV) chains. *J. Biol. Chem.,* 272, 17023-17032.

Kaisho, Y., Yoshiura, K., Nakahama, K. 1990. Cloning and expression of cDNA encoding a novel human neurotrophic factor. *FEBS Lett.,* 266, 187-191.

Kakehata, S., Nakagawa, T., Takasaka, T., Akaike, N. 1992. Glycine response in isolated dorsal cochlear nucleus of C57BL/6J mouse. *Brain Res.,* 574, 21-25.

Kakoi, H., Anniko, M. 1996. Auditory epithelial migration. IV. Light-and scanning electron-microscopic studies of the tympanic membrane and external auditory canal in the mouse. *J. Otorhinolaryngol. Relat. Spec.,* 58, 136-142.

Kalatzis, V., Petit, C. 1998. The fundamental and medical impacts of recent progress in research on hereditary hearing loss. *Hum. Molec. Genet.,* 7, 1589-1597.

Kalluri, R., Cosgrove, D. 2000. Assembly of type IV collagen. Insights from alpha3(IV) collagen-deficient mice. *J. Biol. Chem.,* 275, 12719-12724.

Kalluri, R., Gattone, V. H., Hudson, B. G. 1998. Identification and localization of type IV collagen chains in the inner ear cochlea. *Connect. Tissue Res.,* 37, 143-150.

Kaltenbach, J. A., Falzarano, P. R. 1994. Postnatal development of the hamster cochlea. I. Growth of hair cells and the organ of Corti. *J. Comp. Neurol.,* 340, 87-97.

Kaltenbach, J. A., Falzarano, P. R., Simpson, T. H. 1996. Postnatal development of the hamster cochlea. II. Growth and differentiation of stereocilia bundles. *J. Comp. Neurol.,* 350, 187-198.

Kamin, L. J. (Ed.). (1965). *Temporal and Intensity Characteristics of the Conditioned Stimulus.* Appleton-Century-Crofts, New York.

Kane, E. C. 1974. Synaptic organization in the dorsal cochlear nucleus of the cat: a light and electron microscopic study. *J. Comp. Neurol.,* 155, 301-330.

Kanes, S., Hitzemann, B., Hitzemann, R. 1996. Mapping the genes for haloperidol-induced catalepsy. *J. Pharmacol. Exper. Therap.,* 277, 1016-1025.

Kanzler, B., Foreman, R. K., Labosky, P. A., Mallo, M. 2000. BMP signaling is essential for development of skeletogenic and neurogenic cranial neural crest. *Devel.,* 127, 1095-1104.

Kaplan, D. R., Martin-Zanca, D., Parada, L. F. 1991. Tyrosine phosphorylation and tyrosine kinase activity of the trk proto-oncogene product induced by NGF. *Nature,* 350, 158-160.

Kaplan, J., Gerber, S., Bonneau, D., Rozet, J. M., Delrieu, O., Briard, M. L., Dollfus, H., Ghazi, I., Dufier, J. L., Frezal, J. 1992. A gene for Usher syndrome type I (USH1A) maps to chromosome 14q. *Genomics,* 14, 979-987.

Karjalainen, H., Koskela, M., Luotonen, J., Herva, E., Sipila, P. 1990. Antibodies against *Streptococcus pneumoniae, Haemophilus influenzae* and *Branhamella catarrhalis* in middle ear effusion during early phase of acute otitis media. *Acta Otolaryngol.,* 109, 111-118.

Karjalainen, S., Pakarinen, L., Terasvirta, M., Kaariainen, H., Vartiainen, E. 1989. Progressive hearing loss in Usher's syndrome. *Ann. Otol. Rhinol. Laryngol.,* 98, 863-866.

Kashtan, C. E. 1999. Alport syndrome. An inherited disorder of renal, ocular, and cochlear basement membranes. *Medicine (Baltimore),* 78, 338-360.

Kashtan, C. E., Atkin, C. L., Gregory, M. C., Michael, A. F. 1989. Identification of variant Alport phenotypes using an Alport-specific antibody probe. *Kidney Int.,* 36, 669-674.

Kashtan, C. E., Gubler, M. C., Sisson-Ross, S., Mauer, M. 1998. Chronology of renal scarring in males with Alport syndrome. *Pediatr. Nephrol.,* 12, 269-274.

Kashtan, C. E., Kim, Y. 1992. Distribution of the alpha 1 and alpha 2 chains of collagen IV and of collagens V and VI in Alport syndrome. *Kidney Int.,* 42, 115-126.

Kashtan, C., Fish, A. J., Kleppel, M., Yoshioka, K., Michael, A. F. 1986. Nephritogenic antigen determinants in epidermal and renal basement membranes of kindreds with Alport-type familial nephritis. *J. Clin. Invest.,* 78, 1035-1044.

Kataoka, Y., Haritani, M., Mori, M., Kishima, M., Sugimoto, C., Nakazawa, M., Yamamoto, K. 1991. Experimental infections of mice and pigs with *Streptococcus suis* type 2. *J. Vet. Med. Sci.,* 53, 1043-1049.

Katbamna, B., Bankaitis, A. W., Metz, D. A., Fisher, L. E. 1993. Effects of hyperthermia on the auditory-evoked brainstem responses in mice. *Audiology,* 32, 344-355.

Kawabata, M., Imamura,T., Miyazono, K. 1998. Signal transduction by bone morphogenetic proteins. *Cytokine Growth Factor Rev.,* 9, 49-61.

Kawaguchi, Y., Katsumaru, H., Kosaka, T., Heizmann, C. W., Hama, K. 1987. Fast spiking cells in the rat hippocampus (CA1 region) contain the calcium-binding protein parvalbumin. *Brain Res.,* 416, 369-374.

Kawai, S., Nomura, S., Harano, T., Harano, K., Fukushima, T., Osawa, G. 1996a. The COL4A5 gene in Japanese Alport syndrome patients: spectrum of mutations of all exons. The Japanese Alport Network. *Kidney Int.,* 49, 814-822.

Kawai, S., Nomura, S., Harano, T., Harano, K., Fukushima, T., Wago, M., Shimizu, B., Osawa, G. 1996b. A single-base mutation in exon 31 converting glycine 852 to arginine in the collagenous domain in an Alport syndrome patient. *Nephron,* 74, 333-336.

Kawauchi, H., Ichimiya, I., Kaneda, N., Mogi, G. 1992. Distribution of immunocompetent cells in the endolymphatic sac. *Ann. Otol. Rhinol. Laryngol. (Suppl.),* 157, 39-47.

Kaylie, D. M., Hefeneider, S. H., Kempton, J. B., Siess, D. C., Vedder, C. T., Merkens, L. S., Trune, D. R. 2001. Decreased cochlear DNA receptor staining in MRL. MpJ-*Fas^lpr* autoimmune mice with hearing loss. *Laryngoscope* (In review.)

Kazee, A. M, West, N. R. 1999. Preservation of synapses on principal cells of the central nucleus of the inferior colliculus with aging in the CBA mouse. *Hear. Res.,* 133, 98-106.

Kazee, A. M., Han, L. Y., Spongr, V. P., Walton, J. P., Salvi, R. J, Flood, D. G. 1995. Synaptic loss in the central nucleus of the inferior colliculus correlates with sensorineural hearing loss in the C57BL/6 mouse model of presbycusis. *Hear. Res.,* 89, 109-120.

Keats, B. J., Berlin, C. I. 1999. *Genomics,* and hearing impairment. *Genome Res.,* 9, 7-16.

Keats, B. J., Nouri, N., Pelias, M. Z., Deininger, P. L., Litt, M. 1994. Tightly linked flanking microsatellite markers for the Usher syndrome type I locus on the short arm of chromosome 11. *Am. J. Hum. Genet.,* 54, 681-686.

Keats, B. J., Nouri, N., Huang, J. M., Money, W., Webster, D. B., Berlin, C. I. 1995. The deafness locus (dn) maps to mouse chromosome 19. *Mamm. Genome,* 6, 8-10.

Keats, B. J., Todorov, A. A., Atwood, L. D., Pelias, M. Z., Hejtmancik, J. F., Kimberling, W. J., Leppert, M., Lewis, R. A., Smith, R. J. 1992. Linkage studies of Usher syndrome type 1: exclusion results from the Usher syndrome consortium. *Genomics,* 14, 707-714.

Keeler, C. 1931. *The Laboratory Mouse. Its Origin, Heredity, and Culture.* Harvard University Press, Cambridge, MA.

Keilson, S. E., Richards, V. M., Wyman, B. T., Young, E. D. 1997. The representation of concurent vowels in the cat anesthetized ventral cochlear nucleus: evidence for a periodicity tagged spectral representation. *J. Acoust. Soc. Am.,* 102, 1056-1071.

Keithley, E. M., Chen, M.-C., Linthicum, F. 1998. Clinical diagnoses associated with histologic findings of fibrotic tissue and new bone in the inner ear. *Laryngoscope,* 108, 87-91.

Keithly, E. M., Erkman, L., Bennett, T., Lou, L., Ryan, A. F. 1999. Effects of a hair cell transcription factor, Brn-3.1, gene deletion on homozygous and heterozygous mouse cochleas in adulthood and aging. *Hear. Res.,* 134, 71-76.

Keleman, G. 1966. Hurler's syndrome and the hearing organ. *J. Laryngol. Otol.,* 80, 791-803.

Kelley, M. W., Turner, J. K., Reh, T. A. 1994. Retinoic acid promotes differentiation of photoreceptors *in vitro. Devel.,* 120, 2091-2102.

Kelley, M. W., Talreja, D. R., Corwin, J. T. 1995. Replacement of hair cells after laser microbeam irradiation in cultured organs of Corti from embryonic and neonatal mice. *J. Neurosci.,* 15, 3013-3026.

Kelley, M. W., Xu, X. M., Wagner, M. A., Warchol, M. E., Corwin, J. T. 1993. The developing organ of Corti contains retinoic acid and forms supernumerary hair cells in response to exogenous retinoic acid in culture. *Devel.,* 119, 1041-1053.

Kelley, P. E., Frisina, R. D., Zettel, M. L, Walton, J. P. 1992. Differential calbindin-like immunoreactivity in the brain stem auditory system of the chinchilla. *J. Comp. Neurol.,* 319, 196-212.

Kelley, P. M., Weston, M. D., Chen, Z. Y., Orten, D. J., Hasson, T., Overbeck, L. D., Pinnt, J., Talmadge, C. B., Ing, P., Mooseker, M. S., Corey, D., Sumegi, J., Kimberling, W. J. 1997. The genomic structure of the gene defective in Usher syndrome type Ib (MYO7A). *Genomics,* 40, 73-79.

Kellogg, C. K., Sullivan, A. T., Bitran, D., Ison, J. R. 1991. Modulation of noise-potentiated acoustic startle via the benzodiazepine-γ-aminobutyric acid receptor complex. *Behav. Neurosci.,* 105, 640-646.

Kelly, J., Kavanagh, G., Picton, T. 1989. Brainstem auditory evoked response in the ferret (*Mustela putorius*). *Hear. Res.,* 39, 231-240.

Kelsell, D. P., Dunlop, J., Steven, H. P., Lench, N. J., Liang, J. N., Parry, G., Mueller, R. F., Leigh, I. M. 1997. Connexin 26 mutations in hereditary non-syndromic sensorineural deafness. *Nature,* 387, 80-83.

Kemp, D. T. 1978. Stimulated acoustic emissions from within the human auditory system. *J. Acoust. Soc. Am.,* 64, 1386-1391.

Kemp, D. T. 1979. Evidence of mechanical nonlinearity and frequency selective wave amplification in the cochlea. *Arch. Oto-Rhino-Laryngol.,* 224, 37-45.

Kemp, D. T., Brown, A. M. 1983. An integrated view of cochlear mechanical nonlinearities observable from the ear canal. In de Boer, E., Viergever, M. A. (Eds.), *Mechanisms of Hearing,* Martinus Nijhoff, The Hague, 75-82.

Kemp, D. T., Brown, A. M. 1984. Ear canal acoustic and round window electrical correlates of $2f_1$-f_2 distortion generated in the cochlea. *Hear. Res.,* 13, 39-46.

Kennedy, D. W., Abkowitz J. L. 1997. Kinetics of central nervous system microglial and macrophage engraftment: analysis using a transgenic bone marrow transplantation model. *Blood,* 90, 986-993.

Kerchner, M., Vatza, E. J., Nyby, J. 1986. Ultrasonic vocalizations by male house mice (*Mus musculus*) to novel odors: roles of infant and adult experience. *J. Comp. Psychol.,* 100, 253-261.

Kevetter, G. A., Perachio, A. A. 1989. Projections from the sacculus to the cochlear nuclei in the Mongolian gerbil. *Brain Behav. Evol.,* 34, 193-200.

Kewley-Port, D.,1983. Time-varying features as correlates of place of articulation in stop consonants. *J. Acoust. Soc. Am.,* 73, 322-335.

Keyer, K., Gort, A. S., Imlay, J. A. 1995. Superoxide and the production of oxidative DNA damage. *J. Bacteriol.,* 177, 6782-6790.

Keyer, K., Imlay, J. A. 1996. Superoxide accelerates DNA damage by elevating free-iron levels. *Proc. Natl. Acad. Sci. USA,* 93, 13635-13640.

Khachaturian, Z. S. 1989. The role of calcium regulation in brain aging: reexamination of a hypothesis. *Aging (Milano),* 1, 17-34.

Khan, D. C., DeGagne, J. M., Trune, D. R. 2000. Abnormal cochlear connective tissue mineralization in the Palmerston North autoimmune mouse. *Hear. Res.,* 142, 12-22.

Khan, K. M., Marovitz, W. F. 1982. DNA content, mitotic activity, and incorporation of tritiated thymidine in the developing inner ear of the rat. *Anat. Rec.,* 202, 501-509.

Khanna, S. M., Sherrick, C. E. 1981. The comparative sensitivity of selected receptor systems. In Gualtierotti, T. (Ed.), *The Vestibular System: Function and Morphology.* Springer-Verlag, Berlin, 132-145.

Khanna, S. M., Tonndorf, J. 1977. External and middle ears, the determinants of the auditory threshold curve. *J. Acoust. Soc. Am.,* 61(Suppl. 1), 54.

Khvoles, R., Freeman, S., Sohmer, H. 1999. Transient evoked otoacoustic emissions in laboratory animals. *Audiology,* 38, 121-126.

Kidd, M. 1961. Electron microscopy of the inner plexiform layer of the retina. In *Cytology of Nervous Tissue: Proceedings of the Anatomical Society of Great Britain and Ireland,* November 1961. Taylor and Francis Ltd., London, 88-91.

Kikuchi, K., Hilding, D. 1965a. The development of the organ of Corti in the mouse. *Acta Otolarygol. Suppl.,* 60, 207-222.

Kikuchi, K., Hilding, D. A. 1965b. The defective organ of Corti in shaker-1 mice. *Acta Otolaryngol.,* 60, 287-301.

Kikuchi, K., Hilding, D. A. 1967. The spiral vessel and stria vascularis in shaker-1 mice: Electron microscopic and histological observations. *Acta Otolaryngol.,* 63, 395-410.

Kim, D. O. 1980. Cochlear mechanics: implications of electrophysiological and acoustical observations. *Hear. Res.,* 2, 297-317.

Kim, D. O. 1984. Functional roles of inner-and-outer-hair-cell subsystems in the cochlea and brainstem. In Berlin, C. I. (Ed.), *Hearing Science: Recent Advances.* College-Hill Press, San Diego, CA, pp. 241-262.

Kim, D. O., Molnar, C. E., Matthews, J. W. 1980. Cochlear mechanics: nonlinear behavior in two-tone responses as reflected in cochlear-nerve-fiber responses and in ear-canal sound pressure. *J. Acoust. Soc. Am.,* 67, 1704-1721.

Kim, M., Davis, M. 1993. Electrolytic lesions of the of the amygdala block acquisition and expression of fear-potentiated startle even with extensive training but do not prevent reacquisition. *Behav. Neurosci.,* 107, 1088-1092.

Kimber, I., Dearman, R. J. 1993. Approaches to the identification and classification of chemical allergens in mice. *J. Pharmacol. Toxicol. Meth.,* 29, 11-16.

Kimberley, B. P., Hernadi, I., Lee, A. M., Brown, D. K. 1994. Predicting pure tone thresholds in normal and hearing-impaired ears with distortion product emissions and age. *Ear Hear.,* 15, 199-209.

Kimberling, W. J., Moller, C. G., Davenport, S., Priluck, I. A., Beighton, P. H., Greenberg, J., Reardon, W., Weston, M. D., Kenyon, J. B., Grunkemeyer, J. A. 1992. Linkage of Usher syndrome type I gene (USH1B) to the long arm of chromosome 11. *Genomics,* 14, 988-994.

Kimberling, W. J., Weston, M. D., Moller, C., van Aarem, A., Cremers, C. W., Sumegi, J., Ing, P. S., Connolly, C., Martini, A., Milani, M. 1995. Gene mapping of Usher syndrome type IIa: localization of the gene to a 2.1-cM segment on chromosome 1q41. *Am. J. Hum. Genet.,* 56, 216-223.

Kimberling, W. J., Weston, M. D., Moller, C., Davenport, S. L., Shugart, Y. Y., Priluck, I. A., Martini, A., Milani, M., Smith, R. J. 1990. Localization of Usher syndrome type II to chromosome 1q. *Genomics,* 7, 245-249.

Kimura, M., Ogata, Y., Shimada, K., Wakabayashi, T., Onoda, H., Katagiri, T., Matsuzawa, A. 1992. Nephritogenicity of the lpr[cg] gene on the MRL background. *Immunology,* 76, 498-504.

Kimura, R. S., Bongiorno, C. L., Iverson, N. A. 1987. Synapses and ephapses in the spiral ganglion. *Acta Otolaryngol. (Suppl.),* 438, 1-18.

Kindås-Mügge, I., Steiner, G., Smolen, J. S. 1993. Similar frequency of autoantibodies against 70-kD class heat-shock proteins in healthy subjects and systemic lupus erythematosus patients. *Clin. Exp. Immunol.*, 92, 46-50.

Kinsley, C., Miele, J., Konen, C., Ghiraldi, L., Svare, B. 1986. Intrauterine contiguity influences regulatory activity in adult female and male mice. *Horm. Behav.*, 20, 7-12.

Kishimoto, J., Tsuchiya, T., Cox, H., Emson, P. C., Nakayama, Y. 1998. Age-related changes of calbindin D-28k, calretinin, and parvalbumin mRNAs in the hamster brain. *Neurobiol. Aging*, 19, 77-82.

Kitamura, K., Nomura, Y., Yagi, M., Yoshikawa, Y., Ochikubo, F. 1991. Morphological changes of cochlea in a strain of new-mutant mice. *Acta Otolaryngol.*, 111, 61-69.

Klein, J. O., Tos, M., Casselbrant, M. L., Daly, K. A., Hoffman, H. J., Ingvarsson, L., Karma, P., van Cauwenberge, P. B. 1998. I. Epidemiology and natural history. *Ann. Otol. Rhinol. Laryngol.*, 107(Suppl.) 174, 9-13.

Klein, R., Lamballe, F., Barbacid, M. 1992. The trkB tyrosine protein kinase is a receptor for neurotrophin-4. *Neuron*, 8, 947-956.

Klein, R., Nanduri, V., Jing, S. A., Lamballe, F., Tapley, P., Bryant, S., Cordon-Cardo, C., Jones, K. R., Reichardt, L. F., Barbacid, M. 1991. The trkB tyrosine protein kinase is a receptor for brain-derived neurotrophic factor and neurotrophin-3. *Cell*, 66, 395-403.

Klein, R., Parada, L. F., Coulier, F., Barbacid, M. 1989a. Trk B, a novel tyrosine protein kinase receptor expressed during mouse neural development. *EMBO J.*, 8, 3701-3709.

Klein, R., Smeyne, R. J., Wurst, W., Long, L. K., Auerbach, B. A., Joyner, A. L., Barbacid, M. 1993. Targeted disruption of the trkB neurotrophin receptor gene results in nervous system lesions and neonatal death. *Cell*, 75, 113-122.

Klein, R., Timpl, R., Zanetti, F. R., Plester, D., Berg, P. A. 1989b. High antibody levels against mouse laminin with specificity for galactosyl-(alpha 1-3)galactose in patients with inner ear diseases. *Ann. Otol. Rhinol. Laryngol.*, 98, 537-542.

Kleppel, M. M., Fan, W., Cheong, H. I., Michael, A. F. 1992. Evidence for separate networks of classical and novel basement membrane collagen. Characterization of alpha 3(IV)-Alport antigen heterodimer. *J. Biol. Chem.*, 267, 4137-4142.

Kleppel, M. M., Michael, A. F. 1990. Expression of novel basement membrane components in the developing human kidney and eye. *Am. J. Anat.*, 187, 165-174.

Kleppel, M. M., Santi, P. A., Cameron, J. D., Wieslander, J., Michael, A. F. 1989. Human tissue distribution of novel basement membrane collagen. *Am. J. Pathol.*, 134, 813-825.

Kline, L., Decena, E., Hitzemann, R., McCaughran, J. Jr. 1998. Acoustic startle, prepulse inhibition, locomotion and latent inhibition in the neuroleptic responsive (NR. and neuroleptic non-responsive (NNR). lines of mice. *Psychopharmacology*, 139, 322-331.

Klump, G. M., Dooling, R. J., Fay, R. R., Stebbins, W. C. (Eds.). 1995. *Methods in Comparative Psychoacoustics*, Birkhäuser, Basel.

Knebelmann, B., Breillat, C., Forestier, L., Arrondel, C., Jacassier, D., Giatras, I., Drouot, L., Deschenes, G., Grunfeld, J. P., Broyer, M., Gubler, M. C., Antignac, C. 1996. Spectrum of mutations in the COL4A5 collagen gene in X-linked Alport syndrome. *Am. J. Hum. Genet.*, 59, 1221-1232.

Knebelmann, B., Deschenes, G., Gros, F., Hors, M. C., Grunfeld, J. P., Zhou, J., Tryggvason, K., Gubler, M. C., Antignac, C. 1992. Substitution of arginine for glycine 325 in the collagen alpha 5 (IV) chain associated with X-linked Alport syndrome: characterization of the mutation by direct sequencing of PCR-amplified lymphoblast cDNA fragments. *Am. J. Hum. Genet.*, 51, 135-142.

Knebelmann, B., Forestier, L., Drouot, L., Quinones, S., Chuet, C., Benessy, F., Saus, J., Antignac, C. 1995. Splice-mediated insertion of an Alu sequence in the COL4A3 mRNA causing autosomal recessive Alport syndrome. *Hum. Molec. Genet.*, 4, 675-679.

Knight, R. D., Kemp, D. T. 2000. Indications of different distortion product otoacoustic emission mechanisms from a detailed f1,f2 area study. *J. Acoust. Soc. Am.*, 107, 457-473.

Knipper, M., Gestwa, L., Ten Cate, W.-J., Lautermann, J., Brugger, H., Maier, H., Zimmermann, U., Rohbock, K., Kopschall, I., Wiechers, B., Zenner, H.-P. 1999. Distinct thyroid hormone-dependent expression of TrkB and p75[NGFR] in nonneuronal cells during the criticial TH-dependent period of the cochlea. *J. Neurobiol.*, 38, 338-356.

Knipper, M., Zimmerman, U., Rohbock, K., Kopschall, I. 1996. Expression of neurotrophin receptor trk B in rat cochlear hair cells at the time of rearrangement of innervation. *Cell Tissue Res.*, 283, 339-353.

Knudsen, E. I. 1999. Mechanisms of experience-dependent plasticity in the auditory localization pathway of the barn owls (Rev.). *J. Comp. Physiol., A*, 185, 305-321.

Knusel, B., Beck, K. D., Winslow, J. W., Rosenthal, A., Burton, L. E., Widmer, H. R., Nikolics, K., Hefti, F. 1992. Brain-derived neurotrophic factor administration protects basel forebrain cholinergic but not nigral dopaminergic neurons from degenerative changes after axotomy in the adult rat brain. *J. Neurosci.*, 12, 4391-4402.

Koay, G., Heffner, H. E., Heffner, R. S. 1997. Audiogram of the big brown bat (*Eptesicus fuscus*). *Hear. Res.*, 105, 202-210.

Koay, G., Kearns, D., Heffner, H. E., Heffner, R. S. 1998. Passive sound localization ability of the big brown bat (*Eptesicus fuscus*). *Hear. Res.*, 119, 37-48.

Koch, M., Lingenhöhl, K., Pilz, P. K. D. 1992. Loss of the acoustic startle response following neurotoxic lesion of the caudal pontine reticular formation: possible role of giant neurons. *Neuroscience,* 49, 617-625.

Koch, M. 1996. The septohippocampal system is involved in prepulse inhibition of the acoustic startle response in rats. *Behav. Neurosci.*, 110, 468-477.

Koch, M., Friauf, E. 1995. Glycine receptors in the caudal pontine reticular formation: are they important for the inhibition of the acoustic startle response? *Brain Res.*, 671, 63-72.

Koch, M., Schnitzler, H. U. 1997. The acoustic startle response in rats-circuits mediating evocation, inhibition and potentiation. *Behav. Brain Res.*, 89, 35-49.

Kodama, S., Kurono, Y., Shigemi, H., Mogi, G. 1996. Oral vaccination with outer membrane proteins of nontypable *Haemophilus infuenzae* in mice. In Lim, D. J., Bluestone, C. D., Casselbrant, M., Klein, J. O., Ogra, P. L. (Eds.), *Recent Advances in Otitis Media.* B. C. Decker, Hamilton, 502-503.

Kodsi, M. H., Swerdlow, N. R. 1995. Prepulse inhibition in the rat is regulated by ventral and caudodorsal striato-pallidal circuitry. *Behav. Neurosci.*, 109, 912-928.

Koide, Y., Hando, R., Yoshikawa, Y. 1964. Distribution of some oxidizing enzymes in the cochlea. *Acta Otolaryngol.*, 58, 344-354.

Kolston, J., Osen, K. K., Hackney, C. M., Ottersen, O. P., Storm-Mathisen, J. 1992. An atlas of glycine- and GABA-like immunoreactivity and colocalization in the cochlear nuclear complex of the guinea pig. *Anat. Embryol.*, 186, 443-465.

Kondo, S., Pastore, S., Shivji, G. M., McKenzie, R. C., Sauder, D. N. 1994. Characterization of epidermal cytokine profiles in sensitization and elicitation phases of allergic contact dermatitis as well as irritant contact dermatitis in mouse skin. *Lymphokine Cytokine Res.*, 13, 367-375.

Kondo, T., Reaume, A. G., Huang, T. T., Carlson, E., Murakami, K., Chen, S. F., Hoffman, E. K., Scott, R. W., Epstein, C. J., Chan, P. H. 1997. Reduction of CuZn-superoxide dismutase activity exacerbates neuronal cell injury and edema formation after transient focal cerebral ischemia. *J. Neurosci.*, 17, 4180-4189.

Konigsmark, B. W., Murphy, E. A. 1970. Neuronal populations in the human brain. *Nature,* 228, 1335-1336.

Konigsmark, B. W, Murphy, E. A. 1972. Volume of the ventral cochlear nucleus in man: Its relationship to neuronal population and age. *J. Neuropath. Exp. Neurol.*, 31, 304-316.

Korenberg, J. R., Chen, X. N., Devon, K. L., Noya, D., Oster-Granite, M. L., Birren, B. W. 1999. Mouse molecular cytogenetic resource: 157 BACs link the chromosomal and genetic maps. *Genome Res.*, 9, 514-523.

Kornfeld, S. 1992. Structure and function of the mannose 6-phosphate/insulin-like growth factor II receptors. *Annu. Rev. Biochem.*, 61, 307-330.

Kornguth, S. E., Anderson, J. W., Scott, G. 1968. The development of synaptic contacts in the cerebellum of *Macaca mulatta. J. Comp. Neurol.*, 132, 531-546.

Kornguth, S. E., Scott, G. 1972. The role of climbing fibers in the formation of Purkinje cell dendrites. *J. Comp. Neurol.*, 146, 61-82.

Koyner, J., Demarest, K., McCaughran, J. Jr., Cipp, L., Hitzemann, R. 2000. Identification and time dependence of quantitative trait loci for basal locomotor activity in the BXD recombinant inbred series and a B6D2 F_2 intercross. *Behav. Genet.*, in press.

Kozel, P. J., Friedman, R. A., Erway, L. C., Yamoah, E. N., Liu, L. H., Riddle, T., Duffy, J. J., Doetschman, T., Miller, M. L., Cardell, E. L., Shull, G. E. 1998. Balance and hearing deficits in mice with a null mutation in the gene encoding plasma membrane Ca2+-ATPase isoform 2. *J. Biol. Chem.*, 273, 18693-18696.

Kraus, H.-J., Aulbach-Kraus, K. 1981. Morphological changes in the cochlea of the mouse after the onset of hearing. *Hear. Res.*, 4, 89-102.

Krauter, E. E., Wallace, J. E., Campbell, B. A. 1981. Sensory-motor function in the aging rat. *Behav. Neural Biol.*, 31, 367-392.

Krekorian, T. D., Keithley, E. M., Fierer, J., Harris, J. P. 1991. Type B *Haemophilus influenzae*-induced otitis media in the mouse. *Laryngoscope,* 101, 648-656.

Krekorian, T. D., Keithley, E. M., Takahashi, M., Fierer, J., Harris, J. P. 1990. Endotoxin-induced otitis media with effusion in the mouse. Immunohistochemical analysis. *Acta Otolaryngol.,* 109, 288-299.

Krenning, J., Hughes, L. F., Caspary, D. M., Helfert, R. H. 1998. Age-related subunit changes in the cochlear nucleus of Fischer-344 rats. *Laryngoscope,* 108, 26-31.

Kros, C. J., Marcotti, W., Richardson, G. P., Brown, S. D. M., Steel, K. P. 1999. Electrophysiology of outer hair cells from myosin VIIA mutant mice. *Assoc. Res. Otolaryngol. Abstr.,* 22, 60.

Krzywkowski, P., Potier, B., Billard, J. M., Dutar, P., Lamour, Y. 1996. Synaptic mechanisms and calcium binding proteins in the aged rat brain. *Life Sci.,* 59, 421-428.

Kubisch, C., Schroeder, B., Friedrich, T., Lutnohann, B., El-Amraoui, A., Marlin, S., Petit, C., Jentsch, T. 1999. KCNQ4, a novel potassium channel expressed in sensory outer hair cells, is mutated in dominant deafness. *Cell,* 96, 437-446.

Kulig, J., Willott, J. F. 1984. Frequency difference limens of C57BL/6 and DBA/2 mice: relationship to auditory neuronal response properties and hearing impairment. *Hear. Res.,* 16, 169-174.

Kummer, P., Janssen, T., Arnold, W. 1995. Suppression tuning characteristics of the $2f_1$-f_2 distortion-product otoacoustic emission in humans. *J. Acoust. Soc. Am.,* 98, 197-210.

Kummer, P., Janssen, T., Arnold, W. 1998. The level and growth behavior of the $2f_1$-f_2 distortion product otoacoustic emission and its relationship to auditory sensitivity in normal hearing and cochlear hearing loss. *J. Acoust. Soc. Am.,* 103, 3431-3444.

Kuratani, S., Satokata, I., Blum, M., Komatsu, Y., Haraguchi, R., Nakamura, S., Suzuki, K., Kosai, K., Yamada, G. 1999. Middle ear defects associated with double knock out mutation of murine genes. *Cell. Molec. Biol.,* 45, 589-599.

Kurono, Y., Bakaletz, L. O., Lim, D. J. 1993. Inhibition of the adherence of *Streptococcus pneumoniae* to buccal epithelial cells in BALB/c mice by oral immunization. In Lim, D. J., Bluestone, C. D., Klein, J. O., Nelson, J. D., Ogra, P. L. (Eds.), *Recent Advances in Otitis Media.* Decker Periodicals, Philadelphia, 206-208.

Kurono, Y., Fujihashi, K., McGhee, J. R., Mogi, G., Kiyono, H. 1999b. The role of interferon (IFN)-γ inducing IgA responses against nontypable *Haemophilus influenzae.* Presented at *Seventh International Symposium on Recent Advances in Otitis Media.* June 1-5, Fort Lauderdale, FL, 99.

Kurono, Y., Hirono, T., Watanabe, T., Suzuki, M., Mogi, G. 1998. The role of IL-1 beta in murine model of otitis media with effusion [Japanese]. *Nippon Jibiinkoka Gakkai Kaiho* [*J. Oto-Rhino-Laryngol. Soc. Japan*], 101, 1093-1098.

Kurono, Y., Shimamura, K., Mogi, G. 1992. Inhibition of nasopharyngeal colonization of *Hemophilus influenzae* by oral immunization. *Ann. Otol. Rhinol. Laryngol. (Suppl.),* 157, 11-15.

Kurono, Y., Suzuki, M., Mogi, G., Yamamoto, M., Fujihashi, K., McGhee, J. R., Kiyono, H. 1999a. Effects of intranasal immunization on protective immunity against otitis media. *Int. J. Ped. Otorhinolaryngol.,* 49(Suppl. 1), S227-229.

Kusakari, C., Hozawa, K., Koike, S., Kyogoku, M., Takasaka, T. 1992. MRL/MP-*lpr/lpr* mouse as a model of immune-induced sensorineural hearing loss. *Ann. Otol. Rhinol. Laryngol.,* 101, 82-86.

Kuwabara, N, Zook, J. M. 1991. Classification of the principal cells of the medial nucleus of the trapezoid body. *J. Comp. Neurol.,* 314,707-720.

Kuwabara, N., Zook, J. M. 1992. Projections to the medial superior olive from the medial and lateral nuclei of the trapezoid body in rodents and bats. *J. Comp. Neurol.,* 324, 522-538.

Kuwabara, N., DiCaprio, R. A., Zook, J. M. 1991. Afferents to the medial nucleus of the trapezoid body and their collateral projections. *J. Comp. Neurol.,* 314, 684-706.

Kveton, J. F., Pensak, M. L. 1995. Cochlear implantation. In Lee, J. K. (Ed.), *Essential Otolaryngology.* Appleton and Lange, New Haven, 161-172.

Kwitek-Black, A. E. 2000. The role of rats in functional genomics. *Lab Anim.,* 29, 44-48.

Lacour, M., Rudolphi, U., Schlesier, M., Peter, H.-H. 1990. Type II collagen-specific human T cell lines established from healthy donors. *Eur. J. Immunol.,* 20, 931-934.

Lake, 3rd, G. M., Sismanis, A., Ariga, T., Yamawaki, M., Gao, Y., Yu, R. K. 1997. Antibodies to glycosphingolipid antigens in patients with immune-mediated cochleovestibular disorders. *Am. J. Otol.,* 18, 175-178.

Lalwani, A. K., Walsh, B. J., Reilly, P. G., Muzyczka, N., Mhatre, A. N. 1996. Development of an *in vivo* gene therapy for hearing disorders: introduction of adeno-associated virus into the cochlea of the guinea pig. *Gene Ther.,* 3, 588-592.

Lalwani, A. K, Brister, R., Fex, J., Grundfast, K. M., Pikus, A. T., Ploplis, B., Agustin, T. S., Sharka, H., Wilcox, E. R. 1994. A new nonsyndromic X-linked sensorineural hearing impairment linked to Xp21.2. *Am. J. Hum. Genet.*, 55, 685-694.

Lamballe, F., Klein, R., Barbacid, M. 1991. Trk C A new member of the trk family of tyrosine protein kinases, is a receptor for neurotrophin-3. *Cell*, 66, 967-979.

Lambert, P. R, Schwartz, I. R. 1982. A longitudinal study of changes in the cochlear nucleus in the CBA mouse. *Otolaryngol. Head Neck Surg.*, 90, 787-794.

Lander, E., Kruglyak, L. 1995. Genetic dissection of complex traits: guidelines for interpreting and reporting linkage results. *Nature Genet.*, 11, 241-247.

Lander, E. S., Botstein, E. 1989. Mapping mendelian factors underlying quantitative traits using RFLP linkage maps. *Genetics*, 121, 185-199.

Landis, C., Hunt, W. A. 1939. *The Startle Pattern*. Farrar & Rinehart, New York.

Landis, D. M. D. 1987. Initial junctions between developing parallel fibers and Purkinje cells are different from mature synaptic junctions. *J. Comp. Neurol.*, 260, 513-525.

Lane, P. W. 1987. Deaf waddler (dfw). *Mouse News Lett.*, 77, 129.

Lanford, P. J., Lan, Y., Jiang, R., Lindsell, C., Weinmaster, G., Gridley, T., Kelley, M. W. 1999. Notch signalling pathway mediates hair cell development in mammalian cochlea [see Comments], *Nature Genet.*, 21, 289-292.

Lanford, P. J., Shailam, R., Norton, C. R., Gridley, T., Kelley, M. W. 2000. Expression of Math1 and HES5 in the cochlea of wildtype and Jagged2 mutant mice. *JARO 1*, in press.

Langman, J. 1982. *Medical Embryology*. Williams & Wilkins, Baltimore.

Langner, G. 1992. Periodicity coding in the auditory system (review), *Hear. Res.*, 60, 115-142.

Larget-Piet, D., Gerber, S., Bonneau, D., Rozet, J. M., Marc, S., Ghazi, I., Dufier, J. L., David, A., Bitoun, P., Weissenbach, J. 1994. Genetic heterogeneity of Usher syndrome type 1 in French families. *Genomics*, 21, 138-143.

Larsson, K. 1979. Features of the neuroendocrine regulation of masculine behavior. In Beyer, C. (Ed.), *Endocrine Control of Sexual Behavior*. Raven Press, New York, 63-77.

Lasky, R. 1984. A developmental study on the effect of stimulus rate on the auditory evoked brain-stem response. *Electroenceph. Clin. Neurophysiol.*, 59, 411-419.

Latchman, D. S. 1999. POU family transcription factors in the nervous system. *J. Cell Physiol.*, 179, 126-133.

Lauder, J. M. 1993. Neurotransmitters as growth regulatory signals: role of receptors and second messengers. *Trends Neurosci.*, 16, 233-240.

Lauder, J. M., Han, V. K. M., Henderson, P., Verdoorn, T., Towle, A. C. 1986. Prenatal ontogeny of the GABAergic system in the rat brain: an immunocytochemical study. *Neuroscience*, 19, 465-493.

Lautermann, J., ten Cate, W. J. 1997. Postnatal expression of the alpha-thyroid hormone receptor in the rat cochlea. *Hear. Res.*, 107, 23-28.

Lawrence, M. 1971. The function of the spiral capillaries. *Laryngoscope*, 81, 1314-1322.

Lawrence, M., Nuttall, A. L. 1972. Oxygen availability in tunnel of Corti measured by microelectrode. *J. Acoust. Soc. Am.*, 52, 566-573.

Lazarus, H. S., Sly W. S., Kyle J. W., Hageman G. S. 1993. Photoreceptor degeneration and altered distribution of interphotoreceptor matrix in the mucopolysaccharidosis mouse. *Exp. Eye Res.*, 56, 531-541.

Le Moine, C., Young, W. S. D. 1992. RHS2, a POU domain-containing gene, and its expression in developing and adult rat. *Proc. Natl. Acad. Sci.*, 89, 3285-3289.

Leake, P. A., Hradek, G. T., Rebscher, S. J., Snyder, R. L. 1991. Chronic intracochlear electrical stimulation induces selective survival of spiral ganglion neurons in neonatally deafened cats. *Hear. Res.*, 54, 251-271.

Leaton, R. N., Borscz, G. S. 1985. Potentiated startle: Its relation to freezing and shock intensity in rats. *J. Exp. Psychol. Anim. Behav.*, Process. 11, 421-428.

Lebovitz, R., Zhang, H., Vogel, H., Cartwright, J. J., Dionne, L., Lu, N., Huang, S., Matzuk, M. 1996. Neurodegeneration, myocardial injury, and perinatal death in mitochondrial superoxide dismutase-deficient mice. *Proc. Natl. Acad. Sci.*, 93, 9782-9787.

Le Calvez, S., Avan, P., Gilain, L., Romand, R. 1998a. CD1 hearing-impaired mice. I. Distortion product otoacoustic emission levels, cochlear function and morphology. *Hear. Res.*, 120, 37-50.

Le Calvez, S., Gulhaume, A., Romand, R. Aran, J. M., Avan, P. 1998b. CD1 hearing impaired mice. II. Group latencies and optimal f2/f1 ratios of distortion product otoacoustic emissions, and scanning electron microscopy. *Hear. Res.*, 120, 51-61.

LeDoux, J. E., Iwata, I., Pearl, D., Reis, D. J. 1986. Disruption of auditory but not visual learning by destruction of intrinsic neurons in the rat medial geniculate body. *Brain Res.,* 371, 395-399.

LeDoux, J. E., Sakaguchi, A., Iwata, J., Reis, D. J. 1985. Auditory emotional memories: establishment by projections from the medial geniculate nucleus to the posterior neostriatum and/or dorsal amygdala. *Ann. N.Y. Acad. Sci.,* 463-464.

LeDoux, J. E., Sakaguchi, A., Reis, D. J. 1983. Subcortical efferent projections of the medial geniculate nucleus mediate emotional responses conditioned to acoustic stimuli. *J. Neurosci.,* 4, 683-698.

Lee, A. M., Navaratnam, D., Ichimiya, S., Greene, M. I., Davis, J. G. 1996. Cloning of m-ehk2 from the murine inner ear, an eph family receptor tyrosine kinase expressed in the developing and adult cochlea. *DNA and Cell Bio.,*15, 817-825.

Lee, K., Bachman, K., Landis, S., Jaenish, R. 1994. Dependance on p75 for innervation of some sympathetic targets. *Science,* 11, 1447-1449.

Lee, K. F., Li, E., Huber, L. J., Landis, S. C., Sharpe, A. H., Chao, M. V., Jaenisch, R. 1992. Targeted mutation of the gene encoding the low affinity receptor p75 leads to deficits in the peripheral sensory nervous system. *Cell,* 69, 737-749.

Lee, K.-S., Kimura, R. S. 1994. Ultrastructural changes of the vestibular sensory organs after streptomycin application on the lateral canal. *Scan. Microsc.,* 8, 107-124.

Lefebvre, P. P., Leprince, P., Weber, T., Rigo, J.-M., Delree, P., Moonen, G. 1990. Neuronotrophic effects of the developing otic vesicle on cochleovestibular neurons: evidence for nerve growth factor involvement. *Brain. Res.,* 507, 254-260.

Lefebvre, P. P., Malgrange, B., Staecker, H., Moghadassi, M., Van De Water, T. R., Moonen, G. 1994. Neurotrophins affect survival and neuritogenesis by adult injured auditory neurons *in vitro. NeuroRep.,* 5, 865-868.

Lefebvre, P. P., Van De Water, T. R., Weber, T., Rogister, B., Moonen, G. 1991. Growth factor interactions in cultures of dissociated adult acoustic ganglia: neuronotrophic effects. *Brain Res.,* 567, 306-312.

Legan, K., Goodyear, R., Lukashkina, V., Russell, I., Richardson, G. 2000. Transgenic mice with a deletion in the entactin domain of alpha-tectorin have detached tectorial membranes lacking striated sheet matrix and are deaf. *Assoc. Res. Otolaryngol. Abstr.,*

Legrand, C., Bréhier, A., Clavel, M. C., Thomasset, M., Rabié, A. 1988. Cholecalcin (28-kDa CaBP) in the rat cochlea. Development in normal and hypothyroid animals. An immunocytochemical study. *Devel. Brain Res.,* 38, 121-129.

Leibrock, J., Lottspeich, F., Hohn, A. 1989. Molecular cloning and expression of brain derived neurotrophic factor. *Nature,* 341, 149-152.

Leitner, D. S., Cohen, M. E. 1985. Role of the inferior colliculus in the inhibition of acoustic startle in the rat. *Physiol. Behav.,* 34, 65-70.

Leitner, D. S., Powers, A. S., Hoffman, H. S. 1980. The neural substrate of the startle response. *Physiol. Behav.,* 25, 291-297.

Leitner, D. S., Powers, A. S., Stitt, C. L., Hoffman, H. S. 1981. Midbrain reticular formation involvement in the inhibition of acoustic startle. *Physiol. Behav.,* 26, 259-268.

Lemmink, H. H., Mochizuki, T., van den Heuvel, L. P., Schroder, C. H., Barrientos, A., Monnens, L. A., van Oost, B. A., Brunner, H. G., Reeders, S. T., Smeets, H. J. 1994. Mutations in the type IV collagen alpha 3 (COL4A3) gene in autosomal recessive Alport syndrome. *Hum. Molec. Genet.,* 3, 1269-1273.

Lemmink, H. H., Nillesen, W. N., Mochizuki, T., Schroder, C. H., Brunner, H. G., van Oost, B. A., Monnens, L. A., Smeets, H. J. 1996. Benign familial hematuria due to mutation of the type IV collagen alpha4 gene. *J. Clin. Invest.,* 98, 1114-1118.

Lemmink, H. H., Schroder, C. H., Monnens, L. A., Smeets, H. J. 1997. The clinical spectrum of type IV collagen mutations. *Hum. Mutat.,* 9, 477-499.

Lemmink, H. H., Schroder, C. H., Brunner, H. G., Nelen, M. R., Zhou, J., Tryggvason, K., Haagsma-Schouten, W. A., Roodvoets, A. P., Rascher, W., van Oost, B. A. 1993. Identification of four novel mutations in the COL4A5 gene of patients with Alport syndrome. *Genomics,* 17, 485-489.

Lemmon, S. K., Riley, M. C., Thomas, K. A. 1982. Bovine fibroblast growth factor: comparison of brain and pituitary preparations. *J. Cell Biol.,* 95, 162-169.

LeMoine, C., Young, W. S. III. 1992. RHS2, a POU domain-containing gene and its expression in developing and adult rats. *Proc. Nat. Acad. Sci. USA,* 89, 3285-3289.

Lenn, N. J., Reese, T. S. 1966. The fine structure of nerve endings in the nucleus of the trapezoid body and the ventral cochlear nucleus. *Am. J. Anat.,* 118, 375-390.

Lenoir, M., Puel, J. L., Pujol, R. 1987. Stereocilia and tectorial membrane development in the rat cochlea. A SEM study. *Anat. Embryol.*, 175, 477-487.

Lenoir, M., Shnerson, A., Pujol, R. 1980. Cochlear receptor development in the rat with emphasis on synaptogenesis. *Anat. Embryol.*, 160, 253-262.

Letts, V. A., Felix, R., Biddlecome, G. H., Arikkath, J., Mahaffey, C. L., Valenzuela, A., Bartlett II, F. S., Mori, Y., Campbell, K. P., Frankel, W. N. 1998. The mouse stargazer gene encodes a neuronal Ca^{2+}-channel γ subunit. *Nature Genet.*, 19, 340-347.

Letts, V. A., Gervais, J. L. M., Frankel, W. N. 1994. Remutation at the shaker-1 locus. *Mouse Genome*, 92, 116.

Leuba, G., Kraftsik, R., Saini, K. 1998. Quantitative distribution of parvalbumin, calretinin and calbindin D-28k immunoreactive neurons in the visual cortex of normal and Alzheimer cases. *Exp. Neurol.*, 152, 278-291.

Levi-Montalcini, R., Hamburger, V. 1951. Selective growth stimulating effects of mouse sarcoma on the sensory and sympathetic nervous system of the chick embryo. *J. Exp. Zool.*, 116, 321-362.

Levy, G., Levi-Acobas, F., Blanchard, S., Gerber, S., Larget-Piet, D., Chenal, V., Liu, X. Z., Newton, V., Steel, K. P., Brown, S. D., Munnich, A., Kaplan, J., Petit, C., Weil, D. 1997. Myosin VIIA gene: heterogeneity of the mutations responsible for Usher syndrome type IB. *Hum. Molec. Genet.*, 6, 111-116.

Lewis, A. K., Frantz, G. D., Carpenter, D. A., de Sauvage, F. J., Gao, W. Q. 1998. Distinct expression patterns of notch family receptors and ligands during development of the mammalian inner ear. *Mech. Devel.*, 78, 159-163.

Lewis, J. 1991. Rules for the production of sensory cells. *Ciba Found Symp.* 160, 25-39; discussion 40-53. Review.

Lewis, P. R., Knight, D. P. 1977. Staining methods for sectioned material. In Glauert, A. M. (Series Ed.), *Practical Methods in Electron Microscopy*. North Holland Publishing, Amsterdam, 27.

Lewis, R. A., Otterud, B., Stauffer, D., Lalouel, J. M., Leppert, M. 1990. Mapping recessive ophthalmic diseases: linkage of the locus for Usher syndrome type II to a DNA marker on chromosome 1q. *Genomics*, 7, 250-256.

Li, C. W., Van De Water, T. R., Ruben, R. J. 1978. The fate mapping of the eleventh and twelfth day mouse otocyst: an *in vitro* study of the sites of origin of the embryonic inner ear sensory structures. *J. Morphol.* 157, 249-267.

Li, D., Henley, C. M., O'Malley, B. W., Jr. 1999. Distortion product otoacoustic emissions and outer hair cell defects in the hyt/hyt mutant mouse. *Hear. Res.*, 138, 65-72.

Li, H. S., Borg, E. 1993. Auditory degeneration after acoustic trauma in two genotypes of mice. *Hear. Res.*, 68, 19-27.

Li, H. S., Hultcrantz, M., Borg, E. 1993. Influence of age on noise-induced permanent threshold shifts in CBA/Ca and C57BL/6J mice. *Audiology*, 32, 195-204.

Li, H.-S. 1992a. Influence of genotype and age on acute acoustic trauma and recovery in CBA/Ca and C57BL/6J mice. *Acta Otolaryngol.*, 112, 956-967.

Li, H.-S. 1992b. Genetic influences on susceptibility of the auditory system to aging and environmental factors. *Scand. Audiol. (Suppl.)*, 36, 1-39.

Li, H.-S., Borg, E. 1991. Age-related loss of auditory sensitiity in two mouse genotypes. *Acta Otolaryngol.*, 111, 827-834.

Li, L., Korngut, L. M., Frost, B. J., Beninger, R. J. 1998b. Prepulse inhibition following lesions of the inferior colliculus: prepulse intensity functions. *Physiol. Behav.*, 65, 133-139.

Li, L., Priebe, R. P., Yeomans, J. S. 1998a. Prepulse inhibition of acoustic or trigeminal startle of rats by unilateral electrical stimulation of the inferior colliculus. *Behav. Neurosci.*, 112, 1187-1198.

Li, X. C., Everett, L. A., Lalwani, A. K., Desmukh, D., Friedman, T. B., Green, E. D., Wilcox, E. R. 1998. A mutation in PDS causes non-syndromic recessive deafness. *Nature Genet.*, 18, 215-218.

Li, Y., Huang, T., Carlson, E., Melov, S., Ursell, P., Olson, J., Noble, L., Yoshimura, M., Berger, C., Chan, P., Wallace, D., CJ, E. 1995. Dilated cardiomyopathy and neonatal lethality in mutant mice lacking manganese superoxide dismutase. *Nature Genet.*, 11, 376-381.

Liberman, M. C. 1991. Central projections of auditory-nerve fibers of differing spontaneous rate. I. Anteroventral cochlear nucleus. *J. Comp. Neurol.*, 313, 240-258.

Liberman, M. C., Dodds, L. W. 1984. Single-neuron labeling and chronic cochlear pathology. III. Sterocilia damage and alterations of threshold tuning curves. *Hear. Res.*, 16, 55-74.

Liberman, M. C., Dodds, L. W., Pierce, S. 1990. Afferent and efferent innervation of the cat cochlea: quantitative analysis with light and electron microscopy. *J. Comp. Neurol.*, 301, 443-460.

Liberman, M. C., O'Grady, D. F., Dodds, L. W., McGee, J., Walsh, E. J. 2000. Afferent innervation of outer and inner hair cells is normal in neonatally de-efferented cats. *J. Comp. Neurol.*, 423, 132-139.

Liberman, M. C., Puria, S., Guinan, Jr., J. J. 1996. The ipsilaterally evoked olivocochlear reflex causes rapid adaptation of the $2f_1$-f_2 distortion product otoacoustic emission. *J. Acoust. Soc. Am.*, 99, 3572-3584.

Lim, D. J. 1968a. Tympanic membrane: Electron microscope observation. I. Pars tense. *Acta Otolaryngol.*, 66, 181-198.

Lim, D. J. 1968b. Tympanic membrane. II. Pars flaccida. *Acta Otolaryngol.*, 66, 565-575.

Lim, D. J. 1970. Human tympanic membrane: an ultrastructural observation. *Acta Otolaryngol.*, 70, 176-186.

Lim, D. J. 1986. Functional structures of the organ of Corti: a review. *Hear. Res.*, 22, 117-146.

Lim, D. J. 1987. Development of the tectorial membrane. *Hear. Res.*, 28, 9-21.

Lim, D. J. 1992. Structural development of the cochlea. In Romand, R. (Ed.), *Development of Auditory and Vestibular Systems 2*. Elsevier, Amsterdam, 33-58.

Lim, D. J., Anniko, M. 1985. Developmental morphology of the mouse inner ear. A scanning electron microscopic observation. *Acta. Otolaryngol. (Suppl.)*, 422, 1-69.

Lim, D. J., DeMaria, T. F. 1987. Immunobarriers of the tubotympanum. *Acta Otolaryngol.*, 103, 355-362.

Lim, D. J., DeMaria, T. F., Bakaletz, L. O. 1988. Current concepts of pathogenesis of otitis media: a review. *Acta Otolaryngol. (Suppl.)*, 458, 174-180.

Lim, D. J., Rueda, J. 1992. Structural development of the cochlea. In Romand, R. (Ed.), *Development of the Auditory and Vestibular Systems 2*. Elsevier Science Publ., BV., Amsterdam, 33-58.

Limb, C. J., Ryugo, D. K. 2000. Development of primary axosomatic endings in the anteroventral cochlear nucleus of mice. *J. Assoc. Res. Otolaryngol.*, in press.

Lin, D. W., Trune, D. R. 1997. Breakdown of stria vascularis blood-labyrinth barrier in C3H/*lpr* autoimmune disease mice. *Otolaryngol. Head Neck Surg.*, 117, 530-534.

Lindblad-Toh, K., Winchester, E., Daly, M. J., Wang, D. G., Hirschhorn, J. N., Laviolette, J. P., Ardlie, K., Reich, D. E., Robinson, E., Sklar, P., Shah, N., Thomas, D., Fan, J. B., Gingeras, T., Warrington, J., Patil, N., Hudson, T. J., Lander, E. S. 2000. Large-scale discovery and genotyping of single-nucleotide polymorphisms in the mouse. *Nature Genet.*, 24, 381-386.

Lindsay, K. R., Zuidema, J. J. 1950. Inner ear deafness of sudden onset. *Laryngoscope*, 60, 238-263.

Lingenhöhl, K., Friauf, E. 1992. Giant neurons in the caudal pontine reticular formation receive short latency acoustic input: An intracellular recording and HRP-study in the rat. *J. Comp. Neurol.*, 325, 473-492.

Lingenhöl, K., Friauf, E. 1994. Giant neurons in the rat reticular formation: a sensorimotor interface in the elementary acoustic startle circuit? *J. Neurosci.*, 14, 1176-1194.

Liu, X. Z., Ondek, B., Williams, D. S. 1998b. Mutant myosin VIIa causes defective melanosome distribution in the RPE of shaker-1 mice. *Nature Genet.*, 19, 117-118.

Liu, X. Z., Udovichenko, I. P., Brown, S. D., Steel, K. P., Williams, D. S. 1999. Myosin VIIa participates in opsin transport through the photoreceptor cilium. *J. Neurosci.*, 19, 6267-6274.

Liu, X. Z., Vansant, G., Udovichenko, I. P., Wolfrum, U., Williams, D. S. 1997d. Myosin VIIa, the product of the Usher 1B syndrome gene, is concentrated in the connecting cilia of photoreceptor cells. *Cell Motil. Cytoskeleton*, 37, 240-252.

Liu, X. Z., Hope, C., Walsh, J., Newton, V., Ke, X. M., Liang, C. Y., Xu, L. R., Zhou, J. M., Trump, D., Steel, K. P., Bundey, S., Brown, S. D. 1998a. Mutations in the myosin VIIA gene cause a wide phenotypic spectrum, including atypical Usher syndrome. *Am. J. Hum. Genet.*, 63, 909-912.

Liu, X. Z., Newton, V. E., Steel, K. P., Brown, S. D. 1997a. Identification of a new mutation of the myosin VII head region in Usher syndrome type 1. *Hum. Mutat.*, 10, 168-170.

Liu, X. Z., Walsh, J., Mburu, P., Kendrick-Jones, J., Cope, M. J., Steel, K. P., Brown, S. D. 1997b. Mutations in the myosin VIIA gene cause non-syndromic recessive deafness. *Nature Genet.*, 16, 188-190.

Liu, X. Z., Walsh, J., Tamagawa, Y., Kitamura, K., Nishizawa, M., Steel, K. P., Brown, S. D. 1997c. Autosomal dominant non-syndromic deafness caused by a mutation in the myosin VIIA gene. *Nature Genet.*, 17, 268-269.

Logue, S. F., Owen, E. H., Rasmussen, D. L., Wehner, J. M. 1997. Assessment of locomotor activity, acoustic and tactile startle, and prepulse inhibition of startle in inbred mouse strains and F_1 hybrids: implications of genetic background for single gene and quantitative trait loci analyses. *Neuroscience*, 80, 1075-1086.

Loh, H. H., Smith, A. P. 1990. Molecular characterization of opioid receptors. *Ann. Rev. Pharmacol. Toxicol.*, 30, 123-147.

Lohmann, C., Friauf, E. 1996. Distribution of the calcium-binding proteins parvalbumin and calretinin in the auditory brainstem of adult and developing rats. *J. Comp. Neurol.*, 367, 90-109.

Lohnes, D., Mark, M., Mendelsohn, C., Dolle, P., Dierich, A., Gorry, P., Gansmuller, A., Chambon, P. 1994. Function of the retinoic acid receptors (RARs) during development (I). Craniofacial and skeletal abnormalities in RAR double mutants. *Devel.,* 120, 2723-2748.

Lombard, W. P. 1887. The variations of the normal knee-jerk, and their relation to the activity of the central nervous system. *Am. J. Psychol.,* 1, 2-71.

Lonsbury-Martin, B. L., Harris, F. P., Stagner, B. B., Hawkins, M. D., Martin, G. K. 1990. Distortion product emissions in humans. I. Basic properties in normally hearing subjects. *Ann. Oto.-Rhino.-Laryngol.,* 99(S147), 3-14.

Lonsbury-Martin, B. L., Martin, G. K., Probst, R., Coats, A. C. 1987. Acoustic distortion products in rabbits ear canal. I. Basic features and physiological vulnerability. *Hear. Res.,* 28, 173-179.

Lonsbury-Martin, B. L., Martin, G. K., Whitehead, M. L. 1997. Distortion product otoacoustic emissions. In Robinette, M. S., Glattke, T. J. (Eds.), *Otoacoustic Emissions.* Thieme, New York, 83-109.

Lonsdale, R. N., Roberts, P. F., Vaughan, R., Thiru, S. 1992. Familial oesophageal leiomyomatosis and nephropathy. *Histopathology,* 20, 127-133.

López, D. E., Merchán M. A., Bajo V. M., Saldaña E. 1993. The cochlear root neurons in the rat, mouse and gerbil. In Merchán, M. A. et al. (Eds.), *The Mammalian Cochlear Nuclei: Organization and Function.* Plenum, New York, 291-301.

Lopez-Gonzalez, M. A., Lucas, M., Sanchez, B., Wichmann, I., Garcia-Monge, E., Nuñez-Roldan, A., Delgado, F. 1999. Autoimmune deafness is not related to hyperreactivity to type II collagen. *Acta Otolaryngol.,* 119, 690-694.

Lord, E. M., Gates, W. H. 1929. Shaker, a new mutation of the house mouse (*Mus musculus*). *Am. Naturalist,* 63, 435-442.

Lorente de Nó, R. 1926. Études sur l'anatomie et la physiologie du labyrinthe de l'oreille et du VIII nerf. Deuxième partie: quelques données au sujet de l'anatomie des organes sensoriels du labyrinthe. *Trab. Lab. Recherches Biol. Univ. Madrid,* 24, 53-153.

Lorente de Nó, R. 1933. Anatomy of the eighth nerve. III. General plan of structure of the primary cochlear nuclei. *Laryngoscope,* 43, 327-350.

Lorente de Nó, R. 1981. *The Primary Acoustic Nuclei.* Raven Press, New York.

Louryan, S., Gilineur, R., Dourov, N. 1992. Induced and genetic mouse middle ear ossicular malformations: a model for ossicular diseases and a tool for clarifying their normal ontogenesis. *Surg. Radiol. Anat.,* 14, 227-232.

Lousteau, R. J. 1987. Increased spiral ganglion cell survival in electrically stimulated, deafened guinea pig cochleae. *Laryngoscope,* 97, 836-842.

Lowenheim, H., Furness, D. N., Kil, J., Zinn, C., Gultig, K., Fero, M. L., Frost, D., Gummer, A. W., Roberts, J. M., Rubel, E. W., Hackney, C. M., Zenner, H. P. 1999. Gene disruption of p27(Kip1) allows cell proliferation in the postnatal and adult organ of corti. *Proc. Natl. Acad. Sci., USA,* 96, 4084-4088.

Lowenstein, D. H., Gwinn, R. P., Seren, M. S., Simon, R. P., McIntosh, T. K. 1994. Increased expressiion of mRNA encoding calbindin-D28k, the glucose regulated proteins or the 72kDa heat-shock protein in three models of acute injury. Mol. *Brain Res.,* 22, 299-308.

Lowenstein, D. H., Miles, M. F., Hatam, F., McCabe, T. 1991. Up regulation of calbindin-D28k mRNA in the rat hippocampus following focal stimulation of the perforant path. *Neuron,* 6, 627-633.

Lu, W., Phillips, C. L., Killen, P. D., Hlaing, T., Harrison, W. R., Elder, F. F., Miner, J. H., Overbeek, P. A., Meisler, M. H. 1999. Insertional mutation of the collagen genes Col4a3 and Col4a4 in a mouse model of Alport syndrome. *Genomics,* 61, 113-124.

Luttge, W. G. 1979. Endocrine control of mammalian sex behavior: an analysis of the potential role of androgen metabolites. In Beyer, C. (Ed.), *Endocrine Control of Sexual Behavior.* Raven Press, New York, 341-363.

Lynch, E. D., Lee, M., K., Morrow, J. E., Welcsh, P. L., Leon, P. E., King, M.-C. 1997. Non-syndromic deafness DFNA1 associated with mutation of a human homolog of the Drosophila gene diaphanous. *Science,* 278, 1315-1318.

Ma, Q., Chen, Z., del Barco Barrantes, I., de la Pompa, J. L., Anderson, D. J. 1998. Neurogenin1 is essential for the determination of neuronal precursors for proximal cranial sensory ganglia. *Neuron,* 20, 469-482.

Ma, W., Behar, T., Barker, J. L. 1992a. Transient expression of GABA immunoreactivity in the developing rat spinal cord. *J. Comp. Neurol.,* 325, 271-290.

Ma, W., Behar, T., Maric, D., Maric, L., Barker, J. L. 1992b. Neuroepithelial cells in the rat spinal cord express glutamate decarboxylase immunoreactivity *in vivo* and *in vitro. J. Comp. Neurol.,* 325, 257-270.

Maass, B., Kellner, J. 1984. Hydrogen clearance and cochlear microcirculation at different levels of blood pressure. *Arch. Otorhinolaryngol.*, 240, 295-310.

MacKenzie, A., Ferguson, M. W., Sharpe, P. T. 1991. Hox-7 expression during murine craniofacial development. *Devel.*, 113, 601-611.

Maeda, K., Hirano, T., Suzuki, M., Mogi, G. 1999. Endotoxin induced long-term otitis media with effusion in mice. Presented at: *Seventh International Symposium on Recent Advances in Otitis Media.* June 1-5, Fort Lauderdale, FL, 121.

Maggio, J. C., Maggio, J. H., Whitney, G. 1983. Experience-based vocalization of male mice to female chemosignals. *Physiol. Behav.*, 31, 269-272.

Maggio, J. C., Whitney, G. 1985. Ultrasonic vocalizing by adult female mice (*Mus musculus*). *J. Comp. Psychol.*, 99, 420-436.

Maggirwar, S. B., Dhanraj, D. N., Somani, S. M., Ramkumar, V. 1994. Adenosine acts as an endogenous activator of the cellular antioxidant defense system. *Biochem. Biophys. Res. Commun.*, 201, 508-515.

Maier, H., Zinn, C., Rothe, A., Tiziani, H., Gummer, A. W. 1997. Development of a narrow water-immersion objective for laserinterferometric and electrophysiological applications in cell biology. *J. Neurosci. Meth.*, 77, 31-41.

Maisonpierre, P. C., Belluscio, L., Squinto, S. 1990. Neurotrophin-3: a neurotrophic factor related to NGF and BDNF. *Science,* 247, 1446-1451.

Majorossy, K., Kiss, A. 1976. Specific patterns of neuron arrangement and of synaptic articulation in the medial geniculate body. *Exp. Brain Res.*, 26, 1-17.

Malakoff, D. 2000. The rise of the mouse, biomedicine's model mammal. *Science,* 288, 248-253.

Male, D., Cooke, A., Owen, M., Trowsdale, J., Champion, B. 1996. *Advanced Immunology.* Mosby, London.

Mallo, M. 1997. Retinoic acid disturbs mouse middle ear development in a stage-dependent fashion. *Devel. Biol.*, 184, 175-186.

Mallo, M., Gridley, T. 1996. Development of the mammalian ear: coordinate regulation of formation of the tympanic ring and the external acoustic meatus. *Devel.*, 122, 173-179.

Mandelbrot, B. B. 1982. *The Fractal Geometry of Nature.* W.H. Freeman, New York.

Mandler, R. N., Schaffner, A. E., Novotny, E. A., Lange, G. D., Smith, S. V., Barker, J. L. 1990. Electrical and chemical excitability appear one week before birth in the embryonic rat spinal cord. *Brain Res.*, 522, 46-54.

Manis, P. B. 1989. Responses to parallel fiber stimulation in the guinea pig dorsal cochlear nucleus *in vitro. J. Neurophysiol.*, 61, 149-161.

Manis, P. B., Marx, S. O. 1991. Outward currents in isolated ventral cochlear nucleus neurons. *J. Neurosci.*, 11, 2865-2880.

Manis, P. B., Spirou, G. A., Wright, D. D., Paydar, S., Ryugo, D. K. 1994. Physiology and morphology of complex spiking neurons in the guinea pig dorsal cochlear nucleus. *J. Comp. Neurol.*, 348, 261-276.

Mansergh, F. C., Millington-Ward, S., Kennan, A., Kiang, A. S., Humphries, M., Farrar, G. J., Humphries, P., Kenna, P. F. 1999. Retinitis pigmentosa and progressive sensorineural hearing loss caused by a C12258A mutation in the mitochondrial MTTS2 gene. *Am. J. Hum. Genet.*, 64, 971-985.

Mansour, S., Goddard, J. M., Capecchi, M. R. 1993. Mice homozygous for a targeted disruption of the proto-oncogene INT-2 have developmental defects in the tail and ear. *Devel.*, 117, 13-28.

Manthorpe, M., Skaper, S. D., Barbin, G., Varon, S. 1982. Cholinergic neuronotrophic factors (CNTF's). VII. Concurrent activities on certain nerve growth factor responsive neurons. *J. Neurochem.*, 38, 415-421.

Marangos, N., Laszig, R. 1996. Restoration of hearing with multichannel prostheses: 10 years' experience. *Folia Phoniatr. Logop.*, 48, 131-136.

Mariyama, M., Zheng, K., Yang-Feng, T. L., Reeders, S. T. 1992. Colocalization of the genes for the alpha 3(IV) and alpha 4(IV) chains of type IV collagen to chromosome 2 bands q35-q37. *Genomics,* 13, 809-813.

Mark, M., Lufkin, T., Dolle, P., Dierich, A., LeMeur, M., Chambon, P. 1993. Roles of Hox genes: what we have learnt from gain of function and loss of function mutations in the mouse. *C.R. Acad. Sci. III,* 316, 995-1008.

Markel, P., Shu, P., Ebeling, C., Carlson, G. A., Nagle, D. L., Smutko, J. S., Moore, K. J. 1997. Theoretical and empirical issues for marker-assisted breeding of congenic mouse strains [see Comments]. *Nature Genet.*, 17, 280-284.

Markl, H., Ehret, G. 1973. Die Hörschwelle der Maus (*Mus musculus*). Eine kritische Wertung der Methoden zur Bestimmung der Hörschwelle eines Säugetieres. *Z. Tierpsychol.*, 33, 274-286.

Marks, J. L., King, M. G., Baskin, D. G. 1991. Localization of insulin and type I IGF receptors in rat brain by *in vitro* autoradiography and *in situ* hybridization. In Raizada, M. K., LeRoith, D. (Eds.), *Molecular Biology and Physiology of Insulin and Insulin like Growth Factors*. Plenum Press, New York, 100-120.

Marks, M. J., Stitzel, J. A., Collins, A. C. 1989. Genetic influences on nicotinic responses. *Pharmacol. Biochem. Behav.*, 33, 667-678.

Marovitz, W. F., Shugar, J. M. 1976. Single mitotic center for rodent cochlear duct. *Ann. Otol. Rhinol. Laryngol.*, 85, 225-233.

Marr, J. N., Gardner, L. E., Jr. 1965. Early olfactory experience and later social behavior in the rat: preference, sexual responsiveness and care of young. *J. Genet. Psychol.*, 107, 167-174.

Marsh, R., Hoffman, H. S., Stitt, C. L. 1973. Temporal integration in the acoustic startle reflex of the rat. *J. Comp. Physiol. Psychol.*, 82, 507-511.

Martin, G. K., Lonsbury-Martin, B. L., Kimm, J. 1980. A rabbit preparation for neuro-behavioral auditory research. *Hear. Res.*, 2, 65-78.

Martin, J. F., Bradley, A., Olson, E. N. 1995. The paired-like homeo box gene MHox is required for early events of skeletogenesis in multiple lineages. *Genes Devel.*, 9, 1237-1249.

Martin, M. 1981. Morphology of the cochlear nucleus of the normal and reeler mutant mouse. *J. Comp. Neurol.*, 197,141-152.

Martin, M., Rickets, C. 1981. Histogenesis of the cochlear nucleus of the mouse. *J. Comp. Neurol.*, 197,169-184.

Martin, P., Heiskari, N., Zhou, J., Leinonen, A., Tumelius, T., Hertz, J. M., Barker, D., Gregory, M., Atkin, C., Styrkarsdottir, U., Neumann, H., Springate, J., Shows, T., Pettersson, E., Tryggvason, K. 1998. High mutation detection rate in the COL4A5 collagen gene in suspected Alport syndrome using PCR and direct DNA sequencing. *J. Am. Soc. Nephrol.*, 9, 2291-2301.

Martin-Zanca, D., Barbacid, M., Parada, L. F. 1990. Expression of the trk proto-oncogene is restricted to the sensory cranial and spinal ganglia of neural crest origin in mouse development. *Genes Devel.*, 4, 683-694.

Maruniak, J., Bronson, F. 1976. Gonadotropic responses of male mice to female urine. *Endocrinology*, 99, 963-969.

Massagué, J. 1990. The transforming growth factor-beta family. *Annu. Rev. Cell Biol.*, 6, 597-641.

Massagué, J., Guillette, B. J., Czech, M. P., Morgan, C. J., Bradshaw, R. A. 1981. Identification of a nerve growth factor receptor protein in sympathetic ganglia membranes by affinity labelling. *J. Biol. Chem.*, 256, 9419-9424.

Masterton, R. G., Thompson, G. C., Bechtold, J. K., Robards, M. J. 1975. Neuroanatomical basis of binaural phase-difference analysis for sound localization: a comparative study. *J. Comp. Physiol. Psychol.*, 89, 379-386.

Mathews, K. D., Rapisarda, D., Bailey, H. L., Murray, J. C., Schelper, R. L., Smith, R, 1995. Phenotypic and pathologic evaluation of the *myd* mouse. A candidate for facioscapulohumeral dystrophy. *J. Neuropathol. Exp. Neurol.*, 56, 601-606.

Matochik, J. A., Sipos, M. L., Nyby, J. G., Barfield, R. J. 1994. Intracranial androgenic activation of male-typical behaviors in house mice: motivation versus performance. *Behav. Brain. Res.*, 60, 141-149.

Matsuoka, H., Cheng, K.-C., Krug, M. S., Yazawa, Y., Yoo, T.-J. 1999. Murine model of autoimmune hearing loss induced by myelin protein P0. *Ann. Otol. Rhinol. Laryngol.*, 108, 255-264.

Matsuzawa, A., Moriyama, T., Kaneko, T., Tanaka, M., Kimura, M., Ikeda, H., Katagiri, T. 1990. A new allele of the *lpr* locus, *lpr^{cg}*, that complements the *gld* gene in induction of lymphadenopathy in the mouse. *J. Exp. Med.*, 171, 519-531.

Matthews, J. W., Molnar, C. E. 1986. Modeling intracochlear and ear canal distortion product (2f$_1$-f$_2$). In Allen, J. B., Hall, J. L., Hubbard, A., Meely, S. T., Tubis, A. (Eds.), *Peripheral Auditory Mechanisms*. Springer Verlag, New York, 258-265.

Matzner, U., Von Figura K. R. P. 1992. Expression of the two mannose 6-phosphate receptors is spatially and temporally different during mouse embryogenesis. *Devel.*, 114, 965-972.

Mayes, M. D. 1999. Epidemiologic studies of environmental agents and systemic autoimmune diseases. *Environ. Health Perspect.*, 107, 743-748.

Mazzucco, G., Barsotti, P., Muda, A. O., Fortunato, M., Mihatsch, M., Torri-Tarelli, L., Renieri, A., Faraggiana, T., De Marchi, M., Monga, G. 1998. Ultrastructural and immunohistochemical findings in Alport's syndrome: a study of 108 patients from 97 Italian families with particular emphasis on COL4A5 gene mutation correlations. *J. Am. Soc. Nephrol.*, 9, 1023-1031.

Mburu, P., Liu, X. Z., Walsh, J., Saw, Jr., D., Cope, M. J., Gibson, F., Kendrick-Jones, J., Steel, K. P., Brown, S. D. 1997. Mutation analysis of the mouse myosin VIIA deafness gene. *Genes Funct.*, 1, 191-203.

McCabe, B. F. 1979. Autoimmune sensorineural hearing loss. *Ann. Otol.,* 88, 585-589.

McCaughran, J., Bell, J., Hitzemann, R. 1999. On the relationship of high frequency hearing loss and cochlear pathology to the acoustic startle response (ASR) and prepulse inhibition of the ASR in the BXD recombinant inbred series. *Behav. Genet.,* 29, 21-30.

McCaughran, J. A., Bell, J., Hitzemann, R. J. 2000. Fear-potentiated startle response in mice: genetic analysis of the C57BL/6J and DBA/2J intercross. *Pharmacol. Biochem. Behav.,* 65, 301-312.

McCaughran, Jr., J., Mahjubi, E., Decena, E., Hitzemann, R. 1997. Genetics, haloperidol-induced catalepsy and haloperidol-induced changes in acoustic startle and prepulse inhibition. *Psychopharmacology,* 134, 131-139.

McConnell, S. K. 1995. Strategies for the generation of neuronal diversity in the developing central nervous system. *J. Neurosci.,* 15, 6987-6998.

McCord, J. M. 1993. Human disease, free radicals, and the oxidant/antioxidant balance. *Clin. Biochem.,* 26, 351-357.

McCord, J. M., Fridovich, I. 1969. Superoxide dismutase. An enzymic function for erythrocuprein (hemocuprein). *J. Biol. Chem.,* 244, 6049-6055.

McCord, J. M., Russell, W. J. 1988. Inactivation of creatine phosphokinase by superoxide during reperfusion injury. *Basic Life Sci.,* 49, 869-873.

McCormick, D. P., Uchida, T. 1999. Tobacco smoke, day care, middle-ear surgery, and costs in young children. Presented at *Seventh International Symposium on Recent Advances in Otitis Media.* June 1-5, Fort Lauderdale, FK, P28.

McDermott, H. J., Lech, M., Kornblum, M. S., Irvine, D. R. F. 1998. Loudness perception and frequency discrimination in subjects with steeply sloping hearing loss: possible correlates of neural plasticity. *J. Acoust. Soc. Am.,* 104, 2314-2325.

McDonald, T. J., Zincke, H., Anderson, C. F., Ott, N. T. 1976. Reversal of deafness after renal transplantation in Alport's syndrome. *Laryngoscope,* 88, 38-42.

McDonogh, M. 1986. The middle ear transformer mechanism: man versus mouse. *J. Laryngol. Otol.,* 100, 15-19.

McEvilly, R., Erkman, L., Luo, L., Sawchenko, P., Ryan, A. F., Rosenfeld, M. G. 1996. Requirement for Brn-3.0 in differentiation and survival of sensory and motor neurons. *Nature,* 384, 574-577.

McFadden, S. L., Burkard, R. F., Shero, M., Ding, D. L., Salvi, R. J., Flood, D. G. 2000. Chronic oxidative stress does not exacerbate noise-induced hearing loss in SOD1 mice. *Assoc. Res. Otolaryngol. Abstr.,* 217, 61.

McFadden, S. L., Burkard, R. F., Ohlemiller, K. K., Durand, B. I., Ding, D. L., Flood, D. G., Salvi, R. J. 1999a. Copper/zinc superoxide dismutase deficiency potentiates age-related and noise-induced hearing loss in SOD-1 mice. *Assoc. Res. Otolaryngol. Abstr.,* 132, 33.

McFadden, S. L., Ding, D., Reaume, A. G., Flood, D. G., Salvi, R. J. 1999c. Age-related cochlear hair cell loss is enhanced in mice lacking copper/zinc superoxide dismutase. *Neurobiol. Aging,* 20, 1-8.

McFadden, S. L., Ding, D., Burkard, R. F., Jiang, H., Reaume, A. G., Flood, D. G., Salvi, R. J. 1999b. Cu/Zn SOD deficiency potentiates hearing loss and cochlear pathology in aged 129,CD-1 mice. *J. Comp. Neurol.,* 413, 101-112.

McFadden, S. L., Henselman, L. W. Zheng, X.-Y. 1999d. Sex differences in auditory sensitivity of chinchillas before and after exposure to impulse noise. *Ear Hear.,* 20, 164-174.

McFadden, S. L., Walsh, E. J., McGee, J. 1996. Onset and development of auditory brainstem responses in the Mongolian gerbil (*Meriones unguiculatus*). *Hear. Res.,* 100, 68-78.

McFadden, S. L., Willott, J. F. 1994a. Responses of inferior colliculus neurons in C57BL/6J mice with and without sensorineural hearing loss: effects of changing the azimuthal location of an unmasked pure-tone stimulus. *Hear. Res.,* 78, 115-131.

McFadden, S. L, Willott, J. F. 1994b. Responses of inferior colliculus neurons in C57BL/6J mice with and without sensorineural hearing loss: effects of changing the azimuthal location of a continuous noise masker on responses to contralateral tones. *Hear. Res.,* 78, 132-148.

McGhie, A., Chapman, J. 1961. Disorders of attention and perception in early schizophrenia. *Br. J. Med. Psychol.,* 34, 103-116.

McGill, T. E. 1962. Sexual behavior in three inbred strains of mice. *Behaviour,* 19, 341-350.

McGinn, M. D., Bean-Knudsen, D., Ermel, R. W. 1992. Incidence of otitis media in CBA/J and CBA/CaJ mice. *Hear. Res.,* 59, 1-6.

McHale, J. F., Harari, O. A., Marshall, D., Haskard, D. O. 1999. Vascular endothelial cell expression of ICAM-1 and VCAM-1 at the onset of eliciting contact hypersensitivity in mice: evidence for a dominant role of TNF-alpha. *J. Immunol.,* 162, 1648-1655.

McIntyre, K. R., Ayer-LeLievre, C., Persson, H. 1990. Class II major histocompatibility complex (MHC) gene expression in the mouse brain is elevated in the autoimmune MRL/MP-*lpr/lpr* strain. *J. Neuroimmunol.,* 28, 39-52.

McKernan, R. M., Whiting, P. J. 1996. Which GABAA-receptor subtypes really occur in the brain? *Trends Neurosci.,* 19, 139-143.

McKusick, V. A. 1998. *Mendelian Inheritance in Man. Catalogs of Human Genes and Genetic Disorders.* Johns Hopkins University Press, Baltimore.

McLaren, G. M., Quirk, W. S., Laurikainen, E., Coleman, J. K., Seidman, M. D., Dengerink, H. A., Nuttall, A. L., Miller, J. M., Wright, J. W. 1993. Substance P increases cochlear blood flow without changing cochlear electrophysiology in rats. *Hear. Res.,* 71, 183-189.

McLeod, A. C., McConnell, F. E., Sweeney, A., Cooper, M. C., Nance, W. E. 1971. Clinical variation in Usher's syndrome. *Arch. Otolaryngol.,* 94, 321-334.

McMenomey, S. O., Morton, J. I., Trune, D. R. 1992. Stria vascularis ultrastructural pathology in the C3H/*lpr* autoimmune mouse: a potential mechanism for immune-related hearing loss. *Otolaryngol. Head Neck Surg.,* 106, 288-295.

Meakin, S. O., Shooter, E. M. 1991. Molecular investigations of the high affinity nerve growth factor receptor. *Neuron,* 6, 153-163.

Meakin, S. O., Shooter, E. M. 1992. The nerve growth factor family of receptors. *Trends Neurosci.,* 15, 323-331.

Medd, A. M., Bianchi, L. M. 2000. Analysis of BDNF production in the aging gerbil cochlea. *Exp. Neurol.,* 162, 390-393.

Meek, 3rd, R. B, McGrew, B. M., Cuff, C. F., Berrebi, A. S., Spirou, G. A., Wetmore, S. J. 1999. Immunologic and histologic observations in reovirus-induced otitis media in the mouse. *Ann. Otol. Rhinol. Laryngol.,* 108, 31-38.

Meikle, P. J., Hopwood J. J., Clague A. E. Carey W. F. 1999. Prevalence of lysosomal storage disorders. *J. Am. Med. Assoc.,* 281, 249-254.

Meininger, V., Pol, D., Derer, P. 1986. The inferior colliculus of the mouse. A Nissl and Golgi study. *Neuroscience,* 17, 1159-1179.

Melcher, J. R., Guinan, J. J., Knudson, I. M., Kiang, N. Y. E. 1996b. Generators of brainstem auditory evoked potential in cat. II. Correlating lesion sites with waveform changes. *Hear. Res.,* 93, 28-51.

Melcher, J. R., Kiang, N. Y. E. 1996. Generators of brainstem auditory evoked potential in cat. III. Identified cell populations. *Hear. Res.,* 93, 52-71.

Melcher, J. R., Knudson, I. M., Fullerton, B. C., Guinan, J. J., Norris, B. E., Kiang, N. Y. E. 1996a. Generators of brainstem auditory evoked potential in cat. I. An experimental approach to their identification. *Hear. Res.,* 93, 1-27.

Merchán Pérez, A., Gil-Loyzaga, P., Eybalin, M., Fernandez Mateos, P., Bartolome, M. V. 1994. Choline-acetyltransferase-like immunoreactivity in the organ of Corti of the rat during postnatal development. *Devel. Brain Res.,* 82, 29-34.

Merchán-Pérez, A., Gil-Loyzaga, P., Eybalin, M. 1990a. Immunocytochemical detection of calcitonin gene-related peptide in the postnatal developing rat cochlea. *Int. J. Devel. Neurosci.,* 8, 603-612.

Merchán-Pérez, A., Gil-Loyzaga, P., Eybalin, M. 1990b. Immunocytochemical detection of glutamate decarboxylase in the postnatal developing rat organ of Corti. *Int. J. Devel. Neurosci.,* 8, 613-620.

Merchán-Pérez, A., Gil-Loyzaga, P., Eybalin, M. 1990c. Ontogeny of glutamate decarboxylase and γ-aminobutyric acid immunoreactivities in the rat cochlea. *Eur. Arch. Otorhinolaryngol.,* 248, 4-7.

Merchán-Pérez, A., Gil-Loyzaga, P., López-Sánchez, J., Eybalin, M., Valderrama, F. J. 1993. Ontogeny of gamma-aminobutyric acid in efferent fibers to the rat cochlea. *Devel. Brain Res.,* 76, 33-41.

Mermall, V., Post, P. L., Mooseker, M. S. 1998. Unconventional myosins in cell movement, membrane traffic, and signal transduction. *Science,* 279, 527-533.

Meroni, P. L., D'Cruz, D., Khamashta, M., Youinou, P., Hughes, G. R. 1996. Anti-endothelial cell antibodies: only for scientists or for clinicians too?. *Clin. Exp. Immunol.,* 104, 199-202.

Meuller, M., Smolders, J. W., Meyer zum Gottesberge, A. M., Reuter, A., Zwacka, R. M., Weiher, H., Klinke, R. 1997. Loss of auditory function in transgenic Mpv17-deficient mice. *Hear. Res.,* 114, 259-263.

Meyerhoff, W. L. 1979. Hypothyroidism and the ear: electrophysiological, morphological, and chemical considerations. *Laryngoscope,* 89(S19), 1-25.

Meyerhoff, W. L. 1974. Hearing loss and thyroid disorders. *Minn. Med.,* 57, 897-898.

Meyerson, M. D., Lewis, E., Ill, K. 1984. Facioscapulohumeral muscular dystrophy and accompanying hearing loss. *Arch. Otolaryngol.,* 110, 261-266.

MGD. 2000. *Mouse Genome,* Database: *Mouse Genome,* Informatics Project. Bar Harbor, ME, The Jackson Laboratory.

Michaels, L., Soucek, S. 1991. Auditory epithelial migration. III. Development of the stratified squamous cells layer in the tympanic membrane and external canal in the mouse. *Am. J. Anat.,* 191, 280-292.

Michiels, C., Raes, M., Toussaint, O., Remacle, J. 1994. Importance of Se-glutathione peroxidase, catalase, and Cu/Zn-SOD for cell survival against oxidative stress. *Free Radical Biol. Med.,* 17, 235-248.

Midtgaard, J. 1992. Membrane properties and synaptic responses of Golgi cells and stellate cells in the turtle cerebellum *in vitro. J. Physiol.,* 457, 329-354.

Mikaelian D. O. 1966. Single unit study of the cochlear nucleus in the mouse. *Acta Otolaryngol.,* 62, 545-556.

Mikaelian, D. O. 1979. Development and degeneration of hearing in the C57/bl6 mouse: relation of electro-physiologic responses from the round window and cochlear nucleus to cochlear anatomy and behavioral responses. *Laryngoscope,* 89, 1-15.

Mikaelian, D., Ruben, R. J. 1965. Development of hearing in the normal CBA-J mouse. Correlation of physiological observations with behavioral responses and with cochlear anatomy. *Acta Otolaryng.,* 59, 451-461.

Mikaelian, D. O., Ruben, R. J. 1964. Hearing degeneration in shaker-1 mouse. Correlation of physiological observations with behavioral responses and with cochlear anatomy. *Arch. Otolaryngol.,* 80, 418-430.

Mikaelian, D. O., Warfield, D., Norris, O. 1974. Genetic progressive hearing loss in the C57/bl6 mouse. *Acta Otolaryngol.,* 77, 327-334.

Milbrandt, J. C, Caspary, D. M. 1995. Age-related reduction of [^{3}H]strychnine binding sites in the cochlear nucleus of the Fischer 344 rat. *Neuroscience,* 67, 713-719.

Milbrandt, J. C., Albin, R. L., Turgeon, S. M, Caspary, D. M. 1996. GABAa receptor binding the aging rat inferior colliculus. *Neuroscience,* 73, 449-458.

Milbrandt, J. C., Albin, R. L, Caspary, D. M. 1994. Age-related decrease in GABAb receptor binding in the Fischer 344 rat inferior colliculus. *Neurobiol. Aging,* 15, 699-703.

Milbrandt, J. C., Hunter, C., Caspary, D. M. 1997. Alterations of GABAa receptor subunit mRNA levels in the aging Fischer rat inferior colliculus. *J. Comp. Neurol.,* 379, 455-465.

Miller, D. M. 1994. Physiologic and Histologic Disturbances in the Mouse Mutant, Viable Dominant Spotting. M. A. thesis, Washington University, St. Louis, MO.

Miller, G. A. 1948. The perception of short bursts of noise. *J. Acoust. Soc. Am.,* 20, 160-170.

Miller, J. D., Watson, C. S., Covell, W. P. 1963. Deafening effects of noise on the cat. *Acta Otolaryngol. (Suppl.),* 176.

Miller, J. M., Altschuler, R. A., Dupont, J., Lesperance, M., Tucci, D. 1996. Consequences of deafness and electrical stimulation on the auditory system. In Salvi, R. J., Henderson, D. H., Colletti, V., Fiorino, F. (Eds.), *Auditory Plasticity and Regeneration.* Thieme Medical Publishers, New York, 378-391.

Miller, J. M., Dolan, D. F., Raphael, Y., Altschuler, R. A. 1998. Interactive effects of aging with noise induced hearing loss. *Scand. Audiol. (Suppl.),* 48, 53-61.

Miller, J. M., Nuttall, A. L. 1990. Cochlear blood flow. In Shepherd, A. P., Oberg, A. (Eds.), *Laser Doppler Flowmetry.* Kluwer Academic, Norwell, MA, 319-348.

Millonig, J. H., Millen, K. J., Hatten, M. E. 2000. The mouse Dreher gene Lmx1a controls formation of the roof plate in the vertebrate CNS [see Comments]. *Nature,* 403, 764-769.

Mills, D. M., Norton, S. J., Rubel, E. W. 1993. Vulnerability and adaptation of distortion product otoacoustic emissions to endocochlear potential variation. *J. Acoust. Soc. Am.,* 94, 2108-2122.

Mills, D. M., Rubel, E. W. 1994. Variation of distortion product otoacoustic emissions with furosemide microinjection. *Hear. Res.,* 77, 183-199.

Mills, D. M., Rubel, E. W. 1996. Development of the cochlear amplifier. *J. Acoust. Soc. Am.,* 100, 428-441.

Miner, J. H., Sanes, J. R. 1994. Collagen IV alpha 3, alpha 4, and alpha 5 chains in rodent basal laminae: sequence, distribution, association with laminins, and developmental switches. *J. Cell Biol.,* 127, 879-891.

Miner, J. H., Sanes, J. R. 1996. Molecular and functional defects in kidneys of mice lacking collagen alpha 3(IV): implications for Alport syndrome. *J. Cell Biol.,* 135, 1403-1413.

Minowa, O., Ikeda, K., Sugitani, Y., Oshima, T., Nakai, S., Katori, Y., Suzuki, M. et al. 1999. Altered cochlear fibrocytes in a mouse model of DFN3 nonsyndromic deafness. *Science,* 285, 1408-1411.

Misrahy, G. A., Hildreth, K. M., Shinabarger, E. W., Clark, L. C., Rice, E. A. 1958. Endolymphatic oxygen tension in the cochlea of the guinea pig. *J. Acoust. Soc. Am.,* 30, 247-250.

Mitchell, C. R., Kempton, J. B., Creedon, T. A., Trune, D. R. 1996. Rapid acquisition of auditory brainstem responses with multiple frequency and intensity tone-bursts. *Hear. Res.,* 99, 38-46.

Mitchell, C. R., Kempton, J. B., Creedon, T. A., Trune, D. R. 1999. The use of a 56-stimulus train for rapid acquisition of auditory brainstem responses. *Audiol. Neuro-Otol.*, 4, 80-87.

Mitchell, C. R., Kempton, J. B., Scott-Tyler, B., Trune, D. R. 1997. Otitis media incidence and impact on the ABR in lipopolysaccharide-nonresponsive C3H/HeJ mice. *Otolaryngol. Head Neck Surg.*, 117, 459-64.

Mize, R. R. 1994. Conservation of basic synaptic circuits that mediate GABA inhibition in the subcortical visual system. *Prog. Brain Res.*, 100, 123-132.

Mochizuki, T., Lemmink, H. H., Mariyama, M., Antignac, C., Gubler, M. C., Pirson, Y., Verellen-Dumoulin, C., Chan, B., Schroder, C. H., Smeets, H. J. 1994. Identification of mutations in the alpha 3(IV) and alpha 4(IV) collagen genes in autosomal recessive Alport syndrome. *Nature Genet.*, 8, 77-81.

Mogi, G., Kodama, S., Suzuki, M., Kurono, Y. 1999. Mucosal vaccination for middle ear infection — an animal study. Presented at *Seventh International Symposium on Recent Advances in Otitis Media.* June 1-5, Fort Lauderdale, FL, M10.

Mogi, G., Kurono, Y. 1996. Oral vaccine for otitis media with effusion. In Lim, D. J., Bluestone, C. D., Casselbrant, M., Klein, J. O., Ogra, P. L. (Eds.), *Recent Advances in Otitis Media.* B. C. Decker, Hamilton, 493-495.

Moiseff, A., Konishi, M. 1981. Neuronal and behavioral sensitivity to binaural time differences in the owl. *J. Neurosci.*, 1, 2553-2562.

Møller, A. R. 1974. Function of the middle ear. In Keidel, W. D., Neff, W. D. (Eds.), *Handbook of Sensory Physiology,* Vol. V/1: Auditory System. Berlin, Springer-Verlag, Berlin, 491-517.

Møller, A. R. 1994. Neural generators of auditory evoked potentials, In Jacobson, J. (Ed.), *Principles Applications in Auditory Evoked Potentials.* Allyn & Bacon, Needham Heights, 23-46.

Moller, C. G., Kimberling, W. J., Davenport, S. L., Priluck, I., White, V., Biscone-Halterman, K., Odkvist, L. M., Brookhouser, P. E., Lund, G., Grissom, T. J. 1989. Usher syndrome: an otoneurologic study. *Laryngoscope*, 99, 73-79.

Mom, T., Avan, P., Romand, R., Gilain, L. 1997. Monitoring of functional changes after transient ischemia in gerbil cochlea. *Brain Res.*, 751, 20-30.

Moore, B. C. J. 1997. *An Introduction to the Psychology of Hearing,* 4th ed. Academic Press, New York.

Moore, J. K. 1980. The primate cochlear nuclei: loss of lamination as a phylogenetic process. *J. Comp. Neurol.*, 193, 609-629.

Moore, J. K., Moore, R. Y. 1987. Glutamic acid decarboxylase-like immunoreactivity in brainstem auditory nuclei of the rat. *J. Comp. Neurol.*, 260, 157-174.

Moore, J., Osen, K. 1979. The cochlear nuclei in man. *Am. J. Anat.*, 154, 393-418.

Moore, M. J., Caspary, D. M. 1983. Strychnine blocks bianural inhibition in lateral superior olivary neurons. *J. Neurosci.*, 3, 237-242.

Mooseker, M. S., Cheney, R. E. 1995. Unconventional myosins. *Annu. Rev. Cell Devel. Biol.*, 11, 633-675.

Morell, R. J., Kim, H. J., Hood, L. J., Goforth, L., Friderici, K., Fisher, R., Van Camp, G., Berlin, C. I., Oddoux, C., Ostrer, H., Keats, B., Friedman, T. B. 1998. High prevalence of the 167delT mutation in connexin 26 (GJB2) among Ashkenazi Jews with nonsyndromic recessive deafness. *New Engl. J. Med.*, 339, 1500-1505.

Morest, D. K., Hutson, K., Kwok, S. 1990. Cytoarchitectonic atlas of the cochlear nucleus of the chinchilla, *Chinchilla laniger. J. Comp. Neurol.*, 300, 230-248.

Morest, D. K. 1964. The neuronal architecture of the medial geniculate body of the cat. *J. Anat. (London)*, 98, 611-630.

Morest, D. K. 1968a. The collateral system of the medial nucleus of the trapezoid body of the cat, its neuronal architecture and relation to the olivo-cochlear bundle. *Brain Res.*, 9, 288-311.

Morest, D. K. 1968b. The growth of synaptic endings in the mammalian brain: a study of the calyces of the trapezoid body. *Z. Anat. Entwickl. Gesch.*, 127, 201-220.

Morest, D. K. 1975. Synaptic relationships of Golgi type II cells in the medial geniculate body of the cat. *J. Comp. Neurol.*, 162, 157-194.

Morest, D. K. 1993. The cellular basis for signal processing in the mammalian cochlear nuclei. In Merchan, M. A., Juiz, J. M. Godfrey, D. A. (Eds.), *The Mammalian Cochlear Nuclei: Organization and Function.* Plenum, New York, 1-18.

Morest, D. K., Winer, J. A. 1986. The comparative anatomy of neurons: homologous neurons in the medial geniculate body of the opossum and the cat. *Adv. Anat. Embryol. Cell Biol.*, 97, 1-94.

Morgenstern, C., Kessler, M. 1978. Oxygen consumption and oxygen distribution in the inner ear. *Arch. Otorhinolaryngol.*, 220, 159-62.

Morgret, M. K. 1973. The long-term development of fighting in mice: implications for future research. *Devel. Psychobiol.,* 6, 503-509.

Morgret, M. K., Dengerink, H. A. 1972. The squeal as an indicator of aggression in mice. *Behav. Res. Meth. Instrum.,* 4, 138-140.

Morris-Kay, G. M., Ward, S. J. 1999. Retinoids and mammalian development. *Int. Rev. Cytol.,* 188, 73-131.

Morrison, A., Hodgetts, C., Gossler, A., Hrabe de Angelis, M., Lewis, J. 1999. Expression of Delta1 and Serrate1 (Jagged1) in the mouse inner ear. *Mech. Devel.,* 84, 169-172.

Morrow, E. M., Belliveau, M. J., Cepko, C. L. 1998. Two phases of rod photoreceptor differentiation during rat retinal development. *J. Neurosci.,* 18, 3738-3748.

Morsli, H., Choo, D., Ryan, A., Johnson, R., Wu, D. K. 1998. Development of the mouse inner ear and origin of its sensory organs. *J. Neurosci.,* 18, 3327-3335.

Morsli, H., Tuorto, F., Choo, D., Postiglione, M. P., Simeone, A., Wu, D. K. 1999. Otx1 and Otx2 activities are required for the normal development of the mouse inner ear. *Devel.,* 126, 2335-2343.

Mosig, D. W., Dewsbury, D. A. 1976. Studies of copulatory behavior of house mice. *Behav. Biol.,* 16, 463-473.

Moss, C. F., Schnitzler, H. U. 1996. Behavioral studies of auditory information processing. In Popper, A. N., Fay, R. R. (Eds.), *Hearing by Bats.* Springer-Verlag, New York, 87-145.

Motohashi, H., Hozawa, K., Oshima, T., Takeuchi, T., Takasaka, T. 1994. Dysgenesis of melanocytes and cochlear dysfunction in mutant microphtalmia (mi) mice. *Hear. Res.,* 80, 10-20.

Moulin, A. 2000. Influence of primary frequencies ratio on distortion product otoacoustic emission amplitude. II. Interrelations between multicomponent DPOAEs, tone-burst-evoked OAEs, and spontaneous OAEs. *J. Acoust. Soc. Am.,* 107, 1471-1486.

Mountain, D. C. 1980. Changes in endolymphatic potential and crossed olivocochlear bundle stimulation alters cochlear mechanics. *Science,* 210, 71-72.

Mountcastle, V. B. 1957. Modality and topographic properties of single neurons of cat's somatic sensory cortex. *J. Neurophysiol.,* 20, 408-434.

Mugford, R. A., Nowell, N. W. 1971. Endocrine control over production and activity of the anti-aggression pheromone from female mice. *J. Endocrinol.,* 49, 225.

Mugnaini, E. 1985. GABA neurons in the superficial layers of the rat dorsal cochlear nucleus: light and electron microscopic immunocytochemistry. *J. Comp. Neurol.,* 235, 61-81.

Mugnaini, E., Dino, M. R., Jaarsma, D. 1997. The unipolar brush cells of the mammalian cerebellum and the cochlear nucleus: cytology and microcircuitry. *Prog. Brain Res.,* 114, 131-150.

Mugnaini, E., Floris, A., Wright-Goss, M. 1994. Extraordinary synapses of the unipolar brush cell: an electron microscope study in the rat cerebellum. *Synapse,* 16, 284-311.

Mugnaini, E., Oertel, W. H. 1985. An atlas of the distribution of GABAergic neurons and terminals in the rat CNS as revealed by GAD immunohistochernistry. In Björklund, A., Hökfelt, T. (Eds.), *GABA and Neuropeptides in the CNS,* Part 1, 4. Elsevier Science, New York, 436-608.

Mugnaini, E., Warr, W. B, Osen, K. K. 1980a. Distribution and light microscopic features of granule cells in the cochlear nuclei of cat, rat and mouse. *J. Comp. Neurol.,* 191, 581-606.

Mugnaini, E., Osen, K. K., Dahl, A. L., Friedrich, V. L, Korte, G. 1980b. Fine structure of granule cells and related interneurons (termed Golgi cells) in the cochlear nuclear complex of cat, rat and mouse. *J. Neurocytol.,* 9, 537-570.

Muller, M., Smolders, J. W., Meyer zum Gottesberge, A. M., Reuter, A., Zwacka, R. M., Weiher, H., Klinke, R. 1997. Loss of auditory function in transgenic Mpv17-deficient mice. *Hear. Res.,* 114, 259-263.

Müller-Schwarze, D., Müller-Schwarze, C. 1971. Olfactory imprinting in a precocial mammal. *Nature,* 229, 55-56.

Mulroy, M. J., Curley, F. J. 1982. Stereociliary pathology and noise-induced threshold shift: A scanning electron microscopic study. *Scan. Microsc.,* IV, 1753-1762.

Munck, A., Mendel, D. B., Smith, L. I., Orti, E. 1990. Glucocorticoid receptors and actions. *Am. Rev. Respir. Dis.,* 141, S2-S10.

Munemoto, Y., Kuriyama, H., Doi, T., Sato, K., Matsumoto, A., Sugatani, J., Cho, H., Komeda, M., Altschuler, R. A., Kitajiri, M., Mishina, M., Yamashita, T. 1998. Auditory pathway and auditory brainstem response in mice lacking NMDA receptor epsilon 1 and epsilon 4 subunits. *Neurosci. Lett.,* 251, 101-104.

Munroe, R. J., Bergstrom, R. A., Zheng, Q. Y., Libby, B., Smith, R., John, S. W., Schimenti, K. J., Browning, V. L., Schimenti, J. C. 2000. Mouse mutants from chemically mutagenized embryonic stem cells. *Nature Genet.,* 24, 318-321.

Munyer, P. D., Schulte B. A. 1994. Immunohistochemical localization of keratin sulfate and chondroitin 4- and 6-sulfate proteoglycans in subregions of the tectorial and basilar membranes. *Hear. Res.,* 79, 83-93.

Musicant, A. D., Chan, J. C. K., Hind, J. E. 1990. Direction-dependent spectral properties of cat external ear: new data and cross-species comparisons. *J. Acoust. Soc. Am.,* 87, 757-781.

Musiek et al. 1994. Auditory brainstem response: threshold estimation and auditory screening. In Katz, J. (Ed.), *Handbook of Clinical Audiology,* 4th ed. Williams & Wilkins, Baltimore, 351-374.

Nadol, J. B., McKenna, M. J. 1987. Histopathology of Meniere's disease and otosclerosis. In Veldman, J. E. (Ed.), *Immunobiology, Histophysiology, Tumor Immunology in Otolaryngology.* Kugler Publications, Amsterdam, 165-184.

Nagata, S., Suda, T. 1995. Fas and Fas ligand: lpr and gld mutations. *Immunol. Today,* 16, 39-43.

Nair, T. S., Prieskorn, D. M., Miller, J. M., Dolan, D. F., Raphael, Y., Carey, T. E. 1999. KHRI-3 monoclonal antibody-induced damage to the inner ear: antibody staining of nascent scars. *Hear. Res.,* 129, 50-60.

Nair, T. S., Prieskorn, D. M., Miller, J. M., Mori, A., Gray, J., Carey, T. E. 1997. *In vivo* binding and hearing loss after intracochlear infusion of KHRI-3 antibody. *Hear. Res.,* 107, 93-101.

Nair, T. S., Raphael, Y., Dolan, D. F., Parrett, T. J., Perlman, L. S., Brahmbhatt, V. R., Wang, Y., Hou, X., Ganjei, G., Nuttal, A. L., Carey, T. E. 1995. Monoclonal antibody induced hearing loss. *Hear. Res.,* 83, 101-113.

Naito, I., Kawai, S., Nomura, S., Sado, Y., Osawa, G. 1996. Relationship between COL4A5 gene mutation and distribution of type IV collagen in male X-linked Alport syndrome. Japanese Alport Network. *Kidney Int.,* 50, 304-311.

Naito, I., Nomura, S., Inoue, S., Kagawa, M., Kawai, S., Gunshin, Y., Joh, K., Tsukidate, C., Sado, Y., Osawa, G. 1997. Normal distribution of collagen IV in renal basement membranes in Epstein's syndrome. *J. Clin. Pathol.,* 50, 919-922.

Nakae, S., Tachibana, M. 1986. The cochlea of the spontaneously diabetic mouse. II. Electron microscopic observations of non-obese diabetic mice. *Arch. Otorhinolaryngol.,* 243, 313-316.

Nakanishi, K., Iijima, K., Kuroda, N., Inoue, Y., Sado, Y., Nakamura, H., Yoshikawa, N. 1998. Comparison of alpha5(IV) collagen chain expression in skin with disease severity in women with X-linked Alport syndrome. *J. Am. Soc. Nephrol.,* 9, 1433-1440.

Nakanishi, K., Yoshikawa, N., Iijima, K., Kitagawa, K., Nakamura, H., Ito, H., Yoshioka, K., Kagawa, M., Sado, Y. 1994. Immunohistochemical study of alpha 1-5 chains of type IV collagen in hereditary nephritis. *Kidney Int.,* 46, 1413-1421.

Nakanishi, K., Yoskikawa, N., Iijima, K., Nakamura, H. 1996. Expression of type IV collagen alpha 3 and alpha 4 chain mRNA in X-linked Alport syndrome. *J. Am. Soc. Nephrol.,* 7, 938-945.

Nakashima, T., Nuttall, A. L., Miller, J. M. 1994. Effects of vasodilating agents on cochlear blood flow in mice. *Hear. Res.,* 80, 241-246.

Nakazato, H., Hattori, S., Matsuura, T., Koitabashi, Y., Endo, F., Matsuda, I. 1993. Identification of a single base insertion in the COL4A5 gene in Alport syndrome. *Kidney Int.,* 44, 1091-1096.

Nakazato, H., Hattori, S., Ushijima, T., Matsuura, T., Koitabashi, Y., Takada, T., Yoshioka, K., Endo, F., Matsuda, I. 1994. Mutations in the COL4A5 gene in Alport syndrome: a possible mutation in primordial germ cells. *Kidney Int.,* 46, 1307-1314.

Nance, W. E., Setleff, R., McLeod, A., Sweeney, A., Cooper, C., McConnell, F. 1971. X-linked mixed deafness with congenital fixation of the stapedial footplate and perilymphatic gusher. *Birth Defects: Original Article Series,* 07, 64-69.

Nariuchi, H., Sone, M., Tago, C., Kurata, T., Saito, K. 1994. Mechanisms of hearing disturbance in an autoimmune model mouse, NZB/kl. *Acta Otolaryngol. (Suppl.),* 514, 127-131.

National Institute for Occupational Safety and Health, 1988. A proposed national strategy for the prevention of noise-induced hearing loss. In Proposed National Strategies for the Prevention of Work-Related Diseases and Injuries, Part 2. The Association of Schools of Public Health, Washington, D.C., pp. 51-63.

National Institute for Occupational Safety and Health. 1996. Hearing Loss. National Occupational Research Agenda, Washington, D.C., U.S. Department of Health and Human Services, Public Health Service, Centers for Disease Control and Prevention, 96-115, pp. 14-15.

National Institute for Occupational Safety and Health. 1998. Criteria for a Recommended Standard: Occupational Noise Exposure. Revised Criteria 1998. Cincinnati, OH, U.S. Department of Health and Human Services, Public Health Service, Centers for Disease Control and Prevention, 98-126.

Nebreda, A. R., Martin-Zanca, D., Kaplan, D. R., Parada, L. F., Santos, E. 1991. Induction by NGF of meiotic maturation of Xenopus oocytes expressing the trk proto-oncogene product. *Science,* 252, 558-563.

Nelken, I., Young, E. D. 1994. Two separate inhibitory mechanisms shape the responses of dorsal cochlear nucleus type IV units to narrowband and wideband stimuli. *J. Neurophysiol.,* 71, 2446-2462.

Nelson, S. K., Bose, S. K., McCord, J. M. 1994. The toxicity of high-dose superoxide dismutase suggests that superoxide can both initiate and terminate lipid peroxidation in the reperfused heart. *Free Radical Biol. Med.,* 16, 195-200.

Neri, T. M., Zanelli, P., De Palma, G., Savi, M., Rossetti, S., Turco, A. E., Pignatti, G. F., Galli, L., Bruttini, M., Renieri, A., Mingarelli, R., Trivelli, A., Pinciaroli, A. R., Ragaiolo, M., Rizzoni, G. F., De Marchi, M. 1998. Missense mutations in the COL4A5 gene in patients with X-linked Alport syndrome. *Hum. Mutat.,* Suppl. 1, S106-S109.

Netzer, K. O., Pullig, O., Frei, U., Zhou, J., Tryggvason, K., Weber, M. 1993. COL4A5 splice site mutation and alpha 5(IV) collagen mRNA in Alport syndrome. *Kidney Int.,* 43, 486-492.

Netzer, K. O., Renders, L., Zhou, J., Pullig, O., Tryggvason, K., Weber, M. 1992. Deletions of the COL4A5 gene in patients with Alport syndrome. *Kidney Int.,* 42, 1336-1344.

Neufeld, E. F., Fratantoni J. C. 1970. Inborn errors of mucopolysaccharide metabolism. *Science,* 169, 141-146.

Neumann, P. E. 1990. Two-locus linkage analysis using recombinant inbred strains and Bayes' theorem. *Genetics,* 126, 277-284.

Neumann, P. E. 1992. Three locus linkage analysis of multifactorial traits using recombinant inbred strains of mice. *Behav. Genet.,* 22, 665-676.

Neumann, P. E., Collins, R. L. 1991. Genetic dissection of susceptibility to audiogenic seizures in inbred mice. *Proc. Natl. Acad. Sci., USA,* 88, 5408-5412.

Newlander, J. K., Erway, L. C., Davis, R. R., Cortopassi, G. A. Ling, X-B. 1995. Susceptibility to NIHL and age-related hearing loss in mice. *Assoc. Res. Otolaryngol. Abstr.,* 18, 356.

Newman, S. W. 1999. The medial extended amygdala in male reproductive behavior: a node in the mammalian social behavior network. *Ann. N.Y. Acad. Sci.,* 877, 242-257.

Neyroud, N., Tesson, F., Denjoy, I., Leibovici, M., Donger, C., Barhanin, J., Faure, S., Gary, F., Coumel, P., Petit, C. 1997. A novel mutation in the potassium channel KVLQT1 causes the Jervell and Lang-Nielsen cardioauditory syndrome. *Nature Genet.,* 15, 186-189.

Nguyen-Legros, J., Hicks D. 2000. Renewal of photoreceptor outer segments and their phagocytosis by the retinal pigment epithelium. *Int. Rev. Cytol.,* 196, 245-313.

Nikolopoulos, T. P., O'Donoghue, G. M., Archbold, S. 1999. Age at implantation: its importance in pediatric cochlear implantation. *Laryngoscope,* 109, 595-599.

Nilsson, G. E., Tenland, T., Oberg, P. A. 1980. Evaluation of a laser Doppler flowmeter for measurement of tissue blood flow. *IEEE Trans. Biomed. Eng.,* 27, 597-604.

Nishi, M., Houtani, T., Noda, Y., Mamiya, T., Sato, K., Doi, T., Kuno, J., Takeshima, H., Nukada, T., Nabeshima, T., Yamashita, T., Noda, T., Sugimoto, T. 1997. Unrestrained nociceptive response and disregulation of hearing ability in mice lacking the nociceptin/orphaninFQ receptor. *EMBO J.,* 16, 1858-1864.

Nishizaki, K., Yoshino, T., Orita, Y., Nomiya, S., Masuda, Y. 1999. TUNEL staining of inner ear structures may reflect autolysis, not apoptosis. *Hear. Res.,* 130, 131-136.

Nitecka, L. M., Sobkowicz, H. M. 1996. The GABA/GAD innervation within the inner spiral bundle in the mouse cochlea. *Hear. Res.,* 99, 91-105.

Nitecka, L. M., Sobkowicz, H. M., Shi, X. 1995. The developmental expression of GAD by the neurons of the spiral ganglion. *Assoc. Res. Otolaryngol. Abstr.,* 18, 109.

Noben-Trauth, K., Naggert, J. K., North, M. A., Nishina, P. M. 1996. A candidate gene for the mouse mutation tubby. *Nature,* 380, 534-538.

Noben-Trauth, K., Zheng, Q. Y., Johnson, K. R., Nishina, P. M. 1997. *mdfw*: a deafness susceptibility locus that interacts with deaf waddler (*dfw*). *Genomics,* 44, 266-272.

Noble, W., Byrne, D., Lepage, B. 1994. Effects on sound localization of configuration and type of hearing impairment. *J. Acoust. Soc. Am.,* 95, 992-1005.

Noirot, E. 1972. Ultrasounds and maternal behavior in small rodents. *Devel. Psychobiol.,* 5, 371-387.

Nolan, P. M., Kapfhamer, D., Bucan, M. 1997. Random mutagenesis screen for dominant behavioral mutations in mice. *Methods,* 13, 379-395.

Nolan, P. M., Sollars, P. J., Bohne, B. A., Ewens, W. J., Pickard, G. E., Bucan, M. 1995. Heterozygosity mapping of partially congenic lines: mapping of a semidominant neurological mutation, *Wheels* (*Whl*), on mouse chromosome 4. *Genetics,* 140, 245-254.

Nomura, S., Naito, I., Fukushima, T., Tokura, T., Kataoka, N., Tanaka, I., Tanaka, H., Osawa, G. 1998. Molecular genetic and immunohistochemical study of autosomal recessive Alport's syndrome. *Am. J. Kidney Dis.,* 31, E4.

Nomura, S., Osawa, G., Sai, T., Harano, T., Harano, K. 1993. A splicing mutation in the alpha 5(IV) collagen gene of a family with Alport's syndrome. *Kidney Int.,* 43, 1116-1124.

Nonet, M., Staunton, J., Kilgard, M., Fergestad, T., Hartwieg, E., Horvitz, H., Jorgensen, E., Meyer, B. 1997. Caenorhabditis elegans rab-3 mutant synapses exhibit impaired function and are partially depleted of vesicles. *J. Neurosci.,* 17, 8061-8073.

Nordmann, A. S., Bohne, B. A., Harding, G. W. 2000. Histopathological differences between temporary and permanent threshold shift. *Hear. Res.,* 139, 13-30.

Northern, J. L., Downs, M. P. 1991. *Hearing in Children.* Williams & Wilkins, Baltimore.

Norton, S. J., Rubel, E. W. 1990. Active and passive ADP components in mammalian and avian ears. In Dallos, P., Geisler, C. D., Mathews, J. W., Ruggero, M. A., Steele, C. R. (Eds.), *Mechanics and Biophysics of Hearing.* Springer-Verlag, New York, 219-226.

Nosrat, C. A., Tomac, A., Hoffer, B. J., Olson, L. 1997. Cellular and developmental patterns of expression of Ret and glial cell line-derived neurotrophic factor receptor alpha mRNA's. *Exp. Brain Res.,* 115, 410-422.

Nunez, A. A., Nyby, J., Whitney, G. 1978. The effects of testosterone, estradiol, and dihydrotestosterone on male mouse (*Mus musculus*) ultrasonic vocalizations. *Horm. Behav.,* 11, 264-272.

Nunez, A. A., Pomerantz, S. M., Bean, N. J., Youngstrom, T. G. 1985. Effects of laryngeal denervation on ultrasound production and male sexual behavior in rodents. *Physiol. Behav.,* 34, 901-905.

Nunez, A. A., Tan, D. T. 1984. Courtship ultrasonic vocalizations in male Swiss-Webster mice: effects of hormones and sexual experience. *Physiol. Behav.,* 32, 717-721.

Nuttall, A. L. 1986. Intravital microscopy for measurement of blood cell velocities in the cochlea. *Assoc. Res. Otolaryngol. Abstr.,* 9.

Nuttall, A. L. 1987. Techniques for the observation and measurement of red blood cell velocity in vessels of the guinea pig cochlea. *Hear. Res.,* 27, 111-119.

Nuttall, A. L. 1999. Sound-induced cochlear ischemia/hypoxia as a mechanism of hearing loss. A review. *Noise Health,* 5, 17-31.

Nuttall, A. L., Lawrence, M. 1980. Endocochlear potential and scala media oxygen tension during partial anoxia. *Am. J. Otolaryngol.,* 1, 147-153.

Nyby, J. 1983. Ultrasonic vocalizations during sex behavior of male house mice (*Mus musculus*): a description. *Behav. Neural Biol.,* 39, 128-134.

Nyby, J., Dizinno, G. A., Whitney, G. 1976. Social status and ultrasonic vocalizations of male mice. *Behav. Biol.,* 18, 285-289.

Nyby, J., Dizinno, G., Whitney, G. 1977a. Sexual dimorphism in ultrasonic vocalizations of mice (*Mus musculus*): gonadal hormone regulation. *J. Comp. Physiol. Psychol.,* 91, 1424-1431.

Nyby, J. G., Simon, N. G. 1987. Nonaromatizable androgens may stimulate a male mouse reproductive behavior by binding estrogen receptors. *Physiol. Behav.,* 39, 147-151.

Nyby, J., Matochik, J. A., Barfield, R. J. 1992. Intracranial androgenic and estrogenic stimulation of male-typical behaviors in house mice (*Mus domesticus*). *Horm. Behav.,* 26, 24-45.

Nyby, J., Whitney, G. 1978. Ultrasonic communication by adult myomorph rodents. *Neurosci. Biobehav. Rev.,* 2, 1-14.

Nyby, J., Whitney, G., Schmitz, S., Dizinno, G. 1978. Postpubertal experience establishes signal value of mammalian sex odor. *Behav. Biol.,* 22, 545-552.

Nyby, J., Wysocki, C. J., Whitney, G., Dizinno, G. 1977b. Pheromonal regulation of male mouse courtship. *Anim. Behav.,* 25, 333-341.

Nyby, J., Wysocki, C. J., Whitney, G., Dizinno, G., Schneider, J. 1979. Elicitation of male mouse (*Mus musculus*) ultrasonic vocalizations: I. Urinary cues. *J. Comp. Physiol. Psychol.,* 93, 957-975.

Nyby, J., Zakeski, D. 1980. Elicitation of male mouse ultrasounds: bladder urine and aged urine from females. *Physiol. Behav.,* 24, 737-740.

O'Connor, L., Erway, L. C., Vogler, C. A., Sly, W. S., Nicholes, A., Grubb, J., Holmberg, S. W., Levy, B., Sands, M. S. 1998. Enzyme replacement therapy for murine mucopolysaccharidosis type VII leads to improvements in behavior and auditory function. *J. Clin. Invest.,* 101, 1394-1400.

O'Malley, B. W., Li, D., Turner, D. S. 1995. Hearing loss and cochlear abnormalities in the congenital hypothyroid (hyt/hyt) mouse. *Hear. Res.,* 88, 181-189.

O'Neill, W. E., Ison, J. R. 2000. Gap detection thresholds (GDT) and acoustic startle reflexes (ASR) vary with age, but only weakly with audiometric (ABR) thresholds, in CBA/CaJ mice. *Assoc. Res. Otolaryng. Abstr.,* 23, #538.

O'Neill, W. E., Zettel, M. L., Whittemore, K. R, Frisina, R. D. 1997. Calbindin D-28k immunoreactivity in the medial nucleus of the trapezoid body declines with age in C57BL/6, but not CBA/CaJ mice. *Hear. Res.,* 112, 158-166.

Oertel, D. 1983. Synaptic responses and electrical properties of cells in brain slices of the mouse anteroventral cochlear nucleus. *J. Neurosci.,* 3, 2043-2053.

Oertel, D. 1985. Use of brain slices in the study of the auditory system: spatial and temporal summation of synaptic inputs in cells in the anteroventral cochlear nucleus of the mouse. *J. Acoust. Soc. Am.,* 78, 328-333.

Oertel, D. 1997. Encoding of timing in the brainstem auditory nuclei of vertebrates. *Neuron,* 19, 959-962.

Oertel, D. 1999. The role of timing in the brain stem auditory nuclei of vertebrates. *Annu. Rev. Physiol.,* 61, 497-519.

Oertel, D., Golding, N. L. 1997. Circuits of the dorsal cochlear nucleus. In Syka, J. (Ed.), *Acoustic Signal Processing in the Central Auditory System.* Plenum, New York, 127-138.

Oertel, D., Wickesberg, R. E. 1996. A mechanism for suppression of echoes in the cochlear nuclei. In Ainsworth, W. A., Evans, E. F., Hackney, C. M. (Eds.), *Advances in Speech, Hearing and Language Processing.* JAI, London, 293-321.

Oertel, D., Wu, S.-H., Garb, M. W., Dizack, C. 1990. Morphology and physiology of cells in slice preparations of the posteroventral cochlear nucleus of mice. *J. Comp. Neurol.,* 295, 136-154.

Oertel, W. H., Schmechel, D. E., Mugnaini, E., Tappaz, M. L., Kopin, I. J. 1981. Immunocytochemical localization of glutamate decarboxylase in rat cerebellum with a new antiserum. *Neuroscience,* 6, 2715-2735.

Oexle, K., Herrmann, R., Dode, C., Leturcq, F., Hubner, C. H., Kaplan, J. C., Mizuno, Y., Ozawa, E., Campbell, K. P., Voit, T. 1996. Neurosensory hearing loss in secondary adhalinopathy. *Neuropediatrics,* 27, 32-36.

Ogra, P. L., Barenkamp, S. J., Mogi, G., Pelton, S. I., Juhn, S. K., Karma, P., Bakaletz, L. O., Bernstein, J. M., DeMaria, T. F., Diven, W. F., Faden, H., Giebink, G. S., Hellström, S. O. M., Howie, V. M., Klein, D. L., Kuijpers, W., McInnes, P. M., Prellner, K., Ryan, A. F., Rynnel-Dagöö, B. 1994. Microbiology, immunology, biochemistry, and vaccination. *Ann. Otol. Rhinol. Laryngol.,* 103(Suppl. 164), 27-42.

Ogra, P. L., Barenkamp, S. J., Mogi, G., Murphy, T. F., Bakaletz, L. O., Bernstein, J. M., DeMaria, T. F., Faden, H., Forsgren, J., Garofalo, R., Giebink, G. S., Gu, X. X., Karma, P., Patel, J., Prellner, K., Ryan, A. F. 1998. Microbiology, immunology, and vaccination. *Ann. Otol. Rhinol. Laryngol.,* 107(Suppl. 174), 29-49.

Oh, S.-H., Johnson, R., Wu, D. K. 1996. Differential expression of bone morphogenetic proteins in the developing vestibular and auditory sensory organs. *J. Neurosci.,* 16, 6463-6475.

Ohashi, T., Kenmochi, M., Kinoshita, H., Ochi, K., Kikuchi, H. 1999. Cochlear function of guinea pigs with experimental chronic renal failure. *Ann. Otol. Rhinol. Laryngol.,* 108, 955-962.

Ohga, H., Kawauchi, H., Nagata, T., Katoh, T. 1999. S-carboxymethylcysteine has a suppressive effect on the hydrogen peroxide production of neutrophils. Presented at *Seventh International Symposium on Recent Advances in Otitis Media.* Fort Lauderdale, FL, June 1-5, 95.

Ohinata, Y., Yamasoba, T., Schacht, J., Miller, J. M. 1999. The effect of glutathione monoethylester in the prevention from noise-induced hearing loss. *Assoc. Res. Otolaryngol. Abstr.,* 22, 601.

Ohlemiller, K. K., Dugan, L. L. 1999. Elevation of reactive oxygen species following ischemia-reperfusion in mouse cochlea observed *in vivo. Audiol. Neuro-Otol.,* 4, 219-228.

Ohlemiller, K. K., Hughes, R. M., Mosinger-Ogilvie, J., Speck, J. D., Grosof, D. H., Silverman, M. S. 1995. Cochlear and retinal degeneration in the tubby mouse. *NeuroRep.,* 6, 845-849.

Ohlemiller, K. K., Hughes, R. M., Lett, J. M., Ogilvie, J. M., Speck, J. D., Wright, J. S., Faddis, B. T. 1997. Progression of cochlear and retinal degeneration in the tubby (rd5) mouse. *Audiol. Neuro-Otol.,* 2, 175-185.

Ohlemiller, K., Lear, P., Ho, Y. S. 2000a. Deficiency of cellular glutathione peroxidase increases noise-induced hearing loss in young adult mice. *Assoc. Res. Otolaryngol. Abstr.,* 23, 219.

Ohlemiller, K. K., McFadden, S. L., Ding, D.-L., Reaume, A. G., Hoffman, E. K., Scott, R. W., Wright, J. S., Putcha, G. V. Salvi, R. J. 1999a. Targeted deletion of the cytosolic Cu/Zn-superoxide dismutase gene (Sod1) increases susceptibility to noise-induced hearing loss. *Audiol. Neuro-Otol.,* 4, 237-246.

Ohlemiller, K. K., Vogler, C. A., Roberts, M., Galvin, N. Sands, M. S. 2000b. Retinal function is improved in a murine model of a lysosomal storage disease following bone marrow transplantation. *Exp. Eye Res.,* 71, 469-481.

Ohlemiller, K. K., Wright, J. S., Dugan, L. L. 1999b. Early elevation of cochlear reactive oxygen species following noise exposure. *Audiol. Neuro-Otol.,* 4, 229-236.

Ohlsen, A., Hultcrantz, E., Engstrom, B. 1993. The effect of topical application of vasodilating agents on cochlear electrophysiology. *Acta Otolaryngol. (Stockholm)*, 113, 55-61.

Ohlsen, K. A., Nuttall, A. L., Miller, J. M. 1989. The influence of adrenergic drugs on the cochlear blood flow. *Assoc. Res. Otolaryngol. Abstr.*, 12, 116.

Ohlsen, K. A., Didier, A., Baldwin, D., Miller, J. M., Nuttall, A. L., Hultcrantz, E. 1992. Cochlear blood flow in response to dilating agents. *Hear. Res.*, 58, 19-25.

Ohlsen, K. A., Miller, J. M., Nuttall, A. L. 1990. Enhancing cochlear blood flow. A survey of six vasodilating agents applied locally and systematically. *Assoc. Res. Otolaryngol. Abstr.*, 13, 353.

Ohya, K., Ichimiya, I., Yoshida, K., Suzuki, M., Mogi, G. 1999. The influence of experimental otitis media on the cochlear lateral wall. *In vivo* and *in vitro* studies. Presented at *Seventh International Symposium on Recent Advances in Otitis Media*. June 1-5, Fort Lauderdale, FL, 96.

Okon, E. E. 1972. Factors affecting ultrasound production in infant rodents. *J. Zool. Proc. Zool. Soc. London*, 168, 139-148.

Oliver, D. L. 1984. Dorsal cochlear nucleus projections to the inferior colliculus in the cat: a light and electron microscopic study. *J. Comp. Neurol.*, 224, 155-172.

Oliver, D. L. 1987. Projections of the cochlear nucleus from the anteroventral cochlear nucleus in the cat: possible substrates for binaural interaction. *J. Comp. Neurol.*, 264, 24-46.

Oliver, D. L., Hall, W. C. 1978. The medial geniculate body of the tree shrew, *Tupaia glis:* I. Cytoarchitecture and midbrain connections. *J. Comp. Neurol.*, 182, 423-458.

Oliver, D. L., Huerta, M. F. 1992. Inferior and superior colliculi. In Webster, D. P., Popper, A. N., Fay, R. R. (Eds.), *The Mammalian Auditory Pathway: Neuroanatomy*. Springer-Verlag, New York, 168-221.

Oliver, D. L., Morest, D. K. 1984. The central nucleus of the inferior colliculus in the cat. *J. Comp. Neurol.*, 222, 237-264.

Ollo, C., Schwartz, I. R. 1979. The superior olivary complex in C57BL/6 mice. *Am. J. Anat.*, 155, 349-374.

Omelchenko, I., Shi, X., Nuttall, A. L. 2001. Production of NO and noise-induced hearing loss in nNos knock-out mice. *Assoc. Res. Otolaryngol.*, 24, 114.

Opstelten, D. J., Vogels, R., Robert, B., Kalkhoven, E., Zwartkruis, F., de Laaf, L., Destree, O. H., Deschamps, J., Lawson, K. A., Meijlink, F. 1991. The mouse homeobox gene, S8, is expressed during embryogenes is predominantly in mesenchyme. *Mech. Devel.*, 34, 29-41.

Orita, Y., Nishizaki, K., Sasaki, J., Kanda, S., Kimura, N., Nomiya, S., Yuen, K., Masuda, Y. 1999. Does TUNEL staining during peri-and post-natal development of the mouse inner ear indicate apoptosis? *Acta Otolaryngol.*, (Suppl.) 540, 22-26.

Ornitz, D. M., Bohne, B. A., Thalmann, I., Harding, G. W., Thalmann, R. 1998. Otoconial agenesis in *tilted* mutant mice. *Hear. Res.*, 122, 60-70.

Ornitz, E. M., Lane, S. J., Sugiyama, T., de Traversay, J. 1992. Prestimulation-induced startle modulation in attention deficit hyperactivity disorder and nocturnal enuresis. *Psychophysiology*, 29, 437-451.

Orozco, C. R., Niparko, J. K., Richardson, B. C., Dolan, D. F., Ptok, M. U., Altschuler, R. A. 1990. Experimental model of immune-mediated hearing loss using cross-species immunization. *Laryngoscope*, 100, 941-947.

Orrenius, S., Nicotera, P. 1994. The calcium ion and cell death. *J. Neural Transm.*, Suppl. 43, 1-11.

Osen, K. K. 1969. Cytoarchitecture of the cochlear nuclei in the cat. *J. Comp. Neurol.*, 136, 453-484.

Osen, K. K. 1972. Projection of the cochlear nuclei on the inferior colliculus in the cat. *J. Comp. Neurol.*, 144, 355-372.

Ottaviani, F., Cadoni, G., Marinelli, L., Fetoni, A. R., De Santis, A., Romito, A., Vulpiani, P., Manna, R. 1999. Anti-endothelial autoantibodies in patients with sudden hearing loss. *Laryngoscope*, 109, 1084-1087.

Ou, H. C., Bohne, B. A., Harding, G. W. 2000a. Noise damage in the C57BL/CBA mouse cochlea. *Hear. Res.*, 145, 111-122.

Ou, H. C., Harding, G. W., Bohne, B. A., 2000b. An anatomically based frequency-place map for the mouse cochlea. *Hear. Res.*, 145, 123-129.

Pack, A. K., Slepecky, N. B. 1995. Cytoskeletal and calcium-binding proteins in the mammalian organ of Corti: cell type-specific proteins displaying longitudinal and radial gradients. *Hear. Res.*, 91, 119-135.

Pajari, H., Koskimies, O., Muhonen, T., Kaariainen, H. 1999. The burden of genetic disease and attitudes toward gene testing in Alport syndrome. *Pediatr. Nephrol.*, 13, 471-476.

Pakarinen, L., Karjalainen, S., Simola, K. O., Laippala, P., Kaitalo, H. 1995. Usher's syndrome type 3 in Finland. *Laryngoscope*, 105, 613-617.

Palmer, A. R., Jiang, D., Marshall, D. H. 1996. Responses of ventral cochlear nucleus onset and chopper units as a function of signal bandwidth. *J. Neurophysiol.*, 75, 780-794.

Palombi, P. S., Caspary, D. M. 1992. GABA$_a$ receptor antagonist bicuculline alters response properties of posteroventral cochlear nucleus neurons. *J. Neurophysiol.*, 67, 738-746.

Palombi P. S., Caspary D. M. 1996a. Responses of young and aged Fischer 344 rat inferior colliculus neurons to binaural tonal stimuli. *Hear. Res.*, 100, 59-67.

Palombi P. S., Caspary D. M. 1996b. Physiology of the aged Fischer 344 rat inferior colliculus: responses to contralateral monaural stimuli. *J. Neurophysiol.*, 5, 3114-3121.

Papsin, B. C., Vellodi A., Bailey C. M., Ratcliffe P. C. Leighton S. E. 1998. Otologic and laryngologic manifestations of mucopolysaccharidoses after bone marrow transplantation. *Otolaryngol. Head Neck Surg.*, 118, 30-36.

Parham, K. 1997. Distortion product otoacoustic emission in the C57BL/6J mouse model of age-related hearing loss. *Hear. Res.*, 112, 216-234.

Parham, K., Bonaiuto, G., Carlson, S., Turner, J. G., D'Angelo, L. S. Bross, W. R., Fox, A., Willott, J. F., Kim, D. O. 2000. Purkinje-cell degeneration and control mice: responses of single units in the dorsal cochlear nucleus and the acoustic startle response. *Hear. Res.*, 148, 137-152.

Parham, K., Gerber, A., McKowen, A., Sun, X.-M., Kim, D. O. 1997. Distortion product otoacoustic emissions of the DBA/2J mouse with early-onset progressive hearing loss. *Assoc. Res. Otolaryngol. Abstr.*, 20, 194.

Parham, K., Kim, D. O. 1995. Spontaneous and sound-evoked discharge characteristics of complex-spiking neurons in the dorsal cochlear nucleus of the unanesthetized decerebrate cat. *J. Neurophysiol.*, 73, 550-561.

Parham, K., Sun, X.-M., Kim, D. O. 1999. Distortion product otoacoustic emission in the CBA/J mouse model of presbycusis. *Hear. Res.*, 134, 29-38.

Parham, K., Willott, J. F. 1988. The acoustic startle response in young and aging C57BL/6J and CBA/J mice. *Behav. Neurosci.*, 102, 881-886.

Parham, K., Willott, J. F. 1990. The effects of inferior colliculus lesions on the acoustic startle response. *Behav. Neurosci.*, 104, 831-840.

Park, J. W., Choi, C. H., Kim, M. S., Chung, M. H. 1996. Oxidative status in senescence-accelerated mice. *J. Gerontol. A Biol. Sci. Med. Sci.*, 51, B337-345.

Park, K., Ueno, K., Lim, D. J. 1992. Developmental anatomy of the eustachian tube and middle ear in mice. *Am. J. Otolaryngol.*, 13, 93-100.

Pasteels, B., Parmentier, M., Lawson, D. E. M., Verstappen, A., Pochet, R. 1987. Calcium binding protein immunoreactivity in pigeon retina. *Invest. Opthalmol. Vis. Sci.*, 28, 658-664.

Patel, N. V., Hitzemann, R. 2000. Detection and mapping of quantitative trait loci for haloperidol-induced catalepsy in a C57BL/6J x DBA/2J F$_2$ intercross. *Behav. Genet.*, 29, 303-310.

Paylor, R., Baskall, L., Wehner, J. 1993. Behavioral disociations between C57BL/6 and DBA/2 mice on learning and memory tasks: a hippocampal-dysfunction hypothesis. *Psychobiology*, 21, 11-26.

Paylor, R., Baskall-Balindi, L., Yuva, L., Wehner, J. M. 1996. Developmental differences in place-learning performance between C57BL/6J and DBA/2 mice parallel the ontogeny of hippocampal protien kinase C. *Behav. Neurosci.*, 110, 1415-1425.

Paylor, R., Crawley, J. N. 1997. Inbred strain differences in prepulse inhibition of the mouse startle response. *Psychopharmacology*, 132, 169-180.

Paylor, R., Tracy, R., Wehner, J., Rudy, J. W. 1994. DBA/2 and C57BL/6J mice differ in contextual fear conditioning but not auditory fear conditioning. *Behav. Neurosci.*, 108, 810-817.

Peck, J. E. 1984. Hearing loss in Hunter's syndrome-mucopolysaccharidosis II. Ear Hear. 5, 243-246.

Pedersen, A. D., Morton, J. I., Trune, D. R. 1993. Inner ear basic fibroblast growth factor in CBA/J, C3H/HeJ, and autoimmune Palmerston North mice. *Hear. Res.*, 66, 253-259.

Peissel, B., Geng, L., Kalluri, R., Kashtan, C., Rennke, H. G., Gallo, G. R., Yoshioka, K., Sun, M. J., Hudson, B. G., Neilson, E. G. 1995. Comparative distribution of the alpha 1(IV), alpha 5(IV), and alpha 6(IV) collagen chains in normal human adult and fetal tissues and in kidneys from X-linked Alport syndrome patients. *J. Clin. Invest.*, 96, 1948-1957.

Pekkarinen, J. 1995. Noise, impulse noise, and other physical factors: combined effects on hearing. *Occupat. Med. State Art Rev.*, 10, 545-559.

Peled-Kamar, M., Lotem, J., Wirguin, I., Weiner, L., Hermalin, A., Groner, Y. 1997. Oxidative stress mediates impairment of muscle function in transgenic mice with elevated level of wild-type Cu/Zn superoxide dismutase. *Proc. Natl. Acad. Sci., USA*, 94, 3883-3887.

Pelton, R. W., Hogan, B. L., Miller, D. A., Moses, H. L. 1990. Differential expression of genes encoding TGFs beta 1, beta 2, and beta 3 during murine palate formation. *Devel. Biol.*, 141, 456-460.

Pennisi, E. 2000. A mouse chronology. *Science,* 288, 248-257.

Peris, J., Wehner, J. M., Zahniser, N. R. 1989. [35S]TBPS binding sites are decreased in the colliculi of mice with a genetic predisposition to bicuculline-induced seizures. *Brain Res.,* 503, 288-295.

Perkins, R. E., Morest, D. K. 1975. A study of cochlear innervation patterns in cats and rats with the Golgi method and Nomarski optics. *J. Comp. Neurol.,* 163, 129-158.

Perlmann, T., Evans, R. M. 1997. Nuclear receptors in Sicily: all in the famiglia. *Cell,* 90, 391-397.

Perraud, F., Labourdette, G., Miehe, M., Loret, C., Sensenbrenner, M. 1988. Comparisons of the morphological effects of acidic and basic fibroblast growth factors on rat astroblasts in culture. *J. Neurosci. Res.,* 20, 1-11.

Pettigrew, A. G., Morey, A. L. 1987. Changes in the brainstem auditory evoked response of the rabbit during the first postnatal month. *Brain Res. Devel. Brain Res.,* 33, 267-276.

Pfeiffer, R. R. 1966a. Anteroventral cochlear nucleus: wave forms of extracellularly recorded spike potentials. *Science,* 154, 667-668.

Pfeiffer, R. R. 1966b. Classification of response patterns of spike discharges for units in the cochlear nucleus: tone burst stimulation. *Exp. Brain Res.,* 1, 220-235.

Pfister, M. H., Apaydin, F., Turan, O., Bereketoglu, M., Bilgen, V., Braendle, U., Kose, S., Zenner, H. P., Lalwani, A. K. 1999. Clinical evidence for dystrophin dysfunction as a cause of hearing loss in locus DFN4. *Laryngoscope,* 109, 730-735.

Pfister, M. H., Apaydin, F., Turan, O., Bereketoglu, M., Bylgen, V., Braendle, U., Zenner, H. P., Lalwani, A. K. 1998. A second family with nonsyndromic sensorineural hearing loss linked to Xp21.2: refinement of the DFN4 locus within DMD. *Genomics,* 53, 377-382.

Phelps, P. D., Reardon, W., Pembrey, M., Bellman, S., Luxom, L. 1991. X-linked deafness, stapes gushers and a distinctive defect of the inner ear. *Neuroradiology,* 33, 326-330.

Phillips, R. J. S., Fisher, G. 1978. A screen for X-ray induced mutations. *Mouse News Lett.,* 58, 44.

Phippard, D., Boyd, Y., Reed, V., Fisher, G., Masson, W. K., Evans, E. P., Saunders, J. C., et al. 2000. The sex-linked fidget mutation abolishes Brn4/Pou3f4 gene expression in the embryonic inner ear. *Hum. Molec. Genet.,* 9, 79-85.

Phippard, D. J., Heydemann, A., Lechner, M., Lu, L., Lee, D., Kyin, T., Crenshaw III, E. B. 1998. Changes in the subcellular localization of the *Brn4* gene product precede mesenchymal remodeling of the otic capsule. *Hear. Res.,* 120, 77-85.

Phippard, D., Lihui, L., Lee, D., Saunders, J. C., Crenshaw III, E. B. 1999. Targeted mutagenesis of the POU-domain gene, *Brn4/Pou3f4,* causes development defects in the inner ear. *J. Neurosci.,* 19, 5980-5989.

Piccini, M., Vitelli, F., Bruttini, M., Pober, B. R., Jonsson, J. J., Villanova, M., Zollo, M., Borsani, G., Ballabio, A., Renieri, A. 1998. FACL4, a new gene encoding long-chain acyl-CoA synthetase 4, is deleted in a family with Alport syndrome, elliptocytosis, and mental retardation. *Genomics,* 47, 350-358.

Pickles, J. O., van Heumen, W. R. A. 1997. The expression of messenger RNAs coding for growth factors, their receptors, and eph-class receptor tyrosine kinases in normal and ototoxically damaged chick cochleae. *Devel. Neurosci.,* 19, 476-487.

Pieke-Dahl, S., Moller, C. G., Kelley, P. M., Astuto, L. M., Cremers, C. W., Gorin, M. B., Kimberling, W. J. 2000. Genetic heterogeneity of Usher syndrome type II: localisation to chromosome 5q. *J. Med. Genet.,* 37, 256-262.

Pieke-Dahl, S., Ohlemiller, K. K., McGee, J., Walsh, E. J., Kimberling, W. J. 1997. Hearing loss in the RBF/DnJ mouse, a proposed animal model of Usher syndrome type IIa. *Hear. Res.,* 112, 1-12.

Pieke-Dahl, S., van Aarem, A., Dobin, A., Cremers, C. W., Kimberling, W. J. 1996. Genetic heterogeneity of Usher syndrome type II in a Dutch population. *J. Med. Genet.,* 33, 753-757.

Pierson, M. G., Gray, B. H. 1982. Superoxide dismutase activity in the cochlea. *Hear. Res.,* 6, 141-151.

Pillers, D. M., Bulman, D. E., Weleber, R. G., Sigesmund, D. A., Musarella, M. A., Powell, B. R., Murphey, W. H., Westall, C., Panton, C., Becker, L. E., Worton, R. G., Ray, P. N. 1993. Dystrophin expression in the human retina is required for normal function as defined by electroretinography. *Nature Genet.,* 4, 82-86.

Pillers, D. M., Duncan, N. M., Dwinnell, S. J., Rash, S. M., Kempton, J. B., Trune, D. R, 1999a. Normal cochlear function in *mdx* and *mdx*^{Cv3} Duchenne muscular dystrophy mouse models. *Laryngoscope,* 109, 1310-1312.

Pillers, D. M., Duncan, N. M., Rash, S. M., Dwinnell, S. J., Kempton, J. B., Trune, D. R. 1999b. Hearing loss in laminin-deficient mouse model of muscular dystrophy, *Assoc. Res. Otolaryngol. Abstr.,* 22, 8.

Pirvola, U., Arumae, U., Moshnyakov, M., Palgi, J., Saarma, M., Ylikoski, J. 1994. Coordinated expression and function of neurotrophins and their receptors in the rat inner ear during target innervation. *Hear. Res.*, 75, 131-144.

Pirvola, U., Cao, Y., Oellig, C., Suoqiang, Z., Pettersson, R. F., Ylikoski, J. 1995. The site of action of neuronal acidic fibroblast growth factor is the organ of Corti of the rat cochlea. *Proc. Natl. Acad. Sci., USA*, 92, 9269-9273.

Privola, U., Hallbook, F., Xing-Qun, L., Virkkala, J., Saarma, M., Ylikoski, J. 1997. Expression of neurotrophins and Trk receptors in the developing, adult, and regenerating avian cochlea. *J. Neurobiol.*, 33, 1019-1033.

Pirvola, U., Lehtonen, E., Ylikoski, J. 1991. Spatiotemporal development of cochlear innervation and hair cell differentiation in the rat. *Hear. Res.*, 52, 345-355.

Pirvola, U., Ylikoski, J., Palgi, J., Lehtonen, E., Arumae, U., Saarma, M. 1992. Brain-derived neurotrophic factor and neurotrophin-3 mRNA's in the peripheral target fields of developing inner ear ganglia. *Proc. Natl. Acad. Sci., USA*, 89, 9915-9919.

Plant, K. E., Green, P. M., Vetrie, D., Flinter, F. A. 1999. Detection of mutations in COL4A5 in patients with Alport syndrome. *Hum. Mutat.*, 13, 124-132.

Platzer, J., Schrott-Fischer, A., Stephan, K., Walter, D., Zheng, H., Chen, H., Striessing, J. 2000. The role of the class D-L-type Ca2+ channels for hearing in mice. *Assoc. Res. Otolaryngol. Abstr.*,

Plomin, R., McClearn, G. E. 1993. Quantitative trait loci (QTL) analyses and alcohol related behaviors. *Behav. Genet.*, 23, 197-211.

Podos, S. D., Ferguson, E. L. 1999. Morphogen gradients: new insights from DPP. *Trends Genet.*, 15, 396-402.

Pomerantz, S. M., Nunez, A. A., Bean, N. J. 1983. Female behavior is affected by male ultrasonic vocalizations in house mice. *Physiol. Behav.*, 31, 91-96.

Popelár, J., Erre, J.-P., Aran, J.-M., Cazals, Y. 1994. Plastic changes in ipsi-/contralateral differences of auditory cortex and inferior colliculus evoked potentials after injury to one ear in the adult guinea pig. *Hear. Res.*, 72, 125-134.

Porter, J., Momanics, G., Balaban, C. 1998. The effects of gene deletion of the GABA-A receptor beta-3 subunit on the auditory and vestibular periphery. *Assoc. Res. Otolaryngol. Abstr.*,

Porter, R., Ghosh, S., Lange, G. D., Smith, Jr., T. G., 1991. A fractal analysis of pyramidal neurons in mammalian motor cortex. *Neurosci. Lett.*, 130, 112-116.

Pratt, H., Zaaroor, M., Bleich, N., Starr, A. 1991. Effects of myelin or cell body brainstem lesions on 3-channel Lissajous' trajectories of feline auditory brainstem evoked potentials. *Hear. Res.*, 53, 237-252.

Prazma, J., Carrasco, V. N., Garrett, C. G., Pillsbury, H. C. 1989. Measurement of cochlear blood flow, intravital fluorescence microscopy. *Hear. Res.*, 42, 229-236.

Prazma, J., Vance, S. G., Rodgers, G. 1984. Measurement of cochlear blood flow — new technique. *Hear. Res.*, 14, 21-28.

Price, G. R. 1974. Loss and recovery processes operative at the level of the cochlear microphonic during intermittent stimulation. *J. Acoust. Soc. Am.*, 56, 183-189.

Price, G. R. 1976. Effect of interrupting recovery on loss in cochlear microphonic sensitivity. *J. Acoust. Soc. Am.*, 59, 709-712.

Prieskorn, D. M., Miller, J. M. 2000. Technical report: chronic and acute intracochlear infusion in rodents. *Hear. Res.*, 140, 212-215.

Prieto, J. J., Rueda, J., Merchan, J. A. 1990a. The effect of hypothyroidism on the development of the glycogen content of organ of Corti's hair cells. *Devel. Brain Res.*, 51, 138-141.

Prieto, J. J., Rueda, J., Sala, M. L., Merchan, J. A. 1990b. Lectin staining of saccharides in the normal and hypothyroid developing organ of Corti. *Devel. Brain Res.*, 52, 141-149.

Probst, F. J., Camper, S. A. 1999. The role of mouse mutants in the identification of human hereditary hearing loss genes. *Hear. Res.*, 130, 1-6.

Probst, F. J., Fridell, R. A., Raphael, Y., Saunders, T. L., Wang, A., Liang, Y., Morell, R. J., Touchman, J. W., Lyons, R. H., Noben-Trauth, K., Friedman, T. B., Camper, S. A. 1998. Correction of deafness in shaker-2 mice by an unconventional myosin in a BAC transgene [see Comments] *Science*, 280, 1444-1447.

Propst, F. J., Rosenberg, M. P., Cork, L. C., Kovatch, R. M., Rauch, S., Westphal, H., Khillan, J., Schulz, N. T., Neumann, P. E., Newmann, P. E., Neuropathological changes in transgenic mice carrying copies of a transcriptionally activated Mos protooncogene. *Proc. Natl. Acad. Sci. U.S.A.*, 87, 9703-9707.

Prosen, C. A., Bath, K. G., Vetter, D. E., May, B. J. 2000. Behavioral assessments of auditory sensitivity in transgenic mice. *J. Neurosci. Meth.*, 97, 59-67.

Prosser, S., Tartari, M. C., Arslan, E. 1988. Hearing loss in sports hunters exposed to occupational noise. *Br. J. Audiol.,* 22, 85-91.

Puel, J.-L., d'Aldin, C. G., Saffiedine, S., Eybalin, M., Pujol, R. 1996. Excitotoxic and plasticity of IHC-auditory nerve contributes to both temporary and permanent threshold shift. In Axelsson, A., Borchgrevink, H. M., Hamernik, R. P., Hellström, P-A, Henderson, D. Salvi, R. J. (Eds.), *Scientific Basis of Noise-Induced Hearing Loss.* Theime Medical Publishers, New York, 36-42.

Pujol, R., Abonnenc, M. 1977. Receptor maturation and synaptogenesis in the golden hamster cochlea. *Arch. Otorhinolaryngol.,* 217, 1-12.

Pujol, R., Carlier, E. 1982. Cochlear synaptogenesis after sectioning the efferent bundle. *Devel. Brain Res.,* 3, 151-154.

Pujol, R., Carlier, E., Devigne, C. 1978. Different patterns of cochlear innervation during the development of the kitten. *J. Comp. Neurol.,* 177, 529-536.

Pujol, R., Carlier, E., Devigne, C. 1979. Significance of presynaptic formations in early stages of cochlear synaptogenesis. *Neurosci. Lett.,* 15, 97-102.

Pujol, R., Hilding, D. 1973. Anatomy and physiology of the onset of auditory function. *Acta Otolarygol.,* 76, 1-11.

Pujol, R., Lavigne-Rebillard, M., Lenoir, M. 1997. Development of sensory and neural structures in the mammalian cochlea. In Rubel, E. W., Popper, A. N., Fay, R. R. (Eds.), *Development of the Auditory System.* Springer, New York, 146-192.

Pujol, R., L., M., Ladrech, S., Tribillac, F., Redbillard, G. 1992. Correlation between the length of outer hair cells and the frequency coding of the cochlea. In Casals, Y., Demany, L., Horner, K. C. (Eds.), *Auditory Physiology and Perception.* Pergammon Press, Oxford, 45-52.

Qiu, M., Bulfone, A., Ghattas, I., Meneses, J. J., Christensen, L., Sharpe, P. T., Presley, R., Pedersen, R. A., Rubenstein, J. L. 1997. Role of the Dlx homeobox genes in proximodistal patterning of the branchial arches: mutations of Dlx-1, Dlx-2, and Dlx-1 and -2 alter morphogenesis of proximal skeletal and soft tissue structures derived from the first and second arches. *Devel. Biol.,* 185, 165-184.

Qiu, M., Bulfone, A., Martinez, S., Meneses, J. J., Shimamura, K., Pedersen, R. A., Rubenstein, J. L. 1995. Null mutation of Dlx-2 results in abnormal morphogenesis of proximal first and second branchial arch derivatives and abnormal differentiation in the forebrain. *Genes Devel.,* 9, 2523-2538.

Quadagno, D. M., McQuitty, C., McKee, J., Koelliker, L., Wolfe, G., Johnson, D. 1987. The effects of intrauterine position on competition and behavior in the mouse. *Physiol Behav.,* 41, 639-642.

Quirk, W. S., Seidman, M. D., Laurikainen, E. A., Nuttall, A. L., Miller, J. M. 1994. Influence of calcitonin-gene related peptide on cochlear blood flow and electrophysiology. *Am. J. Otol.,* 15, 56-60.

Rabie, A., Ferraz, C., Clavel, M.-C., Legrand, C. 1988. Gelsolin immunoreactivity and development of the tectorial membrane in the cochlea of normal and hypothyroid rats. *Cell Tissue Res.,* 254, 241-245.

Rabie, A., Thomasset, M., Legrand, C. 1983. Immunocytochemical detection of a calcium binding protein in the cochlear and vestibular hair cells of the rat. *Cell Tissue Res.,* 232, 691-696.

Raine, C. S., Cannella, B., Duijvestijn, A. M., Cross, A. H. 1990. Homing to central nervous system vasculature by antigen-specific lymphocytes. II. Lymphocyte/endothelial cell adhesion during the initial stages of autoimmune demyelination. *Lab. Invest.,* 63, 476-489.

Rajan, R., Irvine, D. R. F., Wise, L. Z., Heil, P. 1993. Effect of unilateral partial lesions in adult cats on the representation of lesioned and unlesioned cochleas in primary auditory cortex. *J. Comp. Neurol.,* 338, 17-49.

Rakic, P., Caviness, Jr., V. S. 1995. Cortical development: view form neurological mutants two decades later. *Neuron,* 14, 1101-1104.

Ralls, K. 1967. Auditory sensitivity in mice: *Peromyscus* and *Mus musculus. Anim. Behav.,* 15, 123-128.

Raman, I. M., Zhang, S., Trussell, L. O. 1994. Pathway-specific variants of AMPA receptors and their contribution to neuronal signaling. *J. Neurosci.,* 14, 4998-5010.

Ramón y Cajal, S. 1909. *Histologie du Système Nerveux de l'Homme et Vertébrés.* Maloine, Paris, chap. 28.

Randolf, H.-B., Haupt, H., Scheibe, F. 1990. Cochlear blood flow following temporary occlusion of cerebellar arteries. *Eur. Arch. Otorhinolaryngol.,* 247, 226-228.

Ranmakers, G. J., Winter, J., Hoogland, T. M., Lequin, M. B., van Hulten, P., van Pelt, J., Pool, C. W. 1998. Depolarization stimulates lamellipodia formation and axonal but not dendritic branching in cultured rat cerebral cortex neurons. *Devel. Brain Res.,* 108, 205-216.

Raphael, Y. 1991. Pure-tone overstimulation protects surviving avian hair cells from acoustic trauma. *Hear. Res.,* 53, 173-184.

Rapisardi, S. C., Miles, T. P. 1984. Synaptology of retinal terminals in the dorsal lateral geniculate nucleus of the cat. *J. Comp. Neurol.,* 223, 515-534.

Rarey, K. E., Yao, X. 1996. Localization of Cu/Zn-SOD and Mn-SOD in the rat cochlea. *Acta Otolaryngol.,* 116, 833-835.

Rasmussen, E. 1999. The Catalepsy Phenotype, Correlated Traits, and Associated QTLs. Ph. D. dissertation, SUNY at Stony Brook.

Rasmussen, E., Hitzemann, R. 1999. Detection of QTLs for haloperidol-induced catalepsy in a BALB/c x LP F_2 intercross. *J. Pharmacol. Exp. Therap.,* 290, 1337-1346.

Rasmussen, G. 1961. A method of staining the statoacoustic nerve in bulk with Sudan black B. *Anat. Rec.,* 139, 465-469.

Rathouz, M., Trussell, L. 1998. A characterization of outward currents in neurons of the nucleus magnocellularis. *J. Neurophysiol.,* 80, 2824-2835.

Rauch, S. D. 1992. Malformation and degeneration in the inner ear of mos transgenic mice. *Ann. Otol. Rhinol. Laryngol.,* 101, 430-436.

Rauch, S. D., Neuman, P. E. 1991. Malformation and degeneration in the inner ear of MOS transgenic mice. *Ann. N.Y. Acad. Sci.,* 630, 268-269.

Rauch, J., Tannenbaum, H., Stollar, B. D., Schwartz, R. S. 1984. Monoclonal anti-cardiolipin antibodies bind to DNA. *Eur. J. Immunol.,* 14, 529-534.

Rauch, S. D., Zurakowski, D., Bloch, D. B., Bloch, K. J. 2000. Anti-HSP70 antibodies in Ménière's disease. *Laryngoscope,* (in review).

Ray, B. A. 1970. Psychophysical testing of neurologic mutant mice. In Stebbins, W. C. (Ed.), *Animal Psychophysics.* Appleton, Century, Crofts, New York.

Raynor, E. M., Mulroy, M. J. 1997. Sensorineural hearing loss in the *mdx* mouse: a model of Duchenne muscular dystrophy. *Laryngoscope,* 107, 1053-1056.

Raz, Y., Kelley, M. W. 1997. Effects of retinoid and thyroid receptors during development of the inner ear. *Semin. Cell. Devel. Biol.,* 8, 257-264.

Raz, Y., Kelley, M. W. 1999. Retinoic acid signaling is necessary for the development of the organ of Corti. *Devel. Biol.,* 213, 180-193.

Reale, R. A., Imig, T. J. 1980. Tonotopic organization in auditory cortex of the cat. *J. Comp. Neurol.,* 192, 265-291.

Reaume, A. G., Elliott, J. L., Hoffman, E. K., Kowall, N. W., Ferrante, R. J., Siwek, D. F., Wilcox, H. M., Flood, D. G., Beal, M. F., Brown, Jr., R. H., Scott, R. W., Snider, W. D. 1996. Motor neurons in Cu/Zn superoxide dismutase-deficient mice develop normally but exhibit enhanced cell death after axonal injury. *Nature Genet.,* 13, 43-47.

Redowicz, M. J. 1999. Myosins and deafness. *J. Muscle Res. Cell Motil.,* 20, 241-248.

Reetz, G., Ehret, G. 1999. Inputs from three brainstem sources to identified neurons of the mouse inferior colliculus slice. *Brain Res.,* 816, 527-543.

Reimer, K., Urbanek, P., Busslinger, M., Ehret, G. 1996. Normal brainstem auditory evoked potentials in Pax5-deficient mice despite morphologic alterations in the auditory midbrain region. *Audiology,* 35, 55-61.

Reiter, L. A., Ison, J. R. 1977. Inhibition of the human eyeblink reflex: an examination of the Wendt-Yerkes method for threshold detection. *J. Exp. Psychol.: Human Perform. Percept.,* 3, 325-336.

Relkin, E. M. 1988. An introduction to the analysis of the middle ear. In Jahn and Santos-Sacchi, J. (Eds.), *Physiology of the Ear.* Raven Press, New York, 103-124.

Relkin, E. M., Saunders, J. C. 1980. The development of tympanic membrane displacements in the hamster. *Acta Otolaryngol.,* 90, 6-15.

Remezal, M., Gil-Loyzaga, P. 1993. Incorporation of D^3H glucosamine to the adult and developing cochlear tectorial membrane of normal and hypothyroid rats. *Hear. Res.,* 66, 23-30.

Ren, T., Brown, N. J., Zhang, M., Nuttall, A. L., Miller, J. M. 1995. A reversible ischemia model in gerbil cochlea. *Hear. Res.,* 92, 30-37.

Ren, T., Lin, X., Nuttall, A. L. 1993a. Polarized-light intravital microscopy for study of cochlear microcirculation. *Microvasc. Res.,* 46, 383-393.

Ren, T., Nuttall, A. L., Miller, J. M. 1993b. Contribution of the anterior inferior cerebellar artery to cochlear blood flow in guinea pig, a model-based analysis. *Hear. Res.,* 71, 91-97.

Renieri, A., Bassi, M. T., Galli, L., Zhou, J., Giani, M., De Marchi, M., Ballabio, A. 1994a. Deletion spanning the 5′ ends of both the COL4A5 and COL4A6 genes in a patient with Alport's syndrome and leiomyomatosis. *Hum. Mutat.,* 4, 195-198.

Renieri, A., Bruttini, M., Galli, L., Zanelli, P., Neri, T., Rossetti, S., Turco, A., Heiskari, N., Zhou, J., Gusmano, R., Massella, L., Banfi, G., Scolari, F., Sessa, A., Rizzoni, G., Tryggvason, K., Pignatti, P. F., Savi, M., Ballabio, A., De Marchi, M. 1996. X-linked Alport syndrome: an SSCP-based mutation survey over all 51 exons of the COL4A5 gene. *Am. J. Hum. Genet.*, 58, 1192-1204.

Renieri, A., Galli, L., De Marchi, M., Li, V. S., Mollica, F., Lupo, A., Maschio, G., Peissel, B., Rossetti, S., Pignatti, P. 1994b. Single base pair deletions in exons 39 and 42 of the COL4A5 gene in Alport syndrome. *Hum. Molec. Genet.*, 3, 201-202.

Renieri, A., Galli, L., Grillo, A., Bruttini, M., Neri, T., Zanelli, P., Rizzoni, G., Massella, L., Sessa, A., Meroni, M. 1995. Major COL4A5 gene rearrangements in patients with juvenile type Alport syndrome. *Am. J. Med. Genet.*, 59, 380-385.

Renieri, A., Meroni, M., Sessa, A., Battini, G., Serbelloni, P., Torri, T. L., Seri, M., Galli, L., De Marchi, M. 1994c. Variability of clinical phenotype in a large Alport family with Gly 1143 Ser change of collagen alpha 5(IV)-chain. *Nephron*, 67, 444-449.

Renieri, A., Seri, M., Myers, J. C., Pihlajaniemi, T., Massella, L., Rizzoni, G., De Marchi, M. 1992a. De novo mutation in the COL4A5 gene converting glycine 325 to glutamic acid in Alport syndrome. *Hum. Molec. Genet.*, 1, 127-129.

Renieri, A., Seri, M., Myers, J. C., Pihlajaniemi, T., Sessa, A., Rizzoni, G., De Marchi, M. 1992b. Alport syndrome caused by a 5′ deletion within the COL4A5 gene. *Hum. Genet.*, 89, 120-121.

Represa, J., Sanchez, A., Miner, C., Lewis, J., Giraldez, F. 1990. Retinoic acid modulation of the early development of the inner ear is associated with the control of c-fos expression. *Devel.*, 110, 1081-1090.

Represa, J., Van de Water, T. R., Bernd, P. 1991. Temporal pattern of nerve growth factor receptor expression in developing cochlear and vestibular ganglia in quail and mouse. *Anat. Embryol.*, 184, 421-432.

Retzius, G. 1884. *Das Gehörorgan der Reptilien, der Vogel und der Saugethiere*. Samson and Wallin, Stockholm.

Reyes, A. D., Rubel, E. W., Spain, W. J. 1994. Membrane properties underlying the firing of neurons in the avian cochlear nucleus. *J. Neurosci.*, 14, 5352-5364.

Rhode, W. S. 1998. Neural encoding of single-formant stimuli in the ventral cochlear nucleus of the chinchilla. *Hear. Res.*, 117, 39-56.

Rhode W. S. 1999. Vertical cell responses to sound in cat dorsal cochlear nucleus. *J. Neurophysiol.*, 82, 1019-1032.

Rhode, W. S., Greenberg, S. 1994. Encoding of amplitude modulation in the cochlear nucleus of the cat. *J. Neurophysiol.*, 71, 1797-1825.

Rhode, W. S., Oertel, D., Smith, P. H. 1983a. Physiological response properties of cells labeled intracellularly with horseradish peroxidase in cat ventral cochlear nucleus. *J. Comp. Neurol.*, 213, 448-463.

Rhode, W. S., Smith, P. H., Oertel, D. 1983b. Physiological response properties of cells labeled intracellularly with horseradish peroxidase in cat dorsal cochlear nucleus. *J. Comp. Neurol.*, 213, 426-447.

Rhode, W. S., Smith, P. H. 1985. Characteristics of tone-pip response patterns in relationship to spontaneous rate in cat auditory nerve fibers. *Hear. Res.*, 18, 159-168.

Rhode, W. S., Smith, P. H. 1986a. Encoding time and intensity in the ventral cochlear nucleus of the cat. *J. Neurophysiol.*, 56, 261-286.

Rhode, W. S., Smith, P. H. 1986b. Encoding time and intensity in the dorsal cochlear nucleus of the cat. *J. Neurophysiol.*, 56, 287-307.

Rice, J. J., May, B. J., Spirou, G. A., Young, E. D. 1992. Pinna-based spectral cues for sound localization in cat. *Hear. Res.*, 58, 132-152.

Richardson, G. P., Forge, A., Kros, C. J., Fleming, J., Brown, S. D., Steel, K. P. 1997. Myosin VIIA is required for aminoglycoside accumulation in cochlear hair cells. *J. Neurosci.*, 17, 9506-9519.

Richardson, G. P., Crossin, K. L., Chuong, C.-M., Edelman, G. M. 1987. Expression of cell adhesion molecules during embryonic induction III. Development of the otic placode. *Devel. Biol.*, 119, 217-230.

Richardson, K. C., Jarrett, L., Finke, E. H. 1960. Embedding in epoxy resin for ultrathin sectioning in electron microscopy. Stain Tech. 35, 313-323.

Ries, P. W. 1985. The demography of hearing loss. In Orlans, H. (Ed.), *Adjustment to Adult Hearing Loss*. College-Hill Press, San Diego, 3-21.

Rinchik, E. M., Carpenter, D. A., Selby, P. B. 1990. A strategy for fine-structure functional analysis of a 6- to 11-centimorgan region of mouse chromosome 7 by high-efficiency mutagenesis. *Proc. Natl. Acad. Sci., USA*, 87, 896-900.

Rines, J. P., Vom Saal, F. S. 1984. Fetal effects on sexual behvior and aggression in young and old female mice treated with estrogen and testosterone. *Horm. Behav.*, 18, 117-129.

Rinkwitz-Brandt, S., Arnold, H.-H., Bober, E. 1996. Regionalized expression of Nkx5-1, Nkx5-2, Pax2 and sek genes during mouse inner ear development. *Hear. Res.,* 99, 129-138.

Rinkwitz-Brandt, S., Justus, M., Oldenettel, I., Arnold, H. H., Bober, E. 1995. Distinct temporal expression of mouse Nkx-5.1 and Nkx-5.2 homeobox genes during brain and ear development. *Mech. Devel.,* 52, 371-381.

Rise, M. T., Frankel, W. N., Coffin, J. M., Seyfried, T. N. 1991. Genes for epilepsy mapped in the mouse. *Science,* 253, 669-673.

Ritter, F. N. 1967. The effects of hypothyroidism upon the ear, nose and throat. A clinical and experimental study. *Laryngoscope,* 77, 1427-1479.

Rivera-Perez, J. A., Mallo, M., Gendron-Maguire, M., Gridley, T., Behringer, R. R. 1995. Goosecoid is not an essential component of the mouse gastrula organizer but is required for craniofacial and rib development. *Devel.,* 121, 3005-3012.

Rivolta, C., Sweklo, E. A., Berson, E. L., Dryja, T. P. 2000. Missense mutation in the USH2A gene: association with recessive retinitis pigmentosa without hearing loss. *Am. J. Hum. Genet.,* 66, 1975-1978.

Rivolta, M. N., Holley, M. C. 1998. GATA3 is down regulated during hair cell differentiation in the mouse cochlea. *J. Neurocytol.,* 27, 637-647.

Roberts, E. 1986. GABA: The road to neurotransmitter status. In Olsen, R. W., Venter, J. C. (Eds.), *Benzodiazepine/GABA Receptors and Chloride Channels: Structural and Functional Properties.* Alan R. Liss, Inc., New York, 1-39.

Roberts, L. H. 1972. Correlation of the respiration and ultrasound production in rodents and bats. *J. Zool., London,* 168, 439-449.

Roberts, L. H. 1975. The rodent ultrasound production mechanism. *Ultrasonics,* 13, 83-88.

Roberts, R. C., Ribak, C. E. 1987. GABAergic neurons and axon terminals in the brainstem auditory nuclei of the gerbil. *J. Comp. Neurol.,* 258, 267-280.

Robertson, D., Irvine, D. R. F. 1989. Plasticity of frequency organization in auditory cortex of guinea pigs with partial unilateral deafness. *J. Comp. Neurol.,* 282, 456-471.

Robertson, N. G., Khetarpal, U., Gutierrez-Espelata, G. A., Bieber, F. R., Morton, C. C. 1994. Isolation of novel and known genes from a human fetal cochlear cDNA library using subtractive hybridization and differential screening. *Genomics,* 23, 42-50.

Robertson, N. G., Skvorak, A. B., Yin, Y., Weremowicz, S., Johnson, K., Kovatch, K. A., Battey, J. F., Bieber, F. R., Morton, C. C. 1997. Mapping and characterization of a novel cochlear gene in human and in mouse: a positional candidate gene for deafness disorder, DFNA9. *Genomics,* 46, 345-354.

Robinson, G. W., Mahon, K. A. 1994. Differential and overlapping expression domains of Dlx-2 and Dlx-3 suggest distinct roles for distal-less homeobox genes in craniofacial development. *Mech. Devel.,* 48, 199-215.

Rodriguez-Tebar, A., Dechant, G., Barde, Y. A. 1990. Binding of brain derived neurotrophic factor to the nerve growth factor receptor. *Neuron,* 4, 487-492.

Rodriquez, M. A., Pesold, C., Liu, W. S., Kriho, V., Guidoti, A., Pappas, G. D., Costa, E. 2000. Colocalization of integrin receptors and reelin in dendritic spine postsynaptic densities of adult nonhuman primate cortex. *Proc. Natl. Acad. Sci., USA,* 97, 3550-3555.

Roitt, I., Brostoff, J., Male, D. 1998. *Immunology.* Mosby, London.

Roitt, I. M. 1997. *Roitt's Essential Immunology.* Blackwell Science, Oxford.

Romand, M. R., Romand, R. 1990. Development of spiral ganglion cells in the mammalian cochlea. *J. Elec. Micro. Tech.,* 15, 144-154.

Romand, R. 1978. Survey of intracellular recording in the cochlear nucleus of the cat. *Brain Res.,* 148, 43-65.

Romand, R., Ehret, G. 1990. Development of tonotopy in the inferior colliculus I. Electrophysiological mapping in house mice. *Devel. Brain Res.,* 54, 221-234.

Romand, R., Ehret, G. 1992. Development of tonotopy, thresholds, latencies and tuning in the mouse inferior colliculus. *J. Physiol.,* 111(Suppl. 2), 181-184.

Romand, R., Sapin, V., Dolle, P. 1998. Spatial distributions of retinoic acid receptor gene transcripts in the prenatal mouse inner ear. *J. Comp. Neurol.,* 393, 298-308.

Rontal, D. A., Echteler, S. M. 1999. Postnatal remodeling of afferent and efferent innervation within the gerbil cochlea: a DiI study. *Assoc. Res. Otolaryngol. Abstr.,* 22, 133.

Rose, J. E., Sobkowicz, H. M., Bereman, B. 1977. Growth in culture of the peripheral axons of the spiral neurons in response to displacement of the receptors. *J. Neurocytol.,* 6, 49-70.

Rose, N. R., Bona, C. 1993. Defining criteria for autoimmune diseases (Witebsky's postulates revisited). *Immunol. Today,* 14, 426-430.

Rosenberg, T., Haim, M., Hauch, A. M., Parving, A. 1997. The prevalence of Usher syndrome and other retinal dystrophy-hearing impairment associations. *Clin. Genet.*, 51, 314-321.

Rosenthal, A., Goeddel, D. V., Lewis, N. M. 1990. Primary structure and biological activity of a novel human neurotrophic factor. *Neuron*, 4, 767-773.

Rosowski, J. J. 1992. Hearing in transitional mammals: predictions from the middle-ear anatomy and hearing capabilities of extant mammals. In Poper, A. N., Fay, R. R., and Webster, D. B. (Eds.), *The Evolutionary Biology of Hearing*. Springer-Verlag, New York, 615-631.

Rosowski, J. J. 1994. Outer and middle ears. In Fay, R. R., Popper, A. N. (Eds.), *Comparative Hearing: Mammals*. Springer-Verlag, New York, 172-247.

Rosowski, J. J. 1996. Models of external-and middle-ear function. In Hawkins, H. L., McMullen, T. A., Popper, A. N., Fay, R. R. (Eds.), *Auditory Computation*. Springer-Verlag, New York, 15-61.

Rosowski, J. J., Greybeal, A. 1991. What did *Morganucodon* hear? *Zool. J. Linnean Soc.*, 101, 131-168.

Ross, M. 1965. The auditory pathway of the epileptic waltzing mouse. II. Partially deaf mice. *J. Comp. Neurol.*, 125, 141-164.

Rossi, D. J., Alford, S., Mugnaini, E., Slater, N. T. 1995. Properties of transmission at a giant glutamatergic synapse in cerebellum: the mossy fiber-unipolar brush cell synapse. *J. Neurophysiol.*, 74, 24-42.

Roth, B., Bruns, V. 1993. Late developmental changes of the innervation densities of the myelinated fibres and the outer hair cell efferent fibres in the rat cochlea. *Anat. Embryol.*, 187, 565-571.

Roth, B., Dannhof, B., Bruns, V. 1991. ChAT-like immunoreactivity of olivocochlear fibres on rat outer hair cells during the postnatal development. *Anat. Embryol.*, 183, 483-489.

Roth, G. L., Aikin, L. M., Andersen, R. A., Merzenich, M. M. 1978. Some features of the spatial organization of the central nucleus of the inferior colliculus of the cat. *J. Comp. Neurol.*, 182, 661-680.

Ruan, R. S., Leong, S. K., Yeoh, K. H. 1997. Localization of nitric oxide synthase and NADPH-diaphorase in guinea pig and human cochleae. *J. Hirnforsch.*, 38, 433-441.

Rubel, E. W. 1978. Ontogeny of structure and function in the vertebrate auditory system. In M. Jacobson (Ed.), *Handbook of Sensory Physiology IX*. Springer-Verlag, New York, 135-237.

Ruben, R. J. 1967. Development of the inner ear of the mouse: a radioautographic study of terminal mitoses. *Acta Otolarygol.*, Suppl. 220, 1-44.

Rubenstein, J. B., Saunders, J. C. 1983. The effects of tympanic membrane perforation on auditory evoked activity and audiogenic seizure behavior in neonatal C57Bl/6J mice. *Trans. Penn. Acad. Opthal. Otolaryngol.*, 36, 52-56.

Ruckenstein, M. J., Gaber, L. L., Marion, T. N. 1999c. Cochlear and renal pathology in the (NZBxW)F1 mouse. *Assoc. Res. Otolaryngol. Abstr.*

Ruckenstein, M. J., Hu, L. 1999. Antibody deposition in the stria vascularis of the MRL-*Fas*[lpr] mouse. *Hear. Res.*, 127, 137-142.

Ruckenstein, M. J., Keithley, E. M., Bennett, T., Powell, H. C., Baird, S., Harris, J. P. 1999b. Ultrastructural pathology in the stria vascularis of the MRL-*Fas*[lpr] mouse. *Hear. Res.*, 131, 22-28.

Ruckenstein, M. J., Milburn, M., Hu, L. 1999a. Strial dysfunction in the MRL-*Fas*[lpr] mouse. *Otolaryngol. Head Neck Surg.*, 121, 452-456.

Ruckenstein, M. J., Mount, R. J., Harrison, R. V. 1993. The MRL-lpr/lpr mouse: a potential model of autoimmune inner ear disease. *Acta Otolaryngol.*, 113, 160-165.

Ruckenstein, M. J., Sarwar, A., Hu, L., Shami, H., Marion, T. N. 1999d. Effects of immunosuppression on the development of cochlear disease in the MRL-*Fas*[lpr] mouse. *Laryngoscope*, 109, 626-630.

Rueda, J., De la Sen, C., Juiz, J., Merchan, J. A. 1987. Neuronal loss in the spiral ganglion of young rats. *Arch. Otolaryngol.*, 104, 417-421.,

Rugh, R. 1968. *The mouse: Its Reproduction and Development*. Burgess Publishing Minneapolis.

Rumpelt, H. J. 1987. Alport's syndrome: specificity and pathogenesis of glomerular basement membrane alterations. *Pediatr. Nephrol.*, 1, 422-427.

Rupprecht, R., Reul, J. M. H. M., van Steensel, B., Spengler, D., Soder, M., Berning, B., Holsboer, F., Damn, K. 1993. Pharmacological and functional characterization of human mineralocorticoid and glucocorticoid receptor ligands. *Eur. J. Pharmacol. Molec. Pharmacol.*, 247, 145-54.

Rusch, A., Erway, L. C., Campos-Barros, A., Faric, J., Vennstrom, B., Forrest, D. 1998a. Thyroid hormone receptor functions in development of the auditory system studied in receptor-deficient mice. *Molec. Biol. Hear. Deafness Abstr.*, 3, 10.

Rusch, A., Erway, L. C., Oliver, D., Vennstrom, B., Forrest, D. 1998b. Thyroid hormone receptor beta-dependent expression of a potassium conductance in inner hair cells at the onset of hearing. *Proc. Natl. Acad. Sci. USA*, 95, 15758-15762.

Russell, L. B., Russell, W. L. 1992. Frequency and nature of specific-locus mutations induced in female mice by radiations and chemicals: a review. *Mutat. Res.*, 296, 107-127.

Ryan, A. F., Axelsson, A., Myers, R., Woolf, N. K. 1988. Changes in cochlear blood flow during acoustic stimulation as determined by ^{14}C-iodoantipyrine autoradiography. *Acta Otolaryngol.*, 105, 232-241.

Ryan, A. F., Catanzaro, A., Wasserman, S. I., Harris, J. P. 1986. Secondary immune response in the middle ear: immunological, morphological, and physiological observations. *Ann. Otol. Rhinol. Laryngol.*, 95, 242-249.

Ryan, A. F., Catanzaro, A. 1983. Passive transfer of immune-mediated middle ear inflammation and effusion. *Acta Otolaryngol.*, 95, 123-130.

Ryan, A. F., Dulon, D., Keithley, E. M., Erkman, L. 1998. A Brn-3.1 promoter element directs gene expression limited to hair cells in postnatal transgenic mice. *Abstr. 3rd Int. Conf. Molec. Biol. Hear. Deafness*, 166.

Ryan, A. F., Goodwin, P., Woolf, N. K., Sharp, F. 1982. Auditory stimulation alters the pattern of 2-deoxy-glucose uptake in the inner ear. *Brain Res.*, 234, 213-225.

Ryan, A. F., Sharp, P. A., Harris, J. P. 1990. Lymphocyte circulation to the middle ear. *Acta Otolaryngol.*, 109, 278-287.

Ryan, A. K., Rosenfeld, M. G. 1997. POU domain family values: flexibility, partnerships, and developmental codes. *Genes Devel.*, 11, 1207-1225.

Ryugo, D. K., Fekete, D. M. 1982. Morphology of primary axosomatic endings in the anteroventral cochlear nucleus of the cat: a study of the endbulbs of Held. *J. Comp. Neurol.*, 210, 239-257.

Ryugo, D. K., Pongstaporn, T., Huchton, D. M., Niparko, J. K. 1997. Ultrastructural analysis of primary endings in deaf white cats: morphologic alterations in endbulbs of Held. *J. Comp. Neurol.*, 385, 230-244.

Ryugo, D. K., Rosenbaum, B. T., Kim, P. J., Niparko, J. K., Saada, A. A. 1998. Single unit recordings in the auditory nerve of congenitally deaf white cats: morphological correlates in the cochlea and cochlear nucleus. *J. Comp. Neurol.*, 397, 532-548.

Ryugo, D. K., Willard, F. H. 1985. The dorsal cochlear nucleus of the mouse: a light microscopic analysis of neurons that project to the inferior colliculus. *J. Comp. Neurol.*, 242, 381-396.

Ryugo, D. K., Willard, F. H., Fekete, D. M. 1981. Differential afferent projections to the inferior colliculus from the cochlear nucleus in the albino mouse. *Brain Res.*, 210, 342-349.

Ryugo, D. K., Wu, M. M., Pongstaporn, T. 1996. Activity-related features of synapse morphology: a study of endbulbs of Held. *J. Comp. Neurol.*, 365, 141-158.

Sadanaga, M., Morimitsu, T. 1995. Development of endocochlear potential and its negative component in mouse cochlea. *Hear. Res.*, 89, 155-161.

Sado, Y., Kagawa, M., Naito, I., Ueki, Y., Seki, T., Momota, R., Oohashi, T., Ninomiya, Y. 1998. Organization and expression of basement membrane collagen IV genes and their roles in human disorders. *J. Biochem. (Tokyo)*, 123, 767-776.

Saga, Y., Yagi, T., Ikawa, Y., Sakakura, T., Aizawa, S. 1992. Mice develop normally without tenascin. *Genes Devel.*, 6, 1821-1831.

Sagara, T., Furukawa, H., Makishima, K., Fujimoto, S. 1995. Differentiation of the rat stria vascularis. *Hear. Res.*, 83, 121-132.

Sahly, I., el-Amraoui, A., Abitbol, M., Petit, C., Dufier, J. L. 1997. Expression of myosin VIIA during mouse embryogenesis. *Anat. Embryol. (Berl.)*, 196, 159-170.

Saint Marie, R. L., Shneiderman, A, Stanforth, D. A. 1997. Patterns of gamma-aminobutyric acid and glycine immunoreactivities reflect structural and functional differences of the cat lateral lemniscal nuclei. *J. Comp. Neurol.*, 389, 264-276.

Saitoh, Y., Hosokawa, M., Shimada, A., Watanabe, Y., Yasuda, N., Murakami, Y., Takeda, T. 1995. Age-related cochlear degeneration in senescence-accelerated mouse. *Neurobiol. Aging*, 16, 129-136.

Saitoh, Y., Hosokawa, M., Shimada, A., Watanabe, Y., Yasuda, N., Takeda, T., Murakami, Y. 1994. Age-related hearing impairment in senescence-accelerated mouse (SAM). *Hear. Res.*, 75, 27-37.

Sakaguchi, N., Spicer, S. S., Thomopoulos, G. N., Schulte, B. A. 1997. Increased laminin deposition in capillaries of the stria vascularis of quiet-aged gerbils. *Hear. Res.*, 105, 44-56.

Sakamoto, N., Kurono, Y., Ueyama, T., Mogi, G. 1996. Detection of *Haemophilus infuenzae* in nasopharyngeal secretions and the adenoids by polymerase chain reaction. In Lim, D. J., Bluestone, C. D., Casselbrant, M., Klein, J. O., Ogra, P. L. (Eds.), *Recent Advances in Otitis Media.* B. C. Decker, Hamilton, 423-424.

Sales, G. D. 1972a. Ultrasound and aggressive behaviour in rats and other small mammals. *Anim. Behav.,* 20, 88-100.

Sales, G. D. 1972b. Ultrasound and mating behaviour in rodents with some observations on other behavioral situation. *J. Zool. London,* 168, 149-164.

Sales, G., Pye, D. 1974. *Ultrasound in Rodents, Ultrasonic Communication by Animals.* Chapman and Hill, London, 149-201.

Salminen, M., Meyer, B. I., Bober, E., Gruss, P. 2000. Netrin 1 is required for semicircular canal formation in the mouse inner ear. *Devel.,* 127, 13-22.

Salvi, R., Ding, D., Burkard, R., McFadden, S. 1998. Knockout mice lacking the Cu-Zn-superoxide dismutase gene exhibit greater age-related sensory cell loss. *Assoc. Res. Otolaryngol. Abstr.,*

Salvi, R. J., Henderson, D., Fiorino, F., Colleti, V. 1996. *Auditory System Plasticity and Regeneration.* Thieme, New York.

Sandell, J. H. 1998. GABA as a developmental signal in the inner retina and optic nerve. *Persp. Devel. Neurobiol.,* 5, 269-278.

Sands, M. S., Barker J. E. 1999. Percutaneous intravenous injection in neonatal mice. Lab. Anim. *Science,* 49, 328-330.

Sands, M. S., Barker, J. E., Vogler, C., Levy, B., Gwynn, B., Galvin, N., Sly, W. S., Birkenmeier, E. 1993. Treatment of murine mucopolysaccharidosis type VII by syngeneic bone marrow transplantation in neonates. *Lab. Invest.,* 68, 676-686.

Sands, M. S. Birkenmeier E. H. 1993. A single-base-pair deletion in the beta-glucuronidase gene accounts for the phenotype of murine mucopolysaccharidosis Type VII. *Proc. Natl. Acad. Sci.,* 90, 6567-6571.

Sands, M. S., Kyle J. W., Grubb J. H., Levy B., Galvin N., Sly, W. S. Birkenmeier E. H. 1994. Enzyme replacement therapy for murine mucopolysaccharidosis Type VII. *J. Clin. Invest.,* 93, 2324-2331.

Sands, M. S., Erway L. C., Vogler C., Sly W. S. Birkenmeier E. H. 1995. Syngeneic bone marrow transplantation reduces the hearing loss associated with murine mucopolysaccharidosis Type VII. *Blood,* 86, 2033-2040.

Sands, M. S., Vogler, C., Torrey, A., Levy, B., Gwynn, B., Grubb, J., Sly, W. S. 1997a. Murine mucopolysaccharidosis Type VII: long term therapeutic effects of enzyme replacement and enzyme replacement followed by bone marrow transplantation. *J. Clin. Invest.,* 99, 1596-1605.

Sands, M. S., Wolfe, J. H., Birkenmeier, E. H., Barker, J. E., Vogler, C., Sly, W. S., Okuyama, T., Freeman, B., Nicholes, A., Muzyczka, N., Chang, P. L. Axelrod, H. R. 1997b. Gene therapy for murine mucopolysaccharidosis Type VII. *Neuromusc. Disord.,* 7, 352-360.

Sanes, J. N. 1984. Voluntary movement and excitability of cutaneous eyeblink reflexes. *Psychophysiology,* 21, 653-664.

Sanford, L. P., Ormsby, I., Gittenberger-de Groot, A. C., Sariola, H., Friedman, R., Boivan, G. P., Cardell, E. L., Doetschman, T. 1997. TGFbeta2 knockout mice have multiple developmental defects that are non-overlapping with other TGFbeta knockout phenotypes. *Devel.,* 124, 2659-2670.

Sankarapandi, S., Zweier, J. L. 1999. Bicarbonate is required for the peroxidase function of Cu, Zn-superoxide dismutase at physiological pH. *J. Biol. Chem.,* 274, 1226-1232.

Sankila, E. M., Pakarinen, L., Kaariainen, H., Aittomaki, K., Karjalainen, S., Sistonen, P., de la Chapelle, A. 1995. Assignment of an Usher syndrome type III (USH3) gene to chromosome 3q. *Hum. Molec. Genet.,* 4, 93-98.

Santi, P. A., Ruggero, M. A., Nelson, D. A., Turner, C. W. 1982. Kanamycin and bumetanide ototoxicity: anatomical, physiological and behavioral correlates. *Hear. Res.,* 7, 261-279.

Saouda, M., Mansour, A., Bou, M. Y., El Zir, E., Mustapha, M., Chaib, H., Nehme, A., Megarbane, A., Loiselet, J., Petit, C., Slim, R. 1998. The Usher syndrome in the Lebanese population and further refinement of the USH2A candidate region. *Hum. Genet.,* 103, 193-198.

Sapolsky, R. J., Hsie, L., Berno, A., Ghandour, G., Mittmann, M., Fan, J. B. 1999. High-throughput polymorphism screening and genotyping with high-density oligonucleotide arrays. *Genet. Anal.,* 14, 187-192.

Sarelius, I. H., Duling, B. R. 1982. A new method for measurement of hematocrit, red cell flux, and capillary transit time. *Microsc. Res.,* 23, 272-273.

Sato, H., Sando, I., Takahashi, H. 1991. Sexual dimorphism and development of the human cochlea. Computer 3-D measurement. *Acta Otolaryngol.,* 111, 1037-1040.

Satoh, H., Kawasaki, K., Kihara, I., Nakano, Y. 1998. Importance of type IV collagen, laminin, and heparan sulfate proteoglycan in the regulation of labyrinthine fluid in the rat cochlear duct. *Eur. Arch. Otorhinolaryngol.*, 255, 285-288.

Satokata, I., Maas, R. 1994. Msx1 deficient mice exhibit cleft palate and abnormalities of craniofacial and tooth development. *Nature Genet.*, 6, 348-356.

Saunders, J. C., Canlon, B. Flock, Å. 1986. Growth of threshold shift in hair-cell stereocilia following overstimulation. *Hear. Res.*, 23, 245-255.

Saunders, J. C., Doan, D. E., Cohen, Y. E. 1993. The contribution of middle-ear sound conduction to auditory development. *Comp. Biochem. Physiol.*, 106A, 7-13.

Saunders, J. C., Dolgin, K. G., Lowry, L. D. 1980. The maturation of frequency selectivity in C57BL/6J mice studied with auditory-evoked response tuning curves. *Brain Res.*, 187, 69-79.

Saunders, J. C., Duncan, R. K., Doan, D. E., Werner, Y. L. 2000. The middle ear of reptiles and birds. In Dooling, R. J., Popper, A. N., and Fay, R. R. (Eds.), *Comparative Hearing: Non-Mammals*. Springer Verlag, New York, 13-69.

Saunders, J. C., Garfinkle, T. 1983. Peripheral Physiology II. In Willott, J. F. (Ed.), *Auditory Psychobiology of the Mouse*. B.C. Thomas, Springfield, IL, 131-168.

Saunders, J. C., Johnstone, B. M. 1972. A comparative analysis of middle-ear function in non-mammalian vertebrates. *Acta Otolaryngol.*, 73, 353-361.

Saunders, J. C., Kaltenback, J. A., Relkin, E. M. 1983. The structural and functional development of the outer and middle ear. In Romand, R. (Ed.), *Development of the Auditory and Vestibular Systems*. Academic Press, New York, 3-25.

Saunders, J. C., Summers, R. M. 1982. Auditory structure and function in the mouse middle ear: an evaluation by SEM and capacitive probe. *J. Comp. Physiol. A*, 146, 517-525.

Savage, C. O., Pottinger, B. E., Gaskin, G., Lockwood, C. M., Pusey, C. D., Pearson, J. D. 1991. Vascular damage in Wegener's granulomatosis and microscopic polyarteritis: presence of anti-endothelial cell antibodies and their relation to anti-neutrophil cytoplasm antibodies. *Clin. Exp. Immunol.*, 85, 14-19.

Sayers, R., Kalluri, R., Rodgers, K. D., Shield, C. F., Meehan, D. T., Cosgrove, D. 1999. Role for transforming growth factor-beta1 in alport renal disease progression. *Kidney Int.*, 56, 1662-1673.

Schanbacher, A., Koch, M., Pilz, P. K., Schnitzler, H. U. 1996. Lesions of the amygdala do not affect the enhancement of the acoustic startle response by background noise. *Physiol. Behav.*, 605, 1341-1346.

Schecterson, L., Bothwell, M. 1994. Neurotrophin and neurotrophin receptor mRNA expression in developing inner ear. *Hear. Res.*, 73, 92-100.

Scheibe, F., Haupt, H., Ludwig, C. 1993. Intensity-related changes in cochlear blood flow in the guinea pig during and following acoustic exposure. *Eur. Arch. Otorhinolaryngol.*, 250, 281-285.

Scheibe, F., Haupt, H., Nuttall, A. L., Ludwig, C. 1990. Laser Doppler measurements of cochlear blood flow during loud sound presentation. *Eur. Arch. Otorhinolaryngol.*, 247, 84-88.

Schiavo, G., Stenbeck, G. 1998. Molecular analysis of neurotransmitter release. *Essays Biochem.*, 33, 29-41.

Schielke, G. P., Yang, G.-Y., Shivers, B. D., Betz, A. L. 1998. Reduced ischemic brain injury in interleukin-1 B converting enzyme-deficient mice. *J. Cereb. Blood. Flow Metab.*, 18, 180-185.

Schimenti, J., Bucan, M. 1998. Functional genomics in the mouse: phenotype-based mutagenesis screens. *Genome Res.*, 8, 698-710.

Schimmang, T., Minichiello, L., Vazquez, E., San Jose, I., Giraldez, F., Klein, R., Represa, J. 1995. Developing inner ear sensory neurons require TrkB and TrkC receptors for innervation of their peripheral targets. *Devel.*, 121, 3381-3391.

Schleidt, W. M., Kickert-Magg, M. 1979. Hearing thresholds of albino house mouse between 1 and 80 kHz by shuttle box training. *J. Aud. Res.*, 19, 37-40.

Schmiedt, R. A. 1986. Acoustic distortion in the ear canal. I. Cubic difference tones: effects of acute noise injury. *J. Acoust. Soc. Am.*, 79, 1481-1490.

Schmitt, J. M., Hwang, K., Winn, S. R., Hollinger, J. O. 1999. Bone morphogenetic proteins: an update on basic biology and clinical relevance. *J. Orthop. Res.*, 17, 269-278.

Schneeberger, P. R., Norman, A. W., Heizmann, C. W. 1985. Parvalbumin and vitamin D-dependent calcium binding proteins (M_r 28,000): comparison of their localization in normal and ruchitic rats. *Neurosci. Lett.*, 59, 97-103.

Schofield, B. R. 1995. Projections from the cochlear nucleus to the superior periolivary nucleus in guinea pigs. *J. Comp. Neurol.*, 360, 135-149.

Schofield, B. R., Cant, N. B. 1996. Origins and targets of commissural connections between the cochlear nuclei in guinea pigs. *J. Comp. Neurol.*, 375, 128-146.

Schofield, B. R., Cant, N. B. 1997. Ventral nucleus of the lateral lemniscus in guinea pigs: cytoarchitecture and inputs from the cochlear nucleus. *J. Comp. Neurol.*, 379, 363-385.

Schonemann, M. D., Ryan, A. K., McEvilly, R. J., O'Connell, S. M., Arias, C. A., Kalla, K. A., Li, P. et al. 1995. Development and survival of the endocrine hypothalamus and posterior pituitary gland requires the neuronal POU domain factor Brn-2. *Genes Devel.*, 9, 3122-3135.

Schorle, H., Meier, P., Buchert, M., Jaenisch, R., Mitchell, P. J. 1996. Transcription factor AP-2 essential for cranial closure and craniofacial development. *Nature*, 381, 235-238.

Schrader, M., Poppendieck, J., Weber, B. 1990. Immunohistologic findings in otosclerosis. *Ann. Otol. Rhinol. Laryngol.*, 99, 349-352.

Schrott, A., Puel, J.-L., Rebillard, G. 1991. Cochlear origin of 2f1-f2 distortion products assessed by using 2 types of mutant mice. *Hear. Res.*, 52, 245-254.

Schubert, J., Felix, H., Weiher, H., Meyer-Zum-Gottesberge, A. 1999. Loss of MPV17 gene alters the ultrastructure and immmunohistochemistry of lateral wall fibrocytes. *Assoc. Res. Otolaryngol. Abstr.*,

Schuknecht, H. F. 1974. *Pathology of the Ear.* Harvard University Press, Cambridge.

Schuknecht, H. F. 1993. *Pathology of the Ear.* Lea and Febiger, Philadelphia.

Schuknecht, H. F., Nadol, Jr., J. B., 1994. Temporal bone pathology in a case of Cogan's syndrome. *Laryngoscope*, 104, 1135-1142.

Schulte, B. A., Steel, K. P. 1994. Expression of α and β subunit isoforms of Na,K-ATPase in the mouse inner ear and changes with mutations at the W^v or Sl^d loci. *Hear. Res.*, 78, 65-76.

Schultze-Bahr, E., Wang, Q., Wedekind, H., Haverkamp, W., Chen, Q., Sun, Y. 1997. KCNE1 mutations cause Jervell and Lang-Nielsen syndrome. *Nature Genet.*, 17, 267-268.

Schwaber, M. K., Garraghty, P. E., Kaas, J. H. 1993. Neuroplasticity of the adult primary auditory cortex following cochlear hearing loss. *Am. J. Otolaryngol.*, 14, 252-258.

Schwartz, G. M., Hoffman, H. S., Stitt, C. L., Marsh, R. R. 1976. Modification of the rat's acoustic startle response by antecedent visual stimulation. *J. Exp. Psychol: Anim. Behav. Proc.*, 2, 28-37.

Schwarz, D. W. F., Schwarz, I. E., Hu, K., Vincent, S. R. 1988. Retrograde transport of [3H]-GABA by lateral olivocochlear neurons in the rat. *Hear. Res.*, 32, 97-102.

Schweitzer, L. 1987. Development of brainstem auditory evoked responses in the hamster. *Hear. Res.*, 25, 249-255.

Scott, J. P. 1966. Agonistic behavior of mice and rats: A review. *Am. Zool.*, 6, 683-701.

Scott, J. P., Fredericson, E. 1951. The causes of fighting in mice and rats. *Physiol. Zool.*, 24, 273-309.

Segal, Y., Peissel, B., Renieri, A., De Marchi, M., Ballabio, A., Pei, Y., Zhou, J. 1999. LINE-1 elements at the sites of molecular rearrangements in Alport syndrome-diffuse leiomyomatosis. *Am. J. Hum. Genet.*, 64, 62-69.

Seidahmed, M. Z., Sundada, Y., Oxo, C. O., Hamid, F., Campbell, K. P., Salih, A. M. 1996. Lethal congenital muscular dystrophy in two sibs with arthrogryposis multiplex: new entity or variant of Cobblestone Lissencephaly syndrome? *Neuropediatrics*, 27, 305-310.

Seidman, M. D., Quirk, W. S., Nuttall, A. L., Schweitzer, V. G. 1991. The protective effects of allopurinol and superoxide dismutase-polyethlyene glycol on ischemic and reperfusion induced cochlear damage. *Otolaryngol. Head Neck Surg.*, 105, 457-463.

Seidman, M. D., Shivapuja, B. G., Quirk, W. S. 1993. The protective effects of allopurinol and superoxide dismutase on noise-induced cochlear damage. *Otolaryngol. Head Neck Surg.*, 109, 1052-1056.

Seki, T., Naito, I., Oohashi, T., Sado, Y., Ninomiya, Y. 1998. Differential expression of type IV collagen isoforms, alpha5(IV) and alpha6(IV) chains, in basement membranes surrounding smooth muscle cells. *Histochem. Cell Biol.*, 110, 359-366.

Seldon, H. L, Clark, G. M. 1991. Human cochlear nucleus: comparison of Nissl-stained neurons from deaf and hearing patients. *Brain Res.*, 551, 185-194.

Self, T., Brown, S., Williams, D., Steel, K. 2000. Role of myosin VIIa in developing hair cells of the mouse. *Assoc. Res. Otolaryngol. Abstr.*, 23, 248.

Self, T., Mahony, M., Fleming, J., Walsh, J., Brown, S. D., Steel, K. P. 1998. Shaker-1 mutations reveal roles for myosin VIIA in both development and function of cochlear hair cells. *Devel.*, 125, 557-566.

Sellick, P. M., Patuzzi, R., Johnstone, B. M. 1982. Measurement of basilar membrane motion in guinea pig using the Mossbauer technique. *J. Acoust. Soc. Am.*, 72, 131-141.

Sendtner, M., Holtmann, B., Kolbeck, R., Thoenen, H., Barde, Y.-A. 1992. Brain-derived neurotrophic factor prevents the death in motoneurons in newborn rats after nerve section. *Nature,* 360, 24-31.

Sewell, G. D. 1967. Ultrasound in adult rodents. *Nature,* 215, 512.

Sewell, G. D. 1968. Ultrasound in rodents. *Nature,* 217, 682-683.

Seymour, J. C. 1954. Observations on the circulation in the cochlea. *J. Laryngol.,* 68, 689-711.

Sha, S.-H., Zajic, G., Schacht, J. 1997. Transgenic mice overexpressing copper-zinc superoxide dismutase are protected from kanamycin-induced ototoxicity. *Assoc. Res. Otolaryngol. Abstr.,*

Shailam, R., Lanford, P. J., Kelley, M. W. 1999. Overexpression of MATH1 results in increased numbers of inner hair cells in the mammalian cochlea. *Assoc. Res. Otolarngol. Abstr.,* 22, 138.

Shatz, C. J. 1990. Impulse activity and the patterning of connections during CNS development. *Neuron,* 5, 45-56.

Shen, J. X., Xu, Z. M, Yao, Y. D. 1999. Evidence for columnar organization in the auditory cortex of the mouse. *Hear. Res.,* 137, 174-177.

Shepherd, A. P., Oberg, P. A. 1990. *Laser-Doppler Blood Flowmetry.* Kluwer Academic, Boston, MA.

Sher, A. E. 1971. The embryonic and postnatal development of the inner ear of the mouse. *Acta Otolaryngol.,* (Suppl.) 285, 1-19.

Shera, C. A., Guinan, Jr., J. J. 1999. Evoked otoacoustic emissions arise by two fundamentally different mechanisms: a taxonomy of mammalian OAEs. *J. Acoust. Soc. Am.,* 105, 782-798.

Sherr, C. J., Roberts, J. M. 1995. Inhibitors of mammalian G1 cyclin-dependent kinases. *Genes Devel.,* 9, 1149-1163.

Shetty, A. K., Turner, D. A. 1998. Hippocampal interneurons expressing glutamic acid decarboxylase and calcium-binding proteins decrease with aging in Fischer 344 rats. *J. Comp. Neurol.,* 394, 252-269.

Shi, X., Ren, T., Nuttall, A. 2000. Nitric oxide distribution and production in the guinea pig cochlea. (Submitted.)

Shimada, T., Lim, D. J. 1971. The fiber arrangement of the human tympanic membrane. *Ann. Otol. Rhinol. Laryngol.,* 80, 210-217.

Shin, S. O., Billings, P. B., Keithley, E. M., Harris, J. P. 1997. Comparison of anti-heat shock protein 70 (anti-hsp70) and anti-68-kDa inner ear protein in the sera of patients with Meniere's disease. *Laryngoscope,* 107, 222-227.

Shnerson, A., Devigne, C., Pujol, R. 1982. Age-related changes in the C57BL/6J mouse cochlea. II. Ultra-structural findings. *Devel. Brain Res.,* 2, 77-88.

Shnerson, A., Lenoir, M., van de Water, T. R., Pujol, R. 1983. The pattern of sensorineural degeneration in the cochlea of the deaf shaker-1 mouse: ultrastructural observations. *Brain Res.,* 285, 305-315.

Shnerson, A., Pujol, R. 1982. Age-related changes in the C57Bl/6J mouse cochlea. I. Physiological findings. *Devel. Brain Res.,* 2, 65-75.

Shnerson, A., Pujol, R. 1983. Development: anatomy, electrophysiology and behavior. In Willott, J. F. (Ed.), *The Auditory Psychobiology of the Mouse.* Charles B. Thomas, Springfield, IL, 395-425.

Shnerson, A., Willott, J. F. 1980. Ontogeny of the acoustic startle response in C57BL/6J mouse pups. *J. Comp. Physiol. Psychol.,* 94, 36-40.

Shone, G., Altschuler, R. A., Miller, J. M., Nuttall, A. L. 1991a. The effect of noise exposure on the aging ear. *Hear. Res.,* 56, 173-178.

Shone, G., Raphael, Y., Miller, J. M. 1991b. Hereditary deafness occurring in cd/1 mice. *Hear. Res.,* 57, 153-156.

Shvarev, Y. N. 1994. Brainstem auditory evoked potentials characteristics in mice: the effect of genotype. *Hear. Res.,* 81, 189-198.

Sidman, M., Ray, B. A., Sidman, R. L., Klinger, J. M. 1966. Hearing and vision in neurological mutant mice: a method for their evaluation. *Exp. Neurol.,* 16, 377-402.

Sidman, R. L., Angevine, J. B. Jr., Taber Pierce, E. 1971. *Atlas of the Mouse Brain and Spinal Cord.* Harvard University Press, Cambridge.

Sidman, R. L., Green, M. C., Appel, S. H. 1965. *Catalog of the Neurological Mutants of the Mouse.* Harvard University Press, Cambridge, MA.

Siegel, J. H., Kim, D. O. 1982. Efferent neural control of cochlear mechanics? Olivocochlear bundle stimulation affects cochlear biomechanical nonlinearity. *Hear. Res.,* 6, 171-182.

Siegel, J. H., Kim, D. O., Molnar, C. E. 1982. Effects of altering organ of Corti on distortion products f_2-f_1 and $2 f_1$-f_2. *J. Neurophysiol.,* 47, 303-328.

Silver, L. M. 1995. *Mouse Genetics.* Oxford University Press, New York.

Simeone, A., Acampora, D., Pannese, M., D'Esposito, M., Stornaiuolo, A., Gulisano, M., Mallamaci, A., Kastury, K., Druck, T., Huebner, K., et al. 1994. Cloning and characterization of two members of the vertebrate Dlx gene family. *Proc. Natl. Acad. Sci., USA,* 91, 2250-2254.

Simmler, M. C., Cohen-Salmon, M., El-Amraoui, A., Guillaud, L., Benichou, J. C., Petit, C., Panthier, J. J. 2000. Targeted disruption of otog results in deafness and severe imbalance [see Comments]. *Nature Genet.,* 24, 139-143.

Simmons, D. D., Bertolotto, C., Kim, J., Raji-Kubba, J., Mansdorf, N. 1998. Choline acetyltransferase expression during a putative developmental waiting period. *J. Comp. Neurol.,* 397, 281-295.

Simmons, D. D., Mansdorf, N. B., Kim, J. H. 1996a. Olivocochlear innervation of inner and outer hair cells during postnatal maturation: evidence for a waiting period. *J. Comp. Neurol.,* 370, 551-562.

Simmons, D. D., Manson-Gieseke, L., Hendrix, T. W., McCarter, S. 1990. Reconstructions of efferent fibers in the postnatal hamster cochlea. *Hear. Res.,* 49, 127-140.

Simmons, D. D., Moulding, H. D., Zee, D. 1996b. Olivocochlear innervation of inner and outer hair cells during postnatal maturation: an immunocytochemical study. *Devel. Brain Res.,* 95, 213-226.

Simon, M. M., Gern, L., Hauser, P., Zhong, W., Nielsen, P. J., Kramer, M. D., Brenner, C., Wallich, R. 1996. Protective immunization with plasmid DNA containing the outer surface lipoprotein A gene of *Borrelia burgdorferi* is independent of an eukaryotic promoter. *Eur. J. Immunol.,* 26, 2831-2840.

Sipos, M. L., Kerchner, M., Nyby, J. G. 1992. An ephemeral sex pheromone in the urine of female house mice (*Mus domesticus*). *Behav. Neural Biol.,* 58, 138-143.

Sipos, M. L., Nyby, J. G., Serran, M. F. 1993. An ephemeral sex pheromone of female house mice (*Mus domesticus*): pheromone fade-out time. *Physiol. Behav.,* 54, 171-174.

Sipos, M. L., Nyby, J. G., Snyder, R. W., Kerchner, M. 1999. Ultrasound-eliciting and aggression-reducing pheromones in female house mouse urine: are they the same? *Physiol. Behav.,* (under review).

Sipos, M. L., Nyby, J. G. 1996. Concurrent androgenic stimulation of the ventral tegmental area and medial preoptic area: synergistic effects on male-typical behaviors in house mice. *Brain Res.,* 729, 29-44.

Sipos, M. L., Nyby, J. G. 1998. Intracranial androgenic activation of male-typical behaviours in house mice: concurrent stimulation of the medial preoptic area and medial nucleus of the amygdala. *J. Neuroendocrinol.,* 10, 577-586.

Sipos, M. L., Wysocki, C. J., Nyby, J. G., Wysocki, L., Nemura, T. A. 1995. An ephemeral pheromone of female house mice: perception via the main and accessory olfactory systems. *Physiol. Behav.,* 58, 529-534.

Sjostrom, B., Anniko, M. 1990. Variability in genetically induced age-related impairment of auditory brainstem response thresholds. *Acta Otolaryngol.,* 109, 353-360.

Sjostrom, B., Anniko, M. 1992a. Genetically induced inner ear degeneration. A structural and functional study. *Acta Otolaryngol.,* S493, 141-146.

Sjostrom, B., Anniko, M. 1992b. Cochlear structure and function in a recessive type of genetically induced inner ear degeneration. *ORL J. Otorhinolaryngol. Relat. Spec.,* 54, 220-228.

Skene, J. H. P. 1989. Axonal growth-associated proteins. *Annu. Rev. Neurosci.,* 12, 127-156.

Slaaf, D. W., Alewijnse, R., Wayland, H. 1981. Telescopic imaging in intravital microscopy. *Bibliotheca Anatomica,* 20, 53-57.

Slaaf, D. W., Alewijnse, R., Wayland, H. 1982. Use of telescopic imaging in intravital microscopy, A simple solution for conventional microscopes. *Int. J. Microcir.,* 1, 121-134.

Slepecky, N. B. 1996. Structure of the mammalian cochlea. In Dallos, P., Popper, A. N., Fay, R. R. (Eds.), *The Cochlea.* Springer-Verlag, New York, 44-129.

Sloviter, R. S. 1989. Calcium-binding protein (calbindin-D28k) and parvalbumin immunocytochemistry: localization in the rat hippocampus with specific reference to the selective vulnerability of hippocampal neurons to seizure activity. *J. Comp. Neurol.,* 280, 183-196.

Sly, W. S., Quinton, B. A., McAlister, W. H. Rimoin, D. L. 1973. Beta glucuronidase deficiency: report of clinical, radiologic, and biochemical features of a new mucopolysaccharidosis. *J. Pediat.,* 82, 249-257.

Smeets, H. J., Melenhorst, J. J., Lemmink, H. H., Schroder, C. H., Nelen, M. R., Zhou, J., Hostikka, S. L., Tryggvason, K., Ropers, H. H., Jansweijer, M. C. 1992. Different mutations in the COL4A5 collagen gene in two patients with different features of Alport syndrome. *Kidney Int.,* 42, 83-88.

Smith, C. A. 1968. Ultrastructure of the organ of Corti. *Adv. Sci.,* 245, 419-433.

Smith, P. H., Joris, P. X., Carney, L. H., Yin, T. C. T. 1991. Projections of physiologically characterized globular bushy cell axons from the cochlear nucleus of the cat. *J. Comp. Neurol.,* 304, 387-407.

Smith, P. H., Joris, P. X., Yin, T. C. T. 1993a. Projections of physiologically characterized spherical bushy cell axons from the cochlear nucleus of the cat: evidence for delay lines to the medial superior olive. *J. Comp. Neurol.*, 331, 245-260.

Smith, P. H., Joris, P. X., Banks, M. I., Yin, T. C. T. 1993b. Responses of cochlear nucleus cells and projections of their axons. In Merchan, M. A., Juiz, J. M., Godfrey, D. A., Mugnaini, E. (Eds.), *The Mammalian Cochlear Nuclei: Organization and Function.* Plenum, New York, 349-360.

Smith, P. H., Rhode, W. S. 1989. Structural and functional properties distinguish two types of multipolar cells in the ventral cochlear nucleus. *J. Comp. Neurol.*, 282, 595-616.

Smith, R. J., Berlin, C. I., Hejtmancik, J. F., Keats, B. J., Kimberling, W. J., Lewis, R. A., Moller, C. G., Pelias, M. Z., Tranebjaerg, L. 1994. Clinical diagnosis of the Usher syndromes. Usher Syndrome Consortium. *Am. J. Med. Genet.*, 50, 32-38.

Smith, R. J., Lee, E. C., Kimberling, W. J., Daiger, S. P., Pelias, M. Z., Keats, B. J., Jay, M., Bird, A., Reardon, W., Guest, M. 1992. Localization of two genes for Usher syndrome type I to chromosome 11. *Genomics*, 14, 995-1002.

Snell, K. B, Frisina, D. R. 2000. Relationships among age-related differences in gap detection and word recognition. *J. Acoust. Soc. Am.*, 107, 1615-1626.

Snell, K. B. 1997. Age-related changes in temporal gap detection. *J. Acoust. Soc. Am.*, 101, 2214-2220.

Snyder, D. L., Salvi, R. J. 1994. A novel chinchilla restraint. *Lab Animal*, 23, 42-44.

Snyder, E. Y., Kim, S. U. 1980. Insulin: is it a nerve survival factor? *Brain Res.*, 196, 565-571.

Sobkowicz, H. M. 1992. The development of innervation in the organ of Corti. In Romand, R. (Ed.), *Development of Auditory and Vestibular Systems II.* Elsevier, Amsterdam, 59-100.

Sobkowicz, H. M., Bereman, B., Rose, J. E. 1975. Organotypic development of the organ of Corti in culture. *J. Neurocytol.*, 4, 543-572.

Sobkowicz, H. M., Emmerling, M. R. 1989. Development of acetylcholinesterase-positive neuronal pathways in the cochlea of the mouse. *J. Neurocytol.*, 18, 209-224.

Sobkowicz, H. M., Loftus, J. M., Slapnick, S. M. 1993. Tissue culture of the organ of Corti. *Acta Otolaryngol.*, S502, 3-36.

Sobkowicz, H. M., Rose, J. E., Scott, GL., Levenick, C. V. 1986. Distribution of synaptic ribbons in the developing orgain of Corti. *J. Neurocytol.*, 15, 693-714.

Sobkowicz, H. M., Slapnick, S. M. 1994. The efferents interconnecting auditory inner hair cells. *Hear. Res.*, 75, 81-92.

Sobkowicz, H. M., Slapnick, S. M., Nitecka, L. M., August, B. K. 1997. Compound synapses within the GABAergic innervation of the auditory inner hair cells in the adolescent mouse. *J. Comp. Neurol.*, 377, 423-442.

Sobkowicz, H. M., Slapnick, S. M., Nitecka, L. M., August, B. K. 1998. Tunnel crossing fibers and their synaptic connections within the inner hair cell region in the organ of Corti in the maturing mouse. *Anat. Embryol.*, 198, 353-370.

Sokolich, W. G. 1977. Improved acoustic system for auditory research. *J. Acoust. Soc. Am.*, Suppl. 62, S12.

Soliman, A. M. 1990. Type II collagen-induced inner ear disease: critical evaluation of the guinea pig model. *Am. J. Otol.*, 11, 27-32.

Sone, M., Nariuchi, H., Saito, K., Yanagita, N. 1995. A substrain of NZB mouse as a animal model of autoimmune inner ear disease. *Hear. Res.*, 83, 26-36.

Sone, M., Schachern, P. A., Paparella, M. M., Morizono, N. 1999. Study of systemic lupus erythematosus in temporal bones. *Ann. Otol. Rhinol. Laryngol.*, 108, 338-344.

Soppet, D., Escandon, E., Maragos, J. 1991. The neurotrophic factors, brain derived neurotrophic factor and neurotrophin-3 are ligands for the trkB tyrosine kinase receptor. *Cell*, 65, 895-903.

Sørensen, M. S., Nielsen, L. P., Bretlau, P., Jorgensen, M. B. 1988. The role of type II collagen autoimmunity in otosclerosis revisited. *Acta Otolaryngol.*, 105, 242-247.

Spear, G. S. 1974. Pathology of the kidney in Alport's syndrome. *Pathol. Annu.*, 9, 93-138.

Spear, G. S., Slusser, R. J. 1972. Alport's syndrome. Emphasizing electron microscopic studies of the glomerulus. *Am. J. Pathol.*, 69, 213-224.

Spector, G. J. 1975. The ultrastructural cytochemistry of lactic dehydrogenase, succinic dehydrogenase, dihydro-nicotinamide adenine dinucleotide diaphorase and cytochrome oxidase activities in hair cell mitochondria of the guinea pig cochlea. *J. Histochem. Cytochem.*, 23, 216-234.

Speidel, C. C. 1948. Correlated studies of sense organs and nerves of the lateral line in living frog tadpoles. II. The trophic influence of specific nerve supply as revealed by prolonged observations of denervated and reinnervated organs. *Am. J. Anat.,* 82, 277-320.

Sperling, N. M., Tehrani, K., Liebling, A., Ginzler, E. 1998. Aural symptoms and hearing loss in patients with lupus. *Otolaryngol. Head Neck Surg.,* 118, 762-765.

Spirou, G. A., Brownell, W. E., Zidanic, M. 1990. Recordings from cat trapezoid body and HRP labeling of globular bushy cell axons. *J. Neurophysiol.,* 56, 261-286.

Spirou, G. A., Young, E. D. 1991. Organization of dorsal cochlear nucleus type IV unit response maps and their relationship to activation by bandlimited noise. *J. Neurophysiol.,* 66, 1750-1768.

Spoendlin, H. 1988. Biology of the vestibulocochlear nerve. In Albert, P. W., Ruben, R. J. (Eds.), *Otol. Med. & Surg.* Vol. 1. Churchill Livingston, New York, 117-150.

Spoendlin, H. H., Balogh, K. 1963. Histochemical localization of dehydrogenases in the cochlea of living animals. *Laryngoscope,* 73, 1061-1083.

Spoerri, P. E. 1987. GABA-mediated developmental alterations in a neuronal cell line in culture of cerebral and retinal neurons. In Redburn, D. A., Schousboe, A. (Eds.), *Neurotrophic Activity of GABA During Development.* Liss, New York, 189-220.

Spongr, V. P., Boettcher, F. A., Saunders, S. S., Salvi, R. J. 1992. Effects of noise and salicylate on hair cell loss in the chinchilla cochlea. *Arch. Otolaryngol. Head Neck Surg.,* 118, 157-164.

Spongr, V. P., Flood, D. G., Frisina, R. D, Salvi, R. J. 1997a. Quantitative measures of hair cell loss in CBA and C57BL/6 mice throughout their life spans. *J. Acoust. Soc. Am.,* 101, 3546-3553.

Spongr, V. P., Walton, J. P., Frisina, R. D., Kazee, A. M., Flood, D. G., Salvi, R. J. 1997b. Hair cell loss and synaptic loss in inferior colliculus of C57Bl/6 mice: relationship to abnormal temporal processing. In Syka, J. (Ed.), *Acoustical Signal Processing in the Central Auditory System,* Plenum Press, New York, 350-380.

Sporn, M. B., Roberts, A. B., Wakefield, L. M., de Crombrugghe, B. 1987. Some recent advances in the chemistry and biology of transforming growth factor-beta. *J. Cell Biol.,* 105, 1039-1045.

Sprenkle, P. M., Walsh, E. J., McGee, J., Bertoni, J. M. 1997. Auditory brainstem response (ABR) abnormalities in hyt/hyt mice indicate early onset of hypothyroid-induced hearing impairment. *Assoc. Res. Otolaryngol. Abstr.,* 20, 135.

Sprenkle, P., McGee, J., Bertoni, J., Walsh, E. J., 2001a. Consequences of hypothyroidism on auditory system function in Tshr^{hyt} mutant (hyt) mice. *J. Assoc. Res. Otolaryngol.,* (submitted).

Sprenkle, P., McGee, J., Bertoni, J., Walsh, E. J., 2001b. Development of auditory brainste responses (ABRs) in Tshr^{hyt} mutant mice derived from euthyroid and hypothyroid dams. *J. Assoc. Res. Otolaryngol.,* (submitted).

Sprenkle, P., McGee, J., Bertoni, J., Walsh, E. J., 2001c. Prevention of auditory dysfunction in hypothyroid Tshr^{hyt} mutant mice by thyroxin treatment during development. *J. Assoc. Res. Otolaryngol.,* (submitted).

Squinto, S. P., Stitt, T. N., Aldrich, T. H. 1991. Trk B encodes a functional receptor for brain derived neurotrophic factor and neurotrophin-3 but not nerve growth factor. *Cell,* 65, 886-893.

Srivastava, D., Thomas, T., Lin, Q., Kirby, M. L., Brown, D., Olson, E. N. 1997. Regulation of cardiac mesodermal and neural crest development by the bHLH transcription factor, dHAND. *Nature Genet.,* 16, 154-160.

St. John, R. D. 1973. Genetic analysis of tail rattling in the mouse. *Nature,* 241, 549-551.

St. John, R. D. 1978. A reexamination of the genetic control of sonic vocalization in mice. *Behav. Genet.,* 8, 169-175.

Staecker, H., Cammer, M., Rubenstein, R., Van De Water, T. R. 1994. A procedure for RT-PCR amplification of mRNA's on histological specimens. *Biotechniques,* 16, 76-80.

Staecker, H., Van De Water, T. R., Lefebvre, P., Liu, W., Moghadassi, M., Galinovic-Schwartz, V., Malgrange, B., Monnen, G. 1996. NGF, BDNF and NT-3 play unique roles in the *in vitro* development and patterning of innervation of the mammalian inner ear. *Devel. Brain Res.,* 92, 49-60.

Starr, A., Picton, T. W., Sininger, Y. S., Hood, L. J., Berlin, C. I. 1996. Auditory neuropathy. *Brain,* 119, 741-753.

Starr, A., Achor, J. 1975. Auditory brainstem responses in neurological disease. *Arch. Neurol.,* 32, 761-786.

Stearns, G. S., Keithley, E. M., Harris, J. P. 1993. Development of high endothelial venule-like characteristics in the spiral modiolar vein induced by viral labyrinthitis. *Laryngoscope,* 103, 890-898.

Stebbins, W. C. 1970. Studies of hearing and hearing loss in the monkey. In Stebbins, W. C. (Ed.), *Animal Psychophysics,* Appleton-Century-Crofts, New York, 41-66.

Steel, K. P. 1991. Similarities between mice and humans with hereditary deafness. *Ann. N.Y. Acad. Sci.,* 630, 68-79.

Steel, K. P. 1995. Inherited hearing defects in mice. *Annu. Rev. Genet.,* 29, 675-701.

Steel, K. P. 1999. Perspectives: biomedicine. The benefits of recycling [Comment]. *Science,* 285, 1363-1364.

Steel, K. P., Bock, G. R. 1983. Hereditary inner-ear abnormalities in animals. Relationships with human abnormalities. *Arch. Otolaryngol.,* 109, 22-29.

Steel, K. P., Brown, S. D. 1994. Genes and deafness. *Trends Genet.,* 10, 428-435.

Steel, K. P., Brown, S. D. 1996. Genetics of deafness. *Curr. Opin. Neurobiol.,* 6, 520-525.

Steel, K. P., Bussoli, T. J. 1999. Deafness genes: expressions of surprise. *Trends Genet.,* 15, 207-211.

Steel, K. P., Erven, A., Kiernan, A. E. 2001. Mice as models for human hereditary deafness. In Keats, B., Popper A., Fay, R. (Eds.), *Genetics and Auditory Disorders.* Springer, New York, 100-130.

Steel, K. P., Harvey, D. 1992. Development of auditory function in mutant mice. In Romand, R. (Ed.), *Development of Auditory and Vestibular Systems 2.* Elsevier Science, Amsterdam, 221-242.

Stein, S. A., Oates, E. L., Hall, C. R., Grumbles, R. M., Fernandez, L. M., Taylor, N. A., Puett, D., Jin, S. 1994. Identification of a point mutation in the thyrotropin receptor of the hyt/hyt hypothyroid mouse. *Molec. Endocrinol.,* 8, 129-138.

Stenberg, A. E., Wang, H., Sahlin, L., Hultcrantz, M. 1999. Mapping of estrogen receptors α and β in the inner ear of the mouse. *Hear. Res.,* 136, 29-34.

Stenfors, L. E., Salen, B., Winblad, B. 1979. The role of pars flaccida in the mechanics of the middle ear. *Acta Otolaryngol.,* 88, 395-416.

Stenkamp, D. L., Barthel, L. K., Raymond, P. A. 1997. Spatiotemporal coordination of rod and cone photo-receptor differentiation in goldfish retina. *J. Comp. Neurol.,* 382, 272-284.

Stewart, R., Erskine, L., McCaig, C. D. 1995. Calcium channel subtypes and intracellular calcium stores modulate electric field-stimulated and -oriented nerve growth. *Devel. Biol.,* 171, 340-351.

Stiebler, I., Ehret, G. 1985. Inferior colliculus of the house mouse. I. A quantitative study of tonotopic organization, frequency representation, and tone-threshold distribution. *J. Comp. Neurol.,* 238, 65-76.

Stiebler, I. 1987. A distinct ultrasound-processing area in the auditory cortex of the mouse. *Naturwissenschaften,* 74, 96-97.

Stiebler, I., Neulist, R., Fishtel, I., Ehret, G. 1997. The auditory cortex of the house mouse: left-right differences, tonotopic organization and quantitative analysis of frequency representation. *J. Comp. Physiol.,* A 181, 559-571.

Stitt, C. L., Hoffman, H. S., Marsh, R. R., Schwartz, G. M. 1976. Modification of the pigeon's visual startle reaction by the sensory environment. *J. Comp. Physiol. Psychol.,* 90, 601-619.

Stockard, J., Stockard, J., Sharbrough, F. 1978. Nonpathologic factors influencing brainstem auditory evoked potentials. *Am. J. EEG Tech.,* 18, 177-209.

Stover, L. J., Neely, S. T., Gorga, M. P. 1999. Cochlear generation of intermodulation revealed by DPOAE frequency functions in normal and impaired ears. *J. Acoust. Soc. Am.,* 106, 2669-2678.

Stover, L. J., Neely, S. T., Gorga, M. P. 1996. Latency and multiple sources of distortion product otoacoustic emissions. *J. Acoust. Soc. Am.,* 99, 1016-1024.

Stover, T., Gong, T. W. L, Cho, Y., Altschuler, R. A., Lomax, M. I. 2000. Expression of the GDNF family members and their receptors in the mature rat cochlea. *Molec. Brain Res.,* 76, 25-35.

Stover, T., Yagi, M., Raphael, Y. 1999. Cochlear gene transfer: round window versus cochleostomy inoculation. *Hear. Res.,* 136, 124-130.

Street, V. A., McKee-Johnson, J. W., Fonseca, R. C., Tempel, B. L., Noben-Trauth, K. 1998. Mutations in a plasma membrane Ca2+-ATPase gene cause deafness in deafwaddler mice. *Nature Genet.,* 19, 390-394.

Strominger, N., Strominger, A. 1971. Ascending brain stem projections of the anteroventral cochlear nucleus in the rhesus monkey. *J. Comp. Neurol.,* 143, 217-241.

Studer, M., Lumsden, A., Ariza-McNaughton, L., Bradley, A., Krumlauf, R. 1996. Altered segmental identity and abnormal migration of motor neurons in mice lacking Hoxb-1. *Nature,* 384, 630-634.

Subramaniam, M., Henderson, D., Henselman, L. 1996. Toughening of the mammalian auditory system: spectral, temporal, and intensity effects. In Salvi, R. J., Henderson, D. H., Colletti, V., Fiorino, F. (Eds.), *Auditory Plasticity and Regeneration.* Thieme Medical Publishers, New York, 128-142.

Sudhof, T. 1995. The synaptic vesicle cycle: a cascade of protein-protein interactions. *Nature,* 375, 645-653.

Suenaga, S., Kodama, S., Ueyama, S., Suzuki, M., Mogi, G. 1999. Single cell analysis of the lymphocyte subsets in middle ear mucosa. Presented at *Seventh International Symposium on Recent Advances in Otitis Media.* Fort Lauderdale, FL, 90.

Sugimoto, M., Oohashi, T., Ninomiya, Y. 1994. The genes COL4A5 and COL4A6, coding for basement membrane collagen chains alpha 5(IV) and alpha 6(IV), are located head-to-head in close proximity on human chromosome Xq22 and COL4A6 is transcribed from two alternative promoters. *Proc. Natl. Acad. Sci., USA,* 91, 11679-11683.

Sumegi, J., Bhattacharya, G., Cosgrove, D., Kimberling, W. 2000. The protein product of the Usher syndrome Type IIa gene localizes to the interphotoreceptor cell matrix. *Assoc. Res. Otolaryngol. Abstr.*, 23, 219.

Summers, C. G., Purple, R. L., Krivit, W., Pineda, R., Copland, G. T., Ramsay, N. K., Kersey, J. H., Whitley, C. B. 1989. Ocular changes in the mucopolysaccharidoses after bone marrow transplantation--preliminary report. *Ophthalmology*, 96, 977-984.

Sun, J. C., van Alphen, A. M., Bohne, B. A., De Zeeuw, C. I. 1999. Shaker-1 mice show an optokinetic reflex, but no vestibulo-ocular reflex. *Assoc. Res. Otolaryngol. Abstr.*, 22, 103.

Sun, X.-M. 1998. Distortion Product Otoacoustic Emissions in Mouse Models of Early-onset and Late-onset Presbycusis. Ph.D. dissertation, University of Connecticut.

Sun, X.-M., Kim, D. O., Jung, M. D., Randolph, K. J. 1996. Distortion product otoacoustic emission test of senorineural hearing loss in humans: comparison of unequal- and equal-level stimuli. *Ann. Otol. Rhinol. Laryngol.*, 105, 982-990.

Sun, X.-M., Kim, D. O. 1999. Adaptation of 2f1-f2 distortion product otoacoustic emission in young-adult and old CBA and C57 mice. *J. Acoustic. Soc. Am.*, 105, 3399-3409.

Sun, X.-M., Kim, D. O., Parham, K. 1998. Effects of stimulus parameters on distortion product otoacoustic emissions in the CBA mouse model of age-related hearing. *Assoc. Res. Otolaryngol. Abst.*, 21, 79.

Sun, X.-M., Parham, K., Kim, D. O. 1997. Effects of stimulus parameters on distortion product otoacoustic emissions in the C57BL/6J mouse with age-related hearing loss. *Assoc. Res. Otolaryngol. Abst.*, 20, 101.

Sundin, V., Turner, J. G., Willott, J. F. 2000. Ameliorative effects of an augmented acoustic environment (AAE) on progressive hearing loss are limited by delayed implementation. *Assoc. Res. Otolaryngol. Abstr.*, 23, 157.

Sutherland, D. P. 1991. A role of the dorsal cochlear nucleus in the localization of elevated sound sources. *Assoc. Res. Otolaryngol. Abstr.*, 14, 33.

Sutjita, M., Peter, J. B., Baloh, R. W., Oas, J. G., Laurent, C., Nordang, L. 1992. Type II collagen antibodies in patients with sensorineural heairng loss. *Lancet*, 339, 559-560.

Sutton, L. A., Lonsbury-Martin, B. L., Martin, G. K., Whitehead, M. L. 1994. Sensitivity of distortion-product otoacoustic emissions in humans to tonal over-exposure: time course of recovery and effects of lowering L_2. *Hear. Res.*, 75, 161-174.

Suzuki, M., Cheng, K.-C., Krug, M. S., Yoo, T.-J. 1998. Successful prevention of retrocochlear hearing loss in murine experimental allergic encephalomyelitis with T cell receptor Vβ8-specific antibody. *Ann. Otol. Rhinol. Laryngol.*, 107, 917-927.

Suzuki, M., Harris, J. P. 1995. Expression of intercellular adhesion molecule-1 during inner ear inflammation. *Ann. Otol. Rhinol. Laryngol.*, 104, 69-75.

Suzuki, T., Iwagaki, T., Hibi, T., Nakashima, T. 2000. Effects of the anterior inferior cerebellar artery occlusion on cochlear blood flow, A comparison between the laser Doppler and microsphere methods. *Assoc. Res. Otolaryngol. Abstr.*, #698.

Suzuki, T., Ren, T., Nuttall, A. L., Miller, J. M. 1998. Age-related changes in cochlear blood flow response to occlusion of anterior inferior cerebellar artery in mice. *Ann. Otol. Rhinol. Laryngol.*, 107, 648-653.

Swedberg, M. D. 1994. The mouse grid-shock analgesia test: pharmacological characterization of latency to vocalization threshold as an index of antinociception. *J. Pharmacol. Exp. Ther.*, 269, 1021-1028.

Swerdlow, N. R., Benbow, C. H., Zisook, S., Geyer, M. A., Braff, D. L. 1993. A preliminary assessment of sensorimotor gating in patients with obsessive compulsive disorder. *Biological Psychiatry*, 33(4), 298-301.

Swerdlow, N. R., Braff, D. L., Taaid, N., Geyer, M. A. 1994. Assessing the validity of an animal model of deficient sensorimotor gating in schizophrenic patients. *Arch. Genet. Psychol.*, 51, 139-154.

Swerdlow, N. R., Braff, D. L., Geyer, M. A. 1999. Cross-species studies of sensorimotor gating of the startle reflex. *Ann. N.Y. Acad. Sci.*, 877, 202-216.

Swerdlow, N. R., Geyer, M. A. 1993. Prepulse inhibition of acoustic startle in rats after lesions of the pedunculopontine tegmental nucleus. *Behav. Neurosci.*, 107, 104-117.

Swerdlow, N. R., Hartman, P. L., Auerbach, P. P. 1997. Changes in sensorimotor inhibition across the menstrual cycle: implications for neuropsychiatric disorders. *Biological Psychiatry*, 41(4), 452-460.

Swiatek, P. J., Lindsell, C. E., del Amo, F. F., Weinmaster, G., Gridley, T. 1994. Notch1 is essential for postimplantation development in mice. *Genes Devel.*, 8, 707-719.

Szpir, M. R., Sento, S., Ryugo, D. K. 1990. The central progections of the cochlear nerve fibers in the alligator lizard. *J. Comp. Neurol.*, 295, 530-547.

Szpiro-Tapia, S., Bobrie, G., Guilloud-Bataille, M., Heuertz, S., Julier, C., Frezal, J., Grunfeld, J. P., Hors-Cayla, M. C. 1988. Linkage studies in X-linked Alport's syndrome. *Hum. Genet.*, 81, 85-87.

Taber Pierce, E. 1967. Histogenesis of the dorsal and ventral cochlear nuclei in the mouse. An autoradiographic study. *J. Comp. Neurol.*, 131, 27-54.

Tachibana, M., Kuriyama, K. 1974. Gamma-aminobutyric acid in the lower auditory pathway of the guinea pig. *Brain Res.*, 69, 370-374.

Tachibana, M., Perez-Jurado, L. A., Nakayama, A., Hodgkinson, C. A., Li, X., Schneider, M., Miki, T., Fex, J., Francke, U., Arnheiter, H. 1994. Cloning of MITF, the human homolog of the mouse microphthalmia gene and assignment to chromosome 3p14.1-p12.3. *Hum. Molec. Genet.*, 3, 553-557.

Tago, C., Yanagita, N. 1992. Cochlear and renal pathology in the autoimmune strain mouse. *Ann. Otol. Rhinol. Laryngol.*, 101, 87-91.

Takahashi, M., Harris, J. P. 1988a. Anatomic distribution and localization of immunocompetent cells in normal mouse endolymphatic sac. *Acta Otolaryngol.*, 106, 409-416.

Takahashi, M., Harris, J. P. 1988b. Analysis of immunocompetent cells following inner ear immunostimulation. *Laryngoscope*, 98, 1133-1138.

Takahashi, M., Harris, J. P. 1993. Secretory component and IgA in the endolymphatic sac. *Acta Otolaryngol.*, 113, 615-619.

Takahashi, M., Hokunan, K. 1992. Localization of type IV collagen and laminin in the guinea pig inner ear. *Ann. Otol. Rhinol. Laryngol.*, (Suppl.) 157, 58-62.

Takahashi, M., Kanai, N. 1992. T cell subsets in round window membrane after middle ear immunostimulation. *Acta Otolaryngol.*, (Suppl.) 493, 147-153.

Takahashi, M., Kanai, N., Watanabe, A., Oshima, O., Ryan, A. F. 1992. Lymphocyte subsets in immune-mediated otitis media with effusion. *Eur. Arch. Oto-Rhino-Laryngol.*, 249, 24-27.

Takahashi, M., Peppard, J., Harris J. P. 1989. Immunohistochemical study of murine middle ear and eustachian tube. *Acta Otolaryngol.*, 107, 97-103.

Takahashi, T., Moiseff, A., Konishi, M. 1984. Time and intensity cues are processed independently in the auditory system of the owl. *J. Neurosci.*, 4, 1781-1786.

Takeda, T., Sudo, N., Kitano, H., Yoo, T. J. 1996. Type II collagen-induced autoimmune ear disease in mice: a preliminary report on an epitope of the type II collagen molecule that induced inner ear lesions. *Am. J. Otol.*, 17, 69-75.

Takemura, T., Sakagami, M., Takebayashi, K., Umemoto, M., Nakase, T., Takaoka, K., Kubo, T., Kitamura, Y., Nomura, S. 1996. Localization of bone morphogenetic protein-4 messenger RNA in developing mouse cochlea. *Hear. Res.*, 95, 26-32.

Talbot, C. J., Nicod, A., Cherny, S. S., Fulker, D. W., Collins, A. C., Flint, J. 1999. High resolution mapping of quantitative trait loci in outbred mice. *Nature Genet.*, 21, 305-308.

Talmadge, C. L., Tubis, A., Long, G. R., Piskorski, P. 1998. Modeling otoacoustic emission and hearing threshold fine structure. *J. Acoust. Soc. Am.*, 104, 1517-1543.

Tamagawa, Y., Kitamura, K., Ishida, T., Ishikawa, K., Tanaka, H., Tsuji, S., Nishizawa, M. 1996. A gene for a dominant form of non-syndromic sensorineural deafness (DFNA11) maps within the region containing the DFNB2 recessive deafness gene. *Hum. Molec. Genet.*, 5, 849-852.

Tassabehji, M., Read, A. P., Newton, V. E., Patton, M., Gruss, P., Harris, R., Strachan, T. 1993. Mutations in the PAX3 gene causing Waardenburg syndrome type 1 and type 2. *Nature Genet.*, 3, 26-30.

Taylor, B. A. 1978. Recombinant inbred strains: use in gene mapping. In Morse, H. C. (Ed.), *Origins of Inbred Mice*. Academic Press, New York, 423-438.

Taylor, B. A. 1989. Recombinant inbred strains. In Lyon, M. F. and Searle, A. G., (Eds.), *Genetic Variants and Strains of the Laboratory Mouse*, 2nd ed. Oxford University Press, Oxford, 773-779.

Taylor, B. A., Navin, A., Phillips, S. J. 1994. PCR-amplification of simple sequence repeat variants from pooled DNA samples for rapidly mapping new mutations of the mouse. *Genomics*, 21, 626-632.

Taylor, B. A., Wnek, C., Kotlus, B. S., Roemer, N., MacTaggart, T., Phillips, S. J. 1999. Genotyping new BXD recombinant inbred mouse strains and comparison of BXD and consensus maps. *Mamm. Genome*, 10, 335-348.

Taylor, D. A., Carroll, J. E., Smith, M. E., Johnson, M. O., Johnston, G. P., Brooke, M. H. 1982. Facioscapulohumeral dystrophy associated with Coats syndrome. *Ann. Neurol.*, 12, 395-398.

Tello, J. F. 1931. Le réticule des cellules ciliées du labyrinthe chez la souris et son indépendance des terminaisons nerveuses de la VIIIe paire. *Trav. Lab. Rech. Biol. Univ. Madrid*, 27, 151-186.

ten Berge, D., Brouwer, A., Korving, J., Martin, J. F., Meijlink, F. 1998. Prx1 and Prx2 in skeletogenesis: roles in the craniofaciel region, inner ear and limbs. *Devel.* 125, 3831-3842.

Teng, X., Ahn, K., Bove, M., Frenz, D., Crenshaw, E. B. 2000. Malformations of the lateral semicircular canal occur in heterozygous Bmp4 knockout mice. *Assoc. Res. Otolaryngol. Abstr.,*

Thalmann, R. 1976. Quantitative biochemical techniques for studying normal and noise-damaged ears. In Henderson, D., Hamernik, R. P., Dosanjh, D. S., Mills, J. H. (Eds.), *Effects of Noise on Hearing.* Raven Press, New York, 129-155.

Theofilopoulos, A. N., Dixon, F. J. 1985. Murine models of systemic lupus erythematosus. *Adv. Immunol.,* 37, 269-390.

Theofilopoulos, A. N., Kofler, R., Singer, P. A., Dixon, F. J. 1989. Molecular genetics of murine lupus models. *Adv. Immunol.,* 46, 61-109.

Thiessen, D. D., Kittrell, E. M. W. 1979. Mechanical features of ultrasound emission in the Mongolian gerbil, *Meriones unguiculatus. Am. Zool.,* 19, 509-512.

Thiessen, D. D., Kittrell, E. M. W., Graham, J. M. 1980. Biomechanics of ultrasound emissions in the Mongolian gerbil, *Meriones unguiculatus. Behav. Neural Biol.,* 29, 415-429.

Thomadakis, G., Ramoshebi, L. N., Crooks, J., Rueger, D. C., Ripamonti, U. 1999. Immunolocalization of bone morphogenetic Protein-2 and -3 and osteogenic Protein-1 during murine tooth root morphogenesis and in other craniofacial structures. *Eur J. Oral Sci.,* 107, 368-377.

Thomas, D. A., Howard, S. B., Barfield, R. J. 1982. Male-produced ultrasonic vocalizations and mating patterns in female rats. *J. Comp. Physiol. Psychol.,* 96, 807-815.

Thomas, H., Tillein, J., Heil, P., Scheich, H. 1993. Functional organization of auditory cortex in the Mongolian gerbil (*Meriones unguiculatus*). I. Electrophysiological mapping of frequency representation and distinction of fields. *Eur. J. Neurosci.,* 5, 882-897.

Thomas, K. A., Rios-Candelore, M., Fitzpatrick, S. 1984. Purification and characterization of acidic fibroblast growth factor from bovine brain. *Proc. Natl. Acad. Sci., USA,* 81, 357-361.

Thompson, G., Heffner, H., Masterton, B. 1974. An automated localization chamber. *Behav. Res. Meth. Instr.,* 6, 550-552.

Thorne, P. R., Nuttall, A. L. 1987. Laser Doppler measurements of cochlear blood flow during loud sound exposure in the guinea pig. *Hear. Res.,* 27, 1-10.

Thorne, P. S., Hawk, C., Kaliszewski, S. D., Guiney, P. D. 1991. The noninvasive mouse ear swelling assay. I. Refinements for detecting weak contact sensitizers. *Fund. Appl. Tox.,* 17, 790-806.

Tilney, L. G., Tilney, M. S., DeRosier, D. J. 1992. Actin filaments, stereocilia, and hair cells: how cells count and measure. *Annu. Rev. Cell Biol.,* 8, 257-274.

Timpl, R. 1989. Structure and biological activity of basement membrane proteins. *Eur. J. Biochem.,* 180, 487-502.

Timpl, R. 1996. Supramolecular assembly of basement membranes. *Bioessays,* 18, 123-132.

Timpl, R., Wiedemann, H., van, D., V, Furthmayr, H., Kuhn, K. 1981. A network model for the organization of type IV collagen molecules in basement membranes. *Eur. J. Biochem.,* 120, 203-211.

Tohyama, Y., Senba, E., Yamashita, T., Kitajiri, M., Kuriyama, H., Kumazawa, T., Ohata, K., Tohyama, M. 1990. Coexistence of calcitonin gene-related peptide and enkephalin in single neurons of the lateral superior olivary nucleus of the guinea pig that project to the cochlea as lateral olivocochlear system. *Brain Res.,* 515, 312-314.

Tolbert, L. P., Morest, D. K. 1982. The neuronal architecture of the anteroventral cochlear nucleus of the cat in the region of the cochlear nerve root: electron microscopy. *Neuroscience,* 7, 3053-3067.

Tomiyama, S., Harris, J. P. 1987. The role of the endolymphatic sac in inner ear immunity. *Acta Otolaryngol.,* 103, 182-188.

Tomiyama, S., Jinnouchi, K., Ikezono, T., Pawankar, R., Yagi, T. 1999. Experimental autoimmune labyrinthitis induced by cell-mediated immune reaction. *Acta Otolaryngol.,* 119, 665-670.

Tomoda, K., Yamawaki, T., Suzuka, Y., Yamashita, T., Kumazawa, T. 1992. Alterations of charge barrier in the inner ear following immune reactions. *Ann. Otol. Rhinol. Laryngol.,* Suppl. 157, 63-66.

Toren, A., Amariglio, N., Rozenfeld-Granot, G., Simon, A. J., Brok-Simoni, F., Pras, E., Rechavi, G. 1999. Genetic linkage of autosomal-dominant Alport syndrome with leukocyte inclusions and macrothrombocytopenia (Fechtner syndrome) to chromosome 22q11-13. *Am. J. Hum. Genet.,* 65, 1711-1717.

Torihara, K., Morimitsu, T., Suganuma, T. 1995. Anionic sites on Reissner's membrane, stria vascularis, and spiral prominence. *J. Histochem. Cytochem.,* 43, 299-305.

Torra, R., Badenas, C., Cofan, F., Callis, L., Perez-Oller, L., Darnell, A. 1999. Autosomal recessive Alport syndrome: linkage analysis and clinical features in two families. *Nephrol. Dial. Transplant.*, 14, 627-630.

Torres, M., Gaomez-Pardo, E., Gruss, P. 1996. Pax2 contributes to inner ear patterning and optic nerve trajectory. *Devel.*, 122, 3381-3391.

Traynor, S. J., Cohen, J. I., Morton, J. I., Trune, D. R. 1992. Immunohistochemical analysis of otic capsule lesions in the Palmerston North autoimmune mouse. *Otolaryngol. Head Neck Surg.*, 106, 196-201.

Trune, D. R., Morgan, C. R. 1988. Influence of developmental auditory deprivation on neuronal ultrastructure in the mouse anteroventral cochlear nucleus. *Devel. Brain Res.*, 42, 304-308.

Trune, D. R. 1982. Influence of neonatal cochlear removal on the development of mouse cochlear nucleus. I. Number, size, and density of its neurons. *J. Comp. Neurol.*, 209, 409-424.

Trune, D. R. 1997. Cochlear immunoglobulin in the C3H/*lpr* mouse model for autoimmune hearing loss. *Otolaryngol. Head Neck Surg.*, 117, 504-508.

Trune, D. R., Craven, J. P., Morton, J. I., Mitchell. C. 1989. Autoimmune disease and cochlear pathology in the C3H/*lpr* strain mouse. *Hear. Res.*, 38, 57-66.

Trune, D. R., DeGagne, J. M., Morton, J. I. 1994. Ultrastructure of otic capsule sclerosis in Palmerston North autoimmune mice. *Am. J. Otolaryngol.*, 15, 114-123.

Trune, D. R., Hertler, C. K., Haun, D. K. Z., Sauter, R. W. 1990. Histochemistry of otic capsule sclerotic lesions in Palmerston North autoimmune strain mice. *Hear. Res.*, 48, 241-246.

Trune, D. R., Kempton, J. B. 2001. Aldosterone and prednisolone control of cochlear function in MRL/MpJ-*Fas*[lpr] autoimmune mice. *Hear. Res.*, (in review).

Trune, D. R., Kempton, J. B., Hefeneider, S. H., Bennett, R. M. 1997. Inner ear DNA receptors in MRL/*lpr* autoimmune mice: potential 30 and 70 kilodalton link between autoimmune disease and hearing loss. *Hear. Res.*, 105, 57-64.

Trune, D. R., Kempton, J. B., Kessi, M. 2000. Aldosterone (mineralocorticoid) equivalent to prednisolone (glucocorticoid) in reversing hearing loss in autoimmune mice. *Laryngoscope*, 110, 1902-1906.

Trune, D. R., Kempton, J. B., Mitchell, C. 1996. Auditory function in the C3H/HeJ and C3H/HeSnJ mouse strains. *Hear. Res.*, 96, 41-45.

Trune, D. R., Kempton, J. B., Mitchell, C. M., Hefeneider, S. H. 1998a. Failure of elevated heat shock protein 70 antibodies to alter cochlear function in mice. *Hear. Res.*, 116, 65-70.

Trune, D. R., Kempton, J. B., Mitchell, C. R. 1996. Decreased auditory function in the C3H/*lpr* autoimmune disease mouse. *Hear. Res.*, 95, 57-62.

Trune, D. R., Kempton, J. B., Vedder, C. T., Bennett, R. M., Hefeneider, S. H. 1998b. Development of autoimmune sensorineural hearing loss in normal mice by inoculation with the DNA binding protein. *Assoc. Res. Otolaryngol. Abstr.*, 21, 194.

Trune, D. R., Morton, J. I., Craven, J. P., Traynor, S. J., Mitchell, C. R. 1991. Inner ear pathology in the Palmerston North autoimmune strain mouse. *Am. J. Otolaryngol.*, 12, 259-266.

Trune, D. R., Wobig, R. J., Kempton, J. B., Hefeneider, S. H. 1999a. Steroid therapy improves cochlear function in the C3H. MRL-*Fas*[lpr] autoimmune mouse. *Hear. Res.*, 137, 160-166.

Trune, D. R., Wobig, R. J., Kempton, J. B., Hefeneider, S. H. 1999b. Steroid treatment in young MRL. MpJ-*Fas*[lpr] autoimmune mice prevents cochlear dysfunction. *Hear. Res.*, 137, 167-173.

Trussell, L. O. 1997. Cellular mechanisms for preservation of timing in central auditory pathways. *Curr. Opin. Neurobiol.*, 7, 487-492.

Trussell, L. O. 1999. Synaptic mechanisms for coding timing in auditory neurons. *Annu. Rev. Physiol.*, 61, 477-496.

Tsukada, N., Koh., C.-S., Yanagisawa, N., Behan, W. M. H., Behan, P. O. 1987. A new model for multiple sclerosis: chronic experimental allergic encephalomyelitis induced by immunization with cerebral endothelial cell membrane. *Acta Neuropathol.*, 73, 259-266.

Tsukada, N., Tanaka, Y., Yanagisawa, N. 1989. Autoantibodies to brain endothelial cells in the sera of patients with human T-lymphotropic virus type I associated myelopathy and other demyelinating disorders. *J. Neurol. Sci.*, 90, 33-42.

Tueting, P., Costa, E., Dwivedi, Y., Guidddotti, A., Imapnatiello, F., Maney, R., Pesold, C. 1999. The phenotypic characteristics of heterozygous reeler mouse. *NeuroRep.*, 10, 1329-1334.

Tumiati, B., Casoli, P. 1995. Sudden sensorineural hearing loss and anticardiolipin antibody. *Am. J. Otolaryngol.*, 16, 220.

Turco, A. E., Bresin, E., Rossetti, S., Peterlin, B., Morandi, R., Pignatti, P. F. 1997. Rapid DNA-based prenatal diagnosis by genetic linkage in three families with Alport's syndrome. *Am. J. Kidney Dis.,* 30, 174-179.

Turco, A. E., Rossetti, S., Biasi, M. O., Rizzoni, G., Massella, L., Saarinen, N. H., Renieri, A., Pignatti, P. F., De Marchi, M. 1995. A novel missense mutation in exon 3 of the COL4A5 gene associated with late-onset Alport syndrome. *Clin. Genet.,* 48, 261-263.

Turner, J. G., Willott, J. F. 1998. Exposure to an augmented acoustic environment alters progressive hearing loss in DBA/2J mice. *Hear. Res.,* 118, 101-113.

Turner, J. G., Willott, J. F. 1999. Exposure to an augmented acoustic environment and plasticity of neural responses in the inferior colliculus of DBA/2J mice. *Assoc. Res. Otolaryngol. Abstr.,* 22, 220.

Turner, N., Mason, P. J., Brown, R., Fox, M., Povey, S., Rees, A., Pusey, C. D. 1992. Molecular cloning of the human Goodpasture antigen demonstrates it to be the alpha 3 chain of type IV collagen. *J. Clin. Invest.,* 89, 592-601.

Tyler, R. S., Summerfield, A. Q. 1996. Cochlear implantation: relationships with research on auditory deprivation and acclimatization. *Ear Hear., (Suppl.)* 17, 38-50.

Uddman, R., Luts, A., Sundler, F. 1985. Occurrence and distribution of calcitonin gene-related peptide in the mammalian respiratory tract and middle ear. *Cell Tissue Res.,* 241, 551-555.

Ueki, Y., Naito, I., Oohashi, T., Sugimoto, M., Seki, T., Yoshioka, H., Sado, Y., Sato, H., Sawai, T., Sasaki, F., Matsuoka, M., Fukuda, S., Ninomiya, Y. 1998. Topoisomerase I and II consensus sequences in a 17-kb deletion junction of the COL4A5 and COL4A6 genes and immunohistochemical analysis of esophageal leiomyomatosis associated with Alport syndrome. *Am. J. Hum. Genet.,* 62, 253-261.

Ueyama, S., Kawauchi, H., Mogi, G. 1988. Suppresion of immune-mediated otitis media by T-suppressor cells. *Arch. Otolaryngol. Head Neck Surg.,* 114, 878-882.

Ulfendahl, M., Lundeberg, T., Scarfone, E., Theodorsson, E. 1993. Substance P in the guinea-pig hearing organ. *Acta Physiol. Scand.,* 148, 357-358.

Unsicker, K., Reichert-Preibsch, Schmidt, R. 1987. Astroglial and fibroblast growth factors have neurotrophic functions for cultured peripheral and central nervous system neurons. *Proc. Natl. Acad. Sci., USA,* 84, 5459-5463.

Uziel, A., Gabrion, J., Ohresser, M., Legrand, C. 1981. Effects of hypothyroidism on the structural development of the organ of Corti in the rat. *Acta Otolaryngol.,* 92, 469-480.

Uziel, A., Legrand, C., Ohresser, M., Marot M. 1983a. Maturational and degenerative processes in the organ of Corti after neonatal hypothyroidism. *Hear. Res.,* 11, 203-218.

Uziel, A., Legrand, C., Rabié, A. 1985a. Corrective effects of thyroxin on cochlear abnormalities induced by congenital hypothyroidism in the rat. I. Morphological study. *Devel. Brain. Res.,* 19, 111-122.

Uziel, A., Marot, M., Rabié, A. 1985b. Corrective effects of thyroxin on cochlear abnormalities induced by congenital hypothyroidism in the rat. II. Electrophysiological study. *Devel. Brain. Res.,* 19, 123-127.

Uziel, A., Pujol, R., Legrand, C., Legrand, J. 1983b. Cochlear synaptogenesis in the hypothyroid rat. *Brain Res. Devel. Brain Res.,* 7, 295-301.

Uziel, A., Rabié, A., Marot, M. 1980. The effect of hypothyroidism on the onset of cochlear potentials in developing rats. *Brain Res.,* 182, 172-175.

Vahava, O., Morell, R., Lynch, E. D., Weiss, S., Kagan, M., Ahituv, N., Morrow, J. E., Lee, M. K., Skvorak, A. B., Morton, C. C., Blumenfeld, A., Frydman, M., Friedman, T. B., King, M.-C., Avraham, K. B. 1998. Mutation in the transcription factor POU4F3 associated with inherited progressive hearing loss in humans. *Science,* 279, 1950-1953.

Van Camp G., Smith, R. J. H. 2000. Hereditary Hearing Loss Homepage. World Wide Web URL: http://dnalab-www.uia.ac.be/dnalab/hhh/.

Van Camp, G., Willems, P. J., Smith, R. J. 1997. Nonsyndromic hearing impairment: unparalleled heterogeneity. *Am. J. Hum. Genet.,* 60, 758-764.

Van Eden, W. 1991. Heat-shock proteins as immunogenic bacterial antigens with the potential to induce and regulate autoimmune arthritis. *Immunol. Rev.,* 121, 5-28.

Van De Water, T. R. 1986. Determinants of neuron-sensory receptor cell interaction during the development of the inner ear. *Hear. Res.,* 22, 265-277.

Van De Water, T. R., Repressa, J. 1991. Tissue interactions and growth factors that control development of the inner ear. Neural tube-otic anlage interaction. *Ann. N.Y. Acad. Sci.,* 630, 116-128.

Van De Water, T. R., Ruben, R. J. 1984. Neurotrophic interactions during *in vitro* development of the inner ear. *Ann. Otol. Rhinol. Laryngol.,* 93, 558-564.

Van der Kraan, P. M., Vitters, E. L., Postma, N. S., Verbunt, J., van den Berg, W. B. 1993. Maintenance of the synthesis of large proteoglycans in anatomically intact murine articular cartilage by steroids and insulin-like growth factor I. *Ann. Rheum. Dis.*, 52, 734-741.

Van Laer, L., Huizing, E. H., Verstreken, M., van Zuijen, D., Wauters, J. G., Bossuyt, P. J., Van de Heyning, P., McGuirt, W. T., Smith, R. J. H., Willems, P. J., Legan, P. K., Richardson, G. P., Van Camp, G. 1998. Non-syndromic hearing impairment is associated with a mutation in DFNA5. *Nature Genet.*, 20, 194-197.

Van Loo, A., Vanholder, R., Buytaert, I., De Paepe, A., Praet, M., Elewaut, A., Lameire, N. 1997. Alport syndrome and diffuse leiomyomatosis with major morbid events presenting at adult age. *Nephrol. Dial. Transplant*, 12, 776-780.

Van Noort, J. 1969. *The Structure and Connections of the Inferior Colliculus.* Van Gorcum & Comp., N. V., Assen.

VanCott, J. L., Marinaro, M., Chatfield, S. N., Roberts, M., Yamamoto, M., Hiroi, T., Fujihashi, K., Kiyono, H., McGhee, J. R. 1996. Importance of vaccine delivery mode on outcome of helper T subsets and cytokines for mucosal IgA responses. In Lim, D. J., Bluestone, C. D., Casselbrant, M., Klein, J. O., Ogra, P. L. (Eds.), *Recent Advances in Otitis Media.* B. C. Decker, Hamilton, 4-7.

Varecka, L., Wu, C. H., Rotter, A., Frostholm, A. 1994. GABAA/benzodiazepine receptor alpha 6 subunit mRNA in granule cells of the cerebellar cortex and cochlear nuclei: expression in developing and mutant mice. *J. Comp. Neurol.*, 339, 341-352.

Vater, M., Braun, K. 1994. Parvalbumin, calbindin D-28k, and calretinin immunoreactivity in the ascending auditory pathway of horseshoe bats. *J. Comp. Neurol.*, 341, 534-558.

Vater, M., Covey, E., Casseday, J. H. 1997. The columnar region of the ventral nucleus of the lateral lemniscus in the big brown bat (*Eptesicus fuscus*): synaptic arrangements and structural correlates of feedforward inhibitory function. *Cell Tissue Res.*, 289, 223-233.

Vater, M., Feng, A. S. 1990. Functional organization of ascending and descending connections of the cochlear nucleus of horseshoe bats. *J. Comp. Neurol.*, 292, 373-395.

Vazquez, A. E., Jimenez, A., Zheng, Q. Y., Lonsbury, B., Luebke, A. 2000. Distortion-Product Otoacoustic Emissions and effects of noise in B6. CAST-Ahl+/+ mouse strain, a congenic strain of C57BL/6J. *Assos. Res. Otolarygol. Abstr.*

Vazquez, E., Van de Water, T. R., Del Valle, M., Vega, J. A., Staecker, H., Giráldez, F., Represa, J. 1994. Pattern of trkB protein-like immunoreactivity *in vivo* and the *in vitro* effects of brain-derived neurotrophic factor (BDNF) on developing cochlear and vestibular neurons. *Anat. Embryol.*, 189, 157-167.

Veenstra, G. J., van der Vliet, P. C., Destree, O. H. 1997. POU domain transcription factors in embryonic development. *Molec. Biol. Rep.*, 24, 139-155.

Verhagen, W. I., Huygen, P. L., Padberg, G. W. 1995. The auditory, vestibular, and oculomotor system in facioscapulohumeral dystrophy. *Acta Otolaryngol., Suppl. 520*, 1, 140-142.

Verhoeven, K., Laer, L. V., Kirschofer, K., Legan, P. K., Hughes, D. C., Schatteman, I., Verstreken, M., Van Hauwe, P., Coucke, P., Chen, A., Smith, R. J. H., Somers, T., Offeciers, F. E., Van de Heyning, P., Richardson, G. P., Wachtler, F., Kimberling, W. J., Willems, P. J., Govaerts, P. J., Van Camp, G. 1998. Mutations in the human alpha-tectorin gene cause autosomal dominant non-syndromic hearing impairment. *Nature Genet.*, 19, 60-62.

Verkhratsky, A., Toescu, E. C. 1998. Calcium and neuronal ageing. *Trends Neurosci.*, 21, 2-7.

Vernon, J. A., Katz, B., Meikle, M. B. 1976. Sound measurement and calibration of instruments. In Smith, C. A., Vernon, J. A. (Eds.), *Handbook of Auditory and Vestibular Research Methods.* Charles C. Thomas, Springfield, IL, 306-356.

Vernon, J., Brummett, R., Brown, R. 1977. Noise trauma induced in the presence of loop-inhibiting diuretics. *Tr. Am. Acad. Ophth. Otol.*, 84, 407-413.

Vernon, M. 1969. Usher's syndrome — deafness and progressive blindness. Clinical cases, prevention, theory and literature survey. *J. Chronic. Dis.*, 22, 133-151.

Vertes, D., Axelsson, A. 1981. Cochlear vascular histology in animals exposed to noise. *Arch. Otorhinolaryngol.*, 230, 285-288.

Vetrie, D., Boye, E., Flinter, F., Bobrow, M., Harris, A. 1992. DNA rearrangements in the alpha 5(IV) collagen gene (COL4A5) of individuals with Alport syndrome: further refinement using pulsed-field gel electrophoresis. *Genomics*, 14, 624-633.

Vetter, D. E., Adams, J. C., Mugnaini, E. 1991. Chemically distinct rat olivocochlear neurons. *Synapse*, 7, 21-43.

Vetter, D. E., Liberman, M. C., Mann, J., Barhanin, J., Boutler, J., Brown, M. C., Saffiote-Kolman, J., Heinemen, S. F., Elgoyhen, A. B. 1999. Role of α-9 nicotinic Ach receptor subunits in the development and function of cochlear efferent innervation. *Neuron*, 23, 93-103.

Vetter, D. E., Mann, J. R., Wangemann, P., Liu, J., McLaughlin, K. J., Lesage, F., Marcus, D. C., Lazdunski, M., Heinemann, S. F., Barhanin, J. 1996. Inner ear defects induced by null mutation of the *isk* gene. *Neuron*, 17, 1251-1264.

Villa, A. M., Anderson, S. F., Abundo, R. E. 1997. Bilateral disc edema in retinitis pigmentosa. *Optom. Vis. Sci.*, 74, 132-137.

Virag, T., Ison, J. R., Hammond, G. R., 2000, Listening for one particular tone reduces detection rate and reaction speed for a rare tone in a one-alternative forced choice test. *Assoc. Res. Otolaryngol. Abst.*, 23, # 532.

Vismara, A., Meroni, P. L., Tincani, A., Harris, E. N., Barcellini, W., Brucato, A., Khamashta, M., Hughes, G. R., Zanussi, C., Balestrieri, G. 1988. Relationship between anti-cardiolipin and anti-endothelial cell antibodies in systemic lupus erythematosus. *Clin. Exp. Immunol.*, 74, 247-253.

Visscher, P. M. 1999. Speed congenics: accelerated genome recovery using genetic markers. *Genet. Res.*, 74, 81-85.

Vitelli, F., Meloni, I., Fineschi, S., Favara, F., Tiziana, S. C., Rocchi, M., Renieri, A. 2000. Identification and characterization of mouse orthologs of the AMMECR1 and FACL4 genes deleted in AMME syndrome: orthology of Xq22.3 and MmuXF1-F3. *Cytogenet. Cell Genet.*, 88, 259-263.

Vitelli, F., Piccini, M., Caroli, F., Franco, B., Malandrini, A., Pober, B., Jonsson, J., Sorrentino, V., Renieri, A. 1999. Identification and characterization of a highly conserved protein absent in the Alport syndrome (A), mental retardation (M), midface hypoplasia (M), and elliptocytosis (E) contiguous gene deletion syndrome (AMME). *Genomics*, 55, 335-340.

Vogelweid, C. M., Johnson, G. C., Besch-Williford, C. L., Basler, J., Walker, S. E. 1991. Inflammatory central nervous system disease in lupus-prone MRL/lpr mice: comparative histologic and immunohistochemical findings. *J. Neuroimmunol.*, 35, 89-99.

Vogler, C., Birkenmeier, E. H., Sly, W. S., Levy, B., Pegors, C., Kyle, J. W., Beamer, W. G. 1990. A murine model of mucopolysaccharidosis VII. *Am. J. Pathol.*, 136, 207-217.

Vogler, C., Levy, B., Galvin, N. J., Thorpe, C., Sands, M. S., Barker, J. E., Baty, J., Birkenmeier, E. H., Sly, W. S. 1999. Enzyme replacement in murine mucopolysaccharidosis Type VII: neuronal and glia response to beta-glucuronidase requires early initiation of enzyme replacement therapy. *Ped. Ther.*, 45, 838-844.

Vogler, C., Levy, B., Kyle, J. W., Sly, W. S., Williamson, J., Whyte, M. P. 1994. Mucopolysaccharidosis VII: postmortem biochemical and pathological findings in a young adult with beta-glucuronidase deficiency. *Modern Pathol.*, 7, 132-137.

Vogler, C., Sands, M., Higgins, A., Levy, B., Grubb, J., Birkenmeier, E. H., Sly, W. S. 1993. Enzyme replacement with recombinant beta-glucuronidase in the newborn mucopolysaccharidosis type VII mouse. *Pediat. Res.*, 34, 837-840.

Vogler, C., Sands, M. S., Levy, B., Galvin, N., Birkenmeier, E. H., Sly, W. S. 1996. Enzyme replacement with recombinant beta-glucuronidase in murine mucopolysaccharidosis Type VII: impact of therapy during the first six weeks of life on subsequent lysosomal storage, growth, and survival. *Ped. Res.*, 39, 1050-1054.

Vogler, C., Sands, M. S., Galvin, N., Levy, B., Thorpe, C., Barker, J., Sly, W. S. 1998. Murine mucopolysaccharidosis Type VII: the impact of therapies on the clinical course and pathology in a murine model of lysosomal storage disease. *J. Inher. Metabol. Dis.*, 21, 575-586.

Voigt, H. F., Young, E. D. 1980. Evidence of inhibitory interactions between neurons in dorsal cochlear nucleus. *J. Neurophysiol.*, 44, 76-96.

Voigt, H. F., Young, E. D. 1990. Cross-correlation analysis of inhibitory interactions in dorsal cochlear nucleus. *J. Neurophysiol.*, 64, 1590-1610.

Voit, T., Lamprecht, A., Lenard, H. G., Goebel, H. H. 1986. Hearing loss in facioscapulohumeral dystrophy. *Eur. J. Pediatr.*, 145, 280-285.

vom Saal, F. S. 1981. Variation in phenotype due to random intrauterine positioning of male and female fetuses in rodents. *J. Reprod. Fert.*, 62, 633-650.

von Bartheld, C. S., Rubel, E. W. 1989. Transient GABA immunoreactivity in cranial nerves of the chick embryo. *J. Comp. Neurol.*, 286, 456-471.

von Bekesy, G. 1960/1930. *Experiments in Hearing*. McGraw Hill, New York, 321-332.

Vosteen, K. H. 1960. The histochemistry of the enzymes of oxygen metabolism in the inner ear. *Laryngoscope*, 70, 351-162.

Vrettakos, P. A., Dear, S. D., Saunders, J. C. 1988. Middle ear structure in the chinchilla: a quantitative study. *Am. J. Otolaryngol.*, 9, 58-67.

Waering, M., Mhatre A. N., Pettis R., Han J. J., Haut T., Pfister M. H. F., Hong K., Zheng W. W. Lalwani A. K. 1999. Cationic liposome mediated transgene expression in the guinea pig cochlea. *Hear. Res.,* 128, 61-69.

Wagenaar, M., van Aarem, A., Huygen, P., Pieke-Dahl, S., Kimberling, W., Cremers, C. 1999. Hearing impairment related to age in Usher syndrome types 1B and 2A. *Arch. Otolaryngol. Head Neck Surg.,* 125, 441-445.

Wagner, E., Klump, G. M., Hamann, I. 2000. Gap detection in Mongolian gerbils. *Assoc. Res. Otolaryngol. Abst.,* 23, # 97.

Wagner, T. 1996. Lemniscal input to identified neurons of the central nucleus of mouse inferior colliculus: an intracellular brain slice study. *Eur. J. Neurosci.,* 8, 1231-1239.

Wakeland, E., Morel, L., Achey, K., Yui, M., Longmate, J. 1997. Speed congenics: a classic technique in the fast lane (relatively speaking). *Immunol. Today,* 18, 472-477.

Walker, S. E. 1988. Defective primary and secondary IgG responses to thymic-dependent antigens in autoimmune PN mice. *J. Immunol.,* 140, 3426-3433.

Walker, S. E., Gray, R. H., Fulton, M., Wigley, R. D., Schnitzer, B. 1978. Palmerston North mice, a new animal model of systemic lupus erythematosus. *J. Lab. Clin. Med.,* 92, 932-945.

Wallace, S. P., Prutting C. A. Gerber S. E. 1990. Degeneration of speech, language, and hearing in a patient with mucopolysaccharidosis Type VII. *Int. J. Ped. Otorhinolaryngol.,* 19, 97-107.

Waller, A. V. 1852. Sur la reproduction des nerfs et sur la structure et les fonctions des ganglions spinaux. *Arch. Anat. Physiol. Wiss. Med.,* 392-401.

Walsh, E. J., Cranfill, L., Gouthro, M., Gratton, M. A., McGee, J. 2000. Distortion product otoacoustic emissions in Tshr mutant mice. *Assoc. Res. Otolaryngol. Abstr.,* 23, 191-192.

Walsh, E. J., McGee, J., McFadden, S. L., Liberman, M. C. 1998a. Long-term effects of sectioning the olivocochlear bundle in neonatal cats. *J. Neurosci.,* 18, 3859-3869.

Walsh, E. J., McGee, J., Song, L., Liberman, M. C. 1998b. Consequences of neonatal OCB transection on the expression of peripheral auditory nonlinearities. *Assoc. Res. Otolaryngol. Abstr.,* 21, 214.

Walsh, E. J., McGee, J. 1987. Postnatal development of auditory nerve and cochlear nucleus neuronal responses in kittens. *Hear. Res.,* 28, 97-116.

Walsh, E. J., McGee, J., Javel, E. 1986a. Development of auditory-evoked potentials in the cat. I. Onset of response and development of sensitivity. *J. Acoust. Soc. Am.,* 79, 712-724.

Walsh, E. J., McGee, J., Javel, E. 1986b. Development of auditory-evoked potentials in the cat. II. Wave latencies. *J. Acoust. Soc. Am.,* 79, 725-744.

Walsh, E. J., McGee, J., Javel, E. 1986c. Development of auditory-evoked potentials in the cat. III. Wave amplitudes. *J. Acoust. Soc. Am.,* 79, 745-754.

Walsh, E. J., McGee, J. 1997. Does activity in the olivocochlear bundle affect development of the auditory periphery? In Lewis, E. R., Long, G. R., Lyon, R. F., Narins, P. M., Steele, C. R., Hecht-Poinar, E. (Eds.), *Diversity in Auditory Mechanics.* World Science Press, Singapore, 376-385.

Walsh, E. J., McGee, J. 1986. The development of function in the auditory periphery of cats. In Altschuler, R. A., Bobbin, R. P., Hoffman, D. W. (Eds.), *Neurobiology of Hearing: The Cochlea.* Raven Press, New York, 247-269.

Walsh, E. J., McGee, J. 1988. Rhythmic discharge properties of caudal cochlear nucleus neurons during postnatal development in cats. *Hear. Res.,* 36, 233-248.

Walsh, E. J., Romand, R. 1992. Functional development of the cochlea and the cochlear nerve. In Romand, R. (Ed.), *Development of Auditory and Vestibular Systems 2.* Elsevier, Amsterdam, 161-219.

Walsh, M. E., Webster, D. B. 1994. Exogenous GM1 ganglioside effects on conductive and sensorineural hearing losses. *Hear. Res.,* 75, 54-60.

Walton, J. P., Frisina, R. D., Ison, J. E, O'Neill, W. E. 1997. Neural correlates of behavioral gap detection in the inferior colliculus of the young CBA mouse. *J. Comp. Physiol.,* A 181, 161-176.

Walton, J. P., Frisina, R. D., Meierhans, L. R. 1995. Sensorineural hearing loss alters recovery from short-term adaptation in the C57BL/6 mouse. *Hear. Res.,* 88, 19-26.

Walton, J. P., Frisina, R. D., O'Neill, W. E. 1998. Age-related alteration in processing of temporal sound features in the auditory midbrain of the CBA mouse. *J. Neurosci.,* 18, 2764-2776.

Waltzman, S. B., Cohen, N. L., Gomolin, R. H., Shapiro, W. H., Ozdamar, S. R., Hoffman, R. A. 1994. Long term results of early cochlear implantation in congenitally and prelingually deafened children. *Am. J. Otol.,* 15, 9-13.

Waltzman, S., Fisher, S., Niparko, J. K., Cohen, N. 1995. Predictors of postoperative performance with cochlear implants. *Ann. Otol. Rhinol. Laryngol. (Suppl.),* 165, 15-18.

Wang, A., Liang, Y., Fridell, R. A., Probst, F. J., Wilcox, E. R., Touchman, J. W., Morton, C. C., Morell, R. J., Noben-Trauth, K., Camper, S. A., Friedman, T. B. 1998. Association of unconventional myosin MYO15 mutations with human non-syndromic deafness DFNB3. *Science*, 280, 1447-1451.

Wang, L. F., Sun, C. C., Wu, J. T., Lin, R. H. 1999. Epicutaneous administration of hapten through patch application augments TH2 responses which can downregulate the elicitation of murine contact hypersensitivity. *Clin. Exp. Allergy*, 29, 271-279.

Wang, W., Van De Water, T., Lufkin, T. 1998. Inner ear and maternal reproductive defects in mice lacking the Hmx3 homeobox gene. *Devel.* 125, 621-634.

Wang, X., Sachs, M. B. 1994. Neural encoding of single-formant stimuli in the cat. II. Responses of anteroventral cochlear nucleus units. *J. Neurophysiol.*, 71, 59-78.

Wang, Y., Kristan, J., Hao, L., Lenkoski, C. S., Shen, Y., Matis, L. A., 2000a. A role for comlement in antibody-mediated inflammation: C5-deficient DBA/1 mice are resistant to collagen-induced arthritis. *J. Immunol.*, 164, 4340-4347.

Wang, Y., Wondisford, F., Liberman, M. C. 2000b. Thyroid hormone b2 receptor knockout prevents age-related hearing loss in mice. *Assoc. Res. Otolaryngol. Abstr.,*

Wangemann, P., Gruber, D. D. 1998. The isolated *in vitro* perfused spiral modiolar artery: pressure dependence of vasoconstriction. *Hear. Res.*, 115, 113-118.

Warburton, D., Wuenschell, C., Flores-Delgado, G., Anderson, K. 1998. Commitment and differentiation of lung cell lineages. *Biochem. Cell Biol.*, 76, 971-995.

Warburton, V. L., Sales, G. D., Milligan, S. R. 1989. The emission and elicitation of mouse ultrasonic vocalizations: the effects of age, sex and gonadal status. *Physiol. Behav.*, 45, 41-47.

Warburton, V. L., Stoughton, R., Demaine, C., Sales, G. D., Milligan, S. R. 1988. Long-term monitoring of mouse ultrasonic vocalizations. *Physiol. Behav.*, 44, 829-831.

Ward, J. M., Houchens, D. P., Collins, M. J., Young, D. M., Reagan, R. L. 1976. Naturally-occurring Sendai virus infection of athymic nude mice. *Vet. Path.*, 13, 36-46.

Ward, W. D., Glorig, A., Sklar, D. L. 1958. Dependence of temporary threshold shift at 4 kc on intensity and time. *J. Acoust. Soc. Am.*, 30, 944-954.

Warr, W. B. 1982. Parallel ascending pathways from the cochlear nucleus: neuroanatomical evidence of functional specialization. In Neff, W. D. (Ed.), *Contributions to Sensory Physiology*. Academic Press, New York, 1-38.

Warr, W. B. 1992. Organization of olivocochlear efferent systems in mammals. In Webster, D. B., Popper, A. N., Fay, R. R. (Eds.), *Mammalian Auditory Pathway: Neuroanatomy, 1.* Springer-Verlag, Berlin, 410-448.

Warr, W. B., Beck, J. E. 1995. A longitudinal efferent innervation of the inner hair cell region may originate from "shell neurons" surrounding the lateral superior olive in the rat. *Assoc. Res. Otolaryngol. Abstr.,* 18, 194.

Warr, W. B., Boche, J. B., Neely, S. T. 1997. Efferent innervation of the inner hair cell region: origins and terminations of two lateral olivocochlear systems. *Hear Res.,* 108, 89-111.

Warr, W. B., Guinan, Jr., J. J., White, J. S. 1986. Organization of the efferent fibers: the lateral and medial olivocochlear systems. In Altschuler, R. A., Hoffman, D. W., Bobbin, R. P. (Eds.), *Neurobiology of Hearing: The Cochlea.* Raven Press, New York, 333-348.

Wassarman, K. M., Lewandoski, M., Campbell, K., Joyner, A. L., Rubenstein, J. L., Martinez, S., Martin, G. R. 1997. Specification of the anterior hindbrain and establishment of a normal mid/hindbrain organizer is dependent on Gbx2 gene function. *Devel.*, 124, 2923-2934.

Wasserman, R. H., Taylor, A. N. 1966. Vitamin D3-induced calcium binding protein in chick intestinal mucosa. *Science*, 152, 791-793.

Watanabe, T., Cheng, K.-C., Krug, M. S., Yoo, T.-J. 1996. Brain stem auditory-evoked potential of mice with experimental allergic encephalomyelitis. *Ann. Otol. Rhinol. Laryngol.*, 105, 905-915.

Watanabe, T., Hirano, T., Suzuki, M., Mogi, G. 1999. The effects and expression of IL-1B in the murine model of otitis media with effusion. Presented at *Seventh International Symposium on Recent Advances in Otitis Media.* June 1-5, Fort Lauderdale, FL, 55.

Watanabe-Fukunaga, R., Brannan, C. I., Copeland, N. G., Jenkins, N. A., Nagata, S. 1992. Lymphoproliferation disorder in mice explained by defects in Fas antigen that mediates apoptosis. *Nature*, 356, 314-317.

Wayland, H. 1975. Intravital microscopy. In Barer, R., Cosslett, V. E. (Eds.), *Advances in Optical and Electron Microscopy.* Academic Press, New York, 1-50.

Wayne, S., Der, K. V., Schloss, M., Polomeno, R., Scott, D. A., Hejtmancik, J. F., Sheffield, V. C., Smith, R. J. 1996. Localization of the Usher syndrome type ID gene (Ush1D) to chromosome 10. *Hum. Molec. Genet.*, 5, 1689-1692.

Wayne, S., Lowry, R. B., McLeod, D. R., Knaus, R., Farr, C., Smith, R. J. 1997. Localization of the Usher syndrome type 1F (USH1F) to chromosome 10. *Am. J. Hum. Genet. (Abstr).*, 61, A300.

Weber, B. A. 1994. Auditory brainstem response: threshold estimation and auditory screening. In Katz, J. (Ed.), *Handbook of Clinical Audiology* (4th ed.), Williams & Wilkins, Baltimore, 375-386.

Webster, D. B., Ackermann, R., Longa, G. 1968. Central auditory system of the kangaroo rat, *Dipodomys merriami. J. Comp. Neurol.*, 133, 477-494.

Webster, D. B., Trune, D. R. 1982. Cochlear nuclear complex of mice. *Am. J. Anat.*, 163, 103-130.

Webster, D. B., Webster, M. 1977. Neonatal sound deprivation affects brain stem auditory nuclei. *Arch. Otolaryngol.*, 103, 393-396.

Webster, W. R., Aitkin, L. M. 1975. Central auditory processing. In Gazzaniga, M. D., Blakemore, C. (Eds.), *Handbook of Psychobiology*. Academic Press, New York, 325-364.

Wecker, J. R., Ison, J. R. 1986a. Visual function measured by reflex modification in rats with inherited retinal dystrophy. *Behav. Neurosci.*, 100, 679-684.

Wecker, J. R., Ison, J. R. 1986b. Effects of motor activity on the elicitation and modification of the startle reflex in rats. *Anim. Learn. Behav.*, 14, 287-292.

Weedman, D. L., Ryugo, D. K. 1996. Projections from auditory cortex to the cochlear nucleus in rats: synapses on granule cell dendrites. *J. Comp. Neurol.*, 371, 311-324.

Wegner, M., Drolet, D. W., Rosenfeld, M. G. 1993. POU-domain proteins: structure and function of developmental regulators. *Curr. Opin. Cell Biol.*, 5, 488-498.

Weidauer, H., Arnold, W. 1976. Morphological changes in the inner ear of alport's syndrome. *Laryngol. Rhinol. Otol. (Stuttgart)*, 55, 6-16.

Weil, D., Blanchard, S., Kaplan, J., Guilford, P., Gibson, F., Walsh, J., Mburu, P., Varela, A., Levilliers, J., Weston, M. D., Kelley, P. M., Kimberling, W. J., Wagenar, M., Levi-Acobas, F., Larget-Piet, D., Munnich, A., Steel, K. P., Brown, S. D. M., Petit, C. 1995. Defective myosin VIIA gene responsible for Usher syndrome 1B. *Nature*, 274, 60-61.

Weil, D., Kussel, P., Blanchard, S., Levy, G., Levi-Acobas, F., Drira, M., Ayadi, H., Petit, C. 1997. The autosomal recessive isolated deafness, DFNB2, and the Usher 1B syndrome are allelic defects of the myosin-VIIA gene. *Nature Genet.*, 16, 191-193.

Weil, D., Levy, G., Sahly, I., Levi-Acobas, F., Blanchard, S., el-Amraoui, A., Crozet, F., Philippe, H., Abitbol, M., Petit, C. 1996. Human myosin VIIA responsible for the Usher 1B syndrome: a predicted membrane-associated motor protein expressed in developing sensory epithelia. *Proc. Natl. Acad. Sci., USA*, 93, 3232-3237.

Weille, F. L., Gargano, S. R., Pfister, R., Martinez, D., Irwin, J. W. 1954. Circulation of the spiral ligament and stria vascularis of living guinea pig. *Arch. Otolaryngol.*, 59, 731-738.

Weinberg, R. J., Rustioni, A. 1987. A cuneocochlear pathway in the rat. *Neuroscience*, 20, 209-219.

Wenngren, B., Anniko, M. 1988. A frequency-specific auditory brainstem response technique exemplified in the determination of age-related auditory thresholds. *Acta Otolaryngol.*, 106, 238-243.

Wenthold, R. J. 1987. Evidence for a glycinergic pathway connecting the two cochlear nuclei: an immunocytochemical and retrograde transport study. *Brain Res.*, 415, 183-187.

Wenthold, R. J., Zempel, J. M., Parakkal, M. H., Reeks, K. A., Altschuler, R. A. 1986. Immunocytochemical localization of GABA in the cochlear nucleus of the guinea pig. *Brain Res.*, 380, 7-18.

West, J. M., Slomianka, L., Gundersen, H. J. G. 1991. Unbiased stereological estimation of the total number of neurons in the subdivisions of the rat hippocampus using the optical fractionator. *Anat. Rec.*, 231, 482-497.

Wester, D. C., Atkin, C. L., Gregory, M. C. 1995. Alport syndrome: clinical update. *J. Am. Acad. Audiol.*, 6, 73-79.

Weston, M. D., Kelley, P. M., Overbeck, L. D., Wagenaar, M., Orten, D. J., Hasson, T., Chen, Z. Y., Corey, D., Mooseker, M., Sumegi, J., Cremers, C., Moller, C., Jacobson, S. G., Gorin, M. B., Kimberling, W. J. 1996. Myosin VIIA mutation screening in 189 Usher syndrome type 1 patients. *Am. J. Hum. Genet.*, 59, 1074-1083.

Wheeler E. F., Bothwell, M., Schecterson, L. C., von Barthold, C. S. 1994. Expression of BDNF and NT-3 mRNA in hair cells of the organ of Corti: quantitative analysis in developing rats. *Hear. Res.*, 73, 46-56.

White, J. K., Auerbach, W., Duyao, M. P., Vonsattel, J. P., Gusella, J. F., Joyner, A. L., MacDonald, M. E. 1997. Huntingtin is required for neurogenesis and is not impaired by the Huntington's disease CAG expansion. *Nature Genet.,* 17, 404-410.

White, J. S., Warr, W. B. 1983. The dual origins of the olivocochlear bundle in the albino rat. *J. Comp. Neurol.,* 219, 203-214.

White, N. R., Barfield, R. J. 1987. Role of the ultrasonic vocalization of the female rat (*Rattus norvegicus*) in sexual behavior. *J. Comp. Psychol.,* 101, 73-81.

White, N. R., Prasad, M., Barfield, R. J., Nyby, J. G. 1998. 40-and 70-kHz vocalizations of mice (*Mus musculus*) during copulation. *Physiol. Behav.,* 63, 467-473.

Whitehead, M. L., Lonsbury-Martin, B. L., Martin, G. K. 1992a. Evidence of two discrete sources of 2f1-f2 distortion-product otoacoustic emission in rabbit. I. Differential dependence on stimulus parameters. *J. Acoust. Soc. Am.,* 91, 1587-1607.

Whitehead, M. L., Lonsbury-Martin, B. L., Martin, G. K. 1992b. Evidence of two discrete sources of $2f_1-f_2$ distortion-product otoacoustic emission in rabbit. II. Differential physiological vulnerability. *J. Acoust. Soc. Am.,* 92, 2662-2682.

Whitehead, M. L., McCoy, M. J., Lonsbury-Martin, B. L., Martin, G. K. 1995. Dependence of distortion-product otoacoustic emissions on primary levels in normal and hearing impaired ears. I. Effects of decreasing L_2 below L_1. *J. Acoust. Soc. Am.,* 97, 2346-2358.

Whitehead, M., Morest, D. 1985. The development of innervation patterns in the avian cochlea. *Neuroscience,* 14, 255-276.

Whitlon, D. S., Rutishauser, U. S. 1990. NCAM in the organ of Corti of the developing mouse. *J. Neurocytol.,* 20, 970-977.

Whitlon, D. S., Sobkowicz, H. M. 1989. GABA-like immunoreactivity in the cochlea of the developing mouse. *J. Neurocytol.,* 18, 505-518.

Whitlon, D. S., Zhang, X., Kasakabe, M. 1999. Tenascin-C in the cochlea of the developing mouse. *J. Comp Neurol.,* 406, 361-374.

Whitlon, D. S., Zhang, X., Pecelunas, K., Greiner, M. A. 2000. A temporospatial map of adhesive molecules in the organ of Corti of the mouse cochlea. *J. Neurocytol.,* 28, 955-968.

Whitney, G. 1969. Vocalization of mice: a single genetic unit effect. *J. Hered.,* 60, 337-340.

Whitney, G. 1970. Ontogeny of sonic vocalizations of laboratory mice. *Behav. Genet.,* 1, 269-273.

Whitney, G. 1973. Vocalization of mice influenced by a single gene in a heterogeneous population. *Behav. Genet.,* 3, 57-64.

Whitney, G., Alpern, M., Dizinno, G., Horowitz, G. 1974. Female odors evoke ultrasounds from male mice. *Anim. Learn. Behav.,* 2, 13-18.

Whitney, G., Coble, J. R., Stockton, M. D., Tilson, E. F. 1973. Ultrasonic emissions: do they facilitate courtship of mice? *J. Comp. Physiol. Psychol.,* 84, 445-452.

Whitney, G., Nyby, J. 1979. Cues that elicit ultrasounds from adult male mice. *Am. Zool.,* 19, 457-463.

Whitney, G., Nyby, J. 1983. Sound communication among adults. In Willott, J. F. (Ed.), *Auditory Psychobiology of the Mouse.* Plenum, New York, 173-192.

Wickesberg, R. E. 1996. Rapid inhibition in the cochlear nuclear complex of the chinchilla. *J. Acoust. Soc. Am.,* 100, 1691-1702.

Wickesberg, R. E., Oertel, D. 1988. Tonotopic projection from the dorsal to the anteroventral cochlear nucleus of mice. *J. Comp. Neurol.,* 268, 389-399.

Wickesberg, R. E., Oertel, D. 1990. Delayed, frequency-specific inhibition in the cochlear nuclei of mice: a mechanism for monaural echo suppression. *J. Neurosci.,* 10, 1762-1768.

Wickesberg, R. E., Whitlon, D., Oertel, D. 1991. Tuberculoventral neurons project to the multipolar cell area but not to the octopus cell area of the posteroventral cochlear nucleus. *J. Comp. Neurol.,* 313, 457-468.

Wickesberg, R. E., Whitlon, D., Oertel, D. 1994. *In vitro* modulation of somatic glycine-like immunoreactivity in presumed glycinergic neurons. *J. Comp. Neurol.,* 339, 311-327.

Wiechers B., Gestwa, G., Mack, A., Carroll, P., Zenner, H. P., Knipper, M. 1999. A changing pattern of brain-derived neurotrophic factor expression correlates with the rearrangement of fibers during cochlear development of rats and mice. *J. Neurosci.,* 19, 3033-3042.

Wightman, F. L., Kistler, D. J. 1989. Headphone simulation of free-field listening. II. Psychophysical validation. *J. Acoust. Soc. Am.,* 85, 868-878.

Wilkinson, D. G., Bhatt, S., McMahon, A. P. 1989. Expression pattern of the FGF-related proto-oncogene int-2 suggests multiple roles in fetal development. *Devel.*, 105, 131-136.

Wilkinson, D. G., Peters, G., Dickson, C., McMahon, A. P. 1988. Expression of the FGF-related proto-oncogene int-2 during gastrulation and neurulation in the mouse. *Embo J.*, 7, 691-695.

Willard, F. H., Ryugo, D. K. 1983. Anatomy of the central auditory system. In Willott, J. F. (Ed.), *The Auditory Psychobiology of the Mouse.* Charles C. Thomas, Springfield, IL, 201-304.

Williams, L. L., Lowery, H. W., Shannon, B. T. 1987. Evidence of persistent viral infection in Meniere's disease. *Arch. Otolaryngol. Head Neck Surg.*, 113, 397-400.

Willott, J. F. 1981. Comparison of response properties of inferior colliculus neurons of two inbred mouse strains differing in susceptibility to audiogenic seizures. *J. Neurophysiol.*, 45, 35-47.

Willott, J. F. 1983. Central nervous system physiology. In Willott, J. (Ed.), *The Auditory Psychobiology of the Mouse*. Thomas, Springfield, IL, 305-339.

Willott, J. F. 1984. Changes in frequency representation in the auditory system of mice with age-related hearing impairment. *Brain Res.*, 309, 159-162.

Willott, J. F. 1986. Effects of aging, hearing loss, and anatomical location on thresholds of inferior colliculus neurons in C57BL/6 and CBA mice. *J. Neurophysiol.*, 56, 391-408.

Willott, J. F. 1991a. *Aging and the Auditory System: Anatomy, Physiology, and Psychophysics.* Singular, San Diego.

Willott, J. F. 1991b. Central physiological correlates of aging and presbycusis in mice. *Acta Otolaryngol.*, 476, 153-156.

Willott, J. F. 1996a. Auditory system plasticity in the adult C57BL/6J mouse. In Salvi, R. J., Henderson, D. H., Colletti, V., Fiorino, F. (Eds.), *Auditory Plasticity and Regeneration*. Thieme Medical Publishers, New York, 297-316.

Willott, J. F. 1996b. Aging and the auditory system. In Mohr, U., Dungworth, D. L., Capen, C. C., Carlton, W. W., Sundberg, J. P., Ward, J. M. (Eds.), *Pathobiology of the Aging Mouse,* ILSI Monographs on the Pathobiology of Aging Animals. ILSI Press, Washington, D.C., 179-204.

Willott, J. F., Aitkin, L. M., McFadden, S. L. 1993. Plasticity of auditory cortex associated with sensorineural hearing loss in adult C57BL/6J mice. *J. Comp. Neurol.*, 329, 402-411.

Willott, J. F., Bross, L. S. 1990. Morphology of the octopus cell area of the cochlear nucleus in young and aging C57BL/6J and CBA/J Mice. *J. Comp. Neurol.*, 300, 61-81.

Willott, J. F., Bross, L. S. 1996. Morphological changes in the anteroventral cochlear nucleus that accompany sensorineural hearing loss in DBA/2J and C57BL/6J mice. *Devel. Brain Res.*, 91, 218-226.

Willott, J. F., Bross, L. S., McFadden, S. L. 1992. Morphology of the dorsal cochlear nucleus in C57BL/6J and CBA mice across the life span. *J. Comp. Neurol.*, 321, 666-678.

Willott, J. F., Bross, L. S., McFadden, S. L. 1994a. Morphology of the inferior colliculus in C57BL/6J and CBA/J mice across the life span. *Neurobiol. Aging,* 15, 175-183.

Willott, J. F., Carlson, S. 1995. Modification of the acoustic startle response in hearing-impaired C57BL/6J mice: prepulse augmentation and prolongation of prepulse inhibition. *Behav. Neurosci.*, 109, 396-403.

Willott, J. F., Carlson, S., Chen, H. 1994b. Prepulse inhibition of the startle response in mice: relationship to hearing loss and auditory system plasticity. *Behav. Neurosci.*, 108, 703-713.

Willott, J. F., Carlson, S., Falls, W. A., Turner, J., Webster, S. 1996. Behavioral correlates of hearing-loss induced (HLI) plasticity in C57BL/6J mice: Increased effectiveness of tones producing fear-potentiated startle. *Soc. Neurosci. Abstr.*, 22.

Willott, J. F., Demuth, R. M. 1986. The influence of stimulus repetition on the acoustic startle response and on responses of inferior colliculus neurons in mice. *Brain Res.*, 386, 105-112.

Willott, J. F. Demuth, R. M., Lu, S. M. 1984. Excitability of auditory neurons in the dorsal and ventral cochlear nuclei of DBA/2 and C57BL/6 mice. *Exp. Neurol.*, 83, 495-506.

Willott, J. F., Demuth, R. M., Lu, S.-M., Van Bergem, P. 1982. Abnormal tonotopic organization in the ventral cochlear nucleus of the hearing-impaired DBA/2 mouse. *Neurosci. Lett.*, 34, 13–17.

Willott, J. F., Erway, L. C. 1998. Genetics of age-related hearing loss in mice. IV. Cochlear pathology and hearing loss in 25 BXD recombinant inbred mouse strains. *Hear. Res.*, 119, 27-36.

Willott, J. F., Erway, L. C., Archer, J. R., Harrison, D. E. 1995. Genetics of age-related hearing loss in mice. II. Strain differences and effects of caloric restriction on cochlear pathology and evoked response thresholds. *Hear. Res.*, 88, 143-155.

Willott, J. F., Henry, K. R. 1974. Auditory evoked potentials: developmental changes of threshold and amplitude following early acoustic trauma. *J. Comp. Physiol. Psychol.,* 86, 1-7.

Willott, J. F., Hunter, K. P., Coleman, J. R. 1988a. Aging and presbycusis: effects on 2-deoxy-D-glucose uptake in the mouse auditory brainstem in quiet. *Exp. Neurol.,* 99, 615-621.

Willott, J. F., Jackson, L. M, Hunter, K. P. 1987. Morphometric study of the anteroventral cochlear nucleus of two mouse models of presbycusis. *J. Comp. Neurol.,* 260, 472-480.

Willott, J. F., Kulig, J., Satterfield, T. 1984. The acoustic startle response in DBA/2 and C57BL/6 mice: relationship to auditory neuronal response properties and hearing impairment. *Hear. Res.,* 16, 161-167.

Willott, J. F., Milbrandt, J. C., Bross, L. S, Caspary, D. M. 1997. Glycine immunoreactivity and receptor binding in the cochlear nucleus of C57BL/6J and CBA/CaJ mice: effects of cochlear impairment and aging. *J. Comp. Neurol.,* 385, 405-414.

Willott, J. F., Mortenson, V. 1991. Age-related cochlear histopathology in C57BL/6J and CBA/J mice. *Assoc. Res. Otolaryngol. Abstr.,* 14, 16.

Willott, J. F., Pankow, D., Paris Hunter, K, Kordyban, M. 1985. Projections from the anterior ventral cochlear nucleus to the central nucleus of the inferior colliculus in young and aging C57BL/6 mice. *J. Comp. Neurol.,* 237, 545-551.

Willott, J. F., Parham, K., Hunter, K. P. 1988b. Response properties of inferior colliculus neurons in young and very old CBA/J mice. *Hear. Res.,* 37, 1-14.

Willott, J. F., Parham, K., Hunter, K. P. 1988c. Response properties of inferior colliculus neurons in middle aged C57 mice with presbycusis. *Hear. Res.,* 37, 15-28.

Willott, J. F., Parham, K., Hunter, K. P. 1991. Comparison of the auditory sensitivity of neurons in the cochlear nucleus and inferior colliculus of young and aging C57BL/6J and CBA/J mice. *Hear. Res.,* 53, 78-94.

Willott, J. F., Shnerson, A. 1978. Rapid development of tuning characteristics of inferior colliculus neurons in mouse pups. *Brain Res.,* 148, 230-233.

Willott, J. F., Shnerson, A., Urban, G. P. 1979. Sensitivity of the acoustic startle response and neurons in subnuclei of the mouse inferior colliculus to stimulus parameters. *Exp. Neurol.,* 65, 625-644.

Willott, J. M., Turner, J. G. 1999. Prolonged exposure to an augmented acoustic environment ameliorates age-related auditory changes in C57BL/6J and DBA/2J mice. *Hear. Res.,* 135, 78-88.

Willott, J. F., Turner, J. G. 2000. Neural plasticity in the mouse inferior colliculus: relationship to hearing loss, augmented acoustic stimulation, and prepulse inhibition. *Hear. Res.,* 147, 275-281.

Willott, J. F., Turner, J. G., Carlson, S., Ding, D., Bross, L. S., Falls, W. M. 1998. The BALB/c mouse as an animal model for progressive sensorineural hearing loss. *Hear. Res.,* 115, 162-174.

Willott, J. F., Turner, J. G., Sundin, V. S. 2000. Effects of exposure to an augmented acoustic environment on auditory function in mice: Roles of hearing loss and age during treatment. *Hear. Res.,* 142, 79-88.

Wilson, J. L., Henson, M. M., Henson, O. W. J. 1991. Course and distribution of efferent fibers in the cochlea of the mouse. *Hear. Res.,* 55, 98-108.

Winer, J. A., Kelly, J. B, Larue, D. T. 1999. Neural architecture of the rat medial geniculate body. *Hear. Res.,* 130, 19-41.

Winfield, J. B., Jarjour, W. N. 1991. Stress proteins, autoimmunity, and autoimmune disease. *Curr. Topics Microbiol. Immunol.,* 167, 161-88.

Winnier, G., Blessing, M., Labosky, P. A., Hogan, B. L. 1995. Bone morphogenetic protein-4 is required for mesoderm formation and patterning in the mouse. *Genes Devel.,* 9, 2105-2116.

Winter, C. A. 1965. Physiology and pharmacology of pain. In de Stevens, G. (Ed.), *Analgetics.* Academic Press, New York, 34-37.

Winter, I. M., Palmer, A. R. 1990. Responses of single units in the anteroventral cochlear nucleus of the guinea pig. *Hear. Res.,* 44, 161-178.

Witebsky E., Rose, N. R., Terplan, K., Paine, J. R., Egan, R. W. 1957. Chronic thyroiditis and autoimmunization. *J. Am. Med. Assoc.,* 164, 1439-1447.

Wobig, R. J., Kempton, J. B., Trune, D. R. 1999. Steroid responsive cochlear dysfunction in the MRL/*lpr* autoimmune mouse. *Otolaryngol. Head Neck Surg.,* 121, 344-347.

Wolfrum, U., Liu, X., Schmitt, A., Udovichenko, I. P., Williams, D. S. 1998. Myosin VIIa as a common component of cilia and microvilli. *Cell Motil. Cytoskeleton,* 40, 261-271.

Wong, M. L., Young, J. S., Nilaver, G., Morton, J. I., Trune, D. R. 1992. Cochlear IgG in the C3H/*lpr* autoimmune strain mouse. *Hear. Res.,* 59, 93-100.

Woodworth, R. S., Schlosberg, H. 1965. *Experimental Psychology,* revised ed. Holt, Rinehart and Winston, New York.

Woolf, N., Jaquish, D., Koehrn, F., Powell, H., Campbell, I. 1997. Auditory nerve pathology and hearing loss in a new interleukin-3 transgenic mouse model of multiple sclerosis. *Assoc. Res. Otolaryngol. Abstr.,*

Woolf, N. K., Koehrn, F. J., Ryan, A. F. 1992. Immunohistochemical localization of fibronectin-like protein in the inner ear of the developing gerbil and rat. *Devel. Brain Res.,* 65, 21-33.

Wotton, J. M., Haresign, T., Ferragamo, M. J., Simmons, J. A. 1996. Sound source elevation and external ear cues influence the discrimination of spectral notches by the big brown bat, *Eptesicus fuscus.* 100, 1764-1776.

Wouterlood, F. G., Mugnaini, E. 1984. Cartwheel neurons of the dorsal cochlear nucleus: a Golgi-electron microscopic study in rat. *J. Comp. Neurol.,* 227, 136-157.

Wouterlood, F. G., Mugnaini, E., Osen, K. K., Dahl, A. L. 1984. Stellate neurons in rat dorsal cochlear nucleus studies with combined Golgi impregnation and electron microscopy: synaptic connections and mutual coupling by gap junctions. *J. Neurocytol.,* 13, 639-664.

Wright, D. D., Ryugo, D. K. 1996. Mossy fiber projections from the cuneate nucleus to the cochlear nucleus in the rat. *J. Comp. Neurol.,* 365, 159-172.

Wu, M. F., Suzuki, S. S., Siegel, J. M. 1988. Anatomical distribution and response patterns of reticular neurons active in relation to acoustic startle. *Brain Res.,* 457, 399-406.

Wu, S. H. 1999 Physiological properties of neurons in the ventral nucleus of the lateral lemniscus of the rat: intrinsic membrane properties and synaptic responses. *J. Neurophysiol.,* 81, 2862-2874.

Wu, S. H., Kelly, J. B. 1993. Response of neurons in the lateral superior olive and medial nucleus of the trapezoid body to repetitive stimulation: intracellular and extracellular recordings from mouse brain slice. *Hear. Res.,* 68, 189-201.

Wu, S. H, Kelly, J. B. 1994. Physiological evidence for ipsilateral inhibition in the lateral superior olive: synaptic responses in mouse brain slice. *Hear. Res.,* 73, 57-64.

Wu, S. H, Kelly, J. B. 1995. Inhibition in the superior olivary complex: pharmacological evidence from mouse brain slice. *J. Neurophysiol.,* 73, 256-269.

Wu, S.-H., Oertel, D. 1984. Intracellular injection with horseradish peroxidase of physiologically characterized stellate and bushy cells in slices of mouse anteroventral cochlear nucleus. *J. Neurosci.,* 4, 1577-1588.

Wu, S.-H., Oertel, D. 1986. Inhibitory circuitry in the ventral cochlear nucleus is probably mediated by glycine. *J. Neurosci.,* 6, 2691-2706.

Wu, T. H., Gu, X. X. 1999. Outer membrane proteins as a carrier for detoxified lipooligosaccharide conjugate vaccines for nontypeable *Haemophilus influenzae. Infect. Immunol.,* 67, 5508-5513.

Wysocki, C. J. 1979. Neurobehavioral evidence for the involvement of the vomeronasal system in mammalian reproduction. *Neurosci. Biobehav. Rev.,* 3, 301-341.

Wysocki, C. J., Lepri, J. J. 1991. Consequences of removing the vomeronasal organ. *J. Steroid Biochem. Molec. Biol.,* 39, 661-669.

Wysocki, C. J., Nyby, J., Whitney, G., Beauchamp, G. K., Katz, Y. 1982. The vomeronasal organ: primary role in mouse chemosensory gender recognition. *Physiol. Behav.,* 29, 315-327.

Xiang, M., Gan, L., Li, D., Chen, Z. Y., Zhou, L., O'Malley, Jr., B. W., Klein, W., Nathans, J. 1997. Essential role of POU-domain factor Brn-3c in auditory and vestibular hair cell development. *Proc. Natl. Acad. Sci., USA,* 94, 9445-9450.

Xiang, M., Gao, W. Q., Hasson, T., Shin, J. J. 1998. Requirement for Brn-3c in maturation and survival, but not in fate determination of inner ear hair cells. *Devel.,* 125, 3935-3946.

Xu, H., Wu, X. R., Wewer, U. M., Engvall, E. 1994. Murine muscular dystrophy caused by a mutation in the laminin alpha 2 (Lama2) gene. *Nature Genet.,* 8, 297-302.

Xu, P. X., Adams, J., Peters, H., Brown, M. C., Heaney, S., Maas, R. 1999. Eya1-deficient mice lack ears and kidneys and show abnormal apoptosis of organ primordia. *Nature Genet.,* 23, 113-117.

Yagi, M., Magal E., Sheng Z., Ang K. A. Raphael Y. 1999. Hair cell protection from aminoglycoside ototoxicity by adenovirus-mediated overexpression of glial cell line-derived neurotrophic factor. *Hum. Gene Ther.,* 10, 813-823.

Yamada, G., Mansouri, A., Torres, M., Stuart, E. T., Blum, M., Schultz, M., De Robertis, E. M., Gruss, P. 1995. Targeted mutation of the murine goosecoid gene results in craniofacial defects and neonatal death. *Devel.,* 121, 2917-2922.

Yamanaka, N., Hotomi, M., Shimada, J., Togawa, A. 1997. Immunolgical deficiency in "otitis-prone" children. *Ann. N.Y. Acad. Sci.,* 830, 70-81.

Yamane, H., Nakai, Y., Takayama, M., Iguchi, H., Nakagawa, T., Kojima, A. 1995a. Appearance of free radicals in the guinea pig inner ear after noise-induced acoustic trauma. *Eur. Arch. Otorhinolaryngol.,* 252, 504-508.

Yamane, H., Nakai, Y., Takayama, M., Konishi, K., Iguchi, H., Nakagawa, T., Shibata, S., Kato, A., Sunami, K., Kawakatsu, C. 1995b. The emergence of free radicals after acoustic trauma and strial blood flow. *Acta Otolaryngol.,* Suppl. 519, 87-92.

Yamanobe, S., Harris, J. P., Keithley, E. M. 1993. Evidence of direct communication of bone marrow cells with the endolymphatic sac in experimental autoimmune labyrinthitis. *Acta Otolaryngol.,* 113, 166-170.

Yamashita, H., Bagger-Sjoback, D., Wersall, J. 1991. The presence of laminin in the fetal human inner ear. *Eur. Arch. Oto.-Rhino.-Laryngol.,* 248, 479-482.

Yamasoba, T., Nuttall, A. L., Harris, C., Raphael, Y., Miller, J. M. 1998. Role of glutathione in protection against noise-induced hearing loss. *Brain Res.,* 784, 82-90.

Yamasoba, T., Suzuki, M., Kaga, K. 1996. Influence of chronic kanamycin administration on basement membrane anionic sites in the labyrinth. *Hear. Res.,* 102, 116-124.

Yang, F. S., Han, J. S., Dong, Y., Liu, D. X. 1990. A technique for temporal bone sections using non-decalcified frozen guinea pig cochleas: a study of succinic dehydrogenases. *Eur. Arch. Oto-Rhino-Laryngol.,* 247, 283-286.

Yang, Y. P., Myers, L. E., McGuinness, U., Chong, P., Kwok, Y., Klein, M. H., Harkness, R. E. 1997. The major outer membrane protein, CD, extracted from *Moraxella (Branhamella) catarrhalis* is a potential vaccine antigen that induces bactericidal antibodies. *FEMS Immunol. Med. Micro.,* 17, 187-199.

Yanz, J. L., Herr, L. R., Townsend, D. W., Witkop, C. J. 1985. The questionable relationship between cochlear pigmentation and noise-induced hearing loss. *Audiology,* 24, 260-268.

Yao, X., Rarey, K. E. 1996. Detection and regulation of Cu/Zn-SOD and Mn-SOD in rat cochlear tissues. *Hear. Res.,* 96, 199-203.

Yeo, S. W., Gottschlich, S., Harris, J. P., Keithley, E. M. 1995. Antigen diffusion from the perilymphatic space of the cochlea. *Laryngoscope,* 105, 623-628.

Yeomans, J. S., Cochrane, K. A. 1993. Collision-like interactions between acoustic and electrical signals that produce startle reflexes in reticular formation sites. *Brain Res.,* 617, 320-328.

Yerkes, R. M. 1905. The sense of hearing in frogs. *J. Comp. Physiol. Psychol.,* 15, 279-304.

Yi, Y., Yang, X., Brunham, R. C. 1997. Autoimmunity to heat shock protein 60 and antigen-specific production of interleukin-10. *Infect. Immun.,* 65, 1669-1674.

Yin, T. C. T., Chan, J. C. K. 1990. Interaural time sensitivity in medial superior olive of cat. *J. Neurophysiol.,* 64, 465-488.

Yim, M. B., Chock, P. B., Stadtman, E. R. 1993. Enzyme function of copper, zinc superoxide dismutase as a free radical generator. *J. Biol. Chem.,* 268, 4099-4105.

Ylikoski, J., Pirvola, U., Eriksson, U. 1994. Cellular retinol-binding protein type I is prominently and differentially expressed in the sensory epithelium of the rat cochlea and vestibular organs. *J. Comp. Neurol.,* 349, 596-602.

Ylikoski, J., Pirvola, U., Happola, O., Panula, P., Virtanen, L. 1989. Immunohistochemical demonstration of neuroactive substances in the inner ear of rat and guinea pig. *Acta Otolaryngol.,* 107, 417-423.

Ylikoski, J., Pirvola, U., Moshnyakov, M., Palgi, J., Arumae, U., Saarma, M. 1993. Expression patterns of neurotrophin and their receptor mRNAs in the rat inner ear. *Hear. Res.,* 65, 69-78.

Ylikoski, J., Pirvola, U., Virkkala, J., Suvanto, P., Liang, X. Q., Magal, E., Altschuler, R., Miller, J. M., Saarma, M. 1998. Guinea pig auditory neurons are protected by glial cell line-derived growth factor from degeneration after noise trauma. *Hear. Res.,* 124, 17-26.

Ylikoski, M. E. 1994. Prolonged exposure to gunfire noise among professional soldiers. *Scand. J. Work. Environ. Health,* 20, 87-92.

Yoo, T. J., Fujiyoshi, T., Cheng, K.-C., Krug, M. S., Kim, N. S., Lee, K. M., Shen, T., Matsuoka, H. 1997. Molecular basis of type II collagen autoimmune ear diseases. *Ann. N.Y. Acad. Sci.,* 830, 221-235.

Yoo, T. J., Takeda, T., Sudo, N., Stuart, J. M., Floyd, R. A., Ha, S. 1987. Collagen-induced autoimmune ear disease (CIAED) in mice. Localization of inner ear disease inducing determinant of type II collagen molecules. In Veldman, J. E. (Ed.), *Immunobiology, Histophysiology, Tumor Immunology in Otolaryngology.* Kugler Publications, Amsterdam, 435-437.

Yoo, T. J., Tomoda, K., Stuart, J. M., Townes, A. S. 1983a. Type II collagen-induced autoimmune otospongiosis. A preliminary report. *Ann. Otol. Rhinol. Laryngol.,* 92, 103-108.

Yoo, T. J., Tomoda, K., Stuart, J. M., Cremer, M. A., Townes, A. S., Kang, A. H. 1983b. Type II collagen-induced autoimmune sensorineural hearing loss and vestibular dysfunction in rats. *Ann. Otol. Rhinol. Laryngol.*, 92, 267-271.

Yorke, Jr., C. H., Caviness, Jr., V. S., 1975. Interhemispheric neocortical connections of the corpus callosum in the normal mouse: a study based on anterograde and retrograde methods. *J. Comp. Neurol.*, 164, 233-246.

Yoshida, N., Hequembourg, S. J., Atencio, C. A., Rosowski, J. J., Liberman, M. C. 2000. Acoustic injury in mice: 129/SvEv is exceptionally resistant to noise-induced hearing loss. *Hear. Res.*, 141, 97-106.

Yoshida, N., Liberman, M. C. 2000. Sound conditioning reduces noise-induced hearing loss in mice. *Hear. Res.*, 148, 213-219.

Yoshida, S., Castles, J. J., Gershwin, M. E. 1990. The pathogenesis of autoimmunity in New Zealand mice. *Sem. Arth. Rheum.*, 19, 224-42.

Yoshioka, K., Hino, S., Takemura, T., Maki, S., Wieslander, J., Takekoshi, Y., Makino, H., Kagawa, M., Sado, Y., Kashtan, C. E. 1994. Type IV collagen alpha 5 chain. Normal distribution and abnormalities in X-linked Alport syndrome revealed by monoclonal antibody. *Am. J. Pathol.*, 144, 986-996.

Young, E. D. 1980. Identification of response properties of ascending axons from dorsal cochlear nucleus. *Brain Res.*, 200, 23-37.

Young, E. D. 1998. Cochlear nucleus. In Sheperd, G. M. (Ed.), *The Synaptic Organization of the Brain*. Oxford University Press, New York, 121-157.

Young, E. D., Brownell, W. E. 1976. Responses to tones and noise of single cells in dorsal cochlear nucleus of unanesthetized cats. *J. Neurophysiol.*, 39, 282-300.

Young, E. D., Nelken, I., Conley, R. A. 1995. Somatosensory effects on neurons in dorsal cochlear nucleus. *J. Neurophysiol.*, 73, 743-765.

Young, J. S., Upchurch, M. B., Kaufman, M. J. Fechter, L. D. 1987. Carbon monoxide exposure potentiates high-frequency auditory threshold shifts induced by noise. *Hear. Res.*, 26, 37-43.

Young, L. S., Fechter, L. D. 1983. Reflex inhibition procedures for animal audiometry: A technique for assessing oto-toxicity. *J. Acoust. Soc. Am.*, 73, 1686-1693.

Young, R. W. 1985. Cell differentiation in the retina of the mouse. *Anatom. Rec.*, 212, 199-205.

Yuste, R., Katz, C. 1991. Control of postsynaptic Ca 2+ influx in developing neocortex by excitatory and inhibitory neurotransmitters. *Neuron*, 6, 333-344.

Zajic, G., Nair, T. S., Ptok, M., Van Waes, C., Altschuler, R. A., Schacht, J., Carey, T. E. 1991. Monoclonal antibodies to inner ear antigens. I. Antigens expressed by supporting cells of the guinea pig cochlea. *Hear. Res.*, 52, 59-71.

Zaroor, M., Starr, A. 1991a. Auditory brain-stem evoked potentials in cat after kainic acid induced neuronal loss. I. Superior olivary complex. *Electroenceph. Clin. Neurophysiol.*, 80, 422-435.

Zaroor, M., Starr, A. 1991b. Auditory brain-stem evoked potentials in cat after kainic acid induced neuronal loss. II. Cochlear nucleus. *Electroenceph. Clin. Neurophysiol.*, 80, 436-445.

Zdanski, C. J., Prazma, J., Petrusz, P., Grossman, G., Raynor, E., Smith, T. L., Pillsbury, H. C. 1994. Nitric oxide synthase is an active enzyme in the spiral ganglion cells of the rat cochlea. *Hear. Res.*, 79, 39-47.

Zeidner, N., Dreitz, M., Belasco, D., Fish, D. 1996. Suppression of acute *Ixodes scapularis*-induced *Borrelia burgdorferi* infection using tumor necrosis factor-alpha, interleukin-2, and interferon-gamma. *J. Infect. Dis.*, 173, 187-95.

Zettel, M. L., Frisina, R. D., Haider, S, O'Neill, W. E. 1997. Age-related changes in calbindin D-28k and calretinin immunoreactivity in the inferior colliculus of CBA/CaJ and C57Bl/6 mice. *J. Comp. Neurol.*, 386, 92-110.

Zhang, S., Oertel, D. 1993a. Cartwheel and superficial stellate cells of the dorsal cochlear nucleus of mice: intracellular recordings in slices. *J. Neurophysiol.*, 69, 1384-1397.

Zhang, S., Oertel, D. 1993b. Giant cells of the dorsal cochlear nucleus of mice: Intracellular recordings in slices. *J. Neurophysiol.*, 69, 1398-1408.

Zhang, S., Oertel, D. 1993c. Tuberculoventral cells of the dorsal cochlear nucleus of mice: Intracellular recordings in slices. *J. Neurophysiol.*, 69, 1409-1421.

Zhang, S., Oertel, D. 1994. Neuronal circuits associated with the output of the dorsal cochlear nucleus through fusiform cells. *J. Neurophysiol.*, 71, 914-930.

Zhang, S., Trussell, L. O. 1994. A characterization of excitatory postsynaptic potentials in the avian nucleus magnocellularis. *J. Neurophysiol.*, 72, 705-718.

Zhang, Y., Marcillat, O., Giulivi, C., Ernster, L., Davies, K. J. 1990. The oxidative inactivation of mitochondrial electron transport chain components and ATPase. *J. Biol. Chem.*, 265, 16330-16336.

Zhang, Z. J., Saito, T., Kimura, Y., Sugimoto, C., Ohtsubo, T., Saito, H. 2000. Disruption of mdr1a p-glycoprotein gene results in dysfunction of blood-inner-ear barrier in mice. *Brain Res.,* 852, 116-126.

Zheng, J. L., Gao, W. Q. 2000. Overexpression of Math1 induces robust production of extra hair cells in postnatal rat inner ears. *Nat. Neurosci.,* 3, 580-586.

Zheng, Q. Y., Erway, L. C., Pelletier, K. M. Johnson, K. R. 1999a. Genetic analysis of nonsyndromic hearing impairment in inbred mouse strains. Abstracts of the 22nd Annual Midwinter Research Meeting, *Assoc. Res. Otolaryngol. Abstr.,*

Zheng, Q. Y., Johnson, K. R., Erway, L. C. 1999b. Assessment of hearing in 80 inbred strains of mice by ABR threshold analyses. *Hear. Res.,* 130, 94-107.

Zheng, X. Y., Henderson, D., McFadden, S. L., Ding, D. L., Salvi, R. J. 1999. Auditory nerve fiber responses following chronic cochlear de-efferentation. *J. Comp. Neurol.,* 406, 72-86.

Zheng, X. Y., Henderson, D., Hu, B. H., Ding, D. L., McFadden, S. L. 1997. The influence of the cochlear efferent system on chronic acoustic trauma. *Hear. Res.,* 107, 147-159.

Zhong, W., Stehle, T., Museteanu, C., Siebers, A., Gern, L., Kramer, M., Wallich, R., Simon, M. M. 1997. Therapeutic passive vaccination against chronic Lyme disease in mice. *Proc. Natl. Acad. Sci.,* 94, 12533-12538.

Zhou, J., Barker, D. F., Hostikka, S. L., Gregory, M. C., Atkin, C. L., Tryggvason, K. 1991. Single base mutation in alpha 5(IV) collagen chain gene converting a conserved cysteine to serine in Alport syndrome. *Genomics,* 9, 10-18.

Zhou, J., Hertz, J. M., Leinonen, A., Tryggvason, K. 1992a. Complete amino acid sequence of the human alpha 5 (IV) collagen chain and identification of a single-base mutation in exon 23 converting glycine 521 in the collagenous domain to cysteine in an Alport syndrome patient. *J. Biol. Chem.,* 267, 12475-12481.

Zhou, J., Hertz, J. M., Tryggvason, K. 1992b. Mutation in the alpha 5(IV) collagen chain in juvenile-onset Alport syndrome without hearing loss or ocular lesions: detection by denaturing gradient gel electro-phoresis of a PCR product. *Am. J. Hum. Genet.,* 50, 1291-1300.

Zhou, J., Mochizuki, T., Smeets, H., Antignac, C., Laurila, P., De Paepe, A., Tryggvason, K., Reeders, S. T. 1993. Deletion of the paired alpha 5(IV) and alpha 6(IV) collagen genes in inherited smooth muscle tumors. *Science,* 261, 1167-1169.

Zhou, N. N., Nikai, S., Kawakita, T., Oka, M., Nagasawa, H., Himeo, K., Nomoto, K. 1994. Combined treatment of autoimmune MRL/MP-lpr/lpr mice with a herbal medicine, Ren-shen-yang-rong-tang (Japanese name:Ninjin-youei-to) plus suboptimal dosage of prednisolone. *Int. J. Immunopharmacol.,* 16, 845-854.

Zhou, R., Abbas, P. J., Assouline, P. G. 1995b. Electrically evoked auditory brainstem response in peripherally myelin-deficient mice. *Hear. Res.,* 88, 98-106.

Zhou, R., Assouline, J. G., Abbas, P. J., Messing, A., Gantz, B. J. 1995a. Anatomical and physiological measures of auditory system in mice with peripheral myelin deficiency. *Hear. Res.,* 88, 87-97.

Zhou, S. L., Pickles, J. O. 1994. Early hair-cell degeneration in the extreme apex of the guinea pig cochlea. *Hear Res.,* 79, 147-160.

Zhou, X., Van De Water, T. R. 1987. The effect of target tissues on survival and differentiation of mammalian statoacoustic ganglion neurons in organ culture. *Acta Otolaryng.,* 104, 90-98.

Zhu, C. C., Yamada, G. Blum, M. 1997. Correlation between loss of middle ear bones and altered *goosecoid* gene expression in the brachial region following retinoic acid treatment of mouse embryos *in vivo*. *Biochem. Biophysics Res. Commun.,* 235, 748-753.

Zhu, D., Kim, Y., Steffes, M. W., Groppoli, T. J., Butkowski, R. J., Mauer, S. M. 1994. Application of electron microscopic immunocytochemistry to the human kidney: distribution of type IV and type VI collagen in normal human kidney. *J. Histochem. Cytochem.,* 42, 577-584.

Zimmerman, L. B., De Jesus-Escobar, J. M., Harland, R. M. 1996. The Spemann organizer signal noggin binds and inactivates bone morphogenetic protein 4. *Cell,* 86, 599-606.

Zuo, J., Treadaway, J., Buckner, T. W., Fritzsch, B. 1999. Visualization of alpha9 acetylcholine receptor expression in hair cells of transgenic mice containing a modified bacterial artificial chromosome. *Proc. Natl. Acad. Sci., USA,* 96, 14100-14105.

Zurek, P. M., Clark, W. W., Kim, D. O. 1982. The behavior of acoustic distortion products in the ear canals of chinchillas with normal or damaged ears. *J. Acoust. Soc. Am.,* 72, 774-780.

Zwicker, E. 1986. Suppression and $(2f_1-f_2)$ difference tone in a nonlinear cochlear processing model with active feedback. *J. Acoust. Soc. Am.,* 80, 163-176.

Index

A

Adh4 gene, 472
Advantages and limitations of mice, 187, 339, 359, 391,
    401, 429, 442, 459, 479; see Preface
Age-related hearing loss (AHL) genes, 430-433
  Ahl gene, 436-438, 481
Aging, 192
  ABRs, 359
  BALB/c mice, 111, 194
  C57/CBA hybrids, 381-387
  C57 mice, 35, 193
  calcium binding proteins, 327, 345, 346, 351
  CBA mice, 192-193, 340-379
  DPOAEs, 54
  GABA, 361-363
  gap detection, 342, 357-359, 381-387
  glycine, 347
  hair cell loss, 192
  inferior colliculus, 341, 352-357, 361-363
  middle ear, 111
  SOC, 359-361
  SOD and, 502
  startle reflex, 382-387
Allelism testing, 422
Alpha9 gene, 468
Alport syndrome, 568
  mouse model, 573
AMPA glutamate receptor, 304
Anatomy, 99
ASR (acoustic startle response), 442; see startle
Audible sounds of adult mice, 14
  squealing, 14-16
  tail rattling, 16
Auditory cortex, 273
  columnar organization, 276
  general topography, 273
  primary auditory cortex, 274
  secondary cortices, 274
Auditory brainstem response (ABR), 37
  age-related changes, 359
  influence of extrinsic factors on, 40
  middle ear function, 39
  neural substrate, 38
  noise-induced hearing loss, 41
  phenotyping auditory function, 39
  Rab3a mice, 604-612
  recording system, 38
Augmented acoustic environment (AAE), 205-214
  duration of effects, 212
  effects on ABR thresholds, 206

  effects on baseline startle amplitude, 208
  effects on prepulse inhibition, 206
  in normal-hearing mice, 209
  limitations, 210
  possible mechanisms, 212
  time course for acquisition, 209
Autoimmune inner ear disease, 512-519
  steroids, 518
AVCN, see cochlear nucleus

B

BALB/c mouse
  aging cochlea, 194
  aging middle ear, 111
  cochlear cell density, 191
  middle ear, 106, 110
Basic helix-loop-helix (bHLH) DNA binding domain, 143,
  144
Behavioral hearing tests, 20
  acoustic startle reflex, 25
  approach the source of a sound, 24
  avoidance conditioning, 23
  conditioned eyeblink, 23
  conditioned suppression/avoidance, 20
  freezing response, 27
  galvanic skin response (GSR) audiometry, 24, 27
  go/no-go, 21
  pinna movements, 27
  prepulse inhibition, 25
Bone morphogenetic protein 4 and *BMP4* gene, 142, 143,
  467, 473
Brain-derived neurotrophic factor (BDNF), 151-154, 468
Brn 3 gene, 147, 471
Brn4 gene, 618-620
Bulla, 103
Bushy cells (in AVCN), 304, 305
BXD recombinant strains, 206-208, 430, 431
  prepulse inhibition and startle, 443-445

C

C57/CBA F1 hybrids
  age-related changes, 381-387
  cochlear histology, 178-181
  cochlear nucleus, 280-295
  startle, 60-67
C57BL/6J mouse
  ABRs, 39,40

age-related changes, 35, 193
augmented acoustic environment, 206-208
cochlear cell density, 190
DPOAEs, 47, 49, 55
fear-potentiated startle, 92-95
middle ear, 106, 110, 112
noise-induced hearing loss, 481, 482
PnC neuronal responses, 332-338
prepulse inhibition, 73-77
sound localization, 31-35
startle reflex, 60-62; 83-90
tonotopic organization, 240
C57BL/10J mouse, 192
Calbindin, 321-329
Calcitonin receptor (CTR) promoter, 472
Calcium binding proteins, 321-329
aging, 327, 345, 346, 351
effect of noise exposure, 320-327
relation to injury and neurodegenerative disorders, 232
Candidate gene identification, 424
Cartwheel cells (in DCN), 312
Caudal pontine reticular nucleus (PnC), 331
prepulse inhibition, 332
responses of neurons in C57 mice, 332
role in startle, 331
CBA mouse
ABRs, 40, 612
aging, 192-193, 340-379
calcium binding proteins, 327
cochlear blood flow, 220, 221
cochlear cell density, 190
DPOAEs, 51,52,55
noise-induced hearing loss, 481, 482
prepulse inhibition, 72
startle reflex, 62, 64-67
Cerumen, 102
Chemoattractive fields and factors, 158
Ciliary neurotrophic factor (CNTF), 162
COCH gene, 397
Cochlear histology, 172
dissection, 173
embedding, 173
evaluation, 175-181
fixation, 172
flat preparations, 174
thin sections, 175
Cochlear nucleus
age-related changes, 339-349
anatomical organization and cytoarchitectonics, 243-245
anteroventral cochlear nucleus (AVCN), 228, 245, 246, 288-293, 299-309, 318, 325-328
atlas, 283-293
comparative differences, 251
comparison with other mammals, 294
development, 228-230, 249-251
doral cochlear nucleus (DCN), 249, 281-285, 310-314, 318, 325-328
posteroventral cochlear nucleus (PVCN), 246-249, 285-288, 299-309, 318, 325-328
response properties, 253

Cochlear blood flow measures, 215
intravital microscopy, 216
laser doppler flowmetry (LDF), 217-221
microelectrode sensors, 215
microsphere, indicator dilution methods, and 2-deoxyglucose, 216
COL4A genes/collagen, 568-577
Conditioning (toughening) by noise, 478
Cytochrome oxidase, 240-242

D

DBA/2J mouse
augmented acoustic environment, 206-208
cochlear cell density, 191
DPOAEs, 46
fear-potentiated startle, 94-95
tonotopic organization, 240
Deaf-wadler (*dfw*) mouse, 431
Deefferentation deafness syndrome (DDS), 537
Delta1 (*Dll1*), 144, 145, 472
Demyelinating diseases, 473
deoxyglucose, 2- (2-DG), 217, 219
Determination of cell fates in developing cochlea, 143-147
DFNA loci, 397
Distortion product otoacoustic emission (DPOAE), 45
aging, 54
auditory phenotyping, 54
efferent-mediated adaptation, 54
group delay, 53
hearing loss, 49
level versus f_2/f_1, 53
measures, 46
morphological correlates, 54
optimal stimulus parameters, 50
recording system, 45
sources, 46
Dix genes, 463

E

Ear canal, 101
Early onset hearing impairment, 433-436
Embryonic stem cells, 458
Endbulbs of Held, 225
development, 227-230, 2234, 235
shaker-2 mouse, 221, 227, 230-232
structure, 225
Endothelin receptor A (*ET_A*) gene, 467
Ephrins, 152
Equal energy hypothesis, 477
External meatus, 102, 103
Eya1 genes, 463

F

Fear-potentiated startle, 91-95
C57BL/6 mice, 92
DBA/2 mice, 94

light versus tones, 92-94
  procedures, 91
  strain differences, 94
fgfr3 mutant mice, 467
Fibroblast growth factors (FGFs), 162
  Fibroblast growth factor receptor 3 (FGFr3), 146
Flash electroretinogram, 588
Fractal analysis of endbulb complexity, 232
Fusiform and giant cells (in DCN), 312

G

Gamma-aminobutyric acid (GABA), 117-136, 310, 312,
    317-320
  AchE-/ChAT- and GABA-/GAD, 123-125
  age-related changes, 361-363
  innervation of tunnel crossing fibers, 129
  innervation within the inner hair cell region, 123
  terminals on spiral ganglion neurons, 123
  transgenic mouse
  transitory expression, 119
Gap detection, 77-80
  aging, 342, 357-359, 381-387
GAP-43, 125
GATA family of zinc-finger transcription factors, 147
Genetic background, 428, 430
GJB2 gene, 398
Glial cell line-derived neurotrophic factor (GDNF), 153
Glutamic acid decarboxylase (GAD), 117-136
  axosomatic synapses of inner hair cells, 126
  developmental expression in afferent innervation in the
      organ of Corti, 117-118
Glycine, 317-320
  age-related changes, 349
Golgi cells (in VCN), 307, 308
Goosecoid gene, 462

H

Head shadow, 100, 101
Hearing-loss-induced (HLI) plasticity, 207, 213, 214
  frequency reorganization in IC, 351-353
  reticular formation, 335-338
Heat shock proteins, 520
HES genes, 145
Hmx homeobox genes, 464
Hox genes, 463, 473
Hypersensitivity immune reactions and diseases, 506-509
Hypothyroidism and deafness, 538-541
Hypothyroid (*hyt/hyt*) mouse, 42, 148, 537-554
  auditory capacity, 546-553
  development, 548, 549

I

Immunologic diseases, 511-523
  external ear, 511, 529, 530
  inner ear, 511
  middle ear, 511, 523-529

Immunologic mouse models, 509-511
Inbred strains of mice, 429
Inferior colliculus (IC), 263, 319
  aging, 341, 352-357, 361-363
  central nucleus (ICC), 264-269
  commissure (CIC), 268
  dorsal cortex (ICDC), 269
  external nucleus, 270
  inhibition, 361
Inheritance, determination of, 420
Inhibitory amino acid neurotransmitters, 317-320
Inner hair cells, 127
  compound synapses, 127-129
  modes of synaptic connections, 131
Insulin, 162
Insulin-like growth factors, 162
Int-2 gene, 467

J

Jagged1 gene (*Jag1*) , 142
Jagged2 gene (*Jag2*), 144, 145

K

Kolliker's organ, 541
  in hypothyroid Tshr mutants, 541-543

L

Laminin-2 defects, 534
Lunatic fringe gene (*Lfng*), 142
Lysosomal storage diseases (LSDs), 581
  bone marrow transplantation, 592
  enzyme replacement therapy, 590
  viral-mediated gene transfer, 595

M

Mapping mutations, 421
Mapping genes, 392
Math1 gene, 144
Medial geniculate body (MGB), 271
  dorsal division (MGBd), 271
  medial division (MGBm), 272
  ventral division (MGBv), 271

Medial superior olivary complex (MSOC), 129
Microphthalmia (mi) gene, 466

Ngn1 genes, 465
Microtype middle ear, 107
  aging, 111
  development, 110
Middle ear, 103
  anatomy, 103-105
Modifying genes, 427
Mos protooncogene, 471

Mouse deafness mutations, 402: see Table 27.1
  early studies, 402
  endolymph homeostasis, 419
  inner ear effects, 403-417
  morphogenetic defects, 418
  myelin and central nervous system defects, 419
  otolith defects, 418
  outer and inner ear defects, 417
  sensory hair cell defects, 419
MPS VII mouse model (*gus^mps*), 582
Mpv17 gene, 471
Msx genes, 462
Muscular Dystrophy mouse models, 533
    dy mouse, 533,534
    mdx mouse, 533
    myd mouse, 533
Mutagenesis programs, 426
Myo15^sh2/sh2, 236: see *Shaker-2*
Myo7a, 395, 560-563; see also, Usher syndrome

N

Neo gene, 473
Nerve growth factor (NGF), 157, 158-160, 162, 165
Neural cell adhesion molecule (NCAN), 151
Neurogenins, 150
Neurotrophic factors, 157
    definition, 157
    effects of neurotrophin withdrawal, 169
    effects on *in vitro* development of auditory neurons, 164
    knockout studies, 167
    role in auditory neuron survival, 163
Neurotrophins, 152-154
    Neurotrophin-3 (NT-3), 151-154, 160, 164, 167
    NT-4/5, 160
New Zealand Black mouse, 516
NMDA glutamate receptor, 306, 308
Noise-induced hearing loss, 180
    cytocochleogram, 180, 181
    experimental procedures, 486-488
    factors affecting, 483-485
    genetic interaction with, 438, 439
    SOD deficiency and, 500-502
Notch genes, 142, 472
Notch signaling pathway, 142
Nuclei of the lateral lemniscus (LL), 260
    dorsal nucleus (DNLL), 261, 319
    intermediate nucleus (INLL), 262
    ventral nucleus (VNLL), 262, 302

O

Octopus cells (in PVCN), 299-303
    age-related changes, 340
Organ of Corti, 137
    cell fate and cellular patterning, 141
    cellular differentiation, 147
    cellular proliferation and terminal mitosis, 139-191
    length and hair-cell density, 179-181, 189-192

    morphological development, 137-139
    prosensory cell population, 142
    three-dimensional structure, 181
    timeline of gene expression, 153
    timeline of neuronal pathfinding, 156
Ossicles, 103, 105
Otitis media, 523-529
Otocyst-derived factor (ODF), 151
otog gene, 470
Otosclerosis, 522
Otxl and *Otx2* genes, 463
Outer ear, 99

P

p27^kip1, 140-141, 471
Palmerston North mouse, 516
Pax2 and *Pax3* genes, 464
Permanent threshold shift (PTS), 479
Pigmentation and noise-induced hearing loss, 484
Pmca2 gene, 469
Positional cloning of new mutations, 424-426
POU-domain transcription factors/genes, 147, 465, 471
    Pou4f3, 396
Prepulse inhibition (PPI) 71-75
    genetics (QTLs), 445-455
    reticular formation, 332-337
Preyer reflex, 99
Prxl and *Prx2* genes, 464

Q

Quantitative trait loci (QTL), 436-438, 441, 445-454

R

Rab3A gene, 471
Rab3a, 603
    knockout mouse, 605
RAR genes, 465
Reactive oxygen species (ROS), 169, 489-494
Retinoic acid, 147, 148

S

Shaker-1 mouse, 560-568; see also, Usher syndrome
Shaker-2 mouse, 226, 227, 470
    ABR data, 230
    cochlear morphology, 231
    endbulb morphology, 232, 236
Short tandem repeats (STRs), 392
Slc12a1 gene, 469
SNARE complex, 603
Sodl knockout mice, 494-504
Sound location, 258, 259
    superior olivary complex, 101
Stains for cochlear histology, 196
    acetylcholinesterase histochemistry, 202

eosin, 202
hematoxylin, 196, 197
osmium tetroxide, 200-202
phalloidin, 199
silver nitrate, 199, 200
succinate dehydrogenase (SDH) histochemistry, 197, 198
Startle reflex, 60-67, 442
  age-related changes, 381-387
  effect of background sound 67-70, 83-90
  effect of light 70
  genetics (QTLs), 445-455
  reticular formation, 331-338
Statoacoustic ganglion (SAG)
  development, 150-152
Superior olivary complex (SOC), 254
  aging, 359-361
  anterolateral periolivary nucleus, 258
  descending pathways, 259
  dorsolateral periolivary nucleus, 258
  lateral superior olive (LSO), 254
  medial nucleus of the trapezoid body (MNTB), 255, 256
  medial superior olive (MSO), 254, 319
  para- and periolivary nuclei, 258
  superior paraolivary nucleus, 258
  ventral and lateral nuclei (VNTB, LNTB), 257

T

T stellate cells (in VCN), 305-307
TECTA gene, 397, 470
Temporal processing in IC and aging, 342, 357-359
Temporary threshold shift (TTS), 479
Tenascin, 151, 470
TGFβ2 null mutants, 467
Thyroid hormone, 148
  and cochlear development, 148
Thyroid receptors/genes
  Trα and *Tr*β, 148, 149, 465
Tonotopic organization, 239
Transgenic mouse models, 460
  cell phenotypes of the inner ear, 464
  channels/transporters, 469
  gene hierarcies, 466
  inner ear, 463-466: (see Table 30.1)
  ligand/receptor binding, 466
  middle ear, 462
  outer ear, 460

structural proteins/matrix molecules, 470
Transgenic technology, 457-459
Trembler mice, 42
TrkB and TrkC receptors, 153, 468
Tshr [hyt] mutant, 537: see *hyt* mouse
Tub mutant mice, 559
Tuberculoventral cells (in DCN), 313
Tympanic membrane, 104, 111-114
  transfer function, 106

U

Ultrasonic vocalizations in male mice
  androgenic regulation, 6-8
  ethographic analysis, 5
  function, 11-13
  genetic basis, 6
  neural regulation, 8
  pheromonal elicitation, 9-11
  sonagraphic analysis, 4
Ultrasonic vocalizations in female mice, 13
  function, 14
  genetics, 14
Unconventional myosins, 397
Usher syndrome, 395-397, 557-567
  categories of, 557

V

Ventral nucleus of the trapezoid body (VNTB), 129
Vestibular organs, 182-184
Vocalizing mechanism in mice, 3

W

Waardenburg syndrome, 419

X

X-linked deafness type III (DFN3), 617

Y

Yeast artificial chromosomes (YACs), 393

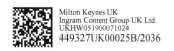

Milton Keynes UK
Ingram Content Group UK Ltd.
UKHW051900071024
449327UK00025B/2036

Kathleen Miranda

Student Solutions Manual

BRIEF CALCULUS: AN APPLIED APPROACH

8th Edition

Michael Sullivan
Chicago State University

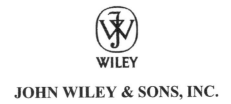

WILEY

JOHN WILEY & SONS, INC.

Cover Photo: ©Photodisc/Getty Images

To order books or for customer service call 1-800-CALL-WILEY (225-5945).

ISBN 0-471-46644-1

10 9 8 7 6 5 4 3 2 1

Contents

Chapter 0   Chapter 0 Review   1

Chapter 1   Functions and Their Graphs   58

Chapter 2   Classes of Functions   114

Chapter 3   The Limit of a Function   171

Chapter 4   The Derivative of a Function   206

Chapter 5   Applications: Graphing Functions; Optimization   285

Chapter 6   The Integral of a Function and Applications   385

Chapter 7   Other Applications and Extensions of the Integral   439

Chapter 8   Calculus of Functions of Two or More Variables   462

Appendix A   Graphing Utilities   510